Child and Adolescent Behavioral Health

Child and Adolescent Behavioral Health

A Resource for Advanced Practice Psychiatric and Primary Care Practitioners in Nursing

Second Edition

Edited by

Edilma L. Yearwood, PhD, PMHCNS-BC, FAAN
Associate Professor and Department Chair
Georgetown University School of Nursing & Health Studies, Washington, DC, USA

Geraldine S. Pearson, PhD, PMHCS-BC, FAAN
Associate Professor Retired
University of Connecticut School of Medicine, Farmington, CT, USA

Jamesetta A. Newland, PhD, FNP-BC, FAANP, DPNAP, FAAN
Clinical Professor Emerita
Rory Meyers College of Nursing, New York University, New York, NY, USA

WILEY Blackwell

Registered Office(s)
John Wiley & Sons, Inc., 111 River Street, Hoboken, NJ 07030, USA

Editorial Office
9600 Garsington Road, Oxford, OX4 2DQ, UK

For details of our global editorial offices, customer services, and more information about Wiley products visit us at www.wiley.com.

Wiley also publishes its books in a variety of electronic formats and by print-on-demand. Some content that appears in standard print versions of this book may not be available in other formats.

Library of Congress Cataloging-in-Publication Data

Names: Yearwood, Edilma Lynch, editor. | Pearson, Geraldine S., editor. |
    Newland, Jamesetta A., editor.
Title: Child and adolescent behavioral health : a resource for advanced
    practice psychiatric and primary care Practitioners in nursing / edited by
    Edilma L. Yearwood, Geraldine S. Pearson, Jamesetta A. Newland.
Description: Second edition. | Hoboken, NJ : John Wiley & Sons, Inc. 2021.
    | Includes bibliographical references and index.
Identifiers: LCCN 2020026986 (print) | LCCN 2020026987 (ebook) | ISBN
    9781119487579 (paperback) | ISBN 9781119487586 (adobe pdf) | ISBN
    9781119487562 (epub)
Subjects: MESH: Mental Disorders–diagnosis | Child | Adolescent | Early
    Diagnosis | Advanced Practice Nursing | Primary Care Nursing |
    Psychiatric Nursing | Case Reports
Classification: LCC RJ499 (print) | LCC RJ499 (ebook) | NLM WS 350.6 |
    DDC 618.92/89–dc23
LC record available at https://lccn.loc.gov/2020026986
LC ebook record available at https://lccn.loc.gov/2020026987

Cover Design: Wiley
Cover Image: School children (8-9) at lunch break © Tetra Images - Jamie Grill / Getty Images, Playing Together at School © FatCamera / Getty Images, Multi-ethnic children at autumn festival © kali9 / Getty Images, WMM - Teenagers hanging out, eating popcorn in urban park © Hero Images / Getty Images

Set in 10.5/12.5pt Minion by SPi Global, Pondicherry, India

SKY10077581_061324

Dedication

This second edition of our textbook is lovingly dedicated first to all the children and families we have worked with, will work with, and are in need of the clinical skills and expertise of advanced practice registered nurses in primary care and psychiatric-mental health specialties. Second, I wish to thank my family, my parents, Dorothy and Edmund, my adult children, Arayna and Matthew, my daughter-in-law Isabella and my new granddaughter Emilia for their continuing love, support, and understanding during the work on this edition. Nurses have an opportunity to meet the crucial mental health needs of one of our most vulnerable populations and this text is intended as a tool to assist in that mission.

Edilma Yearwood

I wish to dedicate this second edition of the textbook first to my family. My husband, Lloyd Pearson, my children, Neal, David, and Elizabeth, and my two grandchildren, Liam and Adalyn, have all contributed in different ways to my thinking about development and mental health. Their support is invaluable to my practice and functioning. Second, I want to dedicate this book to the myriad of children, adolescents, and families I have had the privilege to know in the last 40 years of work as a child psychiatric nurse. They have been the ultimate teachers in my ongoing quest for the most effective and carefully crafted treatment interventions available to optimize mental health.

Geri Pearson

I dedicate this book to my family – my husband Lloyd, my children Kristina, Michael, and Sonya, my granddaughter Maya, my sisters Sharon, Brenda, Sheila, and Michele, and my mother Kather Lene Alexander and mother-in-law Gloria Rerrie Chang. They and many others have supported me in all my professional endeavors. Students confirm my faith in future generations of nurses. Patients enrich my life and give me purpose and direction to always do more. Most importantly, I want to acknowledge the children and adolescents who are the inspiration for writing this text, and to those among them who will benefit by the impact of the book on nursing education and practice.

Jamie Newland

Contents

About the Editors

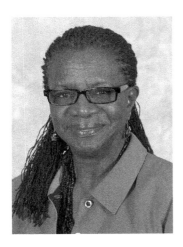

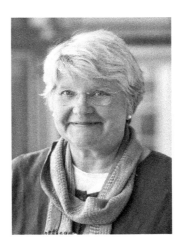

Edilma L. Yearwood, PhD, PMHCNS-BC, FAAN, is Chair, Department of Professional Nursing Practice at Georgetown University School of Nursing & Health Studies where she teaches psychiatric nursing. She is a past president of the International Society of Psychiatric-Mental Health Nursing and is a board member of the Global Alliance for Behavioral Health and Social Justice. She is an associate editor of the journal *Archives of Psychiatric Nursing* and an ANCC certified clinical nurse specialist in child/adolescent psychiatric-mental health nursing. She is the funded director on a project titled, Nurturing Child Well-Being: Educating Communities on Social Determinants of Health (2020-2025).

Geraldine S. Pearson, PhD, PMH-CNS, FAAN, is past co-chairperson of the Committee on Publication Ethics and past president of the International Society of Psychiatric-Mental Health Nurses. She is currently editor-in-chief of the *Journal of the American Psychiatric Nurses Association*. She is a retired associate professor in the Department of Psychiatry at the University of Connecticut School of Medicine. Dr. Pearson is ANCC certified as a clinical nurse specialist in child/adolescent and adult psychiatric-mental health nursing. She is also involved in the Psychiatric Nurse Practitioner Residency at Community Health Center, INC, Middletown, CT.

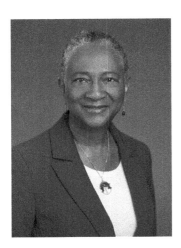

Jamesetta A. Newland, PhD, FNP-BC, FAANP, DPNAP, FAAN, is clinical professor emerita at New York University Rory Meyers College of Nursing. She continues to teach in the family nurse practitioner and Doctor of Nursing Practice programs. She is the editor-in-chief of *The Nurse Practitioner* journal, the first peer-reviewed publication dedicated to the nurse practitioner role. Dr. Newland, an ANCC certified family nurse practitioner, specializes in primary care across the lifespan and maintains clinical practice at a federally qualified health center serving diverse and vulnerable populations.

List of Contributors

Gabrielle Abelard, DNP, PMHNP-BC, RN
Clinical Assistant Professor
Psychiatric Mental Health Nurse Practitioner Program
University of Massachusetts College of Nursing,
    Amherst, MA, USA

Angela F. Amar, PhD, RN, FAAN
Professor and Dean
University of Nevada, Las Vegas School of Nursing,
    Las Vegas, NV, USA

Crystal Marie Bennett, DNP, PMHNP-BC
Child and Adolescent Psychiatric Nurse Practitioner
San Jose, CA, USA

Julie E. Bertram, RN, MSN, PMHCNS-BC, PhD
Assistant Professor of Nursing
University of Missouri, St. Louis, MO, USA

Elizabeth Bonham, PhD, RN, PMHCNS, BC
Associate Professor
University of Southern Indiana College of Nursing,
    Evansville, IN, USA

Susan J. Boorin, PhD, PMHNP-BC
Lecturer
Yale University School of Nursing, Orange, CT, USA

Eve Bosnick, MSN, CRNP
Lecturer, Pediatric Nurse Practitioner Program
University of Pennsylvania School of Nursing,
    Philadelphia, PA, USA

Dawn Bounds, PhD, APRN, PMHNP-BC
Assistant Professor
Rush University College of Nursing, Chicago, IL, USA

Betty Boyle-Duke, DNP, CPNP, RN
Assistant Professor
Long Island University School of Nursing, Brooklyn,
    NY, USA

Patricia K. Bradley, PhD, RN, FAAN
Associate Professor
M. Louise Fitzpatrick College of Nursing, Villanova
    University, Villanova, PA, USA

Bridgette M. Brawner, PhD, MDiv, APRN
Associate Professor
University of Pennsylvania School of Nursing,
    Philadelphia, PA, USA

Judith Coucouvanis, MA, APRN, PMHCNS-BC
Clinical Nurse Consultant and Nurse Practitioner
University of Michigan Health System, Ann Arbor,
    MI, USA

Janiece E. DeSocio, PhD, RN, PMHNP-BC, FAAN
Professor
Seattle University College of Nursing, Seattle,
    WA, USA

Veronica C. Doran, DNP, PMHNP-BC
Assistant Professor
Marymount University, Arlington, VA, USA

Elizabeth Burgess Dowdell, PhD, CRNP, RN, FAAN
Professor
Coordinator of Undergraduate Research
M. Louise Fitzpatrick College of Nursing, Villanova
    University, Villanova, PA, USA

Emma Dundon, MS, RN, CPNP, PhD
Clinical Assistant Professor
University of Massachusetts College of Nursing,
    Amherst, MA, USA

Linda M. Finke, RN, PhD
Professor Emerita
Fort Wayne College of Health & Human Services,
    Indiana University-Purdue University, Fort Wayne,
    IN, USA

Deborah Fisher, PhD, RN, PPCNP-BC, CHPPN
Assistant Professor, School of Medicine and Allied
    Health
George Washington University, Washington,
    DC, USA

Marie Foley, PhD, RN, CNL
Dean and Professor
Seton Hall University College of Nursing, Interpro-
    fessional Health Sciences Campus, Nutley, NJ, USA

Moriah Freeman, DNP, PPCNP-BC, APRN
Pediatric Nurse Practitioner
The New York Foundling Hospital, Astoria, NY, USA

Eileen K. Fry-Bowers, PhD, JD, RN, CPNP, FAAN
Associate Professor
Hahn School of Nursing and Health Science
University of San Diego, San Diego, CA, USA

Judith Fry-McComish, PhD, RN, IMH
Associate Professor Emerita
Wayne State University, Detroit, MI, USA

Pamela Galehouse, PhD, PMHCNS, BC, CNL
Adjunct Professor Graduate Department
Seton Hall University College of Nursing, South
    Orange, NJ, USA

Melissa M. Gomes, PhD, RN, FNAP
Associate Professor
Hampton University School of Nursing, Hampton, VA, USA

Allison Grady, MSN, PNP-BC
Pediatric Nurse Practitioner, Pediatric Oncology,
    Medical College of Wisconsin
Clinical Instructor, University of Wisconsin-Milwaukee,
    College of Nursing, Milwaukee, WI, USA

**Donna Hallas, PhD, PPCNP-BC, CPNP, PMHS,
FAANP, FAAN**
Clinical Professor & Director of the PNP Program
Rory Meyers College of Nursing, New York University,
    New York, NY, USA

Margaret Hardy, RN, MBA, JD
Attorney
Sands Anderson PC, Richmond, VA, USA

Liam C. Hein, PhD, RN, FAAN
Associate Professor
University of South Carolina College of Nursing,
    Columbia, SC, USA

Deborah Johnson, DNP, NP, PMHNP-BC
Assistant Health Sciences Clinical Professor
School of Nursing, University of California San
    Francisco, San Francisco, CA, USA

Joan A. Kearney, PhD, APRN
Associate Professor
Director of Nursing Practice Program
Yale University School of Nursing, Orange, CT, USA

Norman L. Keltner, EdD, RN, CRNP
Professor (Emeritus)
Birmingham School of Nursing, University of Alabama,
    Birmingham, AL, USA

Kathleen Kenney-Riley, EdD, APRN-BC, PNP
Pediatric Nurse Practitioner
Children's Hospital at Montefiore, Bronx, NY, USA
Associate Professor
Mercy College, Dobbs Ferry, NY, USA

Eunjung Kim, PhD, RN, CPNP
Associate Professor, Family and Child Nursing
University of Washington School of Nursing, Seattle,
    Washington, USA

**Jessica Lee Kozlowski, PhD, DNP, RN,
CRNP-PC**
Pediatric Nurse Practitioner and Adjunct Clinical
    Faculty
Brandman University, Irvine, CA, USA

Heeyoung Lee, PhD, PMHNP-BC, CRNP
Associate Professor, School of Nursing
University of Pittsburg, Pittsburg, PA, USA

Necole Leland, DNP, RN, PNP, CPN
Assistant Professor in Residence
University of Nevada, Las Vegas School of Nursing,
    Las Vegas, NV, USA

Cherry Leung, PhD, RN
Assistant Professor
Department of Community Health Systems, University
    of California, San Francisco School of Nursing, San
    Francisco, CA, USA

**Madeleine M. Lloyd, PhD, PMHNP-BC,
FNP-BC**
Psychiatric Nurse Practitioner
Rory Meyers College of Nursing, New York University,
    New York, NY, USA

Pamela Lusk, DNP, RN, FAANP
Clinical Associate Professor
Ohio State University College of Nursing, Columbus,
    OH, USA

Caroline R. McKinnon, PhD, PMHCNS-BC
Associate Professor
Department of Biobehavioral Nursing, College of
    Nursing, Augusta University, Augusta, GA, USA

Mikki Meadows-Oliver, PhD, RN, PNP, FAAN
Associate Professor
Quinnipiac University School of Nursing, Hamden, CT, USA

Lisa Milam, MA, DSW, LCSW
Social Worker and Expansion Director
Our Kids Center, Nashville General Hospital, Nashville, TN, USA

Jamesetta A. Newland, PhD, FNP-BC, FAANP, DPNAP, FAAN
Clinical Professor Emerita
Rory Meyers College of Nursing, New York University, New York, NY, USA

Freida H. Outlaw, PhD, RN, MSN, FAAN
Executive Academic Program Consultant
American Nurses Association, Minority Fellowship Program, Silver Spring, MD, USA

Jose A. Parés-Avila, DNP, MA, NP-C, APRN, FAANP
Associate Professor
University of South Florida College of Nursing, Tampa, FL, USA

Geraldine S. Pearson, PhD, PMHCS-BC, FAAN
Associate Professor Retired
University of Connecticut School of Medicine, Farmington, CT, USA

Sally Raphel, MS, APRN/PMH, FAAN
University of Maryland School of Nursing Emerita, Johns Hopkins University School of Nursing Emerita, Baltimore, MD, USA

Joan B. Riley, MS, MSN, PNP-BC, FAAN
Associate Professor
Georgetown University School of Nursing & Health Sciences, Washington, DC, USA

Patricia Ryan-Krause, MS, RN, MSN, PCPNP-BC
Associate Professor
Yale University School of Nursing, Orange, CT, USA

Naomi A. Schapiro, RN, PhD, CPNP-PC
Professor Emeritus, Family Health Care Nursing
University of California, San Francisco, San Francisco, CA, USA

Kathleen Scharer, PhD, RN, PMHCNS-BC, FAAN
Distinguished Professor Emerita
University of South Carolina, Columbia, SC, USA

Linda Stephan, RN, MSN, PNP
Associate Professor, Family Heath Care Nursing
School of Nursing, University of California San Francisco, San Francisco, CA, USA

Anne M. Teitelman, PhD, FNP-BC, FAANP, FAAN
Associate Professor
Department of Family and Community Health, University of Pennsylvania School of Nursing, Philadelphia, PA, USA

Shannon Vaillancourt D'Alton, MSN, APRN, CPNP, CHPPN
Instructor
College of Nursing
Medical University of South Carolina, Charleston, SC, USA

Sarah B. Vittone, DBe, MSN, RN
Assistant Professor
Georgetown University School of Nursing & Health Sciences, Washington, DC, USA

Stephanie Wright, PhD, FNP-BC, PNP-BC
Associate Professor (Emerita)
George Washington University School of Nursing, Washington, DC, USA

Edilma L. Yearwood, PhD, PMHCNS-BC, FAAN
Associate Professor and Department Chair
Georgetown University School of Nursing & Health Studies, Washington, DC, USA

Forward

I am honored to write a Forward to this impressive volume. The book is especially impressive for its breadth of coverage of topics important not only for nurses but for other healthcare providers as well.

I am struck by the salience of three cross-cutting themes that are of great importance to all healthcare providers. One theme concerns evidence-based practice. It is now widely recognized that healthcare must make better use of empirically based data to apply knowledge that exceeds the experience of individual providers. This book rightly emphasizes the need for trainees and providers to search databases for the latest findings on the effectiveness of interventions. However, it is equally essential to obtain empirically based data on the specific strengths and needs that characterize each child and parent. Although databases contain voluminous information on diagnostic constructs such as attention deficit hyperactivity disorder (ADHD) and autism spectrum disorder (ASD), there are no tests for definitively diagnosing these or most other childhood behavioral, emotional, or social disorders. Instead, appropriate diagnostic formulations require data from people who see the children in various contexts such as home, daycare, and school, as well as in the clinic. To obtain sound empirically based data, it is necessary to use standardized assessment instruments completed by informants such as parents, daycare providers, and teachers, as well as by children regarding their own functioning, plus analogous instruments for assessing parents. It is also necessary for assessment instruments to span broad spectra of functioning and to be supported by published reliability, validity, and normative data. Although diagnostic constructs such as ADHD and ASD are influential, most children display mixtures of problems and strengths that are not fully encapsulated by such constructs. Consequently, providers must avoid prematurely imposing diagnostic labels when integrating empirically based data from multiple sources in order to build a comprehensive picture of the functioning of each child and parent across multiple contexts. As an example, a teacher's report of a child's inattentiveness may argue for ADHD, but parents' reports that the child spends hours on videogames would argue against ADHD. Rather than asking "Who should I believe?" the provider should consider the child's needs for help in attending to schoolwork without being forced to decide whether the child "has" ADHD.

A second cross-cutting theme concerns the need to take account of cultural and societal variations among children and their parents. These include variations characterizing natives of pluralistic societies and variations characterizing migrants to host societies. Despite recent political rhetoric, immigration will continue mixing people from diverse cultural and societal backgrounds. To advance mental health research and practice, assessment must take account of variations associated with cultural and societal differences. This can be done through collaborations with indigenous researchers around the world to advance the use of multicultural assessments that are reliable, valid, and effective with diverse children and parents.

A third cross-cutting theme concerns the need for ongoing multidisciplinary collaboration in research, training, and practice. Just as children's functioning is affected by multiple biological, experiential, and social factors, efforts to help them require multiple kinds of expertise. For effective collaboration, providers from different disciplines – including nurses, psychologists, physicians, and social workers – need to share a common data language for communicating about the children and parents they serve. This can be achieved by using empirically based procedures for assessing the actual functioning of children and parents, in addition to whatever specialized procedures are favored by particular providers. Those who partake of the multiple perspectives represented in this volume will be richly rewarded in their efforts to understand and help children.

Thomas Achenbach, PhD

Professor

President, Research Center for Children, Youth, and Families

The University of Vermont

Burlington, VT

Forward

Child and Adolescent Behavioral Health: A Resource for Advanced Practice Psychiatric and Primary Care Practitioners in Nursing by Edilma Yearwood, Geraldine Pearson and Jamesetta Newland is an outstanding book, one that provides best practices in child and adolescent mental health that are pertinent for both psychiatric mental health and primary care nurse practitioners. The editors have assembled an all-star team of experts to contribute to this book, which is a must read. A unique feature of the book is that each chapter is written by both a psychiatric mental health specialist and a primary care provider, which ensures its relevancy to practice in both mental health and primary care settings. The section on special populations definitely adds value to the text and the case exemplars in the supplementary online materials are an exceptional addition that brings issues to real life.

We are currently living in an era where one out of four to five children and adolescents have a mental health problem, yet less than 25% receive treatment. Wait times for mental health evaluations and treatment in many areas of the United States are 3–6 months, therefore it is imperative that primary care providers become proficient in mental health screening and early interventions for the most common child and adolescent mental health problems. I encourage everyone who reads this book to take action on its terrific content and put the knowledge gained rapidly into practice as all children and adolescents deserve the very best evidence-based care.

Bernadette Mazurek Melnyk, PhD, APRN-CNP, FAANP, FNAP, FAAN

Vice President for Health Promotion, University Chief Wellness Officer, Dean and Professor, College of Nursing Professor of Pediatrics and Psychiatry, College of Medicine Executive Director, The Helene Fuld Health Trust National Institute for Evidence-based Practice in Nursing and Healthcare, The Ohio State University

Preface to Second Edition

As we began revising this second edition of the textbook we remain committed to the goal of developing a useful resource to help advanced practice registered nurses (APRNs) working directly with children and adolescents. As we re-developed the book structure it became evident that since publishing the first edition, we have become better writers, editors, practitioners and nursing scholars. We hope this is reflected in the second edition.

We recognize that nurses are working in various care systems to address the ongoing problem of unmet mental health needs of the pediatric population. The research on health disparities continues to show that early identification, access to care, and early treatment are lacking for vulnerable populations of children and adolescents.

This book recognizes that pediatric populations predominantly access care through their primary care provider, often as a result of school requirements for regular immunizations, physical health exams, and management of common illnesses. There is no such requirement for mental health assessment and treatment and this has led to many children and adolescents going without warranted mental health care. By the time their family seeks services their symptoms have reached an acute or chronic level. Prevention efforts or early interventions might have resulted in a much more positive level of functioning for the child and the family.

Many factors influence seeking mental health care at any level of the continuum. These include geographic availability of specialized pediatric mental health services and absence of stigma associated with mental health symptoms and subsequent need for treatment. The reality is, if a child or adolescent is not treated for their disorder, and the disorder continues into adulthood, it is likely to have a poorer prognosis and more adverse effects on development.

From the beginning we have been committed to developing a book that reflected the collaborative relationship between psychiatric APRNs and primary care APRNs. Most of the chapters have been jointly written by authors who reflect this collaboration. Peer reviewers have reflected the psychiatric and primary care knowledge and each chapter presents state-of-the-art, evidence-based knowledge about specific psychiatric and behavioral health issues presented by children and adolescents in various health care settings.

We hope that any APRN can make use of this book to better understand behavioral disorders and their etiology, assessment guidelines, strategies for treatment in primary care settings, and indications for consultation, collaboration, and referral. The book is developmentally based and proposes strategies for working in partnerships with children, adolescents, families, and other health care providers to improve mental health status with vulnerable populations.

The sections of the book include assessment, treatment, special populations, and special issues. Chapters have been added dealing separately with Child Sexual Development, Adolescent Sexual Identity and Behaviors, Managing the Needs of LGBTQ Youth and Adverse Childhood Events. All chapters from the first edition have been heavily edited and updated to reflect current state of practice.

This book reflects our belief that primary care is at the forefront of meeting the ongoing mental health needs of pediatric populations in the United States and the world. Primary care is the point of entry into health care for many families and can form an effective system of mental health triage, early intervention, and supportive linkages to treatment. It is not the intent of this book to suggest that primary care providers should treat complex mental health presentations. However, APRNs in primary care can be instrumental in initial assessment while continuing to treat simple behavioral presentations, such as ADHD, affective disorders, and anxiety. One purpose of this book is to raise awareness of primary care APRNs in considering behavioral health presentations in their assessment while screening for severity, and then collaborating with psychiatric APRNs to facilitate treatment.

We continue to endorse the view that nursing care is built on trust. Primary care nurses are in the unique position to have long-term relationships with children, adolescents, and their families. They can be the supportive bridge and catalyst to ensure that mental health treatment is both destigmatized and accessed.

We have watched the slow unfolding of health care reform and the burgeoning development of innovative care delivery systems. More recently, the COVID-19 pandemic has challenged and complicated the healthcare delivery system; and all individuals and groups globally. Consequently, mental health of all has been strained, with increased rates of anxiety, depression, isolation, personal loss and self-medication. Given the current uncertainty and crisis, there is an urgent need to integrate behavioral health into primary care treatment and to be mindful of the full range of needs of children, adolescents and their families. We must also be cognizant of providing mental health treatment in non-traditional settings such as in schools, the juvenile justice system and places of worship, to name a few. The ultimate goal remains ensuring that children and adolescents presenting with mental health and behavioral symptoms have access to timely care with the most appropriate health care provider. Healthy People 2020 advocates for all levels of prevention in pediatric care including early identification, access to treatment and increased awareness of mental health needs. Our goal remains facilitation of the work of all APRNs who interact with children and adolescents. We hope that you find this second edition both informative and useful.

Edilma L. Yearwood
Geraldine S. Pearson
Jamesetta A. Newland

Acknowledgment

The Editors wish to express their thanks and gratitude to authors of the chapters in the first edition of this textbook. Their work formed the foundation for this new edition. Thank you!

Angela Amar
Robin Bartlett
Cecily I. Betz
Elizabeth Bonham
Susan Boorin
Eve Bosnick
Penelope R. Buschman-Gemma
Ellen Carroll
Diane M. Caruso
Judith Coucouvanis
Angela A. Crowley
Tammi Damas
Janet Deatrick
Kathleen R. Delaney
Janiece DeSocio
Elizabeth Burgess Dowdell
Edith (Emma) Dundon
Kathryn K. Ellis
Jean Nelson Farley
Linda M. Finke
Marie Foley
Pamela Galehouse
Judith Haber
Donna Hallas
Margaret Hardy
Elizabeth Hawkins-Walsh

Laura C. Hein
Charlotte A. Herrick
Judith Hirsh
M. Katherine Hutchinson
Barbara Schoen Johnson
Kathleen Kenney-Riley
Allison W. Kilcoyne
Maureen Reed Killeen
Eunjung Kim
Carol Anne Marchetti
Natalie McClain
Caroline R. McKinnon
Mikki Meadows-Oliver
Beth Muller
Lois C. Powell
Cathy Quides
Sally Raphel
Amanda Reilly
John B. Riley
Cynda H. Rushton
Patricia Ryan-Krause
Lawrence D. Scahill
Kathleen Scharer
Karen G. Schepp
Carolyn Schmidt
Kelly Ann Sheehy
Deborah Shelton
Sarah B. Vittone
Sandra J. Weiss
Stephanie Wright

About the Companion Website

This book is accompanied by a companion website:

Companion website: www.wiley.com/go/Yearwood

The website includes:

- Case studies
- Further reading
- Weblinks
- Figures and Tables

Scan this QRcode to visit the companion website.

1

Child, Adolescent, and Family Development

Stephanie Wright[1] and Edilma L. Yearwood[2]

[1] George Washington University School of Nursing, Washington, DC, USA
[2] Georgetown University School of Nursing & Health Studies, Washington, DC, USA

Objectives

After reading this chapter, advanced practice registered nurses will be able to:

1. Understand child and adolescent development within biopsychosocial and environmental contexts.
2. Identify characteristics over the developmental continuum that represent age-appropriate social and emotional behaviors of typically developing children and youth.
3. Determine at-risk behaviors in children and youth across the developmental span requiring referral for additional evaluation.
4. Describe behaviors manifested by children and youth with high secure self-esteem, high insecure self-esteem, and low self-esteem.
5. Compare and contrast models of cognitive development and their application to practice.
6. Demonstrate an understanding of common characteristics of language (phonology, morphology, syntax, semantics, and pragmatics) and language development.
7. Identify normal patterns of family development.
8. Identify social determinants of health that impact normal child development.

Introduction

Knowledge of the characteristics of normal development in typically developing infants, children, and youth is a necessary precursor for recognizing characteristics that are considered atypical for the developmental stage. This knowledge is essential for advanced practice psychiatric and primary care practitioners in nursing who screen and monitor for the early signs of developmental abnormalities, mental illness, or behavioral difficulties. These can be indicative of minor developmental issues or of serious diagnostic conditions such as autism spectrum disorder (ASD) that can be ameliorated, although not cured, with intensive early intervention services. Understanding developmental norms aids in early recognition of mental health disorders such as depression in children and youth (American Academy of Child and Adolescent Psychiatry 2015). To identify these, advanced practice registered nurses (APRNs) must have the knowledge of developmental norms applicable to the children and adolescents they treat.

Early assessment, case finding, and treatment of psychiatric disorders in a youngster may preserve the child's sense of self, competence, and relatedness to others and

Child and Adolescent Behavioral Health: A Resource for Advanced Practice Psychiatric and Primary Care Practitioners in Nursing,
Second Edition. Edited by Edilma L. Yearwood, Geraldine S. Pearson, and Jamesetta A. Newland.
© 2021 John Wiley & Sons, Inc. Published 2021 by John Wiley & Sons, Inc.
Companion website: www.wiley.com/go/Yearwood

prevent more serious behavioral and relationship issues. The areas of development chosen for review in this chapter reflect the topics discussed throughout this textbook. Descriptions of early brain development and typical social, emotional, and cognitive development spanning childhood to emerging adulthood are presented. In addition, because child, adolescent, and family development are influenced by contextual and interactional factors, Bronfenbrenner's Bioecological Theory of Human Development is used to illustrate the dynamic nature of these interactions and how individuals and families are either propelled or impeded in their developmental trajectory by these factors. More recently, social scientists are examining the impact of social determinants of health (SDH) on overall wellbeing and vulnerability across multiple groups across the lifespan. SDH are external factors such as socio-economic status, neighborhood conditions, health literacy, educational level attained, early childhood experiences, availability, and access to resources among other things. SDH can affect individuals and families where they live, work and or play. Finally, the family is on a developmental trajectory that can complement or conflict with the trajectory of the child or adolescent while influencing individual and or family outcomes. Therefore, family characteristics and dynamics are discussed here.

Prenatal Development

Child development begins at conception with a basic cell and genetic structure. As the understanding of genetics rapidly increases, the model of how an individual's genetics interacts with human development is changing. Going from a fixed model in which human experience takes place within an individual's genetic context, it begins to be clear that the interaction of genetics and experience is much more nuanced than this, and is transactional and bidirectional in nature (Bjorklund and Causey 2017). This interaction is dynamic, with genes being turned on and off, possibly by other genes or by environmental influences. This fluid and dynamic concept of genetic/environmental interaction is changing our view of the developmental issues and problems encountered as practitioners and, ultimately, in the way in which they are treated (Gottesman and Hanson 2005).

Brain Development

The foundation for understanding child and adolescent development begins with knowledge of early and progressive brain development and environmental, chemical, and biological factors that can interfere with normal brain growth. From conception to age 2, brain development,

while prolific, is uneven. Early brain development is characterized by several processes, including birth of neurons, neuronal migration, neural pathway development, synaptogenesis, and pruning or shedding of unwanted parts. Brain development begins about 2 weeks after conception and continues into adulthood. While prenatal brain development is largely under genetic control, it is clear that there are early environmental influences here (nutrition, hormones, exposure to toxins). Once the early neural tube is formed, neural proliferation proceeds, followed by migration, then differentiation of cells. Many more cells are formed than are needed, so many cells also die off during this process. The development of synapses then proceeds and follows a similar pattern, with an overproduction of synaptic connections and a later pruning of these connections that proceeds into childhood and adolescence (Tierney and Nelson 2009). This ability to form and prune neuronal connections accounts in part for the great plasticity of young brains. Neuronal and synaptic plasticity in the developing brain is believed to be both adaptive and maladaptive. Adaptive plasticity heralds an ability to learn new skills, store and retrieve information, respond to environmental stimuli, repair damage, and maintain an intact memory. Maladaptive plasticity is implicated in neurological disorders, while excessive synaptic pruning is thought to contribute to psychiatric disorders such as schizophrenia (Belsky and Pluess 2009; Johnston 2009; Marsh et al. 2008).

At approximately 2 years of age, the brain is roughly 75% of the weight of the adult brain (Davies 2011). Myelination, a process that enhances nerve impulse transmission, occurs from a posterior to anterior direction, affecting sensory then motor pathways with enhanced myelination supporting greater intellectual functioning (Marsh et al. 2008). The largest part of the brain, the cerebral cortex, has two hemispheres, right and left, each responsible for different functions. The right hemisphere houses our ability to pay attention, intuition, spatial abilities, negative emotions, ability to process environmental challenges, ability to anticipate consequences, and whole to part processing (Berk 2008; Schutz 2005). The left hemisphere is responsible for positive emotions, oral and written language, analytic processing style, and part to whole processing abilities (Berk 2008). The frontal lobe, where executive function originates, is involved with abstract thinking, motor activity, cognition, consciousness, planned behavior regulation, and impulse inhibition (Berk 2008; Yaun and Keating 2007). The temporal lobe is the communication and emotional sensation center of the brain.

Fetal exposure to in utero toxins, exposure to environmental toxins post birth, anoxic trauma, nutritional deficiencies, and genetic vulnerabilities are some of the factors affecting normal brain development and the achievement of normal child and adolescent developmental milestones. While the brain is a unique and complex entity, structural or functional deviations in the brain can have profound emotional, social, intellectual, behavioral, or psychological impact on the developing individual both in the immediate and long term.

Debate continues over when neurogenesis ends (Shen 2018; Snyder 2018). For years neuroscientists believed that most neurogenesis ended at about the end of infancy. More recent research has found possible neurogenesis continuing into adulthood in select areas of the brain, but there are conflicting research findings. Adult brains do not have the plasticity of children's brains, but exactly how those changes occur is not clearly understood (Shen 2018). Current thinking is that neurogenesis gradually slows during childhood and then there is a resurgence at adolescence. Synaptogenesis continues throughout the lifetime, with a burst at adolescence. Synaptogenesis and synaptic pruning occur based on a "use it or lose it" criteria. Synaptic connections that are frequently used are preserved and those that are not are eliminated.

During adolescence, the human brain undergoes significant changes impacting several behaviors that are characteristic of this age group. Neuroplasticity or the ongoing maturation of the structural and functional aspects of the central nervous system (CNS) continues to occur during adolescence as part of normal development, in response to personal experiences and post injury to the brain (Ismail et al. 2017). In a review article examining cerebral plasticity, these authors identified five types of neuroplasticity, developmental, adaptive, reactive, excessive/debilitating, and post injury vulnerability, and reiterated that neuroplasticity can be either adaptive or maladaptive. Abnormal or maladaptive plasticity appears associated with neuropsychiatric disorders such as attention deficit hyperactivity disorder (ADHD), ASD, learning and intellectual disabilities, and schizophrenia (Ismail et al. 2017). The loss of plasticity as we mature is not a completely negative phenomenon, as it allows for greater efficiency and specialization within the brain (Bjorklund and Causey 2017).

Arain et al. (2013) describe a surge in synaptogenesis, in part propelled by the synthesis of sex hormones (estrogen, progesterone, and testosterone) during the teen years. This intense activity is secondary to the surge that occurs in infancy. Consequently, adolescents experience significant changes in the limbic system that impacts self-control, emotions, decision-making, and risk-taking behaviors (p. 450). The amygdala, responsible for our emotions, aggression, and impulsivity, seems to be a significant driver of behavior in this age group.

Neurotransmitters, the chemical messengers of the brain, also have a role in adolescent behavioral presentation. It appears that during the teen years, dopamine and serotonin levels are lower than at other times and melatonin is higher. Low dopamine levels are implicated in mood swings and emotion regulation. Low serotonin levels are associated with mood, anxiety, and poor impulse control behaviors. An increase in melatonin drives a need for more sleep (Arain et al. 2013). Mills et al. (2014) review research indicating a possible developmental mismatch in the maturation of adolescent brains, the subcortical regions developing first and the prefrontal regions lagging slightly behind. They posit that this could explain some of the sensation-seeking and risk-taking behavior of adolescence.

Since 2015, a large multisite study has been in process looking at adolescent brain cognitive development (ABCD Study, 2016). The study coordinating center is located at the University of California at San Diego and extends to 21 additional sites across the United States. To date, they have enrolled over 11 000 children between the ages of 9 and 10 and will track these participants until they are 20 years old.

Impact of Poverty on Brain Development

As will be discussed further in this chapter, poverty as a social determinant of health is a significant factor impacting brain development. In the United States, it is estimated that one in five children live in poverty. The federal poverty level identifies a family of four with an income of $24 600 as living in poverty (US census.gov n.d.). Poverty renders families more vulnerable to access to healthcare, healthy foods, safe and stable living situations, and resources to support child flourishing and developmental needs. Childhood mental, behavioral, and developmental disorders are more prevalent in lower income families and communities when compared to higher income groups (Cree et al. 2018). Johnson et al. (2016) identified material deprivation, stressors, environmental toxins, and poverty as environmental mediators that also impact the developing brains of children and adolescents. Material deprivation includes factors such as living in food deserts which then impacts nutritional status, and having access to experiences/exposure and supplies, such as developmentally appropriate and challenging toys that provide stimulation and promote learning and critical thinking during key stages of development. Health providers are encouraged to screen for poverty, access to services, and the presence of other SDH factors impacting overall health and development at each child healthcare visit.

Stage Theories and Individual Differences

A review of guides to child development reveals a variety of organizational patterns to assist in understanding how children develop. Development is a very complex subject as humans are complex beings with a long developmental trajectory. Development is usually studied by examining behavior and change over time most commonly broken down into physical, social, emotional, and cognitive areas. Many of these approaches to understanding development use stage theories. Children do have commonalities as they progress through their growing and developing which make this helpful (Mercer 2018), but no stage covers all the aspects of development in a given individual. When trying to understand development, the concept of *individual differences* is imposed upon the generalizations of stage theories and the student of development must always seek to marry these two concepts.

The concept of temperament contributes to our ideas about individual differences, particularly in the area of personality. Early research in the areas of temperament and personality developed separately, but most writers and researchers in the area of development link these two (Kagan and Fox 2006). The concept of temperament describes a set of qualities related to reactivity and self-regulation that appear very early and exhibit some stability over time. While parents have described these individual differences in their children for centuries, and other developmental theories had described aspects of temperament, the first developmentalists to describe them in detail were Thomas and Chess as part of the New York Longitudinal Study in the early 1950s (Thomas et al. 1968). Many others have researched and written about temperament since then and have described temperamental characteristics in various ways, but most include some of these:

1. General activity level (physically active versus quiet).
2. Responsiveness to the environment (how sensitive one is to environmental stimuli).
3. Reactivity in terms of approach or withdrawal to new people or new situations.
4. General mood.
5. Rhythmicity: how rapidly one develops a rhythm or pattern.
6. Persistence: attention span.

Some writers have fewer, some have more (Kagan and Snidman 1991; Rothbart 2007; Thomas et al. 1968). These characteristics are not immutable, but are underlying an individual's reaction to their environment and can greatly affect the fit of the child with a parent (and a parent with a child since we all have these temperamental qualities) and within a family.

Social and Emotional Development

Infancy

The period of infancy is characterized by remarkable strides in social and emotional development. For example, beginning at birth through 4 months of age, the infant's behavior evolves from primarily reflexive behaviors. These include primitive infant reflexes (i.e. Moro and parachute reflexes) and the initial manifestations of voluntary or directed behaviors such as turning the head, brief tracking of an object with the eyes, the "freezing" response to an unfamiliar figure, and the emergence of smiling in response to the recognition of familiar caregiving figures (Betz and Sowden 2008; O'Reilly 2007). As infancy concludes, the attachment to primary caregivers is evident by the infant's observable affectionate behaviors and the early use of language to acknowledge parents/primary caregivers (i.e. mama, dada) (Davies 2011).

The insights pertaining to infant social and emotional development were first proposed by Sigmund Freud (1957), who suggested the infant's primary drive was motivated by need for oral satisfaction that could only be met by the mothering figure. This theoretical perspective was largely disregarded later in the work of Erik Erikson (1950, 1959) and subsequent developmental psychologists such as John Bowlby (1980, 1982) and Mary Ainsworth (1989) (Bretherton 1992). Erikson's framework of psychosocial development conceptualized the period of infancy as the stage of *Trust vs. Mistrust*. Erikson (1950, 1959) theorized that the major developmental task to be achieved by the infant was the development of trust with the primary caregiver. This trusting awareness served as the foundation for the development of subsequent relationships. The infant's trust was the product of the primary caregiver's predictable and consistent cycle of response to the infant's needs for food, comfort, and security. In circumstances wherein the infant's needs were not met in this predictable and consistent fashion, then a sense of mistrust evolved instead, with a potential for long-standing struggles with trusting others.

Building on the earlier work of Erik Erikson, John Bowlby formulated additional insights about the process of attachment. Bowlby's work, relying heavily on ethological concepts, viewed attachment between the infant and mother (his focus was directed to the mothering figure) as predicated on instinctual mechanisms found in the imprinting behaviors of lower level species (Lorenz 1937). According to Bowlby (1980, 1982), attachment, an innate survival behavior and as important as feeding and parturition, was described as a reciprocal process of interactions based upon the infant's need for safety, comfort, and protection, and the mother's caregiving responses to address these infant needs. Furthermore, Bowlby suggested that disruptions in the attachment process would increase the risk of negatively affecting the child's psychosocial development.

Subsequent studies examining discordant attachment have supported Bowlby's original propositions (Madigan et al. 2007). Bowlby's work created the foundation for subsequent studies of this nascent mother–child relationship. These studies have attempted to describe the attributes, risk (i.e. maternal depression, extended mother–infant separation), and protective factors (i.e. mind-mindedness, maternal sensitivity) associated with adaptive and maladaptive attachment and the child's subsequent psychosocial development (Arnott and Meins 2007; Finger et al. 2009; Laranjo et al. 2008; Niccols 2008; Strathearn et al. 2009).

Mary Ainsworth, a contemporary of Bowlby, contributed to the study of attachment based upon the Strange Situation methodology that she developed and tested to identify three basic patterns of attachment: securely attached, avoidant, and resistant (Ainsworth et al. 1978). Later, another pattern of attachment was added to the original triad: disorganized/disoriented (Main and Solomon 1990). According to Ainsworth, attachment refers to the affectional bond that develops between the mother and infant. Ainsworth (1989) characterized this bond as dependent on a persistent, consistent, and emotionally important caregiver who provided predictable care responses to meet the needs of the infant. Ainsworth's model has since been tested with divergent populations of children (i.e. premature infants, blind infants) and circumstances (i.e. foster care) to enlarge our understanding of the nature of infant and mother attachment (McMahon et al. 2006; Reyna and Pickler 2009; Van Londen et al. 2007). Other models of attachment have since been developed and refined in an effort to reconceptualize the attachment process as reciprocal rather than a unidimensional process between mother and baby (Goulet et al. 1998; Schenk et al. 2005).

Toddlerhood

The sense of trust the infant develops sets the stage for the new psychosocial developmental challenge of toddlerhood: *Autonomy* versus *Shame and Doubt* (Erikson 1950, 1959). It is during this stage that toddlers learn that the cautious excitement and curiosity of exploring, playing, and learning in new environments, such as at daycare centers, are accompanied by unexpected limitations imposed on their behaviors by parents and other adults. The perceived barriers to pursuing these young desires and satisfying their basic needs create immediate feelings of frustration, bursts of temper, and other displays of unrestrained protest. A mantra ascribed to

toddlers is that they "are long on will and short on skill" (Malley 1991).

It is during this stage of development that physical abilities advance, enabling the obvious progression in gross and fine motor abilities. These advancements include newly acquired gross motor abilities of walking, running, and jumping together with recent fine motor achievements such as simple stacking of blocks and scribbling shapes. The emerging new motor abilities of the toddler, coupled with advances in cognitive development, enable the child to progress socially with noncustodial adults and other peers (California Department of Education [CDE] 2007).

Through their interactions with adults in their enlarging world, as defined in part by their childcare arrangements, toddlers learn to interact with other adult figures by interpreting their social cues. Toddlers engage in the first efforts of social interactions with their peers. They engage in play activities that begin as parallel efforts and eventually loosely resemble cooperative play with the guided assistance of adults (CDE 2007).

Knowledge of typical toddler development is a prerequisite for increasing understanding of this stage of childhood for research, clinical, and parenting purposes. It enables researchers to investigate the behavioral symptomatology and impact associated with chronic conditions and disabilities (Gray and McCormick 2005; Magiati et al. 2007; Peadon et al. 2009). Knowledge of typical development facilitates APRNs' abilities to screen and detect the early manifestations of delays for service referrals (Individuals with Disabilities Education Improvement Act of 2004). Additionally, understanding of typical social and emotional development enables APNs to suggest to parents age-appropriate activities to foster the acquisition of domain-specific milestones.

Preschool Years

The preschool years extend from 3 to 6 years of age. Erikson (1950, 1959) referred to this period of childhood psychosocial development as *Initiative vs. Guilt*. One of the developmental challenges for the preschool child is to begin to learn how to integrate comparisons of his or her efforts that do not correspond to the same level of achievement by his peers. The preschooler's play increasingly evolves with the refinement and development of gross and fine motor skills, enabling more active participation in collective play with peers and evidence of preferred play interests. The preschool child learns to play more cooperatively with peers and is more aware of and sensitive to what are fair and unfair actions toward playmates (Betz and Sowden 2008). Children's play takes on more dramatic overtones, with adaptation of the adult roles of their parents or authority figures into their play and the incorporation of fantasy themes for acting out with their peers.

Knowledge and understanding of the typical psychosocial behaviors expected of preschool children are necessary to properly monitor, screen, and detect behaviors indicative of an actual or potential problem, and for parental guidance regarding their child's development (Hagan et al. 2008). It is during the preschool years that the child begins to move away from an egocentric orientation. The stages of play shown in Table 1.1. illustrate play

Table 1.1 Stages of play

Infancy	Solitary or independent play: infant's play is focused on activities that are dependent on reflexive and sensory actions. Playthings that engage the infant by stimulating sensory motor behaviors are favored. These playthings include: • rattles • mobiles • toys that make sounds • colorful toys • toys that can be mouthed • bodily movements that create pleasurable sensations (i.e. sucking fingers, patting at mobile) • responding to parental bonding and attachment behaviors
Toddler	Toddler play expands beyond the infant's body boundaries. The toddler's developing fine and gross motor abilities enable greater exploration of the environment and manipulation of playthings. The toddler's developing language skills and cognitive skills enable parallel play activities, that is, play that is done in the presence of other children but does not involve other children. • Scribbling and coloring • Riding tricycles • Stacking and nesting toys • Playing with stuffed animals • Playing with dolls • Completing simple, large-sized puzzles
Preschooler	The preschooler is developing social skills that enable the child to move beyond parallel play to play that involves the beginning of interacting with others. The child's developing cognitive abilities result in the emergence of fantasy play involving the adoption of imaginary roles such as storybook characters. Individual interests and preferences in play activities develop. • Playing with pretend toys such as costumes • Playing simple board games • Dancing • Playing with musical toys • Playing with high-tech toys (i.e. video games, movies) • Using wheel toys • Playing group games • Playing fantasy role-playing games • Gender-specific activities are not always evident
School age	School-age children progress in the refinement of gross and fine motor skills associated with play. Their developing social network of classmates and friends provides the context for learning prosocial skills, learning to play by the rules, and making comparisons regarding their competencies in sports activities with their peers. Competitive sports activities emerge and flourish. Individual interests and preferences in play activities continue. • Team sports • Creative hobbies • Crafts • Video and computer games • Board games

Table 1.1 (*cont'd*)

	• Construction activities (making models, art objects, decorative items) • Outdoor sports (swimming, hiking, bicycling) • Special-interest clubs • Technology recreational activities (use of the Internet)
Adolescent	While team sports are focused on gender-specific activities, development of opposite-sex activities can include dancing, music, clubs, and community advocacy/social justice activities. • Competitive team sports (i.e. football, baseball, volleyball, etc.) • Competitive individual sports (i.e. track and field, tennis) • Pleasure reading • Creative hobbies (i.e. drawing) • Collection hobbies (i.e. baseball cards) • Group outings • Technology recreational activities (i.e. surfing the Internet) • Computer games • Outdoor sports (i.e. hiking, swimming)

Source: Cincinnati Children's Hospital Medical Center (2007–2009), Keith (2009), National Parent-Teacher Association (2009), Ramseyer (2007).

activities that the child engages in based on developmental mastery, which also serves to reinforce developmental skills.

School-age Years

Erickson hypothesized that the psychosocial task of the school-age period (7–11 years), entitled *Industry vs. Inferiority*, is the learning and mastery of competencies associated with the child's expanding role expectations. During this stage, the child adopts the role of student, is delegated simple household responsibilities (i.e. making his bed and keeping his bedroom/sleeping area orderly), and engages in sports and recreational activities as a team member or competitor, whether formalized with Little League baseball or soccer teams, or loosely organized with groups of peers (Betz and Sowden 2008). The child's challenge is to achieve proficiency with new skills and knowledge to meet the expectations as a student, team member, and member of a peer group. Failure to do so leads to feelings of inferiority, low self-esteem, social isolation, and depression (Erikson 1950, 1959). Investigating the impact of learning and behavior problems on typical psychosocial development in school-age children has been the focus of research interests. Researchers have also studied the impact of chronic illnesses and disabilities on this school-age developmental domain for the purpose of preventing and ameliorating this psychosocial comorbidity (Grey and Sullivan-Bolyai 1999; Koenning et al. 1995; Sullivan-Bolyai et al. 2003; Woodgate and Degner 2003).

Adolescence

By adolescence, the major psychosocial task of youth is to establish an identity. This identity represents the compilation and integration of intellectual, social, psychological, and physical domains of functioning that the youth has acquired and achieved during the preceding stages of development (Erikson 1950, 1959). In turn, this development has been influenced and shaped by family membership, the social network of peers and adults, and the child- and youth-oriented community (i.e. school, youth groups, etc.).

The youth's developing identity is shaped in part by the company of peers he/she keeps. If the youth has developed an integrated identity without painful and potentially destructive unresolved conflicts from the past, then peers will be chosen who reflect the current psychological and emotional status and future aspirations of the teen. If the conflicts and ensuing intrapersonal and psychosocial turmoil are not resolved appropriately, the adolescent is at risk for associating with other teens who engage in self-destructive, delinquent, and even criminal behavior (Erikson 1950, 1959).

Although teens may espouse the beliefs and values of wanting independence, in truth many seek first and foremost the acceptance of their peers, as evidenced by their conformity in dress styles, physical appearance, colloquial expressions, and recreational and social interests (Bricker et al. 2009; Cin et al. 2009; Santor et al. 2000). Peer-related activities are fortified in their importance by the collective formal and informal group activities that serve to create a group identity, as is found with sports teams, celebrity-worship cults, and recreational interest groups.

For the first time, serious romantic relationships, some of which are based on physical attraction, develop (Nemours Foundation 2008a,b). Formerly, in past generations, these relationships were not seriously entertained until middle to late adolescence. In today's society, younger adolescents engage in sexual relationships as evidenced by the lowering of the age of introduction to sexual intimacy (Abma et al. 2004; Guttmacher Institute 2006). Yet, despite changing trends in adolescence pertaining to earlier initiation of active sexual behavior, the rate of adolescent pregnancy has dropped, due in part to the use of contraceptive options, including delaying sexual intercourse (Guttmacher Institute 2006). Another interesting development is the trend of young adults to delay marriage, childbearing, and entry into the workforce until the late 20s. Formerly, the mean age for these developmental milestones of adulthood occurred earlier in the 20s (Arnett 2000, 2001).

As societal and demographic trends change both nationally and globally, the characteristics associated with social and emotional development as well as all domains of development will be altered and revisited by developmental experts. Astute APRNs in psychiatric and primary pediatric care settings will observe these shifting developmental paradigms in adolescents and respond in their typical clinical expert manner based on the evidence to determine what behaviors represent at-risk or actual concerns that need additional assessment and services.

This section has discussed the social and emotional development of children and youth across the lifespan. Characteristics associated with each developmental stage have been presented to illustrate the age-appropriate behaviors reflective of social emotional behaviors of typically developing children and youth. Knowledge of typical development is a foundation of the knowledge needed to screen, detect, and refer for services those children and youth who require additional evaluation.

Self-esteem

Self-esteem refers to an individual's perception of personal self-worth and it is a mutable view of self whose roots of development begin early in childhood (Rosenberg 1965). A child's self-esteem, as measured by tools such as the Rosenberg Self-Esteem Scale (1965) or the Coopersmith Self-Esteem Inventory (Coopersmith 1981), can be quantified on a continuum from high to low. High levels of self-esteem have been further conceptualized as high secure self-esteem and high insecure self-esteem.

Self-esteem has been described by Robins and Trzesniewski (2005) as having its own developmental trajectory when examining groups of children and adults. Young children are described as having relatively high self-esteem, which declines over the course of childhood and continues to decline in adolescence with a resurgence in adulthood. Children may have a high value of themselves because they have relatively little for comparison. As children have more social experiences in school and develop cognitively, they are able to compare themselves to others and lose the global positive self-regard. This continues into adolescence as adolescents are often highly self-critical and also critical of each other. These are general trends upon which individual experiences are overlaid.

Children who have high self-esteem are confident of their abilities to perform, whereas children with low self-esteem experience hesitancy and doubt about their competencies to function on a par with their peers or as expected by their parents and other responsible adults in their lives. Children with high secure self-esteem perform academically better in school and in athletics, engage in less risky behaviors, are healthier, have more effective coping skills, and are more socially competent (Biro et al. 2006). There are some children with ADHD whose high self-esteem is typified as insecure and who are as at risk for problematic behaviors as children with low self-esteem (Menon et al. 2007). Those who have insecure self-esteem are described as inauthentic with feelings of entitlement narcissism. Children with high insecure self-esteem are particularly sensitive to criticism and react angrily to those who are perceived as criticizing them. They engage in high-risk behavior such as aggression and substance abuse but justify their behavior as appropriate (Menon et al. 2007). In contrast, children with low self-esteem more frequently experience school failure, engage in antisocial, aggressive, and delinquent behaviors, and exhibit more health and mental health problems (Donnellan et al. 2005).

A child's self-esteem can be influenced negatively or positively by maturational, social, and environmental factors. The self-esteem of a child can be adversely affected amid periods of significant changes such as during pubertal growth, transition periods associated with enrollment in new schools (such as progressing from elementary to middle school), and the developmental challenges experienced during adolescence (Adler and Stewart 2008; Biro et al. 2006). Increased levels of anxiety and poor or awkward social skills are additional factors that can contribute to low self-esteem. Researchers have been interested in studying self-esteem in children because it has been associated with adaptive and nonadaptive behaviors and alterable behavioral outcomes.

Additionally, experts have recognized that self-esteem, a perceptual evaluation of our self-worth, is amenable to modification with the use of intervention strategies.

Understanding of self-esteem has evolved from estimates of global self-worth to its association with specific areas of functioning as it pertains to family, school, and peers. For example, researchers found that home and school areas of self-esteem were more strongly associated with teen drug use than was peer self-esteem (Donnelly et al. 2008). Findings from this and other studies suggest that interventions targeting specific aspects of self-esteem may be more effective when the goal is global improvement of self-esteem (Donnelly et al. 2008; Wilkinson 2004; Young et al. 2004).

A number of variables are associated with supporting higher levels of self-esteem. Family and parent variables associated with promoting higher self-esteem in children are secure family attachment, parental acceptance of the child, high parental self-esteem, and intact family structure (Adler and Stewart 2008; Dalgas-Pelish 2006; Donnelly et al. 2008; Edmondson et al. n.d.). The profile of characteristics associated with high self-esteem in children includes productive school participation, protective peer activities, resiliency, and self-perceived physical attractiveness (Adler and Stewart 2008; Donnelly et al. 2008; Edmondson et al. n.d.; Manning 2007; Veselska et al. 2009). Researchers have differed in their explanations of the factors that promote positive levels of self-esteem in children. For example, some argue that achievement outcomes are not the determining factors of self-esteem, but rather the consequence (Menon et al. 2007). That is, children who experience success with academics will, in turn, experience positive feelings about themselves.

The risk factors and consequences associated with low self-esteem have been examined as well. Associations have been reported between maternal and adolescent low self-esteem (Edmondson et al. n.d.). Peer activities may create the medium for at-risk behaviors (Veselska et al. 2009). That is, children and youth may feel encouraged to engage in at-risk activities such as substance abuse if that is an acceptable norm of the peer group (Donnelly et al. 2008). Gender differences have been reported in the behavioral manifestation of low self-esteem. Boys with low esteem exhibit more externalizing behaviors compared to girls with low self-esteem, who have the tendency to internalize problems (Veselska et al. 2009). Lower self-esteem in adolescents was associated with a number of at-risk behaviors including early sexual initiation, unprotected sex, teen substance abuse, and a history of risky partners (i.e. history of AIDS, HIV, and incarceration) in adolescent girls (Ethier et al. 2006). Although self-esteem can serve as a protective factor for at-risk health behaviors, a child who has low self-esteem is at risk for developing psychosocial and psychiatric problems such as social isolation, aggression, and delinquency (Veselska et al. 2009).

Self-esteem in children and youth warrants consideration by APRNs in clinical practice. While it is unlikely that self-esteem would be formally assessed in clinical settings, it is appropriate to acknowledge its importance in determining the extent to which children and youth perceive their self-worth. Those who share feelings and/or demonstrate behaviors indicative of low self-esteem or high insecure self-esteem as described here should be referred for additional evaluations and services.

Cognitive Development

Understanding how cognitive development proceeds in children and being able to judge where a given child is on this timeline are important knowledge and skills for all pediatric healthcare providers. The understanding of aberrations or deviations from the "usual," "common," or "normal" pattern of development is, of course, firmly rooted in having developed an accurate understanding of normative patterns. Cognitive development is particularly challenging because so much of it is either unseen or inferred from a child's actions, language, or other indicators. Despite this, an understanding of how our current knowledge of human cognition developed and how children of various ages are both alike and different will assist readers in increasing knowledge about and skills with children.

Theoretical Considerations

Current developmental theory in the area of cognition is the product of a synthesis of thinking that began in the early part of the twentieth century. Interest in child development in the United States evolved largely out of the child study movement, based in observational studies of child behavior. The development of theory began with the work of Arnold Gesell (1929), who based his descriptions of children's behavior on a theory of maturational unfolding. This unfolding resulted from innate abilities, a genetic template. For Gesell, the environment played a superficial or temporary role in influencing the unfolding of behaviors. While his theory would be regarded as overly simplistic today, what Gesell gave us was a template of development that formed the basis for future work in the field of human development.

Behaviorism developed in contrast to both Gesell's idea of maturationalism and Freud's theories of the mental mechanism, examining so carefully the function of the psyche. For behaviorists, the only important functions of the human organism were those that could be seen and recorded, and these behaviors operated in clear response to certain fundamental rules (Watson 1913). Behaviorist theory reduces cognitive development to learning behaviors without regard for the internal processes that might enable one to learn.

Beginning his writing in the 1920s, Swiss psychologist Jean Piaget (1952) was the most dominant influence on a school of cognitive development commonly referred to as Constructivism. Piaget went largely undiscovered in the United States until the 1950s. His work was the basis for the study of cognitive development versus learning described by the behaviorists. Piaget's work revolves around the idea that individuals "construct" their own understanding of the world around them, organizing and reorganizing the structure of their knowledge. Piaget saw the cognitive structure as a product of the continuous interaction of children's internal abilities and the world around them. Inherent in this thinking is the idea that we all attempt to create a meaning for the world around us and are constantly revising and remaking our interpretations or "schemas." This process takes place by way of the functions of assimilation or accommodation. We take in or assimilate things in our environment that match our internal schema or accommodate our internal schema if the reality does not match our schema.

Best known among Piaget's work are his major stages of development and their characteristics:

1. Sensorimotor period (birth to 2 years). Infants progress from being largely reflex beings to learning to associate their experiences with the outside world through the coordination of sensory input and motor functions. They begin to represent objects mentally and manipulate them.
2. Preoperational thought (ages 2–7). Children in this stage are still primarily dependent upon perception and have little developed logic. They begin to represent the world with words, ideas, and drawings. The period is characterized by egocentric speech and thought, with children unable to appreciate another's point of view.
3. Concrete operations (ages 7–11). Logical thinking replaces intuition and children can perform basic logical operations on concrete objects and perform limited manipulation of mental objects. Piaget's classic tests for this period involved understanding reversibility and conservation.
4. Formal operations (ages 11–15). Individuals begin to think in more abstract ways. They understand hypothetical thinking, multiple causation, and other abstract concepts (Piaget 1952).

Piaget's work with children, largely observational, had a profound impact on the development of modern cognitive psychology. His documentation of how cognition develops and the stages of development is what most who have a passing acquaintance with Piaget remember. Newer research suggests that his stages often underestimated the capabilities of children; however, what endures are his constructivist ideas about how individuals attempt to attach meaning to the external world and how the quality and form of thinking change over time.

Piaget largely ignored the influence of the context within which cognitive development occurred, but the Soviet psychologist Lev Vygotsky (1962) emphasized the importance of the social and cultural environment while maintaining a constructivist approach. He placed great emphasis on the importance of language and social interaction in cognitive development. Education for Vygotsky was a major tool in development, and the function of the adult as "teacher" was to assist the child in learning through the relational interactions. This then contributed to the overall development of the child. His idea of the Zone of Proximal Development proposed that adults as "teachers" provide supports or "scaffolding" for children, enabling them to grow from their basic capabilities to a higher level (Figure 1.1).

A newer approach to the study of cognition is the information processing approach. In some ways an information processing approach is a return to a more reductionistic view of cognitive development, in contrast to the constructivist views which are much more holistic and include the concept of metacognition (Kuhn 1984). Information processing theory compares the functioning of the human mind to a computer model.

Cognitive processes are thus reduced to a list of tasks processed using mechanisms of attention, encoding, representation, execution, decoding, and memory (Bjorklund and Causey 2017). Development is largely a growth in capacity, efficiency, or speed of processing in the individual. Information is taken in through the senses, encoded into electrochemical impulses, and stored in areas of short-term or working and/or long-term memory.

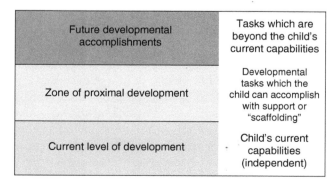

Future developmental accomplishments	Tasks which are beyond the child's current capabilities
Zone of proximal development	Developmental tasks which the child can accomplish with support or "scaffolding"
Current level of development	Child's current capabilities (independent)

Figure 1.1 Vygotsky's Zone of Proximal Development.

Behavior is the result of processing of information by comparison to previous encoded experiences, arriving at a conclusion, and executing a decision via motor output (Figure 1.2).

Information processing theory has been helpful in clarifying some of the relationships between cognitive processes to physiologic mechanisms and states. It is also particularly useful in explaining and understanding some of the learning problems that develop in individuals and explaining where the usual methods of processing might have gone awry.

More recent developments in cognitive developmental theory include revisions of some of Piaget's classic ideas by the neo-Piagetians. Among these is Robbie Case, who relabeled and attempted to more accurately define some of Piaget's stages. Case (1996, p. 2) described the work of neo-Piagetian cognitive theorists in the following passage:

> Theorists began to assert that children's conceptual development was less dependent on the emergence of general logical structures than Piaget has suggested and more dependent on the acquisition of insights or skills that are domain, task, and context specific.

In current thinking, the emergence of cognitive skills is more dependent on social interaction as described by Vygotsky (1962). Neo-Piagetian thinking also includes the idea that the general stages as described by Piaget are more of a "ceiling" or age-linked constraint. Within those constraints, children develop in unique ways more dependent upon their surroundings and interactions. Neo-Piagetian thinking has also included the idea that changes occurring

in children's thinking are less general than originally described by Piaget. Instead, they are more specific or "modular", with children showing growth in cognition in a more piecemeal fashion, first in one area or domain and then in another (Goswami 2008). Although Piaget's ideas have seen modification in recent years, there has been no overarching theory to replace the scope of Piaget's ideas. Bjorklund (2018) argues that developmental biology will have an increasing influence on cognitive development theory, as we learn more about brain development and its profound influence on the development of cognition.

Infant Cognition

If there has been any area in which the capabilities of children have been underestimated over the years, it is in the area of infant development. This is a clearly understandable phenomenon because infants have little in the way of language and motor skills to assist us in our assessment. The testing of infants is considerably more complex and requires some very clever experimental designs.

Infants are born predisposed to social interaction and constantly take in and process the world around them from the moment of birth. Infants are equipped with a set of primitive reflexes to assist them with their initial interactions with their environment, but these are rapidly replaced with reactions based on their developing awareness of the world around them. The sources of their information are their bodies and the senses. Infants, although physically immature, have intact sensory systems. Newborns can see, but have a short focal distance, likely the equivalent of someone quite nearsighted. They prefer

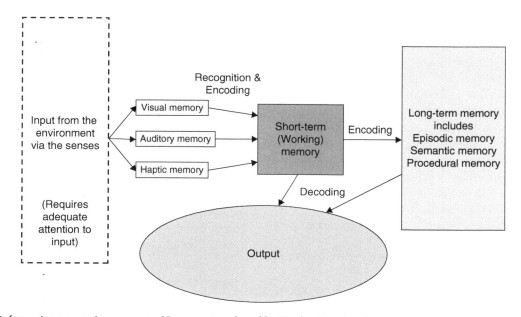

Figure 1.2 Information processing concepts. (*Source:* Developed by Stephanie Wright.)

high contrast and often scan to those areas of the human face. By 2 months of age, the eye has matured sufficiently so that the infant can focus about as well as an adult (McDonough 1999). Depth perception, which requires the brain's coordination of two visual images, first appears around 6–11 months of age and appears to be closely related to crawling (Trawick-Smith 2010).

Touch is a crucial sense for newborns and they are well equipped to use this sense to interact with those caring for them. Newborns also have a well-developed sense of pain. Newborns can distinguish basic tastes and will show this with facial responses. Smell is also well developed in newborns. Hearing is not terribly acute in newborns, likely related to delayed clearing of materials from the ear canal. However, their hearing capabilities are quite sensitive shortly after birth (Trawick-Smith 2010).

Piaget's Sensorimotor Stage describes infants as inadvertently discovering new experiences through their sensual exploration and then trying to repeat those events or actions. This progresses to anticipation of events from cues, and then attempts to repeat interesting events through their own actions. This eventually leads to some goal-directed behavior and some simple problem solving toward the end of the first year of life. Piaget emphasized the importance of the development of object permanence in infants, recognizing that objects exist out of sight. Piaget claimed this appeared at about 8–12 months of age, but current laboratory research indicates that this may appear much earlier, although it is not obvious in everyday events (Goswami 2008). Imitation emerges early in infancy and is likely a primary source of learning for infants. Older infants engage in imitation of complex behaviors of others.

Piaget suggested that infants do not mentally represent their everyday experience until about 18 months of age. Current research largely refutes this, with infant research into memory showing that much younger infants remember events, and later imitate or repeat actions and therefore must have mental representation of them (McDonough 1999). Toward the end of the first year, infants show simple problem solving, such as flipping a light switch to turn on a light, and rapidly progress to problem solving that requires multiple steps.

By the second year, toddlers have well-developed object permanence, searching in multiple locations for objects. They develop excellent skills of deferred imitation of complex behaviors of others. They can actively sort objects.

While we now know that infants have the development of certain cognitive skills earlier than described by Piaget, there is still considerable discussion describing the actual capabilities of infants. Infant development is an area of ongoing rich research.

Early Childhood Cognitive Development

Piaget characterized the Preoperational Stage of development more by what children could not yet do than by what they could do. According to Piaget, the greatest change seen in this age group was the great capacity for mental representation (symbolic function), which permitted young children to separate the physical world from the world of thought. Their play then takes on the characteristics seen so commonly in children of this age: engagement in considerable make-believe and greater complexity in their play. Make-believe play serves a variety of functions for the child, including allowing them to express emotion, anticipate events, and become more socially competent. Children of this age also develop considerable fine motor coordination and use this to represent their ideas. Piaget pointed out several limitations of thought in children of this age. They engage in egocentric thinking, being unable to consider any other point of view or interpretation of the world than their own. Recent research questions this. Gelman and Schatz (1978) point out that young children adapt their language to their audience, at times showing clear appreciation for another's perspective. Several redesigns of Piaget's classic three mountains experiment have shown awareness of others' points of vantage during this preschool (preoperational) period (Borke 1975).

Piaget also held that there were certain limitations of logic for preoperational children. The famous conservation experiments show difficulties of children appreciating the constancy of certain physical characteristics such as volume in the face of changes in appearance (the changing appearance of liquids of the same volume in different containers). Piaget felt this was related to centration, the tendency of preschool children to focus on one characteristic of a situation or object, while ignoring others. As with age-related limitations described by Piaget, preschoolers can overcome appearances and think more logically than he originally described, especially when the materials are familiar to them (Goswami 2008).

Similarly, preschool children appear to be able to categorize with more sophistication than originally described by Piaget. In conclusion, preschool children gradually learn about relationships that involve interpreting appearances of objects, and this understanding is aided by their growing language abilities and their beginning to understand constancy of number. Like infants, preschoolers are considerably more capable than originally described by Piaget, but the steps they must pass through to achieve these milestones were accurately described by him.

Cognition in School-Age Children

Piaget (1952) described the school-age period as characterized by concrete operational thought, with thought becoming more logical and well organized. Children of this age understand concepts of conservation and reversibility, and they grow to be able to perform classifications based on multiple characteristics of the items to be sorted. They can sort according to dimensions and can solve basic inferential problems. They understand spatial relationships and orient themselves in space. This allows them to learn basic directions from one place to another and to draw maps.

The limitation of concrete operations described by Piaget is that the logic of school-age children is limited to what they perceive in the real world around them. They have difficulty considering abstract ideas and thinking about larger principles that might govern the real world.

School and culture heavily influence the growth of cognition in this age group, therefore the achievement of the milestones of concrete operational thinking and the progression to formal operational thinking depend heavily upon the context within which the child grows. Some school-age children show the beginnings of hypothetical thinking and deductive reasoning before Piaget's usual age for formal operational thinking (approximately 11 years), but this greatly depends upon their environment (Goswami 2008).

Adolescent Cognitive Development

At about age 10 or 11, children begin to enter a period of formal operational thinking, according to Piaget. In this stage they develop the ability to think abstractly, going beyond the realm of their everyday experiences. Adolescents develop clear deductive reasoning, allowing them to solve problems based on logic and mental experimentation. The development of language is closely tied to this ability to perform abstract reasoning. Adolescents can consider problems that are counter to their everyday experience and engage in hypothetical thinking about possible outcomes.

Elkind (1967) described limitations on the newly developing cognitive skills of adolescents imposed by their dramatic changes in self-concept. This creates a kind of self-absorption, a new form of egocentrism, which tends to limit some areas of cognitive growth. While Elkind described four characteristics of adolescent egocentrism, his concepts should be examined for applicability within specific cultural contexts. His characteristics include:

Imaginary audience: Adolescents often believe that they are the center of others' attention, creating extreme self-consciousness and making them sensitive to criticism.
Personal fable: Adolescents, because they feel they are the center of others' attention, often feel that they are somehow unique and special, acting out extraordinary lives.

Invulnerability: Because they feel that they are somehow unique, adolescents may feel that are invulnerable to the usual consequences of everyday actions. Their ability to consider the long-term consequences of their actions may be severely limited by their egocentrism.
Idealism: Because they are able to go beyond the limits of reality and into the possible by their cognitive capabilities, adolescents may tend to be very idealistic and become quite critical of others who do not reach these ideals, parents in particular.

Recent research indicates that formal operational thinking is not always attained in all cultures and contexts, indicating that it is educationally and culturally transmitted. In addition, formal operational thinking does not emerge in all areas of thinking at once, but rather appears in relation to specific areas of learning (Keating 2004).

Development and Information Processing Theory

As previously described, information processing theory ascribes the changes in cognition that occur as children grow in terms of growth in processing speed, ability to attend, short- and long-term memory, and organization of thinking. There are few age-related milestones to assist one in tying particular milestones to age. Older children have progressively faster processing speeds and are able to sustain selective attention for longer periods. Short-term memory, that is, retention of information for less than a minute without active memory retention strategies, is usually tested with digit span. Two- to 3-year-olds can usually retain about two digits, 7-year-olds about five digits. This gradually increases to an adult level of about seven to eight digits. Changes in long-term memory may be more related to organization than to capacity, and children's abilities to retrieve information from long-term memory improve with age and with practice. Once children are in formal learning situations, they have many opportunities for improving memory and often learn organization and rehearsal strategies for improving memory (Santrock 2007).

Development of Coping in Children

Responses to stress and imposed change have been extensively studied in adults. Physiologic and psychological response patterns to stress are well documented, but how those patterns develop is still unclear. Coping is defined to include all responses to stressful events. Most stress researchers would consider coping as falling into two categories: instinctive or reflexive reactions and those that are learned responses (Compas 1987). In adult coping literature, there has been much research on coping as an adaptational response as evidenced by studies of coping function and style. As classically described by Lazarus and Folkman (1984), coping functions to both regulate the individual's emotional response and engage in some problem solving around the crisis imposed by the stressor.

Individual variability in coping and the description of coping styles by various researchers (Krohne and Rogner 1982; Miller and Green 1984) lead to the question of how these patterns are developed in individuals and which individual differences and environmental issues play an important part in the development of these patterns. Included in these studies of individual differences is the question of why some children are more resilient and less vulnerable to stress than others (Garmezy 1981).

While coping literature has built upon adult studies of stress psychology, it has important overlaps with traditional areas of child development research, including neurobiology, temperament, cognition, attention, emotion, and parental attachment. Because coping is such a complex phenomenon, no central theory has emerged, but several important principles have been reiterated related to the development of coping in children.

Early coping is embedded in neurobiology and the development of the brain and CNS. Early responses to stress seem to be particularly rooted in the temperamental characteristics related to arousal, reactions to novelty, attention, and affect (Rueda and Rothbart 2009). As the child matures, experience contributes to the development or limiting of coping skills, with different aspects of development playing more important roles at various ages. Early experiences with stress may in turn shape the

development of the brain regions related to emotional regulation (Compas 2009). Early experiences with uncontrollable stress have been associated with changes in the serotonin neurons and a pattern of learned helplessness (Maier and Watkins 2005).

Parents are central figures in the child's development of coping skills, serving as important social support, role models for coping behaviors, and stress-absorbing figures. Parents can make demands on children that are early stressors that children must deal with. How parents support children in coping with their demands is an important variable. The availability and ability of parents to assist children in gaining a sense of control over the demands placed upon them help children develop a sense of mastery and control.

> The development of adaptive coping requires years of deep developmentally attuned interpersonal support for dealing with just-manageable demands. Stressful overarching social conditions, such as poverty, oppression, discrimination, harsh families and parenting, maltreatment, and neglect, pose serious risks to the healthy development of coping.
> (Zimmer-Gembeck and Skinner 2016, p. 3)

Age-graded shifts in coping have been described by Skinner and Zimmer-Gembeck (2007) and serve as a helpful developmental model for coping (Table 1.2). Within the first few months of life, infants progress from largely physiologic and temperamentally based reactions to learning self-soothing and use of distraction as early coping mechanisms. Children learn to regulate their own behavior with a shift occurring at about 18–24 months of

Table 1.2 Broad outlines of possible developmental shifts in means of coping

Developmental period	Approximate ages	Nature of coping	Role of social partners	Nature of regulation
Infancy	Birth to 18 months	From reflexes to coordinated action schema	Carrying out coping actions based on infant's expressed intentions	Interpersonal co-regulation
Preschool age	Ages 2–5	Coping using voluntary direct actions	Availability for direct help and participation	Intrapersonal self-regulation
Middle childhood	Ages 6–8	Coping using cognitive means	Cooperating with and supporting child's coping efforts	Coordinated self-regulation
Early adolescence	Ages 10–2	Coping using metacognitive means	Reminder coping	Proactive self-regulation
Middle adolescence	Ages 14–16	Coping based on personal values	Backup coping	Identified self-regulation
Latef adolescence	Ages 18–22	Coping based on long-term goals	Monitoring coping	Integrated self-regulation

Source: Reprinted from Skinner and Zimmer-Gembeck (2007) with permission from the Annual Review of Psychology. Permission conveyed through Copyright Clearance Center, Inc.

age, as mastery of motor skills and emotion come into play. A second major shift occurs at about 5–7 years of age, when cognitive elements and social relations begin to play important parts in coping. A third shift is described at about age 10–12, marked by changes in patterns of thinking correlated with the growth of more sophisticated cognitive skills represented by formal operational thinking. At 14–16 years of age, autonomy and identity development begin to play salient roles in coping. New patterns again emerge between middle adolescence and the early 20s, when expanding social horizons provide challenging new experiences.

Acute and chronic stresses have been implicated in many physical and mental health problems in both children and adults. Documentation of patterns of coping in children has been a fairly recent field of research and one that will be extremely important as healthcare professionals attempt to understand and better treat the emotional and mental health problems of children as well as understand the behavior of all children.

Language Development

The exact reasons for humans' ability to communicate that is unrivaled by any other species are unclear. Piaget believed that language development was an extension of the intellectual development of humans; we speak because of superior intelligence. Noam Chomsky (1972), on the other hand, argued that humans are prewired for language and have a theoretical "language acquisition device." Regardless of which view is espoused, language development is a critical indicator of normal human development and delays or failure to develop language are an important sign that some pathology exists.

Language is a symbolic form of communication, spoken, written, or, in some cases, signed. Spoken communication can be further broken down into receptive language and expressive language, with expressive language being much easier to assess in children. Although there are many languages in the world, they all have common characteristics, described as phonology, morphology, syntax, semantics, and pragmatics.

Phonology describes the basic sounds of the language. Although there are many similar sounds in languages, there are sounds that are unique to some language structures. Research by Patricia Kuhl (1993) has shown that infants are capable of hearing all possible sounds for the first six months of life, but during the second half of the first year, infants improve their ability to recognize sounds in their own language and gradually lose the ability to hear sounds that do not occur in their native language. This is a prime example of synaptic pruning as neural pathways that are unused are eliminated.

We are more aware of infants developing an understanding of the morphology of language,; that is, learning to recognize the meaning of sounds. During the second half of the first year, infants begin to recognize the boundaries between words in spoken language and to attach meaning to words. By 12 or 13 months, infants recognize about 50 words (Menyuk et al. 1995), many more than they are capable of expressing. This pattern continues with receptive language exceeding expressive language for much of early childhood.

All children, regardless of the language spoken, generally follow a similar pattern of development of expressive language:

- All infants are capable of crying to signal distress and often have distinctive cries as signals for different states.
- Cooing predominantly refers to vowel sounds made by young infants, usually indicating a pleasurable state, but it is also seen in response to an interaction with another.
- Sometime around four to six months, infants begin adding consonant sounds and vocalize consonant–vowel combinations, called babbling.
- Later in infancy, these sounds are strung together and often have the intonation of human speech.

While this is occurring in infancy, infants are learning to communicate in other ways as well, often using gestures and head nods to communicate their wishes. Deaf children at this age often begin learning to sign (Bloom 1998). Signing has also been promoted for hearing children as a method for enhancing their ability to communicate while they are developing spoken language. Daniels (1994) has found that teaching hearing children sign language instruction had a number of benefits, including increased vocabulary among preschoolers. Other small studies have suggested that teaching a version of signing to preverbal infants may enhance communication between parent(s) and child (Thompson et al. 2007) and possibly reduce frustration in preverbal children.

Most children utter their first word sometime between 10 and 15 months of age, usually names of important people, animals, or common objects. While the acquisition of first words is gradual, most children experience a real spurt in growth of vocabulary between 15 and 24 months and achieve a vocabulary of about 50 words (Hoff 2014). During this period, young children often acquire multiple new words each day, a truly amazing feat of learning.

Most children begin to string words together in two-word phrases during the second year, and two-word phrases are expected in normal development by 24 months of age. These two-word phrases often have a characteristic commonly referred to as "telegraphic speech" in which children convey meaning with a very succinct use of words. Thus, a combination of two words expresses the desire to do or have something despite the absence of important nouns, articles, or verbs, such as "Bobby ice cream" to indicate that he wants ice cream or, alternately, that someone else is eating ice cream. Context is important in understanding telegraphic speech.

Children move rapidly from two-word sentences to more complex and longer structures between 2 and 3 years of age. During the entire preschool period, children develop further understanding of the morphology, syntax, semantics, and pragmatics of language. This includes understanding plural and possessive forms, correct word order in sentences, the meaning of sentences, and appropriate use of language in different contexts. Although children make many errors as they attempt to apply language rules, this is part of learning the complex rules of language. By the time children enter 1st grade, they have an extensive expressive vocabulary, estimated at more than 8000 words (Rubin 2006). During elementary school, children refine their grammar and continue a remarkable growth in vocabulary.

Environment influences language development in a number of important ways. Parental and caregiver response to the child in conversation has been shown to be critical in numerous studies. This begins with what is usually referred to as child-directed speech. Adults and older children around a young child alter their speech pattern for the young child, often reducing the number of syllables in words and the number of words in a sentence and changing the pitch of the speech (child-directed speech). This has the important function of capturing the child's attention. Labeling familiar objects for the child serves to expand their vocabulary. In addition, parents and caregivers often use repeating language as reinforcement, recasting something the child said, emphasizing a word, which may include correcting and expanding on what the child said (Hoff 2014). Infants whose mothers speak to them more often have been shown to have larger vocabularies (Huttenlocher et al. 1991). Likewise, adults who read to children and later have their children read to them encourage language development.

The influence of genetic factors on speech and language development has not been clear. Recent findings of several genes related to dyslexia have also found that one of these genes (KIAA0319 on chromosome 6) may be related to speech delay (Rice et al. 2009). Other genes identified related to speech and language disorders include the FOXP2 gene on chromosome 7, which is related to apraxia in children (Medline Plus (n.d.).). These findings simply reinforce the need to identify and treat speech and language disorders early in life, when

neuroplasticity gives children the best outcomes from treatment.

While there is considerable variation in early language milestones, such as the first spoken word, the basic pattern of language learning applies to all children and to all spoken languages. Understanding this basic pattern assists practitioners in knowing when to seek help for children and their families. Emphasizing to parents their important role in language development, the APRN can give them specific suggestions on ways to encourage their child's language development. These include reading to and talking with the child, singing songs to the child while emphasizing particular words or expressions, and providing age-appropriate explanations and descriptions of events.

Bronfenbrenner's Bioecological Theory of Human Development

As stated previously, child, adolescent, and family development is complex and occurs within environmental contexts in which multiple interactions transpire directly or indirectly, affecting the developing individual. In the 1970s, Bronfenbrenner developed and described the Ecology of Human Development Theory (1979). The original theory was composed of the microsystem, mesosystem, exosystem, and macrosystem. He later added the chronosystem. In 1994 he revised his theory and renamed it the Bioecological Theory of Human Development (Bronfenbrenner). Table 1.3 provides concepts from his original model, his evolved thinking, and additions to the model on human development.

The development of each individual is interdependent on multiple factors, genetics, experience, temperament, type, and nature of reciprocal relationships, evolving complexity of interactions, context, time, attachments, quality of environments, and the emotional health of all individuals. A thorough nursing assessment of children, adolescents, and families must pay attention to all of these elements and understand how they affect the growth and development of each family member.

Family Life Cycle Development

As individuals grow and develop, so too does the family in which they are nested. There is no one definition of a family; however, most would agree that a family is how the individuals involved define it and is composed of both biological and nonbiological individuals as determined by the "family" unit. The Committee on the Science of Research on Families of the Institute of Medicine and the National Research Council further described families as, "members with very different

Table 1.3 Bronfenbrenner's evolving model of human development

Ecological Theory of Human Development: Original (individuals and settings)	Bioecological Theory of Human Development: Additional factors operating with original theoretical model
Microsystem: Individual, family, peers, school, and neighborhood; roles; where the individual lives; individual is an active actor in own development	Experience: Subjective feelings that are positive or negative; emotional and motivational in nature
Mesosystem: Connections and relationships between microsystem elements.	Proximal processes: Progressively complex and reciprocal interactions; the higher the levels of positive interactions between the parent/caretaker and the child, the lower the behavioral problems in the child
Exosystem: Connections and relationships between two or more systems, at least one of which does not contain the individual but can indirectly impact processes impacting the individual	Process-person-context-time: Characteristics of the developing person, the environment, changes over time, and developmental outcomes as a result of all interactions
Macrosystem: Customs, culture, ethnicity, beliefs, social fabric impacting the individual	Exposure: Multiple and complex activities must occur over time to promote emotional, social, moral, and intellectual development
Chronosystem: Change over time affecting the individual and the various environments the person experiences	Mutual emotional attachment: Such attachment with parent/caretaker that is internalized motivates child to engage with others
	"Third party": Children growing in environments where they are exposed to more than one caretaker have a greater variety of complex experiences that enriches development
	Future perspective: Psychological development (positive or negative) of caretakers influenced by behavior and development of the child

Source: Bronfenbrenner (1979), Bronfenbrenner (1994), Bronfenbrenner and Ceci (1994), Bronfenbrenner (2005).

perspectives, needs, obligations, and resources. The characteristics of individual family members change over time – within life spans, and across generations. Families exist in a broader economic, social, and cultural context that itself changes over time" (Olson 2011, p. 7).

Contemporary family constellations are influenced by divorce, single parenting, remarriages, older parents, foster and adoptive status, lesbian, gay, bisexual, transgender, and questioning parenting, economics, culture, mores, immigration status, co-parenting, and blended and geographic locations, among other factors (Olson 2011; Wright and Leahey 2013). Regardless of the family structure, family tasks include supporting the development of all its members, socialization, protection, providing food and shelter, communication, transmitting values, beliefs, and cultural norms, role development, and assisting with problem solving.

Two well-known family development models are Duvall (1977) and McGoldrick and Carter (2003). Both models identify developmental stages that families go through over time. Adolescence, adulthood, launching (young adult leaving the nuclear family to live on his own or with a partner), marriage, addition of children (through birth, fostering, or adoption), midlife, and later life are specific times with specific characteristics that comprise the development of the family. While both

models provide the APRN with a foundation for understanding family development, families are increasingly viewed as dynamic, with new configurations and processes that no longer fit into known traditional models. When conducting assessment of the child or adolescent, it is important to understand the factors that the family unit is dealing with because those factors and others beyond the immediate family unit impact the developing child or adolescent.

Positive parent–child relationship and connectedness can serve as a protective factor during child and adolescent development (Viner et al. 2012). APRNs can promote prevention in their practice with families and their children. Preventive efforts include positive behavioral modeling, maintaining a well-child healthcare routine, recommending early childhood programs such as Head Start and Montessori, and home-visiting programs. In addition, stressing with parents the importance of education and attending school and after-school enrichment programs, reducing screen time, reading routinely to the child, and engaging in community events and activities are ways for them to foster learning, stimulation, and connectedness. Educating parents about the importance of their role as teacher, advocate, and protector in their child's development and increasing their health literacy related to normal child and adolescent development and needs will facilitate their understanding of the importance of remaining engaged with their child through presence and active listening (Cprek et al. 2015; Garner et al. 2017; National Academies of Medicine 2016; Simmons et al. 2017; Viner et al. 2012).

Impact of Social Determinants of Health on Child, Adolescent, and Family Development

Discussion of SDH has been part of the social science literature since the early 2000s when Sir Michael Marmot started publishing on health inequalities (2001), subsequently on SDH (2006), and chaired the World Health Organization (WHO) Commission on the Social Determinants of Health. Since 2012, there has been a proliferation of research and published papers on SDH and, by extension, social determinants of mental health (SDMH), looking at the impact of these factors on brain and overall development, relatedness and health/mental health (Allen et al. 2014; Hartman et al. 2017; Li et al. 2017; Viner et al. 2012; WHO and Calouste Gulbenkian Foundation 2014). SDH is defined as "conditions in the environments in which people are born, live, learn, work, play, worship, and age that (in turn) affect a wide range of health, functioning, and quality-of-life outcomes and risks" (Office of Disease Prevention and Health Promotion, 2020). In addition to genetics, SDMH are associated with social inequalities, experiences during critical developmental periods, and environmental factors. Compton and Shim (2015) identified the following factors as influencing mental health status, "social exclusion, adverse early life experiences, poor education, unemployment/underemployment/job insecurity, poverty, income inequality, neighborhood deprivation, poor access to health foods, poor housing quality and instability, adverse features of the built environment and poor access to health care" (p. 421). Additional factors include exposure to violence, residing in a conflict laden or active war zone, exposure to pollutants, dirty water or poor air quality, and gender-based or sexual-orientation-based inequities, among others.

SDH are modifiable factors that will require policy, enforcement, and intentional action across multiple areas impacting people throughout the lifespan course. To ensure opportunity to access factors supporting healthy development for all, healthcare providers, including APRNs, should first assess vulnerabilities and refer to appropriate resources. In addition, APRNs can serve as advocates for strong policies promoting healthy development efforts and for equitable access to resources. The Protocol for Responding to and Assessing Patients' Assets, Risks, and Experiences (PRAPARE) tool is a screening

measure for providers to assist them in gathering data from individuals and families on the SDH factors that may be impeding their health and overall functioning (2016). An Implementation and Action Tool Kit exists along with the screening tool. APRNs are encouraged to review and use the tool as an aide to assist in gathering information about a range of factors impacting children, adolescents, and families, including family income, veteran status of parents, access to transportation, stress, neighborhood conditions, housing, education, language preference, parental employment, material security, social support and social integration, domestic violence, safety, immigrant/refugee status, and parental incarceration history. One very promising program that is being used nationally to assist vulnerable groups with burdensome SDH factors is medical-legal partnerships. These are collaborative practices between clinics, communities, and academic institutions working together to assist community members tackle problems related to housing, healthcare access, legal difficulties, public benefits, and education challenges (Henize et al. 2015).

Assessment Tools

1. The American Academy of Pediatrics Policy Statement on *Identifying Infants and Young Children with Developmental Disorders in the Medical Home: An Algorithm for Developmental Surveillance and Screening* (2006), the American Academy of Child and Adolescent Psychiatry *Practice Parameter for the Assessment of the Family* (2007), and the adapted Calgary Family Assessment Model (CFAM) by Wright and Leahey (2013) are useful documents for both the primary care and child and adolescent APN to use when assessing child, adolescent, and family development.

2. Developmental surveillance is a longitudinal process whereby at each visit the provider assesses and documents the status of the child and family to determine developmental concerns, progress, individual or family risk or protective factors, educational needs, and the effectiveness of prior health promotion or therapeutic regimen recommendations. Historical data,; observation of the child, adolescent, and caretaker(s) alone or during interactions, family structure, functioning, adaptability, and stressors, cultural, gender, and ethnic information, and communication style are specific data that can be gathered using these tools.

3. CFAM looks at three aspects of the family: structural (internal, external, and context), developmental, and functional (instrumental and expressive). Structural

characteristics include gender, ethnicity, class, family composition, and boundaries. Developmental characteristics include stages of family members, tasks performed by family members, and attachments. Functional characteristics include communication, roles, problem solving abilities, power, and beliefs (Wright and Leahey 2013).

4. Hagan et al. Bright Futures: Guidelines for Health Supervision of Infants, Children, and Adolescents, 4th edn (2017). Bright Futures is a series of resources for health supervision in primary care settings. It includes a pocket book, tool and resource kits with screening tools, and a nutrition guide.

Summary

This chapter has provided a focused overview of social, emotional, and cognitive development in children and youth as a basis for understanding age-appropriate and typical behaviors. Major theories of development have been reviewed and discussed in the context of understanding children's individual differences and the importance of social determinants of heath. Bronfenbrenner's Bioecological Theory of Human Development, Family Development Theories, and SDH data remind us that children and adolescents grow in multiple contexts which impact their developmental trajectory. Emphasis was directed to presenting content on the developmental characteristics relevant to clinical understanding for the purposes of screening at-risk and problematic behavior requiring additional evaluation and services. To this end, subject matter on cognitive and social emotional development, self-esteem, coping, and language development was presented. Incorporated within the discussion of these developmental characteristics are the theoretical underpinnings and evidence that support these models of development.

Resources

American Academy of Child and Adolescent Psychiatry. (2016). *Teen Brain: Facts for Families.* Available at http://aacap.org.

Hagan, J.F., Shaw, J.S., and Duncan, P.M. (eds.) (2017). *Bright Futures: Guidelines for Health Supervision of Infants, Children, and Adolescents, (4).* Elk Grove Village, IL: American Academy of Pediatrics.

National Academies of Science, Engineering, Medicine. (2016). *Collaborative on Healthy Parenting in Primary Care.* Available at https://sites.nationalacademies.org/DBASSE/ccab/DBASSE_178080.

National Association of Community Health Centers, Association of Asian Pacific Community Health Organizations, & Oregon Primary Care Association. (2019). *PRAPARE: Protocol for responding to and assessing patient's assets, risks, and experiences tool.* Available at https://www.nachc.org/research-and-data/prapare.

References

Abma, J.C., Martinez, G.M., Mosher, W.D., & Dawson, B.S. (2004). Teenagers in the United States: Sexual activity, contraceptive use, and childbearing, 2002, *Vital and Health Statistics*, Series 23, No. 24.

Adler, N. and Stewart, J. (2008). Self-esteem. In: *In Research: Psychosocial Notebook (Chapter 11), MacArthur Foundation/ Research Network on SES & Health*. San Francisco, CA: The Regents of the University of California Available at https://macses.ucsf.edu/research/psychosocial/selfesteem.php.

ABCD Study. (2016). Adolescent Brain Cognitive Development Study. Available at http://abcdstudy.org.

Ainsworth, M.S. (1989). Attachment beyond infancy. *American Psychologist* 44: 709–716.

Ainsworth, M.S., Blehar, M.C., Waters, E., and Wall, S. (1978). *The Strange Situation: Observing Patterns of Attachment*. Hillsdale, NJ: Erlbaum.

Allen, J., Balfour, R., Bell, R., and Marmot, M. (2014). Social determinants of mental health. *International Review of Psychiatry* 26 (4): 392–407.

American Academy of Child and Adolescent Psychiatry (2007). Practice parameters for the assessment of the family. *Journal of the American Academy of Child and Adolescent Psychiatry* 46 (7): 922–937.

American Academy of Child and Adolescent Psychiatry. (2015). *When to seek help for your child*. Available at https://www.aacap.org/AACAP/Families_and_Youth/Facts_for_Families/FFF-Guide/When-To-Seek-Help-For-Your-Child-024.aspx.

American Academy of Pediatrics (2006). Identifying infants and young children with developmental disorders in the Medical Home: an algorithm for developmental surveillance and screening. *Pediatrics* 118 (1): 405–420.

Arain, M., Haque, M., Johal, L. et al. (2013). Maturation of the adolescent brain. *Neuropsychiatric Disease and Treatment* 9: 449–461.

Arnett, J.J. (2000). Emerging adulthood: a theory of development from the late teens through the twenties. *American Psychologist* 55: 469–480.

Arnett, J.J. (2001). Conceptions of the transition to adulthood: perspectives from adolescence through midlife. *Journal of Adult Development* 8: 133–143.

Arnott, B. and Meins, E. (2007). Links among antenatal attachment representations, postnatal mind-mindedness and infant attachment security: a preliminary study of mothers and fathers. *Bulletin of the Menninger Clinic* 71: 132–149.

Belsky, J. and Pluess, M. (2009). The nature (and nurture?) of plasticity in early human development. *Perspectives on Psychological Science* 4 (4): 345–351.

Berk, L. (2018). Physical development in infancy and toddlerhood. In: *Exploring Lifespan Development*, 4the, Chapter 4, 90–114. Boston, MA: Pearson Education.

Betz, C.L. and Sowden, L. (2008). *Mosby's Pediatric Nursing Reference*, 6e. St. Louis: Mosby.

Biro, F.M., Striegel-Moore, R.H., Franko, D.L. et al. (2006). Self-esteem in adolescent females. *Journal of Adolescent Health* 39: 501–507.

Bjorklund, D.F. (2018). A metatheory for cognitive development (or "Piaget is Dead" revisited). *Child Development* 89 (6): 2288–2302.

Bjorklund, D.F. and Causey, K.B. (2017). *Children's Thinking: Cognitive Development and Individual Differences*. Los Angeles: Sage Publications.

Bloom, L. (1998). Language acquisition in its developmental context. In: *Handbook of Child Psychology, Volume 2: Cognition, perception, and language* (ed. W. Damon), 309–370. Hoboken, NJ: John Wiley & Sons Inc.

Borke, H. (1975). Piaget's mountains revisited: changes in the egocentric landscape. *Developmental Psychology* 11: 240–243.

Bowlby, J. (1980). *Attachment and Loss: Vol. 5*. New York: Basic Books.

Bowlby, J. (1982). *Attachment and Loss: Vol. 1. Attachment*. New York: Basic Books.

Bretherton, I. (1992). The origins of attachment theory: John Bowlby and Mary Ainsworth. *Developmental Psychology* 28 (5): 759–775.

Bricker, J.B., Rajan, K.B., Zalewski, M. et al. (2009). Psychological and social risk factors in adolescent smoking transitions: a population-based longitudinal study. *Health Psychology* 28 (4): 439–447.

Bronfenbrenner, U. (1979). *The Ecology of Human Development*. Cambridge, MA: Harvard University Press.

Bronfenbrenner, U. (1994). Ecological models of human development. *International Encyclopedia of Education* 3 (2): 1643–1647.

Bronfenbrenner, U. (ed.) (2005). *Making Human Beings Human*. Thousand Oaks, CA: Sage.

Bronfenbrenner, U. and Ceci, S. (1994). Nature-nurture reconceptualized in developmental perspective: a bioecological model. *Psychological Review* 101 (4): 568–586.

CDE. (2007). *California infant/toddler learning and developmental foundations*. Available at www.cde.ca.gov/sp/cd/re/itf09intro.asp.

Case, R. (1996). Introduction: Reconceptualizing the nature of children's conceptual structures and their development in middle childhood. In *Monographs of the society for research in child development: Vol. 61. The role of central conceptual structures in the development of children's thought*, R. Case & Y. Okamoto (Eds.), Serial No. 246, 1–2, pp. 1–26. Chicago, IL: University of Chicago Press.

Chomsky, N. (1972). *Language and Mind*. New York: Harcourt Brace.

Cin, S.D., Worth, K.A., Gerrard, M. et al. (2009). Watching and drinking: expectancies, prototypes, and friends' alcohol use mediate the effect of exposure to alcohol use in movies on adolescent drinking. *Health Psychology* 28 (4): 473–483.

Compas, B.E. (1987). Coping with stress during childhood and adolescence. *Psychological Bulletin* 101 (3): 393–403.

Compas, B.E. (2009). Coping, regulation, and development during childhood and adolescence. In: *Coping and the Development of Regulation. New Directions for Child and Adolescent Development*, vol. 124 (eds. E.A. Skinner and M.J. Zimmer-Gemback), 87–99. San Francisco: Jossey-Bass.

Compton, M.T. and Shim, R.S. (2015). The social determinants of mental health. *Focus* 13 (4): 419–425.

Coopersmith, S. (1981). *Self-Esteem inventories (SEI)*. Palo Alto, CA: Consulting Psychologists, Press, Inc.

Cprek, S.E., Williams, C.M., Asaolu, I. et al. (2015). Three positive parenting practices and their correlation with risk of childhood developmental, social, or behavioral delays: an analysis of the national survey of children's health. *Maternal and Child Health Journal* 19 (11): 2403–2411.

Cree, R.A., Bitsko, R.H., Robinson, L.R. et al. (2018). Health care, family, and community factors associated with mental, behavioral, and developmental disorders and poverty among children aged 2-8 years-United States, 2016. *Morbidity and Mortality Weekly Report* 67 (50): 1377–1383.

Dalgas-Pelish, P. (2006). Effects of a self esteem intervention program on school-age children. *Pediatric Nursing* 32: 341–348.

Daniels, M. (1994). The effect of sign language on hearing children's language development. *Communication Education* 43: 291–298.

Davies, D. (2011). *Child Development: A Practitioner's Guide*, 3e. New York: Guilford.

Donnellan, M.B., Trzesniewski, K.H., Robins, R.W. et al. (2005). Low self-esteem is related to aggression, antisocial behavior, and delinquency. *Psychological Science* 16 (4): 328–335.

Donnelly, J., Young, M., Pearson, R. et al. (2008). Area specific self-esteem, values, and adolescent substance use. *Journal of Drug Education* 28: 289–403.

Duvall, E. (1977). *Marriage and Family Development*, 5e. Philadelphia, PA: Lippincott.

Edmondson, J., Grote, L., Haskell, L. et al. (n.d.). Adolescent self-esteem: is there a correlation with maternal self-esteem? *Citations* 3: 1–8.

Elkind, D. (1967). Egocentrism in adolescence. *Child Development* 38 (4): 1025–1034.

Erikson, E. (1950). *Childhood and Society*. New York: Norton.

Erikson, E. (1959). *Identity and the Life Cycle: Selected Papers, Psychological Issues* (Monograph Vol. 1, No. 1). New York: International Press.

Ethier, K.A., Kershaw, T.S., Lewis, J.B. et al. (2006). Self-esteem, emotional distress and sexual behavior among adolescent females: inter-relationships and temporal effects. *Journal of Adolescent Health* 38: 268–274.

Finger, B., Hans, S.L., Bernstein, V.J., and Cox, S.M. (2009). Parent relationship quality and infant-mother attachment. *Attachment and Human Development* 11: 285–206.

Freud, S. (1957). *The Standard Edition of the Complete Psychological Works of Sigmund Freud*, vol. 18 (ed. J. Strachey). London: Hogarth.

Garmezy, N. (1981). Children under stress: perspectives on antecedents and correlates of vulnerability and resistance to psychopathology. In: *Further Explorations in Personality* (eds. A.I. Rabin, J. Aronoff, A.M. Barclay and R.A. Zucker), 196–269. New York: Wiley.

Garner, A.S., Storfer-Isser, A., Szilagyi, M. et al. (2017). Promoting early brain and child development: perceived barriers and the utilization of resources to address them. *Academic Pediatrics* 17 (7): 797–705.

Gelman, R. and Schatz, M. (1978). Appropriate speech adjustments: the operation of conversational constraints on talk in two-year olds. In: *Interaction, Conversation, and the Development of Language* (eds. M. Lewsi and L.A. Rosenblum), 27–61. New York: Wiley.

Gesell, A. (1929). Maturation and infant behavior pattern. *Psychological Review* 36: 307–319.

Goswami, U. (2008). *Cognitive Development: The Learning Brain*. New York: Psychology Press.

Gottesman, I.I. and Hanson, D.R. (2005). Human development: biological and genetic processes. *Annual Review of Psychology* 56: 263–286.

Goulet, C., Bell, L., St-Cyr Tribble, D. et al. (1998). A concept analysis of parent-infant attachment. *Journal of Advanced Nursing* 28: 1071–1081.

Gray, R. and McCormick, M.C. (2005). Early childhood intervention programs in the US: recent advances and future recommendations. *Journal of Primary Prevention* 26 (3): 259–275.

Grey, M. and Sullivan-Bolyai, S. (1999). Key issues in chronic illness research: lessons from the study of children with diabetes. *Journal of Pediatric Nursing: Nursing Care of Children and Families* 14 (6): 351–358.

Guttmacher Institute. (2006). *In brief: Facts on American teen sexual and reproductive health*. Available at http://www.guttmacher.org/pubs/fb_ATSRH.html.

Hagan, J.F., Shaw, J.S., and Duncan, P.M. (eds.) (2008). *Bright Futures: Guidelines for Health Supervision of Infants, Children, and Adolescents*, 3e. Elk Grove Village, IL: American Academy of Pediatrics.

Hagan, JF, Shaw, JS, & Duncan, PM (Eds.). (2017). *Bright Futures Guidelines for health Supervision of Infants, Children and Adolescents*, 4th ed. Elk Grove Village, IL: American Academy of Pediatrics.

Hartman, S., Li, Z., Nettle, D., and Belsky, J. (2017). External-environmental and internal-health early life predictors of adolescent development. *Development and Psychopathology* 29: 1839–1849.

Henize, A.W., Beck, A.F., Klein, M.D. et al. (2015). A road map to address the social determinants of health through community collaboration. *Pediatrics* 136 (4): e993–e1001.

Hoff, E. (2014). *Language Development*, 5e. Belmont, CA: Wadsworth Centage Learning.

Huttenlocher, J., Haight, W., Bruk, A. et al. (1991). Early vocabulary growth: relation to language input and gender. *Developmental Psychology* 27: 236–248.

Individuals with Disabilities Education Act of 2004, 20 U.S.C. § 1400 et seq (2004).

Ismail, F.Y., Fatemi, A., and Johnston, M.N. (2017). Cerebral plasticity: windows of opportunity in the developing brain. *European Journal of Paediatric Neurology* 21 (1): 23–48.

Johnson, S.B., Riis, J.L., and Noble, K.G. (2016). State of the art review: poverty and the developing brain. *Pediatrics* 137 (4): e20153075.

Johnston, M. (2009). Plasticity in the developing brain: implications for rehabilitation. *Developmental Disabilities Research Reviews* 15: 94–101.

Kagan, J. and Fox, N.A. (2006). Biology, culture, and temperamental biases. In: *Handbook of Child Psychology: Social, Emotional, and Personality Development* (eds. N. Eisenberg, W. Damon and R.M. Lerner), 167–225. Hoboken, NJ: Wiley.

Kagan, J. and Snidman, N. (1991). Temperamental factors in human development. *American Psychologist* 46 (8): 856–862.

Keating, D.P. (2004). Cognitive and brain development. In: *Handbook of Adolescent Psychology* (eds. R.M. Lerner and L. Steinberg), 45–84. Hoboken, NJ: Wiley.

Koenning, G.M., Benjamin, J.E., Todaro, A.W. et al. (1995). Bridging the "med-ed gap" for students with special health care needs: a model school liaison program. *Journal of School Health* 65 (6): 207–212.

Krohne, H.W. and Rogner, J. (1982). Repression-sensitization as a central construct in coping research. In: *Achievement, Stress, and Anxiety* (eds. H.W. Krohne and L. Laux), 167–193. Washington: Hemisphere.

Kuhl, P.K. (1993). Infant speech perception: a window on psycholinguistic development. *International Journal of PsychoLinguistics* 9: 33–56.

Kuhn, D. (1984). Cognitive development. In: *Developmental Psychology: An Advanced Textbook* (eds. M.N. Bornstein and M.E. Lamb), 133–180. Hillsdale, NJ: Erlbaum.

Laranjo, J., Bernier, A., and Meins, E. (2008). Associations between maternal mind-mindedness and infant attachment security: investigating the mediating role of maternal sensitivity. *Infant Behavior and Development* 31: 688–695.

Lazarus, R. and Folkman, S. (1984). *Stress, Appraisal and Coping*. New York: Springer.

Li, M., Johnson, S.B., Musci, R.J., and Wiley, A.W. (2017). Perceived neighborhood quality, family processes, and trajectories of child and adolescent externalizing behaviors in the United States. *Social Science & Medicine* 192: 152–161.

Lorenz, K.Z. (1937). The companion in the bird's work. *Auk* 54: 245–273.

Madigan, S., Moran, G., Schuengel, C. et al. (2007). Unresolved maternal attachment representations, disrupted maternal behavior and disorganized attachment in infancy: links to toddler behavior problems. *Journal of Child Psychology and Psychiatry* 48: 1042–1050.

Magiati, I., Charman, T., and Howlin, P. (2007). A two-year prospective follow-up study of community-based early intensive behavioural intervention and specialist nursery provision for children with autism spectrum disorders. *Journal of Child Psychology & Psychiatry & Allied Disciplines* 48 (8): 803–812.

Maier, S.F. and Watkins, L.R. (2005). Stressor controllability and learned helplessness: the roles of the dorsal raphae nucleus, serotonin, and corticotropin-releasing factor. *Neuroscience and Behavioral Reviews* 29: 829–841.

Main, M. and Solomon, J. (1990). Procedures for identifying infants as disorganized/disoriented during Ainsworth strange situation. In: *Attachment in the Preschool Years* (eds. M.T. Greenberg, D. Cicchetti and E.M. Cummings), 120–160. Chicago: University of Chicago Press.

Malley, C. (1991). *Toddler development. National Network for Child Care*. Amherst, MA: University of Massachusetts.

Manning, M.A. (2007). *Self-concept and self esteem in adolescents*. Student Services, 11–15. Available at https://pdfs.semanticscholar.org/5367/523293360cf1fd39a4da7a7f4e7e27bfcbaa.pdf?_ga=2.112261060.1791579078.1596517538-602920245.1596517538.

Marmot, M. (2001). Economic and social determinants of disease. *Bulletin of the World Health Organization*. 79 (10): 988–989.

Marmot, M. (2006). Health in an unequal world [Harveian Oration]. *Lancet* 368: 2081–2094.

Marsh, R., Gerber, A., and Peterson, B. (2008). Neuroimaging studies of normal brain development and their relevance for understanding childhood neuropsychiatric disorders. *Journal of the American Academy of Child & Adolescent Psychiatry* 47 (11): 1233–1251.

McDonough, L. (1999). Early declarative memory for location. *British Journal of Developmental Psychology* 17: 381–402.

McGoldrick, M. and Carter, B. (2003). The family life cycle. In: *Normal Family Processes Growing Diversity and Complexity* (ed. F. Walsh), 375–398. New York, NY: Guilford Press.

McMahon, C.A., Barnett, B., Kowalenko, N.M., and Tennant, C.C. (2006). Maternal attachment state of mind moderates the impact of postnatal depression on infant attachment. *Journal of Child Psychology and Psychiatry* 47: 660–669.

Menon, M., Tobin, D.D., Corby, B.C. et al. (2007). The developmental costs of high self-esteem for antisocial children. *Child Development* 78: 1627–1639.

Medline Plus. (n.d.). FOX P2 gene. Bethesda, MD: National Library of Medicine. Available at :https//Medlineplus.gov/genetics/condition/FOXP2

Mercer, J. (2018). *Child Development Concepts & Theories*. London: Sage.

Menyuk, P., Liebergott, J.W., and Schultz, M.C. (1995). *Early language development in full-term and premature infants*. Hillsdale, NJ: Erlbaum.

Miller, S.M. and Green, M.L. (1984). Coping with stress and frustration: origins, nature, and development. In: *The Socialization of Emotions* (eds. M. Lewsi and C. Saarni), 263–314. New York, NY: Plenum Press.

Mills, K.L., Goddings, A., Clasen, L.S. et al. (2014). The developmental mismatch in structural brain maturation during adolescence. *Developmental Neuroscience* 35: 147–160.

National Academies of Medicine. (2016). *Parenting matters: Supporting parents of children ages 0–8*. Available at http://www.national-academies.org.

National Parent-Teacher Association (2009). *Play at different ages and developmental stages*. Available at http://school.familyeducation.com/games/growth-and-development/38382.html.

Nemours Foundation. (2008a). *Teen health: Sexual attraction and orientation*. Available at http://kidshealth.org/parent/emotions/feelings/sexual_orientation.html.

Nemours Foundation. (2008b). *Teen Health: Am I in a healthy relationship*. Available at http://kidshealth.org/teen/your_mind/relationships/healthy_relationship.html#.

Niccols, A. (2008). "Right from the start": randomized trial comparing an attachment group intervention to supportive home visiting. *The Journal of Child Psychology and Psychiatry* 49: 754–764.

Office of Disease Prevention and Health Promotion. (2020). *Healthy-People 2020: The social determinants of health.* US Department of Health and Human Services. Available at https://www.healthypeople.gov/2020/topics-objectives/topic/social-determinants-of-health.

Olson, S. (2011). *Toward an integrated science of research on families: Workshop Report.* Washington, DC: The National Academies. Available at http://www.nap.edu/catalog/13085.html.

O'Reilly, D. (2007). *Infant reflexes.* Available at http://www.nlm.nih.gov/medlineplus/ency/article/003292.htm.

Peadon, E., Rhys-Jones, B., Bower, C., and Elliott, E.J. (2009). Systematic review of interventions for children with fetal alcohol spectrum disorders. *BMC Pediatrics* 9: 35.

Piaget, J. (1952). *The Origins of Intelligence in Children.* New York: International Universities Press.

PRAPARE. (2016). *Protocol for responding to and assessing patients'assets, risks, and experiences.* Available at http://nachc.org.

Ramseyer, V. (2007). Stages of play. Available at http://ezinearticles.com/?Stages-of-Play&id=900253&opt=print.

Reyna, B.A. and Pickler, R.H. (2009). Mother-infant synchrony. *Journal of Obstetric, Gynecologic, & Neonatal Nursing* 38: 470–477.

Rice, M.L., Smith, S.D., and Gayan, J. (2009). Convergent genetic linkage to language, speech and reading measures in families of probands with Specific Language Impairment. *Journal of Neurodevelopmental Disorders* 1 (4): 264–282.

Robins, R.W. and Trzesniewski, K.H. (2005). Self-esteem development across the lifespan. *Current Directions in Psychological Science* 14 (3): 158–162.

Rosenberg, M. (1965). *Society and the Adolescent Self-Image.* Princeton, NJ: Princeton University Press.

Rothbart, M. (2007). Temperament, development, and personality. *Current Directions in Psychological Science* 16 (4): 207–212.

Rubin, D. (2006). *Gaining Word Power,* 7e. Boston, MA: Allyn & Bacon.

Rueda, M.R. and Rothbart, M.K. (2009). The influence of temperament on the development of coping: the role of maturation and experience. In: *Coping and the Development of Regulation. New Directions for Child and Adolescent Development,* vol. 124 (eds. E.A. Skinner and M.J. Zimmer-Gembeck), 19–31. San Francisco: Jossey-Bass.

Santor, D.A., Messervey, D., and Kusumakar, V. (2000). Measuring peer pressure, popularity, and conformity in adolescent boys and girls: predicting school performance, sexual attitudes, and substance abuse. *Journal of Youth and Adolescence* 29: 163–182.

Santrock, J.W. (2007). *A Topical Approach to Lifespan Development.* Boston: McGraw-Hill.

Schenk, L.K., Kelley, J.H., and Schenk, M.P. (2005). Models of maternal-infant attachment: a role for nurses. *Pediatric Nursing* 31: 514–517.

Schutz, L. (2005). Broad-perspective perceptual disorder of the right hemisphere. *Neuropsychology Review* 15 (1): 11–27.

Shen, H. (2018) Does the adult brain really grow new neurons? *Scientific American.* Available at https://www.scientificamerican.com/article/does-the-adult-brain-really-grow-new-neurons/?print=true.

Simmons, J.G., Schartz, O.S., Bray, K. et al. (2017). Study protocol: families and childhood transitions study (FACTS) – a longitudinal investigation of the role of the family environment in brain development and risk for mental health disorders in community based children. *BMC Pediatrics* 17: 153. https://doi.org/10.1186/s12887-017-0905-x.

Skinner, E.A. and Zimmer-Gembeck, M.J. (2007). The development of coping. *Annual Review of Psychology* 58: 119–144.

Snyder, J.S. (2018). Recalibrating the relevance of adult neurogenesis. *Trends in Neurosciences* https://doi.org/10.1016/j.tins.2018.12.001.

Strathearn, L., Li, J., Fonagy, P., and Montague, P.R. (2009). What's in a smile? Maternal brain responses to infant facial cues. *Pediatrics* 122: 40–51.

Sullivan-Bolyai, S., Deatrick, J., Gruppuso, P. et al. (2003). Constant vigilance: mothers' work parenting young children with type 1 diabetes. *Journal of Pediatric Nursing* 18 (1): 21–29.

Thomas, A., Chess, S., and Birch, H.G. (1968). *Temperament and Behavior Disorders in Children.* New York: New York University Press.

Thompson, R.H., Cotnoir-Bichelman, N.M., McKerchar, P.M. et al. (2007). Enhancing early communication though infant sign training. *Journal of Applied Behavior Analysis* 40: 15–23.

Tierney, A.L. and Nelson, C.A. (2009). Brain development and the role of experience in the early years. *Zero Three* 30 (2): 9–13.

Trawick-Smith, J. (2010). *Early Childhood Development: A Multicultural Perspective.* Upper Saddle River, NJ: Pearson.

US Census (n.d.). *Federal poverty guidelines.* Available at http://census.gov.

Van Londen, W.M., Juffer, F., and van IJzendoorn, M.H. (2007). Attachment, cognitive, and motor development in adopted children: short-term outcomes after international adoption. *Journal of Pediatric Psychology* 32: 1249–1258.

Veselska, Z., Geckova, A.M., Orosova, O. et al. (2009). Self-esteem and resilience: the connection with risky behavior among adolescents. *Addictive Behaviors* 34: 287–291.

Viner, R.M., Ozer, E.M., Denny, S. et al. (2012). Adolescence and the social determinants of health. *Lancet* 379: 1641–1652.

Vygotsky, L. (1962). *Thought and Language.* Cambridge, MA: MIT Press.

Watson, J.B. (1913). Psychology as the behaviorist views it. *Psychological Review* 20 (2): 158–177.

Wilkinson, R.B. (2004). The role of parental and peer attachment in the psychological health and self-esteem of adolescents. *Journal of Youth Adolescents* 33: 479–493.

Woodgate, R.L. and Degner, L.F. (2003). A substantive theory of keeping the spirit alive: the spirit within children with cancer and their families. *Journal of Pediatric Oncology Nursing* 20 (3): 103–119.

WHO and Calouste Gulbenkian Foundation (2014). *Social Determinants of Mental Health.* Geneva, Switzerland: World Health Organization.

Wright, L.M. and Leahey, M. (2013). *Nurses and Families: A Guide to Family Assessment and Intervention,* 6e. Philadelphia, PA: F.A. Davis.

Yaun, A. and Keating, R. (2007). The brain and nervous system. In: *Children with Disabilities,* 6the (eds. M. Batshaw, L. Pellegrino and N. Roizen), 185–202. Baltimore, MD: Paul H. Brookes.

Young, M., Donnelly, J., and Denny, G. (2004). Area specific self-esteem, values and adolescent sexual behavior. *American Journal of Health Education* 35: 282–289.

Zimmer-Gembeck, M.J. and Skinner, E.A. (2016). The development of coping: Implications for psychopathology and resilience. In: *Developmental psychopathology: Risk, resilience, and intervention* (ed. D. Cicchetti), 485–545. Hoboken, NJ: John Wiley & Sons, Inc.

2

Temperament and Self-Regulation

Pamela Galehouse[1] and Marie Foley[2]

[1] Seton Hall University, College of Nursing, South Orange, NJ, USA
[2] Seton Hall University College of Nursing, Interprofessional Health Sciences Campus, Nutley, NJ, USA

Objectives

At the end of this chapter, advanced practice registered nurses (APRNs) will be able to:

1. Identify the key components of temperament and self-regulation.
2. Assess temperament and self-regulation in children.
3. Recognize the importance of "goodness of fit" between temperament and environment.
4. Identify risk factors associated with temperament/self-regulatory abilities and mental health.
5. Determine approaches for managing behaviors related to reduced self-regulatory skills.

Introduction/Overview

The focus of this chapter is on two influential intrinsic constructs: temperament and self-regulation. Each influences how the child interacts with his or her environment and masters developmental tasks. Temperament can be simply described as innate, heritable, not easily changed patterns of behavioral responses to change or stress. Although present at birth, temperament is not believed to be consistent until about 1 year of age, when biological systems are more stabilized (Rothbart 2007). Temperament is shaped by the interactions between multiple factors, including genetics, maturation, and environmental influences (Rothbart 2012). Individual child temperament can influence outcomes related to academic performance (Rothbart 2012; Van Schyndel et al. 2017), social development, and behavior adjustment (Gartstein et al. 2012b). A child's unique temperament and the interaction between temperament and the environment affects the development of self-regulation and, ultimately, developmental task attainment.

Research indicates that children's unique temperament profiles influence the development of self-regulation, with some temperaments increasing the risk for inadequate or rigid self-regulation (Jonas and Kochanska 2018). Unlike temperament, the ability to self-regulate behavior and emotions develops in tandem with the child's brain until hardwiring is completed at about 8 years (Rothbart 2012). While temperament is usually viewed as a continuum of normal behavior that may challenge caretakers, the ability to self-regulate is critical to the individual's capacity to interact and function in society, and can be compromised by factors such as psychological and physiological stress (Lackner et al. 2018). Persistent dysfunctional self-regulation is often associated with specific psychiatric disorders.

Child and Adolescent Behavioral Health: A Resource for Advanced Practice Psychiatric and Primary Care Practitioners in Nursing, Second Edition. Edited by Edilma L. Yearwood, Geraldine S. Pearson, and Jamesetta A. Newland.
© 2021 John Wiley & Sons, Inc. Published 2021 by John Wiley & Sons, Inc.
Companion website: www.wiley.com/go/Yearwood

This chapter will describe both temperament and self-regulation with attention to environmental influences and challenges, assessment, and intervention strategies to enhance self-regulation in young children and to manage dysfunctional self-regulatory skills.

Description of the Issue

Historical Context

Temperament

The concept of temperament is not a new one, but rather has ancient roots in the study of both animals and humans. The premise of child temperament as significant to child-focused clinicians and researchers was introduced in the United States by Thomas and Chess (1977).

In their pioneering work known as the New York Longitudinal Study (NYLS), which began in 1953, these researchers examined individual personality traits of 133 subjects from infancy through adulthood. They defined temperament as constitutional characteristics that interact with the child's environment, are important in the child's development, and present regardless of context, ability, or motivation (Thomas and Chess 1977).

Self-Regulation

Self-regulation as a psychological construct has been traced back as far as William James, who in the eighteenth century included self-control in his principles of psychology. Research and emerging theories in child development over the past 40 years include rigorously studying loss of self-control (Vohs and Baumeister 2016). The seminal work by Barkley (1998) on attention deficit hyperactive disorder (ADHD) has inspired consideration in research and clinical work on specific aspects of attentional regulation or lack thereof. In addition, the work by Rothbart et al. (2014) has led to greater understanding of effortful control as a construct of temperament related to its role in attention and self-regulation. Technological advances have allowed researchers to use neuroimaging to explore differences in brain function of children with differing self-regulation abilities under specific conditions (Choe et al. 2018; Pérez-Edgar et al. 2018; Sánchez-Pérez et al. 2018), thus expanding our knowledge of psychobiology and environment.

Theoretical Approaches

Temperament

Different temperament theorists offer variations in their definitions of temperament. Emphasizing psycho-neuro-biological components, Rothbart and Bates (2006) studied variability in reactivity, both physiological and psychological arousability, and its relationship to effortful control or the regulatory efforts to modulate reactivity. They believe this to be consistent across situations and stable over time. They go on to state that individuals' behavioral responses to change in their environment will vary based on both reactivity and availability of strategies to regulate, by either strengthening or inhibiting these reactions (Rothbart and Bates 2006).

Plomin and Caspi (1999) conceptualized temperament, focusing on the heritable characteristics occurring early in life and being stable across time and circumstances. Kagan (1998) discussed temperament extremes in relation to shyness, which they termed inhibited and uninhibited. They found that the child's environment could moderate these extremely shy behaviors. Through this evolution, most researchers agree that temperament can be defined as a child's behavioral style that he or she consistently exhibits in reaction to the environment. Temperament acts as a screen through which interpretation of the environment occurs.

Self-regulation

The roots of self-regulation are in temperament. It is the counterbalancing "executive attentional system" proposed by Rothbart that begins to develop in late infancy and continues through the early school years (Posner and Rothbart 2000). This allows the individual child to self-regulate by exerting effortful control over the reactive attentional system. Functionally, self-regulation can be described as children's capacities to control reactions to stress, maintain focused attention, and interpret their own mental states and those of others (empathy) (Fonagy and Target 2002).

From a neurobiological perspective self-regulation includes the ability to modulate behavior according to the emotional and social demands of a situation, governed by how the individual takes in, organizes, and uses information (Posner and Rothbart 2000). Neurocognitive research identifies three separate brain network activities relating to attention that evolve during these early years: *orienting*, the selection of information from sensory input, *alerting*, sensitivity to incoming stimulations and maintenance of a vigilant state, and *executive control*, monitoring and resolving thoughts, feelings, and physical responses (Fan and Posner 2004; Posner 2016). Viewed as the result of control of inhibitory and attentional processes, self-regulation consists of both conscious and unconscious processes that exercise control in order to meet certain goals (Calkins and Fox 2002). Because it involves self-monitoring of one's state in relation to one's goal and making the changes and adjustments required to attain that goal, the monitoring and control functions of attention play significant roles in self-regulation (Rothbart and Bates 2006). The most successful self-regulators are children with inherent attention efficacy (Rueda et al. 2004). In other words, children born with certain temperaments tend to have better self-regulation.

Research indicates that the efficiency of executive attention shows marked improvement from ages 2 to 7 (Rothbart et al. 2003; Chang and Burns 2005). Studies of school-age children found increased efficiency in executive attention between 7 and 12 years (Pozuelos et al. 2014). While there appears to be a critical window of opportunity for laying the groundwork for executive attention in early childhood, the attention networks continue to develop in children in supportive environments.

Understanding how the mind directs attention and controls behavior so that children can respond appropriately to challenging situations has been advanced by modern neuroscience. It is beyond the task of this chapter to offer a comprehensive view of the current status of the science (see Chapter 3 for a more detailed account). However, a brief sequence of contemporary understanding of the neuroscience of the development of regulatory capacities will be outlined here, followed by a review of two specific areas of neurophysiology directly related to self-regulation development.

Affective neuroscience describes regulation as complex, hierarchical relations between the three core brains systems (brainstem, limbic, and cortical) that organize behavioral output (Tucker et al. 2000). Feldman (2009) conducted a 5-year study of premature infants that supports a hierarchical and integrative four-stage neurobiological model of physiological, emotional, attentional, and self-regulatory development. These four stages include specific function/system relationships: (i) physiological regulation associated with brain-stem development (late fetal through early neonatal), (ii) emotional regulation (ER), which is limbic mediated and serves to return to homeostasis (first year), (iii) attentional regulation (second year), and (iv) self-regulation, which is determined by cortical control (preschool, 3–5 years). Self-regulation includes behavior adaptation, executive functions, and self-restraint.

Inherent in Feldman's model is evidence that while disruptions in lower level functions may lead to higher system dysfunction resulting in behavior problems at age 5, the system is malleable. With sensitive, responsive care many infants transitioned over the first year of life from highly reactive preemies to toddlers with focused attention, typical to most 2-year-olds. This demonstrates both the dependence of the infant on regulatory context and the openness of regulatory functions to external influences (Bridgett et al. 2009). The process can be further explained by the concept of *attunement*, by which

parents attach to their infants by reading and responding to signals for engagement or disengagement (Stern 1985). Supporting this notion is the work of Schore (1994), who found that the facial expressions of the caregiver (demonstrating transactions) stimulate the production of opiates, which in turn activate dopamine neurons that trigger brain development, particularly in the orbital frontal cortex (OFC). The OFC serves to organize responses to threat by assessing signals of distress/danger, planning behavior, and modulating the timing of emotional responses. The right OFC is believed to be the primary regulator of the limbic system, managing how emotional experiences are handled (Scaer 2005).

The brain's attentional system offers further explanations about how the complex systems of the brain interact and specifically how one system governs the reactions of another, allowing *effortful control*. The part of the brain actively participating in effortful control is the anterior cingulate cortex (ACC), a part of the frontal cortex whose dorsal portion is connected to the executive function center of the prefrontal cortex and whose ventral portion has pathways to the limbic section, where emotion is situated (Bush 2004). This position links cognitive control functions with the emotional center.

From a clinical standpoint differentiation is made among the observed abilities to regulate attention, emotion, and behavior/inhibition (executive function). Although there are complex relationships among the three, each will be described separately.

Emotional Regulation ER is goal oriented and involves monitoring, evaluating, and modifying emotional reactions in order to accomplish goals (Thompson et al. 2008). Goals can be social (pleasing parents or others) or functional (gaining attention or having needs met). It is important to note that the efficiency of efforts to control emotions depends on the strength of the emotional processes against which effort is exerted (Eisenberg et al. 2004). A recent study found that children with temperamental negative affectivity summon more neural resources in order to inhibit prepotent responses when under negative emotional circumstances, thus paying a higher cognitive and emotional price to control emotions and function effectively (Berger and Farbaish, 2018).

Early on parents provide soothing, modeling a repertoire of soothing behaviors, and begin the process of helping the youngster attach names to his or her emotions. As the child matures, the parent or caregiver assists the young child to differentiate between similar feelings (happy:content; sad:nervous; angry:frustrated) and helps the child find ways to verbally express emotions and find suitable outlets for them. Newer studies have explored how a parent's own regulation influences a child's ER abilities (Tan and Smith 2018), and identified key parenting behaviors that buffer the effect of exposures to domestic violence on child ER (Caiozzo et al. 2018).

ER is related to several dimensions of temperament. For example, high effortful control, high empathy, high guilt, and shame have been related to low aggressiveness (Rothbart et al. 2001). Kochanska and others explored effortful control and conscience development and found that fearful preschoolers internalize moral principles, especially when their mothers used gentle discipline. Internalized control is higher in children who have effortful control (Kochanska 1995; Kochanska et al. 1997, 2000). Youngsters with good attentional control are more likely to deal with anger by using nonhostile verbal methods (Eisenberg et al. 1994). When regulation is defective, or emotionally and cognitively based methods such as distraction or relaxation (self-soothing) are ineffective, the child may use certain behaviors to damp down emotions. In these instances, negatively viewed behavioral regulation strategies such as tantrums, striking out, and venting are used by the youngster to reduce the amount of intense affect being experienced (Eisenberg et al. 1997).

Behavioral Regulation The term behavioral regulation is often used interchangeably with inhibition and is also influenced by effortful control. It consists of five domains: attentional shifting, focusing, inhibitory control, low intensity pleasure, and perceptual sensitivity (Rothbart et al. 2001). Generally, regulating behavior requires the ability to suppress a dominant response in favor of a nondominant one.

Clearly, the ability to regulate behavior at an early age has positive consequences for children. For example, kindergarteners with higher levels of behavior regulation have stronger levels of achievement, especially in math, as well as higher teacher ratings of classroom self-regulation at the end of the year (Ponitz et al. 2009). A recent study by Montroy et al. (2016) of a geographically diverse group of 1386 preschool children found that behavioral regulation develops quickly but along three distinct trajectories (early, intermediate, and late) that are marked by periods of rapid gains. They found that the later developers were often 6 months to a year behind the intermediate group, with about 20% of the children making few gains during preschool. This suggests that the timing of behavioral regulation is important to outcomes.

Attentional Regulation Regulation of attention can be considered from two perspectives: (i) modulating negative emotions or states and (ii) facilitating task completion and learning. Attention shifting and focusing is central to modulating internal psychological and physiological reactions and has been discussed previously under ER. Sustained attention, defined as the ability to filter out extraneous information and focus on the task at hand, has demonstrated importance for school readiness and achievement (Gardner-Neblett et al. 2014).

Closely aligned to the temperamental traits of task persistence (McClowry 2003) and effortful control (Rothbart and Bates 2006), attentional regulation skills can be facilitated by environmental inputs, including parental sensitivity and maternal scaffolding (Belskey et al. 2007; Deater-Deckard et al. 2007; Harris et al. 2007). Maternal scaffolding along with physical and verbal cues assist a child in completing a task (Robinson et al. 2009). Within this parent–child learning environment, demonstrated attention regulation in task completion is also influenced by intrinsic child factors: effortful control and motivation (Harris et al. 2007).

In summary, self-regulation is the child's ability to control reactions to stress, maintain focused attention, and interpret mental states in self and others by exercising emotional, behavioral, and attentional control. Whether one believes self-regulation to be rooted in temperament or to *be* temperament there is agreement that its etiology is with two temperament components: reactivity and control (Rothbart and Bates 2006). Development of self-regulation is determined by the strength of these two temperament domains and is enhanced or hindered by individual transactions with the environment (Bridgett et al. 2015; Wang et al. 2016).

Typologies and Variations

Temperament

In their seminal work on temperament, Chess and Thomas (1984) defined nine dimensions of temperament (see Table 2.1). From these nine dimensions of temperament, they found that children tend to cluster in one of three temperamental constellations: "easy," "difficult," and "slow to warm up." The easy child is characterized by high rhythmicity, positive mood, approaches new situations with moderate ease, and is easily adaptable. The "difficult" child is more irregular, has a negative mood, withdraws from new situations, and tends to require much time to adapt to the environment or situations. In contrast, the "slow to warm up" child is more inhibited, withdraws from new situations, has occasional negative moods, and adapts slowly. These constellations represented 65% of their sample population: 10% were difficult, 40% easy, 15% slow to warm up, and the remaining 35% of the subjects did not fall into any of the three constellations (Thomas and Chess 1977).

Building on the theoretical framework of Thomas and Chess, McClowry and her colleagues (1995) examined

Table 2.1 Theoretical approaches to temperament dimensions

Theorist	Dimensions of temperament
Thomas and Chess (1977)	Activity (motor), rhythmicity (regularity), approach/withdrawal (initial response to new stimuli), adaptability (response to situations over time), threshold (intensity of stimulus to evoke response), intensity (energy level), mood (quality of pleasant behavior), distractibility (response to external stimuli), and persistence (continuation of activity through distraction)
Buss and Plomin (1984)	Emotionality (tendency to become psychologically aroused), activity (energy), and sociability (interactions with others)
Goldsmith and Campos (1982)	Activity (motor), anger, fearfulness (moving away), pleasure/joy (smiling/laughing), and interest/persistence (attention)
Posner and Rothbart (2007) Rothbart and Bates (2006)	Surgency-extraversion (activity, positive affect, pleasure, impulsivity, smiling, outgoing), negative affectivity (inhibition, discomfort, fear, sadness, frustration, unable to be soothed), effortful control (attentional shifting, focusing, ability to suppress inappropriate responses, perceptual sensitivity), and sociability/affiliation (social closeness, emotional empathy, empathetic guilt)
Kagan (1998)	Inhibited (shy) and uninhibited (outgoing)
Martin and Bridger(1999)	Negative emotionality (affect), activity (motor), persistence (attention), inhibition (shyness), and impulsivity (speed of response to stimuli)
McClowry (2002a)	Activity (motor), negative reactivity (intensity and frequency of negative affect), approach/withdrawal (initial response to new situations), and task persistence (attention span)

the construct validity of the Middle Childhood Temperament Questionnaire and found four factors emerged from the original nine dimensions (Hegvik et al. 1982) (see Table 2.1). Similar to the work of Thomas and Chess, McClowry (2002a) also identified temperament typologies or profiles based on combinations of dimensions: "high maintenance" and "cautious/slow to warm up." The "high maintenance" child is high in negative reactivity, low in task persistence, and high in activity (8% of the sample). The "cautious/slow to warm up" child is high in negative reactivity and high in withdrawal (8% of the sample). McClowry then took the mirror images of these two profiles and named them "industrious" and "social/eager to try." The "industrious" child is high in task persistence, low in activity, and low in negative reactivity (6% of the original sample) and the "social/eager to try" child is high in approach and low in negative reactivity (9% of the sample). Four percent were both industrious and social/eager to try. Of the remaining 58%, all were found to be either high or low on at least one dimension with the exception of 1.5% of the subjects.

From a psychobiological framework, Putnam and Rothbart (2006) studied child temperament and identified four factors: negative affectivity, surgency/extraversion, effortful control, and sociability/affiliation. The latter, sociability/affiliation, does not present itself until later adolescence and early adulthood.

As temperament theory has evolved, researchers seem to agree that four dimensions emerged, understanding that as a child grows and develops certain traits are no longer salient due to the child's ability to self-regulate themselves and their environments (Rothbart, 2012).

Self-Regulation

Unfortunately, the only available incidence rates related to self-regulation are data collected when individuals lack adequate self-regulation. For example, the incidence of ADHD, depression, anxiety, conduct disorders (CDs), incarceration and schizophrenia could be attributed to an individual's inability to self-regulate. According to the National Health Interview Survey (Child and Adolescent Health Measurement Initiative 2018), in 2014 slightly more than 5% of children aged 4–17 were reported by a parent to have serious difficulties with emotions, concentration, behavior, or being able to get along with other people. Almost twice as many males were reported to have these problems.

Assessment

The following section offers information about assessing infant, preschool, and school-age temperament and self-regulation with the intent of using this information for preventive interventions. In addition, guidelines for assessing the self-regulation abilities of children and adolescents who have diagnosed mental health problems in the context of a treatment or school facility will be presented. Routine temperament assessment of adolescents will not be addressed: temperament in this age group is difficult to separate from personality. There are standardized instruments available for self-regulation measurement with this age group (e.g. Rothbart's); however, they are generally used in research rather than clinical practice.

When performing routine and/or episodic assessments it is important to complete not only physical, but developmental assessments. The import of this is underscored by the similar behaviors presented by both the infant who is a challenge to care for because of health-related problems and the infant whose temperament presents a parenting challenge. Etiology aside, both groups require warm, responsive, soothing parenting and support and education for the parents. Children with difficult temperaments will, however, require more attention throughout childhood.

Assessment of self-regulation in young children should be conducted to inform, assess risk, and consider interventions, as well as to diagnose (Vohs and Baumeister, 2016). This developmental period has critical importance to school and interpersonal success. A comprehensive assessment focusing on strengths/competencies as well as weaknesses/dysfunction is important and in agreement with the notion of health promotion held by nurses (Leddy, 2006; Murdaugh et al. 2018). It is important to remember that there is a wide range of individual variability in the regulatory skills of young children.

Both temperament and self-regulation are measured through parent report questionnaires, teacher report questionnaires, self-report for older children, in-home and laboratory observations, and structured interviews. All of these methods have both strengths and weaknesses for practice and research. The strengths of parent questionnaires include the parent's knowledge of the child and their typical behavior. The parent also knows how the child reacts on rare, but important, occasions and over time. Parent report questionnaires are inexpensive and easy to administer. The weaknesses are parental subjectivity, inaccurate memory of events, desire of acquiescence, and parental interpretation of behaviors (Gartstein et al. 2012a). A historical timeline might be helpful in collecting information.

Teacher questionnaires can be more objective than parent reports, but not as broad reaching. Teachers can only measure a child's temperament and self-regulation within the school environment. Teacher questionnaires are inexpensive and easy to administer but can have the same biases as parent reports in relation to memory and interpretation. The structured Head-Toes-Knees-Shoulders (HTKS; Ponitz et al. 2009) test has been

determined to be a valid measure of self-regulation in preschool children (Graziano et al. 2015) and may be easily administered by clinicians.

The strengths of child observations are their objectivity. However, due to constraints of time and expense they are often limited in number. There also may be a change in the child's behavior due to the presence of the observer. Moreover, the observer has restricted capacity to detect rare events. Laboratory observations, while rarely used by clinicians, allow variable control, but are limited in the range of observations. Dependent upon available time and finances, a combination of techniques is most beneficial to the clinician or researcher in assessing child temperament and self-regulatory abilities. The use of multiple techniques provides an opportunity to obtain historical data as well as a report of child behavior on rare, but important, occasions.

There are many questions about the shortcomings of instruments measuring temperament and self-regulation in relation to validity and reliability (Rothbart and Bates 2006). The researcher and clinician, after choosing a tool based on the theoretical framework that best conceptualizes their research or practice, must be cognizant of any limitations in measurement, in relation to both technique and instrumentation. For a description of tools commonly used to assess temperament and self-regulation, including the reported reliabilities, see Table 2.2.

As indicated in the preceding paragraphs, assessing a child's temperament and self-regulation can provide helpful information to the primary care practitioner who is advising parents and promoting healthy parenting practices. Information gathered will allow targeted parental education and support to be provided for those children most vulnerable to problems. Potential risk for depressive and anxiety symptoms in childhood can be predicted for infants with difficult temperaments before 6 months as well as for future CD with difficult infants (Lahey et al. 2005; Côté et al. 2009). Identifying problems, such as maternal depression, accompanied by appropriate referrals for treatment, has the potential to reduce the risk of the behavioral and mental health problems that develop in early childhood (Nolvi et al. 2016; Rode and Kiel 2016). Considering parental mental health beyond childhood for children at risk is suggested by studies such as the one by Wang et al. (2016), who found low parent positive expressivity (notable with depression) to increase risk for externalizing behavioral problems into adolescence for children with low effortful control (Wang et al. 2016).

While routine temperament assessment in clinical practice is most likely to take place during infancy, practitioners who assess behavior during routine health examinations and acute care episodes may consider

Table 2.2 Tools commonly used to assess temperament and self-regulation

Temperament scale	Age	Description	Reliability
Early Infancy Temperament Questionnaire, EITQ (Medoff-Cooper et al. 1993)	1–4 months	76 items based on Thomas and Chess' nine dimensions of temperament	≤0.42–0.76
Infant Behavior Questionnaire Revised, IBQ-R (Gartstein and Rothbart 2003)	3–12 months	184 items based on Rothbart's neurobiological framework	≤0.70–0.90
Toddler Temperament Scale, TTS (Fullard et al. 1984)	1–3 years	97 items based on Thomas and Chess' framework	≤0.70–0.81
EAS Temperament Survey for Children, EAS[a] (Buss and Plomin 1984)	1–3 years	20 items based on Buss and Plomin's EAS dimensions	≤0.80–0.88
Toddler Behavior Assessment Questionnaire, TBAQ (Goldsmith 1996)	15–36 months	108 items based on the emotion systems approach by Goldsmith and Campos (1982)	≤0.78–0.89
Early Childhood Behavior Questionnaire, ECBQ (Van Schyndel et al. 2017)	18–36 months	267 items based on Rothbart's neurobiological framework	≤0.56–0.90
Colorado Childhood Temperament Inventory, CCTI (Rowe and Plomin 1977)	1–7 years	30 items based on Buss and Plomin's dimensions of EAS	≤0.73–0.88
Dimensions of Temperament Survey Revised, DOTS-R (Windle and Lerner 1986)	Preschool	54 items based on Thomas and Chess' framework	≤0.70–0.84
Temperament Assessment Battery, TAB[a] (Martin and Bridger 1999)	2–7 years	35 items expanded on Thomas and Chess' framework	≤0.65–0.86
Shortened Teacher Temperament Questionnaire, STTQ (Keogh et al. 1982)	3–6 years	23 items based on Thomas and Chess' framework	≤0.62–0.92
EAS Temperament Survey for Children, EAS[a] (Buss and Plomin 1984)	3–9 years	20 items based on Buss and Plomin's EAS dimensions	≤0.65–0.81
Children's Behavior Questionnaire, CBQ (Rothbart et al. 2001)	3–7 years	195 items based on Rothbart's neurobiological framework	≤0.67–0.94
Behavioral Style Questionnaire, BSQ (McDevitt and Carey 1978)	3–7 years	100 items based on Thomas and Chess' framework	≤0.48–0.80
Middle Childhood Temperament Questionnaire, MCTQ (Hegvik et al. 1982)	8–12 years	99 items based on Thomas and Chess' framework	≤0.80–0.93
Dimensions of Temperament Survey Revised, DOTS-R (Windle and Lerner 1986)	School age	54 items based on Thomas and Chess' framework	≤0.54–0.91
The Temperament in Middle Childhood Questionnaire, TMCQ (Simonds and Rothbart 2004).	7–10 years	157 computer-generated items based on Rothbart's neurobiological framework	≤0.50–0.90
School-Age Temperament Inventory, SATI[a] (McClowry 1995; McClowry et al. 2003)	8–12 years	38 items based on Thomas and Chess' framework	≤0.85–0.90
Early Adolescent Temperament Questionnaire-Revised EATQ-R (Ellis and Rothbart 2001)	10–16 years	65 items based on Rothbart's neurobiologic framework	≤0.64–0.81
Self-Regulation Scale	**Age**	**Description**	**Reliability**
Behavior Rating Inventory of Executive Function® Preschool Version, BRIEF®-P[a] (Gioia et al. 2003)	2–5.11 years	63 items, executive functioning (five aspects).	≤0.80–0.95
Behavior Rating Inventory for Executive Function, Brief®[a] (Gioia et al. 2000)	5–18 years	86 items, two broad indexes: behavioral regulation (three scales) and metacognition (five scales) plus a global executive composite	≤0.80–0.98
Behavior Rating Inventory of Executive Function, Second Edition, BRIEF2[a] (Gioia et al. 2015)	5–18 years (parent and teacher reports)	86 items, three regulation indexes: behavioral, emotional, cognitive, 12 scales	$\alpha \geq 0.90$ (parent, teacher)
	11–18 years (self-reports)	55 items, three indexes, 10 scales	$\alpha \geq 0.80$ (self-report indexes)

[a] Parent and teacher versions available.

temperament during preschool and school years as well. As mentioned earlier, child temperament and delays in self-regulation are most apparent in situations that are stressful and during transitional periods, such as entering preschool, moving to a new classroom, or when there are changes in the family structure. Assessing temperament at this time and referring back to earlier assessments and health histories will assist the practitioner to determine if this is a situation that requires referrals to either a parenting program or a mental health provider.

Observations in Context: Children with Serious Emotional or Behavioral Problems

Children and adolescents who require hospitalization or placement in special schools or residential facilities demonstrate behaviors that may be related to underlying deficits in emotional or behavioral self-regulation but are often misunderstood. Nurses, by virtue of their presence and understanding of self-regulation, are in an ideal position to recognize patterns of behavior and to help other treatment team members understand possible underlying self-regulatory behaviors (Delaney 2006a). Delaney (2006b–d) has taken a leading role in developing theoretically based guidelines for inpatient psychiatric observational assessments that consider specific child self-regulatory behaviors in context. In this chapter, we highlight Delaney's guidelines for assessment that are directly related to self-regulation: ER, behavioral regulation/inhibitory control, and coping and stress responses.

Delaney's assessment of ER (2006b) is organized around two areas of inquiry: (i) how well the patient regulates emotions and (ii) how well the patient understands his or her affect. Behavioral signs of ER are provided for each question, along with associated intervention strategies, which are not discussed here. One of six signs of well-regulated emotion is that the ability to "regulate the intensity of an affect, e.g. frustration, does not escalate to intense anger" (Delaney 2006b, p. 179). The behavioral signs of understanding affect include the ability to label affective states and to tie affect to the situation that generates it. Theoretical and empirical support for the individual domains and signs of ER are provided by Rothbart and Bates (2006), Eisenberg (see Diaz and Eisenberg 2015), Izard (see Izard et al. 2011), and Denham (see Feng et al. 2008).

Another part of self-regulation is behavioral control or inhibitory control. It includes the ability to inhibit an action at the idea stage, at the initiation of behavior or to block incoming stimuli that might interfere with completion of the action (Barkley 1998). The concept of inhibitory control is predicated on learning how to control direct attention and developing voluntary control over thoughts and actions (Posner and Rothbart 2000). Delaney's

assessment of behavioral control is organized around a single question that asks how well the patient regulates impulses (Delaney 2006c). Developmentally appropriate behavioral signs are given to differentiate expectations between younger children and latency age and adolescents. An example of the signs of good behavioral control, realistic for the young child, is the ability to contain self during quiet times; more advanced abilities, such as the ability to process troublesome situations, especially their role in a conflict, is expected of older children.

Delaney's third observation assessment guideline related to self-regulation is the managing of stress and use of coping behaviors (Delaney 2006d). Conceptually, coping skill requires multiple conscious efforts to regulate emotion, cognition, and behavior as well as physiological response when faced with stressful events (Compas et al. 2001). This area differs somewhat from the others because of event focus and diversity of coping strategies attempted (Eisenberg et al. 1997, 2004). The observations are centered on a specific question which asks "how well the patient cope[s] with stress and milieu expectations" (Delaney 2006d, p. 200).and include both previously mentioned signs of emotional and behavioral self-regulation as well as items unique to this group. This area highlights the range of coping strategies, some of which are clearly signs of ineffective coping or inability to self-regulate. In addition, specific tendencies may not be evident unless provoked by a stressful situation which tips the balance of control. This phenomenon is explained by several temperament theories, which suggest that as the individual develops strategies, temperament may only be visible in situations of stress (Strelau 2000; McClowry 2003).

Linkages with Behavioral/Psychiatric Profile

Extreme temperamental traits increase the risk for psychopathology, such as ADHD, anxiety, and depression (De Pauw and Mervielde 2011; Martel et al. 2014). The *Diagnostic and Statistical Manual of Mental Disorders 5* (American Psychiatric Association [APA], 2013) identifies temperament as a risk factor for a number of disorders, including ADHD (less behavioral inhibition and effortful control, negative emotionality, elevated novelty seeking), major depression and panic disorder (negative affectivity), general anxiety disorder (less inhibition and negative affectivity), and oppositional defiant disorder (ODD) (problems with ER). The diagnosis of disruptive mood dysregulation disorder was added to the DSM-5 (APA 2013) to identify children who present with symptoms of persistent irritability and frequent episodes of severe behavioral dysregulation.

Children diagnosed with both autistic spectrum disorder (ASD) and ADHD often present with executive dysfunction (inflexibility and disinhibition) and experience comorbid psychopathology; specifically anxiety/depression in children diagnosed with ASD and aggression/oppositionality in children diagnosed with ADHD (Lawson et al. 2015).

Pijl et al. (2019) examined temperament profiles of infants who were at risk for a diagnosis of ASD and found traits of high negative affect and low regulation lead to a diagnosis. These infants were typically diagnosed earlier and tended to have more severe symptoms than high-risk infants, who presented lower on the continuum. Temperamental vulnerabilities in toddlers diagnosed with ASD indicate that attentional and behavioral controls along with affective reactivity contribute to decreased social outcomes in the preschool years and likely put the children at risk for internalizing and externalizing problems in later childhood (Burrows et al. 2016; Macari et al. 2017).

Dysregulation, encompassing under-regulation and/or misregulation (exerting control but making an undesirable response), has been linked to a number of mental health problems, including substance abuse (Moffitt et al. 2011), eating disorders (Van Malderen et al. 2018), sexual abuse (Yates and Kingston 2006), compulsive spending as well as involvement in criminal acts (Zeier et al. 2009; Moffitt et al. 2011). In addition, relationships between self-regulation and personality disorders (Shiner 2009; Ensink et al. 2015), and even schizophrenia (Koren et al. 2006; Rowland et al. 2013), are suggested. Despite seeming theoretical connections, the mechanisms are complex and, in general, unstudied; it is often unclear if self-regulation deficits are causative or the result of the disorder itself. Although clarity is lacking, treatments based on self-regulation assessment and theory are being developed and studied by clinical researchers.

Contributing to the knowledge of developmental psychopathology and the linkage between temperament and self-regulation, and childhood (including adolescence) behavioral and psychiatric problems, prospective, longitudinal studies found that children with extreme temperaments are at higher risk for behavior problems later in childhood (Chess and Thomas 1984; Maziade et al. 1990; Prior et al. 2000). These findings have been supported and expanded upon in contemporary studies which try to tease out the process and pathways of development and enhance understanding of not only how problems develop but, in some instances, to identify protective factors that allow so many of these at-risk children to accomplish successful development.

Research studies illustrate the influence of self-regulation skills on social competence and the ability to function in group settings. As early as preschool, even brief periods of

observed inability to regulate emotions (crying, tantrums) and behavior (aggression, hyperactivity) predict later teacher reports of poor classroom adjustment and peer conflict (Miller et al. 2004).

Rothbart (2007) proposed an explanatory model that outlines the pathways between temperament (including self-regulation) and the development of both internalizing and externalizing problems in children. This model (Figure 2.1) is based upon Rothbart's temperament theory and research. As described earlier, her theory proposes the three dimensions of temperament: extraversion/surgency, negative affectivity, and effortful control. The later, effortful control (the child's ability to control reactive impulses), closely resembles self-regulation, although fear in the form of behavioral inhibition makes some regulatory contributions by controlling approach and aggression (Rothbart and Bates 2006). The linkages are related to current temperament research findings (McClowry et al. 2003; Pérez-Edgar et al. 2018,). As can be noted, anger and fear relate directly to both internalizing problems and externalizing problems, but anger is more strongly related to externalizing problems and fear to internalizing problems (it is low fear that relates to externalizing problems) (Rothbart 2007). Research by Pérez-Edgar et al. (2018) demonstrated that children with high behavioral inhibition (fear) have patterns of right frontal electroencephalography (EEG) asymmetry, a recognized marker of increased risk for anxiety. Using a sample of preschool children, Delgado et al. (2018), in a sample of 364 children, found that extraversion protected against internalizing problems.

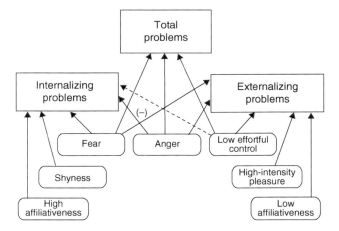

Figure 2.1 Rothbart's model of temperament and problem development. (Source: Reprinted from Rothbart, M.K. Temperament, development, and personality. Current Directions in Psychological Science 16 (4), 207-212. © 2007, SAGE Publication. With permission from SAGE Publication.)

It should be noted that Rothbart's developmental model illustrates direct and distinct relationships between several temperament dimensions and both categories of problems. High affiliativeness and shyness are related to internalizing problems, and high intensity pleasure and low affiliativeness relate to externalizing problems. Affiliativeness, the need for closeness and warmth, in preadolescence predicted problems during adolescence (Ormel et al. 2005). It must be noted that Rothbart's theoretical model, like all such constructions, is general and marks the beginning of work to study the role that temperament and self-regulation play in the development of problems. Clearly, it does not explore the context of the events or the various mediating and moderating factors, such as parenting stress, parental self-regulatory skill, family psychopathology, stressful life events, and intelligence, that influence development.

The inhibited (or shy) temperament has been linked to internalizing problems by many (Hirshfeld-Becker et al. 2004; Gladstone et al. 2005). However, it is important to recognize that the identification of the proposed pathway between temperament and emotional dysregulation to serious anxiety and/or depression is ongoing. Work investigating preschool children provides support and additional detail for Rothbart's model. Temperamental withdrawal (inhibition and low approach) at age 5 and parental internalizing problems predicted internalizing problems at age 11 (Mesman and Koot, 2000) and at 17 (Leve et al. 2005). Another study recognized the centrality of fear, finding that high fear emotionality and low fear regulation predicted internalizing problem behavior (Rydell et al. 2003); another found that functional impairment in young children may be attributed to the inability to refocus attention away from the source (executive attention) of sadness and distress (Cole et al. 2008). The latter is in keeping with the thinking of Kovacs and colleagues (Kovacs et al. 2009), who found that emotional self-regulatory strategies used by children to attenuate sadness can develop atypically, serving to exacerbate rather than relieve distress, resulting in early onset depressive disorders.

A prospective study (Feng et al. 2008) identified the divergent pathways that may influence why some children develop anxiety disorders while others with similar temperament profiles develop depressive disorders. This study uncovered four distinct trajectories in the development of anxiety which were labeled *low, low increasing, high declining* and *high-increasing*. In the presence of maternal negative control and maternal depression, boys who were shy were more likely to have high anxiety in middle childhood. Early shyness (anxiety) is associated with later depression only when it increases over childhood. These findings indicate that primary care nurses should take maternal histories, noting mothers who exhibit or have histories of depression and/or children who display high inhibition or withdrawal. Temperament-focused parent education and/or appropriate referrals to mental health providers may be warranted.

Externalizing behavior problems, ranging from serious misbehaviors to more extreme problems that characterize ODD, CDs, and ADHD, have also been linked to specific temperaments and self-regulation. Young children whose temperaments are highly active, respond negatively to events, and have low task persistence are at higher risk for developing disruptive behavior problems across childhood, and early conduct problems have been associated with delinquency and mental health problems in adolescence (Schaefer et al. 2017). Again, as true with internalizing problems, environmental, contextual, and child characteristics play an important part in determining whether temperamentally vulnerable children fail to develop the self-regulatory skills necessary to avoid disabling behavioral and mental health problems.

Studying developmental pathways to antisocial behaviors in low-income boys, Trentacosta and Shaw (2009) found that the inability to use active distraction as a means to regulate negative emotions in early childhood predicted peer rejection in middle childhood, which in turn predicted antisocial behavior in early adolescence. In another longitudinal, prospective study, Kochanska et al. (2009) looked at the relationship between effortful control, guilt, and disruptive behaviors, and found that children with no sense of guilt and poor effortful control were disruptive. However, those children who displayed a strong sense of guilt avoided disruptive behaviors whether or not they demonstrated effortful control abilities. Well-child visits are an opportune time for primary care nurses to identify young children observed or reported to have difficulties complying with reasonable requests, ruling out sensory or perceptual problems. Preventive actions include referrals to temperament-based parenting programs that focus on providing warmth, structure, consistent rule enforcement, and noncoercive practices. For these youngsters, at each follow-up visit a thorough behavioral history update to track changes as well as ongoing parental guidance and support are necessary. Intractable and pervasive disruptive behaviors require a higher level of intervention.

Much work on temperament and self-regulation has been related to ADHD. Children who are low in self-regulation demonstrate difficulties organizing work, paying attention, and staying on task at home and in school, making and retaining friends, moderating emotions, and controlling impulsive behaviors (De Pauw and Mervielde 2011; Herzhoff et al. 2013). These behaviors are the same symptoms associated with a diagnosis of ADHD.

Karalunas et al. (2018) assert that the temperamental traits of poor attentional focus, low inhibitory control, and high impulsivity (irritable temperament) are associated with and often serve as precursors of symptoms of ADHD. Researchers who examine the theoretical overlap between the constructs of ADHD and temperament conclude that children who are diagnosed with ADHD have temperaments that are high in negative reactivity, activity, and impulsivity, and low in task persistence, attentional focusing, and inhibitory control (Bussing et al. 2006; Foley et al. 2008; Brown et al. 2010). Primary care nurses usually have little difficulty in recognizing the temperaments of children associated with, or at risk for a diagnosis of, ADHD. The challenge is to discern how much can be attenuated by encouraging environmental changes through parent education and parenting programs or when other interventions may be necessary.

Temperament and self-regulation have also been associated with susceptibility for adverse reactions to trauma and stressful situations. For example, a study of children post 9/11 found that temperament had a significant influence on the responses of children residing across the country from the sites of the tragedy (Lengua et al. 2005). They found that children who had poor inhibitory control (low self-regulation) prior to the attacks had higher levels of post-traumatic stress symptoms than their better regulated peers. This remained true after controlling for prior symptomatology, demonstrating the heightened vulnerability of children with poor self-regulatory abilities to traumatic events, even though not directly experienced.

Also important are the temperament traits of behavioral inhibition and negative affect in toddlers and preschool children when associated with maternal depression, anxiety, and exposure to violence. These associations can predict anxiety in the school-age years (Mian et al. 2011). For primary care nurses seeing their patients longitudinally, this implies that they may be able to identify those patients in their caseload most vulnerable to traumatic events and adverse outcomes based on their temperament.

In addition, children with poor self-regulatory skills may be at higher risk for traumatic responses (including post traumatic stress disorder (PTSD)) to abuse and maltreatment (Kruczek et al. 2008; Kim-Spoon et al. 2012); children subjected to maltreatment and abuse are likely to have both altered capacities to regulate emotions and emotional dysregulation due to the abuse (Shipman et al. 2007). This emotional dysregulation is likely to influence cognition and impulse control (Cohen et al. 2006). In the study by Shipman et al. (2007), physically maltreated children received less emotional socialization (emotional coaching, validation) by their mothers than nonmaltreated children, making them less able to implement adaptive ER skills such as self-soothing and attentional control to manage emotional arousal constructively. Nonadaptive self-regulation methods are dependent upon developmental level, and in extreme may include self-mutilation (Mikolajczak et al. 2009), eating disorders, and substance abuse in older children and adolescents (Sloan et al. 2017). Long-term consequences of affect dysregulation associated with childhood maltreatment have been noted in adolescents and adults (Dvir et al. 2014).

Goodness of Fit

A concept in temperament theory that is applicable to advanced practice nursing is goodness of fit. Chess and Thomas (1984) defined goodness of fit as a match between the child's temperament and the expectations or demands of the environment. A good fit would be predictive of favorable outcomes; a poor fit, or incompatible relationship between the child's temperament and the environment, would result in risk of problem development (McClowry et al. 2008; Zentner and Bates 2008; Tsotsi et al. 2019).

The usefulness of this concept is demonstrated in relation to family functioning and behavioral and psychiatric outcomes (Lemery et al. 2002; Keiley et al. 2003) and, more specifically, to later adjustment (Kovacs and Lopez-Duran, 2010). For example, children who were high negative reactors with mothers whose parenting was hostile demonstrated externalizing problems in middle childhood (Garstein, Putnam and Rothbart 2006; Tsotsi et al. 2019); while parents who demonstrated supportive and consistent parenting of their challenging children were more likely to have fewer adjustment problems in later years (Pettit et al. 2007; Chen et al. 2014).

Chess and Thomas (1984) also recognized that the child, along with the parent and/or the environment, interact together and the effects on each are not unidirectional but rather transactional and nested in culture. For example, certain temperamental qualities are more valued in some cultures than others. Inhibition in China is seen positively and inhibited children are viewed favorably, while in Western cultures children's inhibitions are viewed less favorably and efforts are made to teach the child to become more assertive. Likewise, parenting styles are nested within the cultural value system and affect child outcomes (Chen et al. 2015).

For example, Chen et al. (2015) found that inhibition was viewed as relating to emotional difficulties in western societies where value is placed on autonomy and assertiveness yet in eastern society inhibition was not viewed as problematic. Similarly, Gartstein et al. (2012a) found negative affectivity and low levels of self-regulation in infancy were associated with behavioral problems in preschool children, yet the same was not found in Russian children.

Furthermore, the influence of parental temperament and pathology affect the environments they create for their growing children. Depressed parents are often unable to be responsive and model self-regulatory activities for their children, and children who are exposed to maternal depression in the early developmental years are at increased risk for negative outcomes throughout their development (Handley et al. 2017).

Studies using longitudinal data from the National Institute of Child Health and Human Development (NICHD) illustrate the principle of goodness of fit and the importance of environment for children with challenging temperaments. Pleuss and Belsky (2009) found that children described by their parent as difficult in infancy when placed in excellent childcare centers (with warm and encouraging teachers) not only did very well in preschool, but in 5th and 6th grade were better behaved, got along better with their teachers, and had better reading skills. The reverse was true of children who had teachers who did not interact frequently, scolded, and had tense classrooms.

Evidence-Based Implications for Practice

The increased developmental research in temperament and self-regulation has heightened interest in both assessing these areas in young children and integrating treatment strategies that target specific aspects of both temperament and self-regulation. Because parenting practices with children who have extreme temperaments (i.e. challenging, not so easy, high maintenance, slow to warm, feisty, spicy, spirited children) are highly amenable to parental counseling, many pediatricians, nurses, and social workers have integrated temperament work into their clinical practices. Recognition of the effectiveness of early intervention has led to the creation of institutional programs to assess risk and educate parents. An example is a program, originally developed and tested at a large HMO (Preventive Ounce, https://www.preventiveoz.org), which now independently provides online temperament assessments for parents of infants to 6-year-olds along with "forecasts" of common behavior problems and management strategies. Typically, practitioners in HMOs alert new parent participants to this service. Once a profile is obtained, the information may be shared by parents with providers for guidance and/or individualized counseling.

While professionals committed to using temperament as the base of their interventions hold strong beliefs that most children with extreme temperaments will do well with sensitive parenting attuned to the child's individual needs and abilities, there is recognition of the need to distinguish temperament issues from serious emotional and behavioral problems that interfere with functioning and attaining developmental goals, and to refer those children to mental health professionals.

Models of Treatment

Insights

While numerous interventions may be based on temperament theory and research, it is rare to find an intervention whose effectiveness has been empirically studied. One notable exception, the INSIGHTS program developed by McClowry (2003) for parents, teachers, and children, has demonstrated effectiveness in reducing disruptive behavior in young school-age children at home and demonstrated heightened efficacy with children who were at the diagnostic levels of three disruptive disorders: ADHD, ODD, and CDs (McClowry et al. 2005).

Developed over the years as a preventive intervention for nonclinical populations (McClowry and Galehouse 2002; McClowry et al. 2005) INSIGHTS has an established protocol that in the course of a series of group sessions teaches parents and teachers to recognize the advantages and challenges of each temperament domain and utilize strategies to work with the child, as he or she is, in order to gain compliance and foster development. A quartet of puppets representing four common "profiles" of temperament is used to facilitate child understanding of temperament and encourage problem-solving abilities (McClowry 2002b). In addition to the puppets, McClowry has developed CDs to supplement materials and stimulate discussion for all three target groups. McClowry proposes that by helping parents and teachers tailor strategies to the child's unique temperament, goodness of fit is achieved and abilities to self-regulate may be enhanced (McClowry et al. 2008). Responding to the importance of intervention-culture concord, INSIGHTS is being adapted for other cultural groups (New York University Steinhardt 2019).

Using the INSIGHTS intervention in kindergarten and 1st-grade classrooms, O'Connor et al. (2012) found enrollment in the INSIGHTS program assisted children with high maintenance temperaments exhibit decreased disruptive behaviors with more rapid decline when parents and teacher participated in sessions collaboratively. In a later examination of INSIGHTS in the same grades in high-risk school environments, McCormick et al. (2015) found INSIGHTS moderated poor school climate related to social–emotional, behavioral, and academic outcomes.

Empirically supported interventions that specifically target self-regulation abilities are also available but only a few have demonstrated efficacy and each targets different domains of self-regulation. One of these programs, designed for preschool children, is described here. The Emotions Based Prevention Program (originally called the Emotions Course; Izard, 2001) seeks to foster ER abilities. A program focusing on *coparenting*, Family Foundations, has also demonstrated the effectiveness of increasing infants' self-regulation (Feinberg et al. 2009; Solmeyer et al. 2014).

The Emotion Based Prevention Program

Designed for preschool children, The Emotion Based Prevention Program (EBP), which includes the Emotions Course delivered by trained teachers, is based on Izard's conceptual model of emotion utilization (Izard 2001) and endorses adaptive functioning such as substituting self-assertion for anger, identifying reasons, and seeking social support for sadness. The effectiveness of this program has been tested in two randomized cluster studies in Head Start settings (Izard et al. 2008), one rural and the other urban, and was found to increase emotion knowledge and ER in children receiving the Emotions Course. Other program outcomes included greater decreases in negative emotion expressions, aggression, anxious/depressed behavior, and negative peer and adult relationships than the control Head Start group. A follow-up study exclusive to urban Head Start settings (Finlon et al. 2015) demonstrated that the universal EBP intervention was more effective in decreasing expressions of negative emotion and internalizing behavior than a comparison intervention.

Family Foundations

A group program, Family Foundations, targets co-parenting, the way parents coordinate and support each other in the parenting role during the important transitional time surrounding birth (Feinberg 2002, 2003) and has demonstrated success in increasing infant self-regulation (self-soothing behaviors) as well as diminishing parent depression and improving parenting quality (Feinberg et al. 2009). A later post-intervention study (Solmeyer et al. 2014) of toddler behavior noted self-regulation behaviors continued into early childhood. Family Foundations is considered promising by Blueprints for Healthy Youth Development, a registry of evidence-based programs.

Summary

Although child temperament is most easily recognized in infancy and in later situations of change or stress, temperament remains an important intrinsic factor throughout childhood. Children's unique temperaments contribute to self-regulation development and are viewed by many to be the foundation of personality. The ability to self-regulate emotion, behavior, and attention begins in infancy and is influenced by temperament (reactivity and effortful control) and by the warmth, support, modeling, and education provided by caregivers. Culture also plays a part, with some dimensions of temperament fostered by the cultures in which they are valued and those less valued heaped with criticism. Research suggests that there is a critical window of opportunity for regulation development and that capacities are in place by ages 8–10, although it has been suggested that relationships between components of executive function may change as tasks become more complex.

Studies have demonstrated relationships between extreme temperaments and both externalizing and internalizing behaviors. High negative emotionality and high inhibition are two domains that are highly predictive of future problems in early childhood. However, it must be cautioned that the majority of children with these extreme temperaments do not develop behavior or mental disorders. There is some evidence that a lack of task persistence (poor self-regulation) is the strongest predictor of behavior problems in school-age children. It is important to remember that there is some evidence that children from impoverished homes are at most risk from having poor self-regulation skills.

Early assessment of temperament and continued assessment of age-appropriate self-regulatory abilities allow the professional to provide anticipatory guidance to parents and intervene when indicated. Professionals must be cautioned, however, to present differences as unique human qualities, not as defects, and to provide realistic examples of how to secure goodness of fit for the youngster. Several promising new interventions based on temperament or self-regulation theory and research have been designed and are being empirically studied. While these new evidence-based programs focus exclusively on younger children, many professionals have experience working with older children and adolescents whose self-regulatory problems are prominent and dysfunctional. Assessing specific areas of regulatory dysfunction allows the professional to make environmental adjustments to reduce uncontrolled maladaptive behaviors within the setting.

Recommended Resources

Resources for Parents

Carey, W.B. (2005). *Understanding Your Child's Temperament* (Rev. ed.). New York, NY: Macmillan/Simon & Schuster.

Kristal, J. (2004). *The Temperament Perspective: Working with Children's Behavioral Styles*. Baltimore, MD: Brookes. [Viewed by some as more for professionals than parents.

Kurcinka, M.S. (2015). *Raising Your Spirited Child: A Guide for Parents Whose Child Is More Intense, Sensitive, Perceptive, Persistent and Energetic*, 3e. New York, NY: HarperCollins.

Kurcinka, M.S. (2006). *Sleepless in America: Is Your Child Misbehaving or Missing Sleep?* New York, NY: HarperCollins.

McClowry, S.G. (2003). *Your Child's Unique Temperament: Insights and Strategies for Responsive Parenting*. Champaign, IL: Research Press.

Probst, B. (2008). *When the Labels Don't Fit: An Approach to Raising a Challenging Child*. New York, NY: Three Rivers Press.

Siegel, D.J. and Hartzell, M. (2003). *Parenting from the Inside Out*. New York, NY: Penguin.

Resources for Professionals: Evidence-Based and Empirically Tested Prevention Intervention Programs

Insights

Sandee McClowry, PhD, RN
https://insightsintervention.com

Family Foundations
Mark Feldman, PhD
Prevention Treatment Center
Penn State University
http://prevention.psu.edu/projects/Coparenting_Pubs.html

Critical Thinking Questions

1. If interested in assessing temperament and self-regulation in children as a nurse practitioner, what resources do you need to assemble to provide patient/family-centered care?
2. If you are interested in prevention and knowledgeable about temperamental risks, what are the critical areas for assessment prior to planning and prioritizing interventions?
3. Given that temperament falls along a spectrum of behaviors, how may culture and knowledge of child development influence a nurse practitioner's assessment and diagnosis of behavioral challenges?

References

American Psychiatric Association (2013). *Diagnostic and Statistical Manual of Mental Disorders 5*. Washington, DC: American Psychiatric Association.

Barkley, R.A. (1998). *Attention-Deficit Hyperactivity Disorder: A Handbook for Diagnosis and Treatment*. New York, NY: Guilford Press.

Belskey, J., Pasco Fearon, R.M., and Bell, B. (2007). Parenting, attention and externalizing problems: testing mediation longitudinally, repeatedly and reciprocally. *Journal of Child Psychology and Psychiatry* 48 (12): 1233–1242.

Berger, A. & Farbaish, T. (2018, May). *Negative affectivity and inhibitory control: Children's self-regulation in negative emotional challenges*. Paper presented at the Twenty-Second Occasional Temperament Conference, Murcia, Spain.

Bridgett, D.J., Gartstein, M.A., Putnam, S. et al. (2009). Maternal and contextual influences and the effect of temperament development during infancy on parenting in toddlerhood. *Infant Behavior & Development* 32: 103–116.

Bridgett, D.J., Burt, N.M., Edwards, E.S., and Deater-Deckard, K. (2015). Intergenerational transmission of self-regulation: a multidisciplinary review and integrative conceptual framework. *Psychological Bulletin* 142 (2): 602–654. Available at http://dx.doi.org/10.1037/a0038662.

Brown, D.D., Weatherholt, T.N., and Burns, B.M. (2010). Understanding parent reports of children's attention behaviors: role of children's attention skills, temperament, and home environment. *Journal of Early Childhood and Infant Psychology* 6 (2): 41–58.

Burrows, C.A., Usher, L.V., Schwartz, C.B. et al. (2016). Supporting the spectrum hypothesis: self-reported temperament in children and adolescents with high functioning autism. *Journal of Autism Developmental Disorders* 46: 1184–1195. https://doi.org/10.1007/s10803-015-2653-9.

Bush, G. (2004). Multimodal studies of cingulated cortex. In: *Cognitive Neuroscience of Attention* (ed. M.I. Posner), 207–218. New York, NY: Guilford Press.

Buss, A.H. and Plomin, R. (1984). *Temperament: Early Developing Personality Traits*. Mahwah, NJ: Lawrence Erlbaum.

Bussing, R., Lehninger, F., and Eyberg, S. (2006). Difficult child temperament and attention-deficit/hyperactivity disorder in preschool children. *Infants & Young Children* 19 (2), Special Issue: Attention-deficit/hyperactivity disorder: 123–131.

Caiozzo, C.N., Yule, K., and Grych, J. (2018). Caregiver behaviors associated with emotion regulation in high-risk preschoolers. *Journal of Family Psychology* 32 (5): 565–574.

Calkins, S.D. and Fox, N.A. (2002). Self-regulatory processes in early personality development: A multilevel approach to the study of childhood social withdrawal and aggression. *Development and Psychopathology* 14 (3): 477–498.

Chang, F. and Burns, B. (2005). Attention in preschoolers: associations with effortful control and motivation. *Child Development* 76 (1): 247–263.

Chen, N., Deater-Deckard, K., and Bell, M.A. (2014). The role of temperament by family environment interactions in child maladjustment. *Journal of Abnormal Child Psychology* 42: 1251–1262. https://doi.org/10.1007/s10802-014-9872-y.

Chess, S. and Thomas, A. (1984). *Origins and Evolution of Behavior Disorders: From Infancy to Early Adult Life*. Cambridge, MA: Harvard University Press.

Child and Adolescent Health Measurement Initiative (2018). 2014 National Health Interview Survey (NHIS) – Child. Available at http://action.cahmi.org/browse/survey.

Choe, D.E., Deater-Deckard, K., & Bell, M.A. (2018). *Biobehavioral mechanisms and intergenerational continuities in self regulation and emotionality in mother–child dyads*. Paper presented at the Twenty-Second Occasional Temperament Conference, Murcia, Spain.

Cohen, J.A., Mannarino, A.P., and Deblinger, E. (2006). *Treating Trauma and Traumatic Grief in Children and Adolescents*. New York, NY: Guilford Press.

Cole, P.M., Luby, J., and Sullivan, M.W. (2008). Emotions and the development of childhood depression: bridging the gap. *Child Development Perspectives* 2 (3): 141–148.

Compas, B.E., Connor-Smith, J.K., Saltzman, H. et al. (2001). Coping with stress during childhood and adolescence: problems, progress, and potential in theory and research. *Psychological Bulletin* 127: 87–127.

Côté, S., Boivin, M., Liu, X. et al. (2009). Depression and anxiety symptoms: onset, developmental course and risk factors during early childhood. *Journal of Child Psychology & Psychiatry* 50 (10): 1201–1208.

De Pauw, S.S. and Mervielde, I. (2011). The role of temperament and personality in problem behaviors of children with ADHD. *Journal of Abnormal Child Psychology* 39: 277–291. https://doi.org/10.1007/s10802-010-9459-1.

Deater-Deckard, K., Petrill, S.A., and Thompson, L.A. (2007). Anger/frustration, task persistence, and conduct problems in childhood: a behavioral genetic analysis. *Journal of Child Psychology and Psychiatry* 48 (1): 80–87.

Delaney, K.R. (2006a). Learning to observe in context. *Journal of Child and Adolescent Psychiatric Nursing* 19 (4): 170–174.

Delaney, K.R. (2006b). Following the affect: learning to observe emotional regulation. *Journal of Child and Adolescent Psychiatric Nursing* 19 (4): 175–181.

Delaney, K.R. (2006c). Learning to observe cognition, mastery and control. *Journal of Child and Adolescent Psychiatric Nursing* 19 (4): 182–193.

Delaney, K.R. (2006d). Learning to observe relationships in context. *Journal of Child and Adolescent Psychiatric Nursing* 19 (4): 194–202.

Delgado, B., Carrasco, M.A., Gonzalez-Peña, P., and Holgado-Tello, F. (2018). Temperament and behavioral problems in young children: the protective role of extraversion and effortful control. *Journal of Child and Family Studies* 27: 3232–3240. Available at https://doi.org/10.1007/s10826-018-1163-8.

Diaz, A. and Eisenberg, N. (2015). The process of emotion regulation is different from individual differences in emotion regulation: conceptual arguments and a focus on individual differences. *Psychological Inquiry* 26: 37–47. https://doi.org/10.1080/1047840X.2015.959094.

Dvir, Y., Ford, J.D., Hill, M., and Frazier, J.A. (2014). Childhood maltreatment, emotional dysregulation, and psychiatric comorbidities. *Harvard Review of Psychiatry* 22 (3): 150–161. https://doi.org/10.1097/HRP.0000000000000014.

Eisenberg, N., Fabes, R.A., Nyman, M. et al. (1994). The relations of emotionality and regulation to children's anger-related reactions. *Child Development* 65: 109–128.

Eisenberg, N., Fabes, R.A., and Guthrie, J.K. (1997). Coping with stress: the role of regulation and development. In: *Handbook of Children's Coping: Linking the Theory and Intervention* (eds. S.A. Wolchick and I.N. Sandler), 277–306. Mahwah, NJ: Lawrence Erlbaum.

Eisenberg, N., Smith, C., Sadovsky, A., and Spinrad, T.L. (2004). Effortful control: relations with emotional regulation, adjustment and socialization in childhood. In: *Handbook of Self-Regulation: Research, Theory and Applications* (eds. R.F. Baumeister and K.D. Vohs), 259–282. New York, NY: Guilford Press.

Ellis, L.K. & Rothbart, M.K. (2001). *Revision of the early adolescent temperament questionnaire.* Paper presented at the presented at the 2001 biennial meeting of the Society for Research in Child Development, Minneapolis, Minnesota.

Ensink, K., Biberdzic, M., Normandin, L., and Clarkin, J. (2015). A developmental psychopathology and neurobiological model of borderline personality disorder in adolescence. *Journal of Infant, Child and Adolescent Psychotherapy* 14: 46–69. https://doi.org/10.1080/15289168.2015.1007715.

Fan, J. and Posner, M. (2004). Human attentional networks. *Psychiatrische Praxis* 31 (Suppl2): S210–S214.

Feinberg, M.E. (2002). Coparenting and the transition to parenthood: a framework for prevention. *Clinical Child and Family Psychology Review* 5: 173–195.

Feinberg, M. (2003). The internal structure and ecological context of coparenting: A framework for research and intervention. *Parenting, Science and Practice* 3: 95–132.

Feinberg, M.E., Kan, M.L., and Goslin, M.C. (2009). Enhancing coparenting, parenting, and child self-regulation: effects of family foundations 1 year after birth. *Prevention Science* 10: 276–285.

Feldman, R. (2009). The development of regulatory functions from birth to 5 years: insights from premature infants. *Child Development* 80 (2): 544–561.

Feng, X., Shaw, D.S., and Silk, J.S. (2008). Developmental trajectories of anxiety symptoms among boys across early and middle childhood. *Journal of Abnormal Psychology* 117 (1): 32–47.

Finlon, K.J., Izard, C.E., Sidenfeld, A. et al. (2015). Emotion-based preventive intervention: effectively promoting emotion knowledge and adaptive behavior among at-risk preschoolers. *Development and Psychopathology* 27: 1353–1365. https://doi.org/10.1017/S0954579414001461.

Foley, M., McClowry, S., and Castellanos, F. (2008). The relationship between attention deficit hyperactivity disorder and child temperament. *Journal of Applied Developmental Psychology* 29: 157–169.

Fonagy, P. and Target, M. (2002). Early intervention and the development of self-regulation. *Psychoanalytic Quarterly* 22: 307–335.

Fullard, W., McDevitt, S.C., and Carey, W.B. (1984). Assessing temperament in one- to three-year-old children. *Journal of Pediatric Psychology* 9: 205–217.

Gardner-Neblett, N., Decoster, A., and Hamre, B.K. (2014). Linking preschool language and sustained attention with adolescent achievement through classroom self-reliance. *Journal of Applied Developmental Psychology* 35: 457–467. Available at http://dx.doi.org/10.1016/j.appdev.2014.09.003.

Gartstein, M.A., Slobodskaya, H.R., Żylicz, P.O. et al. (2010). A cross-cultural evaluation of temperament development: Japan, United States of America, Poland and Russia. *International Journal of Psychology and Psychological Therapy* 10: 55–75.

Gartstein, M.A., Bridgett, D.J., and Low, C.M. (2012a). Asking questions about temperament: self- and other-report measures across the lifespan. In: *Handbook of Temperament* (eds. M. Zentner and R.L. Shiner), 183–208. New York: Guilford Press.

Gartstein, M.A., Putnam, S.P., and Rothbart, M.K. (2012b). Etiology of preschool behavior problems: contributions of temperament attributes in early childhood. *Infant Mental Health Journal* 33: 197–211.

Gioia, G.A., Isquith, P.K., Guy, S.C., and Kenworthy, L. (2000). Behavior rating inventory of executive function. *Child Neuropsychology* 6 (3): 235–238.

Gioia, G.A., Espy, K.A., and Isquith, P.K. (2003). *The Behavior Rating Inventory for Executive Function – Preschool Version.* Lutz, FL: Psychological Assessment Resources.

Gioia, G.A., Isquith, P.K., Guy, S.C., and Kenworthy, L. (2015). *Brief-2 (Behavior Rating Inventory of Executive Function),* 2nde. Lutz, FL: Psychological Assessment Resources.

Gladstone, G.L., Parker, G.B., Mitchell, P.B. et al. (2005). Relationship between self-reported childhood behavioral inhibition and lifetime anxiety disorders in a clinical sample. *Depression and Anxiety* 22 (3): 103–113.

Goldsmith, H.H. (1996). Studying temperament via construction of the toddler behavior assessment questionnaire. *Child Development* 67: 218–235.

Goldsmith, H.H. and Campos, J.J. (1982). Toward a theory of infant temperament. In: *The Development of Attachment and Affiliative Systems* (eds. R.N. Emde and R.J. Harmon), 161–193. New York: Plenum.

Graziano, P.A., Slavec, J., Ros, R. et al. (2015). Self-regulation assessment among preschoolers with externalizing behavior problems. *Psychological Assessment* 27 (4): 1337–1348. Available at http://dx.doi.org/10.1037/pas0000113.

Handley, E.D., Michl-Petzing, L.C., Rogosch, F.A. et al. (2017). Developmental cascade effects of interpersonal psychotherapy for depressed mothers: longitudinal associations with toddler attachment, temperament, and maternal parenting. *Developmental Psychopathology* 29 (2): 601–615. https://doi.org/10.1017/S0954579417000219.

Harris, R.C., Robinson, J.B., Chang, F., and Burns, B.M. (2007). Characterizing preschool children's attention regulation in parent–child interactions: the role of effortful control and motivation. *Journal of Applied Developmental Psychology* 28: 25–39.

Hegvik, R.L., McDevitt, S.C., and Carey, W.B. (1982). The middle childhood temperament questionnaire. *Journal of Developmental and Behavioral Pediatrics* 3: 197–200.

Herzhoff, K., Tackett, J.L., and Martel, M.M. (2013). A dispositional trait framework elucidates differences between interview and questionnaire measurement of childhood attention problems. *Psychological Assessment* 25 (4): 1079–1090.

Hirshfeld-Becker, D.R., Biederman, J., Fargone, S.V. et al. (2004). Lack of association between behavioral inhibition and psychosocial adversity factors in children at risk for anxiety disorders. *The American Journal of Psychiatry* 161 (3): 547–555.

Izard, C.E. (2001). *The Emotions Course. Helping children understand and manage their feelings: An emotion-centered primary prevention program for Head Start.* Newark, DE: University of Delaware.

Izard, C., Stark, K., Trentacosta, C., and Schultz, D. (2008). Beyond emotion regulation: emotion utilization and adaptive functioning. *Child Development Perspectives* 2 (3): 156–163. https://doi.org/10.1111/j.1750-8606.2008.00058.x.

Izard, C.E., Woodburn, E.M., Finlon, K.J. et al. (2011). Emotion knowledge, emotion utilization, and emotion regulation. *Emotion Review* 3 (1): 44–52. https://doi.org/10.1177/1754073910380972.

Jonas, K. and Kochanska, G. (2018). An imbalance of approach and effortful control predicts externalizing problems: support for extending the dual-systems model into early childhood. *Journal of Abnormal Child Psychology* 46 (8): 1573–1583.

Kagan, J. (1998). Biology and the child. In: *Handbook of Child Psychology*, 5e (ed. W. Damon), 177–235. New York, NY: Wiley.

Karalunas, S.L., Gustafsson, H.C., Fair, D., Musser, E.D. & Nigg, J.T. (2018). Do we need an irritable subtype of ADHD? Replication and extension of a promising temperament profile approach to ADHD subtyping. *Psychological Assessment*. Available at http://dx.doi.org/10.1037/pas000066.

Keiley, M.K., Lofthouse, N., Bates, J.E. et al. (2003). Differential risks of covarying and pure components in mother and teacher reports of externalizing and internalizing behavior across ages 5 to 14. *Journal of Abnormal Child Psychology* 31: 267–283.

Keogh, B.K., Pullis, M.E., and Cadwell, J. (1982). A short form of the teachers temperament questionnaire. *Journal of Educational Measurement* 19: 323–329.

Kim-Spoon, J., Haskett, M.E., Longo, G.S., and Nice, R. (2012). Longitudinal study of self-regulation, positive parenting, and adjustment problems among physically abused children. *Child Abuse & Neglect* 36 (2): 95–107.

Kochanska, G. (1995). Children's temperament, mothers' discipline, and security of attachment: multiple pathways in emerging internalization. *Child Development* 66: 597–615.

Kochanska, G., Murray, K., and Koy, K.C. (1997). Inhibitory control as a contributor to conscience in childhood: from toddler to early school age. *Child Development* 68: 263–277.

Kochanska, G., Murray, K.T., and Harlan, E.T. (2000). Effortful control in early childhood: continuity and change, antecedents, and implications for social development. *Developmental Psychology* 36: 220–232.

Kochanska, G., Barry, R.A., Jimenez, N.B. et al. (2009). Guilt and effortful control: two mechanisms that prevent disruptive developmental trajectories. *Journal of Personality and Social Psychology* 97 (2): 322–333.

Koren, D., Seidman, L.J., Goldsmith, M., and Harvey, P.D. (2006). Real-world cognitive – and metacognitive – dysfunction in schizophrenia: A new approach for measuring (and remediating) more 'right stuff.' *Schizophrenia Bulletin* 32 (2): 310–326.

Kovacs, M. and Lopez-Duran, N.L. (2010). Prodromal symptoms and atypical affectivity as predictors of major depression in juveniles: implications for prevention. *Journal of Child Psychology and Psychiatry* 51 (4): 472–496. Available at https://doi.org/10.1111/j.1469-7610.2010.02230.x.

Kovacs, M., Rottenberg, J., and George, C. (2009). Maladaptive mood repair responses distinguish young adults with early-onset depressive disorders and predict future depression outcomes. *Psychological Medicine* 39 (11): 1841–1854. https://doi.org/10.1017/S0033291709005789.

Kruczek, T., Vitanza, S., and Salsman, J. (2008). Posttraumatic stress disorder in *children*. In: *Handbook of Childhood Behavioral Issues: Evidence-Based Approaches to Prevention and Treatment* (eds. T.P. Gullotta and G.M. Blau), 289–317. New York, NY: Routledge/Taylor & Francis.

Lackner, C.L., Santesso, D.L., Dywan, J. et al. (2018). Adverse childhood experiences are associated with self-regulation and the magnitude of the error-related negativity difference. *Biological Psychology* 132: 244–251. Available at https://doi.org/10.1016/j.biopsycho.2018.01.006.

Lahey, B.B., Van Hulle, C.A., Keenan, K. et al. (2005). Temperament and parenting during the first year of life predict future child conduct problems. *Journal of Abnormal Child Psychology* 36 (8): 1139–1158.

Lawson, R.A., Papadakis, A.A., Higginson, C.I. et al. (2015). Everyday executive function impairments predict comorbid psychopathology in autism spectrum and attention deficit hyperactivity disorders. *Neuropsychology* 29 (3): 445–453. https://doi.org/10.1037/neu0000145.

Leddy, S.K. (2006). *Health Promotion: Mobilizing Strengths to Enhance Health, Wellness, and Well-Being.* Philadelphia, PA: F.A. Davis.

Lemery, K.S., Essex, M.J., and Smider, N.A. (2002). Revealing the relation between temperament and behavior problem symptoms by eliminating measurement confounding: expert rating and factor analyses. *Child Development* 73: 867–882.

Lengua, L.J., Long, A.C., Smith, K.I., and Meltzoff, A.N. (2005). Pre-attack symptomatology and temperament as predictors of children's responses to the September 11 terrorist attacks. *Journal of Child Psychiatry and Psychology* 46 (6): 6331–6645.

Leve, L., Kim, H.K., and Peers, K.C. (2005). Childhood temperament and family environment as predictors of internalizing and externalizing trajectories from ages 5 to 17. *Journal of Abnormal Child Psychology* 33 (5): 505–520.

Macari, S.L., Koller, J., Campbell, D.J., and Chawarska, K. (2017). Temperamental markers in toddlers with autism spectrum disorder. *Journal of Child Psychology and Psychiatry* 58 (7): 819–828. https://doi.org/10.1111/jcpp.12710.

Martel, M.M., Gremillion, M.L., Roberts, B.A. et al. (2014). Longitudinal prediction of the one-year course of preschool ADHD symptoms: implication for models of temperament-ADHD associations. *Personality and Individual Difference* 64: 58–61.

Martin, R. and Bridger, R. (1999). *The Temperament Assessment Battery for Children-Revised*. Athens, GA: University of Georgia.

Maziade, M., Caron, C., Côté, R. et al. (1990). Psychiatric status of adolescents who had extreme temperaments at age 7. *American Journal of Psychiatry* 147 (11): 1531–1536.

McClowry, S.G. (1995). The development of the school-age temperament inventory. *Merrill Palmer Quarterly* 41: 271–285.

McClowry, S.G. (2002a). The temperament profiles of school age children. *Journal of Pediatric Nursing* 17: 3–10.

McClowry, S.G. (2002b). Transforming temperament profile statistics into puppets and other visual media. *Journal of Pediatric Nursing* 17: 11–17.

McClowry, S.G. (2003). *Your Child's Unique Temperament: Insights and Strategies for Responsive Parenting*. Champagne, IL: Research Press.

McClowry, S.G. and Galehouse, P. (2002). A pilot study conducted to plan a temperament-based parenting program for inner city families. *Journal of Child and Adolescent Psychiatric Nursing* 15: 97–108.

McClowry, S.G., Halverson, C.F., and Sanson, A. (2003). A re-examination of the validity and reliability of the school-age temperament inventory. *Nursing Research* 53 (3): 176–182. https://doi.org/10.1097/00006199-200305000-00007.

McClowry, S.G., Snow, D.L., and Tamis-LeMonda, C.S. (2005). An evaluation of the effects of INSIGHTS on the behavior of inner-city primary school children. *Journal of Primary Prevention* 26: 567–584.

McClowry, S.G., Rodriguez, E.T., and Koslowitz, R. (2008). Temperament-based intervention: re-examining goodness of fit. *European Journal of Developmental Science* 2: 120–135.

McCormick, M.P., O'Connor, E.E., Cappella, E., and McClowry, S.G. (2015). Getting a good start in school: effects of INSIGHTS on children with high maintenance temperaments. *Early Childhood Research Quarterly* 30 (A): 128–139. https://doi.org/10.1016/j.ecresq.2014.10.006.

McDevitt, S. and Carey, W.B. (1978). The measurement of temperament in 3-7 year old children. *Journal of Child Psychology and Psychiatry* 19 (3): 245–253.

Medoff-Cooper, B., Carey, W.B., and McDevitt, S.C. (1993). The early infancy temperament questionnaire. *Journal of Developmental and Behavioral Pediatrics* 14 (4): 230–235.

Mesman, J. and Koot, H.M. (2000). Common and specific correlates of preadolescent internalizing and externalizing psychopathology. *Journal of Abnormal Psychology* 109: 367–374.

Mian, N.D., Wainwright, L., Briggs-Gowan, M.J., and Carter, A.S. (2011). An ecological risk model for early childhood anxiety: the importance of early child symptoms and temperament. *Journal of Abnormal Child Psychology* 39 (4): 501–512. https://doi.org/10.1007/s10802-010-9476-0.

Mikolajczak, M., Petrides, K.V., and Hurry, J. (2009). Adolescents choosing self-harm as an emotion regulation strategy: the protective role of trait emotional intelligence. *British Journal of Clinical Psychology* 48: 181–193.

Miller, A.L., Gouley, K.K., Seifer, R. et al. (2004). Emotions and behaviors in the head start classroom: associations among observed dysregulation, social competence and preschool adjustment. *Early Education and Development* 15: 147–165.

Moffitt, T.E., Arseneault, L., Belsky, D. et al. (2011). A gradient of childhood self-control predicts health, wealth, and public safety. *Proceedings of the National Academy of Sciences of the United States of America* 108 (7): 2693–2698.

Montroy, J.J., Bowles, R.P., Skibbe, L.E. et al. (2016). The development of self-regulation across early childhood. *Developmental Psychology* 52 (11): 1744–1762.

Murdaugh, C.L., Parsons, M.A., and Pender, N.J. (2018). *Health Promotion in Nursing Practice*, 8e. New York, NY: Pearson.

New York University Steinhardt. (2019). *INSIGHTS in Jamaica*. Available at https://steinhardt.nyu.edu/insights/jamaica.

Nolvi, S., Karlsson, L., Bridgett, D.J. et al. (2016). Maternal postnatal psychiatric symptoms and infant temperament affect early mother-infant bonding. *Infant Behavior and Development* 43: 13–23. Available at http://dx.doi.org/10.1016/j.infbeh.2016.03.003.

O'Connor, E.E., Rodriguez, E.T., Cappella, E. et al. (2012). Child disruptive behavior and parenting sense of competence: A comparison of the effects of two models of INSIGHTS. *Journal of Community Psychology* 40: 555–572. https://doi.org/10.1002/jcop.21482.

Ormel, A.J., Oldenhinkel, A.J., Ferdinand, R.F. et al. (2005). Internalizing and externalizing problems in adolescence: general and dimension-specific effects of familial loadings and preadolescent temperament traits. *Psychological Medicine* 35 (12): 1825–1835.

Pérez-Edgar, K., Fu, X., & Liu, P. (2018). *The biological underpinnings of attention mechanisms in temperament*. Paper presented at the Twenty-Second Occasional Temperament Conference, Murcia, Spain.

Pettit, G.S., Keiley, M.K., Laird, R.D. et al. (2007). Predicting the developmental course of mother-reported monitoring across childhood and adolescence from early proactive parenting, child temperament, and parents' worries. *Journal of Family Psychology* 21 (2): 206–217.

Pijl, M.K., Bussu, G., Charman, T. et al. (2019). Temperament as an early risk marker for autism spectrum disorders? A longitudinal study of high-risk and low-risk infants. *Journal of Autism Developmental Disorders* https://doi.org/10.1007/s10803-018-3855-8.

Pleuss, M. and Belsky, J. (2009). Differential susceptibility to rearing experiences: the case of childcare. *Journal of Child Psychology and Psychiatry* 50 (4): 396–404.

Plomin, R. and Caspi, A. (1999). Behavioral genetics and personality. In: *Handbook of Personality: Theory and Research*, 2e (eds. L.A. Pervin and O.P. John), 251–276. New York, NY: Guildford Press.

Ponitz, C.C., McClelland, M.M., Matthews, J.S., and Morrison, F.J. (2009). A structured observation of behavioral self-regulation and its contribution to kindergarten outcomes. *Developmental Psychology* 45: 605–619. Available at http://dx.doi.org/10.1037/a0015365.

Posner, M.I. (2016). The orienting of attention: then and now. *The Quarterly Journal of Experimental Psychology* 69 (10): 1864–1875.

Posner, M.I. and Rothbart, M.K. (2000). Developing mechanisms of self-regulation. *Development and Psychopathology* 12: 427–441.

Posner, M.I. and Rothbart, M.K. (2007). Research on attention networks as a model for the integration of psychological science. *Annual Review of Psychology* 58: 1–23. https://doi.org/10.1146/annurev.psych.58.110405.085516.

Pozuelos, J.P., Paz-Alonso, P.M., Castillo, A. et al. (2014). Development of attention networks and their interactions in childhood. *Developmental Psychology* 50 (10): 2405–2415. Available at http://dx.doi.org/10.1037/a0037469.

Prior, M., Sanson, A., Smart, D., and Oberklaid, F. (2000). *Pathways from Infancy to Adolescence: Australian Temperament Project 1983–2000*. Melbourne, Australia: Australian Institute of Family Studies.

Putnam, S.P. and Rothbart, M.K. (2006). Development of short and very short forms of the children's behavior questionnaire. *Journal of Personality Assessment* 87 (1): 102–112.

Robinson, J.B., Burns, B.M., and Davis, D.W. (2009). Maternal scaffolding and attention regulation in children living in poverty. *Journal of Applied Developmental Psychology* 30: 82–91.

Rode, J.L. and Kiel, E.J. (2016). The mediated effects of maternal depression and infant temperament on maternal role. *Archives of Women's Mental Health* 19: 133–140. https://doi.org/10.1007/s00737-015-0540-1.

Rothbart, M.K. (2007). Temperament, development, and personality. *Current Directions in Psychological Science* 16 (4): 207–212.

Rothbart, M. (2012). *Becoming Who We Are: Temperament and Personality in Development*. New York, NY: Guilford Press.

Rothbart, M.K. and Bates, J.E. (2006). Temperament. In: *Handbook of Child Psychology: Vol 3. Social, Emotional, and Personality Development*, 6e (eds. W. Damon, R. Lerner and N. Eisenberg), 99–166. New York: Wiley.

Rothbart, M.K., Ahadi, S.A., Hershey, K., and Fisher, P. (2001). Investigations of temperament at three to seven years: the Children's Behavior Questionnaire. *Child Development* 72 (5): 1394–1408.

Rothbart, M.K., Ellis, L.K., Rueda, M.R., and Posner, M.I. (2003). Developing mechanisms of temperamental effortful control. *Journal of Personality* 71 (6): 1113–1143.

Rothbart, M.K., Sheese, B.E., and Posner, M.I. (2014). Temperament and emotion regulation. In: *Handbook of Emotion Regulation*, 2e (ed. J.J. Gross), 305–320. New York, NY: Guilford Press.

Rowe, D.C. and Plomin, R. (1977). Temperament in early childhood. *Journal of Personal Assessment* 41 (2): 150–156. https://doi.org/10.1207/s15327752jpa4102_5.

Rowland, J.E., Hamilton, M.K., Lino, B.J. et al. (2013). Cognitive regulation of negative affect in schizophrenia and bipolar disorder. *Psychiatry Research* 208 (1): 21–28. https://doi.org/10.1016/j.psychres.2013.02.021.

Rueda, M.R., Posner, M.I., and Rothbart, M.K. (2004). Attentional control and self-regulation. In: *Handbook of Self-Regulation: Research, Theory, and Applications* (eds. R.F. Baumeister and K.D. Vohs), 283–300. New York: Guilford Press.

Rydell, A.M., Berlin, L., and Bohlin, G. (2003). Emotionality, emotion regulation, and adaptation among 5- to 8-year-old children. *Emotion* 3 (1): 30–47.

Sánchez-Pérez, N., Inuggi, A., García Santos, J.M., Fuentes, L.J., & González-Salinas, C. (2018). *Functional brain connectivity in children that differ in temperament-based emotional regulation abilities*. Paper presented at the Twenty-Second Occasional Temperament Conference, Murcia, Spain.

Scaer, R. (2005). *The Trauma Spectrum: Hidden Wounds and Human Resiliency*. New York: W.W. Norton.

Schaefer, J.D., Caspi, A., Belsky, D.W. et al. (2017). Enduring mental health: prevalence and prediction. *Journal of Abnormal Psychology* 126 (2): 212–224.

Schore, A.N. (1994). *Affect Regulation and the Origin of the Self: The Neurobiology of Emotional Development*. Hillsdale, NJ: Erlbaum.

Shiner, R.L. (2009). The development of personality disorders: perspectives from normal personality development in childhood and adolescence. *Development and Psychopathology* 21: 715–734.

Shipman, K., Schneider, R., Fitzgerald, M.M. et al. (2007). Maternal emotion socialization in maltreating and non-maltreating families: implications for children's emotion regulation. *Social Development* 16 (2): 268–285.

Simonds, J. & Rothbart, M.K. (2004). *The Temperament in Middle Childhood Questionnaire (TMCQ): A computerized self-report measure of temperament for ages 7–10*. Poster session presented at the Occasional Temperament Conference, Athens, GA.

Sloan, E., Hall, K., Moulding, R. et al. (2017). Emotion regulation as a transdiagnostic treatment construct across anxiety, depression, substance, eating and borderline personality disorders: A systematic review. *Clinical Psychology Review* 57: 141–163. Available at http://dx.doi.org/10.1016/j.cpr.2017.09.002.

Solmeyer, A.R., Feinberg, M.E., Coffman, D.L., and Jones, D.E. (2014). The effects of the family foundations prevention program on coparenting and child adjustment: A mediation analysis. *Prevention Science* 15: 213–223.

Stern, D. (1985). *The Interpersonal World of the Infant*. New York, NY: Basic Books.

Strelau, J. (2000). *Temperament: A Psychological Perspective*. New York, NY: Plenum.

Tan, L. and Smith, C.L. (2018, September 20). Intergenerational transmission of maternal emotion regulation to child emotion regulation: moderated mediation of maternal positive and negative emotions. *Emotion*: 1–8. https://doi.org/10.1037/emo0000523.

Thomas, A. and Chess, S. (1977). *Temperament and Development*. New York, NY: Brunner & Mazel.

Thompson, R.A., Lewis, M.D., and Calkins, S.D. (2008). Reassessing emotional regulation. *Child Development Perspectives* 2 (3): 124–131.

Trentacosta, C.J. and Shaw, D.S. (2009). Emotional self-regulation, peer rejection, and antisocial behavior: developmental associations from early childhood to early adolescence. *Journal of Applied Developmental Psychology* 30 (3): 356–365.

Tsotsi, S., Broekman, B.F.P., Shek, L.P. et al. (2019). Maternal parenting stress, child exuberance, and preschoolers' behavior problems. *Child Development* 90 (1): 136–146.

Tucker, D.M., Derryberry, D., and Luu, P. (2000). Anatomy and physiology of human emotion: vertical integration of brain stem, limbic and cortical systems. In: *The Neuropsychology of Emotion: Series in Affective Science* (ed. J.C. Borod), 56–79. New York, NY: Oxford University Press.

Van Malderen, E., Goossens, E., Verbeken, S., and Kemps, E. (2018). Unravelling the association between inhibitory control and loss of control over eating among adolescent. *Appetite* 125: 401–409. Available at https://doi.org/10.1016/j.appet.2018.02.019.

Van Schyndel, S., Eisenbert, N., Valiente, C., and Spinrad, T. (2017). Relations from temperamental approach reactivity and effortful control to academic achievement and peer relations in early elementary school. *Journal of Research in Personality* 67: 15–26.

Vohs, K.D. and Baumeister, R.F. (eds.) (2016). *Handbook of Self-Regulation: Research, Theory, and Applications*, 3e. New York, NY: Guilford Press.

Wang, F.L., Eisenberg, N., Valiente, C., and Spinrad, T.L. (2016). Role of temperament in early adolescent pure and co-occurring internalizing and externalizing problems using a bifactor model: moderation by parenting and gender. *Development and Psychopathology* 28: 1487–1504. https://doi.org/10.1017/S0954579415001224.

Windle, M. and Lerner, R.M. (1986). Reassessing the dimensions of temperamental individuality across the life span: the revised dimensions of temperament survey (DOTS-R). *Journal of Adolescent Research* 1: 213–230.

Yates, P.M. and Kingston, D.A. (2006). The self-regulation model of sexual offending: the relationship between offence pathways and static and dynamic sexual offence risk. *Association for the Treatment of Sexual Abusers* 18 (3): 259–270. https://doi.org/10.1177/107906320601800304.

Zeier, J.D., Maxwell, J.S., and Newman, J.P. (2009). Attention moderates the processing of inhibitory information in primary psychopathy. *Journal of Abnormal Psychology* 118 (3): 554–563.

Zentner, M. and Bates, J.E. (2008). Child temperament: an integrative review of concepts, research programs, and measures. *European Journal of Developmental Science* 2: 7–37.

3

Neurobiology and Neurophysiology of Behavioral/Psychiatric Disorders

Susan J. Boorin[1] and Norman L. Keltner[2]

[1] Yale University School of Nursing, Orange, CT, USA
[2] Birmingham School of Nursing, University of Alabama, Birmingham, AL, USA

Objectives

After reading this chapter, advanced practice registered nurses (APRNs) will be able to:

1. Identify the significant neurobiological issues that influence the development of child/adolescent psychiatric disorders.
2. Identify the anatomy of the central nervous system and the brain that are involved in the development of psychiatric disorders.
3. Note influences on the development of the brain.
4. Discuss implications of neurobiological issues on APRN practice, education, and research.

Introduction

The nervous system is composed of several cell types that are assembled into the central and peripheral systems during development. Abnormalities in the organization of the nervous system can occur due to genetic causes, environmental exposures (e.g. in utero or injury), or gene–environment interactions. We are in the early stages of understanding both normal brain development and mental illness, predominantly due to challenges studying the brain. However, science is steadily moving forward incorporating a convergent model of mental illness based on disrupted neural, cognitive, and behavioral systems. In 2010 the National Institute of Mental Health (NIMH) introduced the Research Domain Criteria (RDoC), encouraging a dimensional framework to study the brain and behavior from simple to complex and how individual variations can represent different degrees of health and illness (Insel et al. 2010). Within this framework there is an emphasis on neural circuitry, building on the idea that tightly regulated circuits inform motivation, cognition, and emotion (Insel and Cuthbert 2015). This dimensional approach cuts across our current clinical categories to capture data on psychopathology that in turn will inform new targets for treatment (Insel and Cuthbert 2010; Insel et al. 2010; Carpenter 2016).

Understanding the etiology and treatment of major psychiatric disorders can be strengthened through examination of brain development, structures, and function.

Child and Adolescent Behavioral Health: A Resource for Advanced Practice Psychiatric and Primary Care Practitioners in Nursing,
Second Edition. Edited by Edilma L. Yearwood, Geraldine S. Pearson, and Jamesetta A. Newland.
© 2021 John Wiley & Sons, Inc. Published 2021 by John Wiley & Sons, Inc.
Companion website: www.wiley.com/go/Yearwood

This chapter begins with an examination of neuroanatomy and brain development that forms the foundation of understanding and discourse about the connection of neurobiology and behavior. It goes on to consider neurotransmission and specific neurotransmitters, which offers the possibility to discuss the role of neurobiology in selected psychiatric disorders and the rationale for treatment. The chapter concludes with implications for APRN practice, education, and research.

Anatomy of the Central Nervous System

The central nervous system (CNS) comprises the brain and spinal cord; the peripheral nervous system (PNS) includes the 12 pairs of cranial nerves and all the remaining nerves of the body. The CNS evolves from the neural tube, which emerges about the fourth week of development. In its earliest stage the neural tube consists of three layers: the ectoderm (outside), the mesoderm (middle), and the endoderm (inside). The outer layer will eventually give rise to the CNS and PNS. From the middle layer come the cardiovascular and reproductive systems among others, and from the endoderm arises the gastrointestinal tract, the respiratory system, and other major systems (Johns 2014). The neural tube is organized by a process of cellular folding called neurulation. The adult brain is organized according to its embryonic scheme with the anterior portion of the neural tube developing into the brain and the posterior portion developing into the spinal cord. The fluid-filled cavities within the neural tube develop into ventricles, which contain cerebral spinal fluid (CSF). There are a number of serious neural tube defects, including *spina bifida* (a malformation of the lower spinal cord), *anencephaly* (an absence of parts of the brain and skull), and *encephalocele* (where the membrane-covered brain protrudes through the skull) (National Institute of Child Health and Human Development 2017).

Because the brain grows more rapidly than the membranous skull that contains it, the cerebral hemispheres are forced to grow posteriorly and laterally. This causes the growing brain to crease and fold, producing convolutions that increase the surface area. Kowalski et al. (2019) compare the creasing and folding to the coastline of Norway. If one does not consider the fjords, Norway's coastline is a mere 1600 miles. Taking the fjords into account, Norway's coastline stretches to 15 000 miles. This brain development feature allows more coastline of brain cerebral cortex. Brain development continues rapidly in the postnatal period. By the age of 6 years the total size of the brain is approximately 90% of its adult size. As the child matures into an adolescent, there are age-related changes in white and gray matter volume which continue into young adulthood (Tamnes et al. 2010).

Cranial Vault and Meninges

The brain is protected by hard bones that form the skull and three meningeal layers: pia, arachnoid, and dura. These can be remembered by the mnemonic "PAD" from the interior layer to the outer layer. The word dura means "hard," and like its name the dura is composed of two fibrous layers. The arachnoid is a wispy meningeal layer. The pia adheres closely to the surface of the brain and follows the folds of the brain. The major arteries of the brain run between the arachnoid and pia layers, and this area is called the subarachnoid space (Blumenfeld 2002). Recent advances in diagnostic imaging have enhanced the understanding of neurovascular anatomy. The arterial and venous vascular network is extensive, with notable individual differences (Borden 2007).

Blood–Brain and Blood–CSF Barriers

The blood–brain barrier (BBB) is formed by endothelial cells that line an extensive capillary system in the brain. The BBB has a large surface area, and regulates what enters and exits the CNS. The distinguishing feature of the BBB endothelial cells – compared to endothelial cells in the periphery – is the presence of tight junctions between the cells. Because the BBB has continuous tight junctions, molecules are forced to cross the BBB. Certain drugs and small gases can cross an intact BBB; however, specific transport systems regulate much of the traffic (Deeken and Loscher 2007). Some drug molecules do not penetrate the BBB or do so in small amounts. Thus these agents can have a systemic effect but little to no CNS effect. The BBB is said to have three dimensions (Keltner and Kowalski 2019): an anatomic barrier, a physiologic barrier, and a metabolic barrier. The anatomic barrier is composed of the aforementioned tight junctions between the endothelial cells. The physiologic barrier recognizes some molecules and allows their entry into the brain while other drug molecules are rejected. The third barrier is metabolic. For instance, some drug molecules start their passage through the endothelial walls only to be converted to a nonlipid soluble substance and ferried back out.

The choroids plexus (CP) is located in all four cerebral ventricles and produces CSF. Together with the arachnoid membrane it constitutes the blood–CSF barrier. Increasing evidence indicates that the integrity of the brain tissue–blood barriers plays an important role in brain immune response and neuro-inflammation (Hickey 2001; Szmydynger-Chodobska et al. 2009). For example, oxidative stress, which is a common feature in the pathogenesis of many neuroinflammatory conditions, may contribute to the disruption of the BBB. BBB breakdown plays an important role in the pathogenesis of HIV-1 associated dementia (Chaudhuri et al. 2008).

Cerebral Cortex

The cerebral cortex (Figure 3.1) is the outer layer of the cerebral hemispheres and is responsible for sensory perception, movement, language, thinking, memory, consciousness, and certain aspects of emotion (Hendelman 2006). Comprising billions of neurons and vast interconnections, it is divided into four major lobes (Table 3.1). The majority of the cerebral cortex is composed of neocortex, which has six cell layers labeled I through VI, counting from the surface inward. Neurons in each layer differ in their functional contribution to cerebral processing. The cerebral cor-

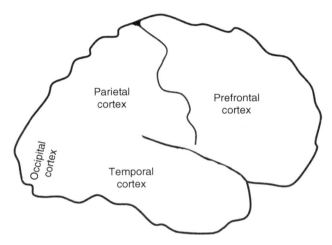

Figure 3.1 Lobes of the cerebral cortex. (*Source:* From Arnsten, A. & Castellanos, F.X. Neurobiology of attention regulation and its disorders. In A. Martin, L. Scahill, & C.J. Kratochvil (Eds.), Pediatric psychopharmacology: Principles and practice (2nd edition; pp. 95–111). © 2011, Oxford University Press. with permission from Oxford University Press.)

tex was mapped out based on 52 cytoarchitectonic regions by the neuroanatomist Brodmann in 1909 (Blumenfeld 2002). Researchers have sought for many years to develop a new map that would provide integrated data on a greater number of brain "parcels" which could be replicated in studies. Advances in imaging have resulted in a new map of the human brain based on data from the Human Connectome Project (Glasser et al. 2016). This new map combines multiple properties to describe 180 parcels per hemisphere which are significantly different from their neighbors. Interestingly, because cortical neurons are not generated within the cortex itself, questions remain regarding how each neuron reaches its appropriate position (Rakic et al. 2009). A visual animation of Rakic's model of neuronal migration in the development of the cerebral cortex can be found at his Yale University website (https://rakichlab.yale.edu).

Cerebral Cortex
Cortical–Subcortical Connections

Over the past 25 years, a substantial amount of research has focused on brain pathways that connect cortical and subcortical structures. Table 3.2 lists the major subcortical structures, primary functions, and connections. Brain circuitry is a vast topic that is beyond the scope of this chapter. However, the principles and structural components can be illustrated through a brief review of dopamine circuits. In a landmark paper, Alexander et al. (1986) described five parallel, minimally overlapping dopamine circuits. These circuits have a common architectural loop from the cortex to the striatum, globus pallidus, thalamus, and back to cortex. The communication

Table 3.1 Major divisions of the cerebral cortex

Lobes	Selected structure	Primary function	Symptoms related to damage
Frontal lobes	Prefrontal cortex	Attention, working memory, impulse control	Deficits in working memory, lack of ability to plan for the future, lack of executive functioning (insight, reasoning, judgment, concept formation)
	Primary motor cortex	Voluntary movement	
	Supplementary motor cortex	Planning movement	
	Broca's area	Speech production	
Parietal lobes	Primary somatosensory cortex	Processing of sensory input, orienting attention	Complex sensory deficits; decreased spatial cognition, sustained attention, and visual selective attention; difficulty understanding actions of others
Occipital lobes	Primary visual cortex	Processing visual input	Decreased visual integration of information, color vision
Temporal lobes	Auditory cortex	Processing auditory input	Deficits in auditory processing, word finding difficulties, impaired language production, prosopagnosia facial (blindness)
	Wernicke's area	Language production	
	Fusiform gyrus	Facial and object recognition	

Table 3.2 Major subcortical structures, primary functions, and connections

Structure	Location	Primary function	Primary connections
Thalamus	Telencephalon	Sensory-motor integration	Cortex, basal ganglia, amygdala
Hypothalamus	Diencephalon	Appetite, temperature regulation, sleep, mood regulation	Pituitary, hippocampus, amygdala
Basal ganglia[a]	Telencephalon	Motor	Cortex, thalamus
Hippocampus	Temporal region	Learning and memory	Cortex, cingulate, amygdala, thalamus
Amygdala	Temporal region, anterior to hippocampus	Emotion regulation, coordination of fear response	Thalamus, cortex, locus coeruleus
Ventral tegmental area	Midbrain (inferior to the diencephalon)	Behavioral reinforcement, motivation	Nucleus accumbens, cortex
Substantia nigra	Midbrain (just inferior to the diencephalon)	Motor	Putamen, caudate

[a] The basal ganglia are gray matter structures that are highly connected to the cortex and other subcortical structures such as the thalamus and hypothalamus.

between the striatum and thalamus is through the globus pallidus, which regulates the connection between the striatum and thalamus. The names of these corticostriatal-thalamic-cortical loops are derived from their cortical origin. For example, the motor circuit arises from the primary motor strip (Figure 3.2). The dorsolateral prefrontal circuit has its origin in the dorsolateral prefrontal region and plays an important role in attention, impulse control, and planning. The circuit emanating from the anterior cingulate plays a role in emotion regulation (Alexander et al. 1986).

Another way to describe dopamine circuits is to trace the pathway from the subcortical origin to the cortex. For example, the nigrostriatal circuit arises from the substantial nigra to the striatum, with connections proceeding to the globus pallidus, thalamus, and motor cortex. Similarly, the mesolimbic circuit has its origin in the ventral tegmental area and courses to the nucleus accumbens (often called the reward circuit). The mesocortical circuit also has its origin in the ventral tegmental area, but it projects directly to the prefrontal cortex (PFC). The tuberoinfundibular pathway is yet another dopamine circuit that warrants mention due to its relevance to antipsychotic medications. Signals from the hypothalamus influence secretion of prolactin. Potent D2 blocking agents such as haloperidol or risperidone result in an increase in prolactin due to blockade of D2 receptors in the tuberoinfundibular system (Keltner and Steele 2019).

Synaptic Organization of the Brain

Brain circuits integrate vast amounts of information to guide biological, behavioral, and cognitive functions.

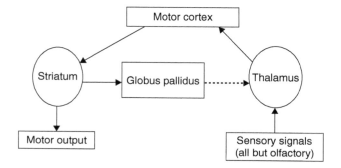

Figure 3.2 The motor circuit, which is one of five dopamine circuits traversing specific regions of the cortex through the striatum, globus pallidus, thalamus, and back to the cortex.

These neural circuits change and develop as a child matures, influenced not only by genetic predispositions but also by unique environmental exposures and experiences. Neurons, dendrites, axons, and supporting glial cells are important components of these neural circuits (Tau and Peterson 2010).

The Neuron

There are 10^{11} (one hundred billion) neurons in the CNS that process information (Kowalski et al. 2019). In turn, among these billions of neurons, a single neuron may make thousands of synaptic connections. Nestler et al. (2015) point out that one monoamine-containing cell in the brainstem may form over 100 000 synapses. Although neurons include the same organelles found in all cells, their structure is specialized to enable intercellular communication. The neuron, which is composed of a cell body, dendrites, and axons, has the ability to receive and integrate information from multiple inputs. In addition, neurons can send information to other neurons, muscles, and organs. Communication between neurons takes place at the synapse via chemical neurotransmitter molecules.

Dendrites and Dendritic Spines

Dendrites, which are the primary target for synaptic input from other neurons, appear as a vast branching structure also known as the dendritic arbor. The arborization of dendrites is not completed until late adolescence or early adulthood. The smallest structural unit of the dendritic arbor is the dendritic spine. These small (1–2 μm) thorn-like projections play a key role in postsynaptic signaling. Spines function as postsynaptic compartments for excitatory synapses that are associated with long-term potentiation (enlarged spine) or long-term depression (shrinkage of spine) (Nakahata and Yasuda 2018). Each spine has multiple potential connections with adjacent axons, and the choice of synaptic partners influences the pattern of neuronal circuitry (Chen and Nedivi 2010). The central role of dendritic spines in learning and memory is illustrated by fragile X, which a genetically inherited mental retardation syndrome characterized by intellectual deficits. In fragile X, dendritic spines are few in number and fail to mature (Dolen and Bear 2008).

Cerebral White Matter, Glia, and Lymphatics

Axons are myelinated fiber pathways that constitute cerebral white matter. White matter tracts can be grouped into five bundles: association fibers, striatal fibers, commissural fibers, thalamic fibers, and pontine fibers. These tracts reflect the anatomical location of the cortical connection. Association fibers are cortical–cortical connections within the hemisphere; commissural fibers are also cortical–cortical connections, but across hemispheres. The names of the other tracts directly refer to location (Schmahmann et al. 2008). During development, axons migrate through the CNS guided by cues from the surrounding cellular environment and follow behind the leading edge of their structure, known as growth cones (Gitai et al. 2003). In addition to linking brain structures that are relatively far apart, axons also form relatively short circuits (interneurons) (Purves et al. 2008). Modern neuroimaging has used functional magnetic resonance imaging (fMRI) to identify functionally distinct networks in the brain (Cao et al. 2017; Cieri and Esposito 2018). In recent years there has been increased interest in studying the association between the microstructure of white matter tracts and psychiatric disorders in youth. Diffusion tensor imaging (DTI) assesses water diffusion within white matter tracts and how well the tracts restrict perpendicular diffusion

(Winklewski et al. 2018). Studies have suggested that white matter tract abnormalities may be associated with antisocial behavior, anorexia nervosa, and emotional dysregulation disorders and are a marker of cognitive decline mediated by metabolic syndrome (Versace et al. 2015; Alfaro et al. 2018; Gaudio et al. 2017; Waller et al. 2017).

Glia astrocytes and oligodendrocytes are the two main types of glial cells in the CNS. Historically, the function of glial cells has been relegated to the provision of support for neurons. Research conducted over the last decade shows that these cells have an important role in synaptic transmission and the modulation of neuronal activity (Halassa et al. 2006). For example, oligodendrocytes provide insulation and support for axons, which improves the efficiency of nerve signals along the axon. Astrocytes play a role in glutamate transmission, which in turn plays an essential role in learning and memory (Halassa et al. 2006). Emerging evidence also suggests that astrocytes play a key role in the integration of neuronal and vascular activity (Barres 2008). Thus, increases in local neuronal activity promote changes in cerebral blood flow to sustain the neuronal activity (Haydon and Carmignoto 2006). This local physiological action is exploited in fMRI. Changes in astrocyte activation may contribute to the pathophysiology of Lyme disease, Alzheimer's disease, and amyotrophic lateral sclerosis (Dotevall et al. 1999; Rossi and Volterra 2009). Microglia, a third type of glial cell, are components of the brain's immune system, an absolutely critical function (Nestler et al. 2015). In 2017, a true lymphatic network was discovered in the brain (Absinta et al. 2017).

Learning and Memory: Synaptic Plasticity

Learning and memory are concepts used to explain how experience influences behavior (Rudy 2008). The brain is able to capture and store the range of content from our experiences. There are two broad types of memory: declarative memory and procedural memory. Declarative memory is specific recall of events, facts, and figures. Procedural memory involves skill acquisition such as riding a bicycle, playing the violin, or pitching a curve ball. Learning and memory involve an impressive array of brain structures and connections including the cortex, medial temporal lobe, striatum, amygdala, cerebellum, and hippocampus (Milner et al. 1998). At the center of learning and memory is the synapse. Bliss and Lomo (1973) showed that synaptic connections can be modified by experience. For example, an isolated weak stimulus evokes commensurate synaptic activity in a specialized region of the hippocampus called the dentate gyrus. When a stronger stimulus is delivered, it evokes a larger synaptic response. If this stronger stimulus is followed by repeated stimuli (even a weaker stimulus) down the same pathway, the evoked response will also be large. This is because repeated neuron-to-neuron connection strengthens the communication (called Hebb's rule). Ultimately, as the connection strengthens, the signal required to "send the message" is reduced (long-term potentiation).

Development of the Central Nervous System

Development is a series of progressive changes that results in elaboration of specialized cell types from a single cell. All types of somatic cells retain all of the genes that are present in the fertilized egg (nuclear equivalence). However, genetically identical cells differentiate over time under the influence of specific genes during development. Genes control development through transcription factors and growth factors (signals from neighboring cells). Transcription factors reside in the neuron cell body and directly facilitate protein transcription. The rare mental retardation syndrome called Rubstein–Taybi syndrome is due to a mutation that interferes with transcription factor activity resulting in dysmorphic features, skeletal abnormalities, and intellectual disability.

The growth factor brain-derived neurotrophic factor (BDNF) is essential for the growth of axons and dendrites. BDNF also plays a role in learning and memory. For many years, there was a commonly held belief that neurons were incapable of regeneration in the adult human brain. Under the influence of BDNF, however, it is clear that neurogenesis does occur in the mature brain, at least in the specialized cells of the dentate gyrus. Recent studies have shown that successful treatment of depression with antidepressant medications promotes neurogenesis in this region (Duman 2009).

Early Gestational Events in the Development of the Nervous System

There is rapid cell proliferation but little gene differentiation following fertilization. Within weeks, however, cells coalesce into the blastocyte to form three primary layers: the endoderm, mesoderm, and ectoderm. This critical stage of development is called gastrulation. Gastrulation involves migration of cells, which permits opportunities for one cell to influence the development of a neighboring cell. Soon after gastrulation, the growing ball of cells begins to fold and extend to form the neural tube. This eventually orients the brain anteriorly and the spinal cord posteriorly. The closure of the tube is subject to environmental impact. For example, folate deficiency in pregnancy increases the risk of spina bifida (De-Regil et al. 2015). By week 4 of gestation, the neural tube is separated into regions called the proencephalon

(forebrain), mesencephalon (midbrain), and rhomben-cephaplon (hindbrain) (Gilbert 2006). It is also known that maternal mental health problems can affect gestational events. For example, maternal depression is directly linked to low birth weight with a concomitant host of effects, i.e. respiratory depression (>90%), retinopathy of prematurity, patent ductus arterious (i.e. failure of this vessel to close possibly leading to heart failure), and others (Habecker and Freeman 2015).

This anterior to posterior scheme for the developing brain is under genetic control (Vaccarino and Leckman 2011). Neuronal migration peaks at gestational weeks 12 and 20 and is largely completed by gestational weeks 26–29 (Tau and Peterson 2010). Newborn neurons migrate to their destination (radial migration) and then initiate dendrite formation (morphogenesis). The switch from migration to morphogenesis is mutually exclusive and highly regulated (Prigge and Kay 2018). As axons continue to grow and synapses are formed, more complex neuronal circuits emerge. Apoptosis, defined as programmed cell death, helps to regulate brain development and specialization.

Brain Development and Synaptogenesis

Total brain volume increases throughout the first years of life and then stabilizes. By the age of 6, the total size of the brain is about 90% of its adult size. Growth in gray matter volume is rapid in early childhood followed by a decline in adolescence (Ostby et al. 2009). This expansion of gray matter in the first few years of life is coincident with intensive axonal growth and dendritic arborization followed by postpubertal loss. By contrast, white matter volume increase follows a more linear path (Tamnes et al. 2010). By late adolescence/early adulthood myelination of the frontal association tracts are complete. White matter organization and refinement, however, continues into adulthood and is influenced by interactions with the environment, paralleling increased cognitive abilities (Sousa et al. 2018). The volume of white matter usually increases with age until the fifth decade of life, with peak around the mid-40s (Gogtay and Thompson 2010).

Synaptogenesis, or formation of synaptic connections in the human cortex, begins in utero and continues during the first two postnatal years. Peak synaptic density is reached at different times throughout the cortex. For example, the PFC achieves maximum density at about 15 months of age; primary sensory areas achieve maximum density at an even younger age (Huttenlocher and Dabholkar 1997). After peaking in the first few postnatal years, synaptic density stabilizes and then starts to decline around 7 years of age. Synaptic density reaches adult levels in the auditory cortex by 12 years and the PFC by mid-adolescence (Tau and Peterson 2010). Early synaptogenesis appears to be intrinsically regulated (controlled by the cell itself). By contrast, the formation of new synapses that occurs later in life is related to learning and memory (Huttenlocher and Dabholkar 1997). In total, it is thought that in the human brain there are over 100 trillion synapses (Nestler et al. 2015).

Development of Neural Circuits: Age-Related Maturation

Brain networks develop from infancy through adulthood and support the brain's evolving capacity for high-level cognition (Menon 2013). Understanding how the millions of synapses in the brain integrate is a central research focus. The Human Connectome Project is a multi-institutional research program launched by the National Institute of Health (NIH) in 2010 to study structural and functional brain connectivity (Sporns 2012). Fundamental brain organization is not static and is refined through development. In infancy connections are shorter and more local, and these dense hubs are located primarily in the primary sensory and motor brain region. As the child develops, connectivity rapidly increases within and across modules (Cao et al. 2017). From middle childhood to adulthood, short-range connections are weakened and long-range connections are strengthened. White matter tracts undergo a prolonged maturation coinciding with local synapse pruning in the gray matter. Three prominent networks that are reconfigured with development are the central executive network (CEN), the salience network (SN), and the default mode network (DMN).

The CEN is activated in tasks that require sustained attention and mental control, utilizing working memory while the SN is activated in orienting attention to salient information and goal-oriented behaviors (Menon 2013). The DMN is defined as the resting state, but it is a metabolically active state with vigorous brain activity. It is activated during undirected times, and consists of daydreaming, thinking about the future and past, and often concerns autobiographical content (Buckner et al. 2008). These three networks work simultaneously during executive tasks, social tasks, and cognitive control task. As the child matures into adulthood, integration of these circuits matures, leading to more advanced cognitive and socio-emotional functioning. By adulthood, engagement of the CEN is generally inversely related to activation of the DMN. Disruption in the development of these networks can be driven by genetic or environmental influences and is associated with neurodevelopmental disorders (Menon 2013; Dégeilh et al. 2018).

Neurotransmission

In the previous sections we examined the gross anatomy of the brain, the architecture of the neuron, and the capacity of the neuron to receive and transmit information. At the center of neurotransmission is the synapse (Shepherd 2004). It is fitting to describe brain connections as circuits that are dedicated to particular brain activities. Although the image of circuitry conjures up a notion of electrical connections, the circuitry of the brain is both electrical and neurochemical. Unlike wiring in a house or in electronic devices, the pathways in the brain do not have "wire-to-wire connection." Indeed, the final transmission of the signal is through a neurochemical. There are several neurochemicals in the brain. In this section, we review the neurotransmitters that are most common to illustrate general principles of neurotransmission and to provide brain–behavior connection. The selected neurotransmitters for this review include dopamine, norepinephrine, serotonin, acetylcholine, gamma-aminobutyric acid (GABA), and glutamate.

Signal Transduction

Before considering these specific neurotransmitter systems, we examine how neurotransmitters carry out their functions. The sequence can be remembered by the mnemonic abbreviation DNA: dentrites > nucleus (cell body) > axon (Kowalski et al. 2019). In this simplified model, the dendrite responds to a neurochemical messenger which, in turn, sends a signal to the cell body from whence "instructions" are sent down the axon for neurotransmitter release. Put more succinctly, neurotransmission begins with the firing of the neuron (e.g. the dopamine firing neurons of the substantia nigra). This causes the stimulus to travel down the axon and release the neurotransmitter at the terminal nerve ending into the synapse. Once released, the neurotransmitter binds to postsynaptic receptors. Binding of the neurotransmitter to the postsynaptic receptor is often the first of many events. For example, binding may promote the passage of ions across the membrane of the postsynaptic receptor, resulting in depolarization and an action potential. Thus, the first, simplest classification of receptors is presynaptic and postsynaptic (Rudy 2008; Heckers et al. 2011) (Figure 3.3).

There are several other systems that need to be considered in this simplified model. For example, once a neurotransmitter is released into the synaptic space, there must be various systems to return that synapse back to its resting state. This is accomplished by several actions. Perhaps the most active method is through reuptake of the released transmitter by the transporter. The transporter resides on the presynaptic nerve end-

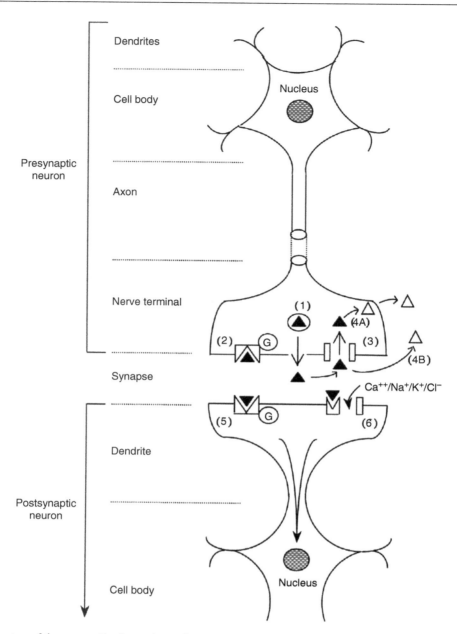

Figure 3.3 Basic structure of the neuron. The figure shows the presynaptic and postsynaptic junction (synapse). The solid triangles illustrate neurotransmitter release from the presynaptic neuron (1), binding at the postsynaptic neuron (5, 6), autoreceptor (2), and reuptake transporter (3); open triangles depict enzymatic degradation (4). The figure also shows the movement of ions into the postsynaptic nerve ending (6) and metabotropic or G-coupled receptor binding (5) (see text for details). (*Source:* From Heckers, S., Konradi, C., & Anderson, G.M. Synaptic function and biochemical neuroanatomy. In A. Martin, L. Scahill, & C.J. Kratochvil (Eds.) Pediatric psychopharmacology: Principles and practice (2nd edition; pp. 23–37). © 2011, Oxford University Press. with permission from Oxford University Press.)

ing and, through active transport, recovers the released neurotransmitter and pulls it back into the presynaptic nerve ending.

Other important regulatory receptors include autoreceptors and enzymatic breakdown. Autoreceptors, typically but not always, serve to inhibit neurotransmitter release in the synapse (Katzung and Trevor 2015). They take readings of the amount of a specific neurotransmitter and send a signal to the cell body whether or not more or less are needed. Clonidine is a good example. As an alpha-2 (autoreceptor) agonist, it tells the neuron that there is enough norepinephrine, thus causing a decline in the release of that monoamine. Clonidine then actually "tricks" the autoreceptor and this is its "secret" for lowering blood pressure.

A familiar example of enzymatic breakdown is monoamine oxidase (MAO), which inactivates dopamine, norepinephrine, and serotonin. MAO resides in the synaptic cleft and in greater amounts inside the presynaptic nerve ending. Many neurotransmitters in the presynaptic nerve ending reside in vesicles, which protect the neurotransmitter from degrading enzymes such as MAO. In addition, they are an effective way to control the amount of released neurotransmitter. When the signal moves down the axon to the terminal end, it causes the vesicle to migrate to the surface of the presynaptic nerve ending and releases its contents into the synapse. Therefore, we expand our simple receptor type 2 postsynaptic and presynaptic to include the transporter and the autoreceptor (Cooper et al. 2003).

Another way to classify receptor subtypes includes ionotropic and metabotropic receptors. Ionotropic, also called ligand gated, receptors are marked by their capacity to mediate rapid effects (several milliseconds) when activated by a neurotransmitter. By far the majority of synapses in the brain utilize ionotropic receptors (Nestler et al. 2015). The ionotropic receptors are directly linked to an ion channel. Ion channels are actual pores that allow specific ions to move across the membrane of the postsynaptic receptor. In the resting state, the intracellular environment is enriched with potassium and the extracellular environment is enriched with sodium. When there is a movement of sodium ions from outside the cell to inside the cell, there is a change in electrical potential. In this example, the change in electric potential is called depolarization (the voltage difference across the cell membrane is less negative compared to the resting state). The general structure is composed of four or five subunits, or leaves. When there is binding to the receptor, there is a conformational change in the receptor, which allows the movement of ions across the membrane. These ions' channels are specific. The biological effects depend on whether the ion is positive or negative. The movement of sodium ions into the intercellular fluid causes depolarization. Hyperpolarization occurs when there is a movement of negative ions into the cell (e.g. chloride ions), which makes the voltage difference between the external environment and the internal environment more negative. Hyperpolarization inhibits signal transduction (Cooper et al. 2003). Benzodiazepines are good examples of drugs that hyperpolarize a neuron by facilitating the movement of chloride into the cell.

The other, and much larger, brain receptor family is the metabotropic type. In contrast to ionotropic receptors, the metabotropic receptors exert biological activity on a slower time course (seconds to minutes). The metabotropic receptors are also called G-coupled protein receptors, reflecting their general structure. The metabotropic receptors have several features in common as well as differences. As with the ionotropic receptors, metabotropic receptors have an extracellular and intracellular terminal. The structure of the internal terminal is complex and composed of so-called alpha, beta, and gamma subunits at rest. These subunits are bound inside the cell membrane and to each other. When there is binding at the receptor, the alpha unit separates away from its companion beta and gamma subunits and begins one or more specific intracellular events. For example, it may initiate the opening of an ion channel as described above with ionotropic receptors. By contrast, the alpha subunit may bind to specific proteins inside the cell and begin a cascade of intracellular activities resulting in turning on a gene for protein synthesis (Cooper et al. 2003).

Neurotransmitters

Dopamine

Tryosine ⊛, Dopa ⊛, Dopamine

The primary neurons that produce dopamine firings are the substantia nigra and ventral tegmental area. The projections on the substantia nigra are central to the motor system, sending projections to the striatum (caudate and putamen). The projections of the ventral tegmental area go to the ventral striatum (nucleus accumbens) and cortical regions. When these dopamine neurons fire, they cause the signal to move along specific axonal pathways organized to carry out specific functions. When the signal makes its way to the terminal end, dopamine is released. As shown in Table 3.3, all dopamine receptors are metabotropic.

Dopamine is central to many functions in the brain, yet of the 100 billion neurons in the brain, only 500 000 produce dopamine (Keltner and Keltner 2019). Perhaps most familiar is its role in movement. The loss of dopamine-firing neurons in the substantia nigra over time is directly related to the onset and course of Parkinson disease. The nigrostrial (*Sambucus nigra* to striatum) pathway plays a central role in the coordination of movement. Other dopaminergic pathways have their origin in the neighboring nuclei of the ventral tegmental area (Green and Ostrander 2009).

There are two main families of dopamine receptors, called D1 type and D2 type. Over time it has been discovered that the D1 type includes D1 and D5 receptor types, and D2 includes D2, D3, and D4 receptors. It is not surprising, given the multiple actions of dopamine in the brain, that these dopamine receptor subtypes are located in specific areas of the brain. For example, D1 and D2 receptors are distributed liberally in the striatum,

Table 3.3 Major families of receptors in the central nervous system

Transmitter	Ionotropic	Metabotropic (or G-coupled)
Dopamine		DA1–5
Norepinephrine		Alpha-1, -2,
		Beta-1, -2, -3
Serotonin	5-HT3	5-HT1, -2, -4, -5, -6, -7
Acetylcholine	Nicotinic	Muscarinic
Glutamate	AMPA, NMDA	mGluR1–5
Gamma-aminobutyric acid	GABAA	GABAB

AMPA, α-amino-3-hydroxy-5-methyl-4-isoxazolepropionic acid; DA1–5, dopamine receptor; GABAA, metabotropic gamma-aminobutyric acid (GABA) type A; GABAB, metabotropic gamma-aminobutyric acid (GABA) type B; 5-HT1, 5-HT3, hydroxytryptamine receptors or serotonin receptors; NMDA, *n*-methyl-D,D-aspartate.

but few are found in the cortex. By contrast, D4 receptors are more commonly found in the cortex.

Alterations in dopamine transmission have been implicated in several major psychiatric disorders, including schizophrenia, substance abuse, and attention deficit hyperactivity disorder (ADHD), and neuropsychiatric conditions such as Tourette syndrome, Parkinson disease, and Huntington chorea. The role of dopamine in these disorders varies by disorder. For example, symptoms of Parkinson disease begin when there is a 70% reduction in dopamine-firing neurons in the substantia nigra (Jankovic and Tolosa 2007). Similarly, the well-known Parkinsonian adverse effects in patients treated with potent D2 blockers such as haloperidol are due to the blockade of D2 receptors in the striatum. In the case of antipsychotic medications, the substantia nigra may be firing, but dopamine is not allowed to bind with these receptors, resulting in a picture that mimics Parkinson disease (Procyshyn et al. 2015).

The evidence of the role of dopamine in schizophrenia emerged primarily from the observation that potent D2 blockers reduce positive symptoms of schizophrenia such as hallucinations and delusions. In addition, repeated use of dopamine-enhancing agents such as amphetamine can mimic the positive symptoms of schizophrenia. As will be discussed later, however, the dopamine hypothesis of schizophrenia does not sufficiently account for the negative symptoms (poverty of thought, low motivation, etc.) of schizophrenia. At the

risk of oversimplification, the negative symptoms of schizophrenia appear to be due to abnormality in the mesocortical circuit and the positive symptoms due to abnormality in the mesolimbic circuit (Khan et al. 2017).

The support for the role of dopamine in drug addiction is emerging as a complex interaction between dopamine and other neurotransmitter systems, especially glutamate. Dopamine is known to play a central role in the reward circuit (the mesolimbic circuit mentioned earlier). Not surprisingly, many drugs of abuse cause a release of dopamine and stimulate the reward circuit. Over the past decade, mounting evidence from animal and human studies indicates that glutamatergic input from the cortex to the striatum appears to play a role in craving and the actual drug-seeking behavior (Kalivas 2009).

The evidence of the supporting role of dopamine in ADHD is substantial. The positive effects of stimulant drugs, which enhance dopamine function in the brain, provide indirect evidence that dopamine plays a role in ADHD. Of particular interest is the dorsolateral prefrontal circuit, which is known to play an important role in the executive functions of attention and planning (Arnsten 2009). Data from more than one MRI study have shown a slight but significant decrease in cortical volume for children with ADHD (Castellanos and Proal 2009). fMRI studies also show reduced activity in the prefrontal region during the performance of neuropsychological tasks of attention and impulse control in children with ADHD compared to controls (Pliszka et al. 2006).

Given the effectiveness of methylphenidate in treating ADHD (MTA Cooperative Group 1999) and the strong evidence supporting the role of dopamine in attention and impulse control, there has been interest in various dopamine genes as candidate genes that could underlie ADHD (Banaschewski et al. 2010). For example, much interest has been focused on the dopamine transporter gene (*DAT1* gene). The action of this gene may influence the efficiency of the dopamine transporter in clearing out dopamine to the synapse. This possibility is supported by the pharmacological action of methylphenidate, which blocks reuptake of dopamine at the transporter. Another gene of interest is the dopamine D4 receptor (*DRD4*) gene. This receptor resides in the cortex and quite likely plays a role in attention and impulse control. Several genetic association studies have shown that individuals with ADHD are more likely to have a particular variant of the gene (Li et al. 2006). However, both genetic and environmental factors play a role in the development of psychiatric disorders, and a monogenetic etiology has not been supported (Ptácek et al. 2011).

In many ways, the term "inattention" is somewhat ambiguous. Presumably it refers to the inability to pay attention. However, discussion with many parents of children with ADHD often results in comments such as, "He can spend hours on playing video games, but can't pay attention in school." This common observation suggests that there is something fundamentally different about the attention required for highly stimulating video games versus the attention required to listen in the classroom or read a book. This difference has been described as bottom-up versus top-down attention. In bottom-up attention, the bright lights and catchy sound effects of video games engage parietal and temporal cortices, which do not require great mental effort. By contrast, a teacher's lecture requires top-down attention and engagement of the PFC (Arnsten 2009). In this model, children with ADHD have difficulty engaging the PFC to select and maintain focus on tasks requiring mental effort (e.g. a teacher's lecture).

Mason and Joshi (2018) have suggestions for dealing with these physiological realities in the classroom:

1. Use clear and concise instruction with visual supplements.
2. Look directly at the student and call by name.
3. Have the student repeat the instructions.
4. Seat the student near the front of the class, close to the teacher.

They find these nonpharmacologic strategies to be helpful bolsters to medications that may be prescribed.

The right inferior PFC is specialized for behavioral inhibition. Impaired functioning in this region presumably contributes to impulsiveness and hyperactivity. The ventral medial PFC is specialized for emotional regulation. At the risk of oversimplification, it might be said that impaired prefrontal cortical function contributes to aggression, obsessional behavior, and perhaps even conduct disorder. The regulation of attention involves the inhibition of external stimuli other than the chosen stimuli, and inhibition of internal stimuli as well.

Norepinephrine

Tyrosine ⊕, Dopa ⊕, Dopamine ⊕, Norepinephrine

The above discussion on ADHD focused on the relevance of dopamine in ADHD. It should be noted, however, that norepinephrine also likely plays an important role in ADHD (Arnsten 2009). The effectiveness of

norepinephrine affecting medications such as guanfacine and atomoxetine further supports the notion that norepinephrine also influences ADHD symptoms (Arnsten 2009).

Norepinephrine-firing neurons are located in the locus coeruleus situated at the top of the brainstem. These neurons send signals to virtually all areas of the brain and are involved in basic physiological functions such as heart rate, blood pressure, breathing, and higher cortical functions (Arnsten 2009). Norepinephrine is known to play a central role in the so-called fight-or-flight reaction. The projections from the locus coeruleus go to the PFC, cingulate, amygdala, hypothalamus, and cerebellum. There are two major types of norepinephrine receptors: alpha-receptors and beta-receptors. Alpha-receptors are further subdivided into alpha-1 and alpha-2 subtypes, each of which also has subtypes. For example, the alpha-2A receptor plays a role in attention and impulse control and is implicated in the action of the medication guanfacine (Arnsten 2009). All norepinephrine receptors belong to the metabotropic family of receptors.

For both dopamine and norepinephrine, there appears to be a "just right" spot for neurotransmitter levels and PFC function. Low levels of norepinephrine are associated with inattention and impaired impulse control. Likewise, high levels of norepinephrine are also associated with decreased attention and decreased working memory. In the fight-or-flight reaction, there is a dramatic rise in the amount of norepinephrine released, which takes the PFC offline (Arnsten 2009).

Practically speaking, threatening situations are not moments for weighing options. Rather, these are times for action. Thus, it makes sense for the PFC to go offline. Given this model, it is clear that norepinephrine function is relevant to ADHD and anxiety disorders. In ADHD, it is possible that a failure to regulate norepinephrine levels in the PFC contributes to difficulties with attention, impulse control, and planning.

Recent evidence suggests that the alpha-2A agonist, guanfacine, stimulates these receptors in the prefrontal brain, which may improve prefrontal function (Arnsten 2009). An extended-release form of the drug is available for the treatment of ADHD in children (Faraone et al. 2013). The potential role of norepinephrine in anxiety disorders such as generalized anxiety, panic, and posttraumatic stress disorder (PTSD) is well accepted (Geracioti et al. 2001; Goddard et al. 2010). For example, perhaps due to genetic vulnerability, environmental exposure, or the interaction of genes and environment, the patient with anxiety disorder is too easily tripped into the fight-or-flight state, mediated by release of norepinephrine. Further support for the role of norepinephrine in anxiety disorders is the direct connection between the locus coeruleus and the amygdala. The amygdala plays an important role in fear and fear conditioning (Davis 1992). Norepinephrine is certainly not the only player in the complex network of circuitry involved in fear and anxiety. However, a reciprocal connection between the amygdala and the locus coeruleus fits with the fight-or-flight reaction.

The neuroscientist Joseph LeDoux has articulated two amygdala pathways that play a role in mammalian fear response (LeDoux 2000). LeDoux's model describes a low road (rapid response) and a high road (slower response). In this model, the sensory input goes to the anterior thalamus, which has a direct connection to the amygdala. The output of the amygdala goes to the hypothalamus and locus coeruleus. This causes direct and rapid physiological effects such as increased heart rate, blood pressure, and increased respiration. The slower mode (or the so-called high road) involves a connection from the thalamus to the cortex. In this mode, the sensory input to the anterior thalamus not only signals the amygdala as discussed previously, but also sends a signal to the cortex. This signal allows consideration of the current threat compared with past events to make an appraisal of threat. The cortex has input to the amygdala, which can then modulate the alarm signals from the amygdala. This is clearly relevant to cognitive behavior therapy, which promotes cortical appraisal of threat to modulate the automatic or rapid mode response.

This idea of perceived threat versus actual threat in generalized anxiety disorder (GAD) also may be relevant to obsessive–compulsive disorder (OCD) and even to some extent PTSD. For many patients with GAD, OCD, or PTSD, life is unpredictable and feels fundamentally unsafe (Woody and Rachman 1994). The perception of threat is high and perception of safety is low. This overestimation of risk gives rise to increased vigilance and avoidance. In the case of GAD, the focus is on worries of upcoming events and situations. In OCD, particular themes often are the focus of potential harm. For example, worries about contamination prompts washing rituals, or concerns about harm coming to the self or others gives rise to checking compulsions and avoidance. In PTSD, a past experience of trauma heightens the perception of threat and decreases the sense of safety.

The circuitry for fear conditioning has been informed greatly through preclinical studies on acoustic startle. Many mammalian species show a startle reaction to loud noises. The startle reaction has been shown to involve a simple three-synapse sequence that is at least partially mediated by norepinephrine (Davis 1986). The auditory nerve fibers signal the cochlea, which sends signals to a specialized area in the temporal lobe. From the temporal lobe, the signal travels directly to facial motor neurons (producing the startled expression) and spinal cord (e.g. arching of the back in the frightened cat) (Davis 1986). Startle can be highly influenced by context. For example, a car backfiring in midday on a busy street would likely induce a startle response for those nearby. The same loud noise at night on a deserted street would produce a larger response. This is called fear-potentiated startle.

Another relevant animal model demonstrates the role of learning in fear responses. In rodents, foot shock produces a characteristic freezing behavior. If a rodent is placed in an environment in which a flash of light (or horn blast) is paired with a foot shock, over time the light flash alone will induce freezing. If the experiment is continued such that the light flash is repeatedly delivered without the foot shock, the freezing behavior in response to the light flash alone will extinguish. Finally, if the light flash is once again paired with the foot shock, the freezing response to the light flash alone will occur after fewer repetitions than the original behavioral response (Rogan et al. 2005).

Serotonin

Tryptophan ⊛, L-tryptophan ⊛, 5-Hydroxytryptamine (Serotonin)

Serotonin (also called 5-hydroxytryptamine or 5-HT) is also a monoamine (like dopamine and norepinephrine). Unlike dopamine and norepinephrine, however, it is not a catecholamine. Serotonin-firing neurons are located in the raphe nucleus, which sits at the top of the brainstem. Examination of the serotonin circuitry shows that it has projection to every area of the brain. Not surprisingly then, it plays a role in several human functions including regulation of mood, emotions, anxiety, memory, aggression, body temperature, sleep, and appetite.

As with the dopamine and norepinephrine receptors, there are multiple types of serotonin receptors. Once again, the location of these receptors is deliberate so that specific serotonin receptor subtypes are dedicated to specific functions. Currently, there are seven major types of serotonin receptors and many of these 5-HT receptors have subtypes. All but one type (5-HT3 receptor) are metabotropic receptors.

A detailed description of these various subtypes and their location is beyond the scope of this discussion. For illustration, however, we note that the serotonin receptor, 5-HT2, resides in the cortex and hippocampus. This receptor subtype is relevant to the action of the atypical antipsychotic medications, which have an antagonist effect at these receptors. The 5-HT7 receptor is located in the thalamus, hippocampus, and amygdala. This receptor is presumed to play a role in fear conditioning and anxiety, as discussed above. Serotonin is believed to play an important role in OCD, depression, and other anxiety disorders. Evidence supporting a role of serotonin in these disorders emanates from the demonstrated effectiveness of the selective serotonin reuptake inhibitor (SSRI) medications in these disorders.

The introduction of the SSRIs revolutionized the treatment of depression, OCD, and other anxiety disorders. As suggested by the name, the SSRIs block reuptake at the serotonin transporter, thereby allowing serotonin to remain in the synapse longer. This pharmacological effect of the SSRIs is evident with the very first dose. However, the benefit of the SSRIs in depression, OCD, or other anxiety disorders in children is generally not evident for several weeks (Geller et al. 2003; Hammerness et al. 2006; Team 2007; Walkup et al. 2008). The explanation of this lag is not clear. The SSRIs have been proposed to be helpful in autism spectrum disorders. When tested in a large-scale, randomized trial, the SSRI citalopram was no better than a placebo in reducing repetitive behavior in children with autism spectrum disorders (King et al. 2009).

Acetylcholine

Acetylcholine is derived from choline and is not an amine. In addition to its role in the CNS, acetylcholine plays a central role in the PNS. There are two major classes of acetylcholine receptors, referred to as muscarinic (metabotropic) and nicotinic (ionotropic). This nomenclature is based on their preferential binding to muscarine (poison in mushrooms) or nicotine. There are five identified subtypes of muscarinic receptors: M1 (nerves), M2 (heart, smooth muscle), M3 (glands), M4 (CNS), and M5 (CNS) (Pappano 2015). There are only two major subtypes of nicotinic receptors: N_M (muscle) and N_N (neuronal type) (Pappano 2015). The organization of the acetylcholine circuitry in the brain is somewhat different from those previously discussed. The primary source of acetylcholine firing is the basal nucleus, which is in the forebrain. It has connections to the PFC and parietal cortex. There are also acetylcholine-firing neurons in the brainstem that project to the thalamus and hypothalamus. Finally, there are specialized interneurons in the striatum that appear to play an important role in regulating movement. Acetylcholine pathways have attracted great interest due to their potential role in Alzheimer's disease (Hardy 2009; Hernandez et al. 2010).

GABA and Glutamate

The two most common neurotransmitters in the CNS are the amino acids glutamate and GABA. Glutamate is the major excitatory neurotransmitter and GABA is a major inhibitory transmitter in the CNS (Gray and Nicoll 2015). Glutamate is synthesized from glucose and GABA is synthesized from glutamate. Glutamate is presumed to play an important role in several disorders, including drug addiction, Tourette syndrome, schizophrenia, and the mental retardation syndrome fragile X (Dolen and Bear 2008; -Dargham et al. 2009; Kalivas 2009; Lombroso et al. 2009). In drug addiction, glutamatergic excitatory signals from the cortex to striatum appear to play a role in craving and drug-taking behavior (Kalivas 2009). Similarly, in Tourette syndrome, signals from the cortex to a different region of striatum may play a role in the dysregulation of the motor circuit and give rise to tic behaviors.

Ionotropic glutamate receptors include NMDA and AMPA receptor types. The NMDA (N-methyl-D-aspartate) receptor is widely distributed in the brain, especially in the cortex and hippocampus, and plays an important role in learning and memory (Berger-Sweeney et al. 2009). Its molecular structure is complicated with multiple binding sites for glutamate as well as drugs such as phencyclidine (PCP) and ketamine. When stimulated, positive sodium and calcium ions move across the cell membrane, resulting in an excitatory effect. When an impulse travels down the axon and causes a release of glutamate, a series of steps follows that involves the movement of first sodium ions and then calcium ions into the cell. The passage of calcium into the postsynaptic cell produces a large action potential which tends to strengthen the connection between the presynaptic and postsynaptic neurons (Cooper et al. 2003). This enhanced connection is now more ready to respond to subsequent stimulation, even signals of lower magnitude.

The potential role of glutamate in psychiatric disorders can be reviewed by examining the role of glutamate in schizophrenia and fragile X. The role of glutamate in schizophrenia is an exciting and still emerging story. First, the compound PCP is an antagonist of the glutamate NMDA receptor. This drug induces both the positive and negative symptoms of schizophrenia. In contrast, as noted above, dopaminergic compounds, such as high doses of amphetamine, mimic the positive but not the negative symptoms of schizophrenia. PCP has now been recognized to promote dopamine release in the mesolimbic circuit (positive symptoms) and decrease dopaminergic tone in the PFC (negative symptoms). These observations suggest an interaction between dopamine and glutamate (Seeman 2009).

Evidence from cerebrospinal fluid studies indicates a decreased amount of glutamate in schizophrenia compared to control subjects. Postmortem studies have also shown decreased glutamate concentration in the PFC and hippocampus in schizophrenia versus controls. Preclinical studies show that NMDA-deficient mice exhibit hyperactivity, stereotypic behavior, and social isolation. These transgenic mice show improvement in hyperactivity and stereotypic behaviors with haloperidol, and show improvement in social isolations when treated with clozapine. These observations have also raised questions about the potential relevance of glutamate in the neurobiology of autism.

The potential role of glutamate in schizophrenia has prompted interest in the development of a glutamate agonist to treat schizophrenia. In a study of 193 adults with schizophrenia, Patil et al. (2007) reported that a novel glutamate agonist was superior to a placebo in reducing both positive and negative symptoms. The positive results of this compound were similar in magnitude to the group that was randomly assigned to olanzapine. These results, although preliminary, show promise that manipulation of the glutamate system could be a useful treatment for schizophrenia. Noting the dynamic interaction of glutamate and dopamine, however, Seeman (2009) proposes dopamine blocking effects (the mechanism of currently available antipsychotics) may also play a role in these observed benefits.

The metabotropic glutamate receptors (mGluRs) include five subtypes (Cooper et al. 2003). Little was known about these mGluRs until the early 1990s. It is now clear that some of these mGluRs play key roles in learning and memory. This is illustrated by recent findings in fragile X syndrome, an inherited syndrome characterized by intellectual deficits caused by a mutation in the X chromosome in which a specific series of DNA nucleotides is expanded in number. This expansion results in a failure to produce the FMR1 protein. FMR1 appears to play a regulatory role in the maturation of dendritic spines (Dolen and Bear 2008). As noted above, the maturation of dendritic spines is essential for learning and memory. Recent work by Dolen and Bear has shown that antagonists to mGluRs remediate deficits in fragile X knockout mice from several of the markers of fragile X syndrome in these animals. These mGluR antagonists are being studied in humans and are an area of great interest (Scharf et al. 2015).

Conclusions and Implications for Primary Care and Mental Health Nursing Practices

The burgeoning of information on neurobiology is extraordinary and will have an increasing impact on nursing practice in the next decade. In the discourse of primary care practice, we can expect to hear discussion about brain circuitry and the mechanisms of action for psychotropic medications. Primary care providers and

mental health clinicians who prescribe medication have an ethical imperative to expand their knowledge about brain function and behavior to practice effectively in this rapidly changing landscape.

The concept of a brain "connectome" (Sporns 2012) and NIH's RDoC (Insel et al. 2010) underscores the move toward understanding psychiatric disorders within a systems perspective, conceptualizing mental illness as a brain disorder. This perspective has a primary focus on neural circuitry, which develops in utero through adulthood (Menon 2013; Cao et al. 2017). Studies have shown that neural circuit development can be impacted by a wide range of factors, both genetic and environmental, which in turn influence behavior. These factors are diverse, and are targets for nursing research and psychosocial treatments. For example, exposure to domestic violence in childhood (Choi et al. 2012) or insulin resistance in adolescence (Nouwen et al. 2017) are associated with decrease white matter tract integrity measured by DTI. To meet the challenges of the coming decade, primary care providers and mental health clinicians in child and adolescent psychiatry have a responsibility to become conversant with clinical neurobiology. This chapter offers an introduction and an invitation for interested readers to learn more.

Thought Questions

1. How much knowledge of neurobiology is necessary for APRNs to safely prescribe psychiatric medication?
2. What are the resources essential for an understanding of neurobiology?
3. How much information about the biologic effects of the psychiatric medications they prescribe should APRNs share and explain to individuals to whom they are prescribing?
4. What information about the individual will influence the level of explanation?

References

Abi-Dargham, A., van de Giessen, E., Slifstein, M. et al. (2009). Baseline and amphetamine-stimulated dopamine activity are related in drug-naïve schizophrenic subjects. *Biological Psychiatry* 65 (12): 1091–1093. https://doi.org/10.1016/j.biopsych.2008.12.007.

Absinta, M., Ha, S.-K., Nair, G. et al. (2017). Human and nonhuman primate meninges harbor lymphatic vessels that can be visualized noninvasively by MRI. *eLife* 6: e29738. https://doi.org/10.7554/eLife.29738.

Alexander, G.E., DeLong, M.R., and Strick, P.L. (1986). Functionally segregated circuits linking basal ganglia and cortex. *Annual Review of Neuroscience* 9: 357–381. https://doi.org/10.1146/annurev.ne.09.030186.002041.

Alfaro, F.J., Gavrieli, A., Saade-Lemus, P. et al. (2018). White matter microstructure and cognitive decline in metabolic syndrome: a review of diffusion tensor imaging. *Metabolism* 78: 52–68. https://doi.org/10.1016/j.metabol.2017.08.009.

Arnsten, A. (2009). Toward a new understanding of attention-deficit hyperactivity disorder pathophysiology: an important role for prefrontal cortex dysfunction. *CNS Drugs* 23 (1): 33–41.

Arnsten, A. and Castellanos, F.X. (2011). Neurobiology of attention regulation and its disorders. In: *Pediatric Psychopharmacology: Principles and Practice*, 2e (eds. A. Martin, L. Scahill and C.J. Kratochvil), 95–111. New York: Oxford University Press.

Banaschewski, T., Becker, K., Scherag, S. et al. (2010). Molecular genetics of attention-deficit/hyperactivity disorder: an overview. *European Child & Adolescent Psychiatry* 19 (3): 237–257.

Barres, B. (2008). The mystery and magic of glia: a perspective on their roles in health and disease. *Neuron* 60: 430–440.

Berger-Sweeney, J., Schaevitz, L., and Frick, K. (2009). Neurochemical systems involved in learning and memory. In: *Neurobiology of Mental Illness*, 3e (eds. D. Charney and E. Nestler), 927–935. New York: Oxford University Press.

Bliss, T.V.P. and Lomo, T. (1973). Long-lasting potentiation of synaptic transmission in the dentate area of the anaesthetized rabbit following stimulation of the perforant path. *Journal of Physiology* 232: 331–356.

Blumenfeld, H. (2002). *Neuroanatomy through Clinical Cases*. Sunderland, MA: Sinauer Associates.

Borden, N. (2007). *3D Angiographic Atlas of Neurovascular Anatomy and Pathology*. New York: Cambridge University Press.

Buckner, R.L., Andrews-Hanna, J.R., and Schacter, D.L. (2008). The brain's default network. *Annals of the New York Academy of Sciences* 1124: 1–38.

Cao, M., Huang, H., and He, Y. (2017). Developmental connectomics from infancy through early childhood. *Trends in Neurosciences* 40 (8): 494–505.

Carpenter, W.T. (2016). The RDoC controversy: alternate paradigm or dominant paradigm? *American Journal of Psychiatry* 173 (6): 562–563.

Castellanos, F.X. and Proal, E. (2009). Location, location, and thickness: volumetric neuroimaging of attention-deficit/hyperactivity disorder comes of age. *Journal of the American Academy of Child and Adolescent Psychiatry* 48 (10): 979–981.

Chaudhuri, A., Duan, F., Morsey, B. et al. (2008). HIV-1 activates pro-inflammatory and interferon-inducible genes in human brain microvascular endothelial cells: putative mechanisms of blood-brain barrier dysfunction. *Journal of Cerebral Blood Flow & Metabolism* 28: 697–711.

Chen, J.L. and Nedivi, E. (2010). Neuronal structural remodeling: is it all about access? *Current Opinions Neurobiology* 20 (5): 557–562.

Choi, J., Jeong, B., Polcari, A. et al. (2012). Reduced fractional anisotropy in the visual limbic pathway of young adults witnessing domestic violence in childhood. *Neuroimage* 59: 1071–1079. https://doi.org/10.1016/j.neuroimage.1022.09.033.

Cieri, F. and Esposito, R. (2018). Neuroaging through the lens of the resting state networks. *BioMed Research International*: 5080981. https://doi.org/10.1155/2018/508098.

Cooper, J., Bloom, F., and Roth, R. (2003). *The Biochemical Basis of Neuropharmacology*, 8e. New York: Oxford University Press.

Davis, M. (1986). Pharmacological and anatomical analysis of fear conditioning using the fear-potentiated startle paradigm. *Behavioral Neuroscience* 100 (6): 814–824.

Davis, M. (1992). The role of the amydala in fear and anxiety. *Annual Review in Neuroscience* 15: 353–375.

Deeken, J. and Loscher, W. (2007). The blood-brain barrier and cancer: transporters, treatment, and Trojan horses. *Clinical Cancer Research* 13 (6): 1663–1674.

Dégeilh, F., Bernier, A., Leblanc, É. et al. (2018). Quality of maternal behaviour during infancy predicts functional connectivity between default mode network and salience network 9 years later. *Developmental Cognitive Neuroscience* 34: 53–62.

De-Regil, L.M., Peña-Rosas, J.P., Fernández-Gaxiola, A.C., and Rayco-Solon, P. (2015). Effects and safety of periconceptional oral folate supplementation for preventing birth defects. *Cochrane Database of Systematic Reviews* (12): CD007950. Available at https://doi.org/10.10.1002/14651858.CD007950.pub3.

Dolen, G. and Bear, M. (2008). Role for metabotropic glutamate receptor 5 (mGluR5) in the pathogenesis of fragile X syndrome. *Journal of Physiology* 586: 1503–1508.

Dotevall, L., Hagberg, L., Karlsson, J., and Rosengren, L. (1999). Astroglial and neuronal in cerebrospinal fluid as markers of CNS involvement in Lyme neuroborreliosis. *European Journal of Neurology* 6 (2): 169–178.

Duman, R. (2009). Neurochemical theories of depression: preclinical studies. In: *Neurobiology of Mental Illness*, 3e (eds. D. Charney and E. Nestler), 413–434. New York: Oxford University Press.

Faraone, S.V., McBurnett, K., Sallee, F.R. et al. (2013). Guanfacine extended release: a novel treatment for attention-deficit/hyperactivity disorder in children and adolescents. *Clinical Therapeutics* 35 (11): 1778–1793.

Gaudio, S., Quattrocchi, C.C., Piervincenzi, C. et al. (2017). White matter abnormalities in treatment-naive adolescents at the earliest stages of anorexia nervosa: a diffusion tensor imaging study. *Psychiatry Research: Neuroimaging* 266: 138–145.

Geller, D., Biederman, J., Stewart, S. et al. (2003). Which SSRI? A meta-analysis of pharmacotherapy trials in pediatric obsessive-compulsive disorder. *American Journal of Psychiatry* 160: 1919–1928.

Geracioti, T., Baker, D., Ekhator, N. et al. (2001). CSF norepinephrine concentrations in posttraumatic stress disorder. *American Journal of Psychiatry* 158: 1227–1230.

Gilbert, S. (2006). *Developmental Biology*, 8e. Sunderland, MA: Sinauer Associates.

Gitai, Z., Yu, T., Lundquist, E. et al. (2003). The netrin receptor UNC-40/DCC stimulates axon attraction and outgrowth through enabled and, in parallel, Rac and UNC-115/AbLIM. *Neuron* 37: 53–65.

Glasser, M.F., Coalson, T.S., Robinson, E.C. et al. (2016). A multimodal parcellation of human cerebral cortex. *Nature* 536 (7615): 171–178.

Goddard, A., Ball, S., Martinez, J. et al. (2010). Current perspectives of the roles of the central norepinephrine system in anxiety and depression. *Depression and Anxiety* 27: 339–350.

Gogtay, N. and Thompson, P.M. (2010). Mapping gray matter development: implications for typical development and vulnerability to psychopathology. *Brain and Cognition* 72 (1): 6–15.

Gray, J.A. and Nicoll, R.A. (2015). Introduction to the pharmacology of CNS drugs. In: *Basic and Clinical Pharmacology* (eds. B.G. Katzung and A.J. Trevor), 355–368. New York: McGraw Hill Lange.

Green, R. and Ostrander, R. (2009). *Neuroanatomy for Students of Behavioral Disorders*. New York: W.W. Norton & Company.

Habecker, E. and Freeman, M.P. (2015). Awareness and management of obstetrical complications of depression. *Current Psychiatry* 14 (12): 39–44.

Halassa, M., Fellin, T., and Haydon, P. (2006). The tripartite synapse: roles for gliotransmission in health and disease. *Trends in Molecular Medicine* 13 (2): 54–63.

Hammerness, P., Vivas, F., and Geller, D. (2006). Selective serotonin reuptake inhibitors in pediatric psychopharmacology: a review of the evidence. *Journal of Pediatrics* 148 (2): 158–165.

Hardy, J.A. (2009). The genetics and pathogenesis of Alzheimer's disease and related dementia. In: *Neurobiology of Mental Illness*, 3e (eds. D. Charney and E. Nestler), 883–895. New York: Oxford University Press.

Haydon, P. and Carmignoto, G. (2006). Astrocyte control of synaptic transmission and neurovascular coupling. *Physiological Reviews* 86: 1009–1031.

Heckers, S., Konradi, C., and Anderson, G.M. (2011). Synaptic function and biochemical neuroanatomy. In: *Pediatric Psychopharmacology: Principles and Practice*, 2e (eds. A. Martin, L. Scahill and C.J. Kratochvil), 23–37. New York: Oxford University Press.

Hendelman, W. (2006). *Atlas of Functional Neuroanatomy*. New York: Taylor and Francis.

Hernandez, C., Kayed, R., Zheng, H. et al. (2010). Loss of α7 nicotinic receptors enhances β-amyloid oligomer accumulation, exacerbating early-stage cognitive decline and septohippocampal pathology in a mouse model of Alzheimer's disease. *Journal of Neuroscience* 30 (7): 2442–2453.

Hickey, W. (2001). Basic principles of immunological surveillance of the normal central nervous system. *Glia* 36: 118–124.

Huttenlocher, P. and Dabholkar, A. (1997). Regional differences in synaptogenesis in human cerebral cortex. *Journal of Comparative Neurology* 387: 167–178.

Insel, T. and Cuthbert, B. (2015). Brain disorders? Precisely. *Science* 328 (6234): 499–500. https://doi.org/10.1126/science.aab2358.

Insel, T., Cuthbert, B., Garvey, M. et al. (2010). Research domain criteria (RDoC): toward a new classification framework for research on mental disorders. *American Journal of Psychiatry* 167 (7): 748–751. https://doi.org/10.1176/appi.ajp.2010.09091379.

Jankovic, J. and Tolosa, E. (2007). *Parkinson's Disease & Movement Disorders*, 5e. Philadelphia: Lippincott Williams & Wilkins.

Johns, P. (2014). *Clinical Neuroscience*. Edinburgh: Churchill Livingstone.

Kalivas, P. (2009). The glutamate homeostasis hypothesis of addiction. *Nature Reviews Neuroscience* 10: 561–572.

Katzung, B.G. and Trevor, A.J. (2015). *Basic and Clinical Pharmacology*. New York: McGraw Hill Lange.

Keltner, N.L. and Keltner, J.G. (2019). Antiparkinsonian drugs. In: *Psychiatric Nursing* (eds. N.L. Keltner and D. Steele), 128–135. St. Louis: Elsevier.

Keltner, N.L. and Kowalski, P.C. (2019). Introduction to psychotropic drugs. In: *Psychiatric Nursing* (eds. N.L. Keltner and D. Steele), 115–127. St. Louis: Elsevier.

Keltner, N.L. and Steele, D. (2019). *Psychiatric Nursing*. St. Louis: Elsevier.

Khan, A.Y., Kalia, R., Ide, G.D., and Ghavami, M. (2017). Residual symptoms of schizophrenia: what are realistic treatment goals? *Current Psychiatry* 16 (3): 35.

King, B., Hollander, E., Sikich, L. et al. (2009). Lack of efficacy of citalopram in children with autism spectrum disorders and high level of repetitive behaviors. *Archives of General Psychiatry* 66 (6): 583–590.

Kowalski, P.C., Dowben, J.S., and Sugerman, R.A. (2019). Psychobiologic bases of behavior. In: *Psychiatric Nursing* (eds. N.L. Keltner and D. Steele), 33–49. St. Louis: Elsevier.

LeDoux, J. (2000). Emotion circuits in the brain. *Annual Review in Neuroscience* 23: 155–184.

Li, D., Sham, P.C., Owen, M.J., and He, L. (2006). Meta-analysis shows significant association between dopamine system genes and attention deficit hyperactivity disorder (ADHD). *Human Molecular Genetics* 15: 2276–2284.

Lombroso, P., Bloch, M., and Leckman, J. (2009). Tourette's syndrome and tic-related disorders in children. In: *Neurobiology of Mental Illness*, 3e (eds. D. Charney and E. Nestler), 1218–1229. New York: Oxford University Press.

Mason, E.J. and Joshi, K.G. (2018). Nonpharmacologic strategies for helping children with ADHD. *Current Psychiatry* 17 (1): 42.

Menon, V. (2013). Developmental pathways to functional brain networks: emerging principles. *Trends Cognitive Sciences* 17 (12): 627–640.

Milner, B., Squire, L., and Kandel, E. (1998). Cognitive neuroscience and the study of memory. *Neuron* 20: 445–468.

MTA Cooperative Group (1999). A 14-Month Randomized Clinical Trial of Treatment Strategies for Attention-Deficit/Hyperactivity Disorder. *Archives of General Psychiatry* 56 (12): 1073–1086. https://doi.org/10.1001/archpsyc.56.12.1073.

Nakahata, Y. and Yasuda, R. (2018). Plasticity of spine structure: local signaling, translation and cytoskeletal reorganization. *Frontiers in Synaptic Neuroscience* 10, 29. https://doi.org/10.3389/fnsyn.2018.00029.

National Institute of Child Health and Human Development. (2017). Neural tube defects (NTDs): Condition Information. US National Institutes of Health. Retrieved 1 August 2018. Available at www.nichd.nih.gov/health/topics/ntds.

Nestler, E.J., Hyman, S.E., Holtzman, D.M., and Malenka, R.C. (2015). *Molecular Neuropharmacology*. New York: McGraw Hill.

Nouwen, A., Chambers, A., Chechlacz, M. et al. (2017). Microstructural abnormalities in white and gray matter in obese adolescents with and without type 2 diabetes. *NeuroImage. Clinical* 16: 43–51. https://doi.org/10.1016/j.nicl.2017.07.004.

Ostby, Y., Tamnes, C., Fjell, A. et al. (2009). Heterogeneity in subcortical brain development: a structural magnetic resonance imaging study of brain maturation from 8 to 30 years. *Journal of Neuroscience* 29 (38): 11772–11782.

Pappano, A.J. (2015). Cholinoceptor-activating & cholinesterase-inhibiting drugs. In: *Basic and Clinical Pharmacology* (eds. B.G. Katzung and A.J. Trevor), 105–120. New York: McGraw Hill Lange.

Patil, S.T., Zhang, L., Martenyi, F. et al. (2007). Activation of mGlu2/3 receptors as a new approach to treat schizophrenia: a randomized phase 2 clinical trial. *Nature Medicine* 13: 1102–1107.

Pliszka, S., Glahn, D., Semrud-Clikeman, M. et al. (2006). Neuroimaging of inhibitory control areas in children with attention deficit hyperactivity disorder who were treatment naïve or in long-term treatment. *American Journal of Psychiatry* 163: 1052–1060.

Prigge, C.L. and Kay, J.N. (2018). Dendrite morphogenesis from birth to adulthood. *Current Opinion in Neurobiology* 53: 139–145.

Procyshyn, R.M., Bezchlibnyk-Butler, K.Z., and Jefferies, J.J. (2015). *Clinical Handbook of Psychotropic Drugs*, 21e. Boston: Hogrefe.

Ptácek, R., Kuzelová, H., and Stefano, G.B. (2011). Dopamine D4 receptor gene DRD4 and its association with psychiatric disorders. *Medical Science Monitor: International Medical Journal of Experimental and Clinical Research* 17 (9): RA215–RA220.

Purves, D., Augustine, G., Fitzpatrick, D. et al. (2008). *Neuroscience*, 4e. Sunderland, MA: Sinauer Associates.

Rakic, P., Ayoub, A., Breunig, J., and Dominguez, M. (2009). Decision by division: making cortical maps. *Trends in Neuroscience* 32 (5): 291–301.

Rogan, M., Leon, K.S., Perez, D., and Kandel, E. (2005). Distinct neural signatures for safety and danger in the amygdale and striatum of the mouse. *Neuron* 46: 309–320.

Rossi, D. and Volterra, A. (2009). Astrocyte dysfunction: insights on the role in neurodegeneration. *Brain Research Bulletin* 80: 224–232.

Rudy, J. (2008). *The Neurobiology of Learning and Memory*. Sunderland, MA: Sinauer Associates.

Scharf, S.H., Jaeschke, G., Wettstein, J.G., and Lindemann, L. (2015). Metabotropic glutamate receptor 5 as drug target for fragile X syndrome. *Current Opinion in Pharmacology* 20: 124–134.

Schmahmann, J., Smith, E., Eichler, F., and Filley, C. (2008). Cerebral white matter. *Annals of the New York Academy of Sciences* 1142: 266–309.

Seeman, P. (2009). Glutamate and dopamine components in schizophrenia. *Journal of Psychiatry & Neuroscience* 34 (2): 143–149.

Shepherd, G. (2004). *The Synaptic Organization of the Brain*, 5e. New York: Oxford University Press.

Sousa, S.S., Amaro, E., Crego, A. et al. (2018). Developmental trajectory of the prefrontal cortex: a systematic review of diffusion tensor imaging studies. *Brain Imaging and Behavior* 12 (4): 1197–1210.

Sporns, O. (2012). *Discovering the Human Connectome*. Cambridge, MA: MIT Press.

Szmydynger-Chodobska, J., Stazielle, N., Zink, B. et al. (2009). The role of the choroid plexus in neutrophil invasion after traumatic brain injury. *Journal of Cerebral Blood Flow & Metabolism* 29: 1503–1516.

TADS Team (2007). The treatment for adolescents with depression study (TADS) long-term effectiveness and safety outcomes. *Archives of General Psychiatry* 64 (10): 1132–1144.

Tamnes, C., Ostby, Y., Fjell, A. et al. (2010). Brain maturation in adolescence and young adulthood: regional age-related changes in cortical thickness and white matter volume and microstructure. *Cerebral Cortex* 20 (3): 534–548.

Tau, G. and Peterson, B. (2010). Normal development of brain circuits. *Neuropsychopharmacology* 35: 147–168.

Vaccarino, F. and Leckman, J. (2011). *Pediatric Psychopharmacology: Principles and Practice*, 2e (eds. A. Martin, L. Scahill and D. Kratchovil), 3–19. New York: Oxford University Press.

Versace, A., Acuff, H., Bertocci, M.A. et al. (2015). White matter structure in youth with behavioral and emotional dysregulation disorders: a probabilistic tractographic study. *JAMA Psychiatry* 72 (4): 367–376.

Walkup, J., Albano, A., Piacentini, J. et al. (2008). Cognitive behavioral therapy, sertaline, or a combination in childhood anxiety. *New England Journal of Medicine* 359 (26): 2753–2765.

Waller, R., Dotterer, H.L., Murray, L. et al. (2017). White-matter tract abnormalities and antisocial behavior: a systematic review of diffusion tensor imaging studies across development. *NeuroImage. Clinical* 14: 201–215.

Winklewski, P.J., Sabisz, A., Naumczyk, P. et al. (2018). Understanding the physiopathology behind axial and radial diffusivity changes-what do we know? *Frontiers in Neurology* 9: 92. https://doi.org/10.3389/fneur.2018.00092.

Woody, S. and Rachman, S. (1994). Generalized anxiety disorder (GAD) as an unsuccessful search for safety. *Clinical Psychology Review* 14 (8): 743–753.

4

Integration of Physical and Psychiatric Assessment

Veronica C. Doran[1] and Jamesetta A. Newland[2]

[1] Marymount University, Arlington, VA, USA
[2] Rory Meyers College of Nursing, New York University, New York, NY, USA

Objectives

After reading this chapter, advanced practice registered nurses (APRN) will be able to:

1. Discuss the elements of psychiatric assessments of children and adolescents by APRNs.
2. Describe the essential elements of a comprehensive medical history and physical examination of children and adolescents seen in primary care to determine presence or absence of medical conditions.
3. Identify common screening tools used to assess mental health and behavioral disorders in children and adolescents.
4. Recognize indications for consultation, referral, and collaboration between primary care and mental health professionals for children and adolescents with mental healthcare needs.

Overview of Chapter

Mental health impacts children's physical health, social relationships, and learning. Early and thorough assessment of children and adolescents with psychiatric-mental health disorders is the most effective way to begin timely treatment, diminish the severity of mental disorders, and decrease the likelihood of chronic mental disorders in adulthood. A landmark report by the National Research Council and Institute of Medicine (2009) reinforced the need for behavioral health screening to take place in primary care settings and for schools to detect risk factors in children and adolescents and the appearance of early symptoms of disorder. Early identification and treatment can ameliorate the effects of mental illness in children and adolescents as well as adults.

This chapter will describe the elements that make up a comprehensive psychiatric-mental health assessment of children and adolescents. This assessment can be used in primary care settings to help identify children and adolescents in need of mental health services. Key areas include history taking, physical examination process, risk, protective factors, teaching needs of the child or adolescent and family, and ways to communicate the assessment findings to the patient and family and, if appropriate, the school so that they are able to pursue appropriate treatment as needed.

Child and Adolescent Behavioral Health: A Resource for Advanced Practice Psychiatric and Primary Care Practitioners in Nursing,
Second Edition. Edited by Edilma L. Yearwood, Geraldine S. Pearson, and Jamesetta A. Newland.
© 2021 John Wiley & Sons, Inc. Published 2021 by John Wiley & Sons, Inc.
Companion website: www.wiley.com/go/Yearwood

Approximately one out of every four or five youths in the United States are estimated to have a mental or behavioral disorder which will impact their functioning throughout their lifetime (Merikangas et al. 2010). This translates to a cost of US$247 billion plus the emotional, social, and economic costs for the child and family (National Research Council and Institute of Medicine 2009). In 2016, it was estimated that 12.8% of adolescents between 12 and 17 years of age had a major depressive episode (MDE) and 9% of all adolescents had an MDE severe enough to cause significant impairment (Substance Abuse and Mental Health Service Administration 2017). Moreover, approximately 15.4% of all US children between the ages of 2 and 8 years had at least one parent-reported diagnosed mental, behavioral, or developmental disorder (Bitsko et al. 2018). While these statistics demonstrate the high rate of mental health disorders in this population, the actual percentage of children with psychiatric disorders who are being diagnosed and/or receiving treatment is low. This is despite the fact that early detection and treatment of child and adolescent mental disorders result in the best outcomes. Furthermore, it is estimated that over half of all visits to a primary care pediatric office involve behavioral, emotional, psychosocial, or developmental concerns and 75% of teenagers with diagnosed mental health disorders are seen in the pediatrician's office (Martini et al. 2012). These statistics help highlight the need for primary care practitioners (PCPs), including advanced practice registered nurses (APRNs), to be able to evaluate children and adolescents for mental health problems and appropriately refer them for services.

A major contributing factor to these startling numbers has been the lack of adequate screening for and identification of mental health problems by PCPs (Ackincigil and Matthews 2017). A review of the 2012–2013 National Ambulatory Medical Care Survey revealed that while the overall rate of depression screening of adults in a primary care setting was only 4.2%, a diagnosis of depression was made in 47% of those screened (Akincigil and Matthews). Citing lack of knowledge and confidence in diagnoses, many PCPs feel that their training did not adequately prepare them to identify behavioral and mental health problems in children and adolescents (Davis et al. 2012; Hampton et al. 2015; Nasir et al. 2016; O'Brien et al. 2016). In fact, despite a 1997 mandate requiring a minimum 1-month rotation in developmental and behavioral pediatrics, many new pediatricians still feel unprepared to both diagnose and treat children and adolescents with mental health issues (Hampton et al. 2015; Stein et al. 2017). Not only do PCPs state that they are unprepared to evaluate children for mental health problems, a US study of adolescents aged 13–17 years found that only

one-third of the adolescents interviewed stated their PCPs had ever had a discussion with them about their emotions and mood during a routine visit (Ozer et al. 2009). Recent studies showed a small number of adolescents, 45%, with any mental health disorder received services for these issues and even less, approximately one out of every four, received services in a specialized mental health setting (Costello et al. 2014). Moreover, in a systematic review of literature examining universal mental health screening in pediatric primary care, Wissow et al. (2013) found that low numbers of providers were explicitly trained in the evaluation of screening results for interpretation and illness management. PCPs must be trained in methods to evaluate children and adolescents for psychiatric problems, as well as recognize that moods and emotions are a mainstay of one's wellbeing and should be incorporated into every primary care visit.

Compounding the problem of so few children and adolescents in need not receiving mental health screening and identification in primary care settings is the severe shortage of physicians, APRNs, and others who are skilled and willing to treat children and adolescents with mental disorders (National Council for Behavioral Health 2017; USDHHS-HRSA 2016; Walker et al. 2015). A recent review of the data in the state of Georgia found that there were only 5.9 child and adolescent psychiatrists per 100 000 youths and 2.9 psychiatric APRNs per 100 000 people working in the field (Walker et al. 2015). Nationwide conservative estimates of data project a 1% decrease in available psychiatrists by 2025 combined with a 6% increase in demand (USDHHS-HRSA 2016). These estimates do project a net increase in available behavioral health nurse practitioners (USDHHS-HRSA 2016), but these numbers do not address the number of psychiatric caregivers that would be needed if all children and adolescents with mental health issues were identified in primary care settings nor do they address the reality of a projected retirement of 55% of the total psychiatrist workforce within the next 10 years (Satiani et al. 2018).

Another discouraging fact in this growing need for mental healthcare providers is the inadequate growth in enrollment of nurses in graduate psychiatry training programs. Recent statistics show that, although the number of students enrolled in masters or doctoral level psychiatric mental health nurse practitioner (PMHNP) programs has experienced a 26% increase in just the past few years, the number of actively working PMHNPs will still only represent about 4.5% of the total licensed nurse practitioners (NPs) (Delaney 2017; Fang et al. 2016). Finally, according to 2012 data, USDHHS-HRSA (2014) showed that 5.6% of practicing NPs worked in the psychiatric-mental health specialty, down from the 6.3% previously reported in 2008 (USDHHS-HRSA 2010).

These realities have generated a growing interest in including and integrating mental health screening into primary care settings. Incorporating mental health assessment into each primary care visit increases the likelihood of identifying children in need earlier and allowing for early intervention to decrease long-term complications from mental health disorders. Assessment during critical periods of a child's or adolescent's development is most likely to result in effective treatment (Jonovich and Alpert-Gilles 2014). The need to provide PCPs with the appropriate knowledge and skills so they are able to screen for mental and behavioral health problems in children and adolescents who present in their practices for routine healthcare has been acknowledged (AACAP 2009; Martini et al. 2012; Nasir et al. 2016; O'Brien et al. 2016; Webb et al. 2016). PCPs must be able to use history taking and the physical examination to differentiate physical problems/conditions from mental health issues in order to offer these children appropriate interventions and support.

The World Health Organization (WHO) and the World Organization of Family Doctors (Wonca 2008) stated, "Certain skills and competencies are required to effectively assess, diagnose, treat, support and refer people with mental disorders: it is essential that primary care workers are adequately prepared and supported in their mental health work" (p. 1). Moreover, clinicians themselves recognize the need for the acquisition of skills that will increase their capability, comfort, and confidence in the management of mental health issues in their patients (Hampton et al. 2015; Horwitz et al. 2015; Nasir et al. 2016).

WHO and Wonca also emphasized how a child's cognitive and emotional developmental levels impact his ability to understand and communicate his mental health issues. Therefore, PCPs/APRNs must receive proper training in order to be cognizant of their expected developmental ability to differentiate normal developmental issues and reactions from mental health problems (Hampton et al. 2015). Additionally, children's and adolescents' responses and reactions are influenced by issues such as fatigue, hunger, and lack of comfort with the people examining them. It is important for PCPs to consider the possibility of drug and alcohol consumption mimicking mental health conditions and should screen children and adolescents for substance use when appropriate.

Finally, the child or adolescent may not be aware of or understand that her feelings or symptoms are related to her mental health, thus she will not tell the PCP that she is depressed, anxious, etc. PCPs should interview the parents as well as the child or adolescent and obtain information from school personnel whenever possible.

Often it is the parents or school personnel who recognize the child or adolescent is having psychiatric symptoms (Biel et al. 2015; Jonovich and Alpert-Gilles 2014). APRNs must be sure to evaluate the child's or adolescent's social environment such as his family dynamics, living situation, friends, and school issues to help evaluate the child fully. These are important sources of information that can help in making a diagnosis.

When caring for children and adolescents in primary care, in addition to the psychiatric-mental health assessment, a thorough medical history and physical examination to determine the presence or absence of underlying medical conditions that might be treatable is warranted. Although the assessment guidelines in this chapter will purposefully be general rather than specific, readers are referred to other chapters in the text that cover each grouping of mental disorders for more in-depth information. The chapter will provide APRNs and other PCPs in primary care and mental health settings with a way to systematically approach the assessment of the behavioral and mental health of their patients.

Integrating Psychiatric and Physical Assessment Approaches

PCPs are often the first individuals who face parents' concerns about their child's mental health. According to data from the National Co-Morbidity Survey, of the 45% of adolescents with psychiatric disorders, approximately 33.7% of those received services in the school or general medical setting (Costello et al. 2014). Often families do not know where to turn when they become aware of their child's behavioral or mental problems; they may realize that "something's not right" with their child, but little else. Importantly, parents who are offered a screening questionnaire during their child's primary care visit were more likely to talk with the provider about mental health concerns (Jonovich and Alpert-Gilles 2014).

Jonovich and Alpert-Gilles (2014) found that parental identification of mental health concerns plays a pivotal role in paving the way for the child's treatment. Bajeux et al. (2018) found that, although parent/child agreement on externalizing mental health factors resulted in 43.83% of mental health contact, parent identification alone of externalizing factors resulted in a significantly higher rate of mental health contact. Biel et al. (2015) found that in instances where the parent felt that the child's behavioral or emotional issues resulted in difficulties, screening scores showing a high level of impairment were found in over half of the cases. These three reports support a strong association between a parent's concern and the presence of mental or behavioral health issues in a child. The PCP's role in detecting behavioral or psychiatric disorders, initiating treatment, and referring for further treatment is paramount in assuring timely and appropriate help for the child.

Alternatively, PCPs are often in the position of having to inform parents who are not aware, ignore, or deny the signs and symptoms of behavioral problems that "something's not right." The long-term relationship developed between child, parent, and PCP can be beneficial in approaching sensitive areas for discussion. PCPs can support parents who do not believe in or trust mental health providers. If the parents have a strong connection with their PCP they are more likely to follow her suggestions, even if they fear or distrust psychiatric healthcare providers. One of this chapter's goals is to assist PCPs with the knowledge and confidence to proceed with their evaluation of the child's history, behavior, complaints, school performance, social skills, family functioning, and available resources for care.

One barrier to asking questions about mental health issues is what to do with the information received. It is, therefore, essential for PCPs to develop strong relationships with mental healthcare providers to whom a child or adolescent and family can be referred or with whom the PCPs can collaborate (Davis et al. 2012; Knutson et al. 2018; O'Brien et al. 2016; Pidano et al. 2014). Pediatric PCPs can also promote protective resilience by building on the child's or adolescent's strengths through reinforcement of competence, confidence, connection to family and community, sense of control over one's actions, and positive coping.

Who Initially Assesses the Child?

Children and adolescents with mental disorders or problems often first appear in the office of their primary care APRN, who might be an NP or other APRN. Many of the "new morbidities," such as attention deficit hyperactivity disorder (ADHD) and learning problems, drug and alcohol abuse, anxiety and mood problems, suicide and homicide, HIV and AIDS, and violence and sexual activity, have been added to the screening responsibilities in pediatrics (Stein et al. 2017). Because PCPs are now being asked to care for children with these chronic conditions it is even more important for mental health evaluations to be a part of routine care. Evans (2009) recommended screening children at risk for mental health problems, particularly children expelled from daycare and preschool settings, children of depressed parents, children with disabling or chronic illnesses, children in military families, and children in foster care or juvenile justice systems. The American Academy of Child and Adolescent Psychiatry (AACAP 2009) supports the initiation of services in primary care by PCPs for emerging developmental and behavioral problems and common mental health

disorders such as ADHD, depression, and anxiety disorders in children and adolescents. The pediatricians, pediatric NPs, and family NPs must possess the necessary skills to complete a thorough and sensitive assessment of the "problem." Primary care practices are the optimal settings for screening for mental health disorders in children and determining the next step in treatment. But just as important, providers must know when mental health specialty care or referral is indicated.

Elements of an Assessment

Several considerations should precede the APRN's gathering of information about the "problem" that prompted the family to seek care for their child or adolescent. The APRN must realize that a thorough assessment does not consist of a checklist to be completed in a robotic way but that the child and family are facing a difficult situation that needs to be approached in a calm, sensitive, and caring manner. The APRN should recognize that screening is often a springboard to discussion and has the potential to increase patient and parent comfort in talking about difficult subjects (Jonovich and Alpert-Gilles 2014). The unknown is generally perceived as frightening and the perceptions of children, adolescents, and families regarding the unknown assessment process are no different. The assessment of these children and adolescents must include a comprehensive medical, environmental, and social history from multiple sources to gain insight into all aspects of the child's problem. Once a comprehensive history has been completed the APRN must complete a full physical assessment. The PCP must take the history, physical examination, and any laboratory tests that are done and consider whether this child or adolescent has a mental health issue that is causing their symptoms. If the APRN or PCP thinks the diagnosis is a mental/behavioral health problem, then she must help the family understand what is going on and connect them with appropriate providers to allow optimal treatment for the child.

Observation of the Child, Adolescent, and Family

The APRN must be skillful in observing and interpreting the child's or adolescent's and family members' verbal behavior and in listening to their spontaneous verbalizations and their answers to questions. Observation includes attention to the family members' interactions, relationships, responses to the child, concerns about the problem at hand, and openness to learn new ways to help their child. It also includes focusing on the child's activity level, interruptions, interaction with parents and siblings, responses to the parents' words and actions, and willingness to separate from the parents to talk privately with the APRN. A family-centered community-based approach provides an integrated assessment of the child (Burns and Duderstadt 2017).

Impact of the Problem or Disorder

The child's or adolescent's mental health problem makes an impact, sometimes a significant one, on all family members. Siblings worry about their troubled brother or sister and may wonder why he or she has this problem and whether they will develop it too. Parents often admit, "We are all affected" or "We are all suffering," when describing the impact of the child's problem on the family. The emotional problem or mental disorder has an impact on the child and her friends, classmates, teachers, grandparents, extended family, and often neighbors. Sometimes the impact seems to be more "internal," such as the suffering of the child or adolescent with anxiety or depression. Other times, the impact is "external" as in children with ADHD, oppositional defiant disorder, conduct disorder, and other disruptive behavior disorders. In any case, the behavior of children and adolescents affects others in their environment, particularly when they have chronic conditions, whether psychiatric or physical (Bitsko et al. 2018). The primary care APRN must encourage open communication with family members and others in the child's life to assess the need for family interventions in order to maximize the child's health and child's and family's quality of life.

Eliciting Information

The most thorough psychiatric-mental health assessments are based on information from all relevant parties, including the child or adolescent, parents/grandparents/guardians, extended family members, school personnel, and past and present treating providers. Often it is not possible to gather information from all these sources and the APRN must proceed with whatever data are available. These data may include emails from teachers, phone calls from other treating professionals (with consent), and testing results from psychologists. It is important for the APRN to attempt to get as much information from as many sources as possible to help in identifying sources of stress or anxiety or the impact the mental health issue is having on the child/adolescent. Each child/adolescent should be interviewed alone to allow him to feel free to speak about any issues or concerns. Parents should also be interviewed without the child present to ensure that they can speak freely and not withhold information because the child is present. During the history taking it is important for the PCP to observe all reactions by the child/adolescent and parents

when being questioned, as well as interactions between them throughout the examination process.

Ways Children and Adolescents Communicate

Children and adolescents communicate in their own ways according to their ages, stages of development, and life circumstances. They use not just verbalizations, but also interactions with others, drawings, play, music, engagement versus withdrawal, appearance, facial expression, eye contact, and other forms of verbal communication. For example, a child may play out feelings of helplessness and fear about being abused; an adolescent may draw pictures of the "devils" he remembers from nightmares or a picture of the torment he wants to inflict on a peer. APRNs should use many forms of communication from the child/adolescent to elicit as much information as possible to aid in making a diagnosis.

Age- and Development-Specific Considerations

When evaluating children of various ages for mental health issues, the APRN must recognize the different developmental stages and how these influence the evaluation process. Mental health assessment must use questioning and other methods appropriate to the child's age and developmental level.

Typically, children and adolescents undergo rapid developmental change. Each age and developmental stage, from a very young age through adolescence, presents its own challenges to the evaluator. When working with toddlers and preschoolers, much of the verbal information is received from parental reports, but the APRN should use multiple sources and resources to gather all the needed information. Research has shown that discrepancies can exist between parent and observer findings of a child's behavior (Moens et al. 2018). Therefore, the APRN can gain more information by watching the parent–child interaction, getting feedback from a preschool teacher, and watching the child's interactions with others. Additionally, there has been recent evidence of the usefulness of the Preschool Age Psychiatric Assessment, both in screening for current pathology in the youngest patients and in prospectively predicting difficulties later in childhood and adolescence (Finsaas et al. 2018). School-age children may not be able to verbalize what they are feeling; rather, they may have physical symptoms that are caused by a mental health issue. Here again, gathering information from the child, parents, teachers, and other resources can help in the evaluation. Adolescents may be able to discuss their feelings, but some adolescents might balk and refuse to talk; trust building may take some time. The use of standardized evaluative tools can assist in the assessment of children of all ages with a range of disorders. APRNs conducting mental health assessments of children and adolescents must consider developmental levels and adapt accordingly.

Personal Factors Influencing the Assessment

No matter what field of practice, APRNs must all recognize the influence of their own biases, anxieties, and fears, life experiences, and needs when working with other people. Whatever their own cultural background, APRNs must be culturally sensitive to the experiences of others. They must accept and celebrate the things that make each child, adolescent, and family unique and capable (Dunn 2010a). In addition, APRNs' views of children as vulnerable makes it especially poignant and difficult when they suffer from either internal challenges, such as heightened anxiety, or external stressors, such as family disruption. These are troublesome concerns for all APRNs to deal with in helping people. One of the most positive messages the APRN can communicate to a child or adolescent and the family is a sense of hopefulness for the child's or adolescent's future.

Areas of Psychiatric Assessment of Children and Adolescents

A thorough assessment of a child presenting with a mental disorder or behavioral problem must include certain points, such as chief complaint, review of systems, developmental history, school history, mental status examination (MSE), physical examination, and formulation of diagnoses and treatment plan. In addition, other elements may need to be assessed in depth in relation to the child's presenting behavior or complaint, such as suicidal behavior and plan, risk for violence, mood lability, or hallucinations. Keep in mind, however, that the child might present to the primary care APRN or other provider with no complaint of psychiatric etiology. Rather, children may present with physical or somatic complaints that mimic a physical problem. The APRN must remember that physical symptoms may represent mental health problems, therefore they should always consider a mental or behavior health diagnosis among the differentials. Many of the following elements of the psychiatric assessment also apply to the medical assessment and will guide additional actions performed in the physical examination (Burns and Duderstadt 2017).

Chief Complaint or Presenting Symptoms and Behaviors

The APRN must first ask, "What brings you in today?" Any complaints or concerns of the child or adolescent and parents should be assessed. A young child may respond, "I don't know," "Because my stomach hurts," or "The teacher yells at me," and thus open the door for reassurance such as, "It sounds like sometimes you get in trouble for your behavior" or another simple explanation. Adolescents may be angry that they were "dragged" to the appointment or they may feel guilty about their problems or too anxious or depressed to be able to express their concerns.

Parents may present a list of complaints or problems which have surfaced recently, or which have been present for many years; they may bring with them a brief or lengthy list of their child's signs and symptoms. Some parents may not recognize that their child is having mental health problems and may not connect their symptoms with their mental wellbeing. The APRN should evaluate all children presenting in the primary care office for any signs of mental or psychiatric distress.

Medically unexplained symptoms, or symptoms that seem out of proportion to the illness, can be an important sign that underlying mental problems exist because emotional distress can cause pain and other physical symptoms (Ames and Leadbeater 2018; Balázs et al. 2018). The primary care APRN also must remember that children or adolescents with chronic illness experience an increased risk of behavioral and emotional problems (Butler et al. 2018; Jones et al. 2017). Repeated screening for depression and anxiety in adolescents with chronic health issues can alert the APRN to treatment needs and can result in more desirable outcomes and decreased impairment (Jones et al. 2017). If the presenting complaint is a medical concern, additional information about onset, location, duration, character, aggravating factors, relieving factors, and current self-treatment measures should be elicited. The APRN should evaluate the child/adolescent for sources of distress to help differentiate medical causes of physical symptoms from emotional sources.

A comprehensive subjective review of systems is helpful in working through physical complaints about the child. Asking questions about general wellbeing, including energy level, excessive fatigue, rashes, eye pain, throat pain, difficulty swallowing, chest pain or palpitations, shortness of breath, abdominal pain, nausea or vomiting, diarrhea or constipation, body aches, or headaches is helpful in working through the differential diagnoses. Addressing possible sources of stress in the child's or adolescent's life is also important when eliciting a history. This includes asking about school, friends, siblings, social activities, and home life.

Prior Treatment

The APRN questions whether and where the child or adolescent has been previously treated for a mental health disorder. The child may have received inpatient care (the most intensive level of treatment), partial hospitalization or day treatment (which is less intensive), and/or outpatient care such as medication management (the least intensive level of care). The child may have been in therapy, sometimes over a period of years and with various therapists. The APRN should also be sensitive to alternative therapy approaches that the child may have had, such as occupational therapy or school-based programs which may indicate an attempt on the part of the parents or school to address difficulties or at-risk behaviors (Arbesman et al. 2013; Bekar et al. 2017). All of the information about prior treatment gives the assessing APRN a picture of the extent to which the family has already sought help for their child and the perceived success or failure of the treatment.

Developmental History

A child's or adolescent's developmental history begins with the mother's age and health during pregnancy and moves on to include any parental health or emotional problems, difficult life circumstances, and drug or alcohol use during pregnancy. This part of the assessment includes information gathering about the labor and birth, any neonatal complications, difficulties in the early weeks and months of life, and whether or not the child met developmental milestones. The APRN must acknowledge that normal development falls somewhere within an identified span of time, with some children meeting developmental milestones earlier or later than others. For younger children, height and weight should be recorded on the Centers for Disease Control and Prevention growth chart to track how his growth compares to previous measurements and standardized norms. With adolescents, it is important to assess the development of secondary sex characteristics. Because of the wide variability in physical appearance and the psychosocial developmental stage of the adolescent, repeated reassurance that she is developing within the normal spectrum might be necessary.

It is imperative that APRNs know normal growth and developmental milestones because often mental health problems may be related to common developmental stages that are not achieved or are not completed. When parents of a child having temper tantrums present to the primary care office it is important for the APRN to recognize that this is a common issue among toddlers as they learn to control their environment or are overwhelmed in a situation. Alternatively, if a child is 7 years old and having temper tantrums, this may represent a mental health issue because by this age the child should be able to communicate her frustrations to others and/or control her emotions better. Parental expectations of the child are also an important part of the developmental assessment. If parents have

expectations of the child that are above what the child can cognitively achieve, they may reprimand the child or punish him inappropriately, causing anxiety or fear.

The importance of understanding growth and development by the PCP cannot be emphasized enough. Lack of achievement of specific milestones or lack of progression along the developmental trajectory may be early signs of mental health problems for the PCP. A comprehensive developmental assessment is a key part of the mental health evaluation (Burns and Duderstadt 2017).

Family History

Assessment of mental health problems in children and adolescents always includes a thorough family history of mental illness. Because the initial reaction of most people is to deny the presence of mental illness in their families, the primary care NP or the psychiatric-mental health APRN (PMH-APRN) must carefully assess whether family members have certain disorders. For example, instead of just asking, "Is there anyone in the family with depression?" it is helpful to ask, "On either side of the biological parents' families, is there anyone who has depression, takes an antidepressant, used to take an antidepressant, should take an antidepressant, committed suicide, or tried to commit suicide?" Instead of asking, "Is there anyone in the family with anxiety," it is helpful to ask, "On either side of the biological parents' families, is there anyone who has anxiety, takes a medication for anxiety, has anxiety attacks, has panic attacks, worries all the time, or can't leave home?"

Comprehensive evaluation of family history with construction of a genogram, pedigree, and/or an ecomap is useful to visually display the structure and pattern of family relationships, medical (and psychiatric) conditions that have affected family members across several generations, and interactions among family members inside and outside the family system (Burns and Duderstadt 2017; Tarini and McInerney 2013). These diagrams can help the APRN and family view the multiple influences on the child's mental and physical health status as well as the child's and family's responses to these influencing factors. The visual revelation may assist in guiding decisions about the appropriate referrals and interventions. Given the time constraints on APRNs in primary care, targeted family histories, based on patient presentation, life stage or age, and viewed as a "living document" that can grow as the child does may be more practical and contribute to positive patient outcomes (Tarini and McInerney 2013).

Medical History

Initial questions the primary care APRN will ask the family when taking the medical history include whether the child's immunizations are up to date; if there is any history of a loss of consciousness or head injury, whether there have been any surgeries or hospitalizations, accidents, chronic illnesses, and recent acute illnesses, and if there are any allergies to medicine, food, or environmental allergens. Chronic illnesses are often associated with mental health issues such as anxiety or depression. If there is a diagnosis, the APRN should ask parents when it was made, what the child/adolescent knows about the diagnosis, and how he is coping with it. Past head trauma is also known to be associated with mental health problems later in life. Children with multiple head injuries should have cognitive testing to evaluate for subtle declines in their mental abilities. Chronic allergies can present as crankiness or moodiness in children. APRNs should evaluate children/adolescents who have mood changes during certain seasons or when exposed to certain environments. Children with histories of trauma and/or abuse are also at increased risk for mental health problems, therefore these questions should be asked when reviewing a child/adolescent's past medical history (Burns and Duderstadt 2017).

Activities of Daily Living

Primary care visits are a time when the PCP should evaluate children's activities of daily living, including nutrition and sleep patterns. Parents might not be aware that their child is overeating or eating too little or consuming unhealthy food and drink. In addition, the family's cultural patterns related to diet and eating must be considered. Eating disorders may include anorexia nervosa and bulimia, overweight or obesity, and severe allergies to foods. Eating patterns, and resultant weight or nutritional imbalances, could be associated with mental health struggles (Banta et al. 2013; Rubio-López et al. 2016; Tevie and Shaya 2015). Children who are hypoglycemic may present with a depressed mood or affect. Conversely, those with diets high in sugar or caffeine may present with symptoms of hyperactivity or anxiety. Obesity in children/adolescents has been associated with depression. APRN must be cognizant of how the child/adolescent feels about her appearance, which influences her emotional wellbeing.

Parents often do not know how much sleep a child needs each day or realize the importance of a regular bedtime, even for older adolescents. Sleep requirements per 24 hours vary according to age, ranging from 16–20 hours for a newborn to 11 hours for a 6-year-old to 8 hours for a 15-year-old. Insufficient sleep can lead to or exacerbate mental health symptoms in children and adolescents (Van Dyk et al. 2016) or even lead to increased risk for self-harm (Liu et al. 2017). Very young children manifest the effects of insufficient sleep with hyperactivity, emotional lability, irritability, and aggressiveness. School-age children may experience inattention, restlessness, emotional lability, or daydreaming at school; symptoms overlap with those of ADHD. Adolescents with inadequate sleep may exhibit excessive sleepiness, difficulties with mood regulation, impaired academic performance, and increased propensity for risky behavior (Hasler et al. 2015). Disordered sleep can lead to physical and mental health issues. Sleep problems may also be related to something that is happening in the family. Children and adolescents with depression or anxiety may be unable to sleep due to worry or obsessive thoughts that keep them awake, which in turn adds to their feelings of fatigue or moodiness.

Medication History

It is important to know past and present medications taken by the child, when they were taken, their effects, side or adverse effects, and why they were discontinued and by whom. Many over-the-counter medications cause symptoms that may be misdiagnosed as anxiety or depression. Pseudoephedrine may cause difficulty in concentrating, palpitations, anxiety, or tremors in children. Asthma medications, including albuterol, may make a child jittery, hyperactive, or aggressive. Benadryl may cause a child/adolescent to appear sad, disinterested, sleepy, or moody. When evaluating children/adolescents for possible psychiatric conditions, the APRN should have parents stop all nonessential medications prior to the evaluation so that the medications have been excreted from the system.

For those children/adolescents for whom psychotropic medications are warranted, parents and children/adolescents must know that all medications have potential side effects and that parents should be responsible for both administering the medication and observing the children for any negative effects. There are certain risk factors to assess when considering specific psychotropic medications, such as the risks associated with the use of stimulant medications in the presence of cardiac structural defect in a child or adolescent or a family member who died of sudden cardiac death at a young age. APRNs must emphasize the importance of taking psychotropic medications as ordered to avoid overdosing and/or decreasing complications from side effects.

Social History

The child's or adolescent's social history should state with whom the child lives and the relationship to the child, the city in which the child lives, whether there has been a recent move, where a separated or divorced parent lives, sources of support from extended family and their proximity to the child, and family dynamics, strengths, and needs. Relationships with parents/grandparents or guardians and with siblings are part of a thorough assessment. In addition, any legal problems or involvement in the juvenile justice system should be included. The occupations of parents, guardians, or primary caretakers, family financial resources, and access to healthcare services are factors that can affect the mental and physical health of a child and family.

Peer relationships, in terms of whether the child has any friends and how she interacts with peers, are important. Sometimes a child or adolescent will report that he has plenty of friends but the parent will report that he is not invited to peers' birthday parties or not asked to join peer activities. Determining how the child views himself in comparison to his peers can help in understanding his view of himself. Children who state "I am not popular" or "I am just a loser" should alert the PCP for possible mental health issues. The APRN should ask the child/adolescent what she likes to do for fun. Asking children/adolescents what they want to do when they grow up can provide a view of how the child/adolescent views her future. Children who say they have no fun, or don't have any activities, or don't think about a future for themselves should be evaluated for depression or mental health challenges. Social relationships and activities are key components of the lives of children/adolescents that often are directly related to their mental wellbeing.

School History

Information to gather about the child's or adolescent's school history includes the school grade, name of the school, and whether the child receives regular education or special education services for a specific learning problem such as ADHD, learning differences, or another behavioral issue that interferes with the educational process. Parents can often identify the years which were "good" for the child related to a particularly excellent teacher versus the year or years which were not as productive. The school-related data must be examined carefully because school is often associated with stressful events for the child and family.

Substance Use/Abuse History

The APRN should ask children and adolescents about drug and alcohol use or abuse. Adolescents, in particular, will often not volunteer information about their use of drugs and alcohol. Some don't consider marijuana a drug. Surprisingly, though, adolescents will often answer direct questions from the APRN assessor honestly and openly. The APRN must not forget that children, even young children, may be using drugs and alcohol, especially when they are part of the parents' lifestyle, therefore they too must be evaluated. Access to medications

in the home should also be part of the evaluation process. Parents who take antidepressants or narcotics should be asked where they keep their medications, if they are locked up, and/or if any of their medications have gone missing. Over-the-counter medications may also be used by children/adolescents who are dealing with mental health issues, so access to these medications should also be included when taking a history (Benotsch et al. 2014).

Risk Behaviors

Every child and adolescent should be assessed for high-risk behaviors involving sex, drugs, alcohol, association with unsavory individuals, and dangerous, thrill-seeking behaviors. Parents may not be aware of their child's behavior and this can be shocking and very upsetting to them. It is important to keep in mind the level of sensitivity and absence of judgment or condemnation needed to discuss risk behaviors.

Abuse and Trauma History

Assessing the child's or adolescent's experience of abuse, whether physical, emotional, or sexual, requires a great deal of sensitivity and care so as not to further traumatize the young patient. It often helps to remark that the abuser's behavior was wrong and that the victim is not to blame. Natural or manmade disasters, family violence, neglect, betrayal, and/or abandonment can also be traumatic. These experiences may contribute to a variety of symptoms, including re-experiencing the trauma, sleep disruptions, and fears, which are collectively known as post-traumatic stress disorder or acute stress disorder.

Mental Status Examination

The MSE provides a snapshot of the child's or adolescent's cognitive functions. The MSE explores psychiatric symptoms and their severity and effect on the patient's and family's lives. The presenting symptoms, such as excessive worries or consuming sadness, and the family history indicate areas to be examined in depth. The MSE can be easily incorporated into primary care visits without adding significant time requirements. This assessment can provide the PCP with an initial evaluation of the mental wellbeing of the child or adolescent during the examination (Lemp et al. 2012).

Initially, the child's or adolescent's appearance is examined; this may include the head size, stature, facial expressions, eye contact, nutritional state, bruising, open sores that have been "picked" by the child, dress, motor mannerisms or tics, signs of anxiety such as chewing on fingernails, or evidences of self-harm such as scratches or knife marks. When a mark is observed, such as a burn on the hand or a scratch on the arm or leg, the child or adolescent should be asked about it ("How did this happen?") to determine if the child was burned by a cigarette, caused himself an "eraser burn," has been cutting herself, etc. Also, initially, during the child's or adolescent's separation from the parent to talk with the APRN privately, the child should be observed to determine if she has excessive difficulty in separating or an inability to do so in relation to her developmental stage. On the other hand, it should be noted if there is too much ease in separating, which is not expected in young children.

The MSE also assesses the child's or adolescent's orientation to time, place, person, and circumstances, although these may be limited in young children. That said, even young children can usually identify a big holiday that is coming up or the season of the year. Impaired orientation may be related to low intelligence, organic brain problems, or thought disorders such as schizophrenic illnesses.

Central nervous system (CNS) functioning is assessed through observing gross (throwing a ball) and fine (copying a circle, cross, triangle) motor coordination, abnormal movements, right–left discrimination, cerebellar functioning (finger-to-nose test), gait (heel-to-toe walking), and symmetry (squeezing hands of examiner). Sensory difficulties may lead to problems in school performance and should be assessed by hearing screening, audiometric testing, and vision screening or other means to determine problems in visual acuity.

Attention span is assessed through the child's ability to focus and follow through, distractibility, and disorganization. Poor attention span can be caused by other factors, such as fatigue, anxiety, language difficulties, disorders on the autism spectrum, and sedation or other effects of medication.

Activity level is a tricky issue to assess because at times a parent or grandparent may comment that a child is "hyperactive," when in fact, she has a developmentally normal activity level. Reports of the child's activity level are most helpful when they come from multiple sources, such as different classes in school and from different parenting figures. Excess activity can be due to anxiety, hypomania or mania, psychosis, or even oppositional behavior.

Academic performance should be assessed by observing the child read and write, evaluating language fluency, and noting the patient's own words about his ability to read, write, and do mathematical computations. Letter and word reversals are common in 1st graders and other young children learning to read and do not necessarily indicate the presence of a learning difference.

Speech and language difficulties may be noted because of a developmentally small vocabulary, overuse of concrete verbs and nouns, underuse of abstract words, or

nodding the head instead of clarifying through speech. Receptive language problems can also be due to a sensory impairment, mental retardation, or a pervasive developmental disorder. Expressive language problems, such as echolalia, misuse of pronouns, or difficulty using language as a means of social interaction, can be due to a language delay or impairment in speech production.

Intelligence is evaluated through the child's or adolescent's use of vocabulary, responsiveness, level of comprehension, curiosity, identification of body parts, and ability to subtract serial sevens or threes for younger children.

Memory difficulties can be due to several causes, including attention problems, anxiety, or organic brain problems. Memory is assessed by having the child repeat three items five minutes after the words are presented. Younger children can be asked what they had for supper yesterday and the names of teachers.

The quality of thinking and perception is related to both thought content and thought process or form. The child's or adolescent's disordered thought content could include hallucinations, delusions, excessive concreteness, or the use of neologisms. His disordered thought process could be seen by slowness of thinking, pressured speech, flight of ideas, muteness, or loose associations. His fantasies and feelings are assessed through his three wishes and spontaneous play or speech, including information offered about dreams and his drawings.

Affect and mood are often misinterpreted terms. When assessing affect, the APRN is looking for the objective manifestation of the child's or adolescent's emotional state, range of affect, predominant affects, and her appropriateness to the situation or content being discussed. Mood, on the other hand, is a subjective internal state and is elicited by asking the child or adolescent directly about feelings and emotions. It may be helpful to have the child or adolescent rate their mood on either a pictorial scale such as with faces or a number scale to assist in validating and objectivizing the mood level (Kennedy et al. 2015).

The risk of harm to self and others is a serious issue to explore in both children and adolescents. Even very young children can have fantasies about their death and not grasp its finality. APRNs must assess any suicidal ideation and behavior, the intent to self-harm, any attempts to self-harm, and self-injurious behavior such as cutting oneself. The APRN can help the patient to differentiate by asking, "Are you cutting to bleed or to die?" In addition, the APRN should assess whether the suicidal attempt was planned versus impulsive, performed out of desperation or depression, and whether it was a lethal act in the child's mind.

The child's or adolescent's typical defenses and ways to cope with conflicts may become evident. For example, is the adolescent's usual response avoidant, angry, phobic, inhibited, depressed, or frustrated? Interests are potential strengths for the child and adolescent. These could be hobbies, sports, favorite subjects in school, and career goals. Nurses must identify positive attributes, which may include coping skills, cooperativeness, cognitive flexibility, friendliness, and social skills, academic success and interests, intelligence, positive self-esteem, and supportive family members. Information is gathered about children's or adolescents' perception of their relationships with family, peers, and teachers and other authority figures.

Subjective Review of Systems

A complete review of systems should be conducted to elicit any report of signs or symptoms consistent with medical conditions: general, skin, head; eyes, ears, nose, and throat; and respiratory, cardiovascular, genitourinary, gastrointestinal, musculoskeletal, neurologic, endocrine. Many physical complaints may be symptoms of a mental health problem. In asking about a child's/adolescent's general health, the APRN should ask what the child's general wellbeing is and how his health compares to children of the same age. Children with various psychiatric conditions may complain of frequent blinking or difficulty swallowing, or they may hear voices. When children complain of shortness of breath the APRN should clarify when these symptoms occur. If the child/adolescent states that she feels short of breath when sitting alone or before a test rather than with activity, the APRN should consider a psychiatric cause rather than a medical one. Children who complain of chest pains and/or palpitations often have issues with anxiety. The longer the symptoms of chest pain or palpitations have been going on, the more likely they are related to mental health problems. Chronic abdominal pain, nausea, vomiting and/or diarrhea, and constipation are frequently related to mental health conditions. The child who has these symptoms with no physical cause should be referred for a psychiatric evaluation. Headaches are another common complaint that may represent mental health problems in children or adolescents.

When conducting a review of systems from children/adolescents, the APRN should ask when these symptoms presented. Physical symptoms that are associated with specific environments such as only during the school week or during testing times should alert the APRN to possible emotional causes. Symptoms that occur more often when people are present than when the child is alone are also concerning for psychosomatic causes. When children with multiple physical complaints are found to have a normal examination and normal laboratory tests, the APRN should consider the

possibility of a psychological cause. Any physical complaints from the child/adolescent should be fully evaluated during the physical examination to determine whether the child's feelings are associated with physical findings in the patient.

Physical Examination

The primary care APRN performs a comprehensive age-appropriate physical examination, recording height, weight, body mass index, and vital signs. Screening tests for hearing and vision and laboratory data are included. Elements of the examination depend on the child's age and information gathered during the review of systems and problems under consideration. A full head-to-toe physical evaluation should be performed by the APRN (Burns et al. 2017). It should include a neurologic evaluation with a developmental assessment. The provider should test reflexes, fine and gross motor skills, and mood. Any complaints the child had during the review of systems such as palpitations should be evaluated during the physical examination, with additional evaluation tools available.

For example, children who complain of chest pain or palpitations should have their heart sound auscultated as well as an electrocardiogram, and if needed a 24-hour halter monitor to be sure there is no cardiac cause for these symptoms. Throughout the physical examination, the APRN should demonstrate to the parents and child the normal findings in order to help them begin to recognize that these symptoms are not related to a physical condition. When appropriate the APRN should order laboratory tests to augment the physical evaluation; such tests might include hematocrit or other blood tests, lead level, and urinalysis.

Data from other disciplines, such as nutrition and social work, should be incorporated with other objective data. The primary care APRN uses her knowledge, experience, and clinical decision-making skills to develop diagnoses that reflect any identified disease states, daily living and developmental needs, and family issues. Evidence-based practice guidelines direct the APRN in the management of the child's physical health within the context of family and culture. Once the APRN has completed the history and physical examination and has collected all the necessary information, he must introduce the possibility of a psychological cause of the child's/adolescent's symptoms. Mental health is managed in collaboration with the PMH-APRN after psychiatric assessments are completed.

Use of Assessment Tools

The purposes of assessment tools are to further the understanding of the child or adolescent experiencing the mental disorder, to accurately diagnose, and to plan treatment recommendations (Mulvaney-Day et al. 2018). Optimal mental health screening tools should be brief and focused on the child's psychosocial functioning and the degree of interference of the child's behaviors and problems in her and the family's life. Assessment tools can augment the history and physical examination for the APRN to aid her in making the diagnosis. In busy pediatric and primary care practices, the use of brief and straightforward assessment tools can help the provider gather a wide variety of data in a relatively short amount of time. Making use of time before and after the visit increases efficiency and effectiveness (Gadomski et al. 2015). Parents and/or children can complete screening tools before the visit, which might help them organize their concerns and questions to maximize time-limited visits. The completed questionnaires can be mailed or sent electronically to the office before the visit, allowing the provider (primary care or psychiatric-mental health) the opportunity to review it in preparation for discussing the results with the parent and child or adolescent. One advantage of using parent-completed questionnaires is that the process might improve parent–provider communication (Biel et al. 2015). Providers benefit when both the children/adolescents and parents complete the forms because they gain information from both sides to optimize their evaluation process. This can be useful even when there is discrepancy between parent and youth reports (Bajeux et al. 2018; Robinson et al. 2018).

Some computer-based screening tools for children/adolescents can be used in primary care settings. Computer or web-based screenings have been shown to be both acceptable and useful for parents and youth to provide comprehensive mental health information in a timely fashion (Fothergill et al. 2013). Perceived ease of use and usefulness of the technological approach to gather sensitive information were significantly associated with satisfaction in both low-risk and high-risk patients and in all topical areas asked (Fothergill et al. 2013; Jakobsen et al. 2017). Primary care settings may choose to have adolescents use these tools while they are waiting to be seen.

Ethnic Differences Using Behavioral Rating Scales

Behavioral rating scales are helpful to the practitioner if the scale is brief, easy to use and interpret, and valid across different ages, genders, and ethnic and racial groups. The normative population, cultural sensitivity, comprehensiveness, utility in medical settings, and attractiveness to children should be considered when selecting assessment tools for use with a specific

population, and not just the established psychometric properties of the tools (Spence 2018). Behavioral rating scales are only useful if they validly reflect the phenomena being examined, i.e. the child's or adolescent's behavior and difficulties.

Review of Specific Evaluation Tools for Use in Primary Care

The following section reviews common tools that can be used in the pediatric and adolescent population in primary care settings as screening tools. They should be used in conjunction with the history and physical findings to aid the PCP to identify children and adolescents who should be referred for psychiatric evaluation and treatment.

Pediatric Symptom Checklist

The Pediatric Symptom Checklist (PSC) (Jellinek and Murphy 1988) is a one-page 35-item questionnaire designed to help the practitioner identify cognitive, emotional, and behavioral problems as perceived by a parent or other caretaker. It is appropriate for children and adolescents aged 4–18 years. Items are rated as "never", "sometimes," or "often" present and scored as 0, 1, and 2, respectively. The PSC is easy to complete and easy to score. The PSC-Youth Report (Y-PSC), a youth self-reported version of the scale, is available for older adolescents. A cutoff score of 28 or higher is indicative of psychological impairment in children and adolescents aged 6 through 16. For children aged 4 and 5, the PSC cutoff score is 24 or higher. For the Y-PSC, the cutoff score is 30 or higher. Items that are left blank are simply ignored; however, the questionnaire is invalid if four or more items are left blank (Jellinek and Murphy 1988; Jellinek et al. 1988).

A positive score suggests the need for further evaluation by a qualified health or mental health professional. Because false positives and false negatives occur, there should be no substitute for interpretation by an experienced clinician; parents and other lay people who administer the form should consult with a licensed professional if their child receives a positive score. However, it is important to note that the use of the Y-PSC continues to show robust association between symptoms and risk for mental health issues in a pediatric population (Murphy et al. 2018; Ratcliff et al. 2018). These scales are in the public domain and can be downloaded for use at http://www2.massgeneral.org/allpsych/psc/psc_home.htm. Users are encouraged to read information about the scales and scoring before first use. Copies of both the PSC and Y-PSC are included at the end of this chapter (Appendix 4.A).

Child Behavior Checklist

Parents or other individuals such as parents, teachers, social workers, or other significant adults in the child's or adolescent's life can use the Child Behavior Checklist (CBCL) (Achenbach 1991) to rate a child's problem behaviors and competencies. This tool can be self-administered or done through an interview with the parent or youth. It can be used for further evaluation if a positive score is found on the PSC. There are two versions, both of which have been revised several times from the original. The most current versions reflex DSM-5 criteria – one for children 18 months to 5 years of age (CBCL/1 1/2–5) (Achenbach 2010a, 2013) (Appendix 4.B) and another for ages 6–18 years (CBCL/6–18) (Achenbach 2010b, 2013) (Appendix 4.C). The CBCL-Youth Self Report (YSR) (Appendix 4.D) can be completed by the adolescents aged 11–18 years (Achenbach 2010c, 2013). Included with the CBCL for preschoolers is a Language Development Survey (LDS), and teacher report forms (TRF) for each age group (version of the CBCL) are also available. The CBCL consists of two sections with items on competence and behavior or emotional problems; the individual completing the scale rates how true each item is now and within the past 6 months (Achenbach and Ruffle 2000). The CBCL has been found to be a valid and reliable tool with African American, Caucasian, and Hispanic/Latino children across all socioeconomic levels (Byck et al. 2013; Rocha et al. 2013; Spencer et al. 2018). Multicultural applications of the Achenbach System of Empirically Based Assessment (ASEBA) can be used for clinical assessment in modules for each age-related CBCL across diverse cultures because problem items have been normed for multiple societies at three different levels. The examiner has the ability to select the norms most appropriate for evaluating each child (Achenbach 2018). Permission is required to use the instrument and several scoring options are available; all can be ordered at www.ASEBA.org.

Strengths and Difficulties Questionnaire

The Strengths and Difficulties Questionnaire (SDQ) is a brief screening tool aimed at assessing for psychological adjustment of adolescents and children (Goodman 1997, 2001). A 25-item questionnaire which focuses on positive and negative attributes of respondents, the SDQ scores respondents in the areas of hyperactivity-inattention, peer issue, emotional symptoms, and conduct problems as well as prosocial behaviors (Goodman 2001). Available in more than 70 languages, the SDQ can be completed by youths from ages 4–16, parents, and teachers in as little as 10–15 minutes (Borg et al. 2014; Goodman 2001). Well validated and reliable as a self-report scale (Goodman 2001), the SDQ also has been shown to have a correlation between parental reports of severity and level of functional impairments (Biel et al. 2015). Furthermore, the SDQ can be used to report out separate scores for the individual areas of assessment (Goodman 1997). The distinct advantages of the SDQ include the brevity of the scale, fitting on one page, and the identicality of the items for all respondents regardless of age or relationship to the patient, as well as its unique inclusion of strength as a factor (Goodman 2001). The SDQ has been used across diverse groups and has had positive results in applicability and prediction (Biel et al. 2015; Borg et al. 2014; Ortuno-Sierra et al. 2018). This tool is free and available for noncommercial purposes. Information for this tool can be found at http://www.sdqinfo.org.

Identifying Risk and Protective Factors

When evaluating children and adolescents for mental health problems, the APRN should assess the child and family for risk factors as well as protective factors. Risk factors are conditions in the child's life, family, environment, or personality that increase the likelihood of negative outcomes, such as the development of mental disorders. Factors that put children and adolescents at higher risk include family history of psychiatric illness and substance abuse, poor physical health, limited intelligence, weak family support, limited family resources, poverty, parental conflict and marital disruption, history of being abused or neglected, community violence (Evans 2009), damaged bonding with primary caregivers, child's temperament, and parental presence of mental health problems (Wlodarczyk et al. 2017). Internal factors such as dissatisfaction with their body and poor response to positive stimulus and external factors, such as bullying, discrimination, and peer pressures, can also predispose adolescents to mental health challenges (Pinto et al. 2014). Although the significance of genetic factors in determining the occurrence of mental illness is recognized, it is important to remember that genetic influences are modulated by environmental factors (Haworth et al. 2017).

An assessment that focuses solely on the weaknesses, problems, and limitations of children and adolescents is not a useful one, for it is their and the families' strengths and abilities which will help them develop the adequate skills needed to build resilience, reduce symptoms, and, if possible, recover from mental disorders. Identifying these protective factors is, therefore, essential. Examples of protective factors, that is, factors that decrease the likelihood of mental illness and help protect the child or adolescent from its negative effects, include healthy parenting, strong family connections, physical health, normal or higher intelligence, strong relationships with parents, and family support and resources.

Teaching Needs

Throughout the assessment process, the APRN should look for and take advantage of opportunities for mental health teaching of the child, adolescent, and family members. This includes clear, concise explanations of the assessment process and findings, reinforcing the positive actions already taken by the child or adolescent and family, and strengthening the competencies of the entire family.

Communicating Findings to Children, Adolescents, and Families

Discussing issues regarding the mental healthcare of children and adolescents can be overwhelming to the PCP. A systematic review of research of PCPs showed that many cited not only a lack of confidence in identification and diagnosis but challenges in establishing the rapport necessary for both drawing out subjective symptomatology from their young patients and for communicating concerns about mental health issues without initiating a negative or defensive response from the patient or parents (O'Brien et al. 2016). Hampton et al. (2015) interviewed 26 pediatric residents who felt that lack of comfort extended beyond concerns about diagnostic formulation and into the stigma associated with mental health. While it is prudent to use caution in placing psychiatric diagnoses on children and adolescents it is also likely that direct and open communication about a diagnosis, one that promotes both education about the diagnosis and family communication about mental health, will produce positive outcomes for the patient (Mueller et al. 2016).

There is nothing magical or mystical about psychiatric assessments, nor should the assessment findings be conveyed to parents as though there is something to be feared or that their child or adolescent is "mental." It is helpful to remember the words of Jensen et al. (1999, p. 118):

> . . .it is all too easy to reify the diagnostic labels and to forget that the labels are temporary abstractions that do not capture the complex presentation of a human being who is suffering from some mental, behavioral, or emotional difficulty within a developmental context.

Parents, grandparents, or guardians should receive clear and accurate explanations of assessment findings in a way that does not alarm them, but rather, offers hopeful ideas about treatment options. Parents must have sufficient information to make informed decisions about which treatment option or options to select.

Establishing Trust with the Child or Adolescent and Family

Bringing a child or adolescent to a psychiatric healthcare provider for a mental health issue is typically an unfamiliar event, wrought with anxiety and fear. The parent, as well as the child or adolescent, may feel defeated, hopeless, and frightened. Parents may believe that their child's problem behavior indicates that they have not been good parents and wonder whether they will be judged as inadequate or weak parents. The child or adolescent may be confused or disheartened by the looming encounter and wonder if they are "bad," "stupid," "in trouble," or whether their parents are angry at them.

On the other hand, the primary care setting is a familiar experience, one that is less likely to be threatening. The primary care APRN is usually already familiar with the family, has a trusting relationship with them, and is knowledgeable of multidisciplinary community resources that can provide further treatment for the child or adolescent and family. The importance of establishing trust cannot be overemphasized. Trust is reinforced when the APRN is calm, supportive, and knowledgeable about the types of disorders children commonly experience and their treatment, including the fact that treatment is available, because many people do not realize that mental health disorders and behavioral problems are treatable.

Referral to Mental Health Professionals

Many children and adolescents with mental health disorders are successfully treated by primary care APRNs, physicians, and others with training in treating certain disorders. The AACAP (2010) has prepared a statement, *When to Seek Referral or Consultation with a Child Adolescent Psychiatrist*, that identifies circumstances under which referral to a trained child and adolescent mental health practitioner is appropriate and preferred. Referrals can be formal, according to procedure, or informal, occurring via telephone, email, or mail consultation.

The decision to refer can be determined by a number of factors such as "the clinical presentation of the patient, training, skill and experience of the practitioner, family and environmental situation, availability of support services and personnel, and availability of a child and adolescent psychiatrist with relevant experience" (AACAP 2010, paragraph 1).

Reporting any of the following behaviors in children and adolescents represents circumstances in primary care that mandate referral (AACAP 2009, p. 6):

1. A significant change in his emotional or behavioral functioning for which there is no obvious or recognized precipitant, e.g. sudden onset of school avoidance.

2. A problem that constitutes a threat to the safety of the child/adolescent or the safety of those around her, e.g. severe aggressive behavior.
3. Significant disruption in day-to-day functioning or reality contact, e.g. repeated severe tantrums with no apparent reason.
4. Difficulty with school performance and no significant improvement after attempts by the PCP and school personnel to remediate the problems.

Emergency situations, such as suicidal behavior or suicide attempt, would not be initially managed in the primary care setting.

Referral to specialized mental health treatment has many variables. Jonovich and Alpert-Gilles (2014) found that patients and parents who voluntarily filled out a mental health questionnaire at their primary care visit were significantly more likely to be referred for counseling services. Hacker et al. (2014) found that PCPs will often refer to psychiatric care when patients ask for help, regardless of screening scores. The ultimate goal is to make sure the children receive the appropriate care from the most qualified professionals to improve long-term outcomes.

After screening in primary care, children and adolescents who have been identified with mental health disorders and behavioral problems should be referred to PMH-APRNs or other qualified mental health professionals for further evaluation and appropriate intervention, as indicated. Interventions might include care that can be directed by the PCP with consultation from the psychiatric experts. Improving patient outcomes requires the integration of collaboration between mental health experts and PCPs working together to promote the wellbeing of the child/adolescent and family (AACAP 2010). Developing efficient and effective referral systems and maintaining open communication with the various specialists, PCPs, and family are integral in assisting families as they attempt to optimize the mental health of their children.

Implications for Nursing Practice, Research, and Education

Assessment of children and adolescents for mental health disorders and behavior problems is within the scope of practice of primary care and PMH-APRNs, and every opportunity to screen should be used, especially during pediatric visits for routine primary care. APRNs must be sure to listen to parental concerns and follow through with the appropriate screening. Easy-to-use scales are available and should be accessible in all pediatric practices. The primary care APRN should refer more complex assessments to the PMH-APRN or another psychiatric provider.

Training for APRNs should include more purposeful content for physical and psychiatric assessments in undergraduate and graduate curricula. A mental health history has significant overlap and commonalities with a child's primary care health history. Teaching more critical observation skills of child behavior to students and practicing APRNs is also key to increasing the numbers of children actually being screened. Studies about child and adolescent mental health by authors from other disciplines far outnumber those conducted by nurses; more nurses must become principal or co-investigators on teams to document how effective nurses are at assessing and identifying children with mental health needs. Testing models in primary care, where nursing takes the lead, might improve access and increase opportunities for screening and early identification of children and adolescents with mental health needs.

Resources for PCPs and Families

This list includes a number of resources available for APRNs in primary care to aid in evaluating children and families. It provides access to the tools discussed in this chapter, and offers some educational and support services for families:

American Academy of Child and Adolescent Psychiatry (AACAP). http://www.aacap.org.

American Academy of Pediatrics (AAP). http://www.aap.org.

American Psychiatric Nurses Association (APNA). http://www.apna.org.

Achenbach System of Empirically Based Assessment (ASEBA). http://www.aseba.org.

Ages and Stages Questionnaire. http://www.agesandstages.com.

Bright Futures. http://www.brightfutures.org.

International Society of Psychiatric-Mental Health Nurses. http://www.ispn-psych.org.

MGH Pediatric Symptom Checklist. http://www2.massgeneral.org/allpsych/psc/psc_home.htm.

National Association of Pediatric Nurse Practitioners (NAPNAP). http://www.napnap.com.

Critical Thinking Questions

1. When assessing a child or adolescent for behavioral or physical health, how does the APRN determine whether observations and findings are within normal variation?

2. The primary care APRN completes the medical examination of a 10-year-old child but the parents will not accept the referral for behavioral health. What does the APRN do?
3. Under what circumstances might a psychiatric and primary care APRN conduct a joint psychiatric and physical assessment?

References

Achenbach, T. (1991). *Integrative Guide to the 1991 CBCL/4–18, YSR, and TRF Profiles*. Burlington, VT: University of Vermont, Department of Psychology.

Achenbach, T. (2010a). *Preschool (Ages 1 1/2–5) assessments*. Available at http://www.aseba.org/preschool.html (accessed 6 November 2010).

Achenbach, T. (2010b). *School-age (Ages 6–11) assessments*. Available at http://www.aseba.org/schoolage.html (accessed 6 November 2010).

Achenbach, T. (2010c). *YSR (Ages 11–18) assessment*. Available at http://www.aseba.org/schoolage.html (accessed 6 November 2010).

Achenbach, T. (2013). *ASEBA DSM-5 oriented scales*. Available at http://www.aseba.org/research/ASEBA DSM-5orientedscales.htm (accessed 11 January 2019).

Achenbach, T. (2018). *Multicultural applications of the ASEBA*. Available at www.Aseba.org/products/multicultural applications.html (accessed 11 January 2019).

Achenbach, T.M. and Ruffle, T.M. (2000). The child behavior checklist and related forms for assessing behavioral/emotional problems and competencies. *Pediatrics in Review* 21: 265–271.

Ackincigil, A. and Matthews, E.B. (2017). National rates and patterns of depression screening in primary care: results from 2012 and 2013. *Psychiatric Services* 68: 660–666. https://doi.org/10.1176/appi.ps.201600096.

American Academy of Child and Adolescent Psychiatry (2009). Improving mental health services in primary care: reducing administrative and financial barriers to access and collaboration. *Pediatrics* 123: 1248–1251.

American Academy of Child and Adolescent Psychiatry. (2010). *When to seek referral or consultation with a child adolescent psychiatrist*. Available at http://www.aacap.org/cs/root/member_information/practice_information/when_to_seek_referral_or_consultation_with_a_child_adolescent_psychiatrist (accessed 2 November 2010).

Ames, M.E. and Leadbeater, B.J. (2018). Depressive symptom trajectories and physical health: persistence of problems from adolescence to young adulthood. *Journal of Affective Disorders* 240: 121–129. https://doi.org/10.1016/j.jad.2018.07.001.

Arbesman, M., Bazyk, S., and Nochajski, S.M. (2013). Systematic review of occupational therapy and mental health promotion, prevention, and intervention for children and youth. *The American Journal of Occupational Therapy* 67 (6): e120–e130. https://doi.org/10.5014/ajot.2013.008359.

Bajeux, E., Klemanski, D.H., Husky, M. et al. (2018). Factors associated with parent-child discrepancies in reports of mental health disorders in young children. *Child Psychiatry and Human Development* https://doi.org/10.1007/s10578-018-0815-7.

Balázs, J., Miklósi, M., Keresztény, A. et al. (2018). Comorbidity of physical and anxiety symptoms in adolescent: functional impairment, self-rated health and subjective well-being. *International Journal of Environmental Research and Public Health* 15 (8) https://doi.org/10.3390/ijerph15081698.

Banta, J.E., Khoie-Mayer, R.N., Somaiya, C.K. et al. (2013). Mental health and food consumption among California children 5–11 years of age. *Nutrition and Health* 22 (3–4): 237–253. https://doi.org/10.1177/0260106015599511.

Bekar, Ö., Shahmoon-Shanok, R., Steele, M. et al. (2017). Effectiveness of school-based mental health playgroups for diagnosable and at-risk preschool children. *American Journal of Orthopsychiatry* 87: 304–316. https://doi.org/10.1037/ort0000173.

Benotsch, E.G., Koester, S., Martin, A.M. et al. (2014). Intentional misuse of over-the-counter medications, mental health, and polysubstance use in young adults. *Journal of Community Health* 39: 688–695. https://doi.org/10.1007/s10900-013-9811-9.

Biel, M.G., Kahn, N.F., Srivastava, A. et al. (2015). Parent reports of mental health concerns and functional impairment on routine screening with the strengths and difficulties questionnaire. *Academic Pediatrics* 15: 412–420.

Bitsko, R.H., Holbrook, J.R., Ghandour, R.M. et al. (2018). Epidemiology and impact of health care provider-diagnosed anxiety and depression among U.S. children. *Journal of Developmental & Behavioral Pediatrics* 39: 395–403. https://doi.org/10.1097/DBP.0000000000000571.

Borg, A.M., Kaukonen, P., Salmelin, R. et al. (2014). Feasibility of the strengths and difficulties questionnaire in assessing childrens' mental health in primary care: Finnish parents', teachers' and public health nurses' experiences with the SDQ. *Journal of Child and Adolescent Mental Health* 26: 229–238. https://doi.org/10.2989/17280583.2014.923432.

Burns, C.E. and Duderstadt, K.G. (2017). Child and family health assessment. In: *Pediatric Primary Care*, 6e (eds. C.E. Burns, A.M. Dunn, M.A. Brady, et al.), 10–32. St. Louis, MO: Elsevier.

Burns, C.E., Dunn, A.M., Brady, M.A. et al. (eds.) (2017). *Pediatric primary care*, 6e. St. Louis, MO: Elsevier.

Butler, A., Van Lieshout, R.J., Lipman, E.L. et al. (2018). Mental disorder in children with physical conditions: a pilot study. *BMJ Open* 8 (1): e019011. https://doi.org/10.1136/bmjopen-2017-019011.

Byck, G.R., Bolland, J., Dick, D. et al. (2013). Prevalence of mental health disorders among low-income African American adolescents. *Social Psychiatry and Psychiatric Epidemiology* 48: 1555–1567. https://doi.org/10.1007/s00127-013-0657-3.

Costello, E.J., He, J., Sampson, N.A. et al. (2014). Services for adolescents with psychiatric disorders: 12-month data from the National Comorbidity Survey–Adolescent. *Psychiatric Services* 65: 359–366. https://doi.org/10.1176/appi.ps.201100518.

Davis, D.W., Honaker, S.M., Jones, V.F. et al. (2012). Identification and management of behavioral/mental health problems in primary care pediatrics: perceived strengths, challenges, and new delivery models. *Clinical Pediatrics* 51: 978–982. https://doi.org/10.1177/0009922812441667.

Delaney, K.R. (2017). Psychiatric mental health nursing advanced practice workforce: capacity to address shortages of mental health professionals. *Psychiatric Services* 68: 952–954. https://doi.org/10.1176/appi.ps.201600405.

Dunn, A.M. (2010a). Cultural perspectives for pediatric primary care. In: *Pediatric Primary Care*, 4e (eds. C.E. Burns, A.M. Dunn, M.A. Brady, et al.), 41–50. St. Louis, MO: Saunders.

Evans, M.E. (2009). Prevention of mental, emotional, and behavioral disorders in youth: the Institute of Medicine report and implications for nursing. *Journal of Child and Adolescent Psychiatric Nursing* 22: 154–159.

Fang, D., Li, Y., Stauffer, D.C., & Trautman, D.E. (2016). *2015–2016 Enrollment and Graduations in Baccalaureate and Graduate Programs in Nursing*. Report from the American Association of Colleges of Nursing. Available at https://cdn.ymaws.com/http://www.nonpf.org/resource/resmgr/docs/NPTables15-16.pdf.

Finsaas, M.C., Bufferd, S.J., Dougherty, L.R. et al. (2018). Preschool psychiatric disorders: homotypic and heterotypic continuity through middle childhood and early adolescence. *Psychological Medicine* 48: 2159–2168. https://doi.org/10.1017/S0033291717003646.

Fothergill, K.E., Gadomski, A., Solomon, B.S. et al. (2013). Assessing the impact of a web-based comprehensive somatic and mental health screening tool in pediatric primary care. *Academic Pediatrics* 13: 340–347. https://doi.org/10.1016/j.acap.2013.04.005.

Gadomski, A.M., Fothergill, K.E., Larson, S. et al. (2015). Integrating mental health into adolescent annual visits: impact of previsit comprehensive screening on within-visit processes. *Journal of Adolescent Health* 56: 267–273. https://doi.org/10.1016/j.jadohealth.2014.11.011.

Goodman, R. (1997). The strengths and difficulties questionnaire: a research note. *Child Psychology & Psychiatry & Allied Disciplines* 38: 581–586. https://doi.org/10.1111/j.1469-7610.1997.tb01545.x.

Goodman, R. (2001). Psychometric properties of the strengths and difficulties questionnaire. *Journal of the American Academy of Child and Adolescent Psychiatry* 40: 1337–1345. https://doi.org/10.1097/00004583-20011000-0015.

Hacker, K., Arsenault, L., Franco, I. et al. (2014). Referral and follow-up after mental health screening in commercially insured adolescents. *Journal of Adolescent Health* 55 (1): 17–23. https://doi.org/10.1016/j.jadohealth.2013.12.012.

Hampton, E., Richardson, J.E., Bostwick, S. et al. (2015). The current and ideal state of mental health training: pediatric resident perspectives. *Teaching and Learning in Medicine* 27: 147–154. https://doi.org/10.1080/10401334.2015.1011653.

Hasler, B.P., Soehner, A.M., and Clark, D.B. (2015). Sleep and circadian contributions to adolescent alcohol use disorder. *Alcohol* 49: 377–387. https://doi.org/10.1016/j.alcohol.2014.06.010.

Haworth, C.M.A., Carter, K., Eley, T.C., and Plomin, R. (2017). Understanding the genetic and environmental specificity and overlap between well-being and internalizing symptoms in adolescence. *Developmental Science* 20 (2) https://doi.org/10.1111/desc.12376.

Horwitz, S.M., Storfer-Isser, A., Kerker, B.D. et al. (2015). Barriers to the identification and management of psychosocial problems: changes from 2004 to 2013. *Academic Pediatrics* 15: 613–620.

Jakobsen, M., Meyer DeMott, M.A., and Heir, T. (2017). Validity of screening for psychiatric disorders in unaccompanied minor asylum seekers: use of computer-based assessment. *Transcultural Psychiatry* 54 (5/6): 611–625. https://doi.org/10.1177/1363461517722868.

Jellinek, M.S. and Murphy, J.M. (1988). Screening for psychosocial disorders in pediatric practice. *American Journal of Diseases of Children* 142: 1153–1157.

Jellinek, M.S., Murphy, J.M., Robinson, J. et al. (1988). Pediatric symptom checklist: screening school-age children for psychosocial dysfunction. *Journal of Pediatrics* 112: 201–209.

Jensen, P.S., Brooks-Gunn, J., and Graber, J.A. (1999). Introduction – dimensional scales and diagnostic categories: constructing crosswalks for child psychopathology assessments. *Journal of American Academy of Child and Adolescent Psychiatry* 38: 118–120.

Jones, L.C., Mrug, S., Elliott, M.N. et al. (2017). Chronic physical health conditions and emotional problems from early adolescence through midadolescence. *Academic Pediatrics* 17 (6): 649–655. https://doi.org/10.1016/j.acap.2017.02.002.

Jonovich, S.J. and Alpert-Gilles, L.J. (2014). Impact of pediatric mental health screening on clinical discussion and referral for services. *Clinical Pediatrics* 53 (4): 364–371. https://doi.org/10.1177/0009922813511146.

Kennedy, H., Unnithan, R., and Wamboldt, M.Z. (2015). Assessing brief changes in adolescents' mood: development, validation, and utility of the Fast Assessment of Children's Emotions (FACE). *Journal of Pediatric Health Care* 29 (4): 335–342. https://doi.org/10.1016/j.pedhc.2015.01.004.

Knutson, K.H., Meyer, M.J., Thakrar, N., and Stein, B.D. (2018). Care coordination for youth with mental health disorders in primary care. *Clinical Pediatrics* 57: 5–10. https://doi.org/10.1177/0009922817733740.

Lemp, T., deLange, D., Radeloff, D., and Bachman, C. (2012). The clinical examination of children, adolescents and their families. In: *IACAPAP e-Textbook of Child and Adolescent Mental Health* (ed. J.M. Rey), 1–25. Geneva, Switzerland: International Association for Child and Adolescent Psychiatry and Allied Professions.

Liu, X., Chen, H., Bo, Q.-G. et al. (2017). Poor sleep quality and nightmares are associated with non-suicidal self-injury in adolescents. *European Child & Adolescent Psychiatry* 26: 271–279. https://doi.org/10.1007/s00787-016-0885-7.

Martini, R., Hilt, R., Marx L., Chenven, M., Naylor, M., Sarvet, B., & Ptakowski, K.K. (2012). *Best principles for integration of child psychiatry into the pediatric health home*. American Academy of Child and Adolescent Psychiatry. Available at https://www.aacap.org/App_Themes/AACAP/docs/clinicalpractice_center/systems_of_care/best_principles_for_integration_of_child_psychiatry_into_the_pediatric_health_home_2012.pdf.

Merikangas, K.R., He, J., Burstein, M. et al. (2010). Lifetime prevalence of mental disorders in U.S. adolescents: results from the national comorbidity survey replication – adolescent supplement (NCS-A). *Journal of the American Academy of Child and Adolescent Psychiatry* 49: 980–989.

Moens, M.A., Weeland, J., Van der Giessen, D. et al. (2018). In the eye of the beholder? Parent-observer discrepancies in parenting and child disruptive behavior assessments. *Journal of Abnormal Child Psychology* 46: 1147–1159. https://doi.org/10.1007/s10802-017-0381-7.

Mueller, J., Callanan, M.M., and Greenwood, K. (2016). Communications to children about mental illness and their role in stigma development: an integrative review. *Journal of Mental Health* 25: 62–70. https://doi.org/10.3109/09638237.2015.1021899.

Mulvaney-Day, N., Marshall, T., Downey Piscopo, K. et al. (2018). Screening for behavioral health conditions in primary care settings: a systematic review of the literature. *Journal of General Internal Medicine* 33: 335–346. https://doi.org/10.1007/s11606-017-4181-0.

Murphy, J.M., Nguyen, T., Lucke, C. et al. (2018). Adolescent self-screening for mental health problems; demonstration of an internet-based approach. *Academic Pediatrics* 18: 59–65. https://doi.org/10.1016/j.acap.2017.08.013.

Nasir, A., Watanabe-Galloway, S., and DiRenzo-Coffey, G. (2016). Health services for behavioral problems in pediatric primary care. *Journal of Behavioral Health Services and Research* 43: 396–401. https://doi.org/10.1007/s11414-014-9450-7.

National Council for Behavioral Health. (2017). *The Psychiatric Shortage: Causes and Solutions*. Available at https://www.thenationalcouncil.org/wp-content/uploads/2017/03/Psychiatric-Shortage_National-Council-.pdf.

National Research Council and Institute of Medicine (2009). *Preventing Mental, Emotional, and Behavioral Disorders Among Young People: Progress and Possibilities*. Washington, DC: The National Academies Press.

O'Brien, D., Harvey, K., Howse, J. et al. (2016). Barriers to managing child and adolescent mental health problems: a systematic review of primary care practitioners' perceptions. *British Journal of General Practice* 66: 693–707. https://doi.org/10.3399/bjgp16X687061.

Ortuno-Sierra, J., Aritio-Solana, R., and Fonseca-Pedrero, E. (2018). Mental health difficulties in children and adolescents: the study of the SDQ in the Spanish National Health Survey 2011-2012. *Psychiatry Research* 259: 236–242. https://doi.org/10.1016/j.psychres.2017.10.025.

Ozer, E.M., Zahnd, E.G., Adams, S.H. et al. (2009). Are adolescents being screened for emotional distress in primary care? *Journal of Adolescent Health* 44: 520–527.

Pidano, A.E., Honigfeld, L., Bar-Halpern, M., and Vivian, J.E. (2014). Pediatric primary care providers' relationships with mental health care providers: survey results. *Child & Youth Care Forum* 43: 135–150. https://doi.org/10.1007/s10566-013-9229-7.

Pinto, A.C.S., Luna, I.T., Sivla, A. et al. (2014). Risk factors associated with mental health issues in adolescents: an integrative review. *Revista da Escola de Enfermagem da USP* 48 (3): 555–564. https://doi.org/10.1590/S0080-623420140000300022.

Ratcliff, M.B., Catlin, P.A., Peugh, J.L. et al. (2018). Psychosocial screening among youth seeking weight management treatment. *Clinical Pediatrics* 57 (3): 277–284. https://doi.org/10.1177/0009922817715936.

Robinson, M., Doherty, D.A., Cannon, J. et al. (2018). Comparing adolescent and parent reports of externalizing problems: a longitudinal population-based study. *British Journal of Developmental Psychology* https://doi.org/10.1111/bjdp.12270.

Rocha, M.M., Rescorla, L.A., Emerich, D.R. et al. (2013). Behavioural/emotional problems in Brazilian children: findings from parents' reports on the child behavior checklist. *Epidemiology and Psychiatric Sciences* 22: 329–338. https://doi.org/10.1017/S2045796012000637.

Rubio-López, N., Morales-Suárez-Varela, M., Pico, Y. et al. (2016). Nutrient intake and depression symptoms in Spanish children: the ANIVA study. *International Journal of Environmental Research and Public Health* 13 (3) https://doi.org/10.3390/ijerph13030352.

Satiani, A., Niedermier, J., Satiani, B., and Svendsen, D.P. (2018). Projected workforce of psychiatrists in the United States: a population analysis. *Psychiatric Services* 69: 710–713. https://doi.org/10.1176/appi.ps.201700344.

Spence, S.H. (2018). Assessing anxiety disorders in children and adolescents. *Child and Adolescent Mental Health* 23: 266–282. https://doi.org/10.1111/camh.12251.

Spencer, A.E., Plasencia, N., Sun, Y. et al. (2018). Screening for attention-deficit/hyperactivity disorder and comorbidities in a diverse, urban primary care setting. *Clinical Pediatrics* 57: 1442–1452. https://doi.org/10.1177/0009922818787329.

Stein, R.E., Storfer-Isser, A., Kerker, B.D. et al. (2017). Does length of developmental behavioral pediatrics training matter? *Academic Pediatrics* 17: 61–67.

Substance Abuse and Mental Health Services Administration. (2017). *Key substance use and mental health indicators in the United States: Results from the 2016 National Survey on Drug Use and Health.* HHS Publication No. SMA 17–5044, NSDUH Series H-52. Rockville, MD: Center for Behavioral Health Statistics and Quality, Substance Abuse and Mental Health Services Administration. Available at https://www.samhsa.gov/data.

Tarini, B.A. and McInerney, J.D. (2013). Family history in primary care pediatrics. *Pediatrics* 132 (Suppl 3): S203–S210. https://doi.org/10.1542/peds.2013-1032D.

Tevie, J. and Shaya, F.T. (2015). Association between mental health and comorbid obesity and hypertension among children and adolescents in the US. *European Child & Adolescent Psychiatry* 24: 497–502. https://doi.org/10.1007/s00787-014-0598-8.

USDHHS-HRSA. (2010). *The registered nurse population: Findings from the 2008 national sample survey of registered nurses.* US Department of Health and Human Services, Health Resources and Services Administration. Available at http://bhpr.hrsa.gov/healthworkforce/rnsurvey/initialfindings2008.pdfhttp://bhpr.hrsa.gov/healthworkforce/rnsurvey/initialfindings2008.pdf.

USDHHS-HRSA. (2014). *Highlights from the 2012 national sample survey of Nurse Practitioners.* US Department of Health and Human Services, Health Resources and Services Administration. Available at https://bhw.hrsa.gov/sites/default/files/bhw/nchwa/npsurveyhighlights.pdf.

USDHHS-HRSA. (2016). *National projections of supply and demand for selected behavioral health practitioners: 2013–2025.* US Department of Health and Human Services, Health Resources and Services Administration. Available at https://bhw.hrsa.gov/sites/default/files/bhw/health-workforce-analysis/research/projections/behavioral-health2013-2025.pdf.

Van Dyk, T.R., Thompson, R.W., and Nelson, T.D. (2016). Daily bidirectional relationships between sleep and mental health symptoms in youth with emotional and behavioral problems. *Journal of Pediatric Psychology* 41: 983–992. https://doi.org/10.1093/jpepsy/jsw040.

Walker, E.R., Berry, F.W., Citron, T. et al. (2015). Psychiatric workforce needs and recommendations for the community mental health system: a state needs assessment. *Psychiatric Services* 66: 115–117. https://doi.org/10.1176/appi.ps.201400530.

Webb, M.J., Kauer, S.D., Ozer, E.M. et al. (2016). Does screening for and intervening with multiple health compromising behaviours and mental health disorders amongst young people attending primary care improve health outcomes? A systematic review. *BMC Family Practice* 17 (104) https://doi.org/10.1186/s12875-016-0504-1.

Wissow, L.S., Brown, J., Fothergill, K.E. et al. (2013). Universal mental health screening in pediatric primary care: a systematic review. *Journal of the American Academy of Child & Adolescent Psychiatry* 52: 1134–1147.

Wlodarczyk, O., Pawils, S., Metzner, F. et al. (2017). Risk and protective factors for mental health problems in preschool-aged children: cross-sectional results of the BELLA preschool study. *Child and Adolescent Psychiatry and Mental Health* 11: 12. https://doi.org/10.1186/s13034-017-0149-4.

World Health Organization (WHO) and World Organization of Family Doctors (WONCA) (2008). *Integrating Mental Health into Primary Care: A Global Perspective.* Geneva, Switzerland: WHO Press.

Appendix 4.A

A Pediatric Symptom Checklist

Emotional and physical health go together in children. Because parents are often the first to notice a problem with their child's behavior, emotions or learning, you may help your child get the best care possible by answering these questions. Please indicate which statement best describes your child.

Please mark under the heading that best describes your child:	NEVER (0)	SOMETIMES (1)	OFTEN (2)
1. Complains of aches and pains			
2. Spends more time alone			
3. Tires easily, has little energy			
4. Fidgety, unable to sit still			
5. Has trouble with teacher			
6. Less interested in school			
7. Acts as if driven by a motor			
8. Daydreams too much			
9. Distracted easily			
10. Is afraid of new situations			
11. Feels sad, unhappy			
12. Is irritable, angry			
13. Feels hopeless			
14. Has trouble concentrating			
15. Less interested in friends			
16. Fights with other children			
17. Absent from school			
18. School grades dropping			
19. Is down on him or herself			
20. Visits the doctor with doctor finding nothing wrong			
21. Has trouble sleeping			
22. Worries a lot			
23. Wants to be with you more than before			
24. Feels he or she is bad			
25. Takes unnecessary risks			
26. Gets hurt frequently			
27. Seems to be having less fun			
28. Acts younger than children his or her age			
29. Does not listen to rules			
30. Does not show feelings			
31. Does not understand other people's feelings			
32. Teases others			
33. Blames others for his or her troubles			
34. Takes things that do not belong to him or her			
35. Refuses to share			

Total score

Does your child have any emotional or behavioral problems for which she/he needs help? _____No _____Yes
Are there any services that you would like your child to receive for these problems? _____No _____Yes

If yes, what type of services? _____

© M.S. Jellinek and J.M. Murphy, Massachusetts General Hospital
English PSC. Gouverneur Revision 01-06-03.

B Pediatric Symptom Checklist – Youth Report

Please mark under the heading that best fits you:

	Never	Sometimes	Often
1. Complain of aches and pains......................................	_____	_____	_____
2. Spend more time alone..	_____	_____	_____
3. Tire easily, little energy..	_____	_____	_____
4. Fidgety, unable to sit still..	_____	_____	_____
5. Have trouble with teacher.......................................	_____	_____	_____
6. Less interested in school.................................	_____	_____	_____
7. Act as if driven by motor..	_____	_____	_____
8. Daydream too much...	_____	_____	_____
9. Distract easily..	_____	_____	_____
10. Are afraid of new situations......................................	_____	_____	_____
11. Feel sad, unhappy..	_____	_____	_____
12. Are irritable, angry..	_____	_____	_____
13. Feel hopeless..	_____	_____	_____
14. Have trouble concentrating...	_____	_____	_____
15. Less interested in friends...	_____	_____	_____
16. Fight with other children...	_____	_____	_____
17. Absent from school..	_____	_____	_____
18. School grades dropping..	_____	_____	_____
19. Down on yourself...	_____	_____	_____
20. Visit doctor with doctor finding nothing wrong.................	_____	_____	_____
21. Have trouble sleeping...	_____	_____	_____
22. Worry a lot...	_____	_____	_____
23. Want to be with parent more than before......................	_____	_____	_____
24. Feel that you are bad...	_____	_____	_____
25. Take unnecessary risks...	_____	_____	_____
26. Get hurt frequently...	_____	_____	_____
27. Seem to be having less fun...	_____	_____	_____
28. Act younger than children your age...............................	_____	_____	_____
29. Do not listen to rules...	_____	_____	_____
30. Do not show feelings..	_____	_____	_____
31. Do not understand other people's feelings....................	_____	_____	_____
32. Tease others..	_____	_____	_____
33. Blame others for your troubles...............................	_____	_____	_____
34. Take things that do not belong to you........................	_____	_____	_____
35. Refuse to share..	_____	_____	_____

Appendix 4.B

Please print.   CHILD BEHAVIOR CHECKLIST FOR AGES 1½-5

For office use only
ID #

CHILD'S FULL NAME	First	Middle	Last

PARENTS' USUAL TYPE OF WORK, even if not working now. Please be specific — for example, auto mechanic, high school teacher, homemaker, laborer, lathe operator, shoe salesman, army sergeant.

CHILD'S GENDER ☐ Boy ☐ Girl	CHILD'S AGE	CHILD'S ETHNIC GROUP OR RACE

PARENT 1 (or MOTHER) TYPE OF WORK _____

PARENT 2 (or FATHER) TYPE OF WORK _____

TODAY'S DATE Mo.____Day____Year____	CHILD'S BIRTHDATE Mo.____Day____Year____

THIS FORM FILLED OUT BY: (print your full name)

_____

Please fill out this form to reflect your view of the child's behavior even if other people might not agree. Feel free to write additional comments beside each item and in the space provided on page 2. **Be sure to answer all items.**

Your relation to child:
☐ Parent 1 (or Mother) ☐ Parent 2 (or Father) ☐ Other (specify):

Below is a list of items that describe children. For each item that describes the child **now or within the past 2 months**, please circle the **2** if the item is **very true or often true** of the child. Circle the **1** if the item is **somewhat or sometimes true** of the child. If the item is **not true** of the child, circle the **0**. Please answer all items as well as you can, even if some do not seem to apply to the child.

0 = Not True (as far as you know)   1 = Somewhat or Sometimes True   2 = Very True or Often True

0 1 2   1. Aches or pains (without medical cause; **do not** include stomach or headaches)
0 1 2   2. Acts too young for age
0 1 2   3. Afraid to try new things
0 1 2   4. Avoids looking others in the eye
0 1 2   5. Can't concentrate, can't pay attention for long
0 1 2   6. Can't sit still, restless, or hyperactive
0 1 2   7. Can't stand having things out of place
0 1 2   8. Can't stand waiting; wants everything now
0 1 2   9. Chews on things that aren't edible
0 1 2   10. Clings to adults or too dependent
0 1 2   11. Constantly seeks help
0 1 2   12. Constipated, doesn't move bowels (when not sick)
0 1 2   13. Cries a lot
0 1 2   14. Cruel to animals
0 1 2   15. Defiant
0 1 2   16. Demands must be met immediately
0 1 2   17. Destroys his/her own things
0 1 2   18. Destroys things belonging to his/her family or other children
0 1 2   19. Diarrhea or loose bowels (when not sick)
0 1 2   20. Disobedient
0 1 2   21. Disturbed by any change in routine
0 1 2   22. Doesn't want to sleep alone
0 1 2   23. Doesn't answer when people talk to him/her
0 1 2   24. Doesn't eat well (describe): _____
0 1 2   25. Doesn't get along with other children
0 1 2   26. Doesn't know how to have fun; acts like a little adult
0 1 2   27. Doesn't seem to feel guilty after misbehaving
0 1 2   28. Doesn't want to go out of home
0 1 2   29. Easily frustrated

0 1 2   30. Easily jealous
0 1 2   31. Eats or drinks things that are not food—**don't** include sweets (describe): _____
0 1 2   32. Fears certain animals, situations, or places (describe): _____
0 1 2   33. Feelings are easily hurt
0 1 2   34. Gets hurt a lot, accident-prone
0 1 2   35. Gets in many fights
0 1 2   36. Gets into everything
0 1 2   37. Gets too upset when separated from parents
0 1 2   38. Has trouble getting to sleep
0 1 2   39. Headaches (without medical cause)
0 1 2   40. Hits others
0 1 2   41. Holds his/her breath
0 1 2   42. Hurts animals or people without meaning to
0 1 2   43. Looks unhappy without good reason
0 1 2   44. Angry moods
0 1 2   45. Nausea, feels sick (without medical cause)
0 1 2   46. Nervous movements or twitching (describe): _____
0 1 2   47. Nervous, highstrung, or tense
0 1 2   48. Nightmares
0 1 2   49. Overeating
0 1 2   50. Overtired
0 1 2   51. Shows panic for no good reason
0 1 2   52. Painful bowel movements (without medical cause)
0 1 2   53. Physically attacks people
0 1 2   54. Picks nose, skin, or other parts of body (describe): _____

Be sure you answered all items. Then see other side.

Please print your answers. Be sure to answer all items.

0 = Not True (as far as you know)   1 = Somewhat or Sometimes True   2 = Very True or Often True

0	1	2	55. Plays with own sex parts too much	0	1	2	79. Rapid shifts between sadness and excitement
0	1	2	56. Poorly coordinated or clumsy				
0	1	2	57. Problems with eyes (without medical cause) (describe): _____	0	1	2	80. Strange behavior (describe): _____ _____
			_____	0	1	2	81. Stubborn, sullen, or irritable
0	1	2	58. Punishment doesn't change his/her behavior	0	1	2	82. Sudden changes in mood or feelings
0	1	2	59. Quickly shifts from one activity to another	0	1	2	83. Sulks a lot
0	1	2	60. Rashes or other skin problems (without medical cause)	0	1	2	84. Talks or cries out in sleep
				0	1	2	85. Temper tantrums or hot temper
0	1	2	61. Refuses to eat	0	1	2	86. Too concerned with neatness or cleanliness
0	1	2	62. Refuses to play active games	0	1	2	87. Too fearful or anxious
0	1	2	63. Repeatedly rocks head or body	0	1	2	88. Uncooperative
0	1	2	64. Resists going to bed at night	0	1	2	89. Underactive, slow moving, or lacks energy
0	1	2	65. Resists toilet training (describe): _____ _____	0	1	2	90. Unhappy, sad, or depressed
				0	1	2	91. Unusually loud
0	1	2	66. Screams a lot	0	1	2	92. Upset by new people or situations (describe): _____
0	1	2	67. Seems unresponsive to affection				_____
0	1	2	68. Self-conscious or easily embarrassed				
0	1	2	69. Selfish or won't share	0	1	2	93. Vomiting, throwing up (without medical cause)
0	1	2	70. Shows little affection toward people	0	1	2	94. Wakes up often at night
0	1	2	71. Shows little interest in things around him/her	0	1	2	95. Wanders away
0	1	2	72. Shows too little fear of getting hurt	0	1	2	96. Wants a lot of attention
0	1	2	73. Too shy or timid	0	1	2	97. Whining
0	1	2	74. Sleeps less than most kids during day and/or night (describe): _____ _____	0	1	2	98. Withdrawn, doesn't get involved with others
				0	1	2	99. Worries
				0	1	2	100. Please write in any problems the child has that were not listed above.
0	1	2	75. Smears or plays with bowel movements				
0	1	2	76. Speech problem (describe): _____ _____	0	1	2	_____
				0	1	2	_____
0	1	2	77. Stares into space or seems preoccupied	0	1	2	_____
0	1	2	78. Stomachaches or cramps (without medical cause)				

Please be sure you have answered all items.
Underline any you are concerned about.

Does the child have any illness or disability (either physical or mental)?   ☐ No ☐ Yes—Please describe:

What concerns you most about the child?

Please describe the best things about the child:

PAGE 2

LANGUAGE DEVELOPMENT SURVEY FOR AGES 18-35 MONTHS

For office use only
ID #

The Language Development Survey assesses children's word combinations and vocabulary. By carefully completing the Language Development Survey, you can help us obtain an accurate picture of the child's developing language. *Please print your answers. Be sure to answer all items.*

I. Was the child born earlier than the usual 9 months after conception?

☐ No   ☐ Yes—how many weeks early? _____ weeks early.

II. How much did the child weigh at birth? _____ pounds _____ ounces; or _____ grams.

III. How many ear infections did the child have before age 24 months?

☐ 0-2   ☐ 3-5   ☐ 6-8   ☐ 9 or more

IV. Is any language beside English spoken in the child's home?

☐ No   ☐ Yes—please list the languages: _____ _____

V. Has anyone in the child's family been slow in learning to talk?

☐ No   ☐ Yes—please list their relationships to the child; for example, brother, father:

_____

VI. Are you worried about the child's language development?

☐ No   ☐ Yes—why? _____

_____

VII. Does the child spontaneously say words in any language? (not just imitates or understands words)?

☐ No   ☐ Yes—if yes, please complete item VIII and page 4.

VIII. Does the child combine 2 or more words into phrases? For example: "more cookie," "car bye-bye."

☐ No   ☐ Yes—please print 5 of the child's longest and best phrases or sentences.

For each phrase that is not in English, print the name of the language.

1. _____

2. _____

3. _____

4. _____

5. _____

Be sure you answered all items. Then see other side.

PAGE 3

Please circle each word that the child says SPONTANEOUSLY (not just imitates or understands). If your child says non-English versions of words on the list, circle the English word and write the first letter of the language (e.g., S for Spanish). Please include words even if they are not pronounced clearly or are in "baby talk" (for example: "baba" for bottle).

FOODS
1. apple
2. banana
3. bread
4. butter
5. cake
6. candy
7. cereal
8. cheese
9. coffee
10. cookie
11. crackers
12. drink
13. egg
14. food
15. grapes
16. gum
17. hamburger
18. hotdog
19. ice cream
20. juice
21. meat
22. milk
23. orange
24. pizza
25. pretzel
26. raisins
27. soda
28. soup
29. spaghetti
30. tea
31. toast
32. water

TOYS
33. ball
34. balloon
35. blocks
36. book
37. crayons
38. doll
39. picture
40. present
41. slide
42. swing
43. teddy bear

OUTDOORS
44. flower
45. house
46. moon
47. rain
48. sidewalk
49. sky
50. snow
51. star
52. street
53. sun
54. tree

ANIMALS
55. bear
56. bee
57. bird
58. bug
59. bunny
60. cat
61. chicken
62. cow
63. dog
64. duck
65. elephant
66. fish
67. frog
68. horse
69. monkey
70. pig
71. puppy
72. snake
73. tiger
74. turkey
75. turtle

BODY PARTS
76. arm
77. belly button
78. bottom
79. chin
80. ear
81. elbow
82. eye
83. face
84. finger
85. foot
86. hair
87. hand
88. knee
89. leg
90. mouth
91. neck
92. nose
93. teeth
94. thumb
95. toe
96. tummy

VEHICLES
97. bike
98. boat
99. bus
100. car
101. motorcycle
102. plane
103. stroller
104. train
105. trolley
106. truck

ACTIONS
107. bath
108. breakfast
109. bring
110. catch
111. clap
112. close
113. come
114. cough
115. cut
116. dance
117. dinner
118. doodoo/poop
119. down
120. eat
121. feed
122. finish
123. fix
124. get
125. give
126. go
127. have
128. help
129. hit
130. hug
131. jump
132. kick
133. kiss
134. knock
135. look
136. love
137. lunch
138. make
139. nap
140. open
141. outside
142. pattycake
143. peekaboo
144. peepee
145. push
146. read
147. ride
148. run
149. see
150. show
151. shut
152. sing
153. sit
154. sleep
155. stop
156. take
157. throw
158. tickle
159. up
160. walk
161. want
162. wash

HOUSEHOLD
163. bathtub
164. bed
165. blanket
166. bottle
167. bowl
168. chair
169. clock
170. crib
171. cup
172. door
173. floor
174. fork
175. glass
176. knife
177. light
178. mirror
179. pillow
180. plate
181. potty
182. radio
183. room
184. sink
185. soap
186. spoon
187. stairs
188. table
189. telephone
190. towel
191. trash
192. T.V.
193. window

PERSONAL
194. brush
195. comb
196. glasses
197. key
198. money
199. paper
200. pen
201. pencil
202. penny
203. pocketbook
204. tissue
205. tooth brush
206. umbrella
207. watch

PLACES
208. church
209. home
210. hospital
211. library
212. park
213. school
214. store
215. zoo

MODIFIERS
216. all gone
217. all right
218. bad
219. big
220. black
221. blue
222. broken
223. clean
224. cold
225. dark
226. dirty
227. dry
228. good
229. happy
230. heavy
231. hot
232. hungry
233. little
234. mine
235. more
236. nice
237. pretty
238. red
239. stinky
240. that
241. this
242. tired
243. wet
244. white
245. yellow
246. yucky

CLOTHES
247. belt
248. boots
249. coat
250. diaper
251. dress
252. gloves
253. hat
254. jacket
255. mittens
256. pajamas
257. pants
258. shirt
259. shoes
260. slippers
261. sneakers
262. socks
263. sweater

OTHER
264. any letter
265. away
266. booboo
267. byebye
268. excuse me
269. here
270. hi, hello
271. in
272. me
273. meow
274. my
275. myself
276. nightnight
277. no
278. off
279. on
280. out
281. please
282. Sesame St.
283. shut up
284. thank you
285. there
286. under
287. welcome
288. what
289. where
290. why
291. woofwoof
292. yes
293. you
294. yumyum
295. any number

PEOPLE
296. aunt
297. baby
298. boy
299. daddy
300. doctor
301. girl
302. grandma
303. grandpa
304. lady
305. man
306. mommy
307. own name
308. pet name
309. uncle
310. name of TV or story character

Other words your child says, including non-English words:

_____
_____
_____
_____

PAGE 4

Source: T. Achenbach & L. Rescorla, ASEBA, University of Vermont, 1 South Prospect St., Burlington, VT 05401-3456, www.ASEBA.org.
© 2000, T. Achenbach & L. Rescorla.

Appendix 4.C

Please print   CHILD BEHAVIOR CHECKLIST FOR AGES 6-18

For office use only
ID #

CHILD'S FULL NAME	First	Middle	Last

PARENTS' USUAL TYPE OF WORK, even if not working now. *(Please be specific — for example, auto mechanic, high school teacher, homemaker, laborer, lathe operator, shoe salesman, army sergeant.)*

PARENT 1 (or FATHER) TYPE OF WORK_____

PARENT 2 (or MOTHER) TYPE OF WORK_____

CHILD'S GENDER ☐ Boy ☐ Girl	CHILD'S AGE	CHILD'S ETHNIC GROUP OR RACE

TODAY'S DATE   Mo. ____ Day ____ Year ____   CHILD'S BIRTHDATE   Mo. ____ Day ____ Year ____

THIS FORM FILLED OUT BY: (print your full name)
_____

GRADE IN SCHOOL_____

NOT ATTENDING SCHOOL ☐

Please fill out this form to reflect *your* view of the child's behavior even if other people might not agree. Feel free to print additional comments beside each item and in the space provided on page 2. *Be sure to answer all items.*

Your gender: ☐ Man ☐ Woman ☐ Other (specify)

Your relation to the child:
☐ Biological Parent ☐ Step Parent ☐ Grandparent
☐ Adoptive Parent ☐ Foster Parent ☐ Other (specify):

I. Please list the sports your child most likes to take part in. For example: swimming, baseball, skating, skate boarding, bike riding, fishing, etc.

☐ None

a. _____
b. _____
c. _____

Compared to others of the same age, about how much time does he/she spend in each?

Less Than Average / Average / More Than Average / Don't Know

Compared to others of the same age, how well does he/she do each one?

Below Average / Average / Above Average / Don't Know

II. Please list your child's favorite hobbies, activities, and games, other than sports. For example: video games, dolls, reading, piano, crafts, cars, computers, singing, etc. (Do *not* include listening to radio, TV, or other media.)

☐ None

a. _____
b. _____
c. _____

Compared to others of the same age, about how much time does he/she spend in each?

Less Than Average / Average / More Than Average / Don't Know

Compared to others of the same age, how well does he/she do each one?

Below Average / Average / Above Average / Don't Know

III. Please list any organizations, clubs, teams, or groups your child belongs to.

☐ None

a. _____
b. _____
c. _____

Compared to others of the same age, how active is he/she in each?

Less Active / Average / More Active / Don't Know

IV. Please list any jobs or chores your child has. For example: doing dishes, babysitting, making bed, working in store, etc. (Include both paid and unpaid jobs and chores.)

☐ None

a. _____
b. _____
c. _____

Compared to others of the same age, how well does he/she carry them out?

Below Average / Average / Above Average / Don't Know

Be sure you answered all items. Then see other side.

Please print. Be sure to answer all items.

V. 1. About how many close friends do you have? (Do *not* include brothers & sisters)

☐ None   ☐ 1   ☐ 2 or 3   ☐ 4 or more

2. About how many times a week do you do things with any friends outside of regular school hours?

(Do *not* include brothers & sisters)   ☐ Less than 1   ☐ 1 or 2   ☐ 3 or more

VI. Compared to others of your age, how well do you:

	Worse	Average	Better	
a. Get along with your brothers & sisters?	☐	☐	☐	☐ I have no brothers or sisters
b. Get along with other kids?	☐	☐	☐	
c. Get along with your parents?	☐	☐	☐	
d. Do things by yourself?	☐	☐	☐	

VII. 1. Performance in academic subjects.   ☐ I do not attend school because _____

Other academic subjects–for example: computer courses, foreign language, business. Do *not* include gym, shop, driver's ed., or other nonacademic subjects.

Check a box for each subject that you take	Failing	Below Average	Average	Above Average
a. English or Language Arts	☐	☐	☐	☐
b. History or Social Studies	☐	☐	☐	☐
c. Arithmetic or Math	☐	☐	☐	☐
d. Science	☐	☐	☐	☐
e. _____	☐	☐	☐	☐
f. _____	☐	☐	☐	☐
g. _____	☐	☐	☐	☐

Do you have any illness, disability, or handicap?   ☐ No   ☐ Yes—please describe:

Please describe any concerns or problems you have about school:

Please describe any other concerns you have:

Please describe the best things about yourself:

PAGE 2   *Be sure you answered all items.*

Please print. Be sure to answer all items.

Below is a list of items that describe children and youths. For each item that describes your child *now or within the past 6 months*, please circle the *2* if the item is *very true or often true* of your child. Circle the *1* if the item is *somewhat or sometimes true* of your child. If the item is *not true* of your child, circle the *0*. Please answer all items as well as you can, even if some do not seem to apply to your child.

0 = Not True (as far as you know)   **1 = Somewhat or Sometimes True**   **2 = Very True or Often True**

0 1 2	1. Acts too young for his/her age	0 1 2	32. Feels he/she has to be perfect
0 1 2	2. Drinks alcohol without parents' approval (describe):	0 1 2	33. Feels or complains that no one loves him/her
0 1 2	3. Argues a lot	0 1 2	34. Feels others are out to get him/her
0 1 2	4. Fails to finish things he/she starts	0 1 2	35. Feels worthless or inferior
0 1 2	5. There is very little he/she enjoys	0 1 2	36. Gets hurt a lot, accident-prone
0 1 2	6. Bowel movements outside toilet	0 1 2	37. Gets in many fights
0 1 2	7. Bragging, boasting	0 1 2	38. Gets teased a lot
0 1 2	8. Can't concentrate, can't pay attention for long	0 1 2	39. Hangs around with others who get in trouble
0 1 2	9. Can't get his/her mind off certain thoughts; obsessions (describe):	0 1 2	40. Hears sound or voices that aren't there (describe):
0 1 2	10. Can't sit still, restless, or hyperactive	0 1 2	41. Impulsive or acts without thinking
0 1 2	11. Clings to adults or too dependent	0 1 2	42. Would rather be alone than with others
0 1 2	12. Complains of loneliness	0 1 2	43. Lying or cheating
0 1 2	13. Confused or seems to be in a fog	0 1 2	44. Bites fingernails
0 1 2	14. Cries a lot	0 1 2	45. Nervous, highstrung, or tense
0 1 2	15. Cruel to animals	0 1 2	46. Nervous movements or twitching (describe):
0 1 2	16. Cruelty, bullying, or meanness to others	0 1 2	47. Nightmares
0 1 2	17. Daydreams or gets lost in his/her thoughts	0 1 2	48. Not liked by other kids
0 1 2	18. Deliberately harms self or attempts suicide	0 1 2	49. Constipated, doesn't move bowels
0 1 2	19. Demands a lot of attention	0 1 2	50. Too fearful or anxious
0 1 2	20. Destroys his/her own things	0 1 2	51. Feels dizzy or lightheaded
0 1 2	21. Destroys things belonging to his/her family or others	0 1 2	52. Feels too guilty
0 1 2	22. Disobedient at home	0 1 2	53. Overeating
0 1 2	23. Disobedient at school	0 1 2	54. Overtired without good reason
0 1 2	24. Doesn't eat well	0 1 2	55. Overweight
0 1 2	25. Doesn't get along with other kids		56. Physical problems *without know medical cause:*
0 1 2	26. Doesn't seem to feel guilty after misbehaving	0 1 2	a. Aches or pains (*not* stomach or headaches)
0 1 2	27. Easily jealous	0 1 2	b. Headaches
0 1 2	28. Breaks rules at home, school, or elsewhere	0 1 2	c. Nausea, feels sick
0 1 2	29. Fears certain animals, situations, or places, other than school (describe):	0 1 2	d. Problems with eyes (*not* if corrected by glasses) (describe):
0 1 2	30. Fears going to school	0 1 2	e. Rashes or other skin problems
0 1 2	31. Fears he/she might think or do something bad	0 1 2	f. Stomachaches
		0 1 2	g. Vomiting, throwing up
		0 1 2	h. Other (describe):

Please print. Be sure to answer all items.

0 = Not True (as far as you know)   1 = Somewhat or Sometimes True   2 = Very True or Often True

0 1 2	57. Physically attacks people		0 1 2	84. Strange behavior (describe):
0 1 2	58. Picks nose, skin, or other parts of body (describe):		0 1 2	85. Strange ideas (describe):
0 1 2	59. Plays with own sex parts in public		0 1 2	86. Stubborn, sullen, or irritable
0 1 2	60. Plays with own sex parts too much		0 1 2	87. Sudden changes in mood or feelings
0 1 2	61. Poor school work		0 1 2	88. Sulks a lot
0 1 2	62. Poorly coordinated or clumsy		0 1 2	89. Suspicious
0 1 2	63. Prefers being with older kids		0 1 2	90. Swearing or obscene language
0 1 2	64. Prefers being with younger kids		0 1 2	91. Talks about killing self
0 1 2	65. Refuses to talk		0 1 2	92. Talks or walks in sleep (describe):
0 1 2	66. Repeats certain acts over and over; compulsions (describe):		0 1 2	93. Talks too much
			0 1 2	94. Teases a lot
0 1 2	67. Runs away from home		0 1 2	95. Temper tantrums or hot temper
0 1 2	68. Screams a lot		0 1 2	96. Thinks about sex too much
0 1 2	69. Secretive, keeps things to self		0 1 2	97. Threatens people
0 1 2	70. Sees things that aren't there (describe):		0 1 2	98. Thumb-sucking
			0 1 2	99. Smokes, chews, or sniffs tobacco
0 1 2	71. Self-conscious or easily embarrassed		0 1 2	100. Trouble sleeping (describe):
0 1 2	72. Sets fires			
0 1 2	73. Sexual problems (describe):		0 1 2	101. Truancy, skips school
0 1 2	74. Showing off or clowning		0 1 2	102. Underactive, slow moving, or lacks energy
0 1 2	75. Too shy or timid		0 1 2	103. Unhappy, sad, or depressed
0 1 2	76. Sleeps less than most kids		0 1 2	104. Unusually loud
0 1 2	77. Sleeps more than most kids during day and/or night (describe):		0 1 2	105. Uses drugs for nonmedical purposes (**don't** include alcohol or tobacco) (describe):
0 1 2	78. Inattentive or easily distracted		0 1 2	106. Vandalism
0 1 2	79. Speech problem (describe):		0 1 2	107. Wets self during the day
			0 1 2	108. Wets the bed
0 1 2	80. Stares blankly		0 1 2	109. Whining
0 1 2	81. Steals at home		0 1 2	110. Wishes to be of opposite sex
0 1 2	82. Steals outside the home		0 1 2	111. Withdrawn, doesn't get involved with others
0 1 2	83. Stores up too many things he/she doesn't need (describe):		0 1 2	112. Worries
				113. Please write in any problems your child has that were not listed above:
			0 1 2	
			0 1 2	
			0 1 2	

PAGE 4   **Please be sure you answered all items.**

Source: T. Achenbach, ASEBA, University of Vermont, 1 South Prospect St., Burlington, VT 05401-3456. HYPERLINK "http://www.ASEBA.org" www.ASEBA.org © 2001, T. Achenbach.

Appendix 4.D

Please print   **YOUTH SELF-REPORT FOR AGES 11-18**   For office use only ID #

YOUR FULL NAME	First	Middle	Last	PARENTS' USUAL TYPE OF WORK, even if not working now. *(Please be specific — for example, auto mechanic, high school teacher, homemaker, laborer, lathe operator, shoe salesman, army sergeant.)*

YOUR GENDER ☐ Boy ☐ Girl	YOUR AGE	YOUR ETHNIC GROUP OR RACE	PARENT 1 (or father) _____

TODAY'S DATE Mo. ____ Date ____ Yr. ____	YOUR BIRTHDATE Mo. ____ Date ____ Yr. ____	PARENT 2 (or mother) _____

GRADE IN SCHOOL _____

NOT ATTENDING SCHOOL ☐

IF YOU ARE WORKING, PLEASE STATE YOUR TYPE OF WORK:

Please fill out this form to reflect *your* views, even if other people might not agree. Feel free to print additional comments beside each item and in the spaces provided on pages 2 and 4. *Be sure to answer all items.*

I. Please list the sports you most like to take part in. For example: swimming, baseball, skating, skate boarding, bike riding, fishing, etc.

☐ None

Compared to others of your age, about how much time do you spend in each?

Compared to others of your age, how well do you do each one?

	Less Than Average	Average	More Than Average		Below Average	Average	Above Average
a. _____	☐	☐	☐		☐	☐	☐
b. _____	☐	☐	☐		☐	☐	☐
c. _____	☐	☐	☐		☐	☐	☐

II. Please list your favorite hobbies, activities, and games, other than sports. For example: video games, cards, reading, piano, cars, computers, crafts, etc. (Do *not* include listening to radio, watching TV, or other media.)

☐ None

Compared to others of your age, about how much time do you spend in each?

Compared to others of your age, how well do you do each one?

	Less Than Average	Average	More Than Average		Below Average	Average	Above Average
a. _____	☐	☐	☐		☐	☐	☐
b. _____	☐	☐	☐		☐	☐	☐
c. _____	☐	☐	☐		☐	☐	☐

III. Please list any organizations, clubs, teams, or groups you belong to.

☐ None

Compared to others of your age, how active are you in each?

	Less Active	Average	More Active
a. _____	☐	☐	☐
b. _____	☐	☐	☐
c. _____	☐	☐	☐

IV. Please list any jobs or chores you have. For example: doing dishes, babysitting, making bed, working in store, etc. (Include *both* paid and unpaid jobs and chores.)

☐ None

Compared to others of your age, how well do you carry them out?

	Below Average	Average	Above Average
a. _____	☐	☐	☐
b. _____	☐	☐	☐
c. _____	☐	☐	☐

Be sure you answered all items. Then see other side.

Please print. Be sure to answer all items.

V. 1. About how many close friends does your child have? (Do *not* include brothers & sisters)

☐ None   ☐ 1   ☐ 2 or 3   ☐ 4 or more

2. About how many times a week does your child do things with any friends outside of regular school hours? (Do *not* include brothers & sisters)   ☐ Less than 1   ☐ 1 or 2   ☐ 3 or more

VI. Compared to others of his/her age, how well does your child:

	Worse	Average	Better	
a. Get along with his/her brothers & sisters?	☐	☐	☐	☐ Has no brothers or sisters
b. Get along with other kids?	☐	☐	☐	
c. Behave with his/her parents?	☐	☐	☐	
d. Play and work alone?	☐	☐	☐	

VII. 1. Performance in academic subjects.   ☐ Does not attend school because _____

Other academic subjects–for example: computer courses, foreign language, business. Do not *include gym, shop, driver's ed., or other nonacademic subjects.*

Check a box for each subject that child takes	Failing	Below Average	Average	Above Average
a. Reading, English, or Language Arts	☐	☐	☐	☐
b. History or Social Studies	☐	☐	☐	☐
c. Arithmetic or Math	☐	☐	☐	☐
d. Science	☐	☐	☐	☐
e. _____	☐	☐	☐	☐
f. _____	☐	☐	☐	☐
g. _____	☐	☐	☐	☐

2. Does your child receive special education or remedial services or attend a special class or special school?

☐ No   ☐ Yes—kind of services, class, or school:

3. Has your child repeated any grades?   ☐ No   ☐ Yes—grades and reasons:

4. Has your child had any academic or other problems in school?   ☐ No   ☐ Yes—please describe:

When did these problems start?

Have these problems ended?   ☐ No   ☐ Yes–when?

Does your child have any illness or disability (either physical or mental)?   ☐ No   ☐ Yes—please describe:

What concerns you most about your child?

Please describe the best things about your child.

Please print. Be sure to answer all items.

Below is a list of items that describe kids. For each item that describes you *now or within the past 6 months*, please circle the **2** if the item is *very true or often true* of you. Circle the **1** if the item is *somewhat or sometimes true* of you. If the item is *not true* of you, circle the *0*.

0 = Not True	1 = Somewhat or Sometimes True	2 = Very True or Often True

0 1 2	1. I act too young for my age	0 1 2	33. I feel that no one loves me
0 1 2	2. I drink alcohol without my parents' approval (describe): _____	0 1 2	34. I feel that others are out to get me
		0 1 2	35. I feel worthless or inferior
		0 1 2	36. I accidentally get hurt a lot
0 1 2	3. I argue a lot	0 1 2	37. I get in many fights
0 1 2	4. I fail to finish things that I start	0 1 2	38. I get teased a lot
0 1 2	5. There is very little that I enjoy	0 1 2	39. I hang around with kids who get in trouble
0 1 2	6. I like animals	0 1 2	40. I hear sounds or voices that other people think aren't there (describe): _____
0 1 2	7. I brag		
0 1 2	8. I have trouble concentrating or paying attention		
0 1 2	9. I can't get my mind off certain thoughts; (describe): _____	0 1 2	41. I act without stopping to think
		0 1 2	42. I would rather be alone than with others
0 1 2	10. I have trouble sitting still	0 1 2	43. I lie or cheat
0 1 2	11. I'm too dependent on adults	0 1 2	44. I bite my fingernails
0 1 2	12. I feel lonely	0 1 2	45. I am nervous or tense
0 1 2	13. I feel confused or in a fog	0 1 2	46. Parts of my body twitch or make nervous movements (describe): _____
0 1 2	14. I cry a lot		
0 1 2	15. I am pretty honest		
0 1 2	16. I am mean to others		
0 1 2	17. I daydream a lot	0 1 2	47. I have nightmares
0 1 2	18. I deliberately try to hurt or kill myself	0 1 2	48. I am not liked by other kids
0 1 2	19. I try to get a lot of attention	0 1 2	49. I can do certain things better than most kids
0 1 2	20. I destroy my own things	0 1 2	50. I am too fearful or anxious
0 1 2	21. I destroy things belonging to others	0 1 2	51. I feel dizzy or lightheaded
0 1 2	22. I disobey my parents	0 1 2	52. I feel too guilty
0 1 2	23. I disobey at school	0 1 2	53. I eat too much
0 1 2	24. I don't eat as well as I should	0 1 2	54. I feel overtired without good reason
0 1 2	25. I don't get along with other kids	0 1 2	55. I am overweight
0 1 2	26. I don't feel guilty after doing something I shouldn't		56. Physical problems *without known medical cause:*
		0 1 2	a. Aches or pains (*not* stomach or headaches)
0 1 2	27. I am jealous of others	0 1 2	b. Headaches
0 1 2	28. I break rules at home, school, or elsewhere	0 1 2	c. Nausea, feel sick
0 1 2	29. I am afraid of certain animals, situations, or places, other than school (describe): _____	0 1 2	d. Problems with eyes (*not* if corrected by glasses) (describe): _____
		0 1 2	e. Rashes or other skin problems
0 1 2	30. I am afraid of going to school	0 1 2	f. Stomachaches
0 1 2	31. I am afraid I might think or do something bad	0 1 2	g. Vomiting, throwing up
0 1 2	32. I feel that I have to be perfect	0 1 2	h. Other (describe): _____

Be sure you answered all items. Then see other side.

Please print. Be sure to answer all items.

0 = Not True	1 = Somewhat or Sometimes True	2 = Very True or Often True

0 1 2   57. I physically attack people

0 1 2   58. I pick my skin or other parts of my body
              (describe): _____
              _____

0 1 2   59. I can be pretty friendly

0 1 2   60. I like to try new things

0 1 2   61. My school work is poor

0 1 2   62. I am poorly coordinated or clumsy

0 1 2   63. I would rather be with older kids than kids my
              own age

0 1 2   64. I would rather be with younger kids than kids
              my own age

0 1 2   65. I refuse to talk

0 1 2   66. I repeat certain acts over and over (describe):
              _____
              _____

0 1 2   67. I run away from home

0 1 2   68. I scream a lot

0 1 2   69. I am secretive or keep things to myself

0 1 2   70. I see things that other people think aren't
              there (describe):_____
              _____

0 1 2   71. I am self-conscious or easily embarrassed

0 1 2   72. I set fires

0 1 2   73. I can work well with my hands

0 1 2   74. I show off or clown

0 1 2   75. I am too shy or timid

0 1 2   76. I sleep less than most kids

0 1 2   77. I sleep more than most kids during day and/or
              night (describe): _____
              _____

0 1 2   78. I am inattentive or easily distracted

0 1 2   79. I have a speech problem (describe): _____
              _____

0 1 2   80. I stand up for my rights

0 1 2   81. I steal at home

0 1 2   82. I steal from places other than home

0 1 2   83. I store up too many things I don't need
              (describe): _____
              _____

0 1 2   84. I do things other people think are strange
              (describe): _____
              _____

0 1 2   85. I have thoughts that other people would think
              are strange (describe):_____
              _____

0 1 2   86. I am stubborn

0 1 2   87. My moods or feelings change suddenly

0 1 2   88. I enjoy being with people

0 1 2   89. I am suspicious

0 1 2   90. I swear or use dirty language

0 1 2   91. I think about killing myself

0 1 2   92. I like to make others laugh

0 1 2   93. I talk too much

0 1 2   94. I tease others a lot

0 1 2   95. I have a hot temper

0 1 2   96. I think about sex too much

0 1 2   97. I threaten to hurt people

0 1 2   98. I like to help others

0 1 2   99. I smoke, chew, or sniff tobacco

0 1 2   100. I have trouble sleeping (describe): _____
               _____

0 1 2   101. I cut classes or skip school

0 1 2   102. I don't have much energy

0 1 2   103. I am unhappy, sad, or depressed

0 1 2   104. I am louder than other kids

0 1 2   105. I use drugs for nonmedical purposes (**don't**
               include alcohol or tobacco) (describe): _____
               _____
               _____

0 1 2   106. I like to be fair to others

0 1 2   107. I enjoy a good joke

0 1 2   108. I like to take life easy

0 1 2   109. I try to help other people when I can

0 1 2   110. I wish I were of the opposite sex

0 1 2   111. I keep from getting involved with others

0 1 2   112. I worry a lot

Please be sure you answered all items.

Please write down anything else that describes your feelings, behavior, or interests:

Source: T. Achenbach, ASEBA, University of Vermont, 1 South Prospect St., Burlington, VT 05401-3456. www.ASEBA.org © 2001, T. Achenbach.

5

Child Sexual Development

Gabrielle Abelard[1] and Emma Dundon[2]

[1] Psychiatric Mental Health Nurse Practitioner Program, University of Massachusetts College of Nursing, Amherst, MA, USA
[2] University of Massachusetts College of Nursing, Amherst, MA, USA

Objectives

After reading this chapter, advanced practice registered nurses (APRNs) will be able to:

1. Discuss development of sexuality from infancy to beginning adolescence.
2. Identify abnormal child sexual development.
3. Assess external influences (social and environmental) that may affect child sexual development.
4. Discuss the role of the APRN in screening for abnormal child sexual development in primary care and psychiatric settings.

Introduction

This chapter will discuss normal and abnormal sexual development during childhood. The advanced practice registered nurse (APRN) will be provided with biological data that will serve as a guide during physical assessment and screening, and will be helpful when conducting child and family psychoeducation. APRNs are frequently at the forefront to intervene with children during times of crisis involving sexual issues and any mental health issues related to these developmental challenges. The authors want to stress the importance of assessment and screening in primary care, of APRN management of minor psychosocial issues associated with sexual development, and of having sensitivity and knowledge of factual information when working with families of children experiencing deviations in sexual development. As will

be stated throughout this text, early case findings of more complex mental health challenges related to sexual development must be referred immediately to a trained mental health professional, including APRNs.

Sexuality in Infancy and Childhood

Healthy parent–child interaction during infancy, toddler-hood, and beyond involves physical contact (hugging, stroking, and kissing) and responsiveness, activities needed for the establishment of trust (Gerlt and Blosser 2016). Normal sexual development begins early with the infant's relationships with primary caregivers (Gleason and Zeanah 2016).

It is estimated that the incidence of genital anomalies could be 1 in 300 births (Rothkopf and John 2014). Called disorders of sexual development (DSD), these

---

generally present in infancy and are largely related to congenital conditions where there is abnormal development of chromosomal, gonadal, or anatomic sex (McCann-Crosby and Sutton 2015). These disorders may present in the newborn when genitalia make sexual assignments ambiguous. The differential diagnosis is difficult and requires complex management of physical, emotional, and family issues. Diagnosing these disorders evident in infancy may require karyotype assessment, hormone levels, urinalysis, imaging, magnetic resonance imaging (MRI), ultrasound, and assessment of sexual chromosomes. Many DSDs are associated with underlying medical issues and require intervention into childhood (Rothkopf and John 2014).

From a psychosocial perspective nurses are key in providing family support and care to parents experiencing DSD in their newborn. Rothkopf and John emphasize that the nurse must be an advocate for the infant given that they cannot express their wishes. Patient-centered care involves focusing on the wellbeing of the child and family by providing education, protection, and advocacy. This extends through childhood and into adolescence.

Preschool and school-age children are curious about their bodies and will engage in self-stimulation and self-exploration without erotic meaning. The fact that their self-stimulation results in a pleasurable feeling prompts repeating the behavior. Parents should be taught that this is normal behavior and that they should not belittle or overreact when this occurs. Instead, they should talk to their youngsters about appropriate names for body parts, one's body being private, good touch/bad touch, and the importance of respectfully conducting self-stimulating activities in private. Children may engage in more provocative behaviors by using language or behaviors centered on sexual exploration to test parental reaction. Parents should be encouraged to minimize reactivity and punishing or condemning these behaviors as that may give the child the impression that there is something wrong with his or her sexual expressions. Parents and primary care APRNs should be open to discussing sexuality and answering any questions children may have without exhaustive and complicated responses. The use of simple language and visual aids to help explain normal sexual development, at age-appropriate times, is helpful in educating children, responding to questions they might have, and minimizing anxiety around their development.

School-age and preadolescent children vacillate between inhibition and disinhibition of their sexual fantasies. Adults may notice more silliness around discussing body parts or gender differences, embarrassment over body changes or new attraction to peers, attentiveness to

media information about sexual development, and a desire for more privacy when changing clothes. During primary care visits, both the child and the parent should be asked questions about normal sexual curiosity and whether the child is engaging in behaviors of concern to the child, parent, or school. If sexual behaviors are worrisome or causing concerns with other peers or the school, further assessment and evaluation may be warranted to rule out an inappropriate sexual event. Often children will be able to use dolls, drawings, or other play therapy techniques to divulge an inappropriate sexual act that they have experienced.

Physical Development in Females

Until puberty the bodies of boys and girls are similar except for the genitalia. The physical, emotional, and hormonal changes of puberty can begin to develop well before a child is chronologically a teenager. The timing of puberty differs between the sexes, with girls starting puberty around the age of 10 and boys following 2 years later. Tanner stages describe the sequence of pubertal development, including breast development for girls, genital development for boys, and the growth of pubic hair for both sexes (Marshall and Tanner 1969, 1970).

The Tanner stages of female puberty begin with Stage 1 in which there is minimal breast development and no public hair, followed by Stage 2 in which there is elevation of breast and papilla with enlarged diameter of areola. Hair growth begins as sparse and downy along labia. In Stage 3 there is further development of the breast and areola with darker, coarser hair spreading over the public junction. In Stage 4 the areola and papilla are enlarged to form a secondary mound above the level of the breast. There is also adult type hair that spreads to the medial surface of the thighs. In Stage 5 there is mature development with adult breasts and hair (Marshall and Tanner 1969).

The sequence of pubertal development in girls generally begins with the emergence of breast buds (thelarche) followed by the appearance of pubic hair (puberache). In a small population of girls puberache will occur before thelarche. Menarche, the initiation of the first menstrual cycle, usually occurs 2 years after the onset of puberty. Historically, this has occurred during mid-adolescence between the ages of 13 and 14. However, the age of menarche has been variable across birth decades over the past 50 years and varies depending on socioeconomic status and race/ethnicity (Krieger et al. 2015; Walvoord 2010). It is not uncommon for a female to have irregular cycles during the initial stages of menarche, especially during the first year after menarche. The first year is often marked with a majority of anovulatory cycles (absence of ovulation) which changes over time. By the third year post menarche, only half of the teen's cycles will be anovulatory, in contrast to year six post menarche when the majority of the cycles will be ovulatory.

Amenorrhea is the absence of menstruation, either transiently or permanently, due to either pregnancy or a variety of endocrine or anatomical anomalies, and can be classified as either primary or secondary. Primary amenorrhea is failure of the menses to occur by either the age of 16 or 2 years after the onset of puberty or absence of menses by age 13 in the absence of secondary sex characteristics. The presence of secondary sexual characteristics indicates normal hormonal function, suggesting that the amenorrhea is ovulatory and due to an obstruction. If secondary sex characteristics are absent, amenorrhea is anovulatory and likely due to a genetic or hormonal disorder.

Secondary amenorrhea is diagnosed when there is an absence of menses for 6 months after previously normal periods and is usually secondary to another disorder. A careful history is necessary to help determine the cause. For example, galactorrhea in the absence of periods may be due to hyperprolactinemia, symptoms of estrogen deficiency (i.e. hot flashes, vaginal dryness, night sweats) may signal premature ovarian failure, and virilization may indicate an androgen excess. The most common causes of amenorrhea are pregnancy (for those of reproductive age), constitutional delay of puberty, functional hypothalamic anovulation, use or abuse of certain medications, breastfeeding, or polycystic ovarian syndrome. Pregnancy should not be ruled out based on history only; testing is required for secondary amenorrhea. Pregnancy can occur prior to the first menstrual period.

Anovulatory amenorrhea is due to a disruption of the hypothalamic–pituitary–ovarian axis. Causes can be due to a hypothalamic or pituitary disorder, ovarian failure, or androgen excess. *Ovulatory amenorrhea* is due to chromosomal abnormalities or other congenital anatomical abnormalities that could cause an obstruction in the menstrual flow. Treatments are based on the underlying cause. A patient with secondary amenorrhea and normal hormonal levels may be given a trial of progesterone to stimulate withdrawal bleeding. If bleeding occurs, amenorrhea suggests a hypothalamic–pituitary dysfunction, ovarian failure, or estrogen excess. If bleeding does not occur, amenorrhea could be due to an obstruction or endometrial lesion. In cases where the provider is concerned regarding hormonal abnormalities affecting menses, the APRN should collaborate with an endocrinologist for proper screening and treatment.

On the opposite end of the spectrum, an adolescent female may present with complaints of *menorrhagia* (heavy menstrual bleeding), which may be caused by organic, endocrine, or anatomical factors. Bleeding disorders, such as von Willebrand disease, should be considered in teens who present with complaints of heavy bleeding since menarche. A detailed history is important to assess for the number of pads used per day on the heaviest day, total pads used during the cycle, length of cycle, quality of life, and number of school days missed. Evaluation should include a von Willebrand profile and complete blood count. If a diagnosis is made, treatment would include intranasal desmopressin (Leebeek and Eikenboom 2016).

The onset of puberty in females varies by individual and between populations. A number of factors, such as race, genetics, and nutritional status, influence the development of secondary sex characteristics. The most prominent genetic factor that affects the onset of puberty is race. African American females tend to start puberty at an earlier age than their Latino and White counterparts (Biro et al. 2006; Chumlea et al. 2003). African American females tend to achieve menarche 2.1 months earlier than White females. Breast development also occurs months earlier in African American and Mexican females compared to White females (Sun et al. 2002). While the most influential environmental factor to affect puberty is nutrition, a model proposed by Ellis and Garber (2000, 2012) suggested that stresses within the family, such as maternal depression or stepfather presence, contributed to earlier pubertal maturation. Research has found increased body fat/elevated body mass index (BMI) leads to an earlier onset of menses and breast development (Kaplowitz et al. 2001; Qing and Karlberg 2001). In a typical 10-year-old girl, the body fat concentration is 6% higher than that of her male counterpart. Overweight children tend to experience puberty early (Wu et al. 2002). On the opposite end of the spectrum, female athletes with a low BMI and increased levels of physical activity have slower rates of puberty. Additionally, poor nutrition in early and middle childhood can lead to a delayed onset of menses, and vegetarian diets consisting of low protein and high dietary fiber are also associated with a delayed onset of menses and puberty. In cases where nutrition is of concern, the APRN should collaborate with a nutritionist to ascertain the best plan of care.

Physical Development in Males

For boys, the first physical sign of puberty is the enlargement of the testes (gonadarche), accompanied by the appearance of pubic hair. Until this time there has been very little growth in the size of the penis since infancy. After the onset of puberty, the testes continue to grow until reaching mature adult size, which usually occurs within 6 years. Within a year after the testes have reached maturity, the length and width of the shaft of the penis grow to adult size, followed by growth of the glans penis. Sperm and hormone production occur about a year after the first signs of puberty. Upon the production of sperm, fertility is reached, occasionally occurring at the age of 13 years.

Shortly after the growth of a male's pubic hair, body and facial hair also begin to grow. This development varies between individuals and populations, with no distinct timeline regarding the growth patterns. The typical order would be axillary, perianal, upper lip, periauricular (sideburns), periareolar, and the beard. Hair growth on the upper and lower extremities along with the abdomen and back tends to grow thicker than the hair on the rest of the body. Facial hair grows thicker over a number of years.

Physical changes occurring during puberty may lead the adolescent male to feel self-conscious and uncomfortable. Gynecomastia (enlargement of breast tissue) occurs in some boys during puberty, lasting 18 to 24 months and then slowly regressing. There is no treatment required unless the condition persists beyond 2 years. This condition may be distressing for the adolescent; reassurance that the symptoms will most likely go away and provision of emotional support are called for. The APRN can also recommend loose-fitting clothing and encourage maintenance of a healthy weight.

Another physical characteristic of pubis is the voice change, which is caused by the hormonal effects on the larynx. Although this effect occurs in both sexes, the effect on the male is more prominent. The longer and thicker vocal cords cause the male's voice to become deeper and drop one octave. The voice change usually occurs during Tanner Stage 3 and reaches full adult level around the age of 15 years. As the male reaches the end of puberty, his skeletal features have grown heavier and he has on average double the muscle mass of a female. The muscular growth will continue even into adulthood. The youth going through the physical changes of puberty need reassurance that they are normal. Youth may be ashamed of their development, whether they are overdeveloped or underdeveloped, compared to their peers. APRNs can help by providing anticipatory guidance regarding the physical and emotional changes that are a normal part of puberty.

Abnormal Puberty

There are two types of abnormal puberty: early puberty and delayed puberty. Early puberty is when puberty begins before age 8 for girls and before age 9 for boys. Delayed puberty occurs when sexual maturation is not evident by 13 years of age in girls and

14 years of age in boys. Puberty is also considered delayed if there is an absence of menarche by the age of 16 or at the 5-year mark of pubertal onset (Rosen and Foster 2001). As a result, it is critical for APRNs to assess the age of onset of pubertal development due to the risk of adjustment problems that may occur in individuals who reach puberty earlier or later than their peer group.

Early Onset

Early puberty is not usually due to an underlying pathological cause if other physical characteristics are within the normal pubertal growth and development. For diagnostic purposes, a radiograph to determine the child's skeletal age is indicated. If the skeletal age is within 2 years of the chronological age, the findings are benign.

Precocious puberty occurs when there is overstimulation of the gonadotropin-releasing hormone (GnRH) hormone. Precocious puberty presents as breast development or menarche in girls younger than 8 years (Kaplowitz, Oberfield, and the Drug and Therapeutics and Executive Committees of the Lawson Wilkins Pediatric Endocrine Society 1999). In boys, signs of precocious puberty include enlarged testicles and penis, facial hair (usually on the upper lip), or a deepening voice. Symptoms that can occur in both genders are pubic or underarm hair, rapid growth in height, acne, or an adult body odor. The potential reason for the cause of these symptoms will determine how the diagnosis is classified. Due to racial disparities in sexual maturation among girls, a provider may revise criteria for referral before diagnosing a child with precocious puberty.

The two types of precocious puberty are central and peripheral. *Central precocious puberty (CPP)*, the most common type, occurs when the entire hypothalamic–pituitary-gonadal (HPG) axis starts too soon. The pattern of growth and development is the same and follows the normal sequence; however, it occurs earlier than normal. Usually the cause of CPP is idiopathic. In a few rare cases, these symptoms are due to a central nervous system (CNS) lesion caused by neurofibromatosis, hydrocephalus, a CNS infection, or an intracranial neoplasm. Other causes of CPP are McCune–Albright syndrome, congenital adrenal hyperplasia, and hypothyroidism. CNS lesions affect both boys and girls equally. However, among children who present with precocious puberty who do not have an underlying pathology, girls are diagnosed 10 to 1 compared to their male counterparts (Carel and Leger 2008).

Peripheral precocious puberty (PPP) is due to the release of estrogen or testosterone into the body as a result of problems with the ovaries, testicles, or adrenal or pituitary glands. GnRH is not involved in the development of PPP. Upon assessment a patient may present with a tumor of the adrenal or pituitary gland, that is secreting either estrogen or testosterone (McCune–Albright syndrome) or exposure to a topical estrogen or testosterone cream. Female patients may be diagnosed with either an ovarian cyst or tumor. Male patients may have a tumor in the germ cells (cells that make sperm) or Leydig cells (cells that make testosterone). A rare gene mutation may also be the result of a disorder called familial gonadotropin-independent sexual precocity, which results in the production of testosterone between the ages of 1 and 4 (Muir 2006).

The prevalence of precocious puberty varies depending on the age limits used by researchers but is approximately 4–5%. Risk factors for developing precocious puberty are being female, African American, and/or obese, having exposure to sex hormones or environmental toxins that disrupt endocrine function, or having a disorder such as McCune–Albright syndrome or congenital adrenal hyperplasia (Cesario and Hughes 2007; Muir 2006). Excessive stress, increase in nutritional intake, and child obesity have been other factors attributable to the accelerated rate of early onset puberty (Rhie and Lee 2015).

Diagnosing the type of precocious puberty may be accomplished with a history, physical examination, and hormonal blood tests. A radiograph to measure bone age may also be indicated. Hormonal blood tests are done following a GnRH injection. Increase in follicle stimulating hormone (FSH) and luteinizing hormone (LH) levels indicates CPP, whereas in PPP the FSH and LH levels will remain constant. If a diagnosis of CPP is made, MRI may be performed to identify potential central nervous system (CNS) lesions. A thyroid test is done to rule out hypothyroidism if a child presents with signs such as sensitivity to cold, dry skin, fatigue, or constipation. Treatment for CPP is focused on medications aimed at preventing further pubertal development. The treatment of choice is a GnRH analog (typically leuprolide). The medication is given monthly to delay the pubertal process until the child reaches the appropriate age. Once the medication is discontinued, the process of puberty resumes.

Complications of precocious puberty may include development of psychological and psychosocial problems, polycystic ovarian syndrome or short stature. Polycystic ovarian syndrome may be recognized at the time of diagnosis of early menarche. Short stature is the result of rapid bone mineralization, which causes decreased linear growth. Experiencing rapid growth, hormonal shift, and monthly body changes can be stressful, especially to the younger developing youth (Kim and Lee 2012).

Clinical Implications

Growth maturation and biological processes are closely tied to the development of our personality and mental health. Self-concept is influenced by social role perception and body awareness, thus the correlation between negative physical development and self-concept is not surprising in the adolescent. There is evidence for the correlation of pubertal status and psychological adjustment in adolescents. If puberty is not progressing at a similar rate to the peer group, mental health issues may develop as any perceived disharmony may potentially affect the ego and the adolescent's social identity. Additionally, adolescents with early- and or late-onset puberty with comorbid environmental stressors such as parental absence, financial barriers, and or social conflicts are at increased risk for mental health issues such as depression, anxiety, social isolation, teasing, and or bullying. Counseling and education regarding body image, environmental stress factors, and normal growth and development can help alleviate and or prevent mental health issues in youth. Knowledge of developmental milestones for both normal and delayed puberty will help the APRN provide the appropriate counseling and intervention for the patient and their family. Assessing the needs of the patient and the family with precocious puberty is important, especially since the family may struggle on how to care for and support the youth. Social support programs for legal guardians of children with precocious puberty have demonstrated decreased stress and guilt among family members (Lee et al. 2019).

Sexual Behaviors

Assessing a child's sexual behavior must be done in the context in which the behavior occurs (Horner 2004). Children's sexual behavior is not intrinsic; it is learned from interactions with adults and other children. A child's home environment plays a significant role in the development of his or her sexual behavior. Certain sexual behaviors are considered normal in young children, such as self-stimulation, invasion of personal boundaries (i.e. standing too close, rubbing against another, or touching the mother's breasts or the father's genitals), and exposing body parts (Davies et al. 2000).

Normal child sexuality is differentiated from adult sexuality by the focus on curiosity and play, whereas adult sexuality presents with a mature understanding of the sexual behavior and its consequences. A child's sexual behavior is open, spontaneous, and sensual, while adult behavior is private, passionate, or erotic. Curiosity, playfulness, spontaneity, and sensuality are all a part of normal sexual development in the child. When caring for children, the APRN must consider normal sexual behavior and view the behavior in context. Johnson (1991) developed a continuum of sexual behaviors, ranging from normal to pathological, which may help APRNs determine their level of concern.

Group I. The majority of children fall into this category and exhibit natural and healthy sexual play. They may play "house" or "doctor" and develop scenarios to include sexual exploration. The play is voluntary, fun, and spontaneous. Neither of the parties feels fear, shame, or anxiety. There is mutual touch and exploration as a way of learning. The child's level of interest in sexuality is not any different than other aspects of their lives. The child should show an equal balance in their interest of sexual matters and other areas and people in their environment.

Group II. Children in this group engage in more sexual behaviors than their counterparts in Group I. They will sometimes admit to feeling guilty and ashamed about their sexuality. These children have usually been either sexually abused or exposed to sexually explicit materials. A parent may complain about their excessive masturbation, conversations about sexual acts, or their overtly sexual behaviors around adults. These may be signs of the child trying to work through their confusion regarding their sexual experiences.

Group III. Children in this group engage in all aspects of adult sexual behaviors with a consenting child partner. These children are usually physically and/or sexually abused. They consent to participating in sexual acts but are private about their sexual behaviors. Due to their betrayal, usually by adults, adults are not a part of their sexual world. Psychologically, these children do not exhibit emotions like the light-heartedness of Group I or the anxiety of Group II. They often present with a blank affect.

Group IV. Unlike the consenting partners in Group III, children in Group IV coerce others into sexual acts. This behavior can be classified as molestation. These children are usually acting out the aggressor role from their own personal experience of being a victim of child molestation in the past. These children have very little impulse control and suffer from a number of social-behavioral problems.

In addition to the four categories that Johnson (1991) classified, she also developed a "RED FLAG" checklist to identify inappropriate sexual behaviors in children. These include:

1. Interest in sex that is out of proportion with their interest in other aspects of the world.
2. Interest in sex that is compulsive, to the exclusion of interest in other developmentally appropriate activities.
3. A level of sexual knowledge that is greater than that of other same-age children from similar socioeconomic backgrounds and neighborhoods.
4. Approaching unfamiliar children instead of peers to engage in sexual acts.
5. Attempting to bribe or force other children to engage in sexual acts.
6. Other children complain about the sexual behavior of the child.
7. When sexual conversations are raised the child becomes anxious, fearful, or angry.

Along with noting the aforementioned symptoms and behaviors, the APRN should also screen patients for other mental health disorders that may also influence sexual behavior, such as disruptive mood disorder, bipolar disorder, and or post-traumatic stress disorder. The DSM-5 Level 1 Symptom Measure published by the American Psychiatric Association (2013) is a reliable tool that assesses mental health domains across psychiatric diagnosis and assists clinicians in identifying further testing needed for psychiatric diagnosis. As APRNs, if any of these symptoms are identified, the family should be counseled to seek professional help. There is also an ethical duty to report any episodes of suspected sexual abuse to the authorities. The following case study illustrates the APRN actions when a child presents with an issue with sexual development.

Summary

Childhood is a time of growth and self-exploration, which may also include an increase in sexual curiosity. Young children may engage in sexual behaviors that may include masturbation, self-exposure, and touching of others. As part of human development, some young children may not fully understand all the changes and boundaries that exist pertaining to their gender and or behaviors. While exploration can be a normal part of development that can result in a healthy relationship with self and others, some behaviors may require further assessment and referral. Early sexual experimentation can lead to an early sexual debut that places the youth at risk for multiple consequences, some of which can have lifelong implications. Behaviors that are aggressive in nature towards the self or others, and/or carry stimulating compulsive attributes should be noted and explored further for intervention. The APRN should rule out abuse or neglect, consider development age and maturity, and understand that atypical sexual behavior may dissipate over time and is not always diagnosable as a clinical disorder (Schwartz et al. 2006). The APRN can be instrumental in identifying and facilitating treatment of disorders of sexual disorders.

Resources on Adolescent Sexual Development

Resources for Patients and Families

Harris, R.H. and Emberley, M. 2014. *It's Perfectly Normal: Changing Bodies, Growing Up, Sex, and Sexual Health*. Massachusetts: Candlewick.

Gravelle, K. and Gravelle, J. 2017. *The Period Book: Everything You Don't Want to Ask but Need to Know*. New York: Bloomsbury.

Mayle, P. 2000. *What's Happening to Me? An Illustrated Guide to Puberty*. Lyle Stuart: Kensington.

American Academy of Pediatrics.
www.healthychildren.org.

Sexuality Information and Education Council of the United States.
www.siecus.org.

Resources for Precocious Puberty

Resources for Patients and Families

Magic Foundation
1327 North Harlem Avenue
Oak Park, IL 60302
Tel 7 083 830 808
www.magicfoundation.org

National Adrenal Diseases Foundation
505 Northern Boulevard
Great Neck, NY 11021
Tel 5 164 874 992
www.nadf.us

National Institute of Child Health and Human Development
http://www.nichd.nih.gov/health/topics/puberty/resources/patients

KidsHealth: Precocious Puberty
http://kidshealth.org/en/parents/precocious.html

Resources for Clinicians

American Academy of Pediatrics
141 Northwest Point Boulevard
Elk Grove Village, IL 60007–1098
Tel 847 434–4000
www.aap.org

NIH/National Institute of Child Health and Human Development
31 Center Drive
Building 31, Room 2A32
MSC2425, Bethesda, MD 20892
Tel 3 014 965 133
http://www.nichd.nih.gov

Society for Adolescent Medicine
1916 Copper Oaks Circle
Blue Springs, MO 64015
Tel 816 224–8010
www.adolescenthealth.org

Other Resources

Advocates for Youth. Advocates for youth and helps them to make informed and responsible decisions about their sexual and reproductive health.
www.advocatesforyouth.org

Sexuality Information and Education Council of the United States
90 John Street Suite 402
New York, NY 10038
Tel 212 819–9770
www.siecus.org

References

American Psychiatric Association (2013). *Diagnostic and Statistical Manual of Mental Disorders 5*. Arlington, VA: American Psychiatric Publishing.

Biro, F.M., Huang, B., Crawford, P.B. et al. (2006). Pubertal correlates in black and white girls. *Journal of Pediatrics* 148: 234–240.

Carel, J.C. and Leger, J. (2008). Precocious puberty. *New England Journal of Medicine* 358: 2366–2377.

Cesario, S.K. and Hughes, S.A. (2007). Precocious puberty: a comprehensive review of literature. *Journal of Obstetric, Gynecologic, and Neonatal Nursing* 36 (3): 263–274.

Chumlea, W.C., Schubert, C.M., Roche, A.F. et al. (2003). Age at menarche and racial comparisons in US girls. *Pediatrics* 111: 110–113.

Davies, S.L., Glaser, D., and Kossoff, R. (2000). Children's sexual play and behavior in pre-school settings: Staff's perceptions, reports, and responses. *Child Abuse & Neglect* 24: 1329–1343.

Ellis, B.J. and Garber, J. (2000). Psychosocial antecedents of variation in girls' pubertal timing: maternal depression, stepfather presence, and marital and family stress. *Child Development* 71: 485–501.

Ellis, B.J. and Garber, J. (2012). Sex-specific pathways to early puberty, sexual debut, and sexual risk taking: tests of an integrated evolutionary-developmental model. *Developmental Psychology* 48 (3): 687–702.

Gerlt, T. and Blosser, C. (2016). Sexuality. In: *Pediatric primary care*, 6e (eds. C. Burns, A. Dunn, M. Brady, et al.), 285–498. St. Louis, MO: Saunders Elsevier.

Gleason, M.M. and Zeanah, C.H. (2016). Assessing infants and toddlers. In: *Dulcan's Textbook of Child and Adolescent Psychiatry*, 2e (ed. M.K. Dulcan), 17–36. Arlington, VA: American Psychiatric Publishing.

Horner, G. (2004). Sexual behavior in children: normal or not? *Journal of Pediatric Healthcare* 18 (2): 57–64.

Johnson, T.C. (1991). Understanding the sexual behaviors of young children. *SIECUS Report*, August/September, pp. 8–15.

Kaplowitz, P.B., Oberfield, S.E., and the Drug and Therapeutics and Executive Committees of the Lawson Wilkins Pediatric Endocrine Society (1999). Reexamination of the age limit for defining when puberty is precocious in girls in the United States: implications for evaluation and treatment. *Pediatrics* 104: 936–941.

Kaplowitz, P.B., Slora, E.J., Wasserman, R.C. et al. (2001). Earlier onset of puberty in girls: relation to increased body mass index and race. *Pediatrics* 108: 347–353.

Kim, E.Y. and Lee, M.I. (2012). Psychosocial aspects in girls with idiopathic precocious puberty. *Psychiatry Investigation* 9 (1): 25–28.

Krieger, N., Kiang, M., Kosheleva, A. et al. (2015). Age at menarche: 50-year socioeconomic trends among US-born Black and White women. *American Journal of Public Health* 105 (2): 388–397.

Lee, J., Kwak, M.J., and Ju, H.O. (2019). Effect of a social support program for mothers of children with precocious puberty: a preliminary quasi-experimental study. *Journal of Pediatric Nursing* 46: E2–E9.

Leebeek, F.W. and Eikenboom, J.C. (2016). Von Willebrand's disease. *New England Journal of Medicine* 375 (21): 2067–2080.

Marshall, W.A. and Tanner, J.M. (1969). Variations in pattern of pubertal changes in girls. *Archives of Disease in Childhood* 44: 291–303.

Marshall, W.A. and Tanner, J.M. (1970). Variations in pattern of pubertal changes in boys. *Archives of Disease in Childhood* 45: 13–23.

McCann-Crosby, B. and Sutton, V.R. (2015). Disorders of sexual development. *Clinical Perinatology* 42: 395–412. https://doi.org/10.1016/j.clp.2015.02.006.

Muir, A. (2006). Precocious puberty. *Pediatrics in Review* 27: 373–381.

Qing, H. and Karlberg, J. (2001). BMI in childhood and its association with height gain, timing of puberty, and final height. *Pediatric Research* 49: 244–251.

Rhie, Y.J. and Lee, K.H. (2015). Overview and treatment of precocious puberty. *Journal of the Korean Medical Association* 58: 1138–1144.

Rosen, D.S. and Foster, C. (2001). Delayed puberty. *Pediatrics* 22: 309–315.

Rothkopf, A.C. and John, R.M. (2014). Understanding disorders of sexual development. *Journal of Pediatric Nursing* 29: e23–e34. https://doi.org/10.1016/j.pedn.2014.04.002.

Schwartz, B.K., Cavanaugh, D., Pimentel, A., and Prentky, R. (2006). Descriptive study of precursors to sex offending among 813 boys and girls: Antecedent life experiences. *Victims & Offenders : An International Journal of Evidence-based Research, Policy, and Practice* 1 (1): 61–77.

Sun, S.S., Schubert, C.M., Chumlea, W.C. et al. (2002). National estimates of the timing of sexual maturation and racial differences among US children. *Pediatrics* 110: 911–919.

Walvoord, E.C. (2010). The timing of puberty: is it changing? Does it matter? *Journal of Adolescent Health* 47 (5): 433–439.

Wu, T., Mendola, P., and Buck, G. (2002). Ethnic differences in the presence of secondary sex characteristics and menarche among US girls: the third national health and nutrition examination survey, 1988–1994. *Pediatrics* 110: 752–757.

6

Adolescent Sexual Behaviors

Bridgette M. Brawner[1] and Anne M. Teitelman[2]

[1] University of Pennsylvania School of Nursing, Philadelphia, PA, USA
[2] Department of Family and Community Health, University of Pennsylvania School of Nursing, Philadelphia, PA, USA

Objectives

After reading this chapter, advanced practice registered nurses will be able to:

1. Identify normal and abnormal adolescent sexual exploration and behaviors.
2. Assess multilevel influences (individual, social, and structural) that may affect adolescent sexual behaviors.
3. Describe the unique challenges faced by youth with mental illnesses and difficulties with emotion regulation.
4. Develop strategies for conducting sexual health assessment, screening, and intervention to reduce sexual risk behaviors.

Introduction

This chapter discusses normal and abnormal sexual exploration and behaviors, as well as unique concerns among youth dealing with mental illnesses, psychological distress, and difficulties with emotion regulation. The advanced practice registered nurse (APRN) is equipped with information to facilitate sexual health assessment, screening, and intervention when conducting adolescent psychoeducation. The chapter includes a discussion of unintended sexual health outcomes, namely unwanted pregnancy and sexually transmitted infections (STIs), including human immunodeficiency virus (HIV). Clinical strategies are also suggested for the APRN during all levels of preventive efforts. Nurses serve at the forefront to intervene with youth during times of crisis involving sexual development and exploration, as well as any mental health issues related to these developmental challenges. Moreover, sexual health assessment and screening are critical for adolescents in both primary and mental healthcare settings. APRNs have a responsibility to manage minor psychosocial issues associated with sexual behaviors and should have sensitivity and knowledge when working with youth with mental illnesses, psychological distress and/or difficulties in emotion regulation. It is important to note that case findings of more complex mental health challenges must be referred immediately to a trained mental health professional, including APRNs, when screening reveals serious emotional, behavioral, or psychological consequences of abnormal sexual behaviors or youth in crisis.

Sexual Exploration

The developmental stage of adolescence can be a time of great confusion as adolescents make the transition from childhood to adulthood. According to Erickson's stages of psychosocial development, adolescents undergo processes of Identity versus Role Confusion (Erikson 1950). At this time, the individual's life comes to a point wherein multiple physical, emotional, social, and other changes take place rapidly and simultaneously. As a result, the

Child and Adolescent Behavioral Health: A Resource for Advanced Practice Psychiatric and Primary Care Practitioners in Nursing,
Second Edition. Edited by Edilma L. Yearwood, Geraldine S. Pearson, and Jamesetta A. Newland.
© 2021 John Wiley & Sons, Inc. Published 2021 by John Wiley & Sons, Inc.
Companion website: www.wiley.com/go/Yearwood

emotional stress of attempting to establish one's identity and place in society is complicated by the physical stress of increasingly complex changes to the body. In today's society, factors such as increased stressors and hormones in food have contributed toward adolescents developing at a faster pace compared to decades prior. Thus, where certain physical characteristics of adolescence were previously reached at a later age, adolescents are undergoing these changes more rapidly at younger ages. To best support their clients and families, APRNs must be knowledgeable of the physical changes and emotional stressors that adolescents experience. According to Erickson's developmental theory, failure to achieve a sense of identity and to stay true to self may lead to a weak sense of self and role confusion. This failure ultimately places adolescents at increased risk for adverse behaviors and health outcomes, such as substance use and violent behaviors. With knowledge of normal sexual development and behaviors, APRNs can more readily identify abnormalities and/or concerns, supporting adolescents and those close to them in achieving healthier sexual futures.

Sexual Development and Behaviors

Biological, psychological, and social influences all play a role in adolescent sexual development. Hormonal changes initiated during adolescence promote physical attraction toward others, a curiosity about relationships, and interest in sexual activity. Adolescents who go through puberty at earlier ages are more likely to have earlier sexual experiences (Pringle et al. 2017). The usual pattern of brain development, which continues through the mid-20s, progressively enhances cognitive control while impulsivity becomes more muted, allowing for more reasoned decision-making (Steinberg 2008). As such, decision-making into late adolescence, in comparison to adults, is more impulsive, more prone to risk-taking, more influenced by peers, and less likely to consider future consequences. As a result, early adolescents may experience various types of experimentation, followed by interest in novel experiences and risk-taking beginning in middle adolescence, and later developing the ability to assess their own risk-taking. Socially, adolescents shift focus from family to include peers and a wider social network. Adolescents' experiences of learning about sex and relationships through observation and discussions from family while growing up continues to exert a strong influence, but is tempered by other sources, such as friends, partners, and media (Lanier et al. 2018; Stevens et al. 2017b). Gender socialization varies for adolescents depending on their gender and sexual identity, and consequently may have an impact on

sexual behavior. Sexual minority youth may face additional challenges given the dominant social narrative of heteronormativity. Personality characteristics can also influence how an adolescent experiences and interprets these changes (Kar et al. 2015).

During early adolescence (ages 10–13 years), feelings of sexual attraction may begin, followed by sexual fantasies. As development continues, the younger adolescent may experience enhanced sexual interest and attractions. The increasing levels of sex hormones that occur through puberty continue to affect feelings of sexual arousal, attraction, and fantasies. The onset of menstruation for girls and nocturnal emissions for boys indicates the adolescent has reproductive capability. By middle adolescence (ages 14–16 years), the physical development associated with puberty is reaching completion while sexual thoughts, feelings, and behaviors continue to grow. In late adolescence (ages 17–19 years), youth are more likely to become involved in relationships and engage in sexual contact than in middle adolescence, as sexual thoughts and attractions continue to magnify. However, there is wide variation in physical and social maturity among youth across developmental stages and associated ages. Individuals may also experience disparate progress in development in various domains, such that physical maturity, in many instances, advances more quickly than social or cognitive maturity, leaving the adolescent open to challenging social and sexual situations.

Sexual Behavior

In early adolescence, sexual behaviors may involve masturbation as well as some physical contact with opposite or same-gender peers. Sexual activity for the younger adolescent may be motivated by curiosity, opportunity, or sexual orientation and is more focused on self-interest than reciprocity. In middle adolescence, sexual activity may increase in frequency. During this time, males often begin masturbating to ejaculation while masturbation among females is more variable. Sexual relationships are associated with more emotional intimacy and reciprocity. Among older adolescents, sexual activity is most likely to occur in the context of a relationship, but casual sexual encounters occur as well. Sexual behaviors among adolescents can include sexual conversations/jokes, flirting, viewing pornography or sexting, hugging, kissing, fondling, oral sex, and vaginal or anal intercourse. It is important to note that some families may have rules that limit these behaviors and some state laws make certain sexual behaviors illegal (National Center on the Sexual Behavior of Youth 2012). Therefore, it is important for APRNs to be familiar with their state laws regarding adolescent sexual behaviors. In the United States, research about the sexual behaviors of adolescents is assessed every 2 years though the Youth Risk Behavior Survey (Centers for Disease Control and Prevention (CDC) 2018a). In 2017, 40% of youth from grades 9 to 12 indicated they had ever had intercourse while only 3% had sexual intercourse before the age of 13 years. These findings suggest that sexual intercourse is common among high school students, but not among younger adolescents. Even still, there may be substantial risks associated with adolescent sexual activity, as described further below. In addition, some teens may present behaviors that are beyond what is generally considered normative behaviors.

Problematic Sexual Behaviors

Problematic sexual behavior involves sexual body parts (e.g. genitals, anus, buttock, breasts) that are inappropriate developmentally or harmful to self or others. These behaviors may include self-stimulation that causes physical damage, preoccupation with nudity or sexually explicit media, public self-touching or self-exposure, and aggressive sexual touching/acts. Alterations in biopsychosocial development along the life course can have an impact on adolescent sexual behavior. For example, problematic sexual behaviors commonly result from the trauma of earlier experiences of sexual abuse, but this is not always the case. Motivations for these behaviors may not be related to sexual enjoyment but rather to other factors such as curiosity, imitation, anxiety, loneliness, or anger (National Center on the Sexual Behavior of Youth 2012).

APRNs can identify concerning adolescent sexual behaviors. They often involve behaviors between youth of widely different age, size, or ability, may be associated with emotional upset (such as fear/anxiety), occur with greater frequency than expected, and occur within a coercive context. They may involve threats or force and may be seen as leading to harm or actually cause harm (National Center on the Sexual Behavior of Youth 2012). There are many gray areas between normal and problematic adolescent sexual behaviors, and each situation must be assessed individually, taking the family and social context into consideration. For example, while masturbation is considered a normative adolescent sexual behavior, in some families this behavior is considered inappropriate.

If an APRN conducts an assessment and does not identify problematic sexual behavior, there is no need for further intervention regarding the behavior. However, the APRN may find significant family conflict, untreated mental health issues or other difficulties. In such situations, other types of treatment/referrals should be considered. If an APRN identifies any concerning or problematic adolescent sexual behavior, the adolescent

and/or family should be counseled to seek further professional help for developmentally appropriate interventions. The APRN can assist the adolescent and/or family with locating evidenced-based interventions available in their locale. Multisystemic therapy (MST) is an evidence-based approach for youth shown to improve problematic sexual behaviors (Letourneau et al. 2004; National Center on the Sexual Behavior of Youth 2012). MST is designed to reduce the risks of criminal behavior and out-of-home placement for youth with serious behavioral issues by providing intensive family and community-based treatment in all of the youth's environments: home, school, and neighborhood. The APRN also has an ethical duty to report any episodes of suspected sexual abuse to the authorities. Meanwhile, the APRN can identify any actions needed to maintain safety and support for all those involved.

While problematic sexual behaviors may not be a diagnosable condition, these behaviors need further assessment to determine if they are transitory in an otherwise well-functioning adolescent, e.g. related to lack of knowledge or awareness of social customs, negative peer influences, or substance use. Some teens with neurodevelopmental disorders, such as attention deficit hyperactivity disorder (ADHD) or autism spectrum disorder, may also experience such transitory behaviors. If, however, the problematic sexual behavior is part of symptom pattern reflective of a disruptive behavioral disorder according to the *Diagnostic and Statistical Manual of Mental Disorders 5* (DSM-5) (American Psychiatric Association 2013), then the APRN will need to make appropriate mental health referrals.

Multilevel Influences on Sexual Behaviors

There are multiple factors that influence adolescents' decisions about sex and relationships. These occur at the individual (e.g. mood affecting sexual decision-making processes), social (e.g. intimate partner violence [IPV]), and/or structural (e.g. concentrated disadvantage in neighborhoods leading to limited health education resources) levels. While sexual exploration is a normal part of adolescent sexual development, the text below outlines ways in which this process may be complicated and contribute to adverse sexual health outcomes. As APRNs, these factors should be taken into account during clinical encounters to improve sexual health among adolescents.

Individual-level Factors

The decisions adolescents make about sex (e.g. whether or not to abstain or use condoms) are influenced by their mood, feelings, and attitudes. Gross (2014) offers a framework that can be used to help explain the tie between affect and sexual behaviors, and it hinges on the concept of emotion regulation. Emotion regulation is believed to require activation of a goal to up- or down-regulate (i) the magnitude of an emotional response or (ii) the duration of an emotional response (Gross 2013). This goal may be activated in oneself by intrinsic emotion regulation as when the individual regulates his/her own emotions, or in someone else by extrinsic emotion regulation as when the individual's emotions are regulated by a sexual partner. Processes are then recruited to accomplish the regulatory goal, and occur on a continuum from conscious, effortful control (trying to look calm although anxious about a sexual encounter) to unconscious, effortless control (turning away from something upsetting) to automatic regulation. Ultimately, and in response to various stimuli, people then work to decrease or increase their negative or positive emotions. Gross' process model identifies five points at which individuals regulate their emotions: situation selection, situation modification, attentional deployment, cognitive change, and response modulation (2014).

Despite this knowledge, affective components in the sexual decision-making process are poorly attended to in clinical practice and sexual health promotion activities. A substantive body of literature suggests that factors such as the psychological sequelae of mental illness, psychological distress, and difficulties with emotion regulation affect sexual behaviors among adolescents (Braje et al. 2015; Brawner et al. 2017; Brown et al. 2017). This is due in part to the fact that symptoms of mental health diagnoses such as loneliness and impulsivity, the experience of psychological distress in response to internal and/or external conflict, and one's ability to regulate his/her emotions can lead adolescents to engage in sexual behaviors that they might otherwise avoid. For example, an adolescent male experiencing depressive symptoms may feel lonely and/or angry without generalized loss or interest in pleasurable activities. To cope with his feelings, he may desire to have intimate, nonsexual connection with another person. However, if the person he seeks connection with wants to have sex, he may decide to have sex to achieve connection and alleviate his underlying feelings of loneliness and isolation. APRNs can play a critical role in identifying adolescents who may be susceptible to such exchange relationships and can provide psychoeducation to help them identify other means of coping with their symptom experience.

Social-level Factors

Adolescents are inexperienced in romantic relationships and as feelings of attraction and companionship develop they may not know how best to express these feelings very well to another person, often leading to awkward encounters. Most adolescents are eager to learn more about romantic relationships through viewing media content, talking to others or by seeking out these experiences. Adults often do not take these relationships very seriously and have sometimes referred to them as "puppy love." However, adolescent relationships are often very important to teens; negative experiences such as disagreements or break-ups can lead to sadness, disappointment, and even depression, especially in earlier adolescence. Conversely, depression in adolescence can negatively affect the quality of romantic relationships (Olson and Crosnoe 2017; Vujeva and Furman 2011).

Many adolescent relationships with intimate partners are healthy ones in which both partners respect each other, make decisions together, and communicate well, but other relationships are unhealthy, involving violence and controlling behaviors. Adolescent partner abuse, more commonly referred to as dating violence or IPV, has many physical and psychological consequences, but the association with STIs, including HIV, and pregnancy has recently gained increasing attention in research and practice. Compared with their nonabused peers, adolescent females who experience IPV are more than 2.5 times more likely to report being infected with HIV or another STI. Young women with a history of physical IPV are more likely to report having had multiple sex partners and sex without condoms, both of which increase the risk of contracting HIV or another STI. Experiencing violence increases a woman's risk of unintended pregnancies (ACOG 2013). Understanding the connections between STIs/HIV and pregnancy and partner abuse can open up additional opportunities to assist adolescents to recognize and manage their exposure to or involvement in risky situations.

Adolescent IPV is common and usually begins to emerge around age 15 years but can also affect middle school youth. IPV can occur in serious or casual relationships and in same-sex or opposite-sex relationships. The National Youth Risk Behavior Survey indicates that the rate of physical IPV victimization among high school-age youth in the general population was 8% in 2017 (9% females, 6.5% males), but rates may vary among certain subgroups. For example, sexual partner violence is also more commonly experienced by females than males (11% females, 3% males) (CDC 2018a). IPV is defined by the CDC as physical, sexual, or psychological harm by a current or former partner or spouse (CDC 2018b). IPV can be directed toward a current or former spouse, boyfriend or girlfriend, or dating partner. IPV is often an indication of imbalances in power within a relationship. In intimate relationships in which one partner dominates, the other partner may be coerced into participating in risky sexual behaviors that increase the risk for HIV/STIs or pregnancy. The imbalance of power may manifest in subtle and overt ways.

Reproductive coercion can be part of a controlling relationship and involves interference with contraception use and pregnancy risk. Examples include hiding, withholding, or destroying a partner's contraceptives, breaking or poking holes in a condom on purpose or removing a condom during sex in an attempt to promote pregnancy, forcing a partner to carry a pregnancy to term against her wishes through threats or acts of violence, or forcing a female partner to terminate a pregnancy when she does not want to terminate (ACOG 2013).

Counseling sexually active adolescents about ways in which they can be protected from unsafe situations is an important aspect in the prevention of IPV and the associated risk for HIV/STIs and pregnancy. The routine discussion of safer-sex and contraceptive practices during wellness visits can assist youth to identify unhealthy partner dynamics that might lead to sexual risk or abuse. However, it takes patience to develop a relationship in which sensitive topics, such as sexual practices or potentially abusive situations, may be discussed openly. In exchanges with an adolescent patient, conditions that enhance disclosure include trust, knowing that the provider will not take action without her/his permission, confidentiality, and support. The use of a straightforward, nonjudgmental approach can foster open communication with adolescents, which aids in the accurate disclosure of their sexual behaviors. By screening adolescent patients for signs of IPV (experiences and perpetration), healthcare providers can assist them to identify and/or control their exposure to risky situations. Before screening for violence and abuse, know your state reporting requirements and inform your patients about any limits to their confidentiality, should they disclose abuse (Center for Adolescent Health and the Law 2014).

Routine screening for IPV should take place whenever adolescents present for healthcare, particularly reproductive health services. This includes annual gynecologic or family planning examinations, STI/HIV screenings, pregnancy testing visits, and prenatal care. Screening questions that ask about specific behaviors are typically more effective at eliciting accurate information than asking whether abuse is present in the relationship because the latter can vary depending on one's perception or definition of the term.

Asking questions, such as "Have you ever been hit, kicked, slapped, intimidated, or threatened?" are important. However, there are more effective ways to assess for coercive situations that directly affect safer-sex practices. Because STI/HIV and pregnancy prevention occurs in the context of a relationship, it is important to talk about how decisions are made in those relationships and determine the adolescent's level of control over safer-sex practices. For example:

- "A lot of young people I see want to use condoms or dams but worry about their partners not wanting to use them. How often does this happen to you?"
- "During this visit, we also like to discuss healthy relationships. We now know that a lot of young people don't always get to decide when they have sex. Their partners decide for them. And that can make them feel uncomfortable or upset. Has anything like that ever happened to you?"

In addition, the patient's reproductive health history can suggest exposure to IPV. Red flags include a frequent history of STI testing or treatment, repeat pregnancy testing or pregnancy history, any prior abuse history, or frequent requests for emergency contraception. Counseling such a patient about healthy relationships, informing them about the potential consequences of their partner's risky behaviors, safety planning, and letting them know that help is available should they want it can empower them to safely protect their health.

In discussing the difference between healthy and unhealthy relationships, a partner in a healthy relationship will usually:

- communicate openly with you when problems exist
- give you space to spend time with your friends and family
- be supportive and respectful.

A partner in an unhealthy relationship may:

- control where you go, what you wear, or what you do
- try to stop you from seeing or talking to family or friends
- call you derogatory names, put you down, or criticize you
- threaten or scare you
- hit, slap, push, or kick you
- force you to do something sexual when you don't want to, including situations that expose you to HIV, other STIs, or pregnancy.

Assist adolescents to identify trusted peers or adults, such as a close friend, parent, teacher, guidance counselor, school nurse, or clergyperson, with whom they could safely discuss relationship problems if they were to emerge. Present a teen dating violence prevention pamphlet or card in case they or a friend might find it useful in the future. Offer contraception that can be used without the partner's knowledge such as injections or implants. Offer condoms or dams; talk about barrier method negotiation and partner issues that may arise. Offer pre-exposure prophylaxis for HIV if they are at increased risk for HIV.

Of special note, social media plays an increasingly important role in messaging that youth are exposed to about sexual behaviors. Recent evidence indicates that youth who are exposed to sexual health messages on social media were nearly three times more likely to have used contraception or a condom at last intercourse (Stevens et al. 2017a). These positive influences of social interactions can be leveraged by APRNs interested in creating factual, positive sexual health information for online dissemination. It is also important to note, however, that it has also been noted that negative social interactions in the geographic neighborhood may be reproduced and amplified on social media (Stevens et al. 2017b). Thus, as part of their assessment, APRNs can identify the nature and content of media exposure experienced by their clients, and provide factual information to counteract pervasive cultural myths.

Structural-level Factors

The neighborhoods in which adolescents live and national policy related to comprehensive sexual health education in schools are among the plethora of structural-level factors that shape adolescent sexual health. While neighborhoods do not directly affect sexual behaviors, studies demonstrate that factors such as poverty and physical disorder or social disorder contribute to psychological distress, which in turn can affect sexual risk behaviors (Latkin et al. 2013). The training of clinical providers who encounter adolescents in these neighborhoods also matters because if they do not ask the right questions, they will not have accurate information to support and/or intervene (Rubin et al. 2018). The inclusion and content of sexual health education varies across states and schools, but some groups are working toward standardizing education initiatives to ensure that adolescents have the knowledge and skills needed to maintain their sexual health (Saul Butler et al. 2018).

Unintended Sexual Health Outcomes

Some adolescents who engage in early sexual experimentation have an early sexual debut. Because cognitive control of those in early through later adolescence is still developing and may not yet balance out concomitant high levels of impulsivity, sexual decision-making is often less than optimal. This can lead to unplanned sexual encounters in which the use of contraception or STI protection is much less likely. As such, adolescents are at greater risk for a variety of consequences that may have lifelong implications, such as pregnancy. Adolescents

with mental health diagnoses including depression, anxiety, or substance use are less likely to practice safe sex. All of these factors explain why rates of STIs and unintended pregnancy are very high during the adolescence period of development. Young people aged 15–24 years account for half of all new STI infections (CDC 2017).

Pregnancy

Teenage pregnancy in the United States continues to be an area of concern for educators, lawmakers, and healthcare professionals due to the adverse consequences associated with a pregnancy during adolescence. Teenagers who give birth are more likely to have a preterm birth compared to older women and their babies are more at risk of dying during infancy (Xu et al. 2018). Extremes of body mass index, smoking, and physiologic immaturity are common risk factors for premature births among for teen mothers (Ferré et al. 2016). In addition, teen mothers are more at risk for interrupting or stopping their education. From 2007 to 2014, the birth rate for females aged 15–19 years declined 42%, from 41.5 to 24.2 per 1000 females (Ferré et al. 2016). In 2017, the teen birth rate dropped another 7% from 2016 to 18.8 births per 1000 females aged 15–19 years, representing a 55% rate decline overall since 2007 (Martin et al. 2018). Research suggests this reduction is due to more teens abstaining from sexual activity and more sexually active teens using birth control, especially long-acting reversible contraception (LARC) such as intrauterine devices (IUDs) and implants, in comparison to previous years (Lindberg et al. 2016). Despite the continued decrease in teen births over the last decade, the United States still has one of the highest teen birth rates in the world (Sedgh et al. 2015). Although racial/ethnic disparities in teen birth rates continue, they have narrowed in recent years. Between 2006 and 2014, the steepest decline in teen births occurred among Hispanics (51%, from 77.4 to 38.0), followed by blacks (44%, from 61.9 to 34.9), and then whites (35%, from 26.7 to 17.3) (Romero et al. 2016). It is now widely recognized that racial and ethnic minorities are disproportionately affected by social determinants associated with teen births, such as limited education and low income levels (Penman-Aguilar et al. 2013).

During all visits with teens, regardless of gender, it is important to discuss sexuality, relationships, sexual behaviors, and ways to prevent STIs and pregnancy. Although most contraception is used by women (except for male condoms) it is important to talk with sexually active male patients who have sex with women about supporting their female partner in using contraception. During these visits, it is best to talk with the teen alone to provide an opportunity to build trust. Teens are often reluctant to talk about their sexual behavior with a provider as they worry about being judged, so it is important for an APRN to establish rapport and discuss confidentiality (Center for Adolescent Health and the Law 2014). If the teen would like a parent or partner to join in the conversation, they can be welcomed in after an initial one-on-one conversation. The role of the APRN in providing comprehensive sexuality education is important (ACOG 2016) and can be augmented by other supportive adults and peers in the teen's social circle. If the teen does not identify supportive others, the APRN may need to take extra time talking about sexuality, relationships, and reproductive health and/or refer the teen for additional educational and support resources.

APRNs in primary care should have a low threshold for screening for a possible pregnancy among sexually active females and among those who may be reluctant to disclose their sexual activity. This may not be a concern raised by the teen during a healthcare visit as many are not aware they may be pregnant, they may be in denial, or they may be unable or fearful to talk about their concerns. The most common cause for amenorrhea among adolescents who have achieved menarche is pregnancy (Deligeoroglou et al. 2010).

Diagnosing pregnancy with adolescents can be challenging since they may not keep track of their menstrual cycle or may be using contraceptives, such as Depo Provera, that interfere with the normal bleeding cycle. In addition, they may not recognize certain symptoms as being related to pregnancy, such as breast tenderness or more frequent urination. APRNs working with adolescent females in primary care need to be prepared to diagnose and monitor pregnancy, provide options counseling, and make appropriate referrals.

Pregnancy testing offers an opportunity to provide the female adolescent with important information and a chance to reflect on their choices and goals regarding their reproductive health. Urine pregnancy tests are very accurate and can easily be performed in an outpatient clinic. The teen may already know their pregnancy test results from a home test kit, but repeat the test in the office to confirm this. While waiting for the test results, discuss possible reactions to a positive and negative test result, exploring their values and choices. If she has symptoms such as vaginal discharge, odor, or dysuria, she should also be assessed for STIs.

With a negative pregnancy test result it is also important to know when the teen last had unprotected intercourse. If in the last 72 hours, emergency contraception can be offered. If more than 72 hours, but within the last two weeks, the pregnancy test should be repeated in two more weeks, since the test only detects human chorionic gonadotropin (HCG) at levels reached at approximately

10–14 days after conception. A serum HCG test can detect levels by day 7 but is costlier and takes longer to know results. Also use this opportunity to talk about STI/HIV prevention, and if the teen is not trying to conceive to also talk about various contraceptive options.

A positive pregnancy test is a major event for any female, but especially so for an adolescent who may or may not desire to be pregnant. Take time to just be with them as they begin to process this information. This can be a real crisis for them, so have a box of tissues handy. Ask them about their initial thoughts and feelings, and who they are likely to talk to about this. Assist them in processing their emotions and respond to their informational questions before dealing with the physical aspects of pregnancy.

Eliciting the first day of the last normal menstrual cycle (LNMP) is important for dating the pregnancy and in determining the due date. Because women can sometimes spot during pregnancy (e.g. due to implantation bleeding), identifying the last normal period is key to an accurate projected due date. A pelvic examination for sizing the uterus is also usually performed at this visit and a handheld ultrasound can be used to listen for a heartbeat at around 12 weeks. Some teens experience their first pelvic examination during a pregnancy, so inquire and provide a detailed explanation of the examination as needed. APRNs working with adolescents need to provide or make a referral for this examination as well as options counseling (Hornberger and AAP Committee on Adolescence 2017). This usually entails discussing her thoughts about continuing the pregnancy or not and the various options she might have. These options can depend on the dating of the pregnancy, so the two often are performed in tandem. Signs of an impending miscarriage include moderate to severe abdominal pain, more than mild cramping, and/or abnormal bleeding, more than infrequent spotting, and would merit immediate referral to an emergency room.

If she knows she wants to continue the pregnancy, the APRN can provide some initial guidance about expected symptoms of pregnancy, healthy diet, prenatal vitamins, and avoidance of alcohol or drugs. Expected symptoms include breast soreness or enlargement, nausea, vomiting, abdominal cramping, urinary frequency, fatigue, appetite changes, or aversion to certain smells. Depending on your practice setting, referrals may need to be made for continued care during the pregnancy. At this time, explain the different types of providers that can care for women during pregnancy such as nurse-midwives, women's health APRNs, family practice providers (physicians and APRNs), and specialists in obstetrics and gynecology. In addition to monitoring for the potential physiologic concerns related to teen pregnancy, the APRN in primary care can also provide ongoing support and guidance for a teen who has chosen to continue the pregnancy since teen motherhood often leads to many social and economic challenges along with many joys.

Sexually Transmitted Infections

In the United States, four in 10 high school-age youth have ever had sexual intercourse, nearly one in 10 have had sex with four or more people in their lifetime, almost half (46.2%) did not use a condom the last time they had sex, and 18% drank alcohol or used drugs before their last sexual encounter (CDC 2018c). These behaviors increase their risk for acquiring STIs, and current epidemiological profiles among youth are alarming. Those aged 15–24 acquire half of all new STIs, and estimates indicate that one in four young females has an STI (CDC 2018c).

Chlamydia, gonorrhea, and primary and secondary syphilis are key concerns, with rates continuing to rise over the years. Most notably, CDC (2018c) data indicate that youth aged 15–24 years accounted for 62.6% of all chlamydia cases, with highest rates reported among females and a 29.1% increase among males from 2013 to 2017. Gonorrhea rates in males aged 15–24 years rose 51.6% from 2013 to 2017, and primary and secondary syphilis rates increased 83.3% among males and 50.9% among females. Other STIs, such as human papilloma virus (HPV) and herpes simplex virus (HSV), also warrant attention. HPV is the most common STI in the United States, and often goes undetected. Complications are serious, however, including cervical cancer and anogenital warts. Common oral sex among youth – sometimes as a pregnancy prevention strategy – may contribute to a rise in HSV-1. These statistics are particularly concerning given evidence that the presence of an STI increases one's risk for HIV. Of note, youth aged 13–24 accounted for 21% of all new HIV diagnoses – the overwhelming majority of these cases (81%) were among young gay and bisexual men (CDC 2018d).

Untreated STIs and repeat reinfections can cause significant, unnecessary health and social concerns for youth such as reproductive complications (e.g. infertility), cancer, and interpersonal conflict at a time when interpersonal relationships are paramount. HIV, if untreated or poorly managed, can lead to premature death from AIDS-related complications. A key take away for APRNs is that STIs can be prevented, which boosts the need for our role in sexual health promotion. Unless an APRN works in an integrated care setting, he/she will not likely have access to onsite testing for STIs, including HIV. However, unique partnerships can be made with local health centers and AIDS service organizations to offer free, confidential services to those in

need. If a positive STI diagnosis is received, the APRN should be available to discuss how the client is coping with the news and develop a plan for moving forward, such as a suicide safety plan, role play notifying sexual partners, and strategies to prevent future STIs.

Strategies for Conducting Sexual Health Assessment and Interventions to Reduce Sexual Risk Behaviors

APRNs play a critical role in helping youth promote and maintain their sexual health. This begins, however, with a thorough and accurate sexual health history. It can be unnerving to have these conversations, especially when APRNs feel unprepared and youth are uncomfortable sharing. With knowledge of key elements of sexual health assessment and intervention, APRNs can at least begin the conversation and then work with (or refer) their clients as appropriate.

Sexual Health Assessment

The CDC (2005) recommends using the five Ps of sexual health as a guide: partners, practices, protection from STIs, past history of STIs, and prevention of pregnancy. Attention should also be given to with whom the adolescent engages in sexual behaviors (e.g. same or opposite sex), knowledge of their partner's five Ps, and how their mood influences their sexual behaviors (Brawner et al. 2016). To enhance truthfulness, most experts recommend directly asking adolescents questions related to sexual behaviors, sexual orientation, and gender identity without parents/guardians in the room. It should be clarified that you ask all clients about their sexual behaviors, sexual orientation, and gender identity to provide the best care possible to minimize feelings of discomfort with the line of questioning.

Questions for APRNs to consider asking during clinical encounters regarding sexual behaviors include:

- Have you had physical attraction to, or desire for, other people? (Probe for whether this is same sex, opposite sex, or other.)
  - If yes: What have you done about these feelings? (Probe for suppression, sexual exploration, current sexual activity.)
- The times when you've engaged in sexual activity, has anyone ever forced you to do it against your will/without your consent? (Probe for rape, molestation, coercion; *be prepared to act accordingly* [i.e. notify police or child protective services].)
- How many sexual partners have you had? (Probe for sequential and concurrent partnerships, including more than one partner during the same sexual act.)

- What types of sexual activities do you engage in with your partners? (Probe for anal, oral, and vaginal sex, mutual masturbation.)
- What, if anything, are you using to prevent unwanted pregnancy, STIs, or other outcomes you might not want from having sex? (Probe for condom use, birth control use, limiting the number of sexual partners, open communication with partners.)
- Describe for me how you are usually feeling/what you are thinking before deciding to have sex (Probe for anger, stress, frustration, sadness.)
- What do you know about your partners' sexual history? (Probe for history of STIs, number of other partners.)

Sexual orientation and gender identity must explicitly be assessed for APRNs to most holistically support their clients. The Fenway Institute have published guidelines for collecting patient data on sexual orientation and gender identity (The Fenway Institute 2018). Researchers have also developed novel items and instruments to capture these factors among sexual and gender minority youth (Katz-Wise et al. 2016). Questions to consider asking include:

- Do you think of yourself as heterosexual or straight, homosexual or gay/lesbian, bisexual or something else? (Note that some youth may describe their sexual orientation as something other than these categories, such as asexual, pansexual, or queer.)
- What sex were you at birth? What is your current gender identity? (Probe for transgender, gender queer.)
- Do you live full-time in your identified gender? Have you accessed any medical interventions or other services to affirm your gender? (Probe for hormones, surgeries.)

It is important to note that many of these questions should be asked multiple times over the course of engagement with the client. This is especially important given rapid changes occurring during this developmental time period, where behaviors can change on a weekly, or even daily, basis. Also, the APRN should be mindful of practice guidelines in his/her state related to adolescents' privacy and confidentiality to ensure that no breaches occur in the sharing of information with parents and guardians. The safest way is to work with clients to help them communicate their sexual health information on their own, without the APRN disclosing information on their behalf. Studies consistently indicate that youth are looking for both quality and quantity in sexual health conversations with providers (Fuzzell et al. 2016), and APRNs are well positioned to support youth in making informed decisions about their sexual health. With advances in technology, young people have greater access to information than at any other point in human history, but this information is not always factual. Thus, APRNs can also help dispel myths or other misgivings youth may have about their bodies and different sexual practices (e.g. false beliefs learned from online videos that STIs cannot be acquired through oral and anal sex).

Sexual Health Interventions

Providers can let adolescents know that there are a variety of ways they can prevent pregnancy and getting STIs/HIV. Even before a teen becomes sexually active, they are eligible to receive a vaccine that can prevent HPV. This vaccine is recommended for all teens aged 11–14 years but can be given as early as age 9 years. The recommended administration schedule depends on the age at time of the first dose. Information can be found on the CDC site. Parental permission may be needed for those under 18 years of age for the HPV vaccine.

As with mental health and substance use issues, in some states adolescents can see a provider without parental permission for reproductive and sexual health issues. A provider can talk with a teen about their readiness to become sexually active and help them think through the decision to determine if it is right for them at this time and does not involve a coercive situation. Once an adolescent decides they are ready to be sexually active, there is an array of prevention options. For example, enjoying touching, holding, kissing, and other nonpenetrative contact are possible ways to express affection. Even for oral sex the use of condoms or dental dams is recommended to prevention transmission of STIs. Once a teen decides to have intercourse, condoms are important for prevention of STIs and HIV, and can also reduce the chances of unwanted pregnancy. Pre-exposure prophylaxis or PrEP (Truvada) is a pill that can be taken every day to prevent acquisition of HIV. Because the rate of HIV is so high among young men who have sex with men (MSM), PrEP is recommended. It does not fully protect against HIV, so condoms still need to be used. Counseling to support adherence for condoms and PrEP is very important since remembering to use these methods routinely is very challenging. This is especially so for adolescents, who have an increased propensity for impulsivity while not yet having full development of cognitive control.

For pregnancy prevention, there are many varieties of contraception that are currently available. There is now strong evidence that long-acting reversible contraceptives (LARCs) are especially well-suited to adolescents and provide more optimal protection for this age group as they reduce the burden of adherence. Contraceptive counseling should include discussing the benefits and disadvantages of the various methods. It is helpful if the adolescent can actually look at the different types of birth control and have an opportunity to ask questions. Continued adherence counseling is very important for supporting an adolescent on contraception as discontinuation rates, especially for non-LARCs is very high, therefore more frequent follow-up visits for teens may be helpful for improved contraceptive adherence.

Conclusion

According to the World Health Organization, "sexual health is a state of physical, mental, and social well-being in relation to sexuality. It requires a positive and respectful approach to sexuality and sexual relationships, as well as the possibility of having pleasurable and safe sexual experiences, free of coercion, discrimination and violence" (World Health Organization 2019). The journey of adolescent sexual development progresses through various stages, with most finding comfort and joy in their sexuality, sexual behaviors, and partner(s). For some, this path is more challenging, resulting in negative health consequences or emotional distress which may have long-lasting effects. APRNs have the opportunity to intervene early with youth and their families to help smooth out the bumps along this road by offering information and access to clinical services, integrating physical, psychosocial, and sexual development, in a safe and supportive manner to achieve maximal wellbeing in relation to their sexual health.

Critical Thinking Questions

1. How can APRNs help adolescents and families distinguish between "normal" and "abnormal" sexual behaviors?
2. In what ways do multilevel factors affect adolescent sexual behavior?
3. How can APRNs support clients to promote sexual health and wellbeing?
4. How can APRNs support adolescent males' healthy involvement in their female partner's contraceptive use?

Resources for Patients and Families

Harris, R.H. and Emberley, M. (2014). *It's Perfectly Normal: Changing Bodies, Growing Up, Sex, and Sexual Health*, 4ee. Boston, MA: Candlewick.

Krieger, I. (2018). *Helping your transgender teen: A guide for parents*, 2ee. Philadelphia, PA: Jessica Kingsley Publishers.

LaRochelle, D. (2014). *Absolutely Positively Not. . .Gay*. New York, NY: Scholastic, Inc.

Nuchi, A. (2017). *Bunk 9's Guide to Growing Up: Secrets, Tips and Expert Advice on the Good, the Bad, and the Awkward*. New York, NY: Workman Publishing.

American Academy of Pediatrics, 141 Northwest Point Boulevard, Elk Grove Village, IL 60007–1098, Tel 847 434–400. www.healthychildren.org.

Parents, Families and Friends of Lesbians and Gays (PFLAG), National Office, 1828 L Street Suite 660, Washington DC 20036, Tel 202 467–8180. http://www.community.pflag.org.

Advocates for Youth. www.advocatesforyouth.org.

Office of Public Health and Science. https://www.hhs.gov/about/agencies/iea/regional-offices/region-6/ophs/index.html.

Sexuality Information and Education Council of the United States, 1012 14th Street NW, Suite 1108, Washington, DC 20005, Tel: 202–265-2405. www.siecus.org.

CDC HIV Testing Locator, https://www.cdc.gov/hiv/testing/index.html.

PrEP Locator. https://preplocator.org.

Planned Parenthood. https://www.plannedparenthood.org.

Resources for Clinicians

Aggleton, P., Cover, R., Leahy, D. et al. (2018). *Youth, Sexuality and Sexual Citizenship*. London: Routledge.

Coffee, G., Fenning, P., and Wells, T.L. (2015). *Promoting Youth Sexual Health: Home, School, and Community Collaboration*. London: Routledge.

Wolfe, D.A. and Temple, J.R. (2018). *Adolescent Dating Violence: Theory, Research and Prevention*. San Diego, CA: Elsevier.

National LGBTQ Task Force. http://www.thetaskforce.org.

Online SO/GI training from the National LGBT Health Education Center. https://www.lgbthealtheducation.org/.

Health Equality Index from the Human Rights Campaign. https://www.hrc.org/hei.

Center of Excellence for Transgender Health. http://www.transhealth.ucsf.edu.

Do Ask, Do Tell, The Fenway Institute and Center for American Progress. http://doaskdotell.org.

American Academy of Pediatrics, 141 Northwest Point Boulevard, Elk Grove Village, IL 60007–1098, Tel 847 434–4000. www.aap.org.

National Institute of Child Health and Human Development (NIH), 31 Center Drive, Building 31, Room 2A32, MSC2425, Bethesda, MD 20892, Tel 3 014 965 133. http://www.nichd.nih.gov.

Society for Adolescent Medicine, 1916 Copper Oaks Circle, Blue Springs, MO 64015, Tel 816 224–8010. www.adolescenthealth.org.

References

ACOG (2013). ACOG Committee opinion no. 554: reproductive and sexual coercion. *Obstetrics and Gynecology* 121(2 Pt 1): 411–415. https://doi.org/10.1097/01.AOG.0000426427.79586.3b.

ACOG. (2016). *Comprehensive sexuality education*. Committee Opinion No. 678, American College of Obstetricians and Gynecologists. Available at https://www.acog.org/Clinical-Guidance-and-Publications/Committee-Opinions/Committee-on-Adolescent-Health-Care/Comprehensive-Sexuality-Education?IsMobileSet=false.

American Psychiatric Association (2013). *Diagnostic and Statistical Manual of Mental Disorders 5*. Washington, DC: American Psychiatric Association.

Braje, S.E., Eddy, J.M., and Hall, G.C.N. (2015). A comparison of two models of risky sexual behavior during late adolescence. *Archives of Sexual Behavior* 45: 73–83. https://doi.org/10.1007/s10508-015-0523-3.

Brawner, B.M., Alexander, K.A., Fannin, E.F. et al. (2016). The role of sexual health professionals in developing a shared concept of risky sexual behavior as it relates to HIV transmission. *Public Health Nursing* 33: 139–150. https://doi.org/10.1111/phn.12216.

Brawner, B.M., Jemmott, L.S., Wingood, G. et al. (2017). Feelings matter: depression severity and emotion regulation in HIV/STI risk-related sexual behaviors. *Journal of Child and Family Studies* 26: 1635–1645. https://doi.org/10.1007/s10826-017-0674-z.

Brown, L.K., Whiteley, L., Houck, C.D. et al. (2017). The role of affect management for HIV risk reduction for youth in alternative schools. *Journal of the American Academy of Child & Adolescent Psychiatry* 56: 524–531. https://doi.org/10.1016/j.jaac.2017.03.010.

Center for Adolescent Health and the Law. (2014). *State Minor Consent Laws: A Summary*, 3rd edn. Available at https://www.cahl.org.

CDC. (2005). *A guide to taking a sexual history.* Centers for Disease Control and Prevention. Available at https://www.cdc.gov/std/treatment/sexualhistory.pdf.

CDC. (2017). *Sexually transmitted diseases: Adolescents and young adults.* Centers for Disease Control and Prevention, Division of STD Prevention, National Center for HIV/AIDS, Viral Hepatitis, STD, and TB Prevention. Available at https://www.cdc.gov/std/life-stages-populations/adolescents-youngadults.htm.

CDC. (2018a). *Youth risk behavior surveillance system (YRBSS).* Centers for Disease Control and Prevention. Available at https://www.cdc.gov/healthyyouth/data/yrbs/index.htm.

CDC. (2018b). *Intimate partner violence.* Centers for Disease Control and Prevention. Available at https://www.cdc.gov/violenceprevention/intimatepartnerviolence/index.html.

CDC. (2018c). *Sexually transmitted disease surveillance 2017: STDs in adolescents and young adults.* Centers for Disease Control and Prevention. Available at https://www.cdc.gov/std/stats17/adolescents.htm.

CDC. (2018d). *HIV among youth.* Centers for Disease Control and Prevention. Available at https://www.cdc.gov/hiv/group/age/youth/index.html.

Deligeoroglou, E., Athanasopoulos, N., Tsimaris, P. et al. (2010). Evaluation and management of adolescent amenorrhea. *Annals of the New York Academy of Sciences* 1205 (1): 23–32. https://doi.org/10.1111/j.1749-6632.2010.05669.x.

Erikson, E.H. (1950). *Childhood and Society.* New York: Norton.

Ferré, C., Callaghan, W., Olso, C. et al. (2016). Effects of maternal age and age-specific preterm birth rates on overall preterm birth rates – United States, 2007 and 2014. *Morbidity and Mortality Monthly Reports (MMWR)* 65 (43): 1181–1184.

Fuzzell, L., Fedesco, H.N., Alexander, S.C. et al. (2016). "I just think that doctors need to ask more questions": Sexual minority and majority adolescents' experiences talking about sexuality with healthcare providers. *Patient Education and Counseling* 99: 1467–1472.

Gross, J.J. (2013). Emotion regulation: taking stock and moving forward. *Emotion* 13: 359–365. https://doi.org/10.1037/a0032135.

Gross, J.J. (2014). Emotion regulation: conceptual and empirical foundations. In: *Handbook of Emotion Regulation*, 2nde (ed. J.J. Gross), 3–20. New York City: Guilford Press.

Hornberger, L.L. and AAP Committee on Adolescence (2017). Options counseling for the pregnant adolescent patient. *Pediatrics* 140: e20172274.

Kar, S.K., Choudhury, A., and Singh, A.P. (2015). Understanding normal development of adolescent sexuality: a bumpy ride. *Journal of Human Reproductive Sciences* 8 (2): 70–74. https://doi.org/10.4103/0974-1208.158594.

Katz-Wise, S.L., Reisner, S.L., Hughto, J.W., and Keo-Meier, C.L. (2016). Differences in sexual orientation diversity and sexual fluidity in attractions among gender minority adults in Massachusetts. *The Journal of Sex Research* 53 (1): 74–84. https://doi.org/10.1080/00224499.2014.1003028.

Lanier, Y., Stewart, J.M., Schensul, J.J., and Guthrie, B.J. (2018). Moving beyond age: an exploratory qualitative study on the context of young African American men and women's sexual debut. *Journal of Racial and Ethnic Health Disparities* 5: 261–270. https://doi.org/10.1007/s40615-017-0366-9.

Latkin, C.A., German, D., Vlahov, D., and Galea, S. (2013). Neighborhoods and HIV: a social ecological approach to prevention and care. *American Psychologist* 68: 210–224. https://doi.org/10.1037/a0032704.

Letourneau, E.J., Schoenwald, S.K., and Sheidow, A.J. (2004). Children and adolescents with sexual behavior problems. *Child Maltreatment* 9 (1): 49–61. https://doi.org/10.1177/1077559503260308.

Lindberg, L.D., Santelli, J.S., and Desai, S. (2016). Understanding the decline in adolescent fertility in the United States, 2007–2012. *The Journal of Adolescent Health* 59: 577–583.

Martin, J.A., Hamilton, B.E., Osterman, M.J.K. et al. (2018). Births: final data for 2017. *National Vital Statistics Report* 67 (8). National Center for Health Statistics, CDC.

National Center on the Sexual Behavior of Youth. (2012). *Sexual behavior: Typical or problematic?* Available at http://www.ncsby.org/content/sexual-behavior-typical-or-problematic.

Olson, J.S. and Crosnoe, R. (2017). Are you still bringing me down?: romantic involvement and depressive symptoms from adolescence to young adulthood. *Journal of Health and Social Behavior* 58 (1): 102–115. https://doi.org/10.1177/0022146516684536.

Penman-Aguilar, A., Carter, M., Snead, M.C., and Kourtis, A.P. (2013). Socioeconomic disadvantage as a social determinant of teen childbearing in the U.S. *Public Health Reports* 128 (suppl 1): 5–22.

Pringle, J., Mills, K.L., McAteer, J. et al. (2017). The physiology of adolescent sexual behaviour: a systematic review. *Cogent Social Sciences* 3 (1): 1368858–1368858. https://doi.org/10.1080/23311886.2017.1368858.

Romero, L., Pazol, K., Warner, L. et al. (2016). Reduced disparities in birth rates among teens aged 15–19 years — United States, 2006–2007 and 2013–2014. *Morbidity and Mortality Weekly Report* 65: 409–414.

Rubin, E.S., Rullo, J., Tsai, P. et al. (2018). Best practices in North American pre-clinical medical education in sexual history taking: consensus from the summits in medical education in sexual health. *The Journal of Sexual Medicine* 15: 1414–1425. https://doi.org/10.1016/j.jsxm.2018.08.008.

Saul Butler, R., Sorace, D., and Hentz Beach, K. (2018). Institutionalizing sex education in diverse U.S. school districts. *Journal of Adolescent Health* 62: 149–156. https://doi.org/10.1016/j.jadohealth.2017.08.025.

Sedgh, G., Finer, L.B., Bankole, A. et al. (2015). Adolescent pregnancy, birth, and abortion rates across countries: levels and recent trends. *The Journal of Adolescent Health* 56: 223–230.

Steinberg, L. (2008). A social neuroscience perspective on adolescent risk-taking. *Developmental Review* 28 (1): 78–106. https://doi.org/10.1016/j.dr.2007.08.002.

Stevens, R., Gilliard-Matthews, S., Dunaev, J. et al. (2017a). Social media use and sexual risk reduction behavior among minority youth: seeking safe sex information. *Nursing Research* 66: 368–377.

Stevens, R., Gilliard-Matthews, S., Dunaev, J. et al. (2017b). The digital hood: social media use among youth in disadvantaged neighborhoods. *New Media & Society* 19: 950–967. https://doi.org/10.1177/1461444815625941.

The Fenway Institute. (2018). *Ready, set, go! Guidelines and tips for collecting patient data on sexual orientation and gender identity*. Available at https://www.lgbthealtheducation.org/wp-content/uploads/2018/03/Ready-Set-Go-publication-Updated-April-2018.pdf.

Vujeva, H.M. and Furman, W. (2011). Depressive symptoms and romantic relationship qualities from adolescence through emerging adulthood: a longitudinal examination of influences. *Journal of Clinical Child and Adolescent Psychology* 40 (1): 123–135. https://doi.org/10.1080/15374416.2011.533414.

World Health Organization. (2019). *Sexual health*. Available at https://www.who.int/topics/sexual_health/en.

Xu, J.Q., Murphy, S.L., Kochanek, K.D. et al. (2018). Deaths: final data for 2016. *National Vital Statistics Reports* 67 (5). National Center for Health Statistics, CDC.

7

Assessing and Managing the Needs of LGBTQ Youth

Liam C. Hein[1] and Jose A. Parés-Avila[2]

[1]University of South Carolina College of Nursing, Columbia, SC, USA
[2]University of South Florida College of Nursing, Tampa, FL, USA

Objectives

After reading this chapter, advanced practice registered nurses will be able to:

1. Acquaint the psych-mental health and primary care advanced practice registered nurse with issues related to sexual orientation and gender identity.

2. Describe the unique challenges sexual minority youth face.
3. Describe best practices on providing care for sexual minority youth.

This chapter discusses issues faced by sexual minority youth, and how to assess their needs and manage care under the *Diagnostic and Statistical Manual of Mental Disorders 5* (DSM-5). It will serve as a guide for advanced practice psychiatric and primary care practitioners who provide care for lesbian, gay, bisexual, transgender, and questioning/queer (LGBTQ) youth. The term youth is used throughout this chapter because recognition of differentness, which is later attributed to nonheterosexuality or gender-incongruence, often begins in early childhood (Zucker 2010). Throughout this chapter issues related to sexual orientation and gender identity will be viewed through the lens of growth and development framed within the broader context of society (Hein et al. 2018).

Definitions

Before proceeding several important terms need to be defined. Gender is defined in the DSM-5 as "public (and usually legally recognized) lived role as a boy or girl, man or woman . . . biological factors are seen as contributing, in interaction with social and psychological factors to gender development." (American Psychiatric Association 2013, p. 451). *Sexual minority* is a synonym for nonheterosexual and/or nontransgender. While there are numerous self-identifications and sexual practices, within the context of this chapter its meaning is limited to gay, lesbian, bisexual, transgender, and queer behaviors and identities. The terms *gay* (♂♀) and *lesbian* (♀) refer to an exclusive physical and emotional attraction to members of one's own sex. In the past, *homosexual* was used to refer to gay and lesbian persons. However, due to the association of this term with the DSM-5, it has acquired pathological connotations and is considered offensive to many LGBTQ people (American Psychological Association:

Committee on Lesbian and Gay Concerns 1991; Lambda Legal 2010). *Bisexual* and *pansexual* people are physically and emotionally attracted to members of both sexes. *Transgender* (gender identity ♂) refers to a person who feels his or her body is not the sex it should be, regardless of transformational hormone or surgical status. Nonbinary (male/female) gender identities include *genderqueer, agender, bigender, gender fluid* and *nonbinary*. It is important to note that youth can be in both a gender and sexual minority, such as a transwoman whose attraction is to other women (lesbian). Table 7.1 records other important definitions.

Table 7.1 Definitions

Term	Definition
Bisexual	Physical and emotional attraction to members of one's own sex, as well as to members of the opposite sex (Kinsey et al. 1948; Nycum 2000).
Cisgender	Expressing a gender consistent to one's sex designation at birth.
Gay	Having an exclusive physical and emotional attraction to members of one's own sex (Kinsey et al. 1948; Nycum 2000). This term may be used for both men and women.
Gender identity	The psychological counterpart of biological sex. The internal sense of male- or femaleness or somewhere on the continuum of male–female (Rafferty et al. 2018).
Heterosexism	An ideological system that denies, denigrates, and stigmatizes any nonheterosexual form of behavior, identity, relationship, or community (Gregory M. Herek and Berrill 1990, p. 315).
Homophobia	A fear of homosexuals.
Homosexual	A pathology-derived term for a person with same-sex attractions and/or behaviors.
Intersex	A person born with biological characteristics of both sexes (Barrow 2008). A contemporary synonym for hermaphrodite.
Lesbian	A woman with an exclusive physical and emotional attraction to other women (Nycum 2000).
LGBTQ	Lesbian, gay, bisexual, transgender, and queer.
Queer	Any category of gender and sexuality other than strictly heterosexual, including gay, lesbian, bisexual and transsexual, and transgender. Queer was historically a derogatory term used by homophobes against nonheterosexual people which has been appropriated and is used affectionately among nonheterosexual people (Nycum 2000, p. 148; Ridge et al. 1997).
Reparative therapy	Reparative or conversion therapy refers to a collection of treatments intended to change the sexual orientation of nonheterosexuals to heterosexual (Hein and Matthews 2010).
Sex work	The performance of sexual acts, in exchange for food, shelter, money, protection or drugs (Greene et al. 1999; McNamara 1994; Rotheram-Borus et al. 1995). Synonyms: survival sex, prostitution, rent.
Straight	Contemporary, nonclinical term for heterosexual.
Transgender	A term inclusive of people who cross-dress for sexual (transvestite) or theatrical (drag queen) reasons, and people who feel his or her body is not the sex it should be (regardless of transformational surgical status) (transsexual) (Barrow 2008; Califia 1997; Nycum 2000).
Transsexual	A person who feels his or her body is not the sex it should be (regardless of transformational surgical status) (Nycum 2000).
Transman	A person with female sex and male gender: A female-to-male (FtM) transsexual (regardless of transformational surgical status). Use the pronoun "he" when referring to this person.
Transwoman	A person with male sex and female gender: A male-to-female (MtF) transsexual (regardless of transformational surgical status). Use the pronoun "she" when referring to this person.

Source: Modified from Hein (2006, p. 14).

Prevalence

The exact prevalence of same-sex behavior, attraction or gender incongruence is unknown. Divergent results have been reported in the literature depending on whether self-identification or sexual behavior is measured. Prevalence of LGBTQ self-identification is lower than the prevalence of sexual behavior. One in five or 21% of males in the United States report either homosexual behavior or homosexual attraction since age 15 (Sell et al. 1995). In another study 5% self-identified as gay, lesbian or bisexual and/or reported same-sex sexual contact (Massachusetts Youth Risk Behavior Survey 2001). Self-identification rates vary from 3% (Massachusetts Youth Risk Behavior Survey 2001) to 6% of adolescent males self-identifying as gay or bisexual (Remafedi et al. 1992). In a large population study, 2.7% identified as transgender/gender nonconforming (Eisenberg et al. 2017).

Many sexual minority youth are very comfortable with their sexuality and gender identity, and move into adulthood uneventfully; others struggle with their sexual orientation/ gender identity and experience myriad obstacles. Over the last 20 years, LGBTQ youth have become more visible. Being comfortable with their sexual orientation and gender identity can be liberating, but can also cause difficulties when concealment is necessary (Rieger et al. 2009; Sylva et al. 2009).

These youth are members of all racial, ethnic, socioeconomic, and religious groups and may be indistinguishable from their heterosexual peers. Savin-Williams and Diamond (2000) describe a new generation of youth who reject all gender categories, and are attracted to and intimate with both same and opposite-sexes without shame or guilt. They point out that the entertainment industry's normalizing of same-sex desire has had a dramatic impact on the ability of adolescents to understand their own emerging sexual desires.

Increasing societal acceptance, the availability of older LGBTQ role models, access to resources for non-heterosexual youth, the internet, television shows that portray positive same-sex relationships, and school and community based gay/straight alliances have played a role in the possibility of youth "coming out" or disclosing that they are LGBTQ at an earlier age (Walls et al. 2010). Despite the probability of successfully navigating childhood while LGBTQ, individual and collective biases have created a minefield of barriers to their success. Heterosexist beliefs and institutions effectively create an inhospitable territory of oppression LGBTQ youth must traverse.

Significant Historical Factors

Oppression: Heterosexism and Homophobia

Although many youth are comfortable with identifying LGBTQ and discuss it openly, some youth are confused and frightened by their same-sex feelings and attractions, sometimes due to feelings of conflict with their family's beliefs and religious values. These youth are often acutely aware of the stigma associated with being lesbian or gay. Historically, the term homophobia was used to describe the loathing of nonheterosexuals. However, inclusion of "phobia" in the term has created a misnomer related to the loci of hating homosexuals. Phobia or fear doesn't play a role in these feelings (Herek 2002). Heterosexism, however, is the belief and the actions related to feeling that being heterosexual is the only acceptable way of existing (Herek 1990). Although some segments of society are more tolerant of sexual minorities, there is a large portion of society that continues to stigmatize and perpetuate hatred (Fish 2010). Tolerance is not acceptance. Sexual minorities have been adversely affected by this hatred and intolerance, at home, in school, in the work place, and in their places of worship (Hatzenbuehler et al. 2010). Although there had been a period of increased acceptance and safety from approximately 2009–2016, the pendulum has now swung in the opposite direction. "Bathroom bills", laws prohibiting (and criminalizing) transgender people from using the restroom that correlates to their gender identity (and possibly appearance), have been considered in 16 US states (Kralik 2017). Although Title IX of the Civil Rights Act had previously been interpreted to protect transgender persons, the US Department of Education has placed a moratorium on investigations of complaints by transgender persons (Balingit 2018, February 12). This has removed a major protection for transgender youth in the school setting. The negative effects can, in many instances, be profound. Fear and stigma may lead youth to resort to non-healthy methods of coping such as drinking, using drugs, engaging in unprotected sex, self-harm behavior, and running away from home. Not all primary care and psychiatric–mental health nurse practitioners are comfortable working with lesbian, gay, bisexual, and questioning youth. They may be conflicted about their own feelings, thoughts, and religious beliefs related to homosexuality. The nurse practitioner must address his or her own ideas, anxieties, lack of knowledge about LGBTQ related issues, and any discomfort about providing care for these youth in order to work effectively with them and their families. The role of the therapist is to understand LGBTQ adolescents' sense of their own sexuality within the context of their own self-labels. This understanding will hopefully enable a healthy integration of the adolescent's sexuality into his or her own identity. If the practitioner is unable to address his or her own issues about adolescent sexuality and sexual identity and is uncomfortable working with sexual minority adolescents, it is best for the practitioner to refer these youth to another provider who is skilled and comfortable working with nonheterosexual youth (Hoffman et al. 2009).

Victimization

Lesbian, gay, bisexual, and transgender youth recognize their vulnerability to victimization and the absence of resources to assist them (Grossman and D'Augelli 2006). Sexual minorities are twice as likely to have been victims of child abuse and traumatic events and to experience PTSD than heterosexual adults (Roberts et al. 2010). Additionally, recent hate crime data have indicated LGBTQ people are proportionally over twice as likely to be victims of hate crimes as any other group (Smith 2010). Being a victim of a hate crime carries longer-lasting psychological feelings of vulnerability than other victimization (Herek 2009; Willis 2008). Perpetrators of hate crimes target individuals based on their biases and their perceptions based on such biases. For many LGBTQ youth attending school feels like torture due to near-constant harassment (Craig et al. 2008; Grossman and D'Augelli 2006; Wyss 2004). Sexual minorities are often the victims of bullying at school (Berlan et al. 2010). Additionally, when LGBTQ youth break rules at school or laws they tend to receive harsher punishments than heterosexual youth (Himmelstein and Bruckner 2011). However, schools with gay-straight alliances (GSA) have more a positive school climate for all children, even those not involved in the GSA (Walls et al. 2010). Additionally, LGBT youth who attend a high school with a GSA experience less distress, less alcohol use, and have more positive school experiences (Heck et al. 2011).

Mental Health

Many gay and lesbian youth live a life of isolation, alienation, depression, and fear because of negative stereotypes, religious taboos regarding homosexuality, family and cultural beliefs about homosexuality, and their own fears about being lesbian or gay. The stress of trying to negotiate and cope with these issues, as a child, puts lesbian, gay, bisexual, and transgender youth in a position of developmental catch-up. These youth are at risk for depression, suicidal ideation, low self-esteem, sexual risk taking, and substance abuse (McCann et al. 2017).

Advanced practice psychiatric and primary care practitioners are in a unique position to provide counseling, support, and healthcare to LGBTQ youth and families.

Although behavioral, psychosocial, and lifestyle problems are major causes of morbidity and mortality, adolescents rarely choose to seek help from mental healthcare providers. They do not see a connection between psychosocial issues such as depression, drug use/abuse, sexual behaviors, family/school problems, victimization and abuse, and mental health. School personnel, law enforcement personnel or other concerned individuals may refer adolescents for mental health evaluations. Parents may express concern about their child's behavior or symptoms to a primary care provider, who in turn might make a referral to a mental health practitioner. Parents can be the greatest advocate for their child (Ryan et al. 2010) or a source of danger (Balsam et al. 2005). The psychiatric–mental health nurse practitioner provides expert care based on current, factual nonjudgmental information in a confidential manner. The most effective tool the nurse practitioner can use when interacting with LGBTQ youth or their parents is compassion and genuineness.

Self-Realization and Coming Out

Realization that one is different from heterosexual peers is a common experience for LGBTQ youth. This perception of difference is often more acute for transgender youth. Transgender youth tend to become consciously aware of their sex-gender incongruence when they enter preschool (Grossman and D'Augelli 2006); for some youth, other-gender play and interests begin around the age of 2 (American Psychiatric Association 2000, p. 536). In a large longitudinal study early childhood (3 years) gender nonconformity has been associated with a non-heterosexual sexual orientation at 15 years of age (Li et al. 2017). Studying prepubescent transgender children Olson et al. (2015) found transgender children had gender cognitions and behaviors that were indistinguishable from cisgender children of the same gender identity (pp. 467). Male-to-female transgender youth tend to come out as preteens or adolescents (Grossman and D'Augelli 2006). Savin-Williams and Diamond (2000) identified slightly different developmental trajectories for lesbian, gay, and bisexual males and females. Girls tended to develop an emotional attachment to another girl, leading to self-identification (around 18 years old). Boys often pursued sexual relations (at around 16 years old) several years before self-identifying as gay (Savin-Williams and Diamond 2000).

All youth are similar in that they must develop a sense of self, individuate, make decisions about their future, social and ethical issues establish independent from their parents, and have a clear sense of their own identity and sexuality. The coming out process is defined as a developmental process in which gay people recognize their sexual orientation and choose to integrate this knowledge into their personal and social lives (Savin-Williams and Diamond 2000). Several theorists describe coming out as a life-long process with stage-like sequencing. There are several models (Coleman 1982; Katz-Wise et al. 2017; Savin-Williams and Diamond 2000) describing the coming-out process as involving three to five interrelated areas of development: (i) a growing awareness of homosexual feelings, (ii) developing intimate same-sex romantic relationships, (iii) developing social ties with gay and lesbian peers or community, (iv) developing a positive evaluation of homosexuality, and (v) self-disclosure and disclosure to others. These theorists describe the coming-out process as occurring in stages. During this coming-out process, the person can go back to a previous stage if issues have not been resolved.

Coming out is stressful under the best of circumstances (Barrow 2008). LGBTQ youth have to cope with not only the complexities of mastering developmental tasks but also the daily stresses of realizing that they are different. A major source of stress is the fear that a parent, friend or teacher might unexpectedly find out about their sexual orientation/gender identity. Katz-Wise et al. (2018) found that better family functioning was associated with better mental health outcomes for transgender youth. There are times when the lesbian or gay youth might experience feelings of conflict or confusion over his or her sexuality. Some youth might experience pressure to disclose their identity because of having inaccurate information about sexual orientation. Practitioners should assess the level of information the youth has regarding homosexuality and coming out, and provide information about the coming-out process and the ramifications of disclosure.

Family Relationships and Disclosure

Some youth have been put out of their homes after coming out, leaving them at risk for depression, suicide, drug abuse, violence, and sexual victimization (Hein 2010). Many youth become targets of bullying and harassment at school and in their communities. They are left to cope with isolation, depression, fear, and rejection. If their parents and community are religious they may be subjected to reparative therapies, also known as conversion therapies (Hein and Matthews 2010). Some youth who disclose their sexual/gender identity to parents or friends are rejected by them and subsequently by their faith communities. Faced with being told they no longer have value to their families or to their God it is no wonder these youth struggle with depression and consider suicide. Ryan et al. (2009) found that youth who experienced high levels of family rejection during adolescence were six times more likely to be depressed and eight times more likely to have attempted suicide. In a 2018 study, 25% of LGBTQ youth identified nonaccepting families as the most important problem they are currently facing (Human Rights Campaign 2018), more than school/bullying problems (21%).

The coming-out process for LGBTQ adolescents is superimposed on top of the developmental tasks of all adolescents. Adolescents need supportive and affirming adults in their lives as they move toward independence. It is important for these youth to establish social ties with peers and to learn to safely interact within their communities. Due to the barriers these youth face at home, in school, and in the community, many of these youth will experience deficits in development. These youth have the same needs and developmental expectations as heterosexual youth. Unfortunately, secondary to environmental constraints, LGBTQ youth may need assistance in revisiting and reintegrating skipped developmental tasks into their current stage. They will need the support and affirmation of adults who are accepting of their sexual orientation. Developing social ties with healthy LGBTQ adults and peers through school and other social activities is important. However, identifying what resources are safe and helpful can sometimes be difficult.

Faith and Religiosity

Issues related to sexual orientation and gender identity may be magnified in LGBTQ youth from faith or religious backgrounds. Many mainstream faiths and religious affiliations rely on interpretations of the Bible, Torah or Quran that traditionally condemn same-sex behavior. Faith or religious beliefs may complicate the coming-out process. For people whose personal, social, racial or ethnic identity is closely tied to their faith communities, "coming out" sometimes carries a different meaning (Pitt 2009; Wheeler 2003). There are specific gender roles, family values, and expectations of community that may orbit one's faith that contribute to the identity development process within different cultural groups.

Although faith may be protective and foster resilience for heterosexual youth, LGBT may experience shame and rejection in faith communities. Besides alienating LGBTQ youth from these sources of support, these youth will often feel alienated and rejected by their higher power (Super and Jacobson 2011).

Intersectionality

Intersectionality is holding multiple vulnerable identities simultaneously, in this context racial and ethnic minority status in addition to LGBTQ status. Racial and ethnic minority LGBTQ youth face challenges that are similar to their white peers, but there are also additional challenges that they must confront. These youth have the burden of not only racism but also homophobia, and religious and cultural condemnation (Worthen 2017). They may also encounter racism in the LGBTQ community (Hunter 2010). Pressured by the cultural expectations of family and community related to marriage and childbearing these young people may experience high levels of stress. These youth do not have the benefit of their families reframing racial or ethnic stereotypes coupled with sexual orientation in order to support healthy development. Racial and ethnic minority youth may decide not to disclose their orientation and/or gender identity due to the heightened stigma of these intersectional identities and as a result they become invisible (Bowleg 2013), experiencing complex identity conflicts (Corsbie-Massay et al. 2017). Identity conflict may make these youth vulnerable to the enticements of reparative therapy.

Reparative or Conversion Therapy

Reparative or conversion therapy refers to a collection of treatments intended to change the sexual orientation of nonheterosexuals to heterosexual (Hein and Matthews 2010). At times, the parent(s) of LGBTQ youth or even the youth themselves might ask a provider to assist in changing the child's sexual orientation or gender identity. In some cases, parents are pressured by their faith leaders so seek reparative/conversion therapies to "cure" their child's same-sex attractions. In other cases, the adolescent becomes frightened by their same-sex attractions and seeks help from a provider to "fix the problem" or make him or her "normal" (Fox

61, 2009). Encouraging adolescents to change their sexual orientation conveys a message that there is something intrinsically wrong with them (Hein and Matthews 2010). Reparative therapy to change one's sexual orientation has been deemed harmful and/ or unethical by most professional organizations (American Psychiatric Association 2000, as cited in American Psychiatric Association 2018; Blackwell 2008; Hein and Matthews 2010; Hein, Powell, and ISPN Diversity and Equity Committee 2008; SAMHSA 2015). The inherent belief is that homosexuality is a mental illness that can be cured. To date, there is no clinical evidence that reparative therapies cure individuals of homosexuality. There is evidence, however, that reparative therapies can have long-term consequences of sexual dysfunction, depression, and suicidality (Haldeman 2001).

However, partially due to the DSM-5 diagnosis of "gender dysphoria" (F64.0) (American Psychiatric Association 2013), therapies to change a person's gender identity continue and are legal in 35 states (Thomsen 2018). There is debate about whether a diagnosis of gender dysphoria carries some benefit related to insurance and transitioning. However, some insurance companies were quick to explicitly exclude treatments for gender dysphoria from pharmaceutical, mental health, and other coverage. Table 7.2 lists diagnoses codes commonly used. Additionally, there is some evidence that gender atypical behavior in childhood is more predictive of being lesbian, gay or bisexual than transgender (Bailey and Zucker 1995).

Table 7.2 Diagnosis codes for gender identity

DSM-5	ICD-10	ICD-11
	Counseling related to sexual attitude, behavior, and orientation Z70.1	Counseling related to sexual attitude, behavior, and orientation QA15.1
		Counseling related to sexuality, unspecified QA15.Z
		Family counseling QA18
Gender dysphoria in children	Gender identity disorder of childhood F64.2	Gender incongruence 17.HA60-HA6Z
Gender dysphoria in adolescents	Gender identity disorder in adolescence and adulthood F64 Gender identity or role, uncertainty F66	Gender incongruence 17.HA60-HA6Z

Source: APA (2013) and WHO (2018, 2019).

Homelessness and Residential Instability

Youth become homeless for various reasons. LGBTQ youth are proportionally overrepresented among homeless unaccompanied minors. A census of the homeless youth in Washington, DC found 43% identified as LGBTQ (Bahrampour 2016). A study of transgender youth in Ontario, CA found 45% with unsupportive parents were inadequately housed (Travers et al. 2012). The effects of LGBTQ homelessness can follow these youth to adulthood in the form of depression, suicidal ideation, substance use, and other health risk behaviors (Pearson et al. 2017).

Although the US Department of Housing and Urban Development regulations now require shelters to be transgender affirming (US Department of Housing and Urban Development 2016), there are few mechanisms for enforcement. Additionally, there is little legal recourse for youth who have been thrown out of their home by their parents. Although child abandonment is illegal, children do not have legal standing to sue their parents (Judge 2015). Additionally, the child's presence on the street is considered a status offense (a crime based on their status as a minor).

Substance Use and the DSM-5

Many youth use alcohol, tobacco, and drugs to cope with stress and depression. Gay and lesbian youth may use substances to manage feelings of depression, isolation, shame, and low self-esteem. A 2018 study found 52% of LGBT youth had experimented with alcohol and drugs compared to the general population (Human Rights Campaign 2018). Bisexual youth reported the highest rates. However, a study of southern LGBT college students found less than 10% had abuse or addiction conditions (Hood et al. 2019) A thorough assessment that includes sexuality issues can assist the youth and the practitioner in opening the door to discussion about sexual identity and this may be the first opportunity for the youth to talk about concerns, confusion, and/or ask questions. However, it is important for the advanced practice registered nurse (APRN) who regularly works with LGBTQ youth to acquaint themselves with same-sex sexual behaviors and any related risks. Additionally, developing a strong referral network within the community will improve their ability to provide quality comprehensive care. Similar to questions about sexual behaviors, the APRN who enquires about use of substances with abuse and dependence potential should familiarize themselves with drugs used in the LGBTQ community and LGBTQ clubs/venues or risk alienating their patients. Harm reduction lends the practitioner space to suspend judgment and explore with youth the role substances may play in negotiating conflict and confusion around sexual orientation and gender identity. Examples of affirming harm-reduction interventions are introducing ideas like the designated driver. Open discussion about not accepting drinks from strangers or not leaving a drink unattended introduces the reality of date rape through gamma hydroxybutyric acid or rophynol.

Sexual Behavior

It is important to ask your patient about sexual activity. The APRN who on assessment discovers that the youth is engaging in sexual behavior should assess the type of behaviors, helping them to understand how premature sexual behavior (before they've concluded the nature of their sexual attractions) complicates their ability to move through the developmental tasks of adolescence and the development of a healthy sense of self. Nonthreatening questions about any symptoms the youth might be experiencing should be asked, and based on those findings appropriate laboratory work should be ordered, e.g. screening for STIs, HPV, and HIV. However, be prepared to comfortably answer questions about any/all sexual activities. For both the sexually active and nonsexually active LGBTQ youth, counseling about protection for sexual activities which put them at risk for STIs, HIV, and possible pregnancy should be provided. Some LGBTQ youth engage in heterosexual sex as a way of coping with pressure they perceive from peers or family members about dating. They may use heterosexual sex as a way of warding off suspicion about their sexuality or to prove to themselves that they are not lesbian or gay if they are in conflict about their sexual identity. Another risk of this behavior is unwanted pregnancy. Pregnancy can occur because of rape, failure to practice safe sex, drug use/abuse or survival sex. It is also important to be particularly sensitive to the needs of transgender youth. If you are unwilling to assist them with halting the onset of puberty (Asscheman 2009) they may find another way to transition, e.g. street hormones, silicone parties, and occasionally self-mutilation (Padilla et al. 2016). Although sexual activity and unconventional transitioning activities can convey HIV, it is important to be clear you do not see the youth as merely a vector of disease.

It is essential that LGBTQ youth are provided with information about adolescent sexuality, sexual and gender identity, and resources that are able to meet their needs. As healthy sexuality and healthy relationships become part of the health promotion a practitioner conducts, preventing sexual violence, including intimate partner violence, must be addressed. The National Intimate Partner and Sexual Violence Survey (NISVS) is an ongoing telephone survey conducted by the CDC with a representative sample of adults 18 and older (Centers for Disease Control 2010). Through that survey, we have learned that intimate partner violence occurs to LGBTQ individuals at the same rates as heterosexuals. However, some forms of sexual violence occur at higher rates to lesbians, gay men, and bisexual women and men with higher rates among bisexuals. These forms of sexual violence include rape, physical violence, and stalking by an intimate partner. Unfortunately, some states (Alabama, South Carolina, and Texas) criminalize teaching about sexual orientation outside of the context of STDs (Comprehensive Health Education Act 1988) and 18 states mandate the teaching that sexual activity should only occur within the context of marriage (Guttmacher Institute 2011). Although the US Supreme Court struck down all state same-sex marriage bans on 26 June 2015, it is still difficult to ascertain whether this landmark decision has changed sex education in those 18 states. So not only does the sexual education provided in some states ignore the existence of sexual minorities through their emphasis on marriage (something these same states are simultaneously denying to sexual minorities), other states overtly vilify nonheterosexual sex. In this context sex education is just another context in which youth are victimized.

Depression, Anxiety, Nonsuicidal Self-Injury, and Suicide

It is important to assess LGBTQ youth for depression, anxiety, nonsuicidal self-injury (NSSI), and suicidal ideation. Inquiring about suicidal ideation and attempts should be part of your assessment. Suicide is the second leading cause of death in youth between 10 and 24 years in the United States (Centers for Disease Control 2018, p. 11). Data on suicide and suicidal ideation in LGBTQ youth indicate an elevated level of suicidal ideation among LGBTQ youth (Lytle et al. 2018; McDonald 2018). Furthermore, higher levels of religiosity elevate this risk (Lytle et al. 2018). There is a heightened risk for suicide attempts among youth with high levels of religiosity during the period of questioning their sexual orientation (Lytle et al. 2018). A relationship has been reported between victimization, gender nonconformity, and suicide attempts (Bouris et al. 2016; Clements-Nolle et al. 2006; D'Augelli et al. 2005). A large Canadian study found 65% of transgender youth seriously considered suicide in the last year (Veale et al. 2017). Parental support is protective of suicidal ideation and attempts, with 70% of unsupported transgender youth considering suicide and 57% attempting suicide (Travers et al. 2012).

NSSI should also be assessed by the APRN. An integrative review on NSSI in LGBTQ populations found an increased risk of NSSI among transgender and nonbinary identities (Jackman et al. 2016). Furthermore, being the victim of LGBTQ-targeted harassment and discrimination as well as being closeted increased the risk for NSSI (Jackman et al. 2016). Interestingly, Durwood et al. (2017) found transgender youth who had socially transitioned were not significantly more depressed or anxious than nontransgender youth.

Lesbian and gay youth who are conflicted about their sexual orientation, who have been subjected to harassment, violence and/or rejection, and have used addictive substances have a greater chance of becoming depressed and experiencing suicidal ideation. The stress of being lesbian or gay can also exacerbate existing problems such as sexual acting out, a significant decrease in school grades, social isolation, and arguments with parents and peers. When these issues are addressed with youth, it helps them to feel safe. Depressed LGBTQ youth tend to be invisible and they do not usually seek help for fear of being discovered and rejected. When they do come to the attention of healthcare providers, they do not announce that they are LGBTQ. Discussion can help them to address the stressors that affect their wellbeing, such as confusion about their sexuality, fear of rejection by family and peers, the stress of leading a double life, and having to hide their sexual identity. Some adolescents who have disclosed their sexual orientation/gender identity or have had it discovered by peers or family become depressed when they sense little support. Conversely, others find disclosure cathartic and freeing.

The APRN and Safe Healthcare

Lesbian, gay, bisexual, and transgender youth may perceive healthcare services and providers as intolerant and consequently unsafe (Grossman and D'Augelli 2006). Transgender youth may be unable to access needed healthcare services due to unavailability, for example providers willing to prescribe hormone treatment to delay puberty or to assist with transitioning, or simply gynecologic services that are not harassing to masculine lesbians. Compounding the general absence of safe services outside of very large urban areas, we are discussing youth: youth without legal standing to provide independent consent to treatment. There are some ways the affirming provider can demonstrate safety in their practice:

- Acknowledge LGBTQ youth exist (Grossman and D'Augelli 2006). Post a sticker of the rainbow flag or other symbol of the LGBTQ community on the door to their office.
- Stay informed about LGBTQ youth (Hoffman et al. 2009).

- Advocate for safe schools for LGBTQ youth (Rafferty, AAP Committee on Psychosocial Aspects of Child and Family Health, AAP Committee on Adolescence, and AAP Section on Lesbians 2018).
- Include LGBTQ-affirming reading material in their waiting room.
- Modify their intake form to include "partnered" beside checkboxes for "married," "single," and "divorced".
- When discussing relationship status with your client ask everyone (whether male or female) if they have a "boyfriend or girlfriend".
- Ask what pronoun he/she/they would like you to use.
- In the event the youth needs referral, be careful where you refer so that you do not make things worse. Confirm the provider is LGBTQ affirming before referring.
- Carefully consider whether parental involvement in your patient's care will be helpful or harmful (Travers et al. 2012). Many youth prefer to receive care without parental involvement (Hoffman et al. 2009). Are their parents aware of their sexual orientation/gender identity? Will you endanger the youth if you disclose their sexual orientation/gender identity (physical safety, housing etc.)?
- Assist the youth to create a safety plan (Barrow 2008): where can they go, who can assist them if their physical safety (abuse) or housing is compromised?

Once the adolescent has decided that he or she is ready to disclose, the nurse practitioner has an important role in the process. The decision to disclose involves several steps.

1. Weighing the risks and benefits, which include parental response. Coming out to parents can be upsetting for parents, siblings, and the disclosing adolescent. The nurse should be prepared to support both the adolescent and the family during their adjustment to the disclosure. Anticipatory guidance for adolescents and parents involves providing information on adolescent sexuality and practices, resources such as gay and lesbian youth centers, school support networks, and support networks for parents such as Parents, Families and Friends of Lesbian and Gays (PFLAG). GLMA: Health Professionals Advancing LGBTQ Equality, an interdisciplinary professional organization of healthcare providers, offers an online directory of gay-affirming healthcare providers.
2. Examining the youth's motivation for disclosure. While some youth may not be able to clearly identify their motives, they need to be explored to determine whether they are out of anger, self-preservation or self-destruction. Assist the youth

to explore what being LGBTQ means to the youth and the resources and social support available.
3. Exploring the youth's relationship with parents and family cultural/ethnic, moral, and religious views. For reasons of safety, it is important to help the youth recognize their social milieu, to gain insight into their situation and environment. Explore with the youth what resources are available outside the home in the event that there is parental, family and peer disapproval and/or rejection.
4. Offering anticipatory guidance will also be helpful. For instance, what do their parents, family, and friends think about homosexuality? How will they respond to negative comments about LGBTQ people when the comments are directed at them? What are some ways that they might respond if these comments are made by someone in authority? Assisting the youth to think through and answer these questions will not only assist with the coming-out process but will help the youth to be safer once out.

The APRN must help the youth consider their parents' reaction in the event they came out. The APRN can be a source of strength and support for the youth if they wish to come out. The practitioner must be careful not to push the youth toward resolution and disclosure, particularly if they express conflict or confusion about their sexuality. Additionally, the youth must be cautioned to seriously consider their parents' potential reaction; they are still minors and consequently very vulnerable. The youth may need encouraged to consider delaying their disclosure until self-supporting and living independently.

Includes take-home points from the chapter to help APRNs work with LGBTQ patients.

Conclusion

LGBTQ youth usually present for therapy for issues other than their sexual orientation. It is important for the APRN to address the presenting problem even if it is known that the youth is LGBTQ. Engaging youth in a nonjudgmental, nonthreatening manner is essential to developing a therapeutic relationship with them. Sexual minority youth need to be able to explore what being nonheterosexual means and how their lives are affected by it. They need to be able to talk about how they are feeling and coping in a safe and open environment. Nurse therapists who work with LGBTQ youth have a responsibility to become knowledgeable about adolescent sexuality and sexual orientation development.

The provision of quality care to sexual minority youth has been difficult to achieve because it tends to engender fear in many heterosexual people due to lack of knowledge and discomfort. Although in recent years there has been emphasis on sexual health, many providers are uncomfortable broaching the subject. There has been much controversy in deciding who should discuss and educate youth about sexuality and sexual health. Additionally, many providers may be unfamiliar with LGBTQ sexual practices. The fact is that today's adolescents engage in sexual behavior, question their own sexuality, and are often less inhibited about discussing sexual issues than the adults around them. The health needs of LGBTQ youth may go unmet due to provider bias or fear of anticipated discrimination or harassment.

Advanced practice primary care and psychiatric–mental health nurses will encounter adolescents who are moving through the different stages of their physical, psychosocial, and sexual development. Some of these youth will be heterosexual, others will be homosexual, and some of them will be questioning their sexual identity. The advanced practice clinician will encounter these youth in a variety of settings, therefore it is important for the clinician to be educated and knowledgeable about the various sexualities and gender identities as well as the issues that arise as youth move through developmental stages. APRNs must be comprehensive in their assessments of adolescent health and illness, which includes assessment of physical, psychosocial, and sexual orientation and gender identity to determine if there are problems or issues that need to be addressed and/or treated. They provide education about prevention of STIs and access to local resources, and they interface with community and local resources to assure that the provision of care meets the needs of the adolescent and family. Advanced practice registered nurses can be pivotal in helping youth to fully integrate all of the developmental tasks of adolescence as they journey to adulthood.

Resources

The Fenway Institute. Best practices and protocols for LGBTQ health, Tel 1 (617) 927–6400. https://fenwayhealth.org/the-fenway-institute.

GLMA: Health Professionals Advancing LGBTQ Equality. Interdisciplinary organization of healthcare professionals providing LGBTQ healthcare, Tel 1 (202) 600–8037. www.glma.org.

Parents and Friends of Lesbians and Gays (PFLAG). Parents/family group for people who support their LGBTQ family member, 400 local chapters in the United States. https://pflag.org

Trans Lifeline. Crisis and suicide hotline for trans people, 24/7, Tel 1 (877) 565–8860 (US), 1 (877) 330–6366 (Canada). https://www.translifeline.org.

The Trevor Project. Crisis and suicide prevention hotline for LGBTQ youth under 25, 24/7, Tel 1 (866) 488–7386. www.thetrevorproject.org.

World Professional Association of Transgender Professionals (WPATH). Publications, resources, and standards of care for transgender health. https://www.wpath.org

References

American Psychiatric Association (2000). *Diagnostic and Statistical Manual of Mental Disorders: DSM-IV-TR*. Washington, DC: American Psychiatric Association.

American Psychiatric Association (2013). *Diagnostic and Statistical Manual of Mental Disorders 5*. Washington, DC: American Psychiatric Association.

American Psychiatric Association (2018). *Position statement on conversion therapy and LGBTQ patients*. Washington, DC: American Psychiatric Association Available at https://www.psychiatry.org/home/policy-finder?k=conversion%20therapy%20and%20LGBTQ%20patients.

American Psychological Association: Committee on Lesbian and Gay Concerns (1991). Avoiding heterosexual bias in language. *American Psychologist* 46 (9): 973–974.

Asscheman, H. (2009). Gender identity disorder in adolescents. *Sexologies* 18 (2): 105–108.

Bahrampour, T. (2016). Nearly half of homeless youth are LGBTQ, first ever city census finds. *The Washington Post*. Available at https://www.washingtonpost.com/local/social-issues/nearly-half-of-homeless-youth-are-lgbtq-first-ever-city-census-finds/2016/01/13/0cb619ae-ba2e-11e5-829c-26ffb874a18d_story.html.

Bailey, J.M. and Zucker, K.J. (1995). Childhood sex-typed behavior and sexual orientation: a conceptual analysis and quantitative review. *Developmental Psychology* 31 (1): 43–55. https://doi.org/10.1037/0012-1649.31.1.43.

Balingit, M. (2018). Education department no longer investigating transgender bathroom complaints. *The Washington Post*, p. 3. Available at https://www.washingtonpost.com/news/education/wp/2018/02/12/education-department-will-no-longer-investigate-transgender-bathroom-complaints/?noredirect=on&utm_term=.57ab0f9d9899.

Balsam, K.F., Rothblum, E.D., and Beauchaine, T.P. (2005). Victimization over the life span: a comparison of lesbian, gay, bisexual, and heterosexual siblings. *Journal of Consulting and Clinical Psychology* 73 (3): 477–487. https://doi.org/10.1037/0022-006X.73.3.477.

Barrow, K.L. (2008). *Achieving optimal gender identity integration for transgender female-to-male adult patients: An unconventional psychoanalytic guide for treatment*. Publication No. 3326610, Doctoral dissertation, The Wright Institute. ProQuest Dissertations Publishing.

Berlan, E.D., Corliss, H.L., Field, A.E. et al. (2010). Sexual orientation and bullying among adolescents in the growing up today study. *Journal of Adolescent Health* 46 (4): 366–371. https://doi.org/10.1016/j.jadohealth.2009.10.015.

Blackwell, C.W. (2008). Nursing implications in the application of conversion therapies on gay, lesbian, bisexual and transgender clients. *Issues in Mental Health Nursing* 29 (6): 651–665.

Bouris, A., Everett, B.G., Heath, R.D. et al. (2016). Effects of victimization and violence on suicidal ideation and behaviors among sexual minority and heterosexual adolescents. *LGBT Health* 3 (2): 153–161. https://doi.org/10.1089/lgbt.2015.0037.

Bowleg, L. (2013). Once you've blended the cake, you can't take the parts back to the main ingredients': black gay and bisexual men's descriptions and experiences of intersectionality. *Sex Roles* 68 (11–12): 754–767. https://doi.org/10.1007/s11199-012-0152-4.

Califia, P. (1997). *Sex Changes: The Politics of Transgenderism*. San Francisco: Cleis Press.

Centers for Disease Control. (2010). *NISVS: An overview of 2010 findings by sexual orientation*. Available at https://www.cdc.gov/violenceprevention/pdf/cdc_nisvs_victimization_final-a.pdf.

Centers for Disease Control (2018). *Deaths: leading causes for 2016. National Vital Statistics Reports* 67 (6): 77.

Clements-Nolle, K., Marx, R., and Katz, M. (2006). Attempted suicide among transgender persons. The influence of gender-based discrimination and victimization. *Journal of Homosexuality* 51 (3): 53–69. https://doi.org/10.1300/J082v51n03_04.

Coleman, E. (1982). Developmental stages of the coming out process. *Journal of Homosexuality* 7 (2): 31–43.

Comprehensive Health Education Act. (1988), SC ST SEC 59–32-30, South Carolina Code of Laws.

Corsbie-Massay, C.L.P., Miller, L.C., Christensen, J.L. et al. (2017). Identity conflict and sexual risk for black and Latino YMSM. *AIDS and Behavior* 21 (6): 1611–1619. https://doi.org/10.1007/s10461-016-1522-7.

Craig, S.L., Tucker, E.W., and Wagner, E.F. (2008). Empowering lesbian, gay, bisexual, and transgender youth: lessons learned from a safe schools summit. *Journal of Gay and Lesbian Social Services* 20 (3): 237–252.

D'Augelli, A.R., Grossman, A.H., Salter, N.P. et al. (2005). Predicting the suicide attempts of lesbian, gay, and bisexual youth. *Suicide and Life-threatening Behavior* 35 (6): 646–660.

Durwood, L., McLaughlin, K.A., and Olson, K.R. (2017). Mental health and self-worth in socially transitioned transgender youth. *Journal of the American Academy of Child and Adolescent Psychiatry* 56 (2): 116–123.e112. https://doi.org/10.1016/j.jaac.2016.10.016.

Eisenberg, M.E., Gower, A.L., McMorris, B.J. et al. (2017). Risk and protective factors in the lives of transgender/gender nonconforming adolescents. *Journal of Adolescent Health* 61 (4): 521–526. https://doi.org/10.1016/j.jadohealth.2017.04.014.

Fish, J. (2010). Conceptualising social exclusion and lesbian, gay, bisexual, and transgender people: the implications for promoting equity in nursing policy and practice. *Journal of Research in Nursing* 15 (4): 303–312. https://doi.org/10.1177/1744987110364691.

Fox 61. (2009), Connecticut church posts controversial gay exorcism video on YouTube. Available at http://www.youtube.com/watch?v=L9v2uk99o2E.

Greene, J.M., Ennett, S.T., and Ringwalt, C.L. (1999). Prevalence and correlates of survival sex among runaway and homeless youth. *American Journal of Public Health* 89: 1406–1409.

Grossman, A.H. and D'Augelli, A.R. (2006). Transgender youth: invisible and vulnerable. *Journal of Homosexuality* 51 (1): 111–128.

Guttmacher Institute. (2011). *State Policies in Brief. Sex and HV Education.* Available at http://www.guttmacher.org/statecenter/spibs/spib_SE.pdf.

Haldeman, D.C. (2001). Therapeutic antidotes: helping gay and bisexual men recover from converstion therapy. *Journal of Gay and Lesbian Psychotherapy* 5 (3/4): 117–130.

Hatzenbuehler, M.L., McLaughlin, K.A., Keyes, K.M., and Hasin, D.S. (2010). The impact of institutional discrimination on psychiatric disorders in lesbian, gay, and bisexual populations: a prospective study. *American Journal of Public Health* 100 (3): 452–459. https://doi.org/10.2105/ajph.2009.168815.

Heck, N.C., Flentje, A., and Cochran, B.N. (2011). Offsetting risks: high school gay-straight alliances and lesbian, gay, bisexual, and transgender (LGBT) youth. *School Psychology Quarterly* 26 (2): 161–174. https://doi.org/10.1037/a0023226.

Hein, L.C. (2006). *Survival among male homeless adolescents.* PhD thesis, Vanderbilt University, Nashville, Tennessee. ProQuest Dissertation Abstracts database (AAT 3230568). doi: https://doi.org/10.1037/a0023226

Hein, L.C. (2010). Where did you sleep last night? Homeless male adolescents: gay, bisexual, transgender and heterosexual compared. *Southern Online Journal of Nursing Research* 10 (1): Article 9. Available at http://snrs.org/publications/SOJNR_articles2/Vol10Num01Art09.pdf.

Hein, L.C. and Matthews, A.K. (2010). Reparative therapy: the adolescent, the psych nurse and the issues. *Journal of Child and Adolescent Psychiatric Nursing* 23 (1): 29–35. https://doi.org/10.1111/j.1744-6171.2009.00214.x.

Hein, L.C., Powell, L., & ISPN Diversity and Equity Committee. (2008). *Position Statement on Reparative Therapy.* Available at http://www.ispn-psych.org/docs/PS-ReparativeTherapy.pdf.

Hein, L.C., Stokes, E., Greenberg, C.S., and Saewyc, E.M. (2018). Policy brief: protecting vulnerable LGBTQ youth. Advocating for ethical health care. *Nursing Outlook* 66 (5): 505–507. https://doi.org/10.1016/j.outlook.2018.08.006.

Herek, G.M. (1990). The context of anti-gay violence: notes on cultural and psychological heterosexism. *Journal of Interpersonal Violence* 5 (3): 316–333. https://doi.org/10.1177/088626090005003006.

Herek, G.M. (2002). Heterosexuals' attitudes toward bisexual men and women in the United States. *The Journal of Sex Research* 39 (4): 264–274. https://doi.org/10.1080/00224490209552150.

Herek, G.M. (2009). Hate crimes and stigma-related experiences among sexual minority adults in the United States. *Journal of Interpersonal Violence* 24 (1): 54–74.

Herek, G.M. and Berrill, K.T. (1990). Documenting the victimization of lesbians and gay men: methodological issues. *Journal of Interpersonal Violence* 5 (3): 301–315. https://doi.org/10.1177/088626090005003005.

Himmelstein, K.E.W. and Bruckner, H. (2011). Criminal-justice and school sanctions against nonheterosexual youth: a national longitudinal study. *Pediatrics* 127 (1), 49–57. https://doi.org/10.1542/peds.2009-2306.

Hoffman, N.D., Freeman, K., and Swann, S. (2009). Healthcare preferences of lesbian, gay, bisexual, transgender and questioning youth. *The Journal of Adolescent Health* 45 (3): 222–229. https://doi.org/10.1016/j.jadohealth.2009.01.009.

Hood, L., Sherrell, D., Pfeffer, C.A., & Mann, E.S. (2019). LGBTQ college students' experiences with university health services: an exploratory study. *Journal of Homosexuality* 66 (6), 797–814. https://doi.org/10.1080/00918369.2018.1484234.

Human Rights Campaign. (2018). *Growing up LGBT in America.* Available at https://assets2.hrc.org/files/assets/resources/Growing-Up-LGBT-in-America_Report.pdf?_ga=2.204309264.1864619854.1536254424-1512363543.1528714880.

Hunter, M.A. (2010). All the gays are white and all the blacks are straight: black gay men, identity, and community. *Sexuality Research and Social Policy: A Journal of the NSRC* 7 (2): 81–92. https://doi.org/10.1007/s13178-010-0011-4.

Jackman, K., Honig, J., and Bockting, W. (2016). Nonsuicidal self-injury among lesbian, gay, bisexual and transgender populations: an integrative review. *Journal of Clinical Nursing* 25 (23–24): 3438–3453. https://doi.org/10.1111/jocn.13236.

Judge, C. (2015). Thrown away for being gay: the abandonment of LGBT youth and their lack of legal recourse. *Indiana Journal of Law and Social Equality* 3 (2): 260–304.

Katz-Wise, S.L., Rosario, M., Calzo, J.P. et al. (2017). Endorsement and timing of sexual orientation developmental milestones among sexual minority young adults in the growing up today study. *Journal of Sex Research* 54 (2): 172–185. https://doi.org/10.1080/00224499.2016.1170757.

Katz-Wise, S.L., Ehrensaft, D., Vetters, R. et al. (2018). Family functioning and mental health of transgender and gender-nonconforming youth in the trans teen and family narratives project. *Journal of Sex Research* 55 (4–5): 582–590. https://doi.org/10.1080/00224499.2017.1415291.

Kinsey, A.C., Pomeroy, W.B., and Martin, C.E. (1948). *Sexual Behavior in the Human Male.* Philadelphia: W.B. Saunders.

Kralik, J. (2017). *Bathroom Bill Legislative Tracking*. Available at http://www.ncsl.org/research/education/-bathroom-bill-legislative-tracking635951130.aspx.

Lambda Legal. (2010). *When Health Care Isn't Caring: Lambda Legal's Survey of Discrimination Against LGBT People and People with HIV*. Available at http://www.lambdalegal.org/sites/default/files/publications/downloads/whcic-report_when-health-care-isnt-caring.pdf.

Li, G., Kung, K.T., and Hines, M. (2017). Childhood gender-typed behavior and adolescent sexual orientation: a longitudinal population-based study. *Developmental Psychology* 53 (4): 764.

Lytle, M.C., Blosnich, J.R., De Luca, S.M., and Brownson, C. (2018). Association of religiosity with sexual minority suicide ideation and attempt. *American Journal of Preventive Medicine* 54 (5): 644–651. https://doi.org/10.1016/j.amepre.2018.01.019.

Massachusetts Youth Risk Behavior Survey. (2001). *Massachusetts high school students and sexual orientation*. Available at http://www.doe.mass.edu/cnp/hprograms/yrbs/01/results.pdf.

McCann, E., Keogh, B., Doyle, L., and Coyne, I. (2017). The experiences of youth who identify as trans* in relation to health and social care needs: a scoping review. *Youth & Society* https://doi.org/10.1177/0044118x17719345.

McDonald, K. (2018). Social support and mental health in LGBTQ adolescents: a review of the literature. *Issues in Mental Health Nursing* 39 (1): 16–29. https://doi.org/10.1080/01612840.2017.1398283.

McNamara, R.P. (1994). *The Times Square Hustler: Male Prostitutes in New York City*. West Port, CT: Praeger.

Nycum, B. (2000). *XY Survival Guide. Everything You Need to Know About Being Young and Gay*. San Francisco: XY Publishing.

Olson, K.R., Key, A.C., and Eaton, N.R. (2015). Gender cognition in transgender children. *Psychological Science* 26 (4): 467–474. https://doi.org/10.1177/0956797614568156.

Padilla, M.B., Rodríguez-Madera, S., Varas-Díaz, N., and Ramos-Pibernus, A. (2016). Trans-migrations: border-crossing and the politics of body modification among Puerto Rican transgender women. *International Journal of Sexual Health* 28 (4): 261–277.

Pearson, J., Thrane, L., and Wilkinson, L. (2017). Consequences of runaway and thrownaway experiences for sexual minority health during the transition to adulthood. *Journal of LGBT Youth* 14 (2): 145–171. https://doi.org/10.1080/19361653.2016.1264909.

Pitt, R.N. (2009). "Still looking for my Jonathan": gay black men's management of religious and sexual identity conflicts. *Journal of Homosexuality* 57 (1): 39–53. https://doi.org/10.1080/00918360903285566.

Rafferty, J. and AAP Committee on Psychosocial Aspects of Child and Family Health, AAP Committee on Adolescence, and AAP Section on Lesbian, Gay, Bisexual, and Transgender Health and Wellness (2018). Ensuring comprehensive care and support for transgender and gender-diverse children and adolescents. *Pediatrics* 142 (4): e20182162. https://doi.org/10.1542/peds.2018-2162.

Remafedi, G., Resnick, M., Blum, R., and Harris, L. (1992). Demography of sexual orientation in adolescents. *Pediatrics* 89 (4): 714–721.

Ridge, D., Minichiello, V., and Plummer, D. (1997). Queer connections: community, "the scene," and an epidemic. *Journal of Contemporary Ethnography* 26: 146–181.

Rieger, G., Linsenmeier, J., Gygax, L. et al. (2009). Dissecting "gaydar": accuracy adn the rold of masculinity-feminity. *Archives of Sexual Behavior*: 1–17.

Roberts, A.L., Austin, S.B., Corliss, H.L. et al. (2010). Pervasive trauma exposure among US sexual orientation minority adults and risk of posttraumatic stress disorder. *American Journal of Public Health* 100 (12): 2433–2441. https://doi.org/10.2105/ajph.2009.168971.

Rotheram-Borus, M.J., Mahler, K.A., and Rosario, M. (1995). AIDS prevention with adolescents. *AIDS Education and Prevention* 7: 320–336.

Ryan, C., Huebner, D., Diaz, R.M., and Sanchez, J. (2009). Family rejection as a predictor of negative health outcomes in white and latino lesbian, gay, and bisexual young adults. *Pediatrics* 123 (1): 346–352.

Ryan, C., Huebner, D., Diaz, R.M., and Sanchez, J. (2010). Family acceptance in adolescence and the health of LGBT young adults. *Journal of Child and Adolescent Psychiatric Nursing* 23 (4): 205–213.

SAMHSA. (2015). *Ending Conversion Therapy: Supporting and Affirmcth*. Available at http://store.samhsa.gov/shin/content//SMA15-4928/SMA15-4928.pdf.

Savin-Williams, R.C. and Diamond, L.M. (2000). Sexual identity trajectories among sexual-minority youths: gender comparisons. *Archives of Sexual Behavior* 29 (6): 607–627.

Sell, R.L., Wells, J.A., and Wypij, D. (1995). The prevalence of homosexual behavior and attraction in the United States, the United Kingdom and France: results of national population-based samples. *Archives of Sexual Behavior* 24 (3): 235–248. https://doi.org/10.1007/BF01541598.

Smith, J. (2010). *Anti-Gay Hate Crimes: Doing the Math*. Available at http://www.splcenter.org/get-informed/intelligence-report/browse-all-issues/2010/winter/anti-gay-hate-crimes-doing-the-math.

Super, J.T. and Jacobson, L. (2011). Religious abuse: implications for counseling lesbian, gay, bisexual, and transgender individuals. *Journal of LGBT Issues in Counseling* 5 (3–4): 180–196. https://doi.org/10.1080/15538605.2011.632739.

Sylva, D., Rieger, G., Linsenmeier, J., and Bailey, J. (2009). Concealment of sexual orientation. *Archives of Sexual Behavior* 39 (1): 141–152. https://doi.org/10.1007/s10508-008-9466-2.

Thomsen, J. (2018). Maine governor vetoes bill that would ban conversion therapy. *The Hill*, p. 1. Available at http://thehill.com/homenews/state-watch/395909-maine-governor-vetoes-bill-to-ban-conversion-therapy.

Travers, R., Bauer, G., Pyne, J., Bradley, K., Gale, L., Papadimitriou, M., . . . Services, D.Y. (2012). *Impacts of strong parental support for trans youth: A report prepared for Children's Aid Society of Toronto and Delisle Youth Services*. Toronto, ON: Trans PULSE. Available at http://transpulseproject.ca/wp-content/uploads/2012/10/Impacts-of-Strong-Parental-Support-for-Trans-Youth-vFINAL.pdf.

US Department of Housing and Urban Development. (2016). *Equal Access for Transgender People. Supporting Inclusive Housing and Shelters*. Washington, DC: US Department of Housing and Urban Development. Available at http://www.lgbtagingcenter.org/resources/download.cfm?r=786.

Veale, J.F., Watson, R.J., Peter, T., and Saewyc, E.M. (2017). Mental health disparities among Canadian transgender youth. *Journal of Adolescent Health* 60 (1): 44–49. https://doi.org/10.1016/j.jadohealth.2016.09.014.

Walls, N.E., Kane, S.B., and Wisneski, H. (2010). Gay straight alliances and school experiences of sexual minority youth. *Youth and Society* 41 (3): 307–322. https://doi.org/10.1177/0044118X09334957.

Wheeler, D.P. (2003). Methodological issues in conducting community-based health and social services research among urban black and African American LGBT populations. *Journal of Gay and Lesbian Social Services* 15 (1): 65–78.

WHO (2018). *ICD-11: International Classification of Diseases for Mortality and Morbidity Statistics*. Geneva: World Health Organization Available at https://www.who.int/classifications/icd/en/.

WHO (2019). *International Statistical Classification of Diseases and Related Health Problems, 10th Revision (ICD-10)*. World Health Organization Available at https://icd.who.int/browse10/2019/en.

Willis, D.G. (2008). Meanings in adult male victims' experiences of hate crime and its aftermath. *Issues in Mental Health Nursing* 29 (6): 567–584. https://doi.org/10.1080/01612840802048733.

Worthen, M.G. (2017). "Gay equals white"? Racial, ethnic, and sexual identities and attitudes toward LGBT individuals among college students at a Bible Belt University. *The Journal of Sex Research* 55 (8): 995–1011. https://doi.org/10.1080/00224499.2017.1378309.

Wyss, S.E. (2004). 'This was my hell': the violence experience by gender non-conforming youth in US high schools. *International Journal of Qualitative Studies in Education* 17 (5): 709–730.

Zucker, K. (2010). The DSM diagnostic criteria for gender identity disorder in children. *Archives of Sexual Behavior* 39 (2) https://doi.org/10.1007/s10508-009-9540-4.

8

Adverse Childhood Experiences: Providing Trauma-informed Care to Promote Resilience in Children and Their Families in Health Settings

Freida H. Outlaw[1], Lisa Milam[2], and Patricia K. Bradley[3]

[1] American Nurses Association, Minority Fellowship Program, Silver Spring, MD, USA
[2] Our Kids Center, Nashville General Hospital, Nashville, TN, USA
[3] M. Louise Fitzpatrick College of Nursing, Villanova University, Villanova, PA, USA

Objectives

After reading this chapter advanced practice registered nurses (APRNs) will be able to:

1. Define adverse childhood experiences (ACEs) and the key findings from the ACEs study.
2. Describe the magnitude of the issue, including the prevalence of ACEs nationally by state and by race/ethnicity.
3. Discuss the equity and disparity issues related to the intersectionality of poverty, race/ethnicity, and place (community) of young children who experience ACEs.
4. Explain the relationship of ACEs to toxic stress and trauma.
5. Identify challenges, issues, and barriers associated with ACEs and trauma-informed care.
6. Describe evidence-informed ACEs and brain science trauma-informed care approaches that APRNs can use to help children and their families develop the social, emotional, and behavioral skills they need to ensure long-term high-quality health and success in life.

Introduction

Science clearly states that children's development early in life matters for the present and for the future, for them and all of us. Healthy childhood development is the foundation of educational achievement, economic productivity, responsible citizenship, and lifelong health. While the awareness that sustained trauma and social experiences in childhood can have a detrimental impact on adult development, the Adverse Childhood Experiences study reported that sustained trauma and social experiences in childhood can adversely impact adult development (Felitti et al. 1998). Significant new findings include (i) there is a link between adverse events in childhood and poor adult health outcomes and (ii) the effects of these adverse events are cumulative, meaning the greater the number of the child's adverse experiences, the more profound the impact and the greater the risk for their adult health (Srivastav et al. 2017; Van Niel et al. 2014). Before

Child and Adolescent Behavioral Health: A Resource for Advanced Practice Psychiatric and Primary Care Practitioners in Nursing,
Second Edition. Edited by Edilma L. Yearwood, Geraldine S. Pearson, and Jamesetta A. Newland.
© 2021 John Wiley & Sons, Inc. Published 2021 by John Wiley & Sons, Inc.
Companion website: www.wiley.com/go/Yearwood

the Adverse Childhood Experiences study the relationship between health risk behavior and disease in adulthood associated with exposure to emotional, physical, and/or sexual abuse and household dysfunction in childhood had not previously been described (Felitti et al. 1998).

Definition of Adverse Childhood Experiences

Adverse childhood experiences (ACE) are defined as stressful or traumatic experiences, such as abuse, neglect, and family dysfunction, that disrupt the safe, stable, nurturing environments that children need to thrive (CDC 2014; Felitti et al. 1998; SAMHSA 2018; Van Niel et al. 2014). ACEs have been found to significantly harm the developing brains of infants and young children. This level of toxic stress resulting from high ACE scores leads to disrupted brain development that is not always outwardly observable but nevertheless causes permanent changes in brain structure and function (Shonkoff et al. 2012).

Description of the ACE Study

In 1985 Felitti, head of the Kaiser Permanente's obesity clinic in San Diego, California, became increasingly concerned and frustrated about the 50% dropout rate of the participants who were 100–600 lbs overweight from the clinic that he started 5 years prior, in spite of successful weight losses (Stevens 2012). Based on this concern, Dr. Felitti interviewed people who had left the program despite their success at actively losing weight. What he had not expected, but learned, was that the majority of those interviewed had had experience with childhood sexual abuse. Felitti hypothesized, based on the data from the interviews, that the patient's weight gain was used by them to cope with the anxiety, depression, and fear associated with their childhood sexual abuse (Stevens 2012). Thus began the scientific inquiry that is causing the paradigm shift in healthcare from "What is wrong with you?" to "What has happened to you?" and "How can I help?" The Adverse Childhood Experiences study provided the science that shifted from blaming the individual who is exhibiting symptoms associated with toxic stress and ACEs to altering the demeanor of healthcare providers making them more compassionate and helpful to someone in pain (Tennessee Commission on Children and Youth 2017).

Felitti's concern turned into more than 25 years of research. The Adverse Childhood Experiences study conducted by Felitti from Kaiser Permanente and Anda from the Centers for Disease Control and Prevention from 1995 to 1997 described the relationship of health risk behaviors and disease in adults (Figure 8.1). This relationship resulted in substantial morbidity and mortality decades later in life. This was a result of their exposure in childhood to adverse experiences such as emotional, physical, or sexual abuse, and/or household dysfunction (CDC 2016; Felitti et al. 1998; Van Niel et al. 2014).

A confidential survey was mailed to Kaiser Permanente patients that asked about 10 types of childhood experiences and their current health and behaviors (Dube et al. 2001; Felitti et al. 1998). Over 17 000 patients responded to the survey, with two-thirds reporting having one ACE, while 12% reported experiencing four or more ACEs. The 10 questions were organized around five types of child abuse or neglect (emotional abuse, emotional neglect, physical abuse, physical neglect, and sexual abuse) and five types of household dysfunction (mother treated violently, household substance abuse, household mental illness, parental separation or divorce, and having an incarcerated household member) (American Academy of Pediatrics 2014). All of the experiences had to have occurred within the first 18 years of the respondent's life. The researchers found that as the number of ACEs experienced during childhood increased (the graded dose–response relationship), the likelihood that the person would experience poor health outcomes also increased. These outcomes include leading causes of death in adults such as ischemic heart disease, cancer, chronic lung disease, skeletal fractures, liver disease, depression, illicit drug use, alcoholism, and alcohol abuse, to name a few. Dube et al. (2001) noted that the number of ACEs experienced in childhood was found to be a risk factor in suicide attempts across the person's lifespan.

Some Key Findings from the Original Adverse Childhood Experiences Study and Beyond

The original Adverse Childhood Experiences study found that 64% of the people in the study had at least one ACE in every category, except for incarceration of a relative. Also, one in eight had experienced four or more ACEs (See Table 8.1). These findings indicate that the prevalence of ACEs was high in this population (CDC 2016; Dube et al. 2001; Felitti et al. 1998). On a scale of 0–10, four or more ACEs was considered the tipping point for substantial risk for poor physical, emotional, behavorial, and social outcomes (Stevens 2017). The study also found ACEs were common and tended to cluster (Felitti et al. 1998; SAMHSA 2018). The fact that ACEs are common is supported by the finding that 28% of study participants reported physical abuse and 21% reported sexual abuse. Additionally, many reported experiencing a divorce or parental separation, or having a parent with a mental and/or substance use disorder. In

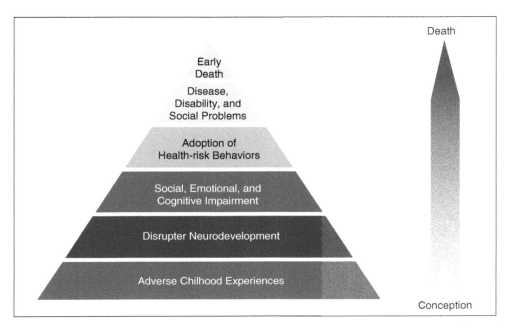

Figure 8.1   The ACE pyramid: mechanisms by which ACEs influence health and wellbeing throughout the lifespan. (*Source:* The CDC–Kaiser Permanente Adverse Childhood Experiences (ACE) Study, ACE Pyramid, CDC. Public Domain. https://www.cdc.gov/violenceprevention/acestudy/ACE_graphics.html.)

the original study, more than half of the respondents reported at least one ACE and almost 40% reported two or more, while 12.5% experienced four or more (Felitti et al. 1998; SAMHSA 2018). What was discovered is that in general ACEs do not occur alone and if the person had one ACE there was an 87% chance that he/she had two or more additional ACEs (Stevens 2017). The finding that ACEs tend to cluster influenced many successive studies to examine the cumulative effects of ACEs rather than the individual effects of each. Finally, ACEs have a dose–response relationship with many health problems, meaning the cumulative ACE score of a person has a strong, graded (i.e. dose–response) relationship to numerous health, social, and behavioral problems throughout their lifespan, and the problems tend to be co-occurring (Fellitti et al. 1998, SAMHSA 2018).

Influence Health and Wellbeing Throughout the Lifespan

Several ACE studies that have been conducted since the original research have found that an ACE score of one to three can be the tipping point at which deleterious risks increase substantially (Sacks and Murphey 2018). Sacks and Murphey posit that many factors need to be considered when accounting for this variation, including individual responses to adversity, biological makeup, and contextual factors. For example, Mersky et al. (2013) derived data from

Table 8.1   Key findings from the CDC–Kaiser Permanente Adverse Childhood Experiences study

- ACEs are common. Nearly two-thirds (64%) of adults have at least one ACE and more than one in five reported three or more ACEs.
- ACEs are cumulative and tend to cluster: if you have one, there's an 87% chance that you have two or more.
- The ACE score, a total sum of the different categories of ACEs reported by participants, is used to assess cumulative childhood stress. People have an ACE score from 0 to 10. Each type of trauma counts as one, no matter how many times it occurs.
- A graded dose–response relationship exists between ACEs and negative health and wellbeing outcomes across the life course such that as one increases (adverse experience) so does the other (negative outcome).
- The more ACEs you have, the greater the risk for chronic disease such as cancer and heart disease, mental illness, violence, and being a victim of violence.
- On a population level, it doesn't matter which four ACEs a person has, the harmful consequences are the same. The brain cannot distinguish one type of toxic stress from another; it's all toxic stress, with the same impact.

Source: The CDC–Kaiser Permanente Adverse Childhood Experiences (ACE) Study, ACE Pyramid, CDC. Public Domain. https://www.cdc.gov/violenceprevention/acestudy/about.html.

the Chicago Longitudinal Study (CLS) of individuals born in 1979 or 1980 to examine the impact of ACEs in childhood on the health, mental health, and substance use of a young, urban, minority sample because there has been very limited ACE research on diverse populations. This is an important deficit to note as most published evidence, clinical interventions, and educational programs have been based on the original ACE research where the demographic and ecological contexts of the population studied (Caucasian, middle class, insured, very educated, and employed) were very different from that of many minority populations. This may have implications for the CLS researchers, who found that their results confirmed the findings of the seminal ACE study. Specifically, they found that increased exposure to adversity in the childhoods of their population was also associated with poor physical and mental health, and substance use outcomes. The CLS researchers also found that the graded dose effect was confirmed in their population. However, they found approximately 80% of their participants reported at least one ACE compared to 64% in the original study, revealing that prevalence was very high in this urban minority group of participants. The urban sample was very poor, with 84% of them eligible for free lunch at school entry, which made them more vulnerable to other demographic and ecological threats than the participants in the original study (Mersky et al. 2013). Dong (2004) found strong evidence that ACEs are interrelated rather than occurring independently, which means that poverty and the associated sequalae were likely to potentiate the impact of the co-occurring ACEs. Finally, the participants in the CLS were much younger people in early adulthood while the participants in the original ACE study were entering middle or late adulthood. The researchers found that the CLS sample by age 24 were experiencing poor health outcomes associated with childhood adversity. This finding has enormous ramifications for addressing the problems faced by minority, urban, young populations associated with the impact of childhood adversity as they are in the productive years for establishing their futures, which can be seriously impacted by negative health, mental health, and social outcomes.

What these findings indicate is that context matters when thinking about what constitutes a tipping point. Gladwell (2002) described the tipping point as the moment when an idea, trend or social behavior crosses a certain line and spreads like an epidemic, where change can happen suddenly. He suggested that the power of small changes in circumstances can be vital in causing individuals to reach a tipping point. The individuals in the original study had more supports, such as employment and health insurance, to serve as buffers against small changes in their circumstances than the poor, young, minority subjects in the CLS study whose entire

circumstances could be altered negatively by a small change such as an increase in the bus fare. Without a buffer such as supports and resources, small changes might cause the latter to reach their tipping point sooner.

Waite et al. (2013) used cross-sectional survey data to examine the association of childhood adversity and poor self-rated health in adulthood among a low-income minority group of patients in a primary healthcare setting. As in the CLS sample, they found that their study participants had much higher ACE scores than the participants in the original study. Their findings also supported the findings of the original study that the more ACEs you have, the greater the risk for chronic diseases, mental illness, and other negative health and social outcomes. Like the CLS study, participants in their study lacked the supportive buffers that the participants in the original study had, thus their tipping points would be lower for experiencing deleterious health, mental health, and social outcomes.

Waite et al. (2013) suggested that providers, researchers, and policy makers need to be more collaborative in their approaches to preventing and mitigating ACEs in minorities served in primary care. Abrams (2018) proposed that collaboration rather than competition is essential when working for a common goal, even when the work involves colleagues who have different and potentially conflicting values and beliefs. Collective impact has elements of collaboration but is different in that the collaboration usually entails entities being involved in a joint effort to solve a common problem, while collective impact involves aligning diverse stakeholders around shared outcomes. Collective impact is a theoretical model developed to help organizations facilitate large-scale social change by employing five conditions that produce true alignment and powerful results guided by the following principles: (i) a common agenda, (ii) a shared measurement system, (iii) continuous communication, (iv) mutually reinforcing activities, and (v) a supportive backbone structure (Kania and Kramer 2011). While a detailed discussion of collective impact is not feasible for this chapter, the model has been recognized as having particular relevance for solving complex social problems where people have traditionally worked in isolation (Grumbach and Davis 2018). It is imperative that the emerging ACE research, clinical interventions, educational programs, and policy strategies continue to evolve by demonstrating a clear understanding of the minority population, especially those of color, whose children are disproportionately poor. This can only be accomplished by integrating practices and working collectively.

Other predictive factors have been added to the list of adverse experiences since the initial Adverse Childhood

Experiences study, including death of a parent, community violence, and poverty and discrimination. While there has been some controversy about poverty as an ACE or as a risk factor for experiencing ACEs, it is important to note that children are more likely than any other age group to live in poverty, and those living in census tracts with poverty rates greater than 50% are children of color who are also the most vulnerable (Bruner 2017). There is disparity in how children of different races and ethnicities experience ACEs (Sacks and Murphey 2018). For example, national data found that 61% of black non-Hispanic children and 51% of Hispanic children had experienced at least one ACE. On the other hand, 40% of white non-Hispanic children and only 23% of Asian children had experienced at least one ACE. The impact of racism on minority children's health and development has been grossly understudied and there are no instruments to date that are normed to measure children's responses to racism (Pachter and Coll 2009). However, there is a critical need to address the impact of racism as a toxic stressor on the development of children of color. The Philadelphia Urban ACE Survey added to their questionnaire items to serve as a proxy for participants feeling discriminated against because of their race, culture, ethnicity, skin color or country of origin (The Research and Evaluation Group: Public Health Management Corporation 2013). Additionally, the Philadelphia Urban ACE Survey included questions that assessed more comprehensive psychosocial stressors of childhood such as if they had witnessed community violence, if they felt safe in their neighborhoods, and whether they had experienced being in foster care (Van Niel et al. 2014).

The survey found that 40.5 adults had witnessed violence during childhood such as hearing someone being beaten, stabbed or shot, while over one-third of adults experienced discrimination based on their race or ethnicity. Additionally, approximately 3 in 10 of the respondents (27.3%) reported having felt unsafe in their neighborhoods, but equally or more disturbing is that they did not trust their neighbors during their childhood (The Research and Evaluation Group: Public Health Management Corporation 2013). The findings from the Philadelphia Urban ACE Survey are compelling and support the urgency of asking questions about race/ethnicity, poverty, culture, and place (neighborhoods) now and going forward if we are truly committed to preventing and mitigating ACEs in all children.

Many ACEs, such as poverty, racism, bullying, gender discrimination, witnessing violence outside of the home, witnessing a sibling being abused as well as other aspects of social determinants of health, have been added to questionnaires since the original study. However, many ACE studies continue to only include the original 10 questions, regardless of the population being treated or studied. As more and more research and advances in the field of inquiry about ACEs is done, questions and discussions about whether the 10 original questions are presently culturally appropriate to capture the breadth and depth of toxic stress and ACEs experienced by diverse populations need to be part of the ongoing discourse. The original ACE study cohort comprised participants who were middle class, with private insurance, and were not likely to have experienced challenges such as invidious discrimination, racism, poverty, or violence in their neighborhoods.

Description of the Magnitude of the Issue

The initial ACE study sparked a growing body of research which has contributed to the body of knowledge confirming that ACEs are a critical public health problem for all populations. They have a negative lasting effect on the health and wellbeing of persons who have experienced trauma and toxic stress during their childhood that continues throughout their lives (Sacks and Murphey 2018). What started as one scientist who had concerns about obesity in a specific population has proliferated into a national interest in understanding the prevalence of ACEs in diverse communities. To this end, the focus is on how to prevent and mitigate ACEs by employing culturally appropriate and community specific strategies and responses (Ellis and Dietz 2017). In the last two decades it has become clear that the high prevalence of people nationally who have experienced one or more ACEs during childhood is creating a massive public health issue. It is a public health issue because childhood adversity has been shown to contribute to leading chronic health diseases as well as mental health and substance use disorders, all of which have a major impact on the economy, community wellbeing, and quality of life for large populations of people. These are also factors associated with enormous human suffering. Sacks and Murphey (2018) posit that some of society's most intractable and growing health issues, such as drug abuse, suicide, obesity, and depression, are linked with ACE scores, providing further evidence that ACEs are a huge public health issue.

Sacks and Murphey (2018) also pointed out that not all children who experience one or more ACEs will have negative health or behavioral consequences, although the reasons are not completely understood. There is emerging evidence that points to the importance of supportive relationships from a committed adult either inside or outside of the home. This supportive relationship can serve as a buffer that profoundly promotes the child's capacity to be resilient (Sacks and Murphey 2018; Shonkoff et al. 2012). Resilience, while often thought of as an internal trait, has been found to be able to be developed by some children who have buffers like safe, stable, nurturing relationships and environments (Center on the Developing Child n.d.a). There is also evidence that some children are biologically more sensitive to stress, causing them to need more support to survive and thrive. Herbert (2011) referred to these children as "orchids" as they need an optimal set of conditions to thrive compared to "dandelions", who can thrive in weeds and less than optimal conditions. The good news is that this knowledge means that all children have the capacity to thrive. The key is to be able to differentiate between the children who are "orchids" and those who are "dandelions" and provide the supports to assist them to be resilient based on their needs, both individual and population based.

The children who are impacted negatively by ACE scores are more likely to struggle in school and experience emotional and behavioral challenges. Therefore, it is important that everyone, including policy makers, researchers, decision makers, helping professionals, and the general public, gets involved in addressing the issues associated with the Adverse Childhood Experiences study (National Technical Assistance Center for Children's Mental Health 2015).

Sacks and Murphey (2018) used data from the 2016 National Survey of Children's Health (NSCH) to describe the prevalence of ACEs among children from birth to 17 years old using data from both the national and state levels. Unlike other ACE studies, including the original, where the adults were asked to respond retrospectively to the questions based on their experiences up to 18 years of age, the answers to the NSCH survey were provided by the parents or guardians of the child. The NSCH survey included nine ACEs but Sacks and Murphey reported on only eight of the nine. They did not report on the ninth item as the parents were asked to report on "How often their child was treated or judged unfairly because of his or her race or ethnicity" (Sacks and Murphey 2018, p. 7). The authors thought that the item was too subjective and that the parents would not have the information needed to answer this question. Additionally, the NSCH survey question about abuse/neglect was worded differently than the original ACE study.

The survey has been conducted at intervals since 2003. The 2018 survey results showed that the most prevalent ACE experienced in children's lifetimes was divorce or separation of a parent (23.4%), followed by living with someone with a drug or alcohol problem (8.0%), and parent or guardian incarceration (7.4%) (USDHHS, 2019). Since the 2016 survey was significantly redesigned, the researchers caution not to attempt to compare data across the years. Conducted in all 50 states and the District of Columbia the survey yielded 50 212 completed surveys using internet-based and mailed paper data instruments. The parent or guardian was instructed to answer questions about only one child per household, as well as questions about themselves.

Overall, Sacks and Murphey (2018) stated that while there is more attention being paid to preventing or mitigating ACEs, they continue to remain common in the United States. The survey found that approximately half of all children nationally, including in most states, had experienced at least one ACE, but the researchers were not willing to generalize about reasons for the findings in those states where the children were more likely to have a high number of ACEs. They did note, however, that Arkansas, New Mexico, and Arizona were among the states with the highest number of ACEs and were three of the 10 states with the highest levels of child poverty. Arkansas was the state with the highest prevalence (56%) of children reporting at least one ACE. Nationally 1 in 10 children had experienced three or more ACEs, meaning they were at a very high risk for negative health outcomes across their lifespan (Sacks and Murphey 2018).

The NSCH found the two most common ACEs identified in all 50 states and the District of Columbia were economic hardship and the separation or divorce of a parent or guardian. Unfortunately, in West Virginia one in three children had experienced economic hardship (Sacks and Murphey 2018). This is not surprising since this state has suffered disproportionately from the demise of the coal industry and in 2016 had the highest rate of opioid-related overdose deaths in the United States (National Institute on Drug Abuse 2018). In contrast, in Minnesota, New Hampshire, and North Dakota, a smaller number of children, one in five, had experienced economic hardship. The NSCH also found that separation or divorce of a parent or guardian was the second highest ACE. Approximately one-third of children in both Arkansas and Kentucky experienced a parental separation or divorce, while a much lower number, 18–19%, of children in Illinois, Maryland, Massachusetts, and Utah had some involvement with this same phenomenon. Nationally, ACEs such as death of a parent or guardian, or being the victim of or witnessing violence in the neighborhood were identified for only 3–4% of children. For those states where these ACEs were more common, their scores were above the national average. Specifically, 6% of children in Arkansas and Georgia had experienced the death of a parent or guardian, while 7% of children in Nevada and Hawaii had been a victim of or witnessed violence in their neighborhoods.

The NSCH survey revealed that disparities exist by race and ethnicity at both national and regional levels on how children experience ACEs. For example, both black non-Hispanic and Hispanic children experienced at least one ACE (61% and 51%, respectively). In comparison, 40% of white, non-Hispanic children and only 23% of Asian children had experienced one ACE (Sacks and Murphey 2018). In most divisions, black non-Hispanic children had the highest prevalence of ACEs, while Asian children had the lowest. Williams and Mohammed (2013) provided an explanation for why black non-Hispanic children and Hispanic children have the highest prevalence of ACEs in the survey, suggesting that racism in its many forms is deeply embedded in American society and disproportionally impacts children of color. Racism is manifested in policies that limit black and brown peoples' access to safe and affordable housing, employment, high-quality educational opportunities, and safe neighborhoods, while exposing them to racial invidious discrimination, a very profound psychological stressor (Williams and Mohammed 2013). All of these factors are associated with toxic stress and ACEs. Public health experts and researchers have documented the connection between poor health and poor communities, especially when the health disparities are so extreme, when compared to more resource rich communities (Harris 2018).

Relationship of Toxic Stress and Trauma to ACEs

About two decades ago the Institute of Medicine and the National Research Council published a report entitled *From Neurons to Neighborhoods: The Science of Early Childhood Development* in which two agendas they thought would address the future of early childhood development were identified (Shonkoff and Levitt 2010). The first agenda item was more broadly focused on how society could use what had been discovered about childhood development to maximize human capital, ensuring the continued vitality of the nation's institutions. The second agenda item was focused on how we as a nation could use knowledge to nurture, protect, and ensure the health and wellbeing of all children (Shonkoff and Levitt 2010). The launching of the Decade of the Brain by the National Institute of Health in the last 10 years of the twentieth century increased government agencies, private foundations, and healthcare professionals' desire to focus more intensity on the architecture of the child's developing brain.

Healthy brain architecture needs to be established early in life because it supports all of the person's future learning (Center on the Developing Child n.d.a;

Fox et al. 2010). Researchers have found that brains are built over time, starting in the earliest years with simple skills coming first and over time more complex skills are built on top of them. When the brain is being built, the foundation is either sturdy or fragile, depending on the experiences a child has early in life when the foundation of all future brain development is being laid. Therefore, a strong foundation increases the likelihood that the child will have positive outcomes in life, including health, while a weak foundation is associated with negative outcomes and poor health, behavorial, and social problems (Center on the Developing Child n.d.a). Children at birth are ready for learning and in the first few years of life are forming one million new neural connections every second (Center on the Developing Child n.d.a). This is a period of rapid growth related to brain development. Therefore, every second counts because by the time the child is 2 their neural connections have proliferated (Center on the Developing Child n.d.a). Although 85% of the brain volume is fully developed by age 3, there is opportunity for new neural connections to be formed throughout the lifespan. In sum, young children who have positive healthy experiences develop brains that are efficient, while children who are exposed to great adversity, such as abuse, neglect, and household dysfunction, can have their brains altered, sometimes for life. Healthy brain architecture can be derailed by toxic levels of stress, such as that experienced by many children with high ACE scores (Center on the Developing Child n.d.a).

Stress as a term is used commonly in popular culture and usually is attached to something that is negative. However, not all stress is negative or toxic. Some stress is positive for everyone, including children. For example, it is positive stress that motivates a child to accomplish a school assignment or some other task which prepares them for future challenges. Positive stress during childhood is also necessary as it is essential for healthy brain development and prepares the brain and body for future stressful events. Tolerable stress is unavoidable and usually is connected to some tragic event like the death of a loved one or experiencing illness or injury. This type of stress is usually episodic and, more importantly, when there are supportive adults available to buffer the stress response, recovery is possible. The key is the nurturing caregiver, who can help the child adapt to a time-limited stress activation, allowing the brain and other organs in the body to recover. However, toxic stress is defined as extreme, frequent, and/or prolonged adversity such as repetitive exposure to abuse, neglect or household dysfunctions, all the ACE categories. Without a supportive, caring adult present in the child's life to help buffer the toxic stress response, chemicals such as cortisol and adrenaline are repeatedly released, damaging the developing structures in the child's brain architecture (Center on the Developing Child n.d.b). Toxic stress leads to increases in heart rate, blood pressure, serum glucose, stress hormones, and inflammatory cytokines that fuel the "fight or flight" response, usually called the hyperarousal or acute stress response (Center on the Developing Child n.d.b). When the acute stress response is prolonged, it can lead to long-term disruptions in brain architecture and other physical illnesses, including cardiovascular disease. Also, when a child is chronically stressed his/her body has trouble returning to a normal state so that over time their reactions to stress are more extreme and immediate. Children who suffer toxic stress are vulnerable to lifelong physical and behavioral health problems as well as cognitive impairment (Center on the Developing Child n.d.b).

Epigenetics is a relatively new field of study of the changes in gene expression without there being changes to the genes. Epigenetic "markers" control where and how protein is made by a gene (Center on the Developing Child n.d.b). In effect, they turn the gene on or off. These modifications happen at the cellular level, which has implications for how structures develop and function. Since genes are vulnerable to modification as a result of a response to toxic stress, the need for a safe, stable, nurturing environment to serve as a buffer for these young children is critical because this is when their brains are most rapidly developing (Center on the Developing Child n.d.b). Although all the mechanisms are not completely understood there is some preliminary evidence that the impact of ACEs and their negative effects can be transmitted from one generation to the other through genetic programming during pregnancy (Buss et al. 2017; Sacks and Murphey 2018). These epigenetic changes in humans are alarming but can be prevented or modified (Monk et al. 2016).

ACEs Informed Care

ACEs informed care begins with awareness that the child's behavior could be secondary to an experience of sexual abuse but could also be related to patterns of parental discipline, communication, conflict, and instability resulting in his/her development of poor social skills, poor impulse control, and emotional dysregulation. Assessment of ACEs is an important step toward treatment planning for children with sexual behavior problems. ACEs informed questioning requires the provider to consider the possibility that the parent may be an adult survivor of traumatic experiences or possibly a nonoffending parent experiencing denial. Using an ACEs informed perspective, the parent will be provided with information and recommendations specific to the child's experience. Some children may require a referral for counseling services. Others may not. Parents must be provided with information about the long-term effects of untreated trauma as they make informed decisions with respect to recommendations for follow-up counseling.

What Can APRNs Do to Prevent or Mitigate ACEs?

Nurses are the largest group of healthcare providers in the United States. They work everywhere, including hospitals, clinics, homeless shelters, prisons, community, and mental health centers (Girouard and Bailey 2017). They are found in federal, regional, and local agencies, where policy is made and implemented. They hold a variety of leadership positions in healthcare institutions and other places where the nursing perspectives are critical to the conversation. For example, the American Academy of Nursing has embarked on a number of critical conversations about toxic stress in children living in poverty. This work has helped make toxic stress in children a national priority (Cox et al. 2018). Because of their positioning, nurses on the front lines where patients present who are suffering from the negative effects of toxic stress, trauma, and adverse events can be a vital resource in the efforts to prevent and mitigate trauma, toxic stress, and ACEs in the lives of children, their families, and the communities in which they live.

The following are some of the ways advanced practice registered nurses (APRNs) can prevent or mitigate ACEs in children, adolescents, and adults:

- Become champions for the need for screening for ACEs in primary health settings. There is a plethora of evidence to support the benefits of screening for ACEs in primary care, yet it is not regularly done (Shafer 2017). One of the challenges, among many, might be that there is no national ACE screening tool that has been recommended for all healthcare providers to use when screening patients (Srivastav et al. 2017). However, Srivastav et al. (2017) believe that the United States Preventive Services Task Force will eventually recognize the importance of including ACE assessments in well-child care. When this happens more healthcare providers will embrace assessing for ACEs as part of their routine care (Srivastav et al. 2017). APRNs can take a leadership role in working on solving the challenges associated with screening for ACEs while championing the benefits of using an established ACE screening tool with a comprehensive clinical interview that assesses for toxic stress and trauma. Glowa et al. (2016) found that screening for ACEs was feasible. They believe they learned from the screening information that provided a more complete and holistic picture of the health determinants of the patient, factors that are not usually assessed.

- Incorporate an assessment of the adult patient's childhood history into their primary care plan even though sometimes it is difficult for the patient to talk about childhood issues. This information is important considering the strong evidence about the impact of ACEs on health, mental health, and addictions (Kalmakis et al. 2017). Information from the assessment can be used to educate patients about the impact of ACEs on their health and social outcomes, such as school achievement. It can also be an opportunity to teach parents ways to create nurturing environments that build resilience in their children (Van Niel et al. 2014). APRNs can teach a simple lesson to parents about the importance of the interaction of "serve and return." Neural connections are developed when adults respond with eye contact, hugs, or words to infants and young children when they babble, gesture, or cry. When parents and other caregivers are responsive in a caring manner to the young child's signals and needs, a caring environment is created that supports rich "serve and return" experiences. This intervention is simple, involves no financial cost to the practitioner or parent, and can be easily learned, yet is a powerful way to help the building of strong brain circuits for each new skill a child has to learn (Center on the Developing Child n.d.a).
- Work to make the clinical setting or organization trauma-informed. This means that all people working in the system including professional and nonprofessionals (i) realize the widespread impact of trauma and understand potential paths for recovery, (ii) recognize the signs and symptoms of trauma in clients, families, staff, and others involved with the system, (iii) respond by fully integrating knowledge about trauma, and (iv) seek to actively resist re-traumatization (SAMHSA 2018).
- Be aware of the six key principles of the trauma-informed approach to patients rather than continuing a prescribed set of procedures. The principles can be operationalized in any setting and include (i) providing safety, (ii) being trustworthy and transparent, (iii) providing peer support, (iv) collaborating and practicing mutuality, (v) empowering and encouraging patient voice and choice, and (vi) being aware of cultural, historical, and gender issues (SAMHSA 2018).
- Learn the signs and symptoms of trauma and toxic stress in clients in the clinical setting. APRNs who are working in academic settings need to work to get ACEs and toxic stress content into the curriculum. This is important as trauma and toxic stress signs and symptoms are often unrecognized and untreated in medical settings (Goldstein et al. 2017), which may be a function of not having been exposed to this content when being educated.
- As part of self-care, nurses need to be aware of their own ACEs. A number of studies have noted that ACEs may be more common among nurses and other health professionals than the general population (Girouard and Bailey 2017). Additionally, research suggests that the stressful nature of the work may exacerbate the stress response in the nurse associated with their ACEs. Therefore, it is important for nurses who are suffering the consequences of toxic stress and ACEs to become aware of their triggers and use techniques like mindfulness-based stress meditation and physical exercise to control their stress responses (Girouard and Bailey 2017). There is evidence that mindfulness meditation may ease anxiety and mental stress, thus reducing the effects of childhood trauma (Ortiz and Sibing 2017). APRNs may also consider having mindfulness training in their toolkit of skills to use with patients. As part of their self-care, in some cases nurses may need to seek professional counseling.
- Bring awareness to educational settings that nursing students at all levels may have experienced trauma and toxic stress that has resulted in their underperforming as students. This can also be the case for practicing nurses. Formal nursing programs or continuing education nursing programs have not given enough attention to this issue (Girouard and Bailey 2017). Given its magnitude in society and the suggestion that nurses may disproportionately experience ACEs, this is a costly oversight for both nurses and the patients they serve.
- Recognize that preventing and mitigating ACEs will have to be a collaborative effort among patients, communities, colleagues, and all healthcare providers, as well as other disciplines (Ellis and Dietz 2017; Girouard and Bailey 2017; Waite et al. 2013). APRNs as well as nurses in general have been taught that a multidisciplinary team approach is optimal for comprehensive care. APRNs can bring team-building skills to fostering collaborative, coordinated care approaches to the prevention and mitigation of ACEs, while leading efforts to build a collective impact model focused on this issue.
- Move beyond healthcare settings to serve in an advocacy role at the local, state, or national level. This can be done in a variety of ways, including becoming active in ACE work at one or all levels, supporting policies that prevent adverse events that profoundly impact communities and families (Girouard and Bailey 2017). Taking active roles in raising awareness about ACEs in institutions where children and families live, work, worship, and play can do this. Campaigns to reduce violence, advocating for evidence-based parenting

skills programs, and other awareness efforts focused on changing the culture of the community away from traumatic events are just some of the advocacy roles that APRNs can do to prevent and mitigate ACEs. Serving on boards that have children, social justice or other issues associated with mitigating and preventing ACEs can also be an effective advocacy tool.

- Be aware of intervention programs like the Family Nurse Partnership program that has proven to be effective in helping first-time parents be successful (www.nursefamilypartnership.org). Research continues to support the finding that interventions which build parents' skills and strengthen the capacities of communities to protect young children from toxic stress and traumas are likely to promote healthier brain development, which is associated with having better physical and mental health as well as better behavioral and social outcomes later in life. There are also a number of other parenting intervention programs, such as Child First (www.childfirst.com).

- Bring awareness to the public that ACEs are a public health problem and encourage all nurses to be involved with primary prevention by raising awareness of the issue, being involved in policy change about factors related to ACEs, including social determinants of health, and changing cultural and healthcare norms from "What is wrong with you?" to "What has happened to you?" and "How can I help?" APRNs can also be extremely helpful at the secondary level providing culturally competent, evidence-based services to those children at risk for ACEs. At the tertiary level there is a need for more APRNs such as psychiatric nurse practitioners and other nurse practitioners who can provide specialty treatment services such as those needed for children and their families who have experienced toxic stress and trauma.

- Be active in professional organizations to create a collective platform for bringing awareness and taking action to increase nursing's voice in preventing and mitigating ACEs, a major public health issue.

Conclusion: Resilience as a Reason for Optimism

Resilience is the process of managing stress and functioning well even when faced with challenges, adversity, and trauma (Center for the Study of Social Policy n.d.). The good news is that resilience can be built and the fact that a child has had trauma, toxic stress, and high ACEs scores does not mean that they are doomed (Stevens 2017). The following are the key components of building resilience in children from the Center on the Developing Child (n.d.c):

- The single most common factor for children who develop resilience is at least one stable and committed relationship with a supportive parent, caregiver, or other adult. These relationships provide the personalized responsiveness, scaffolding, and protection that buffer children from developmental disruption.

- Children who do well in the face of serious hardship typically have a biological resistance to adversity *and* strong relationships with the important adults in their family and community. Resilience is the result of a combination of protective factors. Neither individual characteristics nor social environments alone are likely to ensure positive outcomes for children who experience prolonged periods of toxic stress. It is the interaction between biology and environment that builds a child's ability to cope with adversity and overcome threats to healthy development.

- Research has identified a common set of factors that predispose children to positive outcomes in the face of significant adversity. These counterbalancing factors include (i) facilitating supportive adult–child relationships, (ii) building a sense of self-efficacy and perceived control, (iii) providing opportunities to strengthen adaptive skills and self-regulatory capacities, and (iv) mobilizing sources of faith, hope, and cultural traditions.

- Learning to cope with manageable threats is critical for the development of resilience. Not all stress is harmful. There are numerous opportunities in every child's life to experience manageable stress, and with the help of supportive adults this "positive stress" can be growth promoting.

- The capabilities that underlie resilience can be strengthened at any age. The brain and other biological systems are most adaptable early in life. Yet while this development lays the foundation for a wide range of resilient behaviors, it is never too late to build resilience. Age-appropriate, health-promoting activities can significantly improve the odds that an individual will recover from stress-inducing experiences. For example, regular physical exercise, stress-reduction practices, and programs that actively build executive function and self-regulation skills can improve the abilities of children and adults to cope with, adapt to, and even prevent adversity in their lives. Adults who strengthen these skills in themselves can better model healthy behaviors for their children, thereby improving the resilience of the next generation.

Nurses have a culture of approaching patients and their issues from a strength-based rather than a deficit-based

Tips for Talking to your Child about Sexual Abuse		
As parents we want to say the right things to our children. Over the years at Our Kids, we've noticed there are things parents may say to children when they're worried about sexual abuse that may inadvertently make it more difficult for a child to disclose abuse. Here is a guide that may help:		
What *not* to say	**The reasons why**	**Try saying this instead**
"Don't let anyone touch your private parts." -OR- "No one should ever touch your private parts."	Adults and older children are bigger, stronger and usually able to intimidate or manipulate a child. If you tell your child not to "let" anyone touch their private parts, **children may think they will get in trouble if touching occurs**. Children may be hesitant to talk about the event or may even feel responsible. They may think; "Mom or dad told me not to let this happen. It did, so I will get in trouble."	**"If anyone touches your private parts, it's OK to tell me." -QR- "It's always OK to tell if someone touches your private parts."**
When referring to your child's genital area or private parts, **calling it a "nasty" or "dirty" part of the body.**	It's important that children of all ages know the names for their body parts — and know ALL of their body is OK. **Using substitute names for body parts can be confusing** if a child discloses to another adult and uses the substitute name. Avoid, names that imply shame or something bad about that part of the body.	**"That is your private part." -OR- Refer to the parts of the body as the "vagina" or "penis."**
"Has someone touched you?" -OR- "Has anyone touched you down there?"	**Don't ask your child constantly about being touched.** "Has anyone 'touched' you?" can be a confusing question for younger children. In the literal mind of a child, of course people "touch" them — young children who need assistance with toilet training may be touched "down there" in ways that are appropriate and necessary.	**"Is there anything bothering you?" -OR- "Are you OK?" -OR- "Has anyone done anything that worries or confuses you?"**
"I promise not to tell anyone."	Before a child discloses, they may ask you to promise not to tell anyone about the abuse or abuser. Your child needs to have a trusting relationship with you and **making a promise you'll have to break could be damaging to the child, so don't make one.** If there is abuse, it is always in the best interest of the child to report the abuse — and it's required by law.	**"I cannot promise not to tell, but I can promise that I will do what I can to help you. Let's talk about what is bothering you. I want to help."**
"I'll kill anyone who touches your private parts."	**More than 90% of children who are sexually abused know their abuser** — often it's a relative, caregiver or friend of the family who has a long-term relationship with the child. While your initial reaction to someone touching your child may be very strong, **the child may think they're responsible for the safety or well-being of a person loved by the family.** Children are generally afraid of adult anger and worry it's directed at them, so avoid saying things that fuel that concern.	"My job as your mom (or dad) is to protect you and take care of you. Since I'm not around all the time, I can't always know what's happening. **So if anyone does anything that makes you feel funny or scared or touches you, it's OK to tell me."**
We recommend talking with your child regularly and generally about their activities, people in their life and how they're feeling. If you're concerned something or someone is bothering your child, ask specific questions. Lay the groundwork for open, non-scary, non-threatening conversation and children will be more likely to disclose. If you have concerns about the safety or well-being of a child, you must call 1-877-237-0004 to report your concerns.		

Source: Reprinted with consent from Tips for Talking to Your Kids about Sexual Abuse, Our Kids Centre. © 2015, Our Kids.

perspective. All of the findings about resilience in children from the Center on the Developing Child (n.d.c) are focused on building the strengths of children and their families no matter their circumstances. Nurse practitioners and other APRNs informed by this culture of nursing can be leaders in preventing and mitigating ACEs wherever they are working.

Additional Resources

Centers for Disease Control and Prevention, Violence Prevention Program: ACEs Study. http://www.cdc.gov/violenceprevention/acestudy/about.html.

Robert Wood Johnson Foundation, *The Truth about ACEs.* http://www.rwjf.org/en/library/infographics/the-truth-about-aces.html.

ACEs Connection. http://www.acesconnection.com/blog/aces-101-faqs.

References

Abrams, S. (2018). *Minority Leader. How to Build your Future and Make Real Change.* New York: Holt and Company.

Achenbach, T.M. (2009). *The Achenbach System of Empirically Based Assessment (ASEBA): Development, Findings, Theory, and Applications.* Burlington, VT: University of Vermont Research Center for Children, Youth, & Families.

American Academy of Pediatrics. (2014). *Adverse childhood experiences and the lifelong consequences of trauma.* Available at https://www.aap.org/en-us/Documents/ttb_aces_consequences.pdf.

Bruner, C. (2017). ACE, place, race, and poverty: building hope for children. *Academic Pediatrics* 17 (7S): S123–S129.

Buss, C., Entringer, S., Moog, N.K. et al. (2017). Intergenerational transmission of maternal childhood maltreatment exposure: implications for fetal brain development. *Journal of the American Academy of Child & Adolescent Psychiatry* 56 (5): 373–382.

CDC. (2014). *Essentials for childhood: Steps to create safe, stable, nurturing relationships and environments.* Centers for Disease Control and Prevention. Available at http://www.cdc.gov/violenceprevention/childmaltreatment/essentials.html [accessed 1 January 2019].

CDC. (2016). *About adverse childhood experiences.* Centers for Disease Control and Prevention. Available at https://www.cdc.gov/violenceprevention/acestudy/about.html.

Center for the Study of Social Policy. (n.d.). *Parental Resilience: Protection & Promotion Factors.* Available at https://cssp.org/wp-content/uploads/2018/08/ProtectiveFactorsActionSheets.pdf [accessed 13 January 2019].

Center on the Developing Child. (n.d.a). *Brain Architecture.* Harvard University. Available at https://developingchild.harvard.edu/science/key-concepts/brain-architecture [accessed 13 January 2019].

Center on the Developing Child. (n.d.b). *Gene–Environment Interaction.* Harvard University. Available at https://developingchild.harvard.edu/science/deep-dives/gene-environment-interaction [accessed 13 January 2019].

Center on the Developing Child. (n.d.c). *Resilience.* Harvard University. Available at https://developingchild.harvard.edu/science/key-concepts/resilience [accessed 13 January 2019].

Cox, K.S., Sullivan, C.G., Olshansky, E. et al. (2018). Critical conversation: toxic stress in children living in poverty. *Nursing Outlook* 66 (2): 204–209.

Dong, M.A. (2004). Child interrelatedness of multiple forms of childhood abuse, neglect, and household dysfunction. *Child Abuse and Neglect* 28 (7): 771–784.

DSM-5 (2013). *Diagnostic and Statistical Manual of Mental Disorders 5.* Arlington: American Psychiatric Publishing.

Dube, S.R., Anda, R.F., Felitti, V.J. et al. (2001). Childhood abuse, household dysfunction, and the risk of attempted suicide throughout the life span: findings from the adverse childhood experiences study. *Journal of the American Medical Association* 286 (24): 3089–3096.

Ellis, W.R. and Dietz, W.H. (2017). A new framework for addressing adverse childhood and community experiences: the building community resilience model. *Academic Pediatrics* 17 (7): S86–S93.

Felitti, V.J., Anda, R.F., Nordenberg, D. et al. (1998). Relationship of childhood abuse and household dysfunction to many of the leading causes of death in adults: the adverse childhood experiences (ACE) study. *American Journal of Preventive Medicine* 14 (4): 245–258.

Fox, S.E., Levitt, P., and Nelson, C.A. III (2010). How the timing and quality of early experiences influence the development of brain architecture. *Child Development* 81 (1): 28–40.

Friedrich, W.N. (1997). *Child Sexual Behavior Inventory: Professional Manual.* Lutz, FL: Psychological Assessment Resources Inc.

Girouard, S. and Bailey, N. (2017). ACEs implications for nurses, nursing education, and nursing practice. *Academic Pediatrics* 17 (7): S16–S17.

Gladwell, M. (2002). *The Tipping Point How Little Things Can Make a Big Difference.* Back Bay Books.

Glowa, P.T., Olson, A.L., and Johnson, D.J. (2016). Screening for adverse childhood experiences in a family medicine setting: a feasibility study. *Journal of the American Board of Family Medicine* 29 (3): 303–307.

Goldstein, E., Athale, N., Sciolla, A.F., and Catz, S.L. (2017). Patient preferences for discussing childhood trauma in primary care. *The Permanente Journal* 21: 16–55.

Grumbach, K. and Davis, A. (2018). The imperative for a collective impact approach among family medicine organizations. *The Annals of Family Medicine* 16 (4): 368–369.

Harris, N.B. (2018). *The deepest well: healing the long-term effects of childhood adversity.* Houghton Mifflin Harcourt.

Herbert, W. (2011). *On the trail of the orchid child: One genetic variant leads to the best and worse outcomes in kids.* Available at https://www.scientificamerican.com/article/on-the-trail-of-the-orchid-child.

Kalmakis, K.A., Chandler, G.E., Roberts, S.J., and Leung, K. (2017). Nurse practitioner screening for childhood adversity among adult primary care patients: a mixed-method study. *Journal of the American Association of Nurse Practitioners* 29 (1): 35–45.

Kania, J. &. Kramer, M. (2011). *Collective Impact.* Stanford Social Innovation Reveiw. Available at https://cdn.ymaws.com http://www.lano.org/resource/dynamic/blogs/20131007_093137_25993pdf.

Mersky, J.P., Topitzes, J., and Reynolds, A.J. (2013). Impacts of adverse childhood experiences on health, mental health, and substance use in early adulthood: a cohort study of an urban, minority sample in the US. *Child Abuse and Neglect* 37 (11): 917–925.

Monk, C., Feng, T., Lee, S. et al. (2016). Distress during pregnancy: epigenetic regulation of placenta glucocorticoid-related genes and fetal neurobehavior. *American Journal of Psychiatry* 173 (7): 705–713.

National Institute on Drug Abuse. (2018). Advancing Addiction Science: *West Virginia Opioid Summary.* Available at https://www.drugabuse.gov/drugs-abuse/opioids/opioid-summaries-by-state/west-virginia-opioid-summary [accessed 7 January 2019].

National Technical Assistance Center for Children's Mental Health (2015). *Who needs to pay attention to the ACE study?* Georgetown University Center for Child and Human Development. Available at https://georgetownta.wordpress.com/2015/03/05/who-needs-to-pay-attention-to-the-ace-study.

Ortiz, R. and Sibing, E.M (2017). The role of mindfullness in reducing the adverse effects of childhood in stress and truama. *Children (Basel)* 4 (3): 16. https://doi.org/10.3390/children4030016.

Pachter, L.M. and Coll, C.G. (2009). Racism and child health: a review of the literature and future directions. *Journal of Developmental and Behavioral Pediatrics* 30 (3): 255–262.

Sacks, V. & Murphey, D. (2018). *The prevalence of adverse childhood experiences, nationally, by state, and by race or ethnicity.* Available at http://www.childtrends.org/publications/prevalence-adverse-childhood-experiences-nationally-state-race-ethnicity [accessed 2 January 2019].

SAMHSA. (2018). *Adverse Childhood Experiences.* SAMHSA CAPT Center for the Application of Prevention Technologies. Available at https://www.samhsa.gov/capt/practicing-effective-prevention/prevention-behavioral-health/adverse-childhood-experiences [accessed 2 January 2019].

Shafer, M.B. (2017). *Nurse Practitioner Screening for Adverse Childhood Outcomes in Adult Primary Care.* Available at https://scholar.works.umass.edu/nursing-dnp-capstone/107 [accessed 11 January 2019].

Shonkoff, J.P. and Levitt, P. (2010). Neuroscience and the future of early childhood policy: moving from why to what and how. *Neuron* 67 (5): 689–691.

Shonkoff, J.P., Garner, A.S., Siegel, B.S. et al. (2012). The lifelong effects of early childhood adversity and toxic stress. *Pediatrics* 129 (1): e232–e246.

Srivastav, A., Fairbrother, G., and Simpson, L.A. (2017). Addressing adverse childhood experiences through the affordable care act: promising advances and missed opportunities. *Academic Pediatrics* 17 (7): S136–S143.

Steinberg, A.M., Brymer, M.J., Kim, S. et al. (2013). Psychometric properties of the UCLA PTSD reaction index: part I. *Journal of Traumatic Stress* 26 (1): 1–9.

Stevens, J.E. (2012). The Adverse Childhood Experiences Study – the largest, most important public health study you never heard of–began in an obesity clinic. ACES Too High News, 3. Available at http://www.huffingpost.com/jane-ellen-stevens/theadverse-childhood-exp_1_b_1943647.html.

Stevens, J.E. (2017). *ACEs Science 101. ACEs Science FAQs.* Available at https://acestoohigh.com/aces-101 [accessed 1 January 2019].

Tennessee Commission on Children and Youth. (2017). *Building Strong Brains: Tennessee's ACEs Initiative: The role of life experiences in shaping brain development.* Available at https://www.tn.gov/content/dam/tn/tccy/documents/ace/ACEs-Handout.pdf.

The Research and Evaluation Group: Public Health Management Corporation. (2013). *Findings from the Philadelphia ACE survey.* Available at https://www.rwjf.org/content/dam/farm/reports/reports/2013/rwjf407836.

USDHHS. (2019). *New HRSA data show one in three US children have suffered an adverse childhood experience.* US Department of Health and Human Services, Heath Resources and Services Administration. Available at https://www.hrsa.gov/about/news/press-releases/hrsa-data-national-survey-children-health [accessed 10 August 2020].

Van Niel, C., Pachter, L.M., Wade, R. Jr. et al. (2014). Adverse events in children: predictors of adult physical and mental conditions. *Journal of Developmental & Behavioral Pediatrics* 35 (8): 549–551.

Waite, R.D., Davey, M., and Lynch, L. (2013). Self-rated health and association with ACEs. *Journal of Behavorial Health* 2 (3): 197–205.

Williams, D.R. and Mohammed, S.A. (2013). Racism and health I: pathways and scientific evidence. *American Behavioral Scientist* 57 (8): 1152–1173.

9

Psychopharmacology: Issues in Prescribing Psychiatric Medication to Children and Adolescents

Geraldine S. Pearson[1] and Crystal Marie Bennett[2]

[1] University of Connecticut School of Medicine-retired, Farmington, CT, USA
[2] Child and Adolescent Psychiatric Nurse Practitioner, San Jose, CA, USA

Objectives

After reading this chapter, advanced practice registered nurses (APRNs) will be able to:

1. Identify principles of psychotropic medication management applicable to a pediatric primary care population.
2. Perform mental health assessments in the primary care setting and develop treatment plans that include medication referrals for diagnostic clarity and further treatment.
3. Identify commonly used psychotropic medications, indications for use, dosing, contraindications, and side effect profiles.
4. Discuss collaboration between APRNs in pediatric primary care and child/adolescent psychiatry regarding medication evaluation, medication stabilization, and mediation maintenance strategies.

Introduction

In the United States, it is estimated that 13–20% of children experience a mental health disorder within a given year; an estimated US$247 billion is spent yearly on childhood mental disorders (Centers for Disease Control and Prevention [CDC] 2019). It is likely that the vast majority of children requiring mental health assessment and treatment initially present with these issues to their pediatric primary care provider (PCP) APRNs in primary care settings are frequently the PCP who provided primary care to the child or adolescent. Of all children affected by mental health issues, it is estimated that 80% do not receive specialty mental healthcare in spite of needing it (CDC 2020). This potentially creates a significant negative impact on all aspects of development, including physical, social, cognitive, and emotional health. Untreated mental health conditions have long-term consequences for the child and family. Delays in providing early mental health assessment and treatment lead to exponentially more expensive interventions due to chronic complications from untreated conditions continuing into late adolescence and adulthood.

A chronic lack of mental health providers having direct contact and/or access to these children exists (Delaney 2017). The American Academy of Child and Adolescent Psychiatry (AACAP), in a best principles

Child and Adolescent Behavioral Health: A Resource for Advanced Practice Psychiatric and Primary Care Practitioners in Nursing,
Second Edition. Edited by Edilma L. Yearwood, Geraldine S. Pearson, and Jamesetta A. Newland.
© 2021 John Wiley & Sons, Inc. Published 2021 by John Wiley & Sons, Inc.
Companion website: www.wiley.com/go/Yearwood

document, estimated in 2012 that only 15–25% of children with psychiatric disorders received specialty psychiatry care; 75% of children have contact with their primary care provider (Martini et al. 2012). Opportunities for PCPs to identify, assess, and intervene in childhood mental health problems are significantly higher because they are usually the earliest and primary point of contact for families to the healthcare system. The early identification and treatment of mental health issues lessen the degree of disruption across all domains of development. Therefore, it is imperative that PCPs help children with mental health issues gain access to mental health providers and become more adept at understanding many of the treatment modalities, including medications used to care for children with mental health conditions. Many PCPs feel uncomfortable diagnosing children with complex mental health conditions and believe they do not have the knowledge or skills to prescribe treatments and medications for these children. Legitimately, treatment of some mental health symptoms is outside the scope of their training and practice. The early contact with a pediatric population as part of well-child care, combined with the current national shortage of child psychiatric specialists, has placed the PCP on the frontline of identifying these children, delivering evidence-based care and planning services for young patients with serious mental health problems (Lauerer et al. 2018). While many mental health issues can be addressed with targeted interventions at the individual, family, academic, or community level, the judicious use of psychopharmacological interventions in some child psychiatric disorders is still indicated. This chapter will explore these issues as they apply to prescribing medication for mental health disorders in children and adolescents.

Challenges in Prescribing Psychotropic Medications

Aside from the challenges presented to the advanced practice registered nurse (APRN) considering pediatric pharmacology, there is significant controversy about this intervention that has become central to child and adolescent psychiatric treatment. While there are known developmental hazards to untreated psychiatric illness, the international data suggest that the prescribing rates are increasing (Steinhausen 2015). At the same time there has been an increased reliance on psychotropic medication for symptom management, there are concerns about overtreatment with medication (Rapaport 2013). Prescribing any psychotropic medication requires careful and judicious consideration of the health and developmental risks of this treatment. Full consent and understanding from parents/caregivers and assent/consent from the pediatric

patient are essential. Psychopharmacology interventions may be the treatment of choice for some of the most prevalent disorders, and PCPs must have familiarity with these agents/diagnoses if they plan to treat children in their practice.

The use of stimulants to treat attention deficit hyperactivity disorder (ADHD) marked the beginning of the use of psychotropic medication. ADHD is one of the most common disorders of childhood and the treatment response to stimulants was excellent (Rapaport 2013). This prompted early numerous double-blind, placebo-controlled studies and led the way toward antidepressant medication being used to treat childhood depression and anxiety. Eventually, the combination of drug and nondrug treatment has been found most effective in the treatment of childhood depression, anxiety, and obsessive–compulsive disorders (OCD) (Domino et al. 2008).

While acceptance of psychotropic medication management for a variety of pediatric disorders has slowly grown, among clinicians, physicians, teachers, parents, and children, concerns remain about developmental effects, overuse of medication, and off-label use.

Psychiatric nurse practitioners, family nurse practitioners, pediatric nurse practitioners, and clinical nurse specialists are among an array of people who are prescribing psychotropic medication. Their level of independent practice, from supervisory with a physician to independent practice, is determined by each state's practice laws. Similarly, the ability to write prescriptions for different levels of controlled substances, such as stimulants, is also determined by individual state statutes. Finally, the educational programs of these primary care clinicians often do not include specific information on prescribing psychiatric medications to children and adolescents. Prescribing medications for the treatment of mental health conditions for children requires that the clinician possess the knowledge and skills to assess these children appropriately, identify the condition, and then develop a treatment plan based on their knowledge of psychotropic medication use with a pediatric population.

Assessment

Assessment of a psychiatric disorder in a child or adolescent might occur differently in a pediatric primary care environment versus a more traditional psychiatric service or mental health focused clinic. APRNs tend to provide well-child care and ambulatory acute care to their population. Behavioral health issues will come up during these visits and necessitate action from the primary care provider. Psychiatric evaluation, in its most traditional form, requires knowledge of psychiatric assessment to conduct the evaluation, scheduled time to facilitate this, followed by case formulation, and then treatment planning involving medication choice, dose, and adjunct treatment recommendations. Most pediatric appointments are brief and focused on the physical health issues presented by the patient and/or parent. Few pediatric practices are able to routinely schedule the time needed to conduct a complete psychiatric evaluation; it is not an expectation of the role. Yet primary care pediatric providers, including APRNs, routinely make treatment decisions regarding using stimulants and antidepressants for children in their practice. They also decide when more specialized care and referral are warranted. Primary care practice is influenced by many factors, including limited specialized psychiatric resources for children and adolescents, and family comfort levels and trust with PCPs (Melnyk et al. 2003; Williams et al. 2004). The professional comfort line between treating common conditions related to mental health and managing more complex psychiatric disorders varies by provider and level of training. Prescribing practices of PCPs might also vary according to type of setting, type of community, and degree of access to child psychiatric consultation.

A comprehensive psychiatric assessment integrates information from many sources, including direct interview with the parents/caregivers and child or adolescent and collateral information from daycare providers, schools, medical providers, and other members of the treatment team. Given the time restraints and skills needed by primary care providers, it is not possible to conduct a traditional psychiatric assessment in this setting. The recently developed Pediatric Primary Care Mental Health Specialist (PMHA) certification was developed to validate the skills needed by APRNs in pediatrics to better meet the mental and behavioral health concerns of populations in primary care (Pediatric Nursing Certification Board [PNCB] 2019). The goal of this advanced training is improved assessment and treatment of pediatric primary care populations with mental health needs.

Specifically, the use of evaluation tools can augment the evaluation process in the primary care setting. Tools that have been approved for use and are relatively easy to administer in this setting include structured rating scales such as the Child Behavior Checklist (CBCL), the Vanderbilt Scale, or Conners Rating Scales, used specifically for assessing symptoms of ADHD. Sulik and Sarvet (2016) note that screening tools will improve the identification for children and adolescents with clinical symptoms and functional impairments. It is important for the provider to recognize that rating scales cannot replace a direct interview with a child and parent/guardian, but can be used in conjunction with interviewing to help make a diagnosis.

Performing the Psychiatric Interview

Psychiatric interviews with children and adolescents traditionally involve a comprehensive history and evaluation of the child and parent(s). Reviewing the presenting problem and chief complaint introduces the practitioner to what the child and family perceives is the problem. It is also important to understand what the child and/or parent hope to achieve by a psychiatric evaluation or beginning medication to treat a behavior problem. The evaluation should identify the spheres, including home, school, and/or community, in which the child is having difficulties. Gaining information regarding when and how these problems first presented and what the parents noticed, as well as the child's perceptions of the difficulty, is helpful in formulating a diagnosis. Understanding how long the child has been experiencing problems helps determine whether this is an acute or long-term issue. Finally, gaining an understanding of any preceding or concurrent stressors, trauma, or historical events occurring within the child's environment helps to better understand the issues.

The provider evaluation should include a full psychiatric history, including any related prior treatment. The provider should ask if there is a history of psychiatric hospitalizations or other specialized psychiatric care such as intensive outpatient or partial hospitalization and any prior history of medications used to treat behavior problems. Additionally, the psychiatric history should include a review of any family history of psychiatric diagnoses or treatment. This information will help the provider not only in making the diagnosis but also in understanding the family's past interactions and possible trust/mistrust of mental health treatments.

The child's history must also contain an in-depth medical history, including any chronic conditions, surgeries, cardiac history, head injuries, loss of consciousness, and/or hospitalization. The history should also include a review of any medications the child is or has taken and any allergies to medications.

The developmental history for the child might offer many clues in the diagnostic picture. This history should be comprehensive and include the mother's pregnancy history, birth history, developmental progress up to the current age and developmental delays, history of school performance, including special education status, and any behavioral/developmental areas of concern the parent(s) have had for the child or adolescent.

A social history offers insight into the child's relationships and ability to interact with others and might help identify additional sources of stress or trauma. A comprehensive social history should include discussions about the child's relationships with adults, peers, teachers, and friends, history of arrests or involvement in the juvenile justice system, and involvement in community activities and/or team sports.

Physical Examination

Once the history has been completed, the provider must perform a full physical and mental status examination. The mental status examination includes the child's appearance, behavior, affect, thinking, suicidal/homicidal ideation, ability to relate to others, language, estimation of cognitive issues, and evidence of any sub-stance abuse/use. A full neurological examination, including testing reflexes and gross and fine motor skills, should also be performed to ensure the ability to rule out a physical cause of the child/adolescent's behavior. See Table 9.1 for a list of physical assessment parameters that should be considered before beginning psychotropic medication.

Table 9.1 Physical parameters and laboratory guidelines for medication monitoring in child and adolescent pharmacologic management

Prior to medication initiation: baseline physical examination (within 6–12 months) and medical history

Informed consent and child/adolescent assent (documented in medication record)

Review contraindications of medication to be started and check for interactions with any current medications

Vital signs

Height, weight and body mass index (http://www.cdc.gov/growthcharts)

Consider beta-hCG (in females of child-bearing age who are sexually active)

If not available in prior records:

For age 7 years and under: lead levels beginning at 9–12 months and yearly for high-risk populations

For children with a concern about sexual abuse: consider testing for STIs

PPD and tuberculosis evaluation

Uncomplicated care without medications (provided by the pediatrician):

Every 6 months: VS, Ht, Wt, BMI

Every year: physical, dental, eye, and hearing examinations

The following are protocols for monitoring individual medications:

Psychostimulants

Methylphenidate, dextroamphetamine, mixed amphetamine salts, dexmethylphenidate, lisdexamfetamine, and others:

Baseline: Ht, Wt, and BMI

Every 3 months: Ht, Wt, and BMI

Antidepressants

SSRIs:

Baseline: Ht, Wt, and BMI

Every 6 months: Ht, Wt, and BMI

Venlafaxine (Effexor):

Baseline: VS, Ht, Wt, and BMI

Every visit: VS (monitor for HTN)

Every 3 months: Ht, Wt, and BMI

Bupropion (Wellbutrin):

Baseline: VS, Ht, Wt, and BMI

Every 3 months: VS, Ht, Wt, and BMI

Contraindications: seizure disorder, bulimia, anorexia

Trazadone (Desyrel):

Baseline: Ht, Wt, and BMI

Every year: Ht, Wt, and BMI

(*continued*)

Table 9.1 (cont'd)

Mirtazapine (Remeron):

   Baseline: Ht, Wt, and BMI

   Every year: Ht, Wt, and BMI

Antipsychotics

Typical antipsychotic agents:

   Baseline: VS, Ht, Wt, BMI, CBC, LFTs, AIMS. Baseline ECG for chlorpromazine, thioridazine, haloperidol, pimozide

ECG parameters:

   Sinus rhythm: every QRS complex is preceded by a P wave and a PR interval

   Rate: 60–110 beats per minute

   PR interval <200 ms

   QRS interval <120 ms and no more than 30% over baseline (before drug initiation)

   QTc interval <460 ms

   Stabilizing dose: VS, ECG (chlorpromazine, thioridazine, haloperidol, pimozide)

   Every 3 months: VS, Ht, Wt, and BMI

   Every 6 months: AIMS and ECG (chlorpromazine, thioridazine, haloperidol, pimozide)

   Every year: CBC and LFTs

Atypical antipsychotic agents (all but clozapine):

   Baseline: VS, Ht, Wt, BMI, CBC, LFTs, HgbA1c, fasting lipid panel and glucose, AIMS

   Every visit: Ht, Wt, BMI (http://www.cdc.gov/growthcharts), activity levels and diet. If 7% or greater weight gain on drug relative to baseline, then clinician must address weight loss interventions.

   Every 3–6 months: fasting lipid panel and glucose, LFTs, and AIMS

   Every year: HgbA1c

Clozapine (Clozaril):

   Baseline: VS, Ht, Wt, BMI, CBC (ANC), LFTs, fasting lipid panel and glucose, ECG, and AIMS. Enroll in Clozaril monitoring system through the pharmacy.

   First 6 months: CBC (ANC – www.curehodgekins.com) every week per monitoring system (see below).

   Second 6 months: CBC (ANC) every 2 weeks

   Thereafter: CBC (ANC) every month

   Every visit: VS, Ht, Wt, and BMI

   Every 6 months: LFTs, fasting lipid panel and glucose, ECG, AIMS

Clozapine hematology monitoring for the first 6 months of therapy:

WBC (mm³)	ANC (mm³)	Action
Baseline: ≥3500	Baseline: ≥1500	Weekly monitoring
>3000	>1500	Continue weekly monitoring
Drop in count ≥3000 and total count between 3000 and 3500	>1500	Start twice weekly monitoring
2000–3000	>1500	Discontinue clozapine; start daily blood monitoring; observe for signs/symptoms of flulike illness
≤2000	≤1000	Hematology consult; consider BM aspiration
–	≤500	Agranulocytosis: medical emergency

Mood stabilizers

Lithium (Eskalith, Lithobid):

   Clarify if NSAID is used (will increase lithium level).

Table 9.1 (*cont'd*)

Baseline: VS, Ht, Wt, BMI, CBC, LFTs, electrolytes, BUN, creatinine, TSH, freeT4, urinalysis, and ECG

Stabilizing dose: lithium level

Every 6 months: VS, Ht, Wt, BMI, lithium level, CBC, LFTs, electrolytes, BUN, creatinine, TSH, free T4, and urinalysis

Every year: ECG

Valproate (Depakote, Depakene):

Baseline: VS, Ht, Wt, BMI, CBC, LFTs, electrolytes, and amylase

Stabilizing dose: valproate level, CBC, and LFTs

Every 3 months: VS, Ht, Wt, BMI, valproate level, CBC, and LFTs

Every year: carnitine (free, total, and acyl) and amylase

Carbamezapine (Tegretol):

Baseline: VS, Ht, Wt, BMI, CBC, LFTs, and electrolytes

Stabilizing dose: carbamezapine level, CBC, and LFTs

Every 3 months: VS, Ht, Wt, BMI, carbamzapine level, CBC, and LFTs

Contraindication: concomitant clozapine use (bone marrow suppression)

Oxycarbazepine (Trileptal):

Baseline: VS, Ht, Wt, BMI, CBC, LFTs, electrolytes, BUN, and creatinine

Stabilizing dose (every 1–2 months): VS

Every 3 months: VS, Ht, Wt, BMI, CBC, and electrolytes

Gabapentin (Neurontin):

Baseline: VS, Ht, Wt, BMI, CBC, LFTs, BUN, creatinine, and urinalysis

Stabilizing dose: VS

Every 3 months: VS, Ht, Wt, and BMI

Every year: CBC and LFTs

Lamotrigine (Lamictal):

Baseline: VS, Ht, Wt, BMI, CBC, and LFTs. Clarify if any history of rash reactions to medications.

Stabilizing dose: VS

Every 3 months: VS, Ht, Wt, and BMI

Every year: CBC and LFTs

Note: slow titration decreases risk for rash

Topirimate (Topamax):

Baseline: VS, Ht, Wt, BMI, CBC, LFTs, bicarbonate, and urinalysis. Clarify if any history of preexisting eye disease/glaucoma or kidney stones.

Stabilizing dose: VS

Every 3 months: VS, Ht Wt, BMI, and bicarbonate

Every year: CBC and LFTs

Alpha-2 Agonists

Clonidine (Catapres) and guanfacine (Tenex):

Baseline: VS, Ht, Wt, and BMI

Stabilizing dose: VS

Every 3 months: VS, Ht, Wt, and BMI

Contraindication: history of syncope, cardiovascular disease, Raynaud's syndrome

(continued)

Table 9.1 (*cont'd*)

Anxiolytics

Benzodiazapines and buspirone (Buspar):

> *Baseline:* VS, Ht, Wt, and BMI
>
> *Stabilizing dose:* VS
>
> *Every 6 months:* VS, Ht, Wt, and BMI

Benedryl, Atarax, Vistaril:

> *Baseline:* VS, Ht, Wt, and BMI
>
> *Stabilizing dose:* VS
>
> *Every 6 months:* VS, Ht, Wt, and BMI

Other agents

Non-BZD hypnotics: eszopiclone (Lunestra), zolpidem (Ambien), zaleplon (Sonata):

> *Baseline:* Ht, Wt, and BMI
>
> *Every 6 months:* Ht, Wt, and BMI

Beta blockers:

> *Baseline:* VS, Ht, Wt, BMI, CBC, LFTs, and ECG
>
> *Stabilizing dose:* VS, ECG
>
> *Every 3 months:* VS, Ht, Wt, and BMI
>
> *Every 6 months:* CBC, LFTs, and ECG

Strattera (Atomoxitine):

> *Baseline:* VS, Ht, Wt, and BMI
>
> *Stabilizing dose:* VS
>
> *Every 6 months:* VS, Ht, Wt, and BMI

AIMS, abnormal involuntary movement disorder; ANC, absolute neutrophil count; beta-hCG, beta-human chorionic gonodatropin; BM, bone marrow (aspiration); BMI, body mass index; BUN, blood urea nitrogen; BZD, benzodiazepine; CBC, complete blood cell count; ECG, electrocardiogram; HgbA1c, glycated hemoglobin; Ht, height; HTN, hypertension; LFT, liver function test; NSAID, nonsteroidal anti-inflammatory drugs; PPD, purified protein derivative; SSRI, selective serotonin reuptake inhibitors; STI, sexually transmitted infection; TSH, thyroid stimulating hormone; VS, vital signs; WBC, white blood cell count; Wt, weight.
Source: Adapted from: Connor and Meltzer (2006).

Formulation of a Diagnosis and Plan

Once the provider has accumulated all of the above-mentioned information, he or she must integrate this into a clinical understanding of the child and his or her developmental stage, and then summarize the assessment to guide the treatment planning. This process will lead to a final diagnosis, which will then allow the practitioner to develop a management plan.

Psychiatric diagnoses are organized on the *Diagnostic and Statistical Manual of Mental Disorders 5* (DSM-5; American Psychiatric Association [APA] 2013) or the International Classification of Diseases (ICD) taxonomy created through the World Health Organization (WHO 2005). The diagnoses listed should guide the decisions regarding medication management.

Treatment Plan

The treatment plan should flow from the presenting symptoms and diagnoses. Target symptoms, a problem list, and planning for adjunct clinical services should be included, along with recommendations about type of psychiatric medication. The type or class of medication chosen to treat a disorder needs to follow the evaluation information and the working diagnoses. For example, it is not good practice to give a depressive disorder diagnosis and prescribe stimulant medication. The treatment and choice of medication evolves from the formulation of the problem.

Cultural Considerations

Cultural considerations regarding pharmacological management of pediatric psychiatric problems have to be considered on at least two levels. The growing field of cultural psychopharmacology acknowledges that there is variability among ethnic groups regarding the pharmacokinetics of drug absorption, distribution, metabolism, and excretion (Dell 2010). Further research is needed to better define these ethnic differences. Also, many modern families are a blend of several different cultures and may have differing views of medication management. Equally important as the biochemical considerations regarding using medication is the cultural meaning of psychotropic medication held by parents. Meaning is often linked to bias and stigma regarding mental health issues and to belief systems regarding the efficacy of psychotropic medication (Munoz et al. 2007). Careful assessment of cultural views is essential to effective medication management with a pediatric population.

Decision Making

The decision to begin a medication trial to treat a behavioral health issue is a complex one for pediatric and psychiatric providers. For pediatric providers, the realization that a symptom constellation might benefit from medication requires an assessment of the disorder and type of medication that is most useful for the disorder. For the primary care APRN, the decision regarding which medication would provide the best outcome for the child/adolescent's specific issue should be based upon certain aspects of the medication's profile. Issues to be considered include use of a medication that is expected to be time limited, has a low safety risk defined by evidence-based assessment, and involves a simple treatment plan with clear interventions and follow-up.

Some conditions treated with psychotropic medication in primary care might include:

- ADHD (no comorbid issues identified, such as trauma, anxiety, OCD, or mood disorder).
- Uncomplicated anxiety.
- Depression (without other psychiatric comorbidities).

Conditions that might necessitate referral to a psychiatric APRN or child psychiatrist include:

- Any untoward response to current or past psychotropic medication trial.
- Comorbid symptoms or the presence of two or more psychiatric disorders.
- Trauma history.
- Previous treatment with no improvement in symptoms.
- Any high-risk symptom or behavior such as hallucinations (auditory, visual, tactile, or olfactory) or suicidal or homicidal ideation.
- Substance abuse or addiction.

Need for Consultation

The recognition by the PCP that mental health consultation is needed will likely depend on several factors. The ability to differentiate between situationally driven, lower-level mental health issues versus major mental health disorders or complex symptom clusters will influence referral. The complexity of mental health issues presented by children and adolescents, the interplay between providers, and the need for coordination of multiple systems involved with the child necessitate a team approach to psychotropic prescribing. The psychiatric APRN may be consulting with a variety of other health professionals, including PCPs, psychiatric providers, school systems, and neurology specialists. The process of prescribing is not simple or easy. The skill set necessary for the PCP to appropriately treat mental health issues is complex and requires additional time and knowledge within the primary care setting. A complex skill set encompasses the ability to quickly perform a brief assessment, make an informed diagnosis of the problem, develop a sequential plan of care, facilitate referrals and consultations to appropriate care agencies, and apply knowledge of the various agents that can be used to treat a disorder. When an issue is identified as appropriate to primary care settings, this may include lifestyle interventions, parenting ideas, or psychopharmacological interventions. If presenting symptoms are complex and not appropriate to the primary care setting, the pediatric APRN can assist and support the patient and family in connecting with an available mental health provider to facilitate a positive treatment relationship. Mental health services can run the gamut of traditional psychodynamic individual and family therapy, in-home services, parent management training, or behavioral models such as cognitive behavioral therapy (CBT). The prescriber, whether a PCP or a mental health specialist, must understand how psychotropic medication fits into the other treatment needs presented by a child or adolescent. Rarely does a pill fix the mental health problems of a child presenting to the APRN in a primary or psychiatric care setting. The PCP needs to recognize that along with medications, the child/adolescent and possibly the family require comprehensive treatment: therapy, stress management, and close follow-up care. It is imperative to emphasize that medications alone are not the answer to the mental health issues.

Patient/Family Education

An essential aspect of medication management is the careful patient/family education process that occurs with both primary care and psychiatric APRNs. A clear, focused description of the presenting problem and its possible etiology, trajectory, and possible treatment should be shared with parents and guardians. If the treatment involves medication, there must be written consents from parent/guardian and assent from the pediatric patient. Consent might be noted in the nursing progress note or, depending on the agency, involve a formal document. Whenever possible, medication information should be given to the parent with sensitivity to cultural and language issues. Parents or guardians need to be given an informed choice regarding psychotropic medication management for their child and, if appropriate, the child or adolescent should be included in conversations about medications to be used.

Parents or guardians need to have a time frame for the intervention, a follow-up plan, and a clear explanation of the risks, benefits, and side effects of the proposed medication. Parents need to participate in the decision making regarding seeking a psychiatric opinion when behavior problems are beyond the scope of the pediatric primary care APRN. DiMarco and Melnyk (2009) noted that the mental health needs of children and adolescents could not be met by any one discipline or specialty. They proposed that synergism between primary care and psychiatric APRNs will result in better care and more coordinated services. For those pediatric patients who have been treated with psychiatric medication, the next step is returning to their PCP for continued medication management. The psychiatric APRN remains a consultative and treating back-up if needed.

Review of Common Psychiatric Medications

Stimulants and Nonstimulants for ADHD
Pharmacology

Stimulants are agents that increase norepinephrine and dopamine actions by blocking reuptake and facilitating release (Stahl 2018). This influences the central nervous system (CNS) by activating the level of activity, arousal, and alertness (Spencer et al. 2016). Stimulants can be obtained in short-, intermediate-, and long-acting preparations of methylphenidate and mixed amphetamine salts. Efficacy and safety have been widely studied (Pliszka 2010). They are Schedule II drugs, which are closely regulated and controlled by the US Drug Enforcement Agency (DEA). Stimulants are highly effective when used to treat symptoms of ADHD. Nonstimulant medications include atomoxetine, a norepinephrine reuptake inhibitor, and clonidine and guanfacine, alpha-adrenergic agents.

Indications for Use

Stimulant medication is used for the core ADHD symptoms of inattention and motoric hyperactivity. Nonstimulant medication may be indicated as adjuncts to stimulant treatment or part of monotherapy to reduce hyperactivity, distractibility, and impulsiveness (Leahy 2018).

Contraindications

There are concerns that stimulant treatment might trigger mood instability in patients at risk for mood disorder. The general view is that ADHD can be safely treated with a stimulant provided the mood disorder has been stabilized first (Merkel 2010). Careful psychiatric assessment is imperative given the high prevalence of other comorbid psychiatric disorders in individuals with ADHD. Blood pressure, pulse, and weight/body mass index (BMI) must be monitored regularly.

Side Effects

The only black box warning for stimulant medication involves their abuse potential and risk of dependency (Spencer et al. 2016). The most commonly reported side effects involve appetite suppression and sleep disturbances. Difficulties falling asleep and lack of noontime appetite can be specifically targeted as potential side effects of stimulants. While there have been concerns about the effects of stimulants on growth, research has shown that treatment with stimulant medication into adolescence may lead to only modest delays in growth. The greater deficit tends to involve weight rather than height (Troska et al. 2019). Some children may develop mild and transient behavior tics. The literature suggests that tics are not a serious side effect, and in most instances they will disappear (Merkel 2010). Decisions about continuing or stopping medication should be based on status of tics, how much they concern the parents or the child/adolescent, and a careful consideration of the benefits versus adverse effects of the medications. Atomoxetine has a black box warning for increased suicidal ideation in young children.

Drug–Drug Interactions

While drug–drug interactions between stimulants and other agents tend to be rare, they do exist (Stahl 2018; Wolraich and Doffing 2004). Prescribers are urged to carefully evaluate the interaction of stimulants with other agents using an online prescribing tool or a drug handbook.

Before prescribing a stimulant or any medication to treat ADHD, it is imperative that a list of all medications, including vitamins, herbals, energy drinks, and over-the-counter preparations, be obtained from parents. Monitoring of drug–drug interactions is best done with a complete list of all substances being taken by the child or adolescent and use of drug references or pharmacy consultation.

Monitoring

Stimulant medications have been linked to causing arrhythmias in certain patient populations. Prior to beginning a stimulant, the APRN needs to conduct a thorough screen for any history of sudden death in a first-degree relative or a history of cardiac arrhythmias or abnormalities in the patient. If the patient has a pre-existing cardiac condition, the APRN should consult with a cardiologist before initiating treatment. While an electrocardiogram (ECG) is an effective screen for cardiac symptoms in all patients beginning stimulant treatment, the American Academy of Pediatrics has stated that it is not routinely indicated in otherwise healthy youth (Perrin et al. 2008). This continues to be the current standard of care. Similarly, routine laboratory work is not required prior to beginning stimulant medication.

Dosing

Stimulants are the first line of treatment for children with ADHD and the usual dose range is 0.3–2 mg/kg/day for methylphenidate and half of this for dexedrine derivatives; these agents are approximately twice as potent as methylphenidate (Spencer et al. 2010). These agents have a short half-life and must be given twice a day approximately 4 hours apart. Longer-term agents can be given once a day in the morning. Some children will require a cover dose of a short-acting stimulant after school in addition to the longer-term preparation in the morning. The risk of this afternoon dose is decreased appetite at dinnertime and difficulties falling sleep. Abrupt discontinuation of a stimulant can precipitate transient behavior problems. It is not recommended that "drug holidays" be taken from medication unless carefully discussed with the prescriber, the family, and the patient.

Long-term Use

There is growing evidence that the adverse effects of untreated ADHD on behavior and functioning suggest that long-term stimulant treatment is warranted. While many adolescents eventually stop taking their medication, ADHD symptomatology continues to persist and influence functioning. Risks regarding automobile accidents, academic difficulties, and interpersonal problems related to untreated ADHD in adulthood are well documented (Pliszka 2016). No studies to date suggest that long-term stimulant use has adverse effects on health (Pliszka 2016). See Table 9.2 for stimulant and Table 9.3 for nonstimulant medications.

Antidepressants
Pharmacology

Traditionally, tricyclic antidepressants (TCAs) were the first antidepressants used with children and adolescents, and were characterized by a lack of efficacy, cardiotoxic side effects, and lethal overdose risk (Connor and Meltzer 2006). They have been mostly replaced by the use of selective serotonin reuptake inhibitors (SSRIs), a class of medication with a safer side effect profile. The primary mode of action for SSRIs is thought to be presynaptic inhibition of serotonin reuptake (Emslie et al. 2016). TCAs are generally not used in pediatric populations because of the high side effect profile.

Indications for Use

SSRIs have become the first-line pharmacological treatment for major depressive disorders, OCDs, and other anxiety disorders in pediatric populations (Emslie et al. 2016). They are used in both primary care and child psychiatric settings with positive effectiveness. While there has been controversy in the past regarding the risks of suicidal ideation/suicidal attempts with pediatric use of antidepressants, these risks involve a small percentage of pediatric patients (Emslie et al. 2016). Sharing Food and Drug Administration (FDA) black box warning information with patients and parents is indicated when medication is being considered for treatment (Bridge et al. 2007). Use of rating scales (such as the Beck Depression Inventory) is encouraged prior to initiating SSRI use and during treatment to measure progress in symptom amelioration. Table 9.4 lists FDA-approved indications for use of antidepressant medications.

Contraindications

SSRIs should not be taken with monomine oxidase inhibitor (MAOI) medication or pimozide. Taking tryptophan along with an SSRI can result in headache, nausea, sweating, and dizziness. While a rare side effect, there is documentation of seizures when SSRIs are given with the analgesic tramadol hydrochloride.

Side Effects

The most prominent side effects from SSRI use include gastrointestinal (GI) complaints of nausea or diarrhea, motor restlessness, and behavioral activation (Emslie et al. 2016). Prescribers should watch for symptoms of hypomania and mania, and discontinue the SSRI trial if these occur. Sexual side effects, notable in sexually active adolescents, include erectile dysfunction, delayed ejaculation, and anorgasmia (Block et al. 2018). Adolescents should be informed of these risks.

Monitoring

Before beginning an antidepressant trial, a routine pediatric physical examination is indicated. Baseline assessment of suicide risk and level and severity of depression or anxiety should occur. It takes between 2 and 12 weeks for a positive response to antidepressant treatment and the lowest dose should be given first with gradual increases every 5–7 days. No specific laboratory work is required

Table 9.2 Stimulant medications for ADHD

Drug name (brand)	Active ingredient	Onset of action	Duration of effect	Required number of doses/day	Suggested dosing and titration
Short-acting					
Ritalin® Methylin® Focalin® Metadate®	Methylphenidate	20–60 min Peak effect: 2 h	3–6 h	2–3 doses; occasionally 4 doses	Start with one 5-mg tablet (2.5 mg for Focalin) 2–3× a day Increase by 5 mg (or 2.5 mg for Focalin) until target behavior controlled
Dexedrine® Dextrostat®	D-amphetamine	20–60 min Peak effect: 1–2 h	4–6 h	2–3 doses	Start with one 5-mg tablet 2–3× per day[a]
Adderall®	D,L-amphetamine	30–60 min Peak effect: 1–2 h	4–6 h	2–3 doses	Start with one 5-mg tablet 2–3× per day[a]
First-generation: long-acting					
Ritalin SR® Metadate ER® Methylin ER	Methylphenidate	60–90 min Peak effect: 8 h	5–8 h	1–2 doses	Start with one 10-mg tablet 1–2× per day[a]
Dexedrine Spansules®	D-amphetamine	60–90 min Peak effect: 8 h	6–8 h	1–2 doses	Start with one 5-mg capsule 1–2× per day[a]
Second-generation: long-acting					
Concerta®	Methylphenidate	30 min–2 h	12 h	1 tablet	Start with one 18-mg tablet once per day[a]
Metadate CD® Ritalin LA®	Methylphenidate	30 min–2 h	6–8 h	1–2 capsules	Start with one 10-mg capsule once per day[a]
Daytrana®	Methylphenidate	20–60 min Peak effect: 10 h after single application, 8 h after repeat applications	8–12 h	1 patch	Start 10-mg patch worn 9 h daily Maximum dose: 30 mg patch worn 9 h daily
Focalin XR®	Dexmethylphenidate	1–4 h	8–12 h	1 capsule	Start with one 5-mg capsule once per day[a]
Quillivant XR	Methylphenidate	30 min Peak effect: 5 h	8–12 h	1 liquid dose	Start with 20 mg liquid suspension once per day[a]
Adderall XR	D,L-amphetamine	1–2 h	10–12 h	1 capsule	Start with one 5- or 10-mg capsule once per day[a]
Vyvanse®	L-lysine-dextroamphetamine	2 h Peak effect: 3–4 h	10–12 h	1 capsule	Start with one 30-mg capsule once daily[a]

[a] Titrate upward until target behavior controlled.
CD, controlled delivery; ER and XR, extended release; LA, long acting; SR, sustained release.
Source: Bloch et al. (2018), p. 719. Adapted with permission from Wolters Kluwer Health, Inc.

during an antidepressant trial but weight and vital signs should be regularly evaluated, and the child or adolescent should be seen frequently (at least every 2 weeks) while the dose of medication is being titrated upwards.

Dosing

SSRIs are generally started at the lowest possible dose and slowly titrated upwards with medication increases every 1–2 weeks to optimal dose. Duration of treatment of depression with an SSRI is usually set at 1 year after resolution of symptoms. OCD and anxiety symptoms may require a longer period of treatment (Bloch et al. 2018). When discontinuing the medication, patients and parents need to be cautioned to slowly decrease the dose to avoid SSRI discontinuation syndrome. Abrupt stoppage of an SSRI can result in flu-like symptoms such as dizziness, nausea, vomiting, myalgia, fatigue, and moodiness. See Table 9.5 for a list of antidepressants.

Table 9.3 Nonstimulant medications for ADHD

Medication	Drug name	Frequency	Daily dose range
Atomoxetine	Strattera®	Daily or twice daily	0.5–1.2 mg/kg/day (<70 kg) 40–80 mg/day (≥70 kg)
Clonidine	Clonidine IR®	Twice daily to 4× per day	0.05–0.4 mg/day
	Clonidine ER (Kapvay®)	Daily	0.1–0.4 mg/day
Guanfacine	Guanfacine IR	Twice daily to 4× per day	0.5–0.4 mg/day
	Guanfacine ER (Intuniv®)	Daily	1–4 mg/day
Desipramine	Norpramin®	Twice daily to 3× per day	2–5 mg/kg/day
Bupropion	Wellbutrin®	Twice daily	50–150 mg

Source: Bloch et al. (2018), p. 722. Adapted with permission from Wolters Kluwer Health, Inc.

Table 9.4 FDA-approved indications for use of antidepressant medications

	Age (years)											
	5	6	7	8	9	10	11	12	13	14	15–17	Adult
Selective serotonin reuptake inhibitors												
Citalopram						None						D
Escitalopram				None						D		D, G
Fluoxetine	None		O					O, D				O, D, N
Fluvoxamine		None						O				O
Paroxetine						None						O, D, P, G, S, N
Sertraline	None							O				O, D, P, S, N
Serotonin norepinephrine reuptake inhibitors												
Venlafaxine						None						D, G, S, N
Duloxetine			None					G				D, G
Desvenlafaxine						None						D
Atypical antidepressants												
Bupropion						None						D
Mirtazapine						None						D
Vilazodone						None						D
Vortioxetine						None						D
Trazodone						None						D
Tricyclic Antidepressants												
Clomipramine			None						O			O
Desipramine						None						D
Nortriptyline						None						D

FDA, Food and Drug Administration; O, obsessive–compulsive disorder; D, major depressive disorder; P, posttraumatic stress disorder; G, generalized anxiety disorder; S, social anxiety disorder; N, panic disorder.
Source: Bloch et al. (2018), p. 725. Adapted with permission from Wolters Kluwer Health, Inc.

Table 9.5 Clinical guidance for antidepressant medications utilized in pediatric practice

	Pediatric		Adult		
	Starting dose (mg/day)	Typical dose range (mg/day)	Starting dose (mg/day)	Typical dose range (mg/day)	Half-life
Selective serotonin reuptake inhibitors					
Citalopram	10	20–40	20	40	20 h
Escitalopram	5	10–40	10	20–40	27–32 h
Fluoxetine	10–20	20–80	20	20–80	4–6 days
Fluvoxamine	25–50	50–300	100–300	100–300	16 h
Paroxetine	10	20–60	10–20	40–60	21 h
Sertraline	25–50	100–200	50	150–250	26 h
Serotonin norepinephrine reuptake inhibitors					
Venlaflaxine	37.5	150–225	37.5–75	75–375	10 h
Duloxetine	40	40–60	20–60	20–80	12.5 h
Desvenlafaxine	10	10–100	50	50–400	11 h
Atypical antidepressants					
Bupropion	100	150–300	100–150	150–300	21 h
Mirtazapine	7.5	15–45	15	15–45	20–40 h
Vilazodone	Not studied		10	10–40	25 h
Vortioxetine	Not studied		10	10–80	66 h
Trazodone	25–50	100–150	150	150–300	3–9 h
Tricyclic antidepressants					
Clomipramine	25	50–200	25	100–250	32 h
Desipramine	25	50–200	100–200	150–300	12–27 h
Nortriptyline	30–50	30–150	100	75–150	18–44 h

Source: Bloch et al. (2018), p. 727. Adapted with permission from Wolters Kluwer Health, Inc.

Mood Stabilizers

Pharmacology

Mood stabilizers include lithium and anticonvulsants such as divalproex/valproic acid (Depakote), carbamazepine (Tegretol), oxcarbazepine (Trileptal), lamotrigine (Lamictal), and topiramate (Topomax). Lithium influences neurochemical systems including norepinephrine, dopamine, and serotonin, but effects on intracellular signaling processes comprise its primary action (Block et al. 2018). Exact mechanisms of action for the anticonvulsant agents used in pediatric psychiatry have not been fully established. However, anticonvulsants used for mood stabilization ultimately affect many of the same signaling pathways believed to mediate lithium's therapeutic effects (Manji and Chen 2000).

Indications for Use

Use of mood stabilizers includes symptom management for acute mania, bipolar depression, and aggressive behavior associated with conduct and other behavioral disorders (Gracious et al. 2016). Data for the efficacy for these medications in the pediatric population are mixed. An early open-label trial of the most commonly used mood stabilizers – lithium, divalproex, and carbamazepine – evinced large effect sizes (Cohen's $d > 1.0$) for the treatment of acute pediatric mania (Kowatch et al. 2000). More recent monotherapy trials of lithium, divalproex, and carbamazapine have shown more moderate symptom reduction (Correll et al. 2010). Combination therapy, using two mood stabilizers or a mood stabilizer plus an antipsychotic, has generally demonstrated more significant symptom reduction than the monotherapeutic use of these mood-stabilizing agents (Nandagopal et al. 2009). Lamotrigine may be more effective for bipolar or unipolar depression than for pediatric aggression or acute mania (Gracious et al. 2016). Clinical guidance on mood stabilizers used in pediatric practice is shown in Table 9.6.

Table 9.6 Clinical guidance on mood stabilizers used in pediatric practice

Drug	Mechanism of action	Main indications and clinical uses	Dosage	Schedule	Adverse effects	Comments
Lithium	Inhibition of phosphatidylinositol and protein kinase C signaling pathways; enhancement of serotonergic transmission	Bipolar disorder, manic; prophylaxis of bipolar disorder; MDD aggressive behavior/conduct disorder; adjunct treatment in refractory MDD	10–30 mg/kg/day, dose adjusted to serum levels in the range of 0.6–1.1 mEq/l	Twice a day/three times a day	Polyuria, polydipsia, tremor, ataxia, nausea, diarrhea, weight gain, drowsiness, acne, hair loss; possible effects on thyroid and renal functioning with long-term administration; children prone to dehydration are at higher risk for acute lithium toxicity; lithium levels >2 mEq/l can be life threatening	Therapy requires monitoring of lithium levels, thyroid, and renal function
Divalproex	Inhibition of catabolic enzymes of GABA and of protein kinase C signaling	Bipolar disorder; aggressive behavior; conduct disorder; seizure disorders	15–60 mg/kg/day, dose adjusted to serum levels in the range of 50–125 mcg/l	Twice a day/three times a day	Sedation, nausea, liver toxicity (requires baseline and close monitoring), thrombocytopenia, pancreatitis	Polycystic ovarian disorder has been reported during long-term use for seizure control
Carbamazepine	Inhibition of glial steroidogenesis; inhibition of alpha 2 receptors; blocks sodium	Bipolar disorder; complex partial seizures	10–20 mg/kg/day, dose adjusted to serum levels in the range of 4–14 mcg/l	Twice a day	Bone marrow suppression (requires baseline and close monitoring of blood counts); dizziness, drowsiness, rashes, nausea, liver toxicity, especially under 10 years of age	Potent inductor of CYP3A4, leading to auto-induction requiring periodic dose adjustment
Oxcarbamazepine	Channels block glial calcium influx	Seizure disorders	Maintenance dose of 18.5–48 mg/kg/day, not to exceed 2100 mg/day		No reports of bone marrow suppression; more benign drug interaction profile compared to carbamazepine; no blood level monitoring necessary	No empirical data available for children and adolescents
Lamotrigine	Weak 5HT3 inhibition; release of aspartate and glutamate	Bipolar depression and maintenance therapy; seizure disorders	75–300 mg/day	Every day	Potentially life-threatening rash; Stevens–Johnson syndrome (dose-[direct] and age-[inverse] related event rates)	Slow dose titration (12.5 mg every other week) may reduce risk of skin reactions

5HT3, 5-hydroxtryptamine (receptor antagonists); CYP3A4, cytochrome P450 3A4; GABA, gamma-aminobutyric acid; mcg/l, micrograms per liter; MDD, major depressive disorder; mEq/l, milliequivalents per liter.

Source: Bloch et al. (2018), p. 743. Adapted with permission from Wolters Kluwer Health, Inc.

Contraindications

In general, mood stabilizers should be used with caution in patients with renal, cardiovascular, or hepatic impairment. Lithium uniquely requires cautious use in patients with thyroid dysfunction but may be a good choice for patients with liver disease (Kowatch et al. 2010). Each mood stabilizer has different properties and may be more or less appropriate depending on a patient's medical history and co-occurring medical conditions.

Providers should counsel females of childbearing age regarding the risks and benefits of these medications. Although divalproex has the only US Food and Drug Administration (FDA) black box warning regarding teratogenic effects (FDA 2011), carbamazepine has also demonstrated teratogenic effects (Jones et al. 1989), and lithium has been associated with fetal cardiac defects (Cohen et al. 1994). Although no specific birth defects have been consistently associated with lamotrigine use during pregnancy, caution is warranted (Tennis et al. 2002). Divalproex additionally presents an increased risk of polycystic ovarian syndrome in female patients (Isojarvi and Tapanainen 2000).

Side Effects

Many mood stabilizers have black box warnings (FDA 2011). Carbamazapine has black box warnings for dangerous skin conditions, increased suicidality, and blood dyscrasias. Lamotrigine has black box warnings for dangerous skin conditions and aseptic meningitis. Divalproex has black box warnings for hepatotoxicity, life-threatening pancreatitis, and teratogenic effects. Lithium requires close monitoring due to the risk of lithium toxicity, its only black box warning. Signs of lithium toxicity include nausea, vomiting, slurred speech, altered mental status, and poor motor coordination (Okusa and Crystal 1994).

Common side effects of all mood stabilizers include nausea, vomiting, diarrhea, dizziness, increased appetite, weight gain, sedation, tremor, and headache. Lithium may additionally contribute to acne, hypothyroidism, neurotoxicity, and kidney dysfunction, whereas divalproex use may lead to thrombocytopenia or hyperammonemia (Nandagopal et al. 2009). Although carbamazepine has the only black box warning for increased suicidality, worsening mood and increased thoughts of suicide may be side effects of any of these agents. Hepatotoxicity is also a potential side effect of valproate preparations (Bloch et al. 2018) (see Table 9.7).

Drug–Drug Interactions

Both divalproex and carbamazapine are metabolized by the cytochrome P450 system and therefore interact with many other medications. Unrecognized drug–drug interactions may lead to toxicity or treatment failure and need to be carefully investigated. Mood stabilizers may interact with other antiepileptics, lithium, oral contraceptives, guanfacine, all classes of antidepressants, and some antipsychotics (aripiprazole, haloperidol, and risperidone). Divalproex interacts with other antiepileptic medications – guanfacine, risperidone, TCAs, and salicylates. Lamotrigine interacts with other antiepileptics – desmopressin, olanzapine, and oral contraceptives. Lithium may increase the neurotoxic effects of both TCAs and antipsychotics. Lithium also interacts with carbamazepine, MAOI antidepressants, and nonsteroidal anti-inflammatory drugs (NSAIDs) (Gracious et al. 2016).

Monitoring

Ongoing and careful monitoring is required with all mood stabilizers. Periodically checking serum drug levels may be useful to evaluate patient compliance and possible toxicity for all mood stabilizers, with the exception of lamotrigine. Weight gain and signs/symptoms of suicidality or worsening depression should also be monitored with all mood-stabilizing agents. Prior to beginning mood stabilizers, baseline laboratory tests including complete blood cell count (CBC), liver function tests (LFTs), electrolytes, blood urea nitrogen (BUN), and creatinine should be drawn. They should be repeated after 3 months on the medication and, if within normal limits, yearly (Connor and Meltzer 2006).

Anxiolytics

Introduction

All primary care practitioners will need to address anxiety in their pediatric population at some point in time. Anxiety is the most common mental health issue in childhood and a normative state under many situations. The degree of anxiety and persistence of symptoms under specific conditions are correlated with the individual's hard-wired anxiety traits (temperament), experiences, developmental stage, and parental response sets and expectations. Reactions can result from normative, fear-inducing situations (i.e. medical or dental procedures) to high-intensity responses to typically low-stress phenomenon. There are also the more functionally challenging anxiety response patterns that appear more within the boundary of a mental health condition than a normative response (but of higher intensity) to general life events. As anxiety is a universal, basic emotion experienced by almost everyone at some point in time, the primary care practitioner will be required to evaluate the presenting picture and be confident in addressing the symptoms at the appropriate level. Chapter 11 discusses anxiety seen as a particular mental health disorder and does not address the more transient states that accompany daily caseloads in the primary care setting.

Table 9.7 Mood stabilizers dosing, side effects, and precautions

Medication generic name and (trade)	FDA approved age (years)	Dosing (range)	Side effects	Duration of medication	Pros	Precautions
Lithium carbonate (Lithobid, Eskalith, Cibalith-S)	>12	Start 25 mg/kg/day, twice a day to three times a day Target: 30 mg/kg/day or 900–1200 mg/day divided doses, serum level 0.6–1.2, after meals	Common: nausea, vomiting, diarrhea, increased appetite, weight gain, sedation, tremor, acne Uncommon: hypothyroidism, neurotoxicity, kidney dysfunction, lithium toxicity, nausea, vomiting, slurred speech, altered mental status, ataxia, lack of coordination, polyuria, polydipsia	Half-life 24 h	Good for bipolar mania in adolescence, better choice if liver problems	Initial: BMI %, HCG/UCG, thyroid, chemistry screen, CBS, renal function, ECG, weight, and height check, sun sensitivity, avoid during pregnancy Therapeutic index, blood level absolutely necessary, neurotoxicity
Divalproex sodium and valproic acid (Depokote, Depokote DR, Depokote ER)	>2	Start 15 mg/kg/day, twice a day to three times a day, serum level 50–120 mg/l, range 15–60 mg/kg/day divided doses	Common: nausea, vomiting, diarrhea, constipation, weight gain, sedation, tremor, blurred vision Uncommon: PCOS, hepatotoxicity, pancreatitis, thrombocytopenia, hyperammonemia	Half-life 6–16 h	Good for bipolar in childhood both mania and depression Anticonvulsant, may be useful for aggression	Initial: BMI %, HCG/UCG, thyroid, chemistry screen, CBC with differential, ECG, weight, and height check, BP, P, LFTs, serum ammonia, POCS, hepatotoxic, risk of pancreatitis, teratogenic Depokote ER: no efficacy shown, CYP450 system: lots of interactions
Carbamazepine (Tegretol) Carbamazepine XR (Tegretol XR)	>6	Start 10–20 mg/kg/day, twice a day to three times a day, target: response, serum level 8.9–11 mg/l, range 100–1200 mg/day divided doses	Common: vomiting, diarrhea, weight gain, sedation, tremor, dry mouth, dizziness, trouble urinating Uncommon: increased SI, blood dyscrasias, Steven–Johnson syndrome, renal failure, SAIDH, auto induces own metabolism and many other medications	Half-life 25–65 h	Moderate for BPD in childhood May be useful for rapid cycling, anticonvulsant	BMI %, HCG/UCG, thyroid, chemistry screen, CBC with differential, ECG, weight, and height check, BP, P, LFTs, monitor CYP450 system interactions, teratogenic, black box, caution with Asian children increased risk of hypersensitivity, increased suicidality, blood dyscrasias, bone marrow suppression; warnings around dangerous skin conditions; assess for rash
Lamotrigine (Lamictal)	>16	Start 12.5 mg/wk. up to once a day, range 25–300 mg/day divided doses Titrate carefully and slowly	Common: headache, nausea, vomiting, ataxia, sedation, blurred vision, sedation, dizziness Uncommon: Steven–Johnson syndrome, aseptic meningitis, amnesia, hepatic failure, anemia	Half-life 33 h	Anticonvulsant, may be useful in pediatric BPD and depression, not associated with weight gain, no frequent laboratory tests needed, adult BPD	HCG/UCG, thyroid, chemistry screen, CBC with differential, ECG, weight, and height check, BP, P, LFTs, monitor for aseptic meningitis (anytime), Steven–Johnson syndrome (rash), many drug–drug interactions

(continued)

Table 9.7 (cont'd)

Medication generic name and (trade)	FDA approved age (years)	Dosing (range)	Side effects	Duration of medication	Pros	Precautions
Oxcarbazepine (Trilepal)	No approval for adults and children with BPD	Start 2–20 mg/kg/day twice a day, range 150–1800 mg/day, serum level, Na	Common: nausea, vomiting, ataxia, sedation, blurred vision, sedation, dizziness,, GI upset, tremor Uncommon: rash, hyponatremia, nystagmus, increased risk for URI		No evidence of efficacy for mood in children, no need for frequent blood draws	HCG/UCG, thyroid, chemistry screen, CBC with differential, ECG, weight, and height check, BP, P, LFTs, monitor for hyponatremia
Topiramate (Topamax)	No approval for adults and children with BPD	Start 25–50 mg, twice a day, range 50–400 mg divided doses	Common: nausea, vomiting, sedation, decreased appetite, fatigue, tingling, change in taste, nervousness Uncommon: sudden decreased vision, diaphoresis, fever, suicidal thoughts, agitation, restlessness, insomnia, irritability, anger, aggression, alopecia		No evidence of efficacy for mood in children, anticonvulsant, may facilitate weight loss or be weight neutral	HCG/UCG, chemistry screen, CBC with differential, vision changes, metabolic acidosis, hyperammonemia, cognitive dulling, neurology problems, inattention, word retrieval difficulty, caution with oral contraceptives

BMI%, body mass index percentage; BP, blood pressure; BPD, bipolar personality disorder; CBC, complete blood count; CYP450, cytochrome P450; DR, delayed release; ER and XR, extended release; GI, gastrointestinal; HCG, human chorionic gonadotropin; LFT, liver function test. Na, sodium; P, pulse; PCOS, polycystic ovarian syndrome; POCS, projection onto convex sets (used for magnetic resonance imaging partial Fourier reconstruction); S, solution; SAIDH, syndrome of inappropriate antidiuretic hormone secretion; SI, sacroiliitis; UCG, urine chorionic gonadotropin; URI, upper respiratory infection.

Source: Developed by B. Muller from Connor and Meltzer (2006), Danielyan and Kowatch (2005), Kowatch et al. (2010).

Anxiety that is more trait-dependent, crosses domains and significantly disturbs normal developmental function, and is sustained over time is more appropriately addressed by mental health specialists who would be able to develop comprehensive treatment plans utilizing CBT treatment, desensitization, SSRIs (covered under "Antidepressants"), or a combination of these strategies. Anxiolytics, on the other hand, are the typical choice in primary care to provide short-term intervention for a specific, circumscribed anxiety-provoking situation that is time limited (see Table 9.8). Screening is essential to assess whether the symptoms represent a more embedded pattern of emotional responsiveness or a normative, situation-dependent response that provokes an untoward level of anxiety before prescribing an anxiolytic. Anxiolytics are useful in medical or dental procedures that are fear-inducing or for life events that pose a brief but significant challenge to the coping skills of the child (a death of a family member) or to disrupt a phobic response (i.e. travel by plane). Anxiolytics are also useful for short-term bridging for rapid symptom relief after starting an SSRI, particularly in situations that can rapidly become a mental health crisis such as phobic school refusal. A traumatic event can overwhelm anyone depending on the power of the experience to overturn a child's world. Anxiolytics should only be used in the immediate aftermath of an event and typically should not be used for durations greater than 2 weeks or dependency (e.g. benzodiazepines [BZDs]) or decreased efficacy (e.g. antihistamines) might become problematic.

Assessment

It is necessary to assess the presenting symptoms (internal experience and behavioral manifestations) and whether they are present now or anticipatory. Determining the trigger as specific or diffuse, expected, or out of proportion, the duration, variability across time/environments, intensity (created scale of 1–10) and baseline temperament is the key to deciding to address this within a primary care setting or to refer for more specialized mental health services. Identifying how long the symptoms have been present, what helps (self-soothing strategies), what does not help, and what the child and/or parent believes the behavior/symptom is about (cultural variables and values) is very useful in gathering enough information to justify the use of an anxiolytic. The risk of what could happen if the anxiety is not addressed (i.e. not obtaining a necessary blood test with a needle phobia) should also be heavily factored into the treatment plan. There are many situations that can be addressed, after a good assessment, by providing information and reassurance about the fear-inducing issue. It should be noted that the most typical presentation of

anxiety in the primary care environment is often a somatic picture and frequently does not include affective symptoms in the first round of assessment. For many cultures, anxiety is only expressed through somatic constellations of symptoms, partly because there is no recognition of the connection between the two domains and partly due to stigmatization. Before considering a medication for the symptoms, assess for substance abuse (for child or parent), pregnancy, and medical problems that may mimic anxiety, especially endocrine, cardiac, or autoimmune disorders. The use of caffeine/energy drinks and supplements also can cause anxiety-like symptoms that resolve almost immediately after stopping the offending item.

Anxiety is known to be comorbid with many serious mental health disorders or part of the prodromal trajectory for others. This is a caution about treating anxiety that appears with any other prominent emotional/behavioral symptoms that are not subsumed under the anxiety itself. This is also important when assessing any untoward effects of using an anxiolytic as it may portend complications of another mental health problem that is present or evolving developmentally.

Pharmacology

There are three commonly used groups of anxiolytics used cautiously for short-term anxiety management with children and adolescents: BZDs, antihistamines, and one azaspirone (buspirone). BZDs have been in widespread use since the 1960s as they were less toxic, better tolerated, and safer medications for use in anxiety than the earlier antianxiety agents. They are a Controlled Substance Schedule IV group, which indicates moderate potential for abuse when used with other CNS depressant agents, or used alone in doses that are higher or taken more frequently than prescribed. Tolerance develops rapidly (sometimes in as little as 1–2 weeks), so short-term use is essential and rapid withdrawal is not recommended. BZDs work at the GABA-A receptor sites in the spinal cord (muscle relaxation), brainstem (anticonvulsant effects), brainstem reticular formation (sedation), cerebellum (ataxia), and cortical and limbic CNS (anxiolytic effect) to enhance CNS inhibitory effects. BZDs bind to the GABA-A receptors, facilitating the opening of chloride channels, which reduce cellular excitability, leading to greater general neuronal inhibition throughout the CNS.

Antihistamines have many uses (as do the BZDs) and were developed to suppress anaphylactic shock, for allergies, pruritis, insomnia, nausea, and vomiting, and for preoperative sedation. They are used primarily in primary care for their medical efficacy in a wide variety of problems. The two mostly commonly used antihistamines

Table 9.8 Anxiolytics

Medication generic name and (trade)	FDA approved age	Form	Dosing (range)	Side effects	Duration of medication	Pros	Precautions
Benzodiazepine							
Diazepam (Valium)	>6 months	By mouth, IV, IM	Start 0.1–0.3 mg/kg Start age 5–12 years = 1 mg, age 12+ = 2 mg, range 1–10 mg	Drowsiness, dizziness, sedation, cognitive blunting, ataxia	Onset 15–30 min Long acting 20–100 h half-life, duration 2–3 h	Safe, effective, works rapidly, produces night terrors, less euphoria, somnambulism	Short-term use if possible, behavior disinhibition, consider potential for developing addiction, discontinuation requires gradual taper to avoid seizures or withdrawal high risk for teens
Clonazepam (Klonopin)	2 years	Tabs, melts, wafers	Start 0.25–0.5 mg, dose 0.2–0.8 mg/kg, twice a day to three times a day, range 0.25–2 mg, by mouth, <10 years 0.01–0.03 mg/kg/day in divided doses, maximum 0.05 mg/kg/day		Long-acting 15–50 h half-life, peak 1–2 h, duration 6–12 h	Safe, effective, works rapidly, better for panic disorder and anticonvulsant	Drug–drug interactions: oral contraceptives, antacids, erythromycin, isoniazid
Lorazepam (Ativan)	12 years	By mouth, IV, IM	Start 0.5–1.0 mg twice a day to four times a day every 4–8h, 0.03–0.08 mg/kg, range 0.5–4 mg		Immediate–30 min onset, peak 60–90 min, duration 12–24 h	Safe, effective, works rapidly	Not recommended during pregnancy or breastfeeding
Alprazolam (Xanax)	18 years	By mouth	Start 0.25–0.5 mg, once only 0.25, 0.07–0.08 mg/kg twice a day to three times a day		Immediate–30 min onset, peak 1–2 h, duration 4–6 h, 12–15 h half-life	Safe, effective, works rapidly	Highest risk for abuse
Antihistamines							
Diphenhydramine (Benadryl)	Avoid <2–6 years	Capsules, elixir, IM, IV	<6 years, 12.5 mg at bedtime; 6–12 years, 5 mg/kg/day >12 years, 25–100 mg twice a day to four times a day (up to 300 mg), range, 5–300 mg by mouth	Common: sedation, dizziness, dry mouth, constipation, blurry vision Uncommon: lower seizure threshold, EPS, tachycardia, hypotension, blood dyscrasias, hypotension	Onset 30 min, peak 1–3 h, duration 4–7 h	Not a controlled substance	Taper to avoid cholinergic rebound, not for neonates, tolerance can develop to sedation; urinary obstruction, careful driving and avoid breastfeeding

	Age	Formulation	Dosing	Side effects	Onset/duration	Comments
Hydroxyzine pamoate (Vistaril)	6 years	Capsules, elixir, IM	Start 10–25 mg <6 years, 50 mg/day divided doses >6, 50–100 mg divided doses	Common: sedation, dizziness, dry mouth, constipation, blurry vision Uncommon: lower seizure threshold, EPS, tachycardia, hypotension, blood dysgrasias, hypotension	Onset 15–60 min, duration 4–6 h	Taper to avoid cholinergic rebound, not for neonates, tolerance can develop to sedation; urinary obstruction, careful driving and avoid breastfeeding
Azaspirone						
Buspirone (Buspar)	18 years		Start 2.5–5 mg twice a day Maximum dose <12 years, 40 mg >12 years, 60 mg 0.2–0.6/mg/kg/day, range: 10–60 mg	Dizziness, fatigue, headache, nausea, vomiting, depression, ataxia, nervousness, activation	Onset 1 h, peak 40–90 min, 2–3 h half-life	*Avoid grapefruit juice,* not effective for panic, takes 1–2 weeks for clinical effect, avoid during pregnancy and breastfeeding May help with generalized anxiety disorder, separation anxiety, social phobia, not sedating, not a controlled substance, no muscle relaxation

EPS, extrapyramidal symptoms; IM, intramuscular; IV, intravenous.
Source: Developed by B. Muller and A. Riley, from Connor and Meltzer (2006); Emslie et al. (2016).

for anxiety in children are diphenhydramine (Benadryl) and hydroxyzine hydrochloride or hydroxyzine pamoate (Atarax or Vistaril). The antihistamines act as competitive inhibitors of histamine at H1 receptors both within the CNS and outside the CNS. The anxiolytic effects stem from the effects within the CNS. Side effects are experienced (though generally mild) from within the CNS and peripherally. They are not a controlled substance so the use is much easier as there is no concern about dependency. Tolerability does happen after approximately 2 weeks of consistent use (Scahill et al. 2010).

Azaspirones (Buspirone [Buspar] is the only drug available in the United States) are a more recently derived group of medications developed for mental health conditions. Unlike the previous two groups, the response to buspirone takes 1–4 weeks, so it is not a good choice for immediate problems with anxiety. Buspirone has action as an agonist at presynaptic 5-HT1A autoreceptors, some antagonistic effects on postsynaptic 5-HT1A receptors, and downregulation of 5-HT2 receptors. This is similar to SSRIs approved for anxiety and depression in children. It also has dopaminergic effects at the D2 receptors (although it has not been effective as an antipsychotic agent) and enhances noradrenergic release in the locus coeruleus (it may be helpful for ADHD). It does not have any site of action in the GABA system (though it may have some minor antagonistic effect, leading to possibility of activation).

Indications for Use

BZDs are indicated for short-term use for anxiety in children. Due to the risk for dependency, little research has been done on the use of BZDs for children so few are used. Uses of various agents depend on purpose intended, whether a shorter-acting agent for insomnia or longer-acting agent for temporary anxiety relief is selected. Uses for mental health other than for brief anxiety relief include augmentation for mania and schizophrenia, acute agitation or aggression, somnambulism, sleep terrors (pavor nocturnus), tic disorders, brief sleep induction (less than 2 weeks), or preoperatively for medical or dental procedures. BZDs are approved for seizure disorders and as muscle relaxants as well, which may play a role in some mental health treatment. Significant caution should be used for BZDs in adolescence due to abuse potential, including use with other CNS depressants, which increases risks of overdose and risk of unplanned pregnancy (Connor and Meltzer 2006).

Antihistamines can be used as sedatives, anxiolytics, and to manage extrapyramidal symptoms (EPS). They are not effective in treating chronic anxiety, and toler-

ance builds quickly to sedative effects so daily use is not helpful. They can also be used for angry/aggressive outbursts in an acute situation. Their unpleasant side effects at higher doses make them unlikely agents for abuse. Azaspirones (buspirone/Buspar) currently has no indication for children younger than 18 years. Other agents that have been developed with good efficacy in adults have failed to provide clear evidence of significant effects on anxiety or depression in children and even adolescents. Few studies have been completed at this time as other agents with stronger profiles of efficacy are still in the early stages of being analyzed. Buspirone may be a good candidate for the future, due to its high-safety/low-risk profile, for the treatment of longer-term anxiety. Its timeline of action, however, makes it of minimal use for immediate or acute episodes of anxiety and in general its effectiveness in reducing symptoms of anxiety in children is questionable (Connolly et al. 2016).

Contraindications

BZDs are contraindicated for any child or family with a history of substance abuse. While the use of BZDs alone is relatively safe, many overdose situations involve the combination of BZDs with other CNS depressants. Children who have a history of suicidal ideation, worsening depression, or significant signs of other major mental health disorders should not be treated with BZDs in a primary practice due to risk of worsening of mood and behavioral disinhibition leading to dangerous behavior. Teratogenic effects during pregnancy are known, also infants exposed to BZDs in utero, especially in the third trimester, may experience withdrawal. Birth control must be assessed and a serum pregnancy test (human chorionic gonodatropin [hCG]) should be obtained for females of child-bearing age. Sedative properties can affect driving ability, so special caution is needed with adolescent drivers or with adolescents involved in activities that require high levels of attention. Be aware of the need to taper gradually to avert withdrawal syndrome for use of more than 1–2 weeks.

Antihistamines are relatively safe, but any hypersensitivity to the class of drugs, especially akathesia or history of a paradoxical reaction, should be noted and an agent from a different class of medications would be indicated. Antihistamines are contraindicated for several medical conditions less likely to affect youth but are still unsafe and include narrow-angle glaucoma, urinary outlet obstruction, GI obstruction, acute asthma, and use of other CNS depressants. Use during pregnancy and breastfeeding is not recommended. Contraindications for azaspirones are primarily those associated with other serotonergic agents and include concurrent or recent use of MAOIs, known hypersensitivity to the drug, history of behavioral activation on other serotonergic agents, elevated prolactin levels, and hepatic or renal disease.

Side Effects

Benzodiazepines

Common side effects include sedation, dizziness, ataxia, blurry vision, cognitive dulling, decreased rapid eye movement (REM) sleep, suppression of sleep stage 4, and lack of coordination. Uncommon side effects include paradoxical disinhibition with agitation, activation, insomnia, anxiety, and increased risk behaviors. *Caution:* In combination with other CNS depressants, BZDs can cause fatal respiratory depression.

Antihistamines

Common side effects include sedation, "hangover," dizziness, hypotension, diarrhea, constipation, dry mouth, blurred vision, and urinary retention. Uncommon side effects may include lowered seizure threshold, blood dyscrasias, tachycardia, involuntary movement disorders, and cholinergic rebound/withdrawal symptoms (high doses of antihistamine). The same risk of akathesia and paradoxical response exists with this medication group.

Azaspirones

Common side effects include dizziness, headache, and fatigue/sedation (less than the others). Uncommon side effects include nervousness and increased activation (increased irritability, restlessness, insomnia).

Drug–Drug Interactions

Benzodiazepines

All BZDs are metabolized in the liver by the CYP450 cytochrome enzymatic pathway. They are also highly lipid soluble, quickly cross the blood–brain barrier, and collect readily in lipid tissue. They interact with a variety of agents, especially increased CNS depression in combination with any other CNS depressing agent, leading to increased sedation, decreased cognitive functioning, lack of coordination, and risk of overdose. Commonly prescribed medications that can have drug–drug interactions that decrease metabolism of BZDs are isoniazid (diazepam), erythromycin (diazepam), and oral contraceptives (diazepam). Antacids reduce/delay absorption of BZDs from the GI tract. Bronchodilators can antagonize the effects of diazepam and lorazepam.

Antihistamines

All antihistamines interact with other CNS depressants to increase the symptoms of CNS depression: sedation, lack of coordination, and decreased psychomotor speed. Combined with any other anticholinergic, these agents are also additive in exacerbating anticholinergic side effects.

Azaspirones

Buspirone (Buspar) has a few significant drug–drug interactions. Cimetidine may increase buspirone plasma levels. Buspirone may increase levels of plasma haloperidol when taken together. Caution is advised when using it with trazodone as this may lead to an increase in risk for hepatic toxicity.

Monitoring

Benzodiazepines

For brief treatment (less than 2 weeks) with BZDs, screen for substance use for the child and family, sexual activity, and pregnancy. Otherwise serum or urine hCG, blood pressure, pulse, LFTs, and CBC are standard before beginning a longer-term treatment with BZDs.

Dosing

Dosing should start low and titration should progress very slowly and with clear outcome measures for the anxiety to prevent overshooting the necessary dose for the achievement of the treatment goal. Physiological dependence can occur quite quickly (within 1–2 weeks of steady use). Any requests for additional doses prior to the next anticipated prescription, lost prescriptions, and requests for increased dose without validated need could be an indication that the medication may be misused or that dependency is occurring. Withdrawal should be carefully controlled. If used for any length of time, taper dose at approximately 25% every 5–7 days.

Withdrawal symptoms include dysphoria, anxiety, insomnia, tremor, pain, restlessness, diaphoresis, and hallucinations and disturbances of perception. Signs of overdose (usually in conjunction with other CNS depressants) are drowsiness, ataxia, confusion, slurred speech, tremor, depressed reflexes, diploplia, and, finally, respiratory depression/death. Typically, the protocol involves careful planning to provide a prescription for coverage of a specific number of days with a specific purpose. At the end of the time expected to elicit a particular outcome, the child should be seen again before renewing a prescription for a BZD.

Antihistamines

Initial assessment for any extended use should include blood pressure, pulse, and any history of untoward reactions. If the child has never used an antihistamine and it is being prescribed to manage pre-procedure anxiety, a parent can give a "test" dose prior to the procedure to ensure that the child does not have a paradoxical reaction or akathisia. Caution adolescents using these agents while driving or during the school day when sedative effects can impair cognitive functioning and attention. For longer-standing use (not recommended), a gradual taper is helpful to avoid cholinergic rebound.

Dosing. For children, diphenhydramine (Benadryl) can be given at a dose of 5 mg/kg/day divided into four individual doses every 6 hours.

Azaspirones

There are no indications for short-term use in children (or adults). Obtain a baseline for anxiety before considering a trial of buspirone (Buspar). Typically, other medications that have indications for use in children should be trialed before considering buspirone. The benefit of not being a sedating, addicting, or controlled substance make it appealing, but the lack of firm evidence puts this medication further down the algorithm in treating more global types of anxiety disorders such as separation anxiety, generalized anxiety disorder, or social phobia.

Monitoring

Before initiating this medication, useful laboratory tests would include liver enzymes (serum glutamic-oxaloacetic transaminase and serum glutamic pyruvic transaminase) and a CBC to monitor for a decrease in platelet count or white blood cell count. Like all psychiatric medications, utilizing the start low, go slow strategy is always best. Table 9.8 lists all anxiolytics, dosing, and side effects.

Antipsychotics
Pharmacology

Antipsychotic medication was first introduced to adult populations in the 1950s and since then has evolved for use with pediatric populations (see Tables 9.9 and 9.10). Antipsychotics are classified as typical (first generation) or atypical (second generation) and also according to their potency of dopamine blockade and management of symptoms (Correll 2016). Typical antipsychotics used with pediatric populations are chlorpromazine and haloperidol. Atypical antipsychotics used with children and adolescents are clozapine, olanzapine, risperidone, ziprasidone, quetiapine, asenapine, iloperidone, lurasidone, paliperidone, and aripiprazole (Correll 2016). Typical antipsychotics, while as effective in symptom management as atypical,

have a higher side effect profile, resulting in more movement disorders and tardive dyskinesia.

Atypical antipsychotics are used most often with pediatric populations. They act on the dopamine and serotonin systems. Antipsychotics have an ability to block the dopamine D2 receptor site. This is associated with antimanic, antipsychotic, and antiaggressive effects of this medication (Correll et al. 2010).

Indications for Use

Atypical antipsychotic medication is typically used in children and adolescents to treat psychosis, severe behavioral issues associated with autism and other developmental disorders, along with aggression, bipolar disorder, and tics. They can be used as monotherapy or in conjunction with mood stabilizers. Antipsychotic medication is used in early onset schizophrenia, bipolar disorders, aggressive behaviors, and Tourette syndrome.

Contraindications

Antipsychotics can affect the QTc prolongation of the heart. In patients with a family history of early sudden death, irregular heartbeat, shortness of breath, or dizziness, a cardiac screen is warranted (Correll et al. 2010). Antipsychotics should be used carefully in patients at risk for metabolic syndrome because of either family history or current obesity. These medications can precipitate metabolic syndrome in pediatric patients.

Monitoring

Prior to initiating any antipsychotic medication, the prescriber must obtain baseline physical examination information and do a careful history of metabolic disorders and/or diabetes in the family. Fasting blood glucose, cholesterol, and lipid panel are required prior to initiating therapy. A baseline weight, BMI, and Abnormal Involuntary Movement Disorder (AIMS) scale score should be obtained. Weight must be followed monthly with a follow-up AIMS conducted every 6 months. Psychoeducation regarding weight management and exercise must be part of the treatment process. Other risks involve hyperprolactinemia and neutropenia. Weight and metabolic difficulties can be the outcome of long-term use of psychotropic medication. All should be encouraged to manage weight with diet, exercise, and frequent monitoring. Vital signs, height, weight, and BMI should be measured every 3 months. Fasting metabolic profiles and LFTs should be done every 6 months after obtaining the baseline.

Side Effects

Children and adolescents can be more sensitive to the side effects of antipsychotic medication. These side effects can include sedation, extra pyramidal symptoms,

Table 9.9 FDA-approved indications for use of antipsychotic medications

	Age (y)								
	<1	1–2	3–4	5	6–9	10–11	12	13–17	Adult
Second-generation (atypical) antipsychotics									
Risperidone		None			I	I, M		I, M, S	M, S
Aripiprazole			None		I	I, M		I, M, S	M, S
Quetiapine				None		M		M, S	M, S
Olanzapine			None			D, M		D, M, S	D, M, S
Ziprasidone					None				M, S
Clozapine					None				S
Paliperidone			None				S		S
Lurasidone					None				S
Asenapine			None					M	M, S
Iloperidone					None				S
First-generation (typical) antipsychotics									
Haloperidol		None				H, P, S, T			S, T
Molindone				None			S		S
Pimozide				None			T		T
Chlorpromazine	None				B			None	M, S
Perphenazine				None				S	S
Fluphenazine					None				S
Thioridazine			None				S		S

B, severe behavioral problems marked by combativeness and/or explosive behavior and short-term treatment of hyperactive children who show excessive motor activity with accompanying conduct disorders; D, acute depressive episodes associated with bipolar I disorder (along with fluoxetine); H, hyperactivity; I, irritability associated with autism disorder; M, manic, or mixed episodes associated with bipolar I disorder; P, psychosis; S, schizophrenia; T, Tourette syndrome.
Source: Bloch et al. (2018), p. 733. Adapted with permission from Wolters Kluwer Health, Inc.

dyskenesias (especially at withdrawal), and metabolic effects such as weight gain and prolactin abnormalities (Correll 2016). Prescribers need to review the antipsychotic medication considered for use and identify pertinent side effects and risks.

One of the risks of antipsychotic medication is a rare but serious disorder, neuroleptic malignant syndrome (NMS). It can occur after a single dose of medication but most often occurs within 2 weeks of initiation of antipsychotic medication or a dose increase. This is to be considered a medical emergency with symptoms of severe muscular rigidity, altered mental status, consciousness, stupor, labile pulse and blood pressure, and fever. All antipsychotic medication must be discontinued immediately, and the individual might require hospitalization for supportive measures. Males and young children are considered most at risk (Correll 2016; Connor and Meltzer 2006).

Dosing

The goal is symptom management on the lowest possible dose of antipsychotic medication. It is essential that monitoring of laboratory tests, regular vital signs, height, and weight occur in a documented, systematic manner. Parents and guardians should understand the treatment plan for dosing, the targeted symptoms, and adverse signs and symptoms. Most importantly, the child or adolescent needs to be included in the discussion of medication management and why an antipsychotic medication might be used as treatment.

Summary

This chapter has given an overview of issues of evaluating and treating children and adolescents for psychiatric conditions who present for treatment in primary care and psychiatric settings. Psychiatric medication use with children

Table 9.10 Clinical guidance for antipsychotic medications utilized in pediatric practice

	Pediatric			Adult		
	starting dose (mg/day)	Typical dose range (mg/day)	Number of daily doses	Starting dose (mg/day)	Typical dose range (mg/day)	Number of daily doses
Second-generation (atypical) antipsychotics						
Risperidone	0.5–2	1–6	1–2	2	2–6	1–2
Aripiprazole	2–5	5–30	1	5–15	10–30	1
Quetiapine	25–50	100–800	2–3	50–100	150–800	2–3
Olanzapine	2.5–5	5–20	1	5–10	5–20	1
Ziprasidone	5–20	40–160	2	40–80	80–160	2
Clozapine	12.5–50	300–900	2	25–50	300–900	1–2
Paliperidone	3	3–12	1	3–6	3–12	1
Lurasidone	20	20–160	1	20–40	20–160	1
Asenapine	5	5–20	2	10–20	10–20	2
First-generation (typical) antipsychotics						
Haloperidol	1–10	2–30	2–3	2–15	2–50	2–3
Molindone	25–75	50–225	3–4	50–75	50–225	3–4
Pimozide	0.5–2	1–6	1–2	1–2	2–10	1–2

Source: Bloch et al. (2018), p. 734. Adapted with permission from Wolters Kluwer Health, Inc.

and adolescents has been reviewed. The chapter delineates the different prescribing roles between APRNs in primary care and APRNs in psychiatric practice. The chapter emphasizes the need for collaboration between healthcare providers when psychiatric medication is being considered to treat a psychiatric disorder in a child or adolescent. Involvement of the parent and guardian is essential to the process. Major classes of medication are summarized, and prescribing considerations, side effects, drug interactions, and monitoring are discussed. APRNs in both primary care and psychiatric settings are taking an increasingly important role in prescribing psychiatric medications to children and adolescents. The goal is always evidence-based practice considering the safety and welfare of the pediatric patient based within a professional nursing practice model that provides high-quality care.

Thought Questions

1. What is the prescriptive role in a psychiatric APRN practice and how do nurses ascertain the balance between prescribing and psychotherapy?
2. At what point does the primary care APRN choose to refer children and adolescents to a psychiatric practice for further care?
3. What ideally characterizes the collaborative role psychiatric APRNs take with their psychiatrist colleagues? How does this appear and what influences it?

References

APA (2013). *Diagnostic and Statistical Annual of Mental Disorders*, 5the. Washington, DC: American Psychiatric Association.

Bloch, M.H., Beyer, C., Martin, A., and Scahill, L. (2018). ADHD: stimulant and nonstimulant agents. In: *Pediatric Psychopharmacology*, 2nde (eds. A. Martin, L. Scahill and C. Kratochivil), 718–724. New York, NY: Oxford University Press.

Bridge, J.A., Iyengar, S., Salary, C.B. et al. (2007). Clinical response and risk for reported suicidal ideation and suicide attempts in pediatric antidepressant treatment: a meta-analysis of randomized controlled trials. *Journal of the American Medical Association* 297: 1683–1696.

CDC. (2019). *Key Findings: Children's Mental Health Report*. Available at https://www.cdc.gov/childrensmentalhealth/features/kf-childrens-mental-health-report.html (accessed 27 September 2018).

CDC. (2020). *Improving access to children's mental health care*. Available at https://www.cdc.gov/childrensmentalhealth/access.html.

Cohen, L.S., Friedman, J.M., Jefferson, J.W. et al. (1994). A reevaluation of risk of in utero exposure to lithium. *Journal of the American Medical Association* 271: 146–150.

Connolly, S.D., Suarez, L.M., Victor, A.M. et al. (2016). Anxiety Disorders. In: *Dulcan's Textbook of Child and Adolescent Psychiatry*, 2nde (ed. M.K. Dulcan), 305–343. Washington, DC: American Psychiatric Association Publishing.

Connor, D.F. and Meltzer, B.M. (2006). *Pediatric Psychopharmacology Fast Facts*. New York, NY: W.W. Norton.

Correll, C.U. (2016). Antipsychotic medications. In: *Dulcan's Textbook of Child and Adolescent Psychiatry*, 2nde (ed. M.K. Dulcan), 795–848. Washington, DC: American Psychiatric Association Publishing.

Correll, C.U., Sheridan, E.M., and DelBello, M.P. (2010). Antipsychotic and mood stabilizer efficacy and tolerability in pediatric and adult patients with bipolar I mania: a comparative analysis of acute, randomized, placebo-controlled trials. *Bipolar Disorders* 12: 116–141.

Danielyan, A. and Kowatch, R.A. (2005). Management options for bipolar disorder in children and adolescents. *Paediatric Drugs* 7: 277–294.

Delaney, K.R. (2017). Psychiatric mental health nursing advanced practice workforce: capacity to address shortages of mental health professionals. *Psychiatric Services* 68: 952–954. https://doi.org/10.1176/appi.ps.201600405.

Dell, M.L. (2010). Ethnic, cultural, and religious issues. In: *Dulcan's Textbook of Child and Adolescent Psychiatry* (ed. M.K. Dulcan), 517–529. Washington, DC: American Psychiatric Association Publishing.

DiMarco, M.A. and Melnyk, B. (2009). The mental health needs of children and adolescents. *Archives of Psychiatric Nursing* 23: 334–336.

Domino, M.E., Burns, B.J., Silva, S.G. et al. (2008). Cost-effectiveness of treatments for adolescent depression: results from TADS. *American Journal of Psychiatry* 165: 588–596. https://doi.org/10.1176/appi.ajp.2008.07101610.

Emslie, G.J., Croarkin, P., and Mayes, T.L. (2016). Antidepressants. In: *Dulcan's Textbook of Child and Adolescent Psychiatry*, 2nde (ed. M.K. Dulcan), 737–768. Washington, DC: American Psychiatric Association Publishing.

FDA. (2011). *Drug safety labeling changes*. Available at http://www.fda.gov/Safety/MedWatch/SafetyInformation/Safety-RelatedDrugLabelingChanges/default.htm.

Gracious, B.L., Danielyan, A., and Kowatch, R.A. (2016). Mood stabilizers. In: *Dulcan's Textbook of Child and Adolescent Psychiatry*, 2nde (ed. M.K. Dulcan), 769–794. Washington, DC: American Psychiatric Association Publishing.

Isojarvi, J.I. and Tapanainen, J.S. (2000). Valproate, hyperandrogenism, and polycystic ovaries: a report of 3 cases. *Archives of Neurology* 57: 1064–1068.

Jones, K.L., Lacro, R.V., Johnson, K.A., and Adams, J. (1989). Pattern of malformations in the children of women treated with carbamazepine during pregnancy. *New England Journal of Medicine* 320: 1661–1666.

Kowatch, R.A., Suppes, T., Carmody, T.J. et al. (2000). Effect size of lithium, divalproex sodium, and carbamazepine in children and adolescents with bipolar disorder. *Journal of the American Academy of Child & Adolescent Psychiatry* 39: 713–720.

Kowatch, R.A., Strawn, J.R., and Danielyan, A. (2010). Mood stabilizers: lithium, anticonvulsants, and others. In: *Pediatric Psychopharmacology* (eds. A. Martin, L. Scahill and C. Kratochivil), 297–311. New York, NY: Oxford University Press.

Lauerer, J.A., Marenakos, K.G., Gaffney, K. et al. (2018). Integrating behavioral health in the pediatric medical home. *Journal of Child and Adolescent Psychiatry Nursing* 31: 39–42.

Leahy, L.G. (2018). Diagnosis and treatment of ADHD in children vs adults: what nurses should know. *Archives of Psychiatric Nursing* 32: 890–895. https://doi.org/10.1016/j.apnu.2018.06.013.

Manji, H.K. and Chen, G. (2000). Post-receptor signaling pathways in the pathophysiology and treatment of mood disorders. *Current Psychiatry Reports* 2: 479–489.

Martini, R., Hilt, R., Marx, L., Chenven, M., Nylor, M., Sarvet, B., & Ptakowski, K.K., American Academy of Child and Adolescent Psychiatry (2012). *Best Principles for Integration of Child Psychiatry into the Pediatric Health Home*. Available at www.aacap.org (accessed 1 October 2018).

Melnyk, B.M., Brown, H.E., Jones, D.C. et al. (2003). Improving the mental/psychosocial health of U.S. children and adolescents: outcomes and implementation strategies from the national KySS summit. *Journal of Pediatric Health Care* 17: S1–S24.

Merkel, R.L. (2010). Safety of stimulant treatment in attention deficit hyperactivity disorder: part II. *Expert Opinion on Drug Safety* 9: 917–935.

Munoz, R., Primm, A., and Ananth, J. (2007). *Life in Color: Culture in American Psychiatry*. Chicago, IL: Hilton.

Nandagopal, J.J., DelBello, M.P., and Kowatch, R. (2009). Pharmacologic treatment of pediatric bipolar disorder. *Child and Adolescent Psychiatric Clinics of North America* 18: 455–469.

Okusa, M.D. and Crystal, L.J. (1994). Clinical manifestations and management of acute lithium intoxication. *American Journal of Medicine* 97: 383–389.

Perrin, J.M., Friedman, R.A., and Knilans, T.K. (2008). Cardiovascular monitoring and stimulant drugs for attention-deficit/hyperactivity disorder. *Pediatrics* 122: 451–453.

Pliszka, S.R. (2010). Attention-deficit/hyperactivity disorder. In: *Dulcan's Textbook of Child and Adolescent Psychiatry* (ed. M.K. Dulcan), 205–221. Washington, DC: American Psychiatric Association Publishing.

Pliszka, S.R. (2016). Attention-deficit/hyperactivity disorder. In: *Dulcan's Textbook of Child and Adolescent Psychiatry*, 2nde (ed. M.K. Dulcan), 173–194. Washington, DC: American Psychiatric Association Publishing.

PNCB (2019). *Pediatric Primary Care Mental Health Specialist (PMHS)*. Available at http://pncb.org (accessed 3 February 2019).

Rapaport, J.L. (2013). Pediatric psychopharmacology: too much or too little? *World Psychiatry* 12: 118–123. https://doi.org/10.1002/wps.20028.

Scahill, L., Poncin, Y., and Westphal, A. (2010). Alpha-adrenergics, beta-blockers, benzodiazepines, buspirone, and desmopressin. In: *Dulcan's Textbook of Child and Adolescent Psychiatry* (ed. M.K. Dulcan), 775–785. Washington, DC: American Psychiatric Association Publishing.

Spencer, T.J., Biederman, J., and Wilens, T.E. (2016). Medications used for attention-deficit/hyperactivity disorder. In: *Dulcan's Textbook of Child and Adolescent Psychiatry*, 2e (ed. M.K. Dulcan), 681–700. Washington, DC: American Psychiatric Association Publishing.

Stahl, S.M. (2018). *Stahl's Essential Psychopharmacology Prescriber's Guide: Children and Adolescents*. Cambridge: Cambridge University Press.

Steinhausen, H.-C. (2015). Recent international trends in psychotropic medication prescriptions for children and adolescents. *European Child and Adolescent Psychiatry* 24: 635–640. https://doi.org/10.1007/s00787-014-0631-y.

Sulik, L.R. and Sarvet, B. (2016). Collaborating with primary care. In: *Dulcan's Textbook of Child and Adolescent Psychiatry*, 2e (ed. M.K. Dulcan), 1075–1087. Arlington, VA: American Psychiatric Association.

Tennis, P., Eldridge, R.R., and International Lamotrigine Pregnancy Registry Scientific Advisory Committee (2002). Preliminary results on pregnancy outcomes in women using lamotrigine. *Epilepsia* 43: 1161–1167.

Troksa, K., Kovacich, N., Noro, M., and Chavez, B. (2019). Impact of central nervous system stimulant medication use on growth in pediatric populations with attention-deficit/hyperactivity disorder: A review. *Pharmacotherapy* 39 (6): 665–676. https://doi.org/10.1002/phar.2192.

Williams, J., Klinepeter, K., Pamles, G. et al. (2004). Diagnosis and treatment of behavioral health disorders in pediatric practice. *Pediatrics* 114: 601–606.

Wolraich, M.L. and Doffing, M.A. (2004). Pharmokinetic considerations in the treatment of attention-deficit hyperactivity disorder with methylphenidate. *CNS Drugs* 18: 243–250.

WHO (2005). *Atlas on Child and Adolescent Mental Health Resources—Global Concerns: Implications for the Future*. Geneva, Switzerland: World Health Organization.

10

Attention Deficit Hyperactivity Disorder

Geraldine S. Pearson[1] and Cherry Leung[2]

[1]University of Connecticut School of Medicine-retired, Farmington, CT, USA
[2]Department of Community Health Systems, University of California, San Francisco School of Nursing, San Francisco, CA, USA

Objectives

After reading this chapter, advanced practice registered nurses will be able to:

1. Define the epidemiology and prevalence statistics of attention deficit hyperactivity disorder (ADHD).
2. Discuss theories of etiology associated with ADHD, including family dynamics and neurobiological, genetic, and psychosocial factors.
3. Define and describe the presenting signs and symptoms of ADHD and common comorbid disorders in children and adolescents.
4. Describe evidence-based interventions for children and adolescents diagnosed with ADHD.
5. Describe care management of ADHD and differentiate roles of primary care practitioners and advanced practice psychiatric nurses in the diagnosis and treatment of children and adolescents with ADHD.
6. Discuss implications for nursing practice, research, and education.

Introduction

Attention deficit hyperactivity disorder (ADHD) is a commonly occurring disorder that is observed and treated equally by child psychiatric advanced practice nurses, pediatric nurse practitioners, and all advanced practice registered nurses (APRNs). ADHD is a neurodevelopmental disorder that progresses and changes at different life stages. Treatment options can be dependent on the age of the child and severity of symptoms as well as many other factors, including family stability, support of treatment, and adherence to the treatment (Nagae et al. 2015). APRNs see children and adolescents at all stages of development in a variety of treatment settings and are uniquely positioned to plan care based on developmental needs and symptom presentation.

The diagnosis of ADHD is made after obtaining history and behavior rating scales, carefully listening to caregivers' descriptions of behaviors, and directly observing the child. After careful assessment, the first line of treatment should be psychosocial interventions aimed at promoting parent management of behavior. Medication treatment, the best-studied intervention in child and adolescent psychiatry, should be combined with educational and behavioral interventions depending on the severity and manifestation of the disorder. Some research suggests that stimulant treatment is superior over nondrug interventions

Child and Adolescent Behavioral Health: A Resource for Advanced Practice Psychiatric and Primary Care Practitioners in Nursing, Second Edition. Edited by Edilma L. Yearwood, Geraldine S. Pearson, and Jamesetta A. Newland.
© 2021 John Wiley & Sons, Inc. Published 2021 by John Wiley & Sons, Inc.
Companion website: www.wiley.com/go/Yearwood

and can make a significant difference in symptom presentation (Pliszka 2016). Regardless of this the child and family should be assessed with regards to nonmedication treatment needs and comorbid disorders. Treatment and diagnostic complexity emerges when other disorders are comorbid with ADHD and when behavioral issues presented by the child or adolescent become too psychiatrically based or acute for primary care management.

This chapter discusses historical perspectives of ADHD and reviews presenting signs and symptoms, common comorbid conditions, and evidence-based interventions. The chapter differentiates the roles of primary care pediatric and family nurse practitioners and advanced practice psychiatric nurses, and present indications for referral to a psychiatric provider. The chapter concludes with a case study describing management issues, with implications for nursing practice, research, and education.

Historical Perspective

As noted by Pliszka (2016), the first clinical description of ADHD occurred in 1902 by George Still in which he related problematic behavior to a lack of moral control in children. Early observers of the disorder suggested that behavior disorders, such as hyperkinesis, explosive behavior, fatigability, and attention deficit behaviors,

were related to some biologic etiology such as encephalitis and cerebral trauma in children (Ebaugh and Franklin 1923).

In the 1930s, the term "minimal brain dysfunction" was coined to describe hyperkinesis, impulsivity, learning disability, and short attention span (Spencer et al. 2007). By the 1950s, the terms "hyperactive child syndrome" and "hyperkinetic reaction of childhood" were present in the *Diagnostic Statistical Manual of Mental Disorders 2* (DSM-II) that was published in 1968 (American Psychiatric Association [APA] 1968).

The focus shifted in DSM-III to inattention as a major component of the disorder (Spencer et al. 2007). There was recognition that the disorder could look different at various developmental stages. DSM-III also identified a residual form of ADHD that could continue to cause impairment into adulthood. DSM-IV defined three subtypes of ADHD: predominantly inattentive, predominantly hyperactive–impulsive, and combined. DSM-5 currently has one diagnostic criteria for ADHD with qualifiers for both attention and hyperactivity–impulsivity, predominantly inattentive presentation, and predominantly hyperactive–impulsive presentation. Some symptoms are required to be present before age 12 (previously age 7). The behavior descriptors include behavior of adolescents and adults (Pliszka 2016). Table 10.1 outlines the predominant DSM-5 criteria for ADHD.

Table 10.1 DSM-5 criteria for ADHD

Diagnostic Criteria

A. A persistent pattern of inattention and/or hyperactivity-impulsivity that interferes with functioning or development, as characterized by (1) and/or (2):

1. **Inattention:** Six (or more) of the following symptoms have persisted for at least 6 months to a degree that is inconsistent with developmental level and that negatively impacts directly on social and academic/occupational activities:

- *Note:* The symptoms are not solely a manifestation of oppositional behavior, defiance, hostility, or failure to understand tasks or instructions. For older adolescents and adults (age 17 and older), at least five symptoms are required.

    a. Often fails to give close attention to details or makes careless mistakes in schoolwork, at work, or during other activities (e.g., overlooks or misses details, work is inaccurate).

    b. Often has difficulty sustaining attention in tasks or play activities (e.g., has difficulty remaining focused during lectures, conversations, or lengthy reading).

    c. Often does not seem to listen when spoken to directly (e.g., mind seems elsewhere, even in the absence of any obvious distraction).

    d. Often does not follow through on instructions and fails to finish schoolwork, chores, or duties in the workplace (e.g., starts tasks but quickly loses focus and is easily sidetracked).

    e. Often has difficulty organizing tasks and activities (e.g., difficulty managing sequential tasks; difficulty keeping materials and belongings in order; messy, disorganized work; has poor time management; fails to meet deadlines).

    f. Often avoids, dislikes, or is reluctant to engage in tasks that require sustained mental effort (e.g., schoolwork or homework; for older adolescents and adults, preparing reports, completing forms, reviewing lengthy papers).

    g. Often loses things necessary for tasks or activities (e.g., school materials, pencils, books, tools, wallets, keys, paperwork, eyeglasses, mobile telephones).

    h. Is often easily distracted by extraneous stimuli (for older adolescents and adults, may include unrelated thoughts).

    i. Is often forgetful in daily activities (e.g., doing chores, running errands; for older adolescents and adults, returning calls, paying bills, keeping appointments).

(continued)

Table 10.1 *(cont'd)*

2. **Hyperactivity and impulsivity:** Six (or more) of the following symptoms have persisted for at least 6 months to a degree that is inconsistent with developmental level and that negatively impacts directly on social and academic/occupational activities:

- *Note:* The symptoms are not solely a manifestation of oppositional behavior, defiance, hostility, or a failure to understand tasks or instructions. For older adolescents and adults (age 17 and older), at least five symptoms are required.

   a. Often fidgets with or taps hands or feet or squirms in seat.
   b. Often leaves seat in situations when remaining seated is expected (e.g., leaves his or her place in the classroom, in the office or other workplace, or in other situations that require remaining in place).
   c. Often runs about or climbs in situations where it is inappropriate. (Note: In adolescents or adults, may be limited to feeling restless.)
   d. Often unable to play or engage in leisure activities quietly.
   e. Is often "on the go," acting as if "driven by a motor" (e.g., is unable to be or uncomfortable being still for extended time, as in restaurants, meetings; may be experienced by others as being restless or difficult to keep up with).
   f. Often talks excessively.
   g. Often blurts out an answer before a question has been completed (e.g., completes people's sentences; cannot wait for turn in conversation).
   h. Often has difficulty waiting his or her turn (e.g., while waiting in line).
   i. Often interrupts or intrudes on others (e.g., butts into conversations, games, or activities; may start using other people's things without asking or receiving permission; for adolescents and adults, may intrude into or take over what others are doing).

B. Several inattentive or hyperactive-impulsive symptoms were present prior to age 12 years.

C. Several inattentive or hyperactive-impulsive symptoms are present in two or more settings (e.g., at home, school, or work; with friends or relatives; in other activities).

D. There is clear evidence that the symptoms interfere with, or reduce the quality of, social, academic, or occupational functioning.

E. The symptoms do not occur exclusively during the course of schizophrenia or another psychotic disorder and are not better explained by another mental disorder (e.g., mood disorder, anxiety disorder, dissociative disorder, personality disorder, substance intoxication or withdrawal).

Specify whether:
- **314.01 (F90.2) Combined presentation:** If both Criterion A1 (inattention) and Criterion A2 (hyperactivity-impulsivity) are met for the past 6 months.
- **314.00 (F90.0) Predominantly inattentive presentation:** If Criterion A1 (inattention) is met but Criterion A2 (hyperactivity-impulsivity) is not met for the past 6 months.
- **314.01 (F90.1) Predominantly hyperactive/impulsive presentation:** If Criterion A2 (hyperactivity-impulsivity) is met and Criterion A1 (inattention) is not met for the past 6 months.

Specify if:
- **In partial remission:** When full criteria were previously met, fewer than the full criteria have been met for the past 6 months, and the symptoms still result in impairment in social, academic, or occupational functioning.

Specify current severity:
- **Mild:** Few, if any, symptoms in excess of those required to make the diagnosis are present, and symptoms result in no more than minor impairments in social or occupational functioning.
- **Moderate:** Symptoms or functional impairment between "mild" and "severe" are present.
- **Severe:** Many symptoms in excess of those required to make the diagnosis, or several symptoms that are particularly severe, are present, or the symptoms result in marked impairment in social or occupational functioning.

Source: American Psychiatric Association. Diagnostic and statistical manual of mental disorder, 5th edition. © 2013, American Psychiatric Association. Reprinted with permission from the American Psychiatric Association.

Epidemiology and Prevalence of ADHD

ADHD has a prevalence estimated at 11% of receiving the diagnosis sometime in life up to age 17 with an increase in parent reporting of current history (8.8%) and increased parent reporting of medication management (Visser et al. 2013). In the National Comorbidity Survey, the adult prevalence of ADHD was 4.4% (Kessler et al. 2006). The lifetime prevalence of ADHD implies influence of ADHD at all stages of the life cycle and includes family functioning, academic and occupational success, and the heritable aspects of the disorder.

International prevalence rates of ADHD are estimated at 5.3%, with the highest rates in Africa (8.5%) and South America (11.8%); Asia, Europe, and North America have lower rates. Study method variability and diagnostic accuracy may account for the differences (Polanczyk et al. 2007). Regardless, rates of stimulant prescriptions globally suggest that ADHD is an international problem (Steinhausen 2015).

Males with significant hyperactivity, impulsivity, and disruptiveness as children are more likely to develop substance use and/or adult antisocial behaviors. Adults with ADHD may struggle with finishing high school, be at risk for more automobile accidents, and deal with more unemployment (Spetie and Arnold 2017). Other research showed an increased likelihood of meeting criteria for antisocial disorders (conduct, oppositional defiant), major psychiatric disorders (mood disorders and psychosis), and substance dependence disorders when compared to matched controls at a 10-year follow-up point (Biederman et al. 2006). Having a childhood diagnosis of ADHD puts an individual at risk for developing other comorbid psychiatric diagnoses. This risk of adverse psychiatric outcomes makes it essential that APRNs who encounter ADHD in their young pediatric patients proactively provide effective treatment aimed at reducing the risk of other disorders developing as the child grows and matures.

Etiology

Genetics

The etiology of ADHD is complex and not defined by any single issue. Genetic studies have explored etiology with family/adoption studies, twin studies, and molecular genetics research (Pliszka 2016). While candidate genes have been identified for ADHD, studies have been unable to identify the specific genes responsible for ADHD. It is known that if a child has ADHD, 10–35% of first-degree relatives are likely to also have the disorder (Biederman et al. 1992). Similarly, if a child has a parent with ADHD, the risk of developing the disorder can run as high as 57% (Biederman et al. 1995). ADHD is considered a polygenetic disorder (Pliszka 2016).

Neurobiology

Research suggests that individuals with ADHD may have alterations in specific areas of the brain, including the ventral medial prefrontal cortex, posterior cingulated cortex, and precuneus (Weissman et al. 2006). Other research suggests that adults with ADHD have less functional connectivity between some areas of the brain, resulting in anterior regions failing to suppress the default mode network. This, in turn, results in impaired ability to focus and pay attention (Castellanos et al. 2008).

Research also suggests that atypical consolidation of the brain's default network could be a causative factor of ADHD beginning in childhood (Fair et al. 2010). This shift marks a change in research focused on determining the neurobiological cause of ADHD from a view that regional brain abnormalities caused the disorder to believing it was a dysfunction in distributed network organization. This specifically involves research identifying the dopamine receptors and transporters associated with ADHD (Stergiakouli and Thapar 2010). Additional research is necessary to further define the brain processes that precipitate development of ADHD in children (Konrad and Eickhoff 2010). More research on the structural differences in brains of individuals who have ADHD is ongoing (Spetie and Arnold 2017).

Brain imaging such as positron emission tomography (PET) or magnetic resonance imaging (MRI) is not recommended for the assessment of ADHD (http://archive.psych.org/edu/other_res/lib_archives/archives/200501.pdf). While children with ADHD have an increased number of subtle nonfocal neurological symptoms, these should not determine treatment (Pliszka 2016; Pine et al. 1993). More research is needed in the area of brain imaging used to diagnose ADHD but the best diagnostic tools remain observation, direct interview, and rating scales that measure behavior (Pliszka 2016).

Environmental

A variety of environmental factors are also likely to influence the development of ADHD. These can include severe traumatic brain injury, maternal smoking during pregnancy, prenatal stress and low birth weight, twin births, early social deprivation, and exposure to lead (Pliszka 2016). Greater environmental adversity, including exposure to family conflict, parental psychopathology, and poverty, may influence the development of ADHD but is not thought to contribute to the etiology of ADHD (Pliszka 2016). Research suggests that household chaos could contribute to poor functioning of the child with ADHD (Wirth et al. 2019). Household chaos does not cause ADHD since it is a brain-based disorder that can be mediated by environmental factors but is not directly caused by such factors.

Implications for Adulthood

It is likely that children and adolescents with ADHD continue to show symptoms of the disorder into adulthood and may require pharmacological and psychosocial treatment interventions throughout their lives. The key to adult psychopathology seems to be in identifying comorbid disorders that accompany the ADHD symptomatology along with a degree of impairment that may extend into adulthood.

Adults with a history of ADHD as children tend to have a higher rate of antisocial behavior, injuries and accidents, and employment and marital difficulties (Barkley 2004; Biederman et al. 2006). ADHD symptoms that carry into adulthood have implications for parenting effectiveness and family stability. Assessment of parental history of diagnosed and undiagnosed ADHD should routinely occur when assessing a child for the disorder. ADHD is a disorder whose etiology and presentation are influenced by a complex interplay between genetic and environmental factors. It has a clear influence on adult vocational and social functioning.

Presenting Signs and Symptoms of ADHD

A diagnosis of ADHD is made after careful assessment of the child and family, and determination that inattention, or impulsivity and hyperactivity, or both, is impairing functioning on multiple domains of the child's life for at least 6 months. When diagnosing a child with ADHD it is essential to consider other disorders, including learning disabilities, disruptive behavior disorders, substance abuse disorder, and Tourette's disorder (Pliszka et al. 2007). The child's level of maturity, developmental history, family situation, and physical health, including history of concussion and traumatic brain injury must all be considered. Diagnosing ADHD requires careful attention to assessment details, processing with parents what symptoms they are concerned about, and, most important, understanding the parental attitudes, culture, and potential bias that will influence how they view any type of disorder in their child. Table 10.2 details ADHD symptoms across the life span.

The symptoms of ADHD rarely occur without some other mediating disorder or factor influencing functioning. In the young child, this can include learning disorders, mood disorders, autistic spectrum disorders, and oppositional defiant disorders. In adolescents, the diagnosis of ADHD can be complicated by substance use, learning disorders, and other psychiatric disorders. Table 10.2 describes the diagnostic criteria for ADHD based on DSM-5 criteria (APA 2013).

Assessment tools are useful to use with parents and teachers in identifying the symptoms of ADHD through a normative, well-defined, reliable, and valid scale. It is best to use screening tools that assess across disorders, especially since comorbidity exists between disorders. The cautions of using scales with parents can involve overreporting or underreporting of symptoms based on attitudes about ADHD and stigma around having the disorder. Teacher ratings must be considered in the context of several ratings

Table 10.2 ADHD symptoms across the life span

Developmental stage	Symptoms
Preschool	Excessive motor activity or mobility, low frustration tolerance, impulsivity, inability to sustain attention, distractibility, poorly organized behavior, aggressiveness, noncompliance, inappropriate or demanding behaviors, negative social behavior, less adaptive behaviors
School-age	Symptoms similar to those in preschool-age children, with the emergence of academic difficulties, rejection by peers, oppositional behavior, lying, stealing, poor self-esteem, poor sleep patterns
Adolescence	Inattention, impulsiveness, inner restlessness, continued academic difficulties, problems with authority, increased risky behavior (e.g. smoking, substance abuse, early sexual activity, driving accidents/traffic violations), excessively aggressive and antisocial behavior, overall feelings of worthlessness
Adulthood	Exacerbation of underlying psychiatric conditions, frequent job changes and job losses, marital discord, multiple marriages, problems with the law, substance abuse

Source: Vierhile, A., Robb, A., & Ryan-Krause, P. Attention deficit/hyperactivity disorder in children and adolescents: Closing diagnostic, communication, and treatment gaps. Journal of Pediatric Health Care, 23, S5–S21. © 2009, Elsevier.

involving parents, caregivers, and teachers (Maretl et al. 2015). Rating scales performed before and after treatment intervention can offer APRNs a concrete measurement of change in symptoms and can inform interventions. Table 10.3 gives four common rating scales used in primary care that are also useful in psychiatric settings.

Common Comorbid Conditions and Treatment

Comorbid psychiatric conditions are common in patients with ADHD. Successful management of ADHD involves identification and treatment of comorbid conditions (Pliszka 2016). Comorbid conditions in childhood can include oppositional defiant disorder, conduct disorder, depression, cigarette smoking, anxiety disorder, learning disorders, and tic disorders. In adolescents, the most common comorbidities are substance use disorders, cigarette smoking, conduct disorder, depression, anxiety disorder, and bipolar disorder. In adults with ADHD, the comorbid disorders can include substance use disorders,

Table 10.3 Comparison of common ADHD rating scales used in primary care.

Scale	Age range	Description	Advantages	Disadvantages
Connors Rating Scale Revised (CRS-R)	3–17 years	• Based on DSM-IV criteria • Assesses a wide variety of common behavior problems (e.g. sleep, eating, peer group problems) • Revised scale updates, age, and sex-normative data and factor structure • Available in both short and long, parent, teacher, and self-report versions	• Large normative base • Multiple observer forms • Abbreviated forms aid in treatment monitoring • French version	• Few items regarding comorbidities • Somewhat redundant • Complete version is lengthy
Brown Attention Deficit Disorder Scale for Children and Adolescents (BADDS)	3–12 years, parent and teacher report; 8–12 years self-report; 12–18 years self-report	• Unlike other scales based on DSM-IV criteria, BADDS measures executive functioning associated with ADHD • Also measures developmental impairments • Separate rating scales for 3–7 years, 8–12 years, 12–18 years	• Measures inattentive ADHD • Only scale that accounts for inattentive behavior as a function of age • Strong psychometrics	• Minimal data about use in clinical settings
Vanderbilt ADHD Rating Scale	6–12 years, parent and teacher forms	• Newer scale based on DSM-IV criteria • Both parent and teacher forms • Similar to CRS-R and SNAP-IV • Assesses for comorbidities and school functioning	• Screens for comorbidities (oppositional-defiant disorder, anxiety, depression) • Spanish and German versions • Available online • Psychometrically strong scales	• Newer scales that lack sufficient data to establish their validity • Normative data from only one US region • No self-report scales
Swanson, Nolan, and Pelham IV (SNAP)	5–11 years, parent and teacher rating scale	• One of the first scales based on DSM-IV criteria • Frequently used in ADHD research	• Scoring available online • Same scale used for both parent and teacher • Measures comorbidity	• Lack of published psychometrics and normative data • Brief assessment of comorbidities

Source: Vierhile, A., Robb, A., & Ryan-Krause, P. Attention deficit/hyperactivity disorder in children and adolescents: Closing diagnostic, communication, and treatment gaps. Journal of Pediatric Health Care, 23, S5–S21. © 2009 permission from Elsevier Publishing.

antisocial personality disorder, depression, anxiety disorders, and bipolar disorder (Pliszka 2016).

Oppositional Defiant Disorder and Conduct Disorder

It is estimated that between 30% and 50% of children diagnosed with ADHD also have oppositional defiant disorder or some other form of conduct disorder (Armenteros et al. 2007).

Behavior difficulties in conduct problems include aggression, impulsivity, and oppositional problems beyond the diagnosis of ADHD. However, treating underlying ADHD symptoms with a stimulant medication will help improve the oppositional and aggressive behaviors but is likely not to be the only treatment required (Newcorn et al. 2016)).

If aggression persists even if the ADHD symptoms are improved, bipolar disorder has to be ruled out

(Pliszka 2016). Consideration of an atypical or second-generation antipsychotic medication or mood stabilizer to manage behavior might be considered.

Bipolar Disorder

Bipolar disorder in children with ADHD is difficult to diagnose. Core symptoms of inattention, hyperactivity, impulsivity, and aggression can occur in both disorders (Kowatch and DelBello 2006), yet children with an ADHD diagnosis do not tend to exhibit manic symptoms such as elated mood, grandiosity, decreased need for sleep, or racing thoughts. When children present with symptoms of both ADHD and a mood disorder, it is recommended that initial treatment with medication focus on mood stabilization followed by treatment of the ADHD (Kowatch and DelBello 2006).

Major Depression

The first step in treating a child who meets diagnostic criteria for both major depression and ADHD is determining which disorder is causing the most functional impairment and symptom distress (Pliszka et al. 2006). Depressive symptoms respond best to a combination of cognitive behavioral therapy (CBT) with medication management with a selective serotonin reuptake inhibitor (Dopheide 2006). The APRN must carefully and continuously assess the risk of suicide in any child who suffers from a depressive disorder. Treatment of ADHD symptoms could be considered after some resolution of the depressive symptoms.

Anxiety Disorders

Children with ADHD and comorbid anxiety disorders suffer more impairment when both disorders are present. Research suggests that 25–35% of children with ADHD also have an anxiety disorder (Bowen et al. 2008). APRNs treating ADHD in an anxious child should be aware that the benefits of stimulant treatment might be mixed, causing increased anxiety even if ADHD symptoms have improved (Goez et al. 2007). Anxiety disorders are best treated first with CBT, followed by pharmacologic interventions if CBT is not helpful.

Tic Disorders or Tourette's Disorder

Tic disorders and ADHD are frequently comorbid, with between 21% and 90% of children with Tourette's disorder also suffering from ADHD (Robertson 2006). Research has shown that combination therapy of a stimulant and alpha-agonist resulted in improved ADHD in children with comorbid tic disorders. Studies show that use of methylphenidate and atomoxetine can effectively manage ADHD symptoms without worsening the tic disorder (Pliszka et al. 2006).

Effects of ADHD on Peer Relationships

Recent research has looked at developmental process as it involves peer problems in children diagnosed with ADHD. Compared to a nondiagnosed group, researchers found that, over a 6-year study period, children with ADHD exhibited difficulties with aggression, social skills, inaccurate self-perceptions, and peer rejection (Murray-Close et al. 2010). They found that the peer problems in the children with ADHD reflected their failure to successfully negotiate developmental tasks. The authors described "multiple vicious cycles and cascading effects among areas of functioning across development. These findings suggest that there are a number of indirect effects among overly positive self-perceptions, social skills, aggression, and peer rejection. As a result, failure in one area may have both direct and indirect effects on functioning in other areas across development" (p. 799).

These findings have implications for intervention strategies aimed at better peer relationships for the child with ADHD. The researchers recommend intervening at multiple levels, with a social behavioral curriculum that emphasizes skill building from elementary through high school. The notion that impairments from ADHD have a cascading effect on development is beginning to emerge in the literature and requires more research, especially around effective mediating interventions.

Evidence-based Interventions

Nonpharmacological

Nonpharmacological interventions have been shown to have a positive influence on ADHD symptoms and include behavioral therapy models, including CBT and parent management training. Daley et al. (2014) in their meta-analysis of nonpharmacological treatment for ADHD, noted that behavioral treatment had a stronger effect on parenting behaviors versus core ADHD symptoms. This suggests that the ways parents deal with their children with ADHD can influence the severity of the symptoms. All families with a child with ADHD are at risk for early, damaging, negative relationships with parents and other family members.

For young school-age children, continued indirect models of treatment involving parent training and classroom interventions are recommended. Parent management training specifically helps parents and caregivers learn to manage difficult, impulsive behaviors in a structured, reward-oriented system. Children with learning disabilities require specialized educational programs that consider the role ADHD symptoms play in academic difficulties. Some form of special education services might be needed to maximize use of the classroom.

School-focused interventions include academics, peer relationships, a structured classroom environment, and accommodations such as untimed tests or small class size (Pliszka 2016).

By middle and high school, nonpharmacological treatment becomes more complex, involving parents, classroom, and, for the adolescent, social skills training or CBT. Tutoring support, use of assistive electronic devices, and planning for special accommodations beyond high school in technical school or college are important for the middle and high school patient with ADHD. Until adulthood the recommendation is for a multimodal approach. By adulthood, the recommended psychosocial intervention is CBT (Young and Amarasinghe 2010). By adulthood, most individuals with ADHD will have had at least a trial of stimulant medication. Ideally, this is part of a comprehensive treatment regimen involving psychosocial interventions with parents, teachers, and the patient.

Pharmacological Interventions

Use of stimulant medication has generally been the first-line pharmacological intervention for individuals with diagnosed ADHD. Methylphenidate and amphetamine preparations have been shown to enhance dopaminergic and noradrenergic neurotransmission peripherally and in the central nervous system (Spencer et al. 2016). Clinical trials have consistently shown these medications to be effective and safe in symptom management with children, adolescents, and adults who have ADHD (Pliszka 2016). Stimulant medications come in two formulations (short- and long-acting), based on duration of action and whether the child can swallow pills. While long-acting stimulants are most commonly prescribed in both primary care and specialty clinics, short-acting forms are typically used as the initial treatment in children younger than 6 years (Kaplan and Newcorn 2011). Long-acting preparations are indicated when duration of action longer than 4 hours is necessary or administration of short-acting formulations is inconvenient or stigmatizing (Subcommittee on Attention Deficit/Hyperactivity Disorder 2011). Long-acting forms are also beneficial because they are less likely misused (Wilens et al. 2008). Occasionally, a combination of short- and long-acting formulations is prescribed, where the long-acting stimulant is taken in the morning and the short-acting one may be taken in the afternoon to aid adequate coverage throughout the day (Subcommittee on Attention Deficit/Hyperactivity Disorder 2011).

Other medications have also been used in treating ADHD and include nonstimulant agents (atomoxetine), antidepressants (buproprion), and alpha-agonist preparations (clonidine, guanfacine, guanfacine extended release). These medications tend to be second-line agents and are used if stimulants are poorly tolerated, there is a partial response to stimulant medication, or there are comorbid disorders contraindicating the use of stimulants (Spencer et al. 2016). Medication tables for stimulant and nonstimulant medication are given in Chapter 9.

Approach to Management

Symptoms of ADHD usually emerge as behavioral concerns revealed by parents during well-child primary care visits, or a parent may schedule an appointment to discuss concerns about the child's behavioral issues. With the proliferation of media related to ADHD, parents often present with a question or potential diagnosis of ADHD to explain their child's symptomatology. Teachers frequently encourage parents to seek healthcare assessments and may suggest a diagnosis of ADHD when impulsive and inattentive behavior is observed in the classroom. One of the most important roles of primary care APRN is to accurately diagnose ADHD by gathering an extensive history and assessments, conducting a thorough physical examination, gathering data from multiple sources (school, home, observations), and ruling out other diagnoses.

Once the diagnosis of ADHD is established, the clinician should determine if the patient has a comorbid condition, such as oppositional defiant disorder. Patients with comorbid conditions are more likely to require referral to a child guidance clinic for individual and family therapy. However, the therapist may not be a prescriber and co-management with the primary care provider can be arranged. Best practice advocates that parents and adolescents give written permission so that both clinicians can share confidential information. However, there may be variations across states about the legality of formal consent prior to communication between healthcare providers.

After conducting an evaluation of presenting problem and history, parents, children, and adolescents require at least one full visit to discuss the diagnosis of ADHD and recommended evidence-based management. The clinician should determine the parents' and child's understanding of the diagnosis and the cultural meaning of the disorder (Dell 2010). Previous to diagnosis, parents may view the child's behavior as intentionally "lazy" or difficult. Children in turn are often baffled, sometimes hopeless, and resigned to criticism from parents, teachers, and peers. For some parents the diagnosis is a relief, but others may be fearful that controlled substances will lead to drug dependence. Healthcare providers should speak to parents while fully engaging children and adolescents at their developmental level in the discussion. Adolescents require time alone with the provider to address their specific concerns and in recognition of their growing independence and responsibility to begin managing their healthcare. Despite an in-depth initial discussion, some parents are not prepared to include medication as a component of therapy. The clinician should remain open to the parents' need to explore other options and resources. In many instances, when other therapies have failed, parents will return and accept pharmacotherapy as part of the therapeutic plan. If psychosocial therapies are successful in managing symptoms, medication may not be necessary.

Healthcare providers should explain that effective management of ADHD requires a multifaceted approach, including behavior management at home, at school, and when engaged in other activities, communication with school personnel, and pharmacological therapy. A useful website is www.chadd.org, a comprehensive resource for parents, older children, and adolescents.

Selecting the stimulant dose is not based on weight, which is the standard for most pediatric medications. The provider should start with the lowest dose and explain that the dose will be increased every 1–2 weeks as needed depending on the child's response. Beginning with the lowest dose provides some assurance to parents, who may be reluctant to consider pharmacotherapy. Parents and children should be advised of common side effects, such as anorexia and insomnia, which occur with some but not all patients, and plan accordingly. Parents may prefer to give the first dose on a weekend so they can monitor both positive responses as well as potential side effects. Routine and ongoing visits are critical to monitor progress and reinforce patient and family education about ADHD, pharmacotherapy, and other components of the treatment. Parent and teacher progress forms and observational data can help determine progress in symptom management. Weight, height, blood pressure, and pulse should be monitored at each visit. After 1–2 weeks, if no change in behavior is noted and no significant side effects emerge, the stimulant dose can be increased slowly and incrementally, methylphenidate 18 mg to methylphenidate 27 mg. Once the child has demonstrated positive behavioral changes, the dose can be maintained and periodically reevaluated. Stimulants are Schedule II controlled substances and refills are not allowed. However, the Drug Enforcement Administration rules (http://www.deadiver-sion.usdoj.gov/fed_regs/rules/2006/fr0906.htm) permit prescribers to give multiple prescriptions up to a 90-day supply. This option is appropriate once a child is stabilized on a stimulant dose and the management plan is effective. The importance of monitoring over time as the child grows and develops is countered by the realization that ADHD is a chronic condition. New challenges emerge for the APRN as children mature to adolescence and adulthood, and must make choices about use of medication, dosing, and continuing treatment.

A useful guide for managing ADHD resulted from the Texas Children's Medication Algorithm Project (Pliszka et al. 2006). Revised several times, the project began in 1998 to develop an algorithm for choosing ADHD treatments. Guidelines for treating conditions comorbid with ADHD were also developed.

Role Differentiation between Primary Care and Child Psychiatric Advanced Practice Nurses

Primary care APRNs are educationally well prepared to manage ADHD and it is a practice expectation for the nurse practitioner. The presence of comorbid psychiatric conditions usually requires consultation with a psychiatric APRN. The complexity of the comorbid conditions may determine solo management by the psychiatric nurse practitioner.

The ultimate determination of who manages care is usually based on the presented complexity of ADHD and the response of the child/adolescent and family to the therapeutic plan developed to manage symptoms. The pediatric APRN will usually begin stimulant treatment. If ADHD symptoms do not resolve or if disorders other than ADHD are diagnostically present, it is advised that the pediatric APRN seek referral, with resulting psychiatric evaluation, followed by a management plan. Psychiatric medications, including stimulants, may become the sole responsibility of the psychiatric APRN. They may also transfer back to the pediatric APRN when the child is stable. Either way, the pediatric APRN should continue to monitor progress and treatment. Even if a psychiatric referral occurs, the family or pediatric APRN will still be providing well-child care and would resume management of the ADHD if the child's condition stabilizes.

Implications for Nursing Practice, Research, and Education

ADHD occurs commonly in pediatric populations and is generally responsive to both pharmacological and non-pharmacological interventions. APRNs, who frequently provide physical and mental healthcare to these children, are in an excellent position to practice comprehensive models of care utilizing both primary care and child psychiatry specialties. The seamless transition back and forth between these two nursing specialties as determined by the patient's presenting problems and degree of stability should be the ultimate goal of treatment and will result in improved care outcomes. All pediatric APRNs need to have extensive knowledge of this disorder, its comorbidities, and evidence-based interventions. Nurses are in an excellent position to research the most effective treatment models, especially with ADHD that is comorbid with other conditions requiring combination treatment. The goal is always provision of excellent care resulting in improved functioning.

Critical Thinking Questions

1. What family issues must be considered before choosing to prescribe to a young child with ADHD?
2. What community resources are most helpful to parents of a child with ADHD who is struggling with school performance?
3. How should primary care and psychiatric APRNs respond to critics of pharmacy management of ADHD? How can evidence and data be used to respond to these criticisms?

References

APA (1968). *Diagnostic and Statistical Manual of Mental Disorders II.* Washington, DC: American Psychiatric Association.

APA (2013). *Diagnostic and Statistical Manual of Mental Disorder 5.* Washington, DC: American Psychiatric Association.

Armenteros, J.L., Lewis, J.E., and Davalos, M. (2007). Risperidone augmentation for attention-deficit/hyperactivity disorder. *Journal of the American Academy of Child Adolescent Psychiatry* 46: 558–565.

Barkley, R.A. (2004). Driving impairments in teens and adults with attention-deficit/hyperactivity disorder. *Psychiatric Clinics of North America* 27: 233–260.

Biederman, J., Faraone, S.V., Keenan, K. et al. (1992). Further evidence for family-genetic risk factors in attention deficit hyperactivity disorder: patterns of comorbidity in probands and relatives psychiatrically and pediatrically referred samples. *Archives of General Psychiatry* 49: 728–738.

Biederman, J., Faraone, S.V., Mick, E. et al. (1995). High risk for attention deficit hyperactivity disorder among children of parents with childhood onset of the disorder: a pilot study. *American Journal of Psychiatry* 152: 431–435.

Biederman, J., Monuteaux, M.C., Mick, E. et al. (2006). Young adult outcome of attention deficit hyperactivity disorder: a controlled 10 year follow-up study. *Psychological Medicine* 36: 167–179.

Bowen, R., Chavira, D.A., Baily, K. et al. (2008). Nature of anxiety comorbid with attention deficit hyperactivity disorder in children from a pediatric primary care setting. *Psychiatry Research* 157: 201–208.

Castellanos, F.X., Margulies, D.S., Kelly, C. et al. (2008). Cingulate-precuneus interactions: a new locus of dysfunction in adult attention-deficit/hyperactivity disorder. *Biological Psychiatry* 63: 332–337.

Daley, D., Van der Oord, S., Ferrin, M. et al. (2014). Behavioral interventions in attention-deficit/hyperactivity disorder: a met-analysis of randomized controlled trials across multiple outcome domains. *Journal of the American Academy of Child and Adolescent Psychiatry* 53 (8): 835–847 e1–5. https://doi.org/10.1016/j.jaac.2014.05.013.

Dell, M.L. (2010). Ethnic, cultural, and religious issues. In: *Dulcan's Textbook of Child and Adolescent Psychiatry* (ed. M.K. Dulcan), 517–529. Washington, DC: American Psychiatric Publishing, Inc.

Dopheide, J.A. (2006). Recognizing and treating depression in children and adolescents. *American Journal of Health-System Pharmacy* 63: 233–243.

Ebaugh, F. and Franklin, G. (1923). Neuropsychiatric sequelae of acute epidemic encephalitis in children. *American Journal of Diseases of the Child* 25: 89–97.

Fair, D.A., Posner, J., Nagel, B.J. et al. (2010). Atypical default network connectivity in youth with attention-deficit/hyperactivity disorder. *Biological Psychiatry.* https://doi.org/10.1016/j.biopsych.2010.07.003.

Goez, H., Back-Bennet, O., and Zelnik, N. (2007). Differential stimulant response on attention in children with comorbid anxiety and oppositional defiant disorder. *Journal of Child Neurology* 22: 538–542.

Kaplan, G. and Newcorn, J.H. (2011). Pharmacotherapy for child and adolescent attention-deficit hyperactivity disorder. *Pediatric Clinics of North America* 58 (1): 99–120. https://doi.org/10.1016/j.pcl.2010.10.009.

Kessler, R.C., Adler, L., Barkley, R. et al. (2006). The prevalence and correlates of adult ADHD in the United States: results from the National Comorbidity Survey Replication. *American Journal of Psychiatry* 163: 716–723.

Konrad, K. and Eickhoff, S.B. (2010). Is the ADHD brain wired differently? A review on structural and functional connectivity in attention deficit hyperactivity disorder. *Human Brain Mapping* 31 (6): 904–916.

Kowatch, R.A. and DelBello, M.P. (2006). Pediatric bipolar disorder: emerging diagnostic and treatment approaches. *Child and Adolescent Psychiatric Clinics of North America* 15: 73–108.

Maretl, M.M., Nikolas, M., Schimmack, U., and Nigg, J.T. (2015). Integration of symptom ratings from multiple informants in ADHD diagnosis: a psychometric model with clinical utility. *Psychological Assessment* 27: 1060–1071. https://doi.org/10.1037/pas0000088.

Murray-Close, D., Hoza, B., Hinshaw, S.P. et al. (2010). Developmental processes in peer problems of children with attention-deficit/hyperactivity disorder in the multimodal treatment study of children with ADHD: developmental cascades and vicious cycles. *Development and Psychopathology* 22: 785–802.

Nagae, M., Nakane, H., Honda, S. et al. (2015). Factors affecting medication adherence in children receiving outpatient pharmacotherapy and parental adherence. *Journal of Child and Adolescent Psychiatric Nursing* 28: 109–117. https://doi.org/10.1111/jcap.12113.

Newcorn, J.H., Ivanov, I., Chacko, A., and Javdani, S. (2016). Aggression and violence. In: *Dulcan's Textbook of Child and Adolescent Psychiatry*, 2e (ed. M.K. Dulcan), 603–620. Washington, DC: American Psychiatric Publishing.

Pine, D., Shaffer, D., and Schonfeld, I. (1993). Persistent emotional disorder in children with neurological soft signs. *Journal of the American Academy of Child and Adolescent Psychiatry* 32: 1229–1236.

Pliszka, S.R. (2016). Attention-deficit/hyperactivity disorder. In: *Dulcan's Textbook of Child and Adolescent Psychiatry*, 2e (ed. M.K. Dulcan), 173–193. Washington, DC: American Psychiatric Publishing.

Pliszka, S.R. and AACAP Child and Adolescent Work Group on Quality Issues (2007). Practice parameter for the assessment and treatment of children and adolescents with attention-deficit-hyperactivity disorder. *Journal of the American Academy of Child and Adolescent Psychiatry* 46: 894–921.

Pliszka, S.R., Crismon, M.L., Hughes, C. et al. (2006). The Texas children's medication algorithm project: revision of the algorithm for pharmacotherapy of attention-deficit/hyperactivity disorder. *Journal of the American Academy of Child and Adolescent Psychiatry* 46: 642–657.

Polanczyk, G., de Lima, M.S., Horta, B.L. et al. (2007). The worldwide prevalence of ADHD: a systematic review and metaregression analysis. *American Journal of Psychiatry* 164: 942–948.

Robertson, M.M. (2006). Attention deficit hyperactivity disorder, tics and Tourette's syndrome: the relationship and treatment implications. A commentary. *European Child and Adolescent Psychiatry* 15: 1–11.

Spencer, T.J., Biederman, J., and Mick, E. (2007). Attention-deficit/hyperactivity disorder: diagnosis, lifespan, comorbidities, and neurobiology. *Ambulatory Pediatrics* 7 (1): 73–81.

Spencer, T.J., Biederman, J., and Wilens, T.E. (2016). Medications used for attention-deficit/hyperactivity disorder. In: *Dulcan's Textbook of Child and Adolescent Psychiatry*, 2e (ed. M.K. Dulcan), 709–735. Washington, DC: American Psychiatric Publishing.

Spetie, L. and Arnold, E.L. (2017). Attention-deficit hyperactivity disorder. In: *Lewis's Child and Adolescent Psychiatry: A Comprehensive Textbook*, 5e (eds. A. Marti, M.H. Bloch and F.R. Volkmar), 364–387. Philadelphia, PA: Wolters Kluwer.

Steinhausen, H.C. (2015). Recent international trends in psychotropic medication prescriptions for children and adolescents. *European Child and Adolescent Psychiatry* 24: 635–640. https://doi.org/10.1007/s00787-014-0631-y.

Stergiakouli, E. and Thapar, A. (2010). Fitting the pieces together: current research on the genetic basis of attention-deficit/hyperactivity disorder (ADHD). *Neuropsychiatric Disease and Treatment* 6: 551–560.

Subcommittee on Attention-Deficit/Hyperactivity Disorder, Steering Committee on Quality Management, Wolraich, M., Brown, L. et al. (2011). ADHD: clinical practice guideline for the diagnosis, evaluation, and treatment of attention-deficit/hyperactivity disorder in children and adolescents. *Pediatrics* 128 (5): 1007–1022. https://doi.org/10.1542/peds.2011-2654.

Vierhile, A., Robb, A., and Ryan-Krause, P. (2009). Attention deficit/hyperactivity disorder in children and adolescents: closing diagnostic, communication, and treatment gaps. *Journal of Pediatric Health Care* 23: S5–S21. https://doi.org/10.1016/j.pedhc.2008.10.009.

Visser, S.N., Danielson, M.L., Bitsko, R.H. et al. (2013). Trends in the parent-report of health care provider-diagnosed and medicated attention-deficit/hyperactivity disorder: United States, 2003-2011. *Journal of the American Academy of Child and Adolescent Psychiatry* 53 (1): 34–46.e2. https://doi.org/10.1016/j.jaac.2013.09.001.

Weissman, D.H., Roberts, K.C., Visscher, K.M., and Woldorff, M.G. (2006). The neural bases of momentary lapses in attention. *Nature Neuroscience* 9: 971–978.

Wilens, T.E., Adler, L.A., Adams, J. et al. (2008). Misuse and diversion of stimulants prescribed for ADHD: a systematic review of the literature. *J Am Acad Child Adolesc Psychiatry* 47 (1): 21–31. https://doi.org/10.1097/chi.0b013e31815a56f1.

Wirth, A., Reinelt, T., Gawrilow, C. et al. (2019). Examining the relationship between children's ADHD symptomatology and inadequate parenting: the role of household chaos. *Journal of Attention Disorders* 23: 451–462. https://doi.org/10.1177/1087054716792881.

Young, S. and Amarasinghe, J.M. (2010). Practitioner review: non-pharmacological treatments for ADHD: a lifespan approach. *The Journal of Child Psychology and Psychiatry* 51: 116–133. https://doi.org/10.1111/j.1469-7610.2009.02191.x.

11

Anxiety Disorders

Geraldine S. Pearson[1] and Kathleen Kenney-Riley[2, 3]

[1] University of Connecticut School of Medicine-retired, Farmington, CT, USA
[2] Children's Hospital at Montefiore, Bronx, NY, USA
[3] Mercy College, Dobbs Ferry, NY, USA

Objectives

After reading this chapter, advanced practice registered nurses (APRNs) will be able to:

1. Describe normal developmental stages from infancy through adolescence that are associated with anxiety.
2. Define the epidemiology, prevalence statistics, and theories of etiology related to anxiety disorders.
3. Describe types, common presenting signs, and symptoms of anxiety disorders in children and adolescents.
4. Discuss comorbid conditions associated with anxiety.
5. Define pharmacological and nonpharmacological evidence-based interventions.
6. Differentiate roles of primary care practitioners and advanced practice psychiatric nurses in the diagnosis and treatment of children and adolescents with anxiety.

Introduction

"Anxiety" is a broad term referring to the brain's response to perceived or actual danger. It can be characterized by fear, concern, or dread related to a specific event, or it can be pervasive (Gregory and Eley 2007). The capacity for the basic emotion of anxiety is present in infancy and persists throughout childhood. Anxiety is a normal part of life and is experienced to some degree by all people. Wehry et al. (2015) note that anxiety disorders begin in childhood and adolescence but exhibit homotypic continuity through development and present the risk of secondary anxiety and mood disorders during the lifespan. Anxious reactions can range from mild to severe. Anxiety disorders occur when anxiety becomes so severe that it interrupts and/or disrupts the child's ability to

function. When anxiety disorders present in early childhood, the result may be disruption of the normal growth and developmental trajectory. This sets a course of problems that can extend into adulthood for these children (Connolly et al. 2016). It is challenging for advanced practice registered nurses (APRNs) to differentiate anxiety that is a normal part of development from that which has the potential to disrupt functioning. Anxiety disorders in adulthood have nearly always had their symptomatic roots in childhood or adolescence, lending credence to the need for early identification and intervention.

Anxiety can be characterized by two distinctly different entities of worry and fear. Worry "involves anxious apprehension and thoughts focused on the possibility of

Child and Adolescent Behavioral Health: A Resource for Advanced Practice Psychiatric and Primary Care Practitioners in Nursing,
Second Edition. Edited by Edilma L. Yearwood, Geraldine S. Pearson, and Jamesetta A. Newland.
© 2021 John Wiley & Sons, Inc. Published 2021 by John Wiley & Sons, Inc.
Companion website: www.wiley.com/go/Yearwood

negative future events, while fear is related to the response to threat or danger that is perceived as actual or impending" (Connolly et al. 2016, p. 305). APRNs are likely to see children and adolescents presenting for basic well-child care or psychiatric care who have symptoms of anxiety. Again, the challenge is distinguishing between developmentally normal worries about life and worries that debilitate and inhibit accomplishment of normal developmental milestones.

Anxiety disorders are a common presenting problem in pediatric primary care and within child/adolescent psychiatric practices (Bistko et al. 2018). Many children and adolescents with anxiety disorders are psychosocially complex, with associated family difficulties, exposure to trauma, and/or negative life events. While symptoms can range from transient and mild to extreme and debilitating, they are rarely simple disorders to treat and often are associated with comorbid psychiatric disorders. Conditions such as attention deficit hyperactivity disorder (ADHD), depression, oppositional defiant disorder, and motor tics can be accompanied by varying degrees of anxiety.

Anxiety disorders diagnosed in the Diagnostic and Statistical Manual of Mental Disorders (DSM-5) (American Psychiatric Association 2013) include separation anxiety disorder (SAD), generalized anxiety disorder (GAD), obsessive–compulsive disorder, and social phobia in children and adolescents. Additional categories include specific phobias, agoraphobia, selective mutism (SM), and panic attacks. Post-traumatic stress disorders are also part of the anxiety spectrum of symptoms. There is considerable heterogeneity in diagnostic subsets of anxiety disorders. This can be challenging to the primary care provider (PCP) who is trying to assess the child or adolescent who presents with symptoms of anxiety and to identify its cause and specific manifestation.

This chapter describes anxiety as it is manifested across the pediatric life span. Evidence-based assessments and psychosocial interventions and associated psychopharmacological treatments are presented. The chapter concludes with a case exemplar that illustrates chapter concepts and interventions. Implications for advanced nursing practice, education, and research are discussed.

Normative Anxiety as Part of Development

APRNs who see children with anxiety have to carefully distinguish normative, transient worries and fears that are developmentally appropriate from anxiety disorders that are a constellation of symptoms interfering with functioning. Connolly et al. (2016) noted that common

fears among infants include loud noises, being dropped, stranger anxiety, and, later, separation from the caregiver. Stranger anxiety begins around 7 months of age, when infants are able to recognize persons who are different from their normal caregiver. Separation anxiety represents an infant's inability to recognize that even if his or her parent is not visible, they still exist. Issues such as separation anxiety can be concerning for parents, thus the APRN must be adept at understanding when separation anxiety is part of the normal development of late infancy versus when it becomes pathological. Separation anxiety should be resolved in children around the time of the preschool years before they prepare for school.

As babies move onto toddlerhood, common fears include fears of monsters or darkness. Toddlers who previously seemed fascinated by animals may now become anxious around animals such as dogs, demonstrating significant fear. Preschoolers may worry about physical wellbeing, pleasing their parents and teachers, as well as natural events such as bad weather. Most anxiety reactions are transient and considered a normative part of preschool development (Connolly et al. 2016).

The school-age years bring about a time when children must separate from their parents, spending more and more time away from their main source of support. While some anxiety regarding starting school is normal, school anxiety can become severe in a small subset of children. Anxiety-related school avoidance occurs in school-age children when they are excessively worried about grades, being disliked by others, and/or have persistent separation anxiety. Children who are at risk for significant school anxiety include children with a shy or sensitive temperament, those with overprotective parents, or children who are being teased by other children. Children with social anxiety may be at risk for bullying and for becoming bullies (Pabian and Vandebosch 2016). Bullying is a complex social interaction with destructive effects on children. It should always be assessed in any child or adolescent presenting with anxiety.

Additionally, school-age children are now able to understand what others think of them, which may be different from how they think of or see themselves. This cognitive ability results in fear of what their friends or teachers think of them. They also begin to worry about their appearance and abilities compared to their peers. Older school-age children may also have fears about the dark, peers, school, and sports performance. These children develop anxiety regarding scary things they see on television or hear about from others, such as natural disasters or accidents.

In adolescence, the most common sources of anxiety involve social competence, evaluation, and psychological wellbeing (Connolly et al. 2016). Additional fears include issues regarding sexual development, uncertainty regarding sexual identity, and fear of not being accepted by those they find attractive. Late adolescence is a time when children are told they must begin to think about who they will become later in life. This pressure to choose a career, decide on a college, or get a job can result in adolescent worry and anxiety.

While fear and anxieties are common among different age groups, APRNs must recognize that in certain children and adolescents these fears/anxieties become so great that they interrupt the child's normal activities and development. APRN's should ask children during healthcare visits what they worry about and assess children for signs of distress and anxieties that are overwhelming to them. During the visit, it is important for the provider to ask the child how he or she deals with their anxiety and to whom they turn for help and support. When these anxieties interrupt their daily functioning, it is imperative to provide these children with appropriate evaluation and treatment.

Epidemiology and Prevalence of Anxiety Disorders

Anxiety disorders in children and adolescents are highly prevalent and considered the most common childhood psychiatric disorder. They affect up to 10% of children aged 10–16 and are responsible for approximately a third of all mental health issues in children and adolescents (Bennett et al. 2015). While strongly influenced by assessment and diagnostic variance, lifetime rates across gender and ethnicity for developing any type of anxiety disorder between ages 13 and 18 are estimated to be around 31%, with females having higher rates than males (Bennett et al. 2015). All of these prevalence rates are impacted by the ability of the provider to identify and diagnose patients with anxiety disorders. As the most common psychiatric disorders in children and adolescents, they are also the disorders that can precede manifestation of other developmental and psychiatric difficulties, including disruptive behavior disorders and depression (Connolly et al. 2016). As a precursor to other psychiatric disorders, it is imperative to address pediatric anxiety when it is identified.

Genetics and Environmental Risk Factors

There is documented heritable risk with anxiety in families, along with psychosocial factors that determine the transmission of anxiety disorders in families (Gregory and Eley 2007; Moore et al. 2004). Whaley et al. (1999) found that clinically anxious mothers had higher levels of criticism and a tendency to catastrophize or predict

dire outcomes, modeling a fearful cognitive style for their children. Parents of anxious children were less likely to allow autonomy in their children (Stuart-Parrigon and Kerns 2016). This contributed to parents of anxious children being overprotective. Children with a diminished sense of personal control can become anxious when faced with unpredictable situations (Suarez et al. 2009). The question of whether a child's temperament shaped parental behavior or parental behavior resulted in anxiety among children, suggests that familial anxiety is a complex multifaceted bidirectional process.

Genetics are not the sole cause of anxiety disorders in children. Environmental factors are significant variables that can result in increased rates of anxiety disorders. Parental rearing style can impact the development of anxiety disorders in children. Research has found that children whose parents utilized more coercive and overprotective parenting styles had higher rates of anxiety (Laurin et al. 2015). Leis and Mendelson (2010) found that maternal major depression resulted in greater risk for offspring developing a lifetime mood or anxiety disorder. They suggested that major and minor parental depressive symptoms put offspring at psychiatric risk.

Research has also demonstrated that children who grew up in families with a parent or sibling who was chronically ill had higher rates of anxiety both during childhood and as an adult (Batte et al. 2006). Other risk factors can include temperamental and personality traits and psychosocial adversities such as loss, abuse, or parental divorce (Beesdo et al. 2009), as well as life events such as health problems and poverty (Hirshfeld-Becker et al. 2008). Social risk factors such as being rejected by peers was found to make the child more prone to social anxiety.

Anxiety disorders in children and adolescents are likely the result of a complicated meshing of biologic, personality, and psychosocial risk factors. Ginsburg et al. (2018) found that a childhood diagnosis of anxiety was associated with greater risk of developing a chronic anxiety disability across the life span. They also found that an acute positive response to treatment could result in improved outcomes as the individual ages. Thus, APRNs need to realize that environmental factors also play a significant role in the type of anxiety disorder that may develop, the degree of psychopathology, and the resulting degree of developmental impairment. APRNs should include in-depth assessment of these issues in the primary care setting to assure early identification of potential risks and symptoms of anxiety and provide resources and treatment as soon as possible. It is important to recognize that these disorders can continue throughout the child's life if not addressed early.

Role of Trauma in the Development of Anxiety

Children experiencing childhood adversities, including trauma such as abuse and neglect, have been found to be at risk for developing psychopathology, including anxiety disorders (Benjet et al. 2010). As APRNs evaluate children who have experienced a trauma of any kind, they must recognize the significant impact trauma can have on the development of anxiety disorders, assess for symptoms of anxiety in these children, and provide access to support for these children as early as possible. Children showing symptoms of anxiety need to be carefully assessed to ascertain if the anxiety came after trauma or was present prior to this. Children experiencing trauma and/or anxiety should be referred for psychological care as soon as possible in order to intervene before the anxiety disrupts the child's life and becomes pathological. The APRNs should connect children and families with additional resource and support mechanisms to reduce the likelihood of repeated trauma and abuse, which often can reoccur.

Types and Symptoms of Anxiety Disorders

Anxiety disorders occur within a context that produces various symptoms (Connolly et al. 2016). When assessing symptoms, the APRN must consider whether presenting anxiety symptoms are situation specific or generalized. The most widely identified childhood anxiety disorders are GAD, specific phobia, SM, panic disorder, specific phobia, SAD, social anxiety disorder, and school refusal behavior (APA 2013). Each will be specifically discussed.

Generalized anxiety disorder: GAD is characterized by "chronic, excessive worry in a number of areas such as schoolwork, social interactions, family, health/safety, world events, and natural disasters with at least one associated somatic symptom" (AACAP 2007, p. 268). *Exemplar*: Kate, aged 12, vomits her breakfast on the days she is going to have a written test or oral classroom presentation. She is fearful that she will forget the studied information and fail the test.

Specific phobia: Social phobia involves feeling scared or uncomfortable in one or more social settings or situations where the individual is required to perform. *Exemplar*: Tony, aged 7, refuses to go outside and play with peers. His teacher reports that he is reticent to speak up in class and avoids unstructured, social situations.

Selective mutism: SM, part of social phobia, is a failure to speak aloud in a social situation. These individuals may whisper or gesture with peers or adults. *Exemplar*: Serena, aged 7, has refused to speak at school or at home for the past 2 years. With no clear precipitant or trauma, she communicates in monosyllabic whispers to her parents only.

Panic disorder: Panic disorder involves unexpected but recurrent and intense episodes of fear (AACAP 2007). Panic disorder may occur with or without agoraphobia, an anxiety of social situations or places where escape might be difficult. This agoraphobia may inhibit activities of daily life and restrict the child's or adolescent's environment, causing impairment in functioning. *Exemplar*: Anne, aged 13, is frightened of large groups of people. She refuses to go to the grocery store or mall but manages to go to school, although she is unable to attend large school assemblies. She reports sweating, rapid pulse, and feeling like she will physically die in a group setting.

Specific phobia: Specific phobias involve marked fear or anxiety about a specific situation or object (Connolly et al. 2016) These include reactions that are disproportionate to the situation and are not logical. Insects, blood, clowns, or thunderstorms are all examples of phobia-inducing objects or situations. *Exemplar*: Joe, aged 10, is frightened of elevators and refuses to ride in them. He expresses an extreme fear of being enclosed in a moving "box."

Separation anxiety disorder: SADs involve a high level of fear, worry, and anxiety around separation from home or the primary attachment. The fear of separation must be considered in light of the child's developmental stage. For example, separation anxiety is normative in a very young child (younger than 6 years) but inappropriate or suggestive of anxiety disorder in a teenager (Connolly et al. 2016). *Exemplar*: Tom, aged 15, has not attended school for the past 2 years despite juvenile justice interventions around truancy. His mother has chronic emphysema, and he refuses to leave her.

Social anxiety disorder (previously social phobia): Social anxiety disorder reflects a significant fear of social situations and the fear of being humiliated or embarrassed when is social situations (Kashdan and Herbert 2001). Anxiety is out of proportion to the actual danger or threat in the situation. Exemplar: Jana, aged 10, is terrified to go to church because she is afraid of the large cross in the sanctuary.

School refusal: School refusal is also part of social phobia and involves fear of going to school. This is beyond the occasional fear or anxiety some children exhibit when going to school or being left at school. It is an extreme fear of attending school that impacts the child's ability to attend school. *Exemplar*: Ed, aged 5, cries and clings to his father's leg when taken to kindergarten. Dad has been unsuccessful in getting him to attend a full session of kindergarten.

Agoraphobia: Fear and anxiety about being in public, fear of having no escape, requiring a companion. *Exemplar*: Jane, aged 17, is terrified to leave her house for fear people will look at her and laugh.

Assessment of Anxiety

APRNs must recognize that anxiety disorders may present in primary care offices as common physical or behavioral complaints seen in children and adolescents that represent many actual physical conditions. Therefore, APRNs must become adept at understanding common symptoms that may represent anxiety disorders to ensure that these children are identified and offered treatment as early as possible. Children with anxiety disorders often present with physical symptoms such as headache, abdominal pain, and sleep difficulties. The goal of assessment by any provider is helping the child and parent to understand the meaning of the symptoms and rule out a physical cause unrelated to the anxiety (AACAP 2007).

Common Presenting Signs and Symptoms of Anxiety

Anxiety in childhood can present with many common signs and symptoms seen in primary care offices. The APRN must be able to recognize when symptoms represent somaticizing rather than a specific physical condition. Somatic complaints that interfere with daily functioning are the hallmark features of anxiety disorders in children (Ginsburg et al. 2006). Common symptoms of anxiety include frequent recurrent abdominal pain, muscle aches and pains, chest pain, palpitations, sweating, dizziness, shortness of breath, and headaches even though children and adolescents may not identify these as signs of anxiety. Anxious symptoms can also be manifested as nonspecific complaints such as irritability, somatic complaints, acting out behaviors, and frequent crying (Connolly et al. 2016). Additionally, often these patients have other psychosocial pressures or demands that may make the diagnostic picture cloudy. While many of these symptoms may be signs of an actual physical condition, when the healthcare provider finds no evidence of physical findings consistent with a specific diagnosis, anxiety must be considered as a possible cause.

When children present with any of these complaints along with frequent absences from school and/or an inability to perform routine daily activities, it is of utmost importance that the APRN consider anxiety as a possible cause of the symptoms. Making the diagnosis of anxiety disorders in children and adolescents is not always clear cut. APRNs have to keep in mind that children and young adolescents may not recognize their symptoms of anxiety and may struggle with reporting how they feel. Additionally, many of the physical symptoms, including vomiting, abdominal pain, and/or frequent headaches, are concerning to many providers because of possible physical causes, making the possibility that anxiety is the cause even more difficult to identify.

The goals of assessment by any APRN are to help the child and parent understand the meaning of the symptoms and to rule out a physical cause unrelated to the anxiety (AACAP 2007). When an APRN is presented with these symptoms in the face of a normal physical examination and normal test results, anxiety must be considered. APRNs should be sure to include in all of their assessments a comprehensive history that addresses possible sources of stress and anxiety in the child and/or family.

The following questions can help guide the assessment:

1. What are the symptoms?
2. Are the symptoms stimulus specific, spontaneous, or anticipatory?
3. Are the symptoms out of the realm of normal functioning?
4. When did the presenting symptoms begin to cause problems for the child/adolescent?
5. How is this influencing daily functioning? Assess the specific spheres, including home, school, occupation, interpersonal, and social.
6. Who is expressing concerns about this child or adolescent? Assess teachers, daycare providers, other family members, or probation officers (if the juvenile justice system is involved).

When evaluating these children, the answers to these questions can help guide the APRN in determining the cause of somatic complaints. Symptoms that happen more often on school days than on weekends or those that seem to be stimulus specific should alert the provider to a possible anxiety disorder. Symptoms that appear to be severe in view of a normal physical examination and laboratory tests are concerning for anxiety. Additionally, when symptoms influence the child's or adolescent's daily functioning, an anxiety disorder should be included as a possible diagnosis. In trying to discriminate normal, adaptive, and protective fear from pathological anxiety, the APRN will find that pathological anxiety is more diffuse, lacks specificity, and occurs in the absence of a stimulus (Krain et al. 2007). While many of these symptoms are common complaints among children and adolescents, when the cause is an anxiety disorder, the examination and laboratory results will be normal. APRNs must be aware of the common somatic complaints seen in anxiety disorders in order to accurately identify and diagnose this condition and provide appropriate treatment for these children and adolescents.

Younger children may not be able to verbalize their symptoms of anxiety, therefore the APRN should observe for behavioral symptoms such as crying, irritability, avoidance, clingy behaviors, or somatic complaints (AACAP 2007). Medical causes of anxiety should be ruled out first. Medical conditions that mimic anxiety include hyperthyroidism, asthma, seizure, caffeinism, migraines, hypoglycemia, and lead intoxication. Prescription medications used to treat certain conditions can induce anxiety and should be assessed as anxious children are more likely to have health problems such as asthma, gastrointestinal disorders, and allergies (Connolly et al. 2016).

Diagnostic Screening Instruments

Once the APRN considers that a child or an adolescent patient may be suffering from anxiety, he or she may use one of the available screening tools to aid in making the final diagnosis. Assessment is best accomplished with a careful assessment of all symptoms combined with standardized symptom measures. While a variety of standardized instruments exists for evaluating anxiety in children and adolescents, none are comprehensive enough to fully evaluate this disorder. Beginning with open-ended questions is the best way to begin assessing anxiety in a child or adolescent, followed by use of standardized instruments that confirm or deny a suspected anxiety disorder.

The most commonly used standardized assessments include the Multidimensional Anxiety Scale for Children (MASC), a self-report tool for youngsters aged 8–19 years old that is available for purchase for use with children and parents (March et al. 1997). The parent-reported Preschool Anxiety Scale is for children aged 2.5–6.5 years (available for free from www.wpic.pitt.edu/research). The Screen for Child Anxiety Related Emotional Disorders (SCARED) scale is a 41-item self-report questionnaire that is administered to both the child and parent (Birmaher et al. 1999). This also available for free at www.scaswebsite.com. Also useful in identifying pediatric anxiety and symptom changes is the Child Behavior Checklist (CBCL), available in a parent form, a youth self-report form, and a teacher form (Achenbach 2001). Numerous standardized rating scales are available for use as screening tools but should never be used alone to diagnose anxiety disorders; these are a useful adjunct to open-ended interviewing available to primary providers.

A promising new tool for assessing anxiety disorders in children and adolescents is the Youth Anxiety Measure for DSM-5 (YAM-5). Using the DSM-5 classification system it is constructed in two parts focusing on major anxiety disorders and specific phobias. It is a self and parent report questionnaire showing promise for those working with this population (Muris et al. 2017). Internal consistency and validity are being assessed.

Making the Diagnosis

While APRNs may not feel comfortable making the final diagnosis of anxiety disorder, one should be able to identify those children whose symptoms are related to anxiety and refer them appropriately to a psychiatric provider. In evaluating all children, APRNs must be cognizant of common complaints that may represent anxiety as well as understand the normal developmental anxieties of children. When presented with a child with physical complaints with no identifiable physical diagnosis, anxiety must be part of the differential. Use of approved tools for identifying anxiety can help the provider in assessing these children. Discussion of possible stressors in the child or family can aid in making the diagnosis as well. APRNs should interview the child alone when considering anxiety as a possible diagnosis because children may not feel free to discuss their worries when parents are in the room. Additionally, if abuse is causing the anxiety, the child may be unable to discuss the abuse with the parent present. The primary provider should also interview the parent(s) without the child present to assess for any stressors within or outside the family that may be impacting the child. If no cause is found for any of the child's complaints, APRNs must consider anxiety as a possible diagnosis even if the child and parent deny any source of anxiety.

APRNs providing primary healthcare should refer any child or adolescent with sustained or complex symptoms of anxiety for a full evaluation by a psychiatric clinician. Helping parents understand the importance of seeing a psychiatric clinician is an important part of the diagnostic process as often parents are reluctant to seek psychological help. The relationship between the parent and APRN is an important aspect of the workup as many parents are unable to accept a psychiatric diagnosis as a cause of their child's problem and refuse to follow up when referred. Using the approved diagnostic tools in the primary care setting may help APRNs demonstrate to parents that anxiety is a diagnosis that requires treatment the same way that a throat infection does. The stigma of psychological diagnosis is often a barrier to parents and families seeking and/or following through with treatment. Part of the primary care APRN's role is in connecting the families with the appropriate source for care and helping them recognize the importance of getting psychological help for their child in order to promote the child's optimal health and wellbeing.

Comorbidities of Anxiety Disorder with Other Psychiatric Disorders

The most diagnostically challenging patients are those who present with unclear symptoms of anxiety that are interfering with functioning or anxiety that, while defined, are comorbid with other psychiatric disorders. There is a high rate of comorbidity between anxiety and other psychiatric disorders. Depression, ADHD (MTA Cooperative Group 2001), oppositional defiant disorder, and learning disorders are commonly comorbid with anxiety disorders. Additional comorbid conditions include panic disorders, SM, and SAD. The risk of developing substance abuse in adolescence is increased after experiencing a childhood anxiety disorder (Connolly et al. 2016).

The issue of comorbidity is important from a symptom severity standpoint and from the diagnostic complexities presented by a child who suffers from more than two psychiatric disorders. Overlapping symptoms can make accurate diagnosis difficult (AACAP 2007). Comorbidity, once defined by the APRN in primary care settings, might necessitate a referral for more comprehensive psychiatric evaluation.

Models of Treatment

Psychological Management of Anxiety Disorders

Anxiety disorders in childhood are predictors of psychiatric disorders in adolescence and later in life (Connolly et al. 2016). A multimodal treatment approach for pediatric anxiety disorders involves parent and child education about the disorder, consultation with all involved school, healthcare, and community professionals, and a treatment plan that considers behavioral interventions (AACAP 2007). The severity and degree of impairment from anxiety symptoms will determine the use of medication management as an adjunct to behavioral/psychological treatment. Anxiety can be a lifelong impairment and may require long-term treatment.

From an evidence-based perspective, the treatment of choice for anxiety in children and adolescents is cognitive-behavioral therapy (CBT) (Beidel and Reinecke 2016). Originally, behavior therapy resulted from theoretical frameworks involving classical and operant conditioning. Over time it was increasingly recognized that person–environment interactions were influenced by thinking. The premise of behavior therapy was that changing behaviors would result in altering distressing thoughts and feelings

(Compton et al. 2004). Cognitive models work to connect negative self-talk and negative cognitive schemas, while correcting cognitive distortions. Psychiatric APRNs teach children a new set of adaptive coping skills for specific symptoms of anxiety. These new coping skills include relaxation training, feeling identification, confronting rather than avoiding fears, and decreasing emotional arousal of anxiety cues (Kendall 2018). This can include social skills training, assertiveness training, and positive reinforcement. Systematic desensitization, problem-solving skills, and extinction are all part of the skill set that can be taught to an anxious child.

CBT is a term that encompasses several models of treatment. Nevertheless, there are five shared premises among most CBT treatment models:

1. Adherence to the scientist–clinician model, whereby treatments are chosen based on demonstrated evidence or are applied within a case evaluation format to determine efficacy.
2. A thorough idiographic assessment (e.g. functional analysis) of target behaviors and the situational, cognitive, and behavioral factors that have established or are managing the symptoms of interest.
3. An emphasis on psychoeducation that identifies the specific triggers to the anxiety and the meaning of the anxious symptoms to physical and emotional health.
4. Problem-specific treatment interventions designed to ameliorate the symptoms of concern.
5. Relapse prevention and generalization training at the end of treatment (Compton et al. 2004, p. 930).

Models of CBT treatment are a good choice for managing pediatric anxiety (Cresswell et al. 2014). The common targets of these interventions, cognitive interventions, social and behavioral interventions, and environmental interventions assist in understanding symptoms in the context of the child's life (Connolly et al. 2016). The goal of treatment is normal child development that is not hindered by anxiety symptoms. There are specific interventions for trauma-based anxiety in children and adolescents. A number of manualized treatments have developed and generally include psychoeducation, parenting skills, relaxation skills, affect expression, and development of coping skills through writing a trauma narrative. Research has found that this model is highly effective in youth with post-traumatic stress disorders. A popular and useful example of this is the Coping Cat Workbook (Kendall 1992), developed by Philip Kendall. This program lasts 16–20 weeks and can be used by APRNs as they provide outpatient care. It has demonstrated excellent results for treating anxiety in children and adolescents.

Psychotropic Medication Management of Anxiety Disorders

It is strongly recommended that a course of psychosocial treatment be considered for patients with mild to severe symptoms of anxiety prior to initiating medication management. If the patient has had 6–8 weeks of behavior therapy with no resolution of symptoms, symptoms worsen, has comorbid psychiatric disorders, or has daily impairment of functioning, medication should be considered. Spheres of child assessment include home, school, occupational, interpersonal, and social. Impairment of functioning in three or more of these spheres might necessitate consideration of a medication trial. Consideration of psychotropic medication for anxiety disorders generally occurs after the child and family have participated in CBT or other behavior therapy or if the symptoms of anxiety are severe and unrelenting and unresponsive to less invasive treatment. Medication is ideally used as an adjunct to CBT and should not be used in isolation (Connolly et al. 2016).

While APRNs and other healthcare providers may be pressured by family members to prescribe medications for pediatric anxiety disorder symptoms, the decision to medicate anxiety requires careful consideration of several factors. Ideally medication is used as part of a multimodal treatment plan. Children with some symptoms of anxiety alone should not be medicated; rather, only children who meet the criteria for an anxiety disorder and those involved in CBT or having only partial resolution of symptoms should be prescribed medications. Like most disorders, anxiety requires a combination of pharmacologic and nonpharmacologic treatment to be most effective (Connolly et al. 2016).

When making the decision of whether or not to medicate, a number of questions should be asked. Are there associated medical conditions that could precipitate the anxiety? Is the anxiety related to a medical condition or is the medical condition part of a GAD? What medication, herbal supplements, and over-the-counter preparations are the child taking? Herbal supplements and over-the-counter medications may cause symptoms that mimic anxiety, such as heart palpitations or restlessness. Always carefully assess all over-the-counter, herbal, and prescribed medication being taken by the child. Additionally, healthcare providers must inform parents of the potential interactions between antianxiety medications and herbs or over-the-counter medications for those children requiring medications to treat their anxiety. Is there any current or past substance use by the child or family members living in the immediate household? Medications used to treat anxiety disorders can have a high abuse/misuse potential (Hernandez and Nelson 2010); other family members may access the child's prescribed medication for illicit use.

A thorough physical examination is needed for the anxious child or adolescent to rule out cardiac problems or seizure disorder. These conditions and other disorders could be influencing the presence of anxiety symptoms (Jha 2016). Before undertaking any pharmacologic intervention any child with a history of congenital heart defects or rhythm disturbances should be evaluated by a cardiologist prior to starting medications for medical clearance.

An additional key aspect to medication management is determining the family attitudes to the use of psychotropic medication. Certain cultural and family beliefs do not condone the use of psychotropic medications. Salloum et al. (2016) found that while anxiety disorders are the most common psychiatric disorder among children in the United States, many children do not receive medication. Common barriers to receiving care included parents not knowing where to go to seek care, stigma, and cultural beliefs. They recommended development of interventions that addressed these barriers by helping parents access care/treatment that was cost-effective, addressing cultural beliefs, and minimizing stigma.

Cultural beliefs are essential issues for APRNs when considering pediatric anxiety. The family's beliefs and level of trust in the mental health field have a strong impact on a child's treatment. Many families are a composite of several cultures and their response to psychiatric issues may not be predictable or normative for a specific culture. Addressing the family's concerns and repeatedly answering questions are important in helping to ensure adherence with the prescribed treatment plan. The effect that cultural beliefs have on the diagnosis and treatment of children with anxiety disorders cannot be ignored. APRNs, who have likely fostered a level of trust with parents, often are able to work closely with the psychiatric provider to support choice of treatment options. This collaboration may increase the likelihood of the family following through with the plan of care.

If the family does decide to allow the child to be treated with medication, other considerations include the following: Does the family have sufficient organization to safely manage giving and storing a psychiatric medication? If the anxiety disorder is comorbid with depression, is suicide a risk? This makes development of a safety plan with the family and safe storing of medication even more essential.

Medications

The most studied and widely used medications for anxiety are selective serotonin reuptake inhibitors (SSRIs). These include Prozac (fluoxetine), Zoloft (sertraline), Celexa (citalopram), and Paxil (paroxetine). The general side effects of these medications include nausea, vomiting, diarrhea, headaches, dizziness, sleep disorders, weight changes (gain and loss), and skin rashes. Side effects can vary by individual (Emslie et al. 2016). SSRIs may also carry a risk of increased suicidal thinking and behavior. Psychoeducation must focus on the side effects and potential risk of these medications. See Chapter 9 for a description of medications used to treat anxiety disorders.

Benzodiazepines are a class of medication usually used to treat adult anxiety disorders; they are rarely used to manage long-term pediatric anxiety given the lack of evidence-based efficacy and the abuse potential for both the patient and family members. Benzodiazepines may be administered for short-term use as well as with event-specific sources of anxiety such as medical procedures to help alleviate anxiety or for severe panic disorder. Similarly, tricyclic antidepressants, while effective with pediatric anxiety, are rarely used because of their side effect profile and adverse cardiac effects. Currently, SSRIs are the first pharmacological choice for treating pediatric anxiety disorders (Emslie et al. 2016).

Combined CBT and SSRI treatment is an effective, evidence-based strategy for treating children and adolescents with anxiety disorder. Walkup et al. (2008) evaluated 488 children and adolescents with SAD, GAD, or social phobia who received either 14 sessions of CBT, sertraline, combined CBT and sertraline, or a placebo for 12 weeks. Results showed those who received the combined therapy of CBT and sertraline had an 80% improvement on the Clinical Global Improvement Scale compared to 59% for the CBT-alone group and 54% for the sertraline-alone group. The placebo group had a 23% ratio of improvement in symptoms of anxiety.

Integration with Primary Care and Referral

The role of the APRN in primary care is to identify those children or adolescents with symptoms of an anxiety disorder. While the APRN may not be able to make the actual diagnosis, he or she must be able to identify those patients who present with symptoms of anxiety that are outside of the normal developmental anxieties of childhood and are causing ongoing stress that interferes with normal developmental tasks. Once a patient has been identified with symptoms of a possible anxiety disorder, he or she should be referred for further evaluation and testing by an appropriate child psychiatric APRN or other psychiatric provider. The APRN can play an integral role in helping parents understand the importance of seeking out psychiatric care for their child because of the relationship they have developed over time with the families. APRNs can help with facilitating the connection with a child psychiatric specialist and with continued evaluation and care of the child throughout their treatment.

Management of Anxiety Disorders and Implications for Practice, Research, and Education

Anxiety in children and adolescents is a common presentation to pediatric primary care practices. Psychiatric resources are essential for referring patients to psychiatric care when their anxiety becomes debilitating and interferes with functioning and development. Primary care APRNs are likely to see these children first during well-child visits. They have an opportunity to evaluate and intervene in a potentially debilitating disorder. The high rate of anxiety disorders among children makes it imperative that APRNs understand the disorder, how to evaluate symptoms, and how to plan care. The challenge comes in ensuring that primary care APRNs have the basic assessment skills and the clinical time to assess anxiety while also having access to child psychiatric services that will support their assessment and provide needed psychiatric treatment. The partnership between primary care APRNs and child psychiatric APRNs will result in more comprehensive care for children and adolescents presenting with anxiety that disrupts their development.

Summary

This chapter has given an overview of anxiety in children and adolescents, focusing on normal development, epidemiology, theories of etiology, and the types of anxiety disorders that children and adolescents present when seen in pediatric primary care. Comorbid conditions and evidence-based assessments and interventions have been presented, along with the role differentiation between APRNs focused on psychiatric treatment versus those focused on primary care management. Whenever possible, behavior interventions such as CBT should be used to treat symptoms of anxiety. Implications for research and practice were also discussed.

Resources for Practitioners and Families

Anxiety Disorders Association of American. https://adaa.org.

Mental Health American (Children's Mental Health Resource List). http://www.mentalhealthamerica.net/conditions/adhd-and-kids).

National Institute of Mental Health (Anxiety Disorders). https://www.nimh.nih.gov/health/topics/anxiety-disorders/index.shtml.

International OCD Foundation. https://iocdf.org.

Thought Questions

1. At what point in the treatment should the primary care APRN seek additional psychiatric care for a child who initially presented with an anxiety

disorder but seems to be struggling with a more complex problem?

2. What are the indicators that there is a need for collaboration?

3. What relationships should the primary care APRN have with psychiatric providers prior to making a referral for care?

References

Achenbach, T.M. (2001). *Manual for the Child Behavior Checklist/4–18 and 1991 Profile*. Burlington, VT: University of Vermont Department of Psychiatry.

AACAP (2007). Practice parameter for the assessment and treatment of children and adolescents with anxiety disorders. *Journal of the American Academy of Child and Adolescent Psychiatry* 46: 267–283.

APA (2013). *Diagnostic and Statistical Manual of Mental Disorders 5*. Washington, DC: American Psychiatric Association.

Batte, S., Watson, A.R., and Amess, K. (2006). The effects of chronic renal failure on siblings. *Pediatric Nephrology* 21: 246–250.

Beesdo, K., Knappe, S., and Pine, D.S. (2009). Anxiety and anxiety disorders in children and adolescents: developmental issues and implications for DSM-V. *Psychiatric Clinics of North America* 32: 483–524.

Beidel, D.C. and Reinecke, M.A. (2016). Cognitive-behavioral treatment for anxiety and depression. In: *Dulcan's Textbook of Child and Adolescent Psychiatry*, 2e (ed. M. Dulcan), 973–991. Arlington, VA: American Psychiatric Association.

Benjet, C., Borges, G., and Medina-Mora, M.E. (2010). Chronic childhood adversity and onset of psychopathology during three life stages: childhood, adolescence and adulthood. *Journal of Psychiatric Research* 44: 732–740.

Bennett, K., Manassis, K., Duda, S. et al. (2015). Preventing child and adolescent anxiety disorders: overview of systematic reviews. *Focus on Treatment Response Predictors* 32: 909–918.

Birmaher, B., Brent, D.A., Chiappetta, L. et al. (1999). Psychometric properties of the Screen for Child Anxiety Related Emotional Disorders (SCARED): a replication study. *Journal of the American Academy of Child and Adolescent Psychiatry* 38: 1230–1236.

Bistko, R., Holbrook, J., Ghandour, R. et al. (2018). Epidemiology and impact of health care provider-diagnosed anxiety and depression among US children. *Journal of Developmental & Behavioral Pediatrics* 39 (5): 395–403.

Compton, S.N., March, J.S., Brent, D. et al. (2004). Cognitive-behavioral psychotherapy for anxiety and depressive disorders in children and adolescents: an evidence-based medicine review. *Journal of the American Academy of Child and Adolescent Psychiatry* 8: 930–959.

Connolly, S.D., Suarez, L.M., Victor, A.M. et al. (2016). Anxiety disorders. In: *Dulcan's Textbook of Child and Adolescent Psychiatry*, 2e (ed. M. Dulcan), 305–343. Arlington, VA: American Psychiatric Association.

Cresswell, C., Waite, P., and Cooper, P.J. (2014). Assessment and management of anxiety disorders in children and adolescents. *Archives of Disease in Childhood* 99: 674–678.

Emslie, G.J., Croarkin, P., Chapman, M.R., and Mayes, T.L. (2016). Antidepressants. In: *Dulcan's Textbook of Child and Adolescent Psychiatry* (ed. M. Dulcan), 737–768. Arlington, VA: American Psychiatric Association.

Ginsburg, G.S., Riddle, M.A., and Davies, M. (2006). Somatic complaints in children and adolescents with anxiety disorders. *Journal of the American Academy of Child and Adolescent Psychiatry* 45: 1179–1187.

Ginsburg, G.S., Becker-Haimes, E.M., Keeton, C. et al. (2018). Results from the child/adolescent anxiety multimodal extended long-term study (CAMELS): primary anxiety outcomes. *Journal of the American Academy of Child and Adolescent Psychiatry* 57: 471–480.

Gregory, A.M. and Eley, T.C. (2007). Genetic influences on anxiety in children: what we've learned and where we're heading. *Clinical Child and Family Psychology* 10: 199–212.

Hernandez, S.H. and Nelson, L.S. (2010). Prescription drug abuse: insight into the epidemic. *Clinical Pharmacology and Therapeutics* 88: 307–317.

Hirshfeld-Becker, D.R., Micco, J.A., Simoes, N.A., and Henin, A. (2008). High risk studies and developmental antecedents of anxiety disorders. *American Journal of Medical Genetics* 148C: 99–117.

Jha, P. (2016). Assessing the elementary school-age child. In: *Dulcan's Textbook of Child and Adolescent Psychiatry*, 2e (ed. M. Dulcan), 57–71. Arlington, VA: American Psychiatric Association.

Kashdan, T.B. and Herbert, J.D. (2001). Social anxiety disorder in childhood and adolescence: current status and future directions. *Clinical Child and Family Psychology Review* 4 (1): 37–61.

Kendall, P.C. (1992). *Coping Cat Workbook*. Ardmore, PA: Workbook Publishing.

Kendall, P. (ed.) (2018). *Cognitive Therapy with Children and Adolescents: A Casebook for Clinical Practice*, 3e. New York, NY: Guilford Press.

Krain, A., Ghaffari, M., Freeman, J. et al. (2007). Anxiety disorders. In: *Lewis' Child and Adolescent Psychiatry: A Comprehensive Textbook*, 4e (eds. A. Martin and F.R. Volkman), 538–547. Philadelphia, PA: Lippincott Williams & Wilkin.

Laurin, J., Joussemet, M., Tremblay, R., and Bolvin, M. (2015). Early forms of controlling parenting and the development of childhood anxiety. *Journal of Child and Family Studies* 24: 3279–3292.

Leis, J.A. and Mendelson, T. (2010). Intergenerational transmission of psychopathology: minor versus major parental depression. *Journal of Nervous and Mental Disorders* 198: 356–361.

March, J.S., Parker, J.D., Sullivan, K. et al. (1997). The Multidimensional Anxiety Scale for Children (MASC): factor structure, reliability, and validity. *Journal of the American Academy of Child and Adolescent Psychiatry* 36: 1645–1646.

Moore, P.S., Whaley, S.E., and Sigman, M. (2004). Interactions between mothers and children: impacts of maternal and child anxiety. *Journal of Abnormal Psychology* 113: 471–476.

MTA Cooperative Group (2001). ADHD comorbidity findings from the MTA study: comparing comorbid subgroups. *Journal of the American Academy of Child and Adolescent Psychiatry* 40: 147–158.

Muris, P., Simon, E., Lijphart, H. et al. (2017). The youth anxiety measure for DSM-5 (YAM-5): development and first psychometric evidence of a new scale for assessing anxiety disorders symptoms of children and adolescents. *Child Psychiatry and Human Development* 48: 1–17. https://doi.org/10.1007/s10578-016-0648-1.

Pabian, S. and Vandebosch, H. (2016). An investigation of short-term longitudinal associations between social anxiety and victimization and perpetration of traditional bullying and cyberbullying. *Journal of Youth and Adolescence* 45: 328–339. https://doi.org/10.1007/s10964-015-0259-3.

Salloum, A., Johnco, C., Lewin, A.B. et al. (2016). Barriers to access and participation in community mental health treatment for anxious children. *Journal of Affective Disorders* 196: 54–61. https://doi.org/10.1016/j.jad.2016.02.026.

Stuart-Parrigon, K.L. and Kerns, K.A. (2016). Family processes in child anxiety: the long-term impact of fathers and mothers. *Journal of Abnormal Child Psychology* 44: 1253–1266.

Suarez, L.M., Bennett, S.M., Goldstein, C.R., and Barlow, D.H. (2009). Understanding anxiety disorders from a "triple vulnerability" framework. In: *Oxford Handbook of Anxiety and Related Disorders* (eds. M.M. Anthony and M.B. Stein), 153–172. New York, NY: Oxford University Press.

Walkup, J.T., Albano, A.M., Piacentini, J. et al. (2008). Cognitive behavioral therapy, sertraline, or a combination in childhood anxiety. *New England Journal of Medicine* 359: 2753–2766.

Wehry, A.M., Beesdo-Baum, K., Hennelly, M.M. et al. (2015). Assessment and treatment of anxiety disorders in children and adolescents. *Current Psychiatry Reports* 17: 52. https://doi.org/10.1007/s11920-015-0591-z.

Whaley, S.E., Pinto, A., and Sigman, M. (1999). Characterizing interactions between anxious mothers and their children. *Journal of Consulting Clinical Psychology* 67 (6): 826–836. https://doi.org/10.1037//0022-006x.67.6.826.

12

Mood Dysregulation Disorders

Mikki Meadows-Oliver[1] and Edilma L. Yearwood[2]

[1]Quinnipiac University School of Nursing, Hamden, CT, USA
[2]Georgetown University School of Nursing & Health Studies, Washington DC, USA

Objectives

After reading this chapter, advanced practice registered nurses (APRNs) will be able to:

1. Describe clinical presentations of children and adolescents experiencing a variety of mood dysregulation disorder challenges.
2. Examine neurobiological, environmental, relational, and other etiological risk factors associated with disorders of mood.
3. Analyze the evidence related to assessment and management of mood dysregulation disorders in children and adolescents.
4. Identify potential consequences of untreated mood dysregulation disorders.
5. Differentiate between the roles and responsibilities of primary care practitioners and child and adolescent psychiatric-mental health APRNs in managing the range of mood dysregulation disorders in children and adolescents.

Introduction

It is estimated that there are 2.5 billion youth (children and adolescents) world-wide (UN Department of Economic and Social Affairs 2015). Nearly 20% of these youth will have an emotional, mental, or behavioral disorder at some time during their formative years, with symptoms preceding the diagnosis of a disorder by up to 4 years (Skokauskas et al. 2018; World Health Organization [WHO] 2019). The World Economic Forum estimates that the cost of mental illness between 2011 and 2030 will be US$16 trillion and that untreated anxiety and depression will cost US$1.15 trillion annually (Bloom et al. 2011; Chisholm et al. 2016). In a recently reported study on insurance claims from 2012 to 2013 reported in Academic Pediatrics, children and adolescents with coexisting chronic medical conditions and mental health and substance use disorders had 2.4 times higher healthcare payment cost than those with only a chronic health condition. They further estimated that in the United States US$8.8 billion is spent annually on coexisting mental health and substance use disorders in youth (Perrin et al. 2019). In the United States, approximately 10% of pediatric inpatient hospitalizations were due to a mental health diagnosis, with the most frequent and costly diagnosis being depression followed by bipolar disorder and then psychosis, with an associated cost of over US$2.5 billion (Bardach et al. 2014).

Child and Adolescent Behavioral Health: A Resource for Advanced Practice Psychiatric and Primary Care Practitioners in Nursing,
Second Edition. Edited by Edilma L. Yearwood, Geraldine S. Pearson, and Jamesetta A. Newland.
© 2021 John Wiley & Sons, Inc. Published 2021 by John Wiley & Sons, Inc.
Companion website: www.wiley.com/go/Yearwood

Of the 74.5 million children and adolescents in the United States, there are approximately 17 million with a diagnosable mental or behavioral health concern (Centers for Disease Control and Prevention n.d.; Ghandour et al. 2019). In addition, 1.9 million or 3.2% of 3–17-year-olds have a diagnosis of depression (Ghandour et al. 2019), with depression one of the leading causes of illness and disability in 15–19-year-olds worldwide (WHO 2019). The WHO identifies mental health conditions as responsible for 16% of the Global Burden of Disease (GBD) and injury in people aged 10–19, with half of mental health conditions commencing by age 14 (2019). Pediatric bipolar, now more commonly referred to as disruptive mood dysregulation disorder (DMDD), is estimated to impact between 0.8% and 4.3% of youth (Tang and Pinsky 2015). Adolescent girls are twice as likely to be diagnosed with depression than boys while boys are more likely to be diagnosed with DMDD compared to girls (Child Mind Institute n.d.). Mood dysregulation disorders are a leading contributor to suicide attempts and suicide completion in youth, with suicide now the third cause of death in the adolescent population worldwide (WHO 2019).

This chapter provides an overview of several *Diagnostic and Statistical Manual of Mental Disorders*, 5th edition (DSM-5) (American Psychiatric Association [APA] 2013) mood or affective disorders, including major depression (MD), DMDD, and persistent mood disorder (PMD). In addition, severe mood disorder, described by the National Institute of Mental Health [NIMH], and pediatric bipolar disorder (PBD) will be described briefly (NIMH n.d.). In children and adolescents, depression is one of the three most common psychological symptoms. If left untreated, mood symptoms can progress to a diagnosable disorder with possible engagement in self-destructive activities such as substance use, self-harm, aggression, and isolation. For the purposes of this chapter, mood dysregulation disorders refer to behavioral, psychological, and physiological impairment in the normal regulatory mechanisms associated with mood/affective states. These disorders are dynamic, influenced by internal and external stimuli, and can be reactive to real-life settings and contextual events, whether real or perceived (Ebner-Priemer and Trull 2009; Siever and Davis 1985).

In adolescence, peer pressure, struggles for a sense of autonomy and belonging, relationships within and outside of the family, academic pressures, identity challenges, and exposure to violence and social media can all pose threats to psychological wellbeing (WHO 2019). When mood dysregulation disorders first occur in childhood or adolescence, they can have a long-term impact on quality of life, relationships, academic achievements, self-esteem, and emotional and psychological integrity. Symptom management is dependent on motivation to

seek treatment, availability of human and structural treatment resources, active engagement in treatment, and the success of treatment efforts. Mood disorders are common globally, usually present in late adolescence to early adulthood, impact females at twice the rate of men, and are characterized by low treatment seeking behaviors (Kessler and Bromet 2013). The WHO estimates that unipolar depressive disorders will rise from having been the third cause of GBD to become the leading cause of GBD by 2030 (WHO 2019).

Furthermore, what is concerning is that approximately 50% of children and adolescents experience a depressive episode relapse and 70% have a recurrence of symptoms within 5 years, a harbinger of a potential cycle of worrisome chronicity (Jeffrey et al. 2005). Depression rates between boys and girls under the age of 12 are comparable. However, at puberty there is a dramatic shift, with girls experiencing mood disorders at a 2 : 1 ratio when compared to boys (Costello et al. 2006; Steingard n.d.). It is difficult to accurately assess how many children and adolescents under the age of 18 experience nondiagnosable mood symptoms and to determine the impact of these symptoms on their normal developmental trajectory and quality of life.

This chapter includes specific DSM-5 diagnostic symptoms of MD, persistent depressive disorder (PDD), and DMDD in children and adolescents. Additionally, PBD and the NIMH researched severe mood dysregulation (SMD) disorder descriptors are presented (Stringaris et al. 2018). Associated risk factors and etiology, screening and assessment tools for use in primary care, evidence-based management strategies, roles for the APRN, consequences of untreated mood dysregulation disorders, and implications for conducting and using nursing research in practice with this population are also presented. What is abundantly clear from the data on these disorders is that prevention, early detection, and evidence-based treatment can positively influence the quality of life of those at risk for or affected by these disorders and their long-term prognosis.

Symptom Recognition in Children and Adolescents

Accurately diagnosing mood dysregulation disorders in childhood and adolescence can be difficult due to the potential for comorbid disorders and symptoms in this population, and the rapid growth and maturational shifts characteristic of individuals under the age of 18 years. Mood disorders can be viewed as variable and on a spectrum of symptoms that range from mild to severe. In addition, they reflect challenges with regulation and span internalizing and externalizing behaviors. One cardinal symptom associated with mood/affective disorders appears to be irritability. Irritability has been defined as a heightened anger/aggressive response relative to peers at the same developmental level (Brotman et al. 2017a), and as "easy annoyance that results in anger and temper outbursts" (Noller 2016, p. 25). Researchers at NIMH have been conducting numerous studies aimed at unpacking the neurocognitive drivers, behavioral presentations, and treatment efficacy associated with irritability and other mood dysregulation disorders (Brotman et al. 2017a,b; Stringaris et al. 2018). APRNs are encouraged to stay informed about the latest evidence on these disorders and treatments from the NIMH, the DSM-5 (and future versions of the DSM), the American Academy of Pediatrics (AAP), systematic reviews and current findings from robust randomized clinical trials and evidence-based research. Tables 12.1a–c for MD, PDD, and DMDD, respectively, are discussed in this chapter.

The APRN should be alert for reported and assessed prodromal symptoms, which are the early signs of a disorder seen before an acute episode, which precede the appearance of the full range of symptoms associated with the diagnoseable condition by weeks to months (Fava and Tossani 2007). It is also important for the APRN to keep in mind the difference between a cluster of mood symptoms and the presence of enough symptoms to meet the diagnostic threshold. APRNs must rule out the possibility that the symptoms are due to a medical condition such as hypothyroidism which can mimic symptoms of depression, substance use with use of a

Table 12.1 DSM-5 diagnostic criteria for (a) major depression, (b) persistent depressive disorder (dysthymia), and (c) disruptive mood dysregulation disorder

(a) DSM-5 diagnostic criteria for major depression

A. Five (or more) of the following symptoms have been present during the same 2-week period and represent a change from previous functioning; at least one of the symptoms is either (1) depressed mood or (2) loss of interest or pleasure.

Note: Do not include symptoms that are clearly attributable to another medical condition.

1. Depressed mood most of the day, nearly every day, as indicated by either subjective report (e.g. feels sad, empty, hopeless) or observation made by others (e.g. appears tearful). (*Note:* In children and adolescents, can be irritable mood.)
2. Markedly diminished interest or pleasure in all, or almost all, activities most of the day, nearly every day (as indicated by either subjective account or observation).
3. Significant weight loss when not dieting or weight gain (e.g. a change of more than 5% of body weight in a month), or decrease or increase in appetite nearly every day. (*Note:* In children, consider failure to make expected weight gain.)
4. Insomnia or hypersomnia nearly every day.
5. Psychomotor agitation or retardation nearly every day (observable by others, not merely subjective feelings of restlessness or being slowed down).
6. Fatigue or loss of energy nearly every day.
7. Feelings of worthlessness or excessive or inappropriate guilt (which may be delusional) nearly every day (not merely self-reproach or guilt about being sick).
8. Diminished ability to think or concentrate, or indecisiveness, nearly every day (either by subjective account or as observed by others).
9. Recurrent thoughts of death (not just fear of dying), recurrent suicidal ideation without a specific plan, or a suicide attempt or a specific plan for committing suicide.

B. The symptoms cause clinically significant distress or impairment in social, occupational, or other important areas of functioning.

C. The episode is not attributable to the physiological effects of a substance or to another medical condition.

Note: Criteria A–C represent a major depressive episode.

Note: Responses to a significant loss (e.g. bereavement, financial ruin, losses from a natural disaster, a serious medical illness, or disability) may include the feelings of intense sadness, rumination about the loss, insomnia, poor appetite, and weight loss noted in Criterion A, which may resemble a depressive episode. Although such symptoms may be understandable or considered appropriate to the loss, the presence of a major depressive episode in addition to the normal response to a significant loss should also be carefully considered. This decision inevitably requires the exercise of clinical judgment based on the individual's history and the culture norms for the expression of distress in the context of loss.

D. The occurrence of the major depressive episode is not better explained by schizoaffective disorder, schizophrenia, schizophreniform disorder, delusional disorder, or other specific and unspecified schizophrenia spectrum, and other psychotic disorders.

E. There has never been a manic episode or a hypomanic episode.

Note: This exclusion does not apply if all of the manic-like or hypomanic-like episodes are substance-induced or are attributable to the physiological effects of another medical condition.

Table 12.1 (cont'd)

(b) DSM-5 diagnostic criteria for persistent depressive disorder (dysthymia)

This disorder represents a consolidation of DSM-5-defined chronic major depressive disorder and dysthymic disorder

A. Depressed mood for most of the day, for more days than not, as indicated by either subjective account or observation by others, for at least 2 years.

Note: In children and adolescents, mood can be irritable and duration must be at least 1 year.

B. Presence, while depressed, of two (or more) of the following:

1. Poor appetite or overeating.
2. Insomnia or hypersomnia.
3. Low energy or fatigue.
4. Low self-esteem.
5. Poor concentration or difficult making decisions.
6. Feelings of hopelessness.

C. During the 2-year period (1 year for children or adolescents) of the disturbance, the individual has never been without the symptoms in Criteria A and B for more than 2 months at a time.

D. Criteria for a major depressive disorder may be continuously present for 2 years.

E. There has never been a manic episode or hypomanic episode, and criteria have never been met for cyclothymic disorder.

F. The disturbance is not better explained by a persistent schizoaffective disorder, schizophrenia, delusional disorder, or other specific or unspecified schizophrenia spectrum and other psychotic disorder.

G. The symptoms are not attributable to the physiological effects of a substance (e.g. a drug of abuse, a medication) or another medical condition (e.g. hypothyroidism).

H. The symptoms cause clinically significant distress or impairment in social, occupant, or other important areas of functioning.

(c) DSM-5 diagnostic criteria for disruptive mood dysregulation disorder

A. Severe recurrent temper outbursts manifested verbally (e.g. verbal rages) and/or behaviorally (e.g. physical aggression toward people or property) that are grossly out of proportion in intensity or duration to the situation or provocation.

B. The temper outbursts are inconsistent with developmental level.

C. The temper outbursts occur, on average, three or more times per week.

D. The mood between temper outbursts is persistently irritable or angry most of the day, nearly every day, and is observable by others (e.g. parents, teachers, peers).

E. Criteria A–D have been present for 12 or more months. Throughout that time, the individual has not had a period lasting 3 or more consecutive months without all of the symptoms in Criteria A–D.

F. Criteria A and D are present in at least two of three settings (i.e. at home, at school, with peers) and are severe in at least one of these.

G. The diagnosis should not be made for the first time before age 6 years or after age 18 years.

H. By history or observation, the age at onset of Criteria A–E is before 10 years.

I. There has never been a distinct period lasting more than 1 day during which the full symptom criteria, except duration, for a manic or hypomanic episode have been met.

Note: Developmentally appropriate mood elevation, such as occurs in the context of a highly positive event or its anticipation, should not be considered as a symptom of mania or hypomania.

J. The behaviors do not occur exclusively during an episode of major depressive disorder and are not better explained by another mental disorder (e.g. autism spectrum disorder, post-traumatic stress disorder, separation anxiety disorder, persistent depressive disorder [dysthymia]).

Note: The diagnosis cannot coexist with oppositional defiant disorder, intermittent explosive disorder, or bipolar disorder, though it can coexist with others, including major depressive disorder, attention-deficit/hyperactivity disorder, conduct disorder, and substance use disorders. Individuals whose symptoms meet criteria for both disruptive mood dysregulation disorder and oppositional defiant disorder should only be given the diagnosis of disruptive mood dysregulation disorder. If an individual has ever experienced a manic or hypomanic episode, the diagnosis of disruptive mood dysregulation disorder should not be assigned.

central nervous system (CNS) depressant such as alcohol (again consistent with some symptoms associated with depression), use of a stimulant such as cocaine or amphetamines (associated with irritability, insomnia, mania/hypomania), head trauma (associated with depression or hypomania/mania), hyperthyroidism (associated with symptoms of hypomania/mania), or side effects from *prescribed* medications such as an anticonvulsant, oral contraceptive, or alpha adrenergic agonists like clonidine (associated with depressive symptoms) (Hamrin and Magorno 2010; WebMd n.d.).

Depressive Disorders

Major Depression

Unipolar depression is an affective disorder characterized by chronic feelings of sadness and worthlessness, dark moods, and inability to find enjoyment in things (Child Mind Institute n.d.). Many adults trace the start of their mood symptoms to their childhood. For a diagnosis of MD to be made, there has to be a change from previous functioning, a 2-week duration of symptoms accompanied by five or more of the nine behavioral criteria for the disorder, and presence of either depressed mood *or* anhedonia (APA 2013).

Common comorbid psychiatric diagnoses include anxiety (25–50%), substance use, enuresis or encopresis, conduct disorder, eating disorder, and attention deficit hyperactivity disorder (ADHD) (Anderson and Hope 2008; Forman-Hoffman et al. 2016; Mullen 2018). Somatization symptoms including headaches, stomachaches, and pain along with psychosocial experiences such as trauma, par-

ent–child difficulties, and poor academic achievement may also be part of the child or adolescent presentation (Batelaan 2016; Jeffrey et al. 2005; Mullen 2018). Other comorbidities can include chronic health conditions such as obesity, asthma, and diabetes (Forman-Hoffman et al. 2016). Table 12.2 provides the APRN with symptoms of depressed mood that may be seen or reported by the parent, caretaker, or child or adolescent themselves.

Depression in children and adolescents is usually classified as mild, moderate, or severe. In mild depression, there are fewer symptoms experienced or seen, scores on standardized screening tools are lower (closer to normal scores), and duration of symptoms may be brief, with minimal impact on the individual's functioning. If the depression is assessed as moderate, there are more symptoms which are usually accompanied by functional impairment. In severe depression, the individual has significant impairment in functioning and is considered to be in an acute state with symptoms exceeding those needed to make the diagnosis (APA 2013). The individual may present as actively suicidal, significantly regressed, with significant psychomotor retardation, or psychotic (Hamrin and Magorno 2010; Jeffrey et al. 2005).

Disruptive Mood Dysregulation Disorder

DMDD was added to the DSM-5 in 2013 in response to the controversy over whether children could be diagnosed early as meeting the criteria for bipolar disorder. The cardinal symptom of this dysregulation disorder is chronic and severe irritability accompanied by frequent

Table 12.2 Common symptoms associated with depressed mood

Young children	Adolescents	Both
Somatization (headaches, gastrointestinal disturbances, stomachaches, malaise)	Anhedonia	Suicidal ideation or attempt
	Apathy	Irritability/anger
Sad affect	Hopelessness	Insomnia/hypersomnia
Social withdrawal	Delusions	Poor concentration
Soft spoken/quiet	Psychomotor retardation	Appetite disturbance
Poor self-esteem	Neglect of hygiene	Fatigue/lethargy
Helplessness	Suicidal ideation and/or attempt(s)	Impaired academic functioning
Auditory hallucinations	Behavioral problems	Impaired social functioning
		Rumination
		Negative self-talk/negative self-attributes
		Verbal outbursts/tantrums
		Social isolation

Source: Adapted from Sadock, B.J. & Sadock, V.A. (2009). Kaplan & Sadock's Concise Textbook of Child and Adolescent Psychiatry. Philadelphia, PA: Wolters Kluwer; United States Preventive Services Task Force (2016). Depression in Children and Adolescents: Screening. Retrieved from: https://www.uspreventiveservicestaskforce.org/Page/Document/UpdateSummaryFinal/depression-in-children-and-adolescents-screening1.

temper outbursts (APA 2013) and angry mood states in between temper outbursts. The outbursts are inconsistent with the situation and do not match the child's developmental age. The diagnosis should not be applied to youngsters before the age of 6 or after 18 but occurs before age 10. The prevalence rate is estimated at between 2% and 5% of the childhood population. A differential with pediatric bipolar is that children with DMDD do not exhibit mania or hypomania (NIMH n.d.). Symptoms must be present for more than 1 year and occur more frequently in boys than girls (Child Mind Institute n.d.).

Persistent Depressive Disorder

PDD (also referred to as dysthymia) reflects symptoms of depression that are *less severe but long-standing*. Symptoms include depressed mood most of the day for at least 1 year, irritability, moodiness, sadness, and pessimism. PDD in the DSM-5 combines and replaces the two diagnoses of dysthymia and chronic major depressive disorder (MDD) that were found in the DSM-IV. Children with PDD have intermittent problems with social situations and relationships, low self-esteem, and academic performance. The DSM-5 includes numerous specifiers and severity levels with this diagnosis (APA 2013; Child Mind Institute n.d.). Bernaras et al. (2019) and Mullen (2018) provide good reviews of MDD in children and adolescents.

Pediatric Bipolar Disorder

Bipolar disorder is an affective disorder which in the DSM-5 has been removed from inclusion in the chapter on depressive disorders and placed in its own chapter between depressive disorders and schizophrenia spectrum disorders (APA 2013). At times children exhibit what has been termed "affective storms," which are severe violent outbursts of irritability, anger, and attacking behaviors (Stahl 2008). PBD has been described as, "discrete episodes of elevated mood for multiple days with rapid thoughts, decreased need for sleep, persisting high energy, and unusual risk taking" (Hilt and Nussbaum 2016). The diagnosis of PBD in children has remained controversial and has resulted in inclusion of DMDD as a diagnostic option for youth under the age of 10 in the DSM-5 with the hope that the number of children diagnosed with bipolar disorder would decrease. Controversy has centered on difficulty identifying duration of episodes (this is often difficult to accurately pinpoint from reporting from the child and/or caretakers) to meet the diagnostic criteria in youth and the similarity of several symptoms that are also seen in other disorders such as ADHD and oppositional defiant disorder (ODD). In an effort to capture the variability of behaviors seen in children and adolescents who appear to have bipolar disorder but do not meet the DSM-5 criteria for diagnosis and to distinguish pediatric symptoms from adult

bipolar disorder, researchers, including those at the NIMH, have been conducting longitudinal and randomized clinical trials for over 20 years. The team at the NIMH has written extensively on DMDD and SMD, syndromes presenting as distinct profiles from PBD (Leibenluft 2011; Linke et al. 2019; Stringaris et al. 2018). This team recently conducted a study on 118 youngsters aged 11–21 years. The sample included 44 youth with a diagnosis of DMDD, 36 with a diagnosis of PBD, and 38 healthy youth. Brain imaging and multiple age and disorder specific rating scales were administered to participants. Of significance, brain imaging results found alteration in white matter myelination in subjects with bipolar disorder when compared to subjects with DMDD (Linke et al. 2019).

SMD, which was not included in the DSM-5, was characterized by chronic nonepisodic irritability and hyperarousal (insomnia, distractibility, pressured speech, agitation, racing thoughts, flight of ideas, and intrusiveness) (Brotman et al. 2017b). Given the overlap of these symptoms with ADHD, ADHD replaced SMD as the preferred diagnostic label.

Prevalence rates of bipolar disorder in children and adolescents are difficult to accurately identify because of the lack of good epidemiological studies and the ongoing controversy over using the diagnosis in this population. However, estimates in children under the age of 12 are believed to be approximately 0.1%, with rates during adolescence increasing to between 1% and 3% (Merikangas et al. 2010; NIMH n.d.). Table 12.3 illustrates the symptoms associated with DSM-5 bipolar I and bipolar II disorders.

Bipolar disorder with mixed episodes was eliminated from DSM-5. In DSM-5, mixed episodes are now used as specifiers and as in the past refer to the presence of both high and low symptoms at the same time or in rapid sequence. Mixed symptoms are a more severe form of bipolar disorder, result in a worse course and prognosis, and may present with a higher incidence of comorbid psychiatric disorders (Sole et al. 2017).

The acronym FIND can be used by the APRN during assessment of PBD:

Frequency (symptoms occur most days in a week).
Intensity (severe symptoms that significantly impact one domain or moderately affect two or more domains).
Number (symptoms occur three or more times each day).
Duration (symptoms occur four or more hours per day) (Kowatch et al. 2005).

Etiology

The science behind the etiology of mood disorders points to multiple factors interacting at critical times on vulnerable individuals to cause affective dysregulation. While the causation in children and adolescents appears

Table 12.3 Criteria for DSM-5 bipolar disorders

(a) Bipolar I

Manic episode

A. A distinct period of abnormally and persistently elevated, expansive, or irritable mood and abnormally and persistently increased goal-directed activity or energy, lasting at least 1 week and present most of the day, nearly every day (or any duration if hospitalization is necessary).

B. During the period of mood disturbance and increased energy or activity, three (or more) of the following symptoms (four if the mood is only irritable) are presented to a significant degree and represent a noticeable change from usual behavior:

1. Inflated self-esteem or grandiosity.
2. Decreased need for sleep (e.g. feels rested after only 3 hours of sleep).
3. Flight of ideas or subjective experience that thoughts are racing.
4. Distractibility (i.e. attention too easily drawn to unimportant or irrelevant external stimuli) as reported or observed.
5. Increase in goal-directed activity (either socially, at work or school, or sexual) or psychomotor agitation (i.e. purposeless nongoal-directed activity).
6. Excessive involvement in activities that have a high potential for painful consequences (e.g. engaging in unrestrained buying sprees, sexual indiscretions, or foolish business investments).

C. The mood disturbance is sufficiently severe to cause marked impairment in social or occupational functioning or to necessitate hospitalization to prevent harm to self or others, or there are psychotic features.

D. The episode is not attributable to the physiological effects of a substance (e.g. a drug of abuse, a medication, other treatment) or to another medical condition.

Note: A full manic episode that emerges during antidepressant treatment (e.g. medication, electroconvulsive therapy) but persists at a fully syndromal level beyond the physiological effect of that treatment is sufficient evidence for a manic episode and therefore a bipolar I diagnosis.

Note: Criteria A–D constitute a manic episode. At least one lifetime manic episode is required for the diagnosis of bipolar I disorder.

(b) Bipolar II

Hypomanic episode

A. A distinct period of abnormally and persistently elevated, expansive, or irritable mood and abnormally and persistently increased activity or energy, lasting at least 4 consecutive days and present most of the day, nearly every day.

B. During the period of mood disturbance and increase energy and activity, three (or more) of the following symptoms (four if the mood is only irritable) have persisted, represent a noticeable change from usual behavior, and have been present to a significant degree:

1. Inflated self-esteem or grandiosity.
2. Decreased need for sleep (e.g. feels rested after only 3 hours of sleep).
3. More talkative than usual or pressure to keep talking.
4. Flight of ideas or subjective experience that thoughts are racing.
5. Distractibility (i.e. attention too easily drawn to unimportant or irrelevant external stimuli), as reported or observed.
6. Increase in goal-directed activity (either socially, at work or school, or sexually) or psychomotor agitation.
7. Excessive involvement in activities that have a high potential for painful consequences (e.g. engaging in unrestrained buying sprees, sexual indiscretions, or foolish business investments).

C. The episode is associated with an unequivocal change in functioning that is uncharacteristic of the individual when not symptomatic.

D. The disturbance in mood and the change in functioning are observable by others.

E. The episode is not severe enough to cause marked impairment in social or occupational functioning or to necessitate hospitalization. If there are psychotic features, the episode is, by definition, manic.

F. The episode is not attributable to the physiological effects of a substance (e.g. a drug of abuse, a medication, other treatment).

Note: A full hypomanic episode that emerges during antidepressant treatment (e.g. medication, electroconvulsive therapy) but persists at a fully syndromal level beyond the physiological effect of that treatment is sufficient evidence for a hypomanic episode diagnosis. However, caution is indicated so that one or two symptoms (particularly increased irritability, edginess, or agitation following antidepressant use) are not taken as sufficient for diagnosis of a hypomanic episode, nor necessarily indicative of a bipolar diathesis.

Note: Criteria A–F constitute a hypomanic episode. Hypomanic episodes are common in bipolar I disorder but are not required for the diagnosis of bipolar I disorder.

Source: American Psychiatric Association. Diagnostic and Statistical Manual of Mental Disorders, 5th edition. © 2013, American Psychiatric Association. Reprinted with permission from the American Psychiatric Association.

to be similar to the causation in adults, onset before age 18 and symptoms that are left untreated pose a risk for both the presence of comorbidities and recurrence in adulthood. The Agency for Healthcare Research and Quality (2018), Bernaras et al. (2019), Rocha et al. (2013), and Sadock and Sadock (2009) provide excellent reviews of the biological, genetic, cognitive, personality, and environmental (internal, external, and relational) factors that have been implicated in the development and maintenance of mood disorders. The type and severity of factors, combination of factors, genetic/familial vulnerabilities, intensity, chronicity, and onset during critical developmental periods impact the disease pathway (Siu and USPSTF 2016).

Biological Evidence

The monoamine hypothesis of depression identifies three neurotransmitters as playing a key role in depression. Signaling problems and inefficient or dysregulated serotonin, norepinephrine, and dopamine activity in the amygdala, prefrontal cortex, nucleus accumbens, and hypothalamus explain the symptoms of depressed mood, difficulty with information processing, psychomotor retardation or agitation, emotion regulation, and sleep disturbances (Kraus et al. 2017; Neuroscience Educational Institute 2009; Stahl 2008). Antidepressants target specific neurotransmitters to alleviate these problematic presenting symptoms in children and adolescents presenting with MD.

Dysregulation of the hypothalamic–pituitary–adrenal (HPA) axis has long been identified as a factor in depression. In response to physical or psychological stress, the adrenal gland releases the hormone cortisol and the hypothalamus releases corticotropin-releasing hormone, which triggers a further increase in the production of cortisol. Hypercortisolism is believed to cause the cognitive impairment seen in depressed individuals (Hankin et al. 2010; Howland 2010).

Hypothyroidism

Hypothyroidism occurs when the thyroid gland fails to respond to thyroid-stimulating hormone (TSH) and increases levels of circulating T_3 (triiodothyronine) and T_4 (thyroxine). Primary hypothyroidism can mimic some of the classic symptoms seen in depression such as hypersomnia, fatigue, psychomotor and cognitive slowing, anxiety, mood instability, weight gain, constipation, and depression. The individual with severe hypothyroidism presents with aggression, agitation, and paranoia. Blood serum T_3 and T_4 levels are usually low but TSH is elevated above 3.5 mlU/ml. In subclinical hypothyroidism, T_3 and T_4 are within normal range but TSH is elevated (Bathia et al. 2016; Geracioti 2006; Harvard Mental Health Letter 2007).

Family/Genetic Evidence

Children and adolescents who have one first-degree biological relative with unipolar or bipolar disorder have up to a 24% chance of also having a mood/affective disorder (APA 2013), and the chances increase if both parents have a mood or bipolar disorder. Luby et al. (2006) conducted a 6-month (Time 1 and Time 2) study on 119 preschool-age children (3 years to 5 years and 7 months old) looking at risk factors for preschool depression. Data obtained included family history of psychiatric disorders, caregiver interviews to obtain a structured diagnostic assessment of the child's depression severity score, child assessment, and caregiver response to a stressful life events tool aimed at capturing stressful events experienced by the child within the past year. The researchers found that both family history and stressful life events predicted depression scores at Time 2. In 2012, Luby et al. published a paper on a study entitled "Maternal Support in Early Childhood Predicts Larger Hippocampal Volumes at School-Age". These researchers, who have been conducting longitudinal studies on preschool depression, were able to perform MRI brain imaging on 92 children between the ages of 7 and 13 years for whom they had been tracking mother–child interactions. What they found was that in nonclinically depressed children, those who received support from their mother had a higher hippocampus volume secondary to increased dendritic branching and neurogenesis when compared to depressed youngsters. The hippocampus is the part of the brain responsible for memory and stress modulation. The results of this work highlight the need to work with and enhance positive parent–child interactions during pregnancy and in the critical first few years of the child's life to minimize depression and provide the child with support to be able to handle stress appropriately. Children with negative temperament characteristics are also at-risk for mood and affective disorders. Child temperament styles are discussed further in Chapter 2.

Cognitive Evidence

Maladaptive negative cognitive factors have been implicated in mood dysregulation and appear to be a learned pattern of distorted thinking triggered by stressful events that then activate a cascade of negative thought processes. Beck (1967) first identified cognitive vulnerabilities, which he associated with depression, as including a negative interpretation of events, perceived incompetence, poor self-schema, helplessness, hopelessness, and a pessimistic view of the world. In more recent research, Beck (2008) and Clark and Beck (2010) stated that "dysfunctional schemas about the self are due to early adverse childhood events such as parental loss, rejection or neglect that sensitizes the individual to later losses" (p. 419). Individuals in whom this negative schema is continuously activated develop entrenched and more elaborate negative self-schemas that become more easily triggered by mild stressors. ARPNs are urged to evaluate cognitive distortions within the context of pervasiveness, intensity, and developmental sense of self (Horowitz and Marchetti 2009). Garber (2006) and Jacobs et al. (2008) provide a good review of the evidence related to cognitive susceptibilities in the pediatric population.

Environmental Evidence

Environmental factors have also been implicated in the development of mood dysregulation disorders in children and adolescents. These include adverse childhood experiences, family and peer relationships, maltreatment, school performance, and real or perceived neighborhood threats or risk exposure (Child Mind Institute n.d.; Waite and Ryan 2019). Bronfenbrenner's ecological systems theory is a useful framework for understanding systems with which human beings interact and that contribute to proximal processes involved with development, including development of psychopathology (Bronfenbrenner 1979, 1994). For example, the microsystem is made up of the individual, family, peers, school, and neighborhood. The relationships (attachment and support) and interactions (teasing or bullying) that a child has with individuals within that system during development will affect not only mood but also self-esteem and ability to successfully navigate developmental tasks. The risk for mood psychopathology in the developing child or adolescent may also be affected by linkages and processes occurring between two or more settings (mesosystem), one of which includes the developing child. An example would include conflicts between the school and the parents over the child's behavior at school or the impact of community violence on the developing child.

Mrug and Windle (2010) conducted a longitudinal study with a community sample of 603 boys and girls recruited at the 5th grade and followed for 16 months. At baseline the Birmingham Youth Violence Study Violence Exposure self-report tool was administered. The tool measures witnessing violence, being the victim of violence, or having been threatened by violence, including when a weapon was involved. The context of the violence was also assessed at baseline. At Time 2 of the study, the participants completed a self-report measure of aggression assessing for pure, reactive, and instrumental overt aggression on a Likert 4-point scale. The researchers found that violence exposure in more than one setting, such as at home and at school, was a predictor of adjustment problems, witnessing violence at school and victimization at home was related to depression, witnessing violence and victimization at home was associated with aggression (externalizing symptom), and witnessing violence in the community predicted delinquency. A more detailed discussion of Bronfenbrenner's theory can be found in Chapter 1.

Internalizing and Externalizing Symptoms in the Context of Mood and Dysregulation Disorders

The Child Behavior Checklist (CBCL) developed by Achenbach has proved reliable across cultures and assesses two distinct youth behavioral profiles: internalizing and externalizing. Externalizing youth have been described as undercontrolled with inadequate regulation in that they are aggressive, hostile, and irritable, having low frustration tolerance and having a tendancy to break rules. Internalizing youth have been referred to as overcontrolled in that they exhibit symptoms of anxiety, depression, social withdrawal, more psychosomatic distress, and rumination (Achenbach 1991; Matos et al. 2017; Tackett 2010; Verhulst et al. 2003). Matos et al. (2017) conducted a study on 1590 Portuguese adolescents and 1580 parents. The adolescents were administered the Child Depressive Inventory (CDI) and the parents were asked to complete the CBCL assessing for internalizing and externalizing symptoms in their youngsters. Researchers found that higher levels of externalizing symptoms, such as opposition and immaturity in girls, is a risk factor for internalizing symptoms and that girls in the sample had higher levels of internalizing symptoms. Recommendations included treating both types of symptoms together and not minimizing internal symptom presentation by gender.

Risk Factors for Mood Dysregulation Disorders

As stated previously, risk factors for mood dysregulation disorders are extensive and include family history of depression or bipolar disorder, female gender, comorbid anxiety, being a victim of abuse, stressful life experiences, health problems, one or more traumatic events, negative cognitions, loss, subsyndromal depression, negative affect temperament style, exposure to family or environmental violence, substance use, and interpersonal conflicts (Garber 2006; Moldenhauer 2006; Prager 2009). Factors contributing to mood dysregulation are complex and multifactorial, often posing a challenge to the APRN who works with children and adolescents and may have limited access to resources aimed at providing scaffolding for the child and family. The child's presentation, history, significant current and past experiences, relationships at home and at school, blood serum levels, and physiological status are important components of the comprehensive assessment that must be conducted.

Riehm et al. (2019) conducted a study with over 6500 12–15-year-old adolescent participants looking at their social media use and its relationship to mental health symptoms. Findings show that youth who were engaged in more than 3 hours a day of social media use exhibited more internalizing symptoms, including depression. Excessive social media use has also been implicated in social isolation, sleep disturbance, anxiety, and exposure to negative coping behaviors (Kimball and Cohen 2019).

In a study conducted in Canada on a sample of 2014 children aged 12 and 13 years, researchers wanted to identify the most salient risk factors for depression in youth from among common predictors (MacPhee and Andrews 2006). Researchers looked at self-report data from nine measures available from the National Longitudinal Survey of Children and Youth (NLSCY) study, which collects data on health and wellbeing every 2 years on a randomly selected group of children, following them into adulthood. The most salient risk factors for depression in this sample were low self-esteem and harsh and rejecting parental child-rearing behaviors. The researchers recommended centering prevention efforts around developing and maintaining healthy self-esteem/self-concept in children and supporting effective parenting behaviors. This strengthens the parent–child bond, which is a strong protective factor in healthy development of child self-concept (MacPhee and Andrews).

A thorough, and still timely, review of family risk factors contributing to and maintaining youth depressive symptoms was conducted by Restifo and Bogels (2009). These researchers later concluded that there is a lack of randomized clinical trials related to treatment efforts aimed at addressing family risk factors. In 2010 they conducted a small pilot study in which they taught mindfulness strategies to 10 parents in their sample, meeting once per week with the parents for 3-hour education and mindfulness practice activities. In addition, parents were given mindfulness homework. Findings included a decrease in parental rejection of the child, reduction in parental stress and reactivity, and improvement in marital functioning and co-parenting (Bogels et al. 2010). Bogels and Restifo have subsequently written a text, *Mindful Parenting: A Guide for Mental Health Practitioners*, which includes education about mindfulness and exercises for use during an 8-week intervention with parents (2014).

Child Protective Factors

Research has shown that there are several protective factors against the development of mood dysregulation disorders. One of the most studied protective factors is participation in sports. As sports participation increased, the odds of suffering from depression decreased by 25% among adolescents, and the odds of suicidal ideation decreased by 12%. Adolescents who participated in sports were at decreased risk for substance abuse, which has been associated with both depression and suicidal ideation. Participation in sports also increases physical activity, which has been shown to be protective against depression, suicidal ideation, and obesity. The protective effects were mediated by increases in self-esteem and perceived and experienced social support (Babiss and Gangwisch 2009).

Assessing Mood Dysregulation Disorders in Primary Care

The importance of assessing and treating mood dysregulation disorders early in the pediatric population cannot be stressed enough. Recognition of pediatric mood disorders often presents a challenge for pediatric APRNs, who often lack sufficient time, training, and/or referral sources for management of more complex presentations by these youngsters. As a result, mood dysregulation disorders are often underdiagnosed and undertreated in pediatric primary care settings (Pinfield 2017). The typical duration of pediatric office visits can be a barrier to completing a comprehensive psychiatric screen. The amount of time required to perform a psychiatric interview with both a child and a parent would be difficult to find in a busy pediatric primary care practice.

Mood disorders significantly affect a child's emotional, cognitive, relational, and social development. Unfortunately, such disorders can have a long-lasting negative impact on quality of life. Evidence shows that screening for mood disorders improves the identification of depressed patients and that effective follow-up and treatment decrease clinical morbidity and associated psychosocial complications such as substance use, self-injuring behaviors, suicide, school difficulties, and eating disorders (Leslie and Chike-Harris 2018). APRNs are in an ideal position to conduct routine screening, recognize the warning signs of mild to SMD, and provide initial management and referrals as needed (Bhatta et al. 2018).

Families may be more likely to present to the primary care setting with a complaint about a mental health problem because they may have a long-term relationship with their healthcare provider and the primary care office is a place where they are comfortable (Zuckerbrot et al. 2018). Depressive illnesses, bipolar disorder, and other mood disorders presenting in primary care settings may be less severe than those directly admitted to mental health settings. Thus, the response to treatment, the short-term prognosis, and the chance of recovery may be greater in those children and adolescents who are identified initially in primary care settings early during in course of their symptoms.

Pediatric healthcare providers frequently encounter youths who exhibit symptoms of or are at risk for mood dysregulation. For example, families may present to the pediatric APRN with concerns about childhood sleep problems or adolescent complaints of fatigue, both of which may be symptoms of depression. Unfortunately, without proper knowledge, tools, and support, it may be more feasible (and convenient) to recommend a sleep aid or to order blood tests than to diagnose an underlying and often treatable mental health disorder. This approach, while expedient, does not address the underlying problem and further delays appropriate interventions.

In order to appropriately screen for and diagnose mood disorders in the primary care setting, APRNs need to conduct a comprehensive history and complete physical examination.

History

A detailed and thorough history is essential to create an accurate timeline for onset of symptoms that may be related to a mood disorder and to help guide treatment decisions. For the pediatric patient, multiple informants – such as the child, parents, teachers, and other caregivers – are needed to gather adequate information to determine symptoms, severity, and course of illness (Garzon 2017). When the APRN is assessing a child for a mood disorder, the history can be structured similarly to a well-child history. After determining the chief complaint, a complete history should include a history of the present illness, a past medical and surgical history (including a list of medications and allergies), a family medical history, a psychosocial history, and a review of systems (including diet, sleep, and elimination).

In addition, a comprehensive physical examination, including laboratory blood work, is needed to determine the child/adolescent's general health status and to rule out medical conditions that may mimic mood disorders such as hypothyroidism and chronic fatigue syndrome. When working with children and adolescents who present with symptoms of a mood disorder, the APRN should remember that they may often have comorbid psychiatric conditions such as ADHD, ODD, substance abuse disorders, and/or anxiety disorders. Successful treatment of mood disorders requires effective treatment for the co-occurring conditions (Romain et al. 2018). An additional comorbidity that may present with PBD is overweight and obesity. Overweight/obesity among youth with bipolar disorder may be associated with increased psychiatric burden (Shapiro et al. 2017).

History of the Present Illness

When conducting a history of the present symptoms, it is important to note the duration and severity of symptoms. It is also important to determine what, if anything, triggers or improves the symptoms. APRNs should be aware that in children and adolescents, the presenting symptoms for mood disorders may differ from those seen in adults (Pinfield 2017). The age and developmental level of the pediatric patient must be considered when assessing for these disorders. Again, while the core symptoms of MDD in adolescents are similar to those in adults, younger children are less likely to identify sadness and more commonly present with irritability or auditory hallucinations compared with adults (Tables 12.1–12.3). PBD also differs from the adult form of the disorder. In children, bipolar disease may be marked by longer episodes, rapid cycling, prominent irritability, and high rates of comorbid ADHD and anxiety disorders (Aedo et al. 2018).

It is clear that children with mood disorders may present differently than adults. However, even within the pediatric population, there are differences in presentation based on the child's age, developmental status, and severity of symptoms. An adolescent will likely have a different presentation of a mood disorder than a younger child. For example, adolescents may engage in risky behaviors such as alcohol and drug use, dangerous driving, and/or promiscuous sex. Adolescents may also present with antisocial behavior exemplified by stealing, vandalism, and/or running away from home. Adolescents may also commonly present with severe mood swings, hypersexuality, irritability, distractibility, decreased need for sleep, impulsivity, and racing thoughts (Pinfield 2017). Younger children may present with somatic complaints such as a headache or upset stomach, causing the APRN to treat these symptoms without fully realizing that they may be initial signs of a mood disorder such as depression (Garzon 2017). Regarding the presentation of PBD, the manic and depressive symptoms that occur in young children often occur simultaneously, as in a mixed state, or they cycle several times within a day (Aedo et al. 2018). A child or adolescent who presents to the primary care setting with recurrent depressive symptoms, persistently irritable or agitated behaviors, hyperactivity, labile mood, reckless or aggressive behaviors, or psychotic symptoms may be experiencing the initial symptoms of bipolar disorder.

In infancy and early childhood, depression may present to the primary care setting with a variety of symptoms, including failure to thrive, speech and motor delays, decreased ability to interact, and poor attachment. The child may also display repetitive self-soothing behaviors, withdrawal from social contact, and a loss of previously learned skills (e.g. self-soothing skills). An increase in temper tantrums or irritability, separation anxiety, and phobias may also be noted (Garzon 2017). Older children and adolescents may present with poor self-esteem, reckless and destructive behavior (e.g. unsafe sexual activity, substance abuse), somatic complaints, poor social and academic functioning, hopelessness, boredom, emptiness, and loss of interest in activities (Garzon 2017).

It is known that manic symptoms characterized as elevated, expansive, or irritable are key features of bipolar disorder. However, manic symptoms present differently during childhood. In children, a persistently irritable mood may be noted more than a euphoric mood. Children may also have aggressive uncontrollable outbursts and agitated behaviors with hyperactivity and impulsivity. Extreme fluctuations in mood may be noted. These mood fluctuations can occur on the same day over the course of days or weeks. Children with PBD may also present with reckless behaviors, dangerous play, and inappropriate sexual behaviors. Adolescents with bipolar disorder may present to the primary care office with sleep disturbances, labile mood, agitated behaviors, and pressured speech. They may also have racing thoughts and reckless behaviors such as dangerous driving, substance abuse, and sexual indiscretions. Adolescents may also report illicit activities such as impulsive stealing or fighting, spending sprees, and psychotic symptoms (e.g. hallucinations, delusions, irrational thoughts) (Stebbins and Corcoran 2016).

Past Medical History

When gathering information regarding the past medical history, pertinent birth history information should be obtained. The APRN should be sure to inquire about any history of psychiatric conditions, hospitalizations, surgeries, and/or medical disorders/chronic illnesses since conditions such as diabetes and obesity have been associated with depressive symptoms in children and adolescents (Morrison et al. 2015; Lu et al. 2017). The ages at which conditions occurred should be noted. It should also be noted whether the child is up to date on immunizations. Included in the history should be an assessment of medications that the child or adolescent is taking, since some medications may cause depression-like symptoms such as sedation (Garzon 2017). The medication history should also note not only prescription medications but over-the-counter and herbal medications as well. The APRN should assess allergies to medications, foods, or the environment.

Family Medical History

Children are at higher risk of developing a mood disorder at an earlier age if there is a history of a mood disorder in the family (Garzon 2017). The APRN should inquire about the family's mental health history (e.g. anxiety/mood disorders). Ideally, the family medical history should be obtained for three generations of family members (the child [and his or her siblings], the parents [and their siblings], and the grandparents). A family history of parental mental health diagnoses should be determined. A history of parental depression has been associated with depression in their children (Liskola et al. 2018). If a parent has been diagnosed with a mental health condition and confirms taking prescribed medications, the APRN should record parental responses to those psychiatric medications. A family history of medical conditions such as headaches, chronic illness (obesity, diabetes, dyslipidemia, and cardiovascular disease), or recurrent pain should also be noted.

Psychosocial History

When a child or adolescent presents to the primary care office with symptoms of a mood disorder, a thorough psychosocial history should be obtained. The psychosocial history can take the form of a HEADDSS assessment for adolescents (Home, Education/Employment, Activities, Diet/Drugs, Sexuality/Suicide [or depression]; Cohen et al. 1991; Hagel et al. 2009). This section of the history should describe members of the current household, their relationships to the child, and the familial sources of stress and support. If the visit involves an adolescent, consider gathering this information separately from both the adolescent and the parent. The adolescent should be assured that what is shared in the healthcare encounter is confidential and that only certain information will be shared. Information that cannot be held confidential includes if the adolescent reveals that he or she is considering harming him- or herself, that someone is harming him or her, or if he or she is or is planning to harm someone else. The questioning during this portion of the history should proceed from least to most sensitive questions, giving the APRN a chance to first establish rapport with the patient.

In addition to the HEADDSS assessment, family risk factors such as marital and family conflict and parent stress should be noted. Such factors have been shown to impact the nature of the parent–child relationship. Family conflict has been shown to be associated with adolescent depression (Fosco et al. 2016). Parent–child relationships may also have a significant effect on children with pediatric mood disorders and these relationships may, in turn, be affected by the child's illness. A parent with an active mood disorder may have a negative effect on family interactions. The mood disorder may interfere with the parent's ability to nurture, show affection, and support the child. Compared to controls, parent–child relationships in the mood disorders group were characterized by significantly less warmth, affection, and intimacy, and more quarreling and forceful punishment. Living in a single-parent home was also associated with greater parent–child relationship difficulties (Daryanani et al. 2017). Furthermore, stressful life events such as parental loss through death, incarceration, or substance use may put children at greater risk for developing psychological or behavioral disorders (Garzon 2017).

Peer relationships should be explored, as well as information about the child's social environment. Children with mood dysregulation disorders may have trouble relating to peers. Problematic peer relationships should be noted, with particular attention paid to negative interactive patterns such as ongoing bullying or hurtful teasing, social exclusion, physical violence or threats, sexual and racial harassment, and public humiliation. Anhedonia in the child may limit engagement in social activities, which may interfere with mastery of social and peer-relatedness skills. Irritability may make children difficult to be around and tends to push others away. Disruptive behavior can cause safety problems and interfere with group activities. A history of victimization, including polyvictimization and cyber-bullying, should also be obtained as these types of bullying activities are more pervasive and may lack a clearly defined source, resulting in increased anxiety and depression (Pontes et al. 2018; Reed et al. 2016). A history of social media use should be obtained because a high frequency of social media use has been associated with depressive symptoms in adolescents (Shensa et al. 2018).

Information regarding school and daycare should be gathered since children and adolescents spend more time in daycare and school than in any other setting outside of the home. When conducting a history about school, be sure to inquire about academic, athletic, social, relational, and behavioral functioning. The APRN should also note the child's pattern of attendance and school nurse visits. Children and adolescents with mood disorders may experience difficulty in school, since successful school performance requires concentration, alertness, proper behavior, and teamwork. Poor concentration, irritability, disorganization, and a lack of self-confidence may interfere with academic work. Low academic achievement and poor school attendance have been shown to be related to depression during adolescence (Finning et al. 2019; Rahman et al. 2018). A slow or precipitous drop in school grades, difficulty managing school-related activities, and behavior problems in the classroom may be indicators that students might be experiencing mood dysregulation. These symptoms may also be associated with other health-related

problems and often will not trigger evaluation for a mood disorder. It is important for the APRN to try to determine the cause of these issues since school-related problems often escalate and may lead to academic failure and dropping out of school along with social isolation (Rahman et al.).

In addition to affecting the ability to relate to peers, symptoms of mood dysregulation may interfere with the adolescent's capacity to develop intimate relationships and to manage responsibilities, important tasks for the transition to adulthood. Obtaining occupational preparation and holding a consistent job may be challenges for these youth. APRNs can and should play an important role in helping families plan for educational and occupational preparation of these youngsters (Garzon 2017).

Adolescence is a time when the development and maintenance of peer relationships are of the utmost importance. Adolescents with mood dysregulation often have difficulty in establishing close relationships, which may, in turn, interfere with the development of healthy sexuality. Both girls and boys may succumb to intimidation, bullying, or aggression by their partners to engage in behavior they may not be comfortable with. This may be secondary to fear, anxiety, or a poor sense of self associated with concern about losing the relationship. In adolescents with bipolar disorder, manic episodes may be associated with poor judgment and may lead to impulsive sexual behavior. Adolescents with impulsive sexual behaviors may not use condoms or other contraception and be at increased risk for unwanted pregnancy and sexually transmitted infections (STIs). During the visit, the APRN should be sure to discuss dating and sexual behavior while also providing early contraception education. Testing for pregnancy and STIs should be available as needed.

Review of Systems

The review of systems can provide a comprehensive and methodical overview of the child's health. This structured approach provides an additional opportunity to identify signs and symptoms that may be associated with mood disorders. This approach can cover topics such as diet, sleep, and elimination. This process will also assist the APRN in covering important areas related to safety and anticipatory guidance. When discussing the child's or adolescent's diet, it is important to note that changes in eating patterns may occur with mood dysregulation. Both an increase and a decrease in appetite can be an early symptom associated with mood disorders. Excessive eating may signal an attempt to self-soothe. During mania, children may be "too busy" to stop for a meal. This may result in an inadequate intake of calories and nutrients. The APRN should inquire about a history of hoarding or binge eating. Poor nutrition may result from binge eating because the child may be filling up on junk foods and sweets. Increases or decreases in appetite may be important clues and require additional evaluation.

Asking questions about sleep or elimination is important when conducting the history. The APRN should elicit an account of the child's or adolescent's recent sleep patterns, including any changes from their usual pattern. Sleep disturbances are noteworthy and may include hypersomnia, insomnia, disrupted sleep, or poor quality of sleep. These sleep disturbances may contribute to irritability, agitation, and poor school performance. It is also important for the APRN to ask about changes in elimination patterns. Problems with bedwetting and soiling may present in children with mood disorders (Garzon 2017).

Safety and Anticipatory Guidance

Discussions of safety and anticipatory guidance play an important role when dealing with a child or adolescent with symptoms of a mood disorder. The APRN must assess the child's potential for self-injury secondary to poor judgment and risky behavior. Driving violations, such as speeding, place the adolescent at risk for self-injury and harming others. The use of seat belts in children of all ages should be encouraged at all times. For children already taking psychotropic medications, there may be additional safety considerations. The risk of overdose and potential for adverse medication reactions require that the APRN provide education regarding medications at every healthcare encounter. For children with medical conditions taking psychotropic medications, the APRN must monitor for medication compliance and potential interactions. For example, concurrent use of some antidepressants and nonsteroidal anti-inflammatory (NSAID) medications has been shown to increase bleeding risk.

During primary care encounters, an assessment of substance use is especially important in those youth at risk for a mood dysregulation. The APRN should ask about drug and alcohol use since youth with symptoms of mood disorders may attempt to self-medicate. When inquiring about drugs, the APRN must ask about prescription medications as well as illicit drugs. It is important to remember that substance use can mask symptoms of mood disorders while simultaneously placing youth at risk for overdose, social withdrawal, accidents, impulsive sexual activity, sexual assault, and aggression toward others (Garzon 2017).

Anticipatory guidance regarding mood disorders consists of education and information that will assist families in preparing for expected changes during their child's or adolescent's assessment and treatment. It will

be important to provide information regarding discipline since children with symptoms of a mood disorder may have interaction problems with parents, guardians, or older siblings. A child with depressive symptoms may be quiet and withdrawn. However, these behaviors may be viewed as uncooperative. Children with PBD may demonstrate aggressive behaviors and outbursts. These behaviors may serve to alienate them from other children and adults. Irritability displayed by a child with mood dysregulation symptoms may be seen as a lack of cooperation and lack of respect. In these cases, discipline will not be effective if the underlying disorder is not addressed. Also, inappropriate discipline may intensify undesired behaviors. Consistent limit setting and clear explanation of behavioral contingencies are appropriate discipline strategies for youth with symptoms of mood disorders. Enforcing rules regarding safety is critical (Garzon 2017).

Physical Examination

Mood disorders are not associated with specific alterations in normal physical growth and development, therefore regular age-appropriate growth screening is recommended for these youth. Vital signs, including height, weight, and blood pressure, should be monitored at each visit. A body mass index (BMI) should also be calculated. Height, weight, and BMI should be plotted on the appropriate growth chart. Screenings should be done for hearing and vision to ensure that impaired attention, irritability, distractibility, and low self-esteem are not caused by impaired sight or hearing. When conducting the physical examination, it is important to assess for objective signs of depression such as weight gain or loss and hypoactivity or hyperactivity. A complete physical examination should be conducted, including a thorough neurological examination.

Importance of Differentials

Several problems that have overlapping presentations with mood disorders present to APRNs in primary care settings (Bekhuis et al. 2016). If a mood disorder is suspected from information gathered in the history, there are several medical diagnoses that should be ruled out. Examples include weight loss, somatic complaints, fatigue, recurrent injuries, and school failure. Weight loss and reduced appetite might present similarly to anorexia nervosa. Binge eating or poor food intake may occur with mania. While somatic complaints may be expressions of emotional distress, they may also be signs of a physical illness or a medical problem. For example, a child presenting to the primary care clinic with a stomach ache may have an emotional issue or a gastrointestinal disorder. Fatigue is associated with depression but it is also associated with many physical illnesses. Before attributing a physical symptom to mood disorder, the APRN should be sure to investigate possible physical causes of the complaints (Bekhuis et al. 2016).

Youth presenting with recurrent injuries require not only a thorough evaluation but also safety education. Such education might include information on impulsiveness, a propensity for self-injurious behaviors, abuse, or a physical problem such as neurological disorders. Poor school performance may be the result of a learning or developmental disorder or may be caused by an exacerbation of a mood disorder (Garzon 2017). Sleep problems may also be indicative of either a physical or emotional disorder. School-age children who are depressed may present with hyperactivity, restlessness, or irritability that can be misdiagnosed as ADHD (Garzon 2017).

Laboratory tests may help the APRN rule out other medical conditions that cause symptoms similar to those of a mood disorder. If a patient presents with fatigue, consider ordering thyroid function tests and a complete blood count (with differential) to rule out hypothyroidism and anemia. Mononucleosis can be ruled out by ordering a monospot or heterophile test or Epstein–Barr virus antibody titers, in correlation with clinical symptoms. Although there is no definitive laboratory test for chronic fatigue syndrome, this condition should be included in the differential. Diabetes can also cause fatigue. If the patient is thought to have diabetes, obtain a fasting blood glucose level. If substance use or withdrawal is suspected, the APRN may order a toxicology screen. Sudden behavioral changes may indicate head trauma or a CNS lesion. Lead intoxication may also be associated with behavior changes. A blood lead level should be obtained if lead intoxication is suspected. If the youth is taking any medications, the APRN should review medication side effects to ensure that the youth is not suffering from adverse effects (Garzon 2017).

Surveillance and Screening

Any youth who presents to primary care or psychiatric-mental health APRNs with an emotional problem as the primary complaint should be screened for a mood disorder. After the initial history and review of symptoms, a formal screening can be conducted. When screening for a mood disorder, it is important to remember that depressed mood falls along a continuum. Short periods of sadness or irritability in response to disappointment or loss are a normal developmental reaction in youth. In a supportive environment, these feelings typically resolve promptly. However, some children and adolescents experience intense or long-lasting sadness or irritability that may interfere with self-esteem, friendships, family life, or school performance. Youths who experience long-lasting or intense feelings of sadness may be depressed and should be monitored and further evaluated.

Children and adolescents with depression or depressive symptoms who present to primary care offices often have a greater chance of receiving treatment, responding to that treatment, and achieving recovery if primary care providers screen for depression during the office visit (Zuckerbrot et al. 2018). The AAP and the US Preventive Services Task Force (USPSTF) recommend annual screening for depression in adolescents and youth beginning at the age of 12 years (AAP 2019; USPSTF 2016; Zuckerbrot et al. 2018). The USPSTF states that there is insufficient evidence to recommend routine depression screening of children 11 years of age and younger (USPSTF 2016). Surveillance and screening can begin with open-ended questions such as "How are things at home?" and "How are things at school?" After asking these questions, consider using a validated depression screening instrument to screen for depressive symptoms. There are several validated screening instruments that can be used to screen children and adolescents for depressive symptoms. The *Children's Depression Inventory (CDI)* (Kovacs 1992) was developed for use with children aged 7–17 years. It is written at the 1st-grade level, the lowest of any measure of depression for children. There are 27 multiple choice self-report items that take 10–15 minutes to complete. A short form with 10 items can be used when a quick screening is necessary. While both forms are reported to give comparable results, the longer form generally gives a more robust description of the child's symptoms. Internal consistency reliability has been found to be good, with alpha coefficients ranging from 0.71 to 0.89 with various samples. The CDI was developed from the Beck Depression Inventory (BDI).

The *BDI II* (Beck et al. 1996) is a 21-item self-report questionnaire, written at a 6th-grade reading level, that measures depressive symptoms. The BDI II includes the three subdomains of somatic, cognitive, and affective symptoms and has been found to accurately discriminate between depressed and nondepressed youth based on diagnostic criteria. Disadvantages of the tool are that it does not measure school functioning and there are no accompanying teacher or parent forms.

The *Center for Epidemiologic Studies – Depression Scale (CES-D)* (Radloff 1977) is a reliable and valid instrument that may be used to screen adolescents for depression (Wilcox et al. 1998). The CES-D is a 20-item self-report questionnaire designed for the general population, with an administration time of 5–10 minutes. With responses ranging from 0 ("rarely") to 3 ("most of the time"), participants rate the frequency with which each of the 20 items occurs. Total scores range from 0 to 60, with scores of 16 or higher indicating possible depression.

The *Center for Epidemiological Studies – Depression Scale for Children (CES-DC)* (Weissman et al. 1980) was adapted from the adult version to be more easily understood by children and adolescents (Faulstich et al. 1986). Also a 20-item self-report questionnaire, the responses range from 0 ("not at all") to 3 ("a lot") and yield total scores ranging from 0 to 60. A score of 15 or higher may indicate possible depression. Alpha coefficients for this scale used in adolescent samples range from 0.84 to 0.90 (Faulstich et al.).

The *Reynolds Child/Adolescent Depression Scales (RCDS/RADS)* are 10-minute self-report scales for children aged 7–12 years (RCDS) and adolescents aged 11–20 years (RADS). The screening tool assesses cognitive, somatic, psychomotor, and interpersonal symptoms. While the tool is brief and psychometrically sound, it is not as robust as the BDI-II (Elmquist et al. 2010).

The *Mood and Feelings Questionnaire (MFQ)* (30–35 items) and the *Mood and Feelings Short Form (SMFQ)* (13 items) are self-report tools that assess for symptoms of depression, loneliness, feeling unloved and ugly, and cognitive/affective symptoms. The tool is psychometrically sound with a brief administration time of between 5 and 15 minutes (Elmquist et al. 2010).

The *Patient Health Questionnaire-Adolescent Version (PHQ-9)* is a nine-item self-administered screening tool for depression among 13–17-year-olds. The tool uses DSM-IV-TR criteria for depression and is highly sensitive and specific. Items receive a score of from 0 ("not at all") to 3 ("nearly every day"). A score of 11 or higher correlates with the DSM criteria for MD (Richardson et al. 2010).

While formal screening tools are available for screening for depression, it has been found that screening with two questions about mood and anhedonia may be as effective as using a longer screening instrument (Whooley et al. 1997): (i) Over the past 2 weeks, have you been down, depressed, or hopeless? (ii) Have you felt little interest or pleasure in doing things?

The *Mood Disorders Questionnaire (MDQ)* is a valid, reliable instrument that screens for bipolar spectrum disorder (Hirschfeld et al. 2000). When screening for PBD, the MDQ has been shown to predict risky behavior and poor social adjustment in adolescents. Parents may be asked to complete the *Parent Mood Disorder Questionnaire (P-MDQ)*. The P-MDQ has been shown to have good validity and reliability in detecting bipolar disorder in outpatient health settings (Pavuluri 2007). Additionally, the *Child Behavior Checklist – Pediatric Bipolar Disorder (CBCL-PBD)* profile has been shown to

help identify children at high risk for developing bipolar disorder (Yule et al. 2018).

Treatment Evidence

Treatment effectiveness is variable and inconsistent between children and adolescents with mood dysregulation disorders. In general, the data on effectiveness is more positive in older children and adolescents when compared to younger children. The Treatment for Adolescent Depression Study (TADS) indicates that use of cognitive behavioral therapy (CBT) along with selective serotonin reuptake inhibitors (SSRIs) in teens presenting with depression shows greater symptom improvement that SSRI medications alone (Cheung et al. 2018). Group or individual CBT focuses on challenging cognitive distortions, teaching problem-solving skills, and assisting the youngster to regulate rapid and intense emotional experiences. Another evidence-based treatment, interpersonal psychotherapy (IPT), teaches communication skills, strategies to manage interpersonal conflicts, and problem solving (MacPherson and Fristad 2014; Weersing et al. 2017).

PBD treatment includes parent management training (PMT), CBT or IPT and medication use including antipsychotics, antiepileptics, or lithium (Kircanski et al. 2018; Stringaris et al. 2018). Chapter 9 contains additional psychopharmacological information on treating mood dysregulation disorders in youth.

Additional treatment recommendations include integrative patient-centered care across environments, inclusive of the child or adolescent, the parent or caregiver, clinician and relevant school personnel well known to the child. PMT calls for work directly with the parent(s) to increase their knowledge of the child or adolescent's disorder, teach and model limit setting, encourage prosocial behaviors, teach positive reinforcement, and provide and review assigned homework on managing specific child behavioral presentations (McMahon 2015). More recently, treatment interventions have also focused on lifestyle changes, including healthy eating, incorporation of exercise and endorsement of sleep hygiene, and adequate number of sleep hours (MacPherson and Fristad 2014; Sarris et al. 2014).

Role of APRNs

In the primary care office, APRNs need to promote mental health, engage the family early and effectively in order to address emerging problems, and collaborate with mental health specialists when needed (Cheung et al. 2018). APRNs should be able to recognize the signs and symptoms of mood disorders and establish a basic plan that provides for safety, a therapeutic relationship, and ongoing social support for the child, adolescent, and family. The APRN must find out from the family how they perceive the problem. This may help to address potential and actual barriers (e.g. stigma) that the family may experience when deciding to seek mental health services. It is important to remember that any treatment plan for youth with mood disorders must involve active participation of the whole family. APRNs may instruct youth and/or their caregivers to keep a daily record of the level of depressive and/or manic symptoms ("mood charting") to help monitor symptom presence and patterns. Mood charting via mobile phone may be useful for adolescents (Matthews et al. 2008). Families of youth with depressive symptoms must also be educated about the signs and risk of suicide and other self-injurious behaviors. Families with youth at risk for suicide should be told about the need to remove weapons and other means of carrying out lethal intentions (e.g. ropes, medications, poisons, alcohol) from the home (Stockburger and Omar 2017).

Children with mood disorders may require special accommodations in the school setting, as required by federal law. The APRN may assist the child's school with the development of an individualized education plan (IEP). IEPs are discussed further in Chapters 28 and 32 of this text. In addition, the APRN may be asked to participate in school planning meetings to develop behavioral care plans. Primary care APRNs should become familiar with the child and adolescent psychiatric APRNs in their area in order to facilitate referrals when needed. A transitional meeting between the APRNs, the child or adolescent in need of more intensive treatment, and the family may facilitate a smoother transfer and help to define the unique differences in the two practice roles.

When the youth with symptoms of a mood disorder has problems falling asleep or staying asleep, the APRN can encourage the youth or family members to keep a sleep diary. The implementation of good sleep habits, such as a regular bedtime, avoidance of caffeine products in the evening, and instituting a relaxing routine before sleep, may assist in normalizing sleep patterns. Nutritional counseling may be needed to ensure that the child or adolescent maintains an adequate dietary intake.

APRNs should connect youth and their families with needed services and also coordinate their care. APRNs should be aware of resources and referral sources that are available in the community. They should also be aware of insurance sources and know how to code and bill for mental health services. Referral to psychiatric practitioners to initiate medication use and to provide periodic evaluation is essential for youth with symptoms of mood disorders (Cheung et al. 2018).

Implications for Practice and Nursing Research

The increased morbidity and mortality associated with mood disorders call for APRNs to be involved as a central part of the healthcare team. APRNs play an important role in screening for mood disorders in the primary care setting and for treating minor mood dysregulation in children and adolescents across a variety of settings. Primary care APRNs are instrumental in working with mental health APRNs and making appropriate referrals for behavioral and psychiatric disorders that are beyond the management strategies of their scope of practice. Establishing collaborative treatment partnerships with mental health providers can ensure timely and appropriate treatment of youth, and reduce the treatment wait times and difficulty with access that currently exists. Adhering to recommended routine screening for mental, emotional, and behavioral disorders during primary care visits will result in early case-finding and appropriate referrals for care. Building on a previously established relationship with children and their parents, knowledge of the patient's background, and being among the first line of care that children routinely access, APRNs can bring about positive outcomes for youth with mental health challenges, including mood disorders (National Association of Pediatric Nurse Practitioners [NAPNAP] 2013). APRNs working with youth should work to foster and fortify relationships with mental health advocates, school officials, human services agencies, mental health and substance abuse providers, and developmental specialists. The best results for youth and their families are obtained when screening for mood disorders occurs early in care and is linked to collaborative and comprehensive models of care (NAPNAP 2013).

Most of the randomized controlled trials and large-sample research on mood dysregulation in youth have been conducted by providers in other disciplines. Therefore, more nursing research is needed in the area of pediatric mood dysregulation, especially with preschool, school-age, and preadolescent populations. Table 12.4 provides examples of nursing research conducted with adolescents experiencing or diagnosed with mood dysregulation disorders.

While mental health screening is strongly recommended in primary care, APRNs are in a unique position to conduct research related to assessment and treatment of minor symptoms by primary care APRNs. They are positioned to test the effectiveness of collaborative efforts, and to collect longitudinal data on the well-being of children with mood dysregulation who are able to be maintained in "real world" environments. It is also an opportunity to design collaborative empirical and naturalistic research between primary care APRNs and

Table 12.4 Examples of nursing research on mood disorders

Researcher (s)	Title and source	Year published	Type of study	Findings
Bhatta et al.	Outcomes of depression screening among adolescents accessing school-based pediatric primary care clinic services *Pediatric Nursing*, 38, 8–14	2018	Quantitative	Implementation of PHQ-9 depression screening protocol identified major depressive disorder among adolescents (*n* = 256) accessing pediatric school-based primary care clinic services. Screening facilitated referrals to mental health providers, potentially improving morbidity and mortality among adolescents.
Garmy et al.	Evaluation of a School-Based Program Aimed at Preventing Depressive Symptoms in Adolescents *Journal of School Nursing, 31,* 117–125	2015	Quantitative	62 students (aged 14) and seven tutors participated. Students rated their depressed symptoms as significantly lower after the course, and for the females this was maintained 1 year post intervention. The implementation costs for the initial 2 years were about US$300 per student.
Ladores and Corcoran	Investigating post-partum depression in the adolescent mother using three potential qualitative approaches *Clinical Medicine Insights: Pediatrics,* 13, 1–6	2019	Qualitative	Of 69 studies meeting inclusion criteria for this PRISMA, only two were qualitative studies (*n* = 15; *n* = 19). A qualitative approach was used to better understand the phenomenon under study from the participants directly. Ethnography, phenomenology, and participatory action research were identified as the best methods to use when engaging fully with participants.
Pontes et al.	Additive interactions between gender and bullying victimization on depressive symptoms and suicidality: Youth Risk Behavior Survey 2011–2015 *Nursing Research*, 67, 430–438	2018.	Quantitative	Analyses of pooled data from the 2011, 2013, and 2015 Youth Risk Behavior Survey (*n* = 44 632) were performed to examine whether the relationship between bullying victimization and depressive symptoms or suicidality significantly varied by gender. The relationship between bullying victimization and depressive symptoms or suicidality was significantly greater among female than male individuals.
Stafford et al.	Getting a grip on my depression: How Latina adolescents experience, self-manage, and seek treatment for depressive symptoms *Qualitative Health Research*, 29(12), 1725–1738	2019	Qualitative	25 participants were included in this grounded theory study. Researchers concluded that to best develop culturally sensitive treatment strategies for successful work with this population, they first had to understand participant experience of depression and depression management directly.
Williams et al.	Adolescents transitioning to high school: Sex differences in bullying victimization associated with depressive symptoms, suicide ideation, and suicide attempts *Journal of School Nursing*, 33(6), 467–479	2017	Quantitative	This study looked at sex differences in bullying victimization and the impact on depressive symptoms and suicidal behaviors in 9th-grade students. In a sample of 233 students, females reported significantly more verbal/social and cyberbullying than male students. Male students who reported physical bullying victimization were more likely to experience depressive symptoms. Verbal/social bullying predicted depressive symptoms in males and females. Females who reported being victims of cyberbullying were more likely to report depressive symptoms, suicide ideation, and suicide attempts.

(continued)

Table 12.4 (cont'd)

Young et al.	Testing the feasibility of a mindfulness-based intervention with underserved adolescents at risk for depression *Holistic Nursing Practice,* 32, 316–323	2018	Quantitative	This study tested the feasibility, acceptability, and preliminary effects of a mindfulness-based intervention with at-risk adolescents from a predominantly Hispanic/Latino community. Seven adolescents completed the mindfulness-based intervention, demonstrating feasibility, and reported acceptability as well as sustained improvements in depressive symptoms, perceived stress, and self-esteem.

child and adolescent mental health APRNs to advance the science within the discipline of nursing.

Additional nursing research on mood disorders in children and adolescents is called for, especially in the areas of collaborative practice, effectiveness of randomized clinical trials, effectiveness of translating science into practice, prevention efforts, culture-specific interventions, and alternative models of treatment with high-risk populations. With the proliferation of mood disorders in youth, and the associated risk of ill-fated outcomes such as self-harm, suicide, and poor quality of life, APRNs in primary care and child and adolescent psychiatric-mental health are in a unique position to conduct this research and make positive contributions in a significant public health concern.

The following are resources of guidelines for identifying and treating adolescents with depression in primary care (Cheung et al. 2018; Zuckerbrot et al. 2018).

Conclusion

This chapter has described the symptoms, etiology, and management of mood dysregulation in children and adolescents with a focus on depression, DMDD, PDD, and PBD. The chapter also acknowledges the unique opportunity for pediatric primary care APRNs to become even more pivotal in the screening, early case finding, and referral process for children in need of mental health treatment. All too often there has been a time frame of 2–4 years between onset of symptoms, diagnosis, and initiation of treatment. During that gap, mood symptoms can interfere with normal development, relationships, academic performance, self-esteem, and the safety of the child who is at risk for engaging in self-injurious behaviors. APRNs who have a sound knowledge base regarding recognizing pediatric mood dysregulation and when to refer to mental health providers will improve the mental healthcare that children and adolescents receive when they access the primary care system.

Resources

American Academy of Child and Adolescent Psychiatry www.aacap. org.

Behavioral assessment tools available for purchase at www.pearson-assesments.com.

Guidelines for Adolescent Depression in Primary Care (GLAD-PC), 3rd version. (2018). Tool kit available to download at www. TheResearchInstitute.org. Contains screening tools and psychoeducation materials (depression facts, medications, counseling, self-management, etc.) and treatment referral resources for healthcare providers to use with children, adolescents and parents.

Hagan, J.F., Shaw, J.S., and Duncan, P.M. (eds.) (2017). *Bright Futures: Guidelines for Health Supervision of Infants, Children and Adolescents,* 4the. Elk Grove Village, IL: American Academy of Pediatrics.

Melnyk, B. and Moldenhauer, Z. (2006). *KYSS Guide to Child and Adolescent Mental Health Screening, Early Intervention and Health Promotion.* Cherry Hill, NJ: NAPNAP.

Neuroscience Educational Institute. Continuing Medical Education on psychiatric and neurologic diseases. Annual membership fee to access materials. Annual conferences offered. www.neiglobal.com.

Siu, A. and USPSTF (2016). Screening for depression in children and adolescents: US Preventive Services Task Force recommendation statement. *Annals of Internal Medicine* 164: 360–366.

TeenScreen National Center for Mental Health Checkups at Columbia University. cdn.ymaws.com.

References

Achenbach, T. (1991). *Manual for the Youth Self-Report and 1991 Profiles.* Burlington, VT: University of Vermont Department of Psychiatry.

Aedo, A., Murru, A., Sanchez, R. et al. (2018). Clinical characterization of rapid-cycling bipolar disorder: association with attention deficit hyperactivity disorder. *Journal of Affective Disorders* 240: 187–192.

Agency for Healthcare Research and Quality. (2018). *Evidence-based practice center systematic review protocol on Depression in Children Systematic Review.* Available at https://effectivehealthcare.ahrq. gov>childhood-depression>protocol.

AAP. (2019). *Recommendations for preventive pediatric health care.* American Academy of Pediatrics. Available at https://www.aap. org/en-us/Documents/periodicity_schedule.pdf.

APA (2013). *Diagnostic and Statistical Manual of Mental Disorders 5.* Arlington, VA: American Psychiatric Association.

Anderson, E. and Hope, D. (2008). A review of the tripartite model for understanding the link between anxiety and depression in youth. *Clinical Psychology Review* 28: 275–287.

Babiss, L. and Gangwisch, J. (2009). Sports participation as a protective factor against depression and suicidal ideation in adolescents as mediated by self-esteem and social support. *Journal of Developmental & Behavioral Pediatrics* 30: 376–384.

Bardach, N.S., Coker, T.R., Zima, B.T. et al. (2014). Common and costly hospitalizations for pediatric mental health disorders. *Pediatrics* 133: 602–609.

Batelaan, N. (2016). Childhood trauma predicts onset and recurrence of depression, and comorbid anxiety and depressive disorders. *Evidence-Based Mental Health* 19 (3) https://doi.org/10.1136/eb-2015-102106.

Bathia, M., Singh, M., and Relan, P. (2016). Prevalence of anxiety and depressive symptoms among patients with hypothyroidism. *Indian Journal of Endocrinology and Metabolism* 20 (4): 468–474.

Beck, A. (1967). *Depression: Clinical, Experiential, and Theoretical Aspects*. New York, NY: Harper& Row.

Beck, A. (2008). The evolution of the cognitive model of depression and its neurobiological correlates. *American Journal of Psychiatry* 165 (8): 969–977.

Beck, A., Steer, R., and Brown, G. (1996). *BDI-II manual*. San Antonio, TX: Psychological Corporation.

Bekhuis, E., Boschloo, L., Rosmalen, J. et al. (2016). The impact of somatic symptoms on the course of major depressive disorder. *Journal of Affective Disorders* 205: 112–118.

Bernaras, E., Jaureguizar, J., and Garaigordobil, M. (2019). Child and adolescent depression: a review of theories, evaluation instruments, prevention programs, and treatments. *Frontiers in Psychology* 10: 543. https://doi.org/10.3389/fpsyg.2019.00543.

Bhatta, S., Champion, J., Young, C., and Loika, E. (2018). Outcomes of depression screening among adolescents accessing school-based pediatric primary care clinic services. *Pediatric Nursing* 38: 8–14.

Bloom, D.E., Cafiero, E.T., Jané-Llopis, E. et al. (2011). *The Global Economic Burden of Noncommunicable Diseases*. Geneva, Switzerland: World Economic Forum.

Bogels, S. and Restifo, K. (2014). *Mindful Parenting: A Guide for Mental Health Practitioners*. New York, NY: Springer.

Bogels, S., Lehtonen, A., and Restifo, K. (2010). Mindful parenting in mental health care. *Mindfulness* 1: 107–120.

Bronfenbrenner, U. (1979). *The Ecology of Human Development: Experiments by Nature and Design*. Cambridge, MA: Harvard University Press.

Bronfenbrenner, U. (1994). Nature-nurture reconceptualized in developmental perspective: a bioecological model. *Psychological Review* 101 (4): 568–586.

Brotman, M., Kircanski, N.K., Stringaris, A. et al. (2017a). Irritability in youths: a translational model. *American Journal of Psychiatry* 174 (6): 520–532.

Brotman, M., Kircanski, K., and Leibenluft, E. (2017b). Irritability in children and adolescents. *Annual Review of Clinical Psychology* 13: 317–341.

Centers for Disease Control and Prevention. (n.d.). *Data and statistics on children's mental health*. Available at https://www.cdc.gov/childrensmentalhealth/data.html.

Cheung, A.H., Zuckerbrot, R.A., Jensen, P.S. et al. (2018). Guidelines for adolescent depression in primary care (GLAD_PC): Part II: Treatment and ongoing management. *Pediatrics* 141 (3): e20174082.

Child Mind Institute. (n.d.). Mood Disorders Center. Available at https://childmind.org/center/mood-disorders-center/.

Chisholm, D., Sweeny, K., Sheehan, P. et al. (2016). Scaling-up treatment of depression and anxiety: a global return on investment analysis. *The Lancet Psychiatry* 3 (5): 415–424. https://doi.org/10.1016/s2215-0366(16)30024-4.

Clark, D. and Beck, A. (2010). Cognitive theory and therapy of anxiety and depression: convergence with neurobiological findings. *Trends in Cognitive Sciences* 14: 418–424.

Cohen, E., MacKenzie, R.G., and Yates, G.L. (1991). HEADSS, a psychosocial risk assessment instrument: implications for designing effective intervention programs for runaway youth. *Journal of Adolescent Health* 12 (7): 539–544.

Costello, E.J., Erkanli, A., and Angold, A. (2006). Is there an epidemic of child or adolescent depression? *Journal of Child Psychology and Psychiatry* 47 (12): 1263–1271.

Daryanani, I., Hamilton, J., McArthur, B. et al. (2017). Cognitive vulnerabilities to depression for adolescents in single-mother and two-parent families. *Journal of Youth and Adolescence* 46: 213–227.

Ebner-Priemer, U. and Trull, T. (2009). Ecological momentary assessment of mood disorders and mood dysregulation. *Psychological Assessment* 21 (4): 463–475.

Elmquist, J., Melton, T., Croarkin, P., and McClintock, S. (2010). A systematic overview of measurement-based care in the treatment of childhood and adolescent depression. *Journal of Psychiatric Practice* 16 (4): 217–234.

Faulstich, M., Carey, M., Ruggiero, M. et al. (1986). Assessment of depression in childhood and adolescence: an evaluation of the center for epidemiological studies of depression scale for children (CES-DC). *American Journal of Psychiatry* 143: 1024–1027.

Fava, G. and Tossani, E. (2007). Prodromal stage of major depression. *Early Intervention in Psychiatry* 1: 9–18.

Finning, K., Ukoumunne, O., Ford, T. et al. (2019). The association between child and adolescent depression and poor attendance at school: a systematic review and meta-analysis. *Journal of Affective Disorders* 245: 928–938.

Forman-Hoffman, V.L., McClure, E., McKeeman, J., Wood, C.T., Middleton, J.C., Skinner, A.C., Perrin, E.M., & Viswanathan, M. (2016). *Screening for major depressive disorder among children and adolescents: A systematic review for the US Preventive Services Task Force*. Evidence Synthesis No. 116. AHRQ Publication No. 13–05192-EF-1. Rockville, MD: Agency for Healthcare Research and Quality.

Fosco, G., Connell, A., Van Ryzin, M., and Stormshak, E. (2016). Preventing adolescent depression with the family check-up: examining family conflict as a mechanism of change. *Journal of Family Psychology* 30: 82–92.

Garber, J. (2006). Depression in children and adolescents: linking risk research and prevention. *American Journal of Preventive Medicine* 31: S104–S125.

Garmy, P., Jakobsson, U., Carlsson, K. et al. (2015). Evaluation of a school-based program aimed at preventing depressive symptoms in adolescents. *Journal of School Nursing* 31: 117–125.

Garzon, D. (2017). Coping and stress tolerance: mental health and illness. In: *Pediatric Primary Care*, 6e (eds. C. Burns et al.), 355–385. St. Louis, MO: Elsevier.

Geracioti, T. (2006). Identifying hypothyroidism's psychiatric presentations. *Current Psychiatry Online* 5 (11) Available at http://www.currentpsychiatry.com/article_pages.asp?AID=4545&UID=Overflow.

Ghandour, R.M., Sherman, L.J., Vladdutiu, C.J. et al. (2019). Prevalence and treatment of depression, anxiety, and conduct problems in US children. *Journal of Pediatrics* 206: 256–267.

Hagel, L.D., Mainieri, A.S., Zeni, C.P., and Wagner, M.B. (2009). Brief report: accuracy of a 16-item questionnaire based on the HEADSS approach (QBH-16) in the screening of mental disorders in adolescents with behavioral problems in secondary care. *Journal of Adolescence* 32: 753–761.

Hamrin, V. and Magorno, M. (2010). Assessment of adolescents for depression in the pediatric primary care setting. *Pediatric Nursing* 36 (2): 103–111.

Hankin, B.L., Badanes, L.S., Abela, J.R.Z., and Watamura, S.E. (2010). Hypothalamic-pituitary-adrenal axis dysregulation in dysphoric children and adolescents: cortisol reactivity to psychosocial stress from preschool through middle adolescence. *Biological Psychiatry* 68: 484–490.

Harvard Mental Health Letter (2007). Thyroid deficiency and mental health. *Harvard Mental Health Letter* 23 (11): 4–5.

Hilt, R.J. and Nussbaum, A.M. (2016). *DSM-5 Pocket Guide for Child and Adolescent Mental Health*. Arlington, VA: American Psychiatric Association.

Hirschfeld, R., Williams, J., Spitzer, R. et al. (2000). Development and validation of a screening instrument for bipolar spectrum disorder: the mood disorder questionnaire. *American Journal of Psychiatry* 157: 1873–1875.

Horowitz, J. and Marchetti, C. (2009). Mood disorders. In: *Primary Care of the Child with a Chronic Condition*, 5e (eds. P. Jackson-Allen, J. Vessey and N. Schapiro), 627–653. St. Louis, MO: Mosby Elsevier.

Howland, R. (2010). Use of endocrine hormones for treating depression. *Journal of Psychosocial Nursing* 48 (12): 13–16.

Jacobs, R., Reinecke, M., Gollan, J., and Kane, P. (2008). Empirical evidence of cognitive vulnerability for depression among children and adolescents: a cognitive science and developmental perspective. *Clinical Psychology Review* 28: 759–782.

Jeffrey, D., Sava, D., and Winters, N. (2005). Depressive disorders. In: *Child and Adolescent Psychiatry: The Essentials* (eds. K. Cheng and K. Myers), 169–189. Philadelphia:, PA: Lippincott Williams & Wilkins.

Kessler, R.C. and Bromet, E.J. (2013). Epidemiology of depression across cultures. *Annual Review of Public Health* 34: 119–138.

Kimball, H. and Cohen, Y. (2019). *Children's Mental Health Report: Social Media, Gaming and Mental Health*. New York: Child Mind Institute.

Kircanski, K., Clayton, M.E., Leibenluft, E., and Brotman, M.A. (2018). Psychosocial treatment of irritability in youth. *Current Treatment Options in Psychiatry* 5 (1): 129–140. https://doi.org/10.1007/s40501-018-0140-5.

Kovacs, M. (1992). *Children Depression Inventory (CDI)*. North Tonawanda, NY: Multi-Health Systems.

Kowatch, R.A., Fristad, M., Birmaher, B. et al. (2005). Treatment guidelines for children and adolescents with bipolar disorder. *Journal of the American Academy of Child and Adolescent Psychiatry* 44 (3): 213–235.

Kraus, C., Castren, E., Kasper, S., and Lanzenberger, R. (2017). Serotonin and neuroplasticity-links between molecular, functional and structural pathophysiology in depression. *Neuroscience and Biobehavioral Reviews* 77: 317–326.

Ladores, S. and Corcoran, J. (2019). Investigating postpartum depression in the adolescent mother using 3 qualitative approaches. *Clinical Medicine Insights: Pediatrics* 13: 1–6.

Leibenluft, E. (2011). Severe mood dysregulation, irritability, and the diagnostic boundaries of bipolar disorder in youths. *American Journal of Psychiatry* 168 (2): 129–142.

Leslie, K. and Chike-Harris, K. (2018). Patient administered screening tool may improve detection and diagnosis of depression among adolescents. *Clinical Pediatrics* 57: 457–460.

Linke, J., Adleman, N.E., Sarlis, J. et al. (2020). White matter microstructure in pediatric bipolar and disruptive mood dysregulation disorder. *Journal of the American Academy of Child and Adolescent Psychiatry*, 59(10), 1135–1145.

Liskola, K., Raaska, H., Lapinleimu, H., and Elovainio, M. (2018). Parental depressive symptoms as a risk factor for child depressive symptoms; testing the social mediators in internationally adopted children. *European Child & Adolescent Psychiatry* 27: 1585–1593.

Lu, M., Juan, C., Koo, M., and Lai, N. (2017). Higher incidence of psychiatrist-diagnosed depression in Taiwanese female school-age children and adolescents with Type 1 diabetes: a nationwide, population-based, retrospective cohort study. *Journal of Child and Adolescent Psychopharmacology* 27: 281–284.

Luby, J., Belden, A., and Spitznagel, E. (2006). Risk factors for preschool depression: the mediating role of early stressful life events. *Journal of Child Psychology and Psychiatry* 47 (12): 1292–1298.

Luby, J.L., Barch, D., Belden, A. et al. (2012). Maternal support in early childhood predicts larger hippocampal volumes at school-age. *Proceedings of the National Academy of Sciences of the United States of America* 109 (80): 2854–2859.

MacPhee, A. and Andrews, J. (2006). Risk factors for depression in early adolescence. *Adolescence* 41 (163): 435–466.

MacPherson, H.A. and Fristad, M.A. (2014). Evidence-based psychosocial treatments for pediatric mood and anxiety disorders. *Current Treatment Options in Psychiatry* 1 (1): 48–65.

Matos, A.P., Salvador, M., Costa, J. et al. (2017). The relationship between internalizing and externalizing problems in adolescence: does gender make a difference? *Canadian International Journal of Social Science Education* 8: 45–63.

Matthews, M., Doherty, G., Sharry, J., and Fitzpatrick, C. (2008). Mobile phone mood charting for adolescents. *British Journal of Guidance and Counselling* 36: 113–129.

McMahon, R. (2015). Parent management training interventions for preschool-age children. In: *Encyclopedia of Early Childhood Development* (eds. R.E. Tremblay, M. Bolvin and R.D. Peters). Available at http://www.child-encyclopedia.com/parenting-skillsaccording-experts/parent-management-training-interventions-preschool-age-children.

Merikangas, K., He, J., Burstein, M. et al. (2010). Lifetime prevalence of mental disorders in U.S. adolescents: results from the national comorbidity survey replication adolescent supplement (NCS-A). *Journal of the American Academy of Child and Adolescent Psychiatry* 49 (10): 980–989.

Moldenhauer, Z. (2006). Mood disorders. In: *The KySS (Keep your Children/Yourself-Safe and Secure) Guide to Child and Adolescent Mental Health Screening, Early and Health Promotion* (eds. B. Melnyk and Z. Moldenhauer), 141–172. Cherry Hill, NJ: NAPNAP.

Morrison, K., Shin, S., Tarnopolsky, M., and Taylor, V. (2015). Association of depression and health related quality of life with body composition in children and youth with obesity. *Journal of Affective Disorders* 172: 18–23.

Mrug, S. and Windle, M. (2010). Prospective effects of violence exposure across multiple contexts on early adolescents' internalizing and externalizing problems. *Journal of Child Psychology and Psychiatry* 51 (8): 953–961.

Mullen, S. (2018). Major depressive disorder in children and adolescents. *Mental Health Clinician* 8 (6): 275–283.

NAPNAP (2013). NAPNAP position statement on the integration of mental health care in pediatric primary care settings. *Journal of Ediatric Health Care* 27: 15A–16A.

NIMH. (n.d.). Disruptive mood dysregulation disorder. National Institute of Mental Health. Available at https://www.nimh.nih.gov/

health/topics/disruptive-mood-dysregulation-disorder-dmdd/
disruptive-mood-dysregulation-disorder.shtml.

NEI (2009). *Understanding and Managing the Pieces of Major Depressive Disorder*. Carlsbad, CA: Neuroscience Educational Institute.

Noller, D.T. (2016). Distinguishing disruptive mood dysregulation disorder from pediatric bipolar disorder. *Journal of the American Academy of Physician Assistants* 29 (6): 25–28.

Pavuluri, M. (2007). Parental version of the mood disorder questionnaire for adolescents has good sensitivity and specificity for diagnosing bipolar disorder in psychiatric outpatient clinics. *Evidence-Based Mental Health* 10: 9–9.

Perrin, J.M., Asarnow, J.R., Stancin, T. et al. (2019). Mental health conditions and health care payments for children with chronic medical conditions. *Academic Pediatrics* 19 (1): 44–50.

Pinfield, J. (2017). Recognising and diagnosing depression in children and young people. *Nursing Standard* (48): 51–63.

Pontes, N., Ayres, C., and Pontes, M. (2018). Additive interactions between gender and bullying victimization on depressive symptoms and suicidality: Youth Risk Behavior Survey 2011–2015. *Nursing Research* 67: 430–438.

Prager, L. (2009). Depression and suicide in children and adolescents. *Pediatrics in Review* 30: 199–206.

Radloff, L.S. (1977). The CES-D scale: a self-report depression scale for research in the general population. *Applied Psychological Measurement* 1: 385–401.

Rahman, M., Todd, C., John, A. et al. (2018). School achievement as a predictor of depression and self-harm in adolescence: linked education and health records study. *British Journal of Psychiatry* 212: 215–221.

Reed, K., Cooper, R., Nugent, W., and Russell, K. (2016). Cyberbullying: a literature review of its relationship to adolescent depression and current intervention strategies. *Journal of Human Behavior in the Social Environment* 26: 37–45.

Restifo, K. and Bogels, S. (2009). Family processes in the development of youth depression: translating the evidence to treatment. *Clinical Psychology Review* 29: 294–316.

Richardson, L., McCauley, E., Grossman, D. et al. (2010). Evaluation of the patient health questionnaire: 9-item for detecting major depression among adolescents. *Pediatrics* 126: 1117–1123.

Riehm, K.E., Feder, K.A., and Tormohlen, K.N. (2019). Associations between time spent using social media and internalizing and externalizing problems among US youth. *JAMA Psychiatry* 11: 1–9. https://doi.org/10.1001/jamapsychiatry.2019.2325.

Rocha, T., Zeni, C., Caetano, S., and Kieling, C. (2013). Mood disorders in childhood and adolescence. *Brazilian Journal of Psychiatry* 35: S22–S31.

Romain, A., Marleau, J., and Baillot, A. (2018). Impact of obesity and mood disorders on physical comorbidities, psychological well-being, health behaviours and the use of health services. *Journal of Affective Disorders* 225: 381–388.

Sadock, B.J. and Sadock, V.A. (2009). *Kaplan & Sadock's Concise Textbook of Child and Adolescent Psychiatry*. Philadelphia, PA: Wolters Kluwer.

Sarris, J., O'Neill, A., Coulson, C.E. et al. (2014). Lifestyle medicine for depression. *BMC Psychiatry* 14: 107.

Shapiro, J., Mindra, S., Timmins, V. et al. (2017). A controlled study of obesity among adolescents with bipolar disorder. *Journal of Child and Adolescent Psychopharmacology* 27: 95–100.

Shensa, A., Sidani, J., Dew, M. et al. (2018). Social media use and depression and anxiety symptoms: a cluster analysis. *American Journal of Health Behavior* 42: 116–128.

Siever, L.J. and Davis, K.L. (1985). Overview: toward a dysregulation hypothesis of depression. *American Journal of Psychiatry* 142: 1017–1031.

Siu, A. and USPSTF (2016). Screening for depression in children and adolescents: US Preventive Services Task Force recommendation statement. *Annals of Internal Medicine* 164: 360–366.

Skokauskas, N., Lavelle, T., Munir, K. et al. (2018). The cost of child and adolescent mental health services. *Lancet Psychiatry* 5 (4): 299–300.

Sole, E., Garriga, M., Valleti, M., and Vieta, E. (2017). Mixed features in bipolar disorder. *CNS Spectrums* 22 (2): 134–140.

Stafford, A.M., Aaisma, M.C., Bigatti, S. et al. (2019). Getting a grip on my depression: how Latina adolescents experience, self-manage, and seek treatment for depressive symptoms. *Qualitative Health Research* 29 (12): 1725–1738.

Stahl, S. (2008). *Stahl's Essential Psychopharmacology: Neuroscientific Basis and Practical Applications*, 3e. New York, NY: Cambridge University Press.

Stebbins, M. and Corcoran, J. (2016). Pediatric bipolar disorder: the child psychiatrist's perspective. *Child & Adolescent Social Work Journal* 33: 115–122.

Steingard, R.J. (n.d.). *Mood disorders and teenage girls*. Child Mind Institute. Available at http://childmind.org.

Stockburger, S. and Omar, H. (2017). Youth suicide prevention: an example. *International Journal of Child Health & Human Development* 10: 397–400.

Stringaris, A., Vidal-Ribas, P., Brotman, M., and Leibenluft, E. (2018). Practitioner review: definition, recognition, and treatment challenges of irritability in young people. *Journal of Child Psychology and Psychiatry* 59 (7): 721–739.

Tackett, J. (2010). Toward an externalizing spectrum in DSM-V: incorporating developmental concerns. *Child Development Perspectives* 4 (3): 161–167.

Tang, M.H. and Pinsky, E.G. (2015). Mood and affect disorders. *Pediatrics in Review* 36 (2): 52–61.

UN Department of Economic and Social Affairs Population Division World Population Prospects. (2015). *World Population Prospects: Key Findings & Advance Tables*. Available at https://esa.un.org/unpd/wpp/publications/files/key_findings_wpp_2015.pdf.

USPSTF. (2016). *Depression in children and adolescents: Screening*. Available at https://www.uspreventiveservicestaskforce.org/Page/Document/UpdateSummaryFinal/depression-in-children-and-adolescents-screening1.

Verhulst, F., Achenbach, T., Ende, J. et al. (2003). Comparison of problems reported by youths from seven countries. *American Journal of Psychiatry* 160 (8): 1479–1485.

Waite, R. and Ryan, R. (2019). *Adverse Childhood Experiences: What Students and Health Professionals Need to Know*. London, England: Routledge.

WebMD. (n.d.). *Clonidine HCl ER side effects by likelihood and severity*. Available at www.webmd.com.

Weersing, V.R., Jeffreys, M., Do, M.-C.T. et al. (2017). Evidence-base update of psychosocial treatments for child and adolescent depression. *Journal of Clinical Child and Adolescent Psychology* 46 (1): 11–43.

Weissman, M., Orvaschel, H., and Padian, N. (1980). Children's symptoms and social function self-report scales: comparison of mothers' and children's reports. *Journal of Nervous and Mental Disease* 168: 736–740.

Whooley, M., Avins, A., Miranda, J., and Browner, W. (1997). Case-finding instruments for depression: two questions are as good as many. *Journal of General Internal Medicine* 12: 439–445.

Wilcox, H., Field, T., Prodromidis, M., and Scafidi, F. (1998). Correlations between the BDI and CES-D in a sample of adolescent mothers. *Adolescence* 33: 565–574.

Williams, S., Langhinrichsen-Rohling, J., Wornell, C., and Finnegan, H. (2017). Adolescents transitioning to high school: sex differences in bullying victimization associated with depressive symptoms, suicide ideation, and suicide attempts. *Journal of School Nursing* 33: 467–479.

World Health Organization. (2019). *Adolescent Mental Health: Key Facts*. Available at https://www.who.int/news-room/fact-sheets/detail/adolescent-mental-health.

Young, C., Minami, H., Aguilar, R., and Brown, R. (2018). Testing the feasibility of a mindfulness-based intervention with underserved adolescents at risk for depression. *Holistic Nursing Practice* 32: 316–323.

Yule, A., Fitzgerald, M., Wilens, T. et al. (2018). Further evidence of the diagnostic utility of the child behavior checklist for identifying pediatric bipolar disorder. *Journal of the American Academy of Child & Adolescent Psychiatry, Supplement* 57: S185–S185.

Zuckerbrot, R., Cheung, A., Jensen, P. et al. (2018). Guidelines for adolescent depression in primary care (GLAD-PC) part 1: practice preparation, identification, assessment and initial management. *Pediatrics* 141 (3): e20174081.

13

Deliberate Self-harm: Nonsuicidal Self-injury and Suicide in Children and Adolescents

Edilma L. Yearwood[1] and Eve Bosnick[2]

[1]Georgetown University School of Nursing & Health Studies, Washington, DC, USA
[2]University of Pennsylvania School of Nursing, Philadelphia, PA, USA

Objectives

After reading this chapter, advanced practice registered nurses (APRNs) will be able to:

1. Differentiate between the etiologies and processes involved in various deliberate self-harm (DSH) behaviors such as suicidal ideation (SI), nonsuicidal self-injury (NSSI), and suicide in children and adolescents.
2. Identify internalizing, externalizing, and psychosocial factors that place children and adolescents at risk for engaging in a range of self-harming behaviors.
3. Describe evidence-based pharmacological and nonpharmacological care management models for use by

primary care and child and adolescent psychiatric-mental health APRNs who work with self-harming youth.
4. Identify evidence-based treatment strategies to use with children and adolescents who self-harm and their families/caregivers.
5. Describe the DSM-5 conditions for further study related to suicidal behavior and NSSI.
6. Discuss responsibilities of APRNs in the identification and care of self-harming and suicidal children and adolescents.

Introduction

This chapter will focus on a variety of deliberate self-harm (DSH) behaviors, differentiate between nonsuicidal self-injury (NSSI) and suicidal self-injurious (SSI) behaviors, identify youth at risk for engaging in these behaviors, describe etiologies attributed to DSH behaviors, and present evidence-based management strategies for use when working with these youth. The accuracy of prevalence rates of NSSI in adolescents is difficult to ascertain because of the secrecy that often accompanies these behaviors. However, it is estimated to range

between 12% and 40% in community populations with and without a psychiatric diagnosis and between 38% and 67% in inpatient adolescent psychiatric populations (Cipriano et al. 2017; Gilles et al. 2018; Monto et al. 2018; Muehlenkamp et al. 2009).

In 2016, suicide was the second leading cause of death in youth and young adults aged 10–24 years of age in the United States (Centers for Disease Control and Prevention [CDC] 2016) and the second leading cause of death in 15–29 year-olds world-wide (World Health Organization [WHO] 2019). In 2017, the CDC identified

Child and Adolescent Behavioral Health: A Resource for Advanced Practice Psychiatric and Primary Care Practitioners in Nursing, Second Edition. Edited by Edilma L. Yearwood, Geraldine S. Pearson, and Jamesetta A. Newland.
© 2021 John Wiley & Sons, Inc. Published 2021 by John Wiley & Sons, Inc.
Companion website: www.wiley.com/go/Yearwood

3013 deaths by suicide in youth aged 5–19 (CDC 2017). Since 2011, suicide has surpassed homicide as a cause of injury-related deaths in youth (Carbone et al. 2018). The Youth Risk Behavior Surveillance (YRBS) data obtained between September 2016 and December 2017 on 14765 youth in grades 9–12 found that 17.2% of these youth considered suicide, 13.6% had developed a plan, and 7.4% had made one or more suicidal gestures (CDC 2018). Furthermore, of those who had made a gesture of self-injury by poisoning or overdose, 2.4% required treatment by a nurse or physician (CDC 2018). Self-inflicted gunshot wounds, hanging, suffocation using plastic bags, overdosing, and self-poisoning continue to be the most frequently used methods for suicide in youth (Kidshealth 2015). Males remain twice as likely to be successful in committing suicide when compared to females (Kidshealth 2015).

NSSI, also referred to as self-mutilation, self-injury, self-injurious behaviors, or para-suicide, has been analyzed and discussed in the psychiatric literature for well over 60 years. Initially, these behaviors were thought to be strongly linked to suicide. However, recent evidence points to these behaviors being a distinct and separate phenomena with different motivations. There are youngsters who engage in "common" NSSI behaviors with *no intent* to kill themselves, a second group of youngsters who are suicide attempters, and a third, believed to be the most pathologically entrenched group, who engage in both SSI and NSSI behaviors (Cloutier et al. 2010).

This chapter will highlight the increasing crisis associated with self-harm and suicide behaviors in youth and describe etiologies believed to be the drivers of these behaviors. In addition, factors that put youth at risk for engaging in these behaviors will be identified, along with clinical behaviors frequently seen, assessment tools used for screening at-risk and self-harming youth, and nursing management strategies for use with this population.

Suicidal Ideation and Nonsuicidal Self-Injury

It is not uncommon for children and adolescents to experience suicidal ideation (SI), especially during stressful times when they feel that there is no good solution to their dilemma. SI is the "consideration of or desire to end one's life and can exist as passive (general thought only without specific plan) or active (thinking of committing a specific action)," (Cha et al. 2017, pp. 460–461). Children should not be made to feel guilty about having SI, but instead need to recognize and understand that all people experience a range of thoughts and emotions, and should be taught that it is what people do with these emotions that guides the particular outcome.

DSH and NSSI will be used interchangeably in this chapter. There has been some discrepancy as to whether these terms are similar or different (McDougall et al. 2010; Muehlenkamp et al. 2012). Descriptions of both terms stress the fact that the individual does not preplan the act.

Youngsters who engage in NSSI do not intend to die; they engage in the behaviors to feel better (Favazza 1998). During the act of self-injury, the individual engages in a "socially unacceptable repetitive behavior that causes minor to moderate physical injury. When self-mutilating, the individual is in a psychologically disturbed state but is not attempting suicide or responding to a need for self-stimulation or a stereotypic behavior characteristic of mental retardation or autism" (Suyemoto 1998, p. 532). When NSSI behaviors begin in childhood and continue throughout adolescence, these youngsters are viewed as more entrenched in the ritual and cycle of self-harming behaviors. Common descriptors used to explain the pattern of NSSI include compulsive, ritualistic, episodic, and repetitive. The level of the injury or the amount of harm to the body is usually described as mild, moderate, or extreme. Table 13.1, which was adapted from Favazza (1998), Nock (2010), Suyemoto (1998), and Wells et al. (1998), contains a list of self-harm behaviors rated from mild to extreme. Cutting of the skin is a common act and the most common sites are the arms, legs, inner thighs, and the abdomen. Practitioners should question youth who consistently wear long-sleeved shirts and sweaters or multiple layers of clothing in warm weather and youth who are reluctant to expose certain body surface areas during physical examinations. The APRN needs to keep in mind that NSSI is a quick act that can occur in multiple contexts; it is usually performed in private with the individual having access to inexpensive and readily available tools.

NSSI usually begins between the ages of 12 and 14, with adolescent prevalence rates three to four times greater than adult rates (Klonsky et al. 2003). NSSI is *deliberate, repetitive,* and *direct destruction or alteration* of body tissue that is done without conscious suicidal intent but can result in severe tissue damage (Favazza 1998). Unfortunately, while the intent is not suicide, some who engage in NSSI inadvertently do kill themselves due to the potential lethality of the method chosen, miscalculation associated with intensity of self-harm behavior, or the fact that they fail to access medical treatment in a timely manner. NSSI can be a culturally sanctioned behavior, a pathological act against the self in order to manage perceived intolerable tension, an attempt to avoid suicide (and therefore can be considered a poor coping strategy), or a drastic attempt to communicate needs and feelings to others. It is not uncommon for self-injurers to use multiple methods

Table 13.1 Examples of NSSI/DSH behaviors

Mild to moderate behaviors	Extreme behaviors
Head banging	Object insertion (risk for infection and other trauma)
Self-biting	Branding or carving words or symbols into skin
Skin picking	Deep skin cutting
Burning (first degree)	Ingesting toxic substances (poisoning)
Superficial skin cutting	Burning (second and third degree)
Trichotillomania	Severe onychophagia (nail biting that results in bleeding, infection, and mutilation)
Needle sticking	
Some forms of body piercing	
Hitting walls and objects to induce pain	
Breaking bones	
Preventing wound healing	Eye enucleation and self-castration are usually secondary to a psychotic experience
Excessive rubbing	Self–stabbing

Source: Adapted from Favazza (1998), Nock (2010), Suyemoto (1998), and Wells et al. (1998).

Table 13.2 Factors associated with increased risk of engaging in NSSI

1. History of NSSI
2. Chronic feeling of hopelessness
3. Female gender
4. History of being bullied
5. Social contagion (others engaging in the behavior)
6. Identifying with youth subcultures (gothic or emo)
7. Nonheterosexual orientation
8. Experiencing adverse childhood experiences
9. Vulnerability to social media/internet influence
10. Alleviate intense negative emotions
11. Intense self-anger

Source: Belfort and Miller (2018), Fox et al. (2016, 2018), and Victor and Klonsky (2018).

and more than one body location during the span of time that they engage in self-harm activities. Prevalence rates of NSSI are similar between males and females (American Psychiatric Association 2013).

Two factors clearly evident from the literature chronicling the development of the science of NSSI are that (i) NSSI and suicidal behavior are distinct phenomena with different intent and expected outcome, and (ii) NSSI in its purest form is best understood in the absence of developmental or intellectual impairment and psychosis (American Psychiatric Association 2013; Favazza 1998; Mangnall and Yurkovich 2008). Reportedly, nearly 80% of those who engage in NSSI stop the behavior within 5 years (Whitlock, Eckenrode & Silverman, 2006).

The Diagnostic and Statistical Manual for Mental Disorders, 5th edition (American Psychiatric Association 2013), identified suicidal behavior disorder and NSSI as conditions for further study and have not identified them at this time as specific disorders. This is in response to awareness of the increase in these behaviors, especially during the adolescent years. Proposed criteria for Suicidal Behavior Disorder include suicide attempt within the last 2 years, where the attempt was not an act of NSSI and not associated with ideation, confusion, delirium, or a political driver (American Psychiatric Association 2013). Suicidal behavior disorder is proposed to be associated with comorbid mental disorders such as bipolar disorder, major depression, and personality disorders, among others. The proposed criteria for NSSI includes, among other criteria, engaging in self-injury five or more times in the past year in order to gain relief from overwhelming negative feelings, to prompt a positive feeling state or in reaction to difficulty with others, the behavior is not socially sanctioned (such as tattooing) and the behavior results in distress or interferes with functioning (American Psychiatric Association 2013).

Etiology of NSSI

Over the years, several theories have been offered to explain why people engage in NSSI (Table 13.2). These include engaging in the act to (i) change or influence negative personal affect and emotions such as anger or depression, (ii) punish self, (iii) influence the thoughts and behaviors of others, (iv) interrupt dissociative experiences, (v) experience excitement, and (vi) cope with suicidal thoughts (Klonsky 2007). Engaging in NSSI seems to meet both intrapersonal and interpersonal needs (Klonsky et al. 2015). The initial four-factor model of NSSI offered insight in the drivers of NSSI. The factors included intrapersonal or automatic cessation of feelings which can be positive (sense of release or connection with a feeling state) or negative (release of built up tension) or interpersonal social positive (where sought-after attention from others is obtained as a result of the act) or social negative (a way to escape interactions perceived as unpleasant) (Nock and Prinstein 2004, 2005). Klonsky et al. (2015) reviewed and critiqued the four-factor model and proposed a two-factor structure based on their own research and that of others (Bildik et al. 2013; Klonsky and Glenn 2009). They identified NSSI as having an intrapersonal (to decrease negative emotions) and social (to influence others) function.

Influencing Affect Regulation

Ample research data indicate that individuals engage in NSSI behaviors as a means of modifying negative and highly charged emotions due to their inability to tolerate these intense emotional states (Andover and Morris 2014; Cipriano et al. 2017; Klonsky et al. 2003; Suyemoto 1998). The emotions usually include anger, fear of abandonment or rejection, despair, guilt, or anxiety. Gratz and Roemer (2004) identified four components of *emotion regulation* that are precursors to understanding adaptation to emotional distress and the individual's attempts at self-regulation. First, one must be aware of and understand various emotional states commonly experienced by human beings. Second, the individual must be capable of engaging in goal-directed activities while inhibiting the experience of negative emotions. Third, the individual must have the ability to use one or more strategies to manage intense or negative emotions instead of disconnecting from the emotion. Last, the individual must be willing to experience negative emotions and work through them rather than engaging in maladaptive behavioral responses. As Gratz (2007) pointed out, interventions with individuals who engage in NSSI must include teaching about a range of emotions as this may have been lacking during their formative years, promoting understanding and acceptance of the experience of different emotional states, and teaching management strategies and skills to use during emotionally charged times.

Individuals who engage in NSSI as a form of affect regulation may also be trying to externalize, through physical pain, their affective experience, thereby taking control of the situation. You et al. (2018) conducted a meta-analysis of 42 studies done with adult and adolescent participants, looking at the relationship between emotion regulation and NSSI. They found eight separate categories associated with emotion regulation. These included lack of emotional awareness, lack of emotional clarity, nonacceptance of personal emotional responses, lack of access to effective strategies to manage emotions,

problems controlling impulses, problems in ability to engage in goal-directed behaviors, problems expressing emotions, and problems with emotional reactivity. Of these, emotional reactivity and limited access to effective emotion regulation strategies were most strongly associated with acts of NSSI. These findings point to a potential role of cognitive behavioral therapy (CBT), dialectic behavioral therapy (DBT), and skills modeling and training in work with youth experiencing emotion dysregulation.

As an Act of Self-punishment

Some self-injurers appear to be more self-critical and self-loathing than nonself-injurers and this schema, in combination with low self-esteem, results in NSSI as a form of self-punishment (Andover and Morris 2014; Hooley and St. Germain 2014; Klonsky 2007; Klonsky and Muehlenkamp 2007). Nock (2009) and Glassman et al. (2007) described NSSI as self-directed abuse that becomes a learned behavior secondary to a history of physical or sexual abuse or emotional neglect.

To Influence Others

NSSI behavior has also been associated with attempts to influence the emotions and reactivity of others, call attention to personal distress states, and reactivity secondary to perceived lack of social support, including secondary to bullying victimization (Brown and Plener 2017; Cipriano et al. 2017; Hornor 2016; 2018; Klonsky et al. 2014; Muehlenkamp et al. 2013; Victor and Klonsky 2018). Interventions with youngsters who self-injure to influence others may include being taught socially appropriate relationship development and maintenance and communication and social skills.

To Interrupt Dissociation

NSSI has also been seen as a negative coping behavior used to end dissociative experiences. Dissociation has long been associated with childhood trauma, borderline personality disorder, and exposure to severe or prolonged traumatic events. The individual uses dissociation as a defense mechanism to protect against pain from the trauma. During dissociative states, the individual either feels nothing or experiences derealization or depersonalization. Experiencing a different type of pain (physical) and seeing blood or injury to the skin is believed to interrupt the dissociative state and return the person to a "current or real" and grounded state (Cipriano et al. 2017; Mangnall and Yurkovich 2008; Zetterqvist et al. 2013). In essence, the act of self-injury serves to regulate affect.

As an Experience of Excitement

Self-injurers have also reported engaging in NSSI in order to feel "high" or obtain a sense of "excitement" from the act itself. Klonsky and Muehlenkamp (2007) point out that this group of self-injurers tend to engage in the act with others and report feeling an excitement comparable to that felt when bungee jumping. This is a different profile from most other self-injurers, who tend to be secretive or "loners" when self-mutilating. What chronic self-injurers seem to have in common, however, is that the behavior releases neurochemical endorphins, which serve to impact or regulate their affective state (Klonsky 2014; Klonsky and Muehlenkamp 2007).

Associated with Increased Suicide Risk

While NSSI is a distinct behavior from suicide, long-standing NSSI behavior is a risk factor for suicide and when initiated in adolescence can be a predictor of later suicide behaviors (Chesin et al. 2017; Grandclerc et al. 2016; Kiekens et al. 2018). Engaging in self-harm behaviors over a period of time is viewed as a gateway learned behavior that increases capacity for suicide ideation and attempts and success in adulthood.

Neurochemical Influence

Research has also explored the neurochemical bases of NSSI as there appears to be a correlation between low serotonin (5-hydroxytryptamine [5-HT]) levels and depression, impulsivity, aggression, and DSH behaviors (Crowell et al. 2008). Postmortem autopsies conducted on victims of successful suicides revealed lower levels of serotonin in the ventral prefrontal cortex. In addition, low serotonin blood serum levels have been found in suicide attempters (Currier and Mann 2008; Mann 2003). A properly functioning (adequate amounts of neurotransmitters, transporter sites, and receptors) prefrontal cortex is responsible for decision-making, action, and impulse inhibition. Dysregulation of the site-specific neurotransmitter process or injury to the ventral prefrontal cortex results in disinhibition and may explain the reactive and impulsive act of self-injury. Engaging in NSSI has also been attributed to a decrease in cortisol level secondary to increased stress. It is believed that initially increased cortisol level triggers the act of self-injury, which in turn diminishes the individual's arousal level and decreases cortisol levels while increasing endorphins. This increase in endorphins results in the experience of a calm and relaxed state post self-harm (Nock and Mendes 2008). This frequent experience of elevated endorphins after the self-harm act is thought to become addictive, prompting the individual to repeat the act to achieve a calm and peaceful state (Blasco-Fontecilla et al. 2016; Plener et al. 2017).

Additional Diagnostic Considerations

Rule Out Other Disorders

Engaging in DSH behaviors is one criterion associated with several psychiatric disorders found in the *Diagnostic and Statistical Manual of Mental Disorders 5* (American Psychiatric Association 2013). Therefore, when conducting a complete assessment of these youngsters, it is important for the clinician to first rule out the following disorders: dissociative disorder, borderline personality disorder (routinely diagnosed after age 18), and conduct or antisocial personality disorder (the latter diagnosed after age 18). If the youngster does not meet the criteria for any of the aforementioned disorders, NSSI must be considered. However, NSSI behaviors can co-occur with substance use, mood disorders, anxiety disorders, eating disorders, posttraumatic stress disorder, and dissociative and borderline personality. Youngsters who have a pervasive developmental disorder or psychosis may also exhibit self-injuring behaviors that are frequently associated with those disorders and would not meet the criteria for DSH NSSI.

Rule Out Culturally Endorsed Body Modifications

Throughout history, cultures have engaged in body modification rituals as an expression of their beliefs, as a component of religious practices, to mark a group's identity, to indicate an individual's membership in a group, to promote healing, to identify with a spirit, or to reinforce control and social order (Favazza 1998, 2009, 2011). Culturally endorsed body modifications can range from barbaric and painful actions such as female genital mutilation, branding, or skin scarring to more benign ritualistic acts such as piercing and tattooing. While some of these activities are self-inflicted, many are done to the individual by members of the family or cultural community as part of a rites of passage ritual. While the intent is not to contribute to the demise of the individual, physical and psychological injury can and does occur and can be more devastating the younger the child. Culturally endorsed body modifications are not considered NSSI and do not meet the criteria included in conditions for further study identified in the DSM-5.

Other Factors to Consider/Assess

Suicide and Self-harming Behaviors in LGBTQ Youth

Lesbian, gay, bisexual, transgender and queer (LGBTQ) or sexual minority youth are at increased risk for engaging in self-harm, suicide attempts, and suicide completion when compared with their peer group of non-LGBTQ youth (Fox et al. 2018; Hong et al. 2011; National Action Alliance for Suicide Prevention 2015;

Ream 2019). These youth are at higher risk for bullying, discrimination, violence, isolation, depression and anxiety, and rejection from both peers and family members (Bostwick et al. 2014; Willging et al. 2016), all risk factors that can contribute to self-injurious behaviors.

Nurses can be strong advocates and support for LGBTQ youth who present in primary care, the school, and/or in mental health treatment facilities. Nurses should include assessment of sexual preference, experiences, and relationships with all youth during routine assessment. In addition, creating a welcoming, safe, and inclusive environment in the office and practice site may facilitate openness and willingness by the youth to discuss any self-harm intent based on discrimination and bullying as a result of LGBTQ status. Hong et al. (2011) encourage providers to use a social-ecological model when intervening with LGBTQ youth in order to best address and respond to the complex environmental experiences that these youth encounter and the multiple intersectionality of the health, mental health, and identities of these youth. The APRN can provide professional development education for others in the work environment, family members, and all youth on topics such as diversity and inclusion, implicit bias, sexual orientation, gender identity, and gender expression. The APRN should also be knowledgeable of health and mental health community resources that work specifically with this population for referrals as needed. One resource that provides 24-hour crisis intervention and suicide prevention services for LGBTQ youth is the Trevor Project (n.d.) (info@thetrevorproject.org). The reader is encouraged to review Chapters 7 and 24 for additional information on the needs of LGBTQ youth.

The Internet and NSSI

The internet can be both a positive and a negative tool for youngsters who engage in NSSI (Whitlock, Powers & Eckenrode, 2006). The internet offers anonymity and provides an avenue for social interaction for youth who engage in self-harm behaviors. They learn that they are not alone and that there are countless others globally who also self-injure. Unfortunately, the Internet also contains sites that endorse and provide details on how to self-injure and may endorse the use of certain sites or peers instead of professionals when dealing with their mental health symptoms or urges to self-injure (Belfort and Miller 2018). Youngsters who only use the internet to deal with their self-harm behaviors avoid working through emotions and avoid examining triggers to these behaviors (Whitlock et al. 2007).

Brown et al. (2017) and Koreno et al. (2016) conducted research on Instagram posts and pictures. Findings from this social media source included pictures posted of wounds caused by self-injury, pictures of multiple methods of cutting, the hashtag #cat (indicative of a cutting action), and other methods of inflicting self-injury. The Instagram sites on NSSI were freely available, warnings about the content did not deter from accessing the site, and there were minimal screening actions by Instagram administrators. In working with youth who self-injure and their parents, the APRN should assess for use of the internet and specific sites visited while trying to gain understanding about the influence that this media may have in the life of the youngster. Specific sites to ask about include blogs like xanga.com, myspace.com, and facebook.com. In addition, the APRN should question the sites visited on Youtube.com, whether the youth visits message boards or receives instant messages or text messages from others, and the content of those messages. Frequent bombardment with messages on "how to engage in the act" may place a vulnerable youngster at risk for following through when experiencing overwhelming emotions.

More recently, Marchant et al. 2017 conducted a systematic review of studies conducted between 2011 and 2015. The researchers examined internet use and self-harm behaviors in individuals under the age of 25. Of the 51 studies that met the inclusion criteria,18 provided negative influences, 11 provided positive influences, and 17 were mixed. High levels of internet use, internet addiction, and frequenting sites containing self-harm and suicide content was associated with higher rates of self-harm behaviors. However, findings also indicated that internet use decreased social isolation and could be a source of help for numerous youths. They recommended that given the popularity of social media in young people, efforts should focus on placing more positive messages on social media to provide adolescents with positive alternative messages along with social support.

Maintenance of NSSI Behaviors

Nock (2009) constructed an integrated theoretical model that depicts how NSSI behavior develops and is maintained. The model depicted in Figure 13.1 identifies risk factors such as childhood history of physical or sexual abuse, poor impulse control, high reactivity, and parents or caretakers who are hostile and critical. Bully victimization, self-harm by peers, difficulties at school, and health problems are additional risk factors. The model also identifies vulnerabilities in the individual and in the environment that also influence behavior. When stressed, the individual engages in NSSI to regulate affect or impact the social situation. Nock argues that self-injuring behaviors are maintained by either positive or negative intrapersonal and interpersonal reinforcement. In assessing and working with this population, it would be important for the APRN to be knowledgeable about distal or underlying behavioral drivers, youth vulnerabilities,

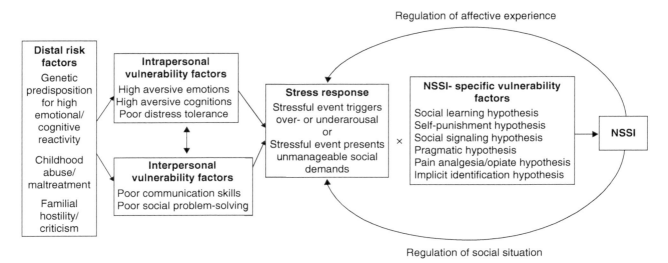

Figure 13.1 Integrated theoretical model of the development and maintenance of self-injury. (*Source:* Reprinted from Nock (2009), with permission from SAGE Publications.)

proximal or immediate precipitating triggers, and patterns of social and affective regulation.

Assessment of Self-injury in Primary Care

Routine assessment for NSSI behaviors should occur at all primary care health maintenance visits in conjunction with assessment for mood disorders, anxiety, depression, SI, and other psychiatric symptoms. At illness visits or episodic care, the review of systems for the chief complaint may include an assessment for psychiatric symptoms and risk for NSSI. Chief complaints that may trigger this assessment would be unexplained injuries or histories that are inconsistent with the presentation. Adolescents may present with vague complaints of headache, sleep disturbances, or other functional symptoms related to anxiety or depression. In attempting to access help, teens may present with a "hidden agenda," which may only be revealed in a confidential interview.

The APRN is in the unique position of having a trusted relationship with the patient and can be the first person the patient may choose to disclose to. In accordance with the recommendations of the American Academy of Pediatrics (Bridgemohan et al. 2018; www.aap.org) and the Society of Adolescent Health and Medicine (Ford et al. 2004; www.adolescenthealth.org), a confidential history should be conducted to provide adolescents with the best opportunity to disclose risk behaviors that may be injurious to them. Typically, some SI and all suicidal gestures or behaviors are exclusionary criteria to confidentiality and require that the APRN inform a caretaker or parent and secure support for urgent or immediate mental health services. Differentiating between NSSI and

SSI is essential for proper triage and management by the APRN. Any patient who poses an immediate life-threatening risk requires immediate transport by police or ambulance to a psychiatric emergency center for evaluation, possible hospitalization, and treatment of suicidal behavior. Those who present with an injury without suicidal intent should be sent to an emergency department for assessment and treatment of any significant wounds related to self-injury. Some patients can receive assessment and treatment in primary care and then be referred to APRNs in mental health for psychological counseling, treatment, and ongoing monitoring.

Most providers will screen youth routinely for concerns about troubling mood symptoms, including overwhelming anxiety and increased depressive and hopeless thoughts, or thoughts about hurting themselves or others. Youths who use NSSI to cope often experience a great deal of shame and are unwilling to disclose their behavior readily. On occasion, the provider will recognize wounds that may represent NSSI and should question the patient about them. To obtain sensitive information of this nature, APRNs must use empathic and compassionate communication, active listening, and reflection. APRNs should begin the assessment of NSSI by normalizing and validating the behavior in certain populations and making statements such as "Being a teenager can be a difficult time with many pressures" or "Sometimes teens may experiment with behaviors like hurting themselves to see if they can improve their mood, reduce bad feelings, or get rid of sad feelings" and "People who hurt themselves to cope with difficult times can be helped by talking to someone." Muehlenkamp (2006), Kerr et al. (2010), and Nafisi and Stanley (2007) focused their interventions with self-injurers around the therapeutic relationship, validating the distress experienced prior to and during the self-harm act, helping the youngster understand the behavior in context, challenging negative beliefs, teaching new coping skills, and empowering the youngster to change the cycle of self-destructive behaviors.

"Normalizing" the youngster's behavior within the context of his or her peer group allows the youth to disclose behavior with less shame or stigma. Initially, a skilled practitioner may assess whether the teen knows anyone who might be engaging in these behaviors, including close friends, and then ask if the patient has ever tried any form of self-injury. By slowly increasing the intensity of this inquiry, patients feel more comfortable offering information from their experience. In addition, disclosure should be seen as a means to access help to deal with the patient's problems, not necessarily to stop the behavior. Kerr et al. (2010) suggest using the mnemonic STOPS FIRE (Table 13.3) as a means of assessing a patient's self-injury and to help guide referral and management strategies.

Another screening tool for use in primary care for quantifying and describing the purpose and effectiveness of self-injurious behavior is the Inventory for Statements about Self Injury (ISAS). There are three sections to the questionnaire: intentional self-harm behaviors, functions of the behaviors (13 categories) and two

Table 13.3 STOPS FIRE evaluation

Suicidal ideations (Assess frequency and quality)

Types (Assess types of self-injury behaviors)

Onset (When did self-injurious behaviors begin? What were precipitants?)

Place/location (What areas of the body are targeted?)

Severity of damage (Presence of bleeding, was hospitalization needed? Infection?)

Functions (What were effects of the behavior on patient and on others?)

Intensity of the urges (On a scale of 0–10, with 10 being relentless urges)

Repetition (How often is the youngster engaging in the behavior?)

Episodic frequency (How many times per day/week/month does youth engage in behavior?)

Source: Reprinted from Kerr, P.L., Muehlenkamp, J.J., & Turner, J.M. Non-suicidal self injury: A review of current research for family medicine and primary care physicians. Journal of the American Board of Family Physicians. 23(2), 240–259. © 2010, American Board of Family Medicine. With permission from the American Board of Family Medicine.

optional open-ended questions (Glenn and Klonsky 2011; Klonsky et al. 2015; Klonsky and Glenn 2009; Klonsky and Olino, 2008). Section I includes behaviors such as severe scratching, swallowing dangerous substances, and hair pulling. Section II (Functions) includes intend options in response to the statement, "When I self-harm, I am . . .calming myself down, punishing myself, bonding with peers, etc." Lastly, the open-ended questions allow for inclusion of information not addressed in the questionnaire. The complete inventory can be accessed at www2.psych.ubc.ca/~klonsky/publications/ISASmeasure.pdf.

The Physical/Comprehensive Examination

During the physical examination, the APRN may notice unusual cuts, burns, nonhealing wounds, or bruises and should ask about them with respectful curiosity. A clue to self-injury is that injuries typically occur on the nondominant arm or hand. The extent and location of the wounds may signal the stage of addiction to the behavior. New users are more likely to use exposed areas like thighs and arms that are visible and easily accessed. The wounds of more committed users may be hidden, under arms, between the toes, and occasionally in insertions under the skin (Favazza 1998; Nock 2010; Whitlock 2010). Some patients may engage in elaborate rituals that include inserting pieces of metal, wood, or plastic under the skin, which may not be immediately noticeable and are only picked up on careful palpation or radiography. The location of injury, especially if found in the genital or face region, is considered significant and would warrant earlier referral. Patients may often minimize the wounds and attempt to distract the provider from investigating them. APRNs should gently interview the patient about the nature of the wounds using the above assessment. Early identification and disclosure of NSSI can prevent progression to higher levels of dependence on the behavior and result in prompt mental health referral as needed.

When a teen discloses that he or she has tried NSSI, the practitioner has a duty to assess the purpose and intent of the injury. In Figure 13.2, Williams et al. (2010) provide an algorithm for assessing the nature and extent of nonsuicidal self-injury behaviors using an approach adapted from an adolescent substance abuse assessment developed by Macdonald (1988).

Table 13.4 provides an explanation for each of the stages, from 0 (no NSSI behaviors) to 4 (pervasive thinking about self-injury and engagement) (Williams et al. 2010). Once the stage is determined, the provider can offer patient-centered messages and plans to address each stage, as shown in Table 13.5 (Williams et al.). Some teens may be experimenting with self-injuring behaviors as a result of peer

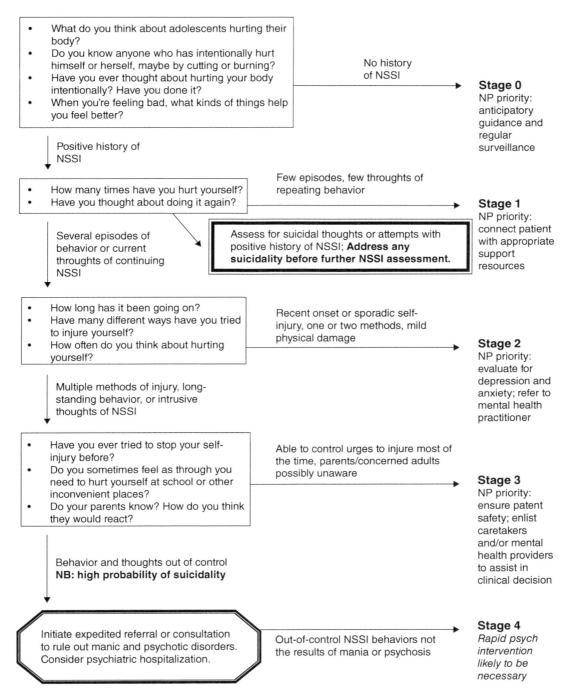

Figure 13.2 Adolescent self-injurious behaviors: assessment algorithm. (*Source:* Reprinted from Williams et al. (2010), with permission from the American Journal for Nurse Practitioners.)

influence and have not established a dependence or identity as real "cutters." They may be experimenting (Stage 1), trying to belong to a group of cutters, or exploring new coping mechanisms. They are not entrenched in the cycle of NSSI behavior, experience no cravings, and do not exhibit an inability to control their behavior. It is important for the primary care APRN to maintain a trusting and supportive relationship with these youths and refer to a child

and adolescent mental health colleague if this youngster moves to Stage 2 (Exploration).

Early recognition and management of youngsters who engage in NSSI behaviors is important in order to prevent the behaviors from escalating and becoming an entrenched coping strategy. APRNs in primary care are in a unique position during well- or sick-child/adolescent visits to assess for evidence of these behaviors.

Table 13.4 Stages of NSSI behaviors in adolescents

Stage 0 No NSSI behavior	• All adolescents "at risk" because of age, cultural context, and developmental level. • Factors that elevate risk include family status, level of behavior in peer group, psychiatric comorbidities, and academic performance.
Stage 1 Experimentation	• Trial period of self-injury. • Learns about how NSSI affects the self. • Decides whether he or she likes NSSI enough to continue.
Stage 2 Exploration	• Physical signs of injury more readily identified. • Adolescent perceives behavior as an effective coping mechanism. • Subtle signs of distress may be detected in appearance, family relationships, scholastic performance, and peer group affiliation.
Stage 3 Encapsulation	• Preoccupation with behavior to the clear detriment of other aspects of the adolescent's life. • Urge strikes at school, in public, or at other inconvenient times. • Adolescent is likely to have tried several methods of self-injury, such as cutting, scratching, burning, or self-hitting.
Stage 4 Pervasive dysfunction	• Most aspects of the adolescent's life can be considered dysfunctional. • Enormity of problems leads to further escalation of NSSI behavior. • Physical or psychological decompensation may ensue, with severe psychiatric symptoms or death as possible outcomes.

Source: Reprinted from Williams, E., Daley, M., & Iennaco, J. Assessing nonsuicidal self-injurious behaviors in adolescents. American Journal of Nurse Practitioners, 14(5), 18–26. © 2010, American Journal for Nurse Practitioners. With permission from the American Journal for Nurse Practitioners.

Table 13.5 Messages to convey to self-injuring patients according to stage of NSSI behavior

These messages help balance the patient–practitioner relationship with the requirement to provide safe care. They can be conveyed verbally, through body language, or in communicating clinical decisions.

All stages
- I don't think you're weird or crazy.
- Most people benefit from talking through their worries with a supportive person.
- I'm concerned for your wellbeing.
- My job is to keep you safe.

Stage 1
- We should decide together what to do about this situation.
- Your preferences are central in deciding what to do next.

Stage 2
- We should decide together what to do about this situation.
- Your preferences are central in deciding what to do next.

Stage 3
- Your preferences are important, but we need to have a plan today.
- There are programs and counselors who specialize in treating kids who harm themselves.
- We need to get your parents/caretakers involved, and I want you to be part of it.

Stage 4
- Your preferences are important, but your safety is more important.
- There are programs and counselors who specialize in treating kids who harm themselves.
- We need to get your parents/caretakers involved, and I want you to be a part of it.

Source: Reprinted from Williams, E., Daley, M., & Iennaco, J. Assessing nonsuicidal self-injurious behaviors in adolescents. American Journal of Nurse Practitioners, 14(5), 18–26. © 2010, American Journal for Nurse Practitioners. With permission from the American Journal for Nurse Practitioners.

Suicide

Suicide is a serious and growing public health concern and remains the second cause of death in youth worldwide (WHO 2019). In the United States, approximately 4600 children and adolescents successfully commit suicide annually (CDC 2017), with a steady increase in suicide rates occurring across different racial and ethnic youth groups. In a review of the literature on psychosocial risk factors for suicidality in youth, 44 studies meeting the inclusion criteria were synthesized. The researchers identified three factors that increased the risk for suicide: (i) psychological factors such as depression, anxiety, substance use, and previous suicidal attempt, (ii) stressful life events such as experiencing bullying, family and peer conflicts, trauma and academic difficulties, and (iii) behaviors associated with personality traits such as impulsivity, low self-esteem, and high level of self-criticism and perfectionism (Carballo et al. 2019).

Chavira et al. (2010) conducted interviews and collected questionnaire data at baseline and 2 years later on 1057 youth aged 11–18 in five public sector care systems (child welfare, juvenile justice, special education, alcohol and other drug treatment, and county mental health). Nearly 30% of their sample screened positive for SI and 20% had attempted suicide one to four or more times. Children in special education had the highest levels of SI and gestures. The researchers strongly recommended screening and using evidence-based interventions across all public sector care environments providing services to children.

Table 13.6 contains risk factors frequently attributed to those who pose the highest risk for suicide. Needless to say, youngsters with multiple risk factors and psychiatric or behavioral comorbidities should be carefully screened for immediate intervention, as may be warranted. Among youngsters, the most frequent methods used in suicide attempts and completed suicides are firearms, suffocation/hanging, medication overdose (analgesics and use of multiple central nervous system depressants), jumping, and poisoning via ingestion of pesticides (CDC 2017; Cha 2017). As discussed earlier in this chapter, neurotransmitter and neuroendocrine dysregulation are also implicated in self-harm behaviors. Pfeffer et al. (1998) found that their prepubertal sample of children aged 6–12 who had attempted suicide had significantly lower blood levels of the enzyme tryptophan, a precursor of serotonin, than a nonsuicidal control group. Crowell et al. (2008) found lower peripheral blood levels of 5-HT in 20 self-injuring adolescents compared to a matched control group. Mann (1998, 2003, 2013) has researched and written extensively for over 20 years on the association between low levels of serotonin and impulsivity and suicidality. Excessive cortisol levels due to acute stress and abnormal

Table 13.6 Risk factors for suicide in youth

Mood disorders (depression and bipolar)[a]

Psychosis

Anxiety

Perceived stressful life events

Poor impulse control

Neurotransmitter and neuroendocrine systems dysfunction (low serotonin levels; HPA dysregulation)[a]

Hopelessness

Previous attempt(s)[a]

Family history

History of victimization

LGBTQ

Multiple out-of-home placements (foster care, group homes, incarceration)

Exposure to peer suicide (cluster suicides)

Substance abuse (addiction)

[a] Access to high lethal methods (guns, analgesics, height, pesticides)

Romantic/idealized portrayal of suicide in the media

[a] Older adolescent (16 years or older)

[a] Male

[a] Ethnicity (Native Americans, Hispanics, and Caucasians at highest risk)

[a] Increases risk, and multiple risk-factors further increases vulnerability and risk.
Source: Adapted from Borowsky et al. (2001), Carballo et al. (2019), Cha et al. (2017), and Dervic et al. (2008).

or hyperactive hypothalamic–pituitary–adrenal (HPA) axis functioning has also been implicated as a component of suicidal behaviors (Currier and Mann 2008; Mann 2003). More recently, research has been reviewed on the role of inflammatory biomarkers cytokine and chemokine on major depression and suicidality (Black and Miller 2014; Brundin et al. 2017). Cytokines are proteins such as interferon and interleukin that serve as signaling molecules that regulate inflammation and immunity. Chemokines are a type of cytokine that serve to attract white blood cells to an infection site (Turner et al. 2014a). Findings point to an association between inflammatory conditions such as traumatic brain injury, infections and autoimmune conditions, and dysregulation of tryptophan, the HPA axis, and monoamine metabolism which impacts behaviors and mood. However, small sample sizes, some inconsistencies across studies, and the presence of some moderating variables warrant some caution in fully endorsing these findings. Longitudinal studies with larger sample sizes are recommended along with anti-inflammatory treatments such as antidepressants (Galecki et al. 2018).

Of note, in addition to the risk factors found in Table 13.6, the American Academy of Child and Adolescent Psychiatry (AACAP) identified aggressive/disruptive behaviors, access to firearms, being a victim of bullying, experiencing a perceived significant loss, perceived rejection, and violence exposure as additional risk factors for suicide (AACAP 2017).

Protective factors that mitigate against suicidal behaviors include emotional wellbeing, engagement in religious life/activities, sense of connectedness with parents at home and with peers at school, academic achievement, engagement in personally meaningful activities, perceived social support, and problem-solving skills (Armstrong and Manion 2015; Borowsky et al. 2001; Cha et al. 2017; O'Connor and Nock 2014).

The terminology most often used when discussing suicide includes ideation, threat, gesture, and attempt. *Ideation* refers to thinking about suicide, including thoughts of being dead, when and how to carry out the act, and imagining the reaction of others to one's death. Suicidal *ideation* is a common phenomenon in youth as indicated by YRBS, which are collected every 2 years. Suicidal *threat* refers to verbalizing a wish to kill oneself, while suicidal *gesture* is a specific behavior signaling intent (AACAP 2001; Cha et al. 2017; Nock 2010). *Threats* and *gestures* may be reactive to environmental events such as disciplinary responses from adults or discord with family and peers. Suicidal *attempt* refers to engaging in actions, which, while they may be rooted in ambivalence, have the intent of causing death (Miller et al. 2007). The most significant predictor of a successful suicide is previous attempt(s). If attempts do not require medical intervention, they may be kept from the healthcare provider, who would be unaware of this most significant risk factor. Given the troubling rates of self-harm in youth, all providers should assess for ideation, attempts, and intent using direct but gentle and supportive questioning and screening tools that are reliable, valid, and culturally and developmentally appropriate.

Suicide Screening

Examples of direct questions that should be asked of youth during screening include, "Did you ever feel so hopeless, sad, or upset that you wanted to die?" and "Have you ever tried to hurt yourself or spent time thinking of ways to hurt yourself?" Positive responses must be followed with an assessment of intended method and availability, which helps the APRN determine imminent risk, lethality, and level of intervention required.

There are numerous evidence-based screening tools available for APRNs to use when assessing youth at risk for suicide. The Child-Adolescent Suicide Potential Index (CASPI) is a 30-item yes/no self-report questionnaire for 8- to 17-year-olds that assesses for early-onset suicidal risk (Pfeffer et al. 2000). The CASPI assesses three behavioral categories: anxiety–impulsivity–depression, SI and threats, and family distress. A total score of 11 or more differentiates suicidal from nonsuicidal youngsters. One of the most widely used and globally tested screening tools with diverse populations is the Columbia Suicide Severity Rating Scale (C-SSRS) for teens. It is a 32-item tool for 11- to 18-year-olds that screens for suicidal risk, ideation, and behaviors (Shaffer et al. 2004). The tool was originally developed and administered to 1729 diverse 9th to 12th graders from 1991 to 1994. Those who screened positive were then administered the Diagnostic Interview Schedule for Children (DISC) to further assess the validity of the C-SSRS. Youngsters screen positive if they endorse any of the following: (i) SI within the past 3 months, (ii) one or more prior suicide attempts, (iii) at least three of the following are rated as bad or very bad: unhappiness, social withdrawal, irritability, anxiety, or substance abuse, and (iv) expressing a desire to speak to a professional about feelings identified in item (iii). Additional screening with both the CASPI and the C-SSRS have proven to be valid and reliable across youth of different ages, genders, and ethnicities. The easy to use abbreviated C-SSRS Screener tool (2018) is included here as Table 13.7.

Suicide Prevention Efforts Joshi et al. (2015) conducted a review of common school-based suicide prevention education curricula and peer leader strategies. The authors concluded that presenting this content in schools is an efficient and cost-effective way to increase mental health literacy related to suicide and suicide prevention in elementary, middle and high school-age populations. Curricular content should include health promotion, prevention education, intervention strategies, and specific postvention activities should a successful suicide occur in a school attending youngster. In another review, Calear et al. (2016) examined the literature on suicide prevention interventions for youth. There were 29 papers that met their review inclusion criteria. The researchers concluded that both universal and selective preventative education programs are most effective in preventing suicide in youth and that including comprehensive individual, group, and family treatment strategies had a positive impact in reducing SI and attempts. While numerous programs show some positive benefits, many lack rigor and consistent use/application, and did not meet best practice/evidence-based standards. Prevention programs with promising evidence-based outcomes are presented in Table 13.8.

Table 13.7 Columbia suicide severity rating scale 2018 screen version-recent

COLUMBIA SUICIDE SEVERITY RATING SCALE		
Screen Version – Recent		
	Past month	
Ask questions that are bolded and <u>underlined</u>.	YES	NO
Ask Questions 1 and 2		
1) *Have you wished you were dead or wished you could go to sleep and not wake up?*		
2) *Have you actually had any thoughts of killing yourself?*		
If YES to 2, ask questions 3, 4, 5, and 6. If NO to 2, go directly to question 6.		
3) *Have you been thinking about how you might do this?* E.g. *"I thought about taking an overdose but I never made a specific plan as to when where or how I would actually do it. . .and I would never go through with it."*		
4) *Have you had these thoughts and had some intention of acting on them?* As opposed to *"I have the thoughts but I definitely will not do anything about them."*		
5) *Have you started to work out or worked out the details of how to kill yourself? Do you intend to carry out this plan?*		
6) *Have you ever done anything, started to do anything, or prepared to do anything to end your life?*	YES	NO
Examples: Collected pills, obtained a gun, gave away valuables, wrote a will or suicide note, took out pills but didn't swallow any, held a gun but changed your mind or it was grabbed from your hand, went to the roof but didn't jump; or actually took pills, tried to shoot yourself, cut yourself, tried to hang yourself, etc.		
If YES, ask: *Was this within the past three months?*		

Low Risk
Moderate Risk
High Risk

Table 13.8 Prevention programs with promising evidence-based outcomes

Name of program	Citation	Description
Surviving the Teens® Suicide Prevention and Depression Awareness Program	Strunk et al. (2014)	Education intervention delivered in 4 days in health education class. Each session is 50 minutes and includes topics such as suicide, substance abuse, risk factors for depression, communication skills, and anger management/conflict resolution
Randomized control trial conducted with good evidence of success 1. Signs of Suicide (SOS) Universal program 2. Good Behavior Game (GBG) Universal program	Katz et al. (2013)	Focus of SOS is on suicide awareness, education, and screening. Students are taught to acknowledge, care, and tell someone if they are concerned about a peer or have SI themselves. Proven effective in decreasing suicidal attempts but not SI. GBG is a Substance Abuse and Mental Health Services Administration-supported intervention that fosters a positive classroom environment, team work, and decreased aggression and behavioral disruption. Proven to be effective in reducing suicidal attempts and ideation.

In 2016, youth suicide prevention researchers reviewed current evidence on prevention efforts. They concluded that future research in this area must improve research design and analysis, and strengthen the competence and expertise of both the research and practice communities. Specific recommendations for researchers included the need to:

- design studies that are multifaceted (longitudinal and across various environments)
- design studies that link to other studies and integrate data
- use valid missing data techniques to minimize elimination of all missing data elements
- develop studies that utilize a variety of rigorous data collection techniques
- promote collaboration across researchers, practice partners, policy makers, healthcare professionals, community members, and law enforcement to strengthen research and intervention efforts related to youth suicide prevention
- disseminate best practice research, education, and training strategies (Little et al. 2016).

Primary care and psychiatric-mental health APRNs are in an excellent practice position to (i) detect youth at risk for suicide early, (ii) educate youth and family about suicide risk factors, (iii) advocate for positive parenting and youth wellbeing, and (iv) initiate preventative interventions. In a longitudinal study conducted by Gould et al. (2009), the researchers followed 317 youth with positive SI screens for 2 years. At the time of the initial screen, 71% of the youth were not receiving any mental health treatment and referrals for further evaluation or treatment were made on those who met screening criteria for serious ideation or past attempts. Two years later, two-thirds of those who were referred for treatment had accessed and used treatment services. These researchers endorsed the President's New Freedom Commission on Mental Health (Department of Health and Human Services 2003) recommendations, which supported placing mental health screening and services within school-based health programs to reach students who would otherwise not ordinarily receive or access services. This is in line with both the American Academy of Pediatrics (Shain and Committee on Adolescents 2016) and the AACAP (2001, 2019; Brahmbhatt 2018) endorsing routine suicide screening by all clinicians during clinical encounters.

Suicide Assessment Tools

APRNs working with children and adolescents who self-injure are encouraged to become familiar with some of the tools available for assessment and which frequently guide the most appropriate intervention based on presenting symptoms and severity of DSH behaviors. For example, the University of Washington (n.d.) Behavioral Research and Therapy Clinics (http://depts.washington.edu/brtc) makes available a range of tools that practitioners can download and use to assess both NSSI and suicidal behaviors. Other tools have been included throughout this chapter.

The Achenbach System of Empirically Based Assessment (ASEBA) contains two questions relevant to issues of self harm, Question 18 which assesses DSH or suicide attempts and Question 91, which assesses for "Talking about killing self." Use of these two screening questions provides a fast and reliable way to assess suicidal risk when the items are fully endorsed or endorsed as sometimes true by the child or adolescent (Achenbach and Rescorla 2011; Van Meter et al. 2018).

A little-discussed prevention tool but a powerful cornerstone of psychiatric-mental health nursing is the relationship that the APRN develops and builds with children and adolescents in their practice. This relationship should be based on trust, honesty, caring, and advocacy. APRNs in primary care often see these youngsters over a period of time in their practice and are equally involved in a long-term relationship. Attentive and reflective listening, presence, validation of contextual feelings, and respect for the youngster and his or her experiences convey a sense of caring without rushing to judge or condemn the NSSI acts. Over-reactivity (shock, pity, blaming, or lecturing) may serve as a barrier in the relationship between the APRN and youth (Deiter et al. 2000).

Additional Treatment Recommendations/ Considerations

Working with self-injuring and suicidal youth is best done using an interdisciplinary or multidisciplinary approach and may require consistent interventions over a long period of time. The treatment team may include the APRN in primary care, the child and adolescent psychiatric nurse, parents, the youth, a trusted teacher or guidance counselor, and a psychiatrist or psychologist. During treatment, both the child and adolescent and the primary care APRN should anticipate the potential for relapse in self-harm behaviors secondary to the stress of working through emotions, while developing alternative coping behaviors. Minimizing the frequency and severity of self-harm behaviors may be a more realistic goal than total cessation of the behaviors. Because of the more intense nature of the reparative work required with these youngsters, the primary care APRN should make a referral to mental health colleagues.

As discussed earlier, there is strong evidence that CBT and DBT are frequent and effective interventions used with self-harming youth. CBT is discussed in detail in Chapter 20, and the reader is referred to that chapter for details about the method. DBT will be discussed briefly here. Extensive research has been done showing the effectiveness of DBT with individuals with borderline personality disorders and with suicidal and other self-harming behaviors (Fleischhaker et al. 2011; Katz et al. 2004; Rathus and Miller 2002).

DBT is an intensive treatment strategy used with severe psychiatric and behavioral presentations. The initial stage of DBT involves stabilizing the individual and eliminating behavioral or environmental barriers to treatment. In stage 2, the focus is on treating any past trauma experienced. Stage 3 focuses on self-esteem development and managing problems of daily living. In stage 4, the last stage of the process, the therapist works with the individual to increase capacity for learning from new experiences. Specific skills as developed by Linehan (1993a,b) include core mindfulness (increasing capacity for observation, description, and participation while increasing mindfulness), regulating emotions and increasing positive emotions, developing effective interpersonal skills, learning how to tolerate distressful emotions through distractions and self-soothing activities, and learning to walk the middle path through validation and dialectic thinking and actions. *Dialectics* is defined as change through persuasion or validation, and *mindfulness* is developing an ability to realistically (wisely) see and understand a situation or an experience without becoming overwhelmed with emotions that distort or confuse reality (Linehan 1993b; Miller et al. 2007). Adrian et al. (2018) conducted research on youth at high risk for suicide over a 6-month period. Specifically, they examined parental validation and invalidation to determine if it was a factor in predicting self-harm. The study was part of a larger randomized control study looking at efficacy of DBT versus individual and group supportive therapy to decrease self-harm behaviors. The researchers found that there were fewer self-harm behaviors in youth when parents validated their youngsters' emotional state, gave unambiguous messages, and avoided invalidation of the teen's experiences and feelings.

Trust and open communication will be important aspects of treatment along with exploration of stressors or triggers to self-harm behaviors. Working around increasing self-esteem, helping youngsters identify feeling states, developing tolerance for distressing feelings, improving decision-making skills, and learning alternate communication behaviors are all important components of treating self-harming youth. Parents and youth should be educated about the importance of social connectedness and participation in normal child and adolescent group activities to promote social skills, relationship building, and emotional wellbeing, and to minimize isolation.

Medications

The use of medications must be viewed as adjunctive to other treatment modalities. Chapter 9 contains additional information about medication use in children and adolescents. Several categories of medications have been used to assist in treating self-harming youngsters. Antidepressants (specifically selective serotonin reuptake inhibitors [SSRIs]) and mood-stabilizing medications are the most frequently prescribed medications for youngsters with mood dysregulation who engage in self-harming behaviors. As noted in the chapter on psychopharmacology, there is a black box warning associated with antidepressant use in children and adolescents related to controversy over the possibility of SSRIs inducing SI and suicidal behaviors (Neuroscience Education Institute 2009). However, reviews of the analyses conducted on large SSRI treatment trials do not support excessive concerns over use of SSRIs with youth. Antidepressants remain the medications of choice in managing major depression, a risk factor for engaging in self-harm behaviors. What is clear is that medications are frequently adjunctive, prescribed to support the success of other interventions. Failure to intervene aggressively, if warranted, will likely result in poor outcomes. Mood-stabilizing agents such as valproic acid (Depakote) and carbamazepine (Tegretol) may be used instead of SSRIs if there is a family history of bipolar disorder or if the mood presentation by the youngster is erratic or unusual, leading to questions about the diagnosis (AACAP 2001; Mann et al. 2005).

A review for pharmacological agents used in treating self-harm behaviors in youth was conducted and found that there is a paucity of studies on this topic conducted with adolescents (Brown and Plener (2017) and Plener et al. 2016). Turner et al. (2014b) conducted a systematic review and found 40 studies with ranges of evidence from Level 1 to Level II-3. Atypical SSRIs and serotonin-norepinephrine reuptake inhibitors were found to have some efficacy in reducing NSSI in conjunction with emotion regulation group therapy and manually assisted CBT. Lastly, Hawton et al. in their Cochrane Database of Systematic Review (2015) found no evidence of the effectiveness of antidepressants, antipsychotics, mood stabilizers or natural products in preventing subsequent self-harm behaviors in adults.

APRNs are advised to adhere to best practices regarding assessment, prescribing, consenting, assenting, and monitoring, when making referrals, and when engaging in collaborative practice with peers. In addition, APRNs must actively engage youth and parents as partners in the treatment process to support success and to minimize risk of untoward events.

Implications for Practice, Education, and Research

Only 27% of primary care providers consistently ask about NSSI in health maintenance visits (Taliferro et al. 2013). These low rates are thought to be a result of lack of training, competence, and comfort in screening for NSSI and related suicidality. APRNs in practice must include an assessment of self-injurious behaviors in their work with all children and adolescents. Assessment of self-injurious behaviors can and should occur when assessing for mood and other feeling states in the youngster. Including this in the psychosocial part of a comprehensive assessment must become as commonplace as assessing for use of substances, eating patterns, and sleep history. Early case finding with these youngsters is important as early intervention can result in early treatment and a reversal of self-injury as a means of coping. School-based APRNs are in a unique position to screen for NSSI/SA due to ready access to students on a consistent basis.

Educators teaching primary care APRNs (family nurse practitioners, pediatric nurse practitioners, etc.) are encouraged to inform their students about the trends regarding self-injuring behaviors in children and adolescents so that they too begin to incorporate this information in their assessment and primary prevention efforts with this population. In the practice setting, APRNs can teach youngsters in their practice appropriate management strategies for their feelings, empower youth to talk about their feelings, and work with parents to support and promote self-esteem in their children and adolescents. APRNs are also in a unique position to conduct longitudinal research on a variety of troubling issues affecting children and adolescents. Research on NSSI and youth suicide has proliferated over the past 10 years, but most of it is not being conducted by nurses. What we do know is that more research is needed on the long-term efficacy of the various treatments used with this population. APRNs in primary care are in a unique position of having strong and long-lasting relationships with the youngsters they see, some of whom engage in DSH behaviors. Qualitative data on the impact of the nurse–patient relationship and the course of NSSI behaviors would highlight the strength of how nurses' practice, and would provide needed strategies for all practitioners in primary care. In addition, as we are advocating for a collaborative practice relationship between primary care APRNs and advanced practice mental health nurses, data about the

prognosis of children and adolescents co-managed by these two practitioners would be useful in developing best practice treatment guidelines. One model that may work would be a treatment group for DSH youngsters led by both a primary care and a psychiatric-mental health APRN. The primary care APRN would bring the relational and medical expertise to the process while the psychiatric-mental health APRN would bring expertise regarding knowledge of group process and knowledge of theories behind self-injuring behaviors and management strategies like CBT, among others. Other models could involve working with both the youth and parents/caretakers or conducting education campaigns in schools and communities about the prevalence of these behaviors among youth and strategies to prevent or minimize their occurrence.

Summary

This chapter presents DSH behaviors of children and adolescents with a focus on nonsuicidal and suicidal self-injuring behaviors. Etiology of self-injury, assessment and management of these behaviors, and the roles that both the primary care and mental health APRNs can have when interfacing with these children and adolescents is presented. In addition, the existing evidence on how best to intervene and the need for nursing research in this area is highlighted. Numerous resources are also provided to guide nursing practice with the youngsters themselves and their families.

Resources

Screening and Other Tools

Bill of Rights for People Who Self-Harm, available at http://www.selfinjury.org/docs/brights.html.

Common Myths about Self-Injury, available at http://www.selfinjury.

Deliberate Self-Harm Inventory (DSHI) (Gratz 2001). A self-report 17-item questionnaire to measure nonsuicidal self-harm behaviors.

Emotion Reactivity Scale (ERS): 21-item self-report that measures emotion sensitivity, intensity, and persistence. (Nock et al. 2008).

Ottawa Self-Injury Inventory (OSI-Clinical) (Cloutier and Nixon 2003). A 33-item self-report questionnaire to identify clinical and psychosocial causes of self-injury.

Self-Harm Inventory (Sansone and Sansone 2010). A 22-item yes or no self-report questionnaire that looks at the history of self-harm in the individual. All yes responses are considered pathological and the maximum score is 22.

Self-Injurious Thoughts and Behavior Interview (SITBI) (Nock et al. 2007). A 72 (short form) or 169 (long form) item structured interview that assesses both NSSI and SI and behaviors.

TeenScreen National Center for Mental Health, available at http://www.teenscreen.org.

Web-Based Injury Statistics Query and Reporting System, available at http://www.cdc.gov/injury/wisqars/index.html (accessed 1 August 2010).

Programs or Websites

American Academy of Pediatrics. www.aap.org.

American Foundation for Suicide Prevention. http://www.afsp.org.

Centers for Disease Control and Prevention.

Cornell Research Program on Self-Injurious Behavior. http://www. crpsib.com/whatissi.asp.

Life Signs: Self Injury Guidance and Network Support. www.lifesigns. org.uk.

S.A.F.E. Alternatives. www.selfinjury.com.

Society for Adolescent Health and Medicine. www.adolescenthealth.org.

Trevor Project, LGBTQ support site. www.thetrevorproject.org.

University of Washington, Behavioral Research and Therapy Clinics. http://depts.washington.edu/brtc

University of Washington, Behavioral Research and Therapy Clinics. http://depts.washington.edu/brtc.

References

Achenbach, T.M. and Rescorla, L.A. (2011). The Achenbach system of empirically based assessment (ASEBA) for ages 1.5 to 18 years. In: *The Use of Psychological Testing for Treatment Planning and Outcomes Assessment*, 3rde, vol. 2 (ed. M.E. Maruish), 179–213. London: Lawrence Erlbaum Associates.

Adrian, M., Berk, M.S., Korslund, K. et al. (2018). Parental validation and invalidation predict adolescent self-harm. *Professional Psychology Research and Practice* 49 (4): 274–281.

AACAP. (2017). *Suicide in children and teens*. American Academy of Child and Adolescent Psychiatry. Available at www.aacap.org.

AACAP. (2019). *Policy Statement on Suicide Prevention*. American Academy of Child and Adolescent Psychiatry. Available at aacap.org.

AACAP (2001). Practice parameters for the assessment and treatment of children and adolescents with suicidal behavior. *Journal of the American Academy of Child and Adolescent Psychiatry* 40 (7 Suppl): 24S–51S.

American Psychiatric Association (2013). *Diagnostic and Statistical Manual of Mental Disorders*, 5e. Washington, DC: American Psychiatric Association.

Andover, M.S. and Morris, B.W. (2014). Expanding and clarifying the role of emotion regulation in nonsuicidal self-injury. *Canadian Journal of Psychiatry* 59 (11): 569–575.

Armstrong, L.L. and Manion, I.G. (2015). Meaningful youth engagement as a protective factor for youth suicidal ideation. *Journal of Research on Adolescence* 25 (1): 20–27.

Belfort, E.L. and Miller, L. (2018). Relationship between adolescent suicidality, self-injury, and social media habits. *Child and Adolescent Psychiatric Clinics of North America* 27: 159–169.

Bildik, T., Somer, O., Basay, B.K. et al. (2013). The validity and reliability of the Turkish version of the inventory of statements about self-injury. *Turkish Journal of Psychiatry* 24: 49–57. Available at http://turkpsikiyatri.com/Data/UnpublishedArticles/4065u9.pdf.

Black, C. and Miller, B.J. (2014). Meta-analysis of cytokines and chemokines in suicidality: distinguishing suicidal versus nonsuicidal patients. *BiologicalPsychiatry* 78: 28–37.

Blasco-Fontecilla, H., Fernandez-Fernandez, R., Colino, L. et al. (2016). The addictive model of self-harming (non-suicidal and suicidal) behavior. *Frontiers in Psychiatry* https://doi.org/10.3389/fpsyt.2016.00008.

Borowsky, I., Ireland, M., and Resnick, M. (2001). Adolescent suicide attempts: risk and protectors. *Pediatrics* 107 (3): 485–493.

Bostwick, W.B., Meyer, I., Aranda, F. et al. (2014). Mental health and suicidality among racially/ethnically diverse sexual minority youths. *American Journal of Public Health* 104 (6): 1129–1136.

Brahmbhatt, K. (2018). 71.1 a clinical pathway: identification, assessment and management in suicide risk screening. *Journal of the American Academy of Child and Adolescent Psychiatry* 57 (10): S103.

Bridgemohan, C., Bauer, N.S., Nielse, B.A. et al. (2018). A workforce survey on developmental-behavioral pediatrics. *Pediatrics* 141 (3): e20172164. https://doi.org/10.1542/peds.2017-2164.

Brown, R.C. and Plener, P.L. (2017). Non-suicidal self-injury in adolescence. *Current Psychiatry Reports* 19: 20. https://doi.org/10.1007/s11920-017-0767-9.

Brown, R.C., Fischer, T., Goldwich, A.D. et al. (2017). #cutting: non-suicidal self-injury (NSSI) on Instagram. *Psychological Medicine* 48: 337–346.

Brundin, L., Bryleva, E., and Rajamani, K.T. (2017). Role of inflammation in suicide: from mechanisms to treatment. *Neuropsychopharmacology Reviews* 42: 271–283.

Calear, A.L., Christensen, H., Freeman, A. et al. (2016). A systematic review of psychosocial suicide prevention interventions for youth. *European Child & Adolescent Psychiatry* 25: 467–482.

Carballo, J.J., Llorente, C., Kehrmann, L. et al. (2019). Psychosocial risk factors for suicidality in children and adolescents. *European Child & Adolescent Psychiatry* https://doi.org/10.1007/s00787-018-01270-9.

Carbone, J., Holzer, K.J., and Vaughn, M.G. (2018). Child and adolescent suicidal ideation and suicide attempts: evidence from the healthcare cost and utilization project. *Journal of Pediatrics* https://www.sciencedirect.com/science/article/abs/pii/S002234761831429X.

CDC. (2018). *CDC releases 2017 youth risk behavior survey (YRBS) results*. Centers for Disease Control and Prevention. Available at https://www.cdc.gov/nchhstp/dear_colleague/2018/dcl-061418-YRBS.html.

CDC. (2017). *Web-based injury statistics query and reporting system*. Centers for Disease Control and Prevention. Available at https://www.cdc.gov/injury/wisqars/fatal_injury_reports.html.

Cha, C.B., Franz, P.J., Guzman, E.M. et al. (2017). Annual research review: suicide among youth-epidemiology, (potential) etiology, and treatment. *Journal of Child Psychology and Psychiatry* 59 (4): 460–482.

Chavira, D., Accurso, E., Garland, A., and Hough, R. (2010). Suicidal behavior among youth in five public sectors of care. *Child and Adolescent Mental Health* 15 (1): 44–51.

Chesin, M.S., Galfavy, H., Sonmez, C.C. et al. (2017). Nonsuicidal self-injury is predictive of suicide attempts among indiviuals with mood disorders. *Suicide and Life Threatening Behaivors* 47 (5): 567–579. https://doi.org/10.1111/sltb.12331.

Cipriano, A., Cella, S., and Cotrufo, P. (2017). Non suicidal self-injury: a systematic review. *Frontiers in Psychology* 8 https://doi.org/10.3389/Fpsyg.2017.01946.

Cloutier, P. and Nixon, M. (2003). The Ottawa self-injury inventory: a preliminary evaluation. *European Child & Adolescent Psychiatry* 12 (Suppl. 1): I/94.

Cloutier, P., Martin, J., Kennedy, A. et al. (2010). Characteristics and co-occurrence of adolescent nonsuicidal self-injury and suicidal behaviors in pediatric emergency crisis services. *Journal of Youth and Adolescence* 39: 259–269.

Crowell, S., Beauchaine, T., McCauley, E. et al. (2008). Parent-child interactions, peripheral serotonin, and self-inflicted injury in adolescents. *Journal of Consulting and Clinical Psychology* 76 (1): 15–21.

Currier, D. and Mann, J. (2008). Stress, genes and the biology of suicidal behavior. *Psychiatric Clinics of North America* 31 (2): 247–269.

Deiter, P., Nicholls, S., and Pearlman, L. (2000). Self-injury and self capacities: assisting an individual in crisis. *Journal of Clinical Psychology* 56 (9): 1173–1191.

Department of Health and Human Services (2003). *New Freedom Commission on Mental Health, Achieving the Promise: Transforming Mental Health Care in America.* Rockville, MD: Department of Health and Human Services.

Dervic, K., Brent, D., and Oquendo, M. (2008). Completed suicide in childhood. *Psychiatric Clinics of North America* 31: 271–291.

Favazza, A. (1998). The coming of age of self-mutilation. *Journal of Nervous and Mental Disease* 186 (5): 259–268.

Favazza, A. (2009). A cultural understanding of nonsuicidal self-injury. In: *Understanding Nonsuicidal Self-Injury* (ed. M. Nock), 19–35. Washington, DC: American Psychological Association.

Favazza, A. (2011). *Bodies Under Siege: Self-Mutilation, Nonsuicidal Self-Injury, and Body Modification in Culture and Psychiatry*, 3e. Baltimore, MD: Johns Hopkins University Press.

Fleischhaker, C., Bohme, R., Six, B. et al. (2011). Dialectical behavioral therapy for adolescents (DBT-A): a clinical trial for patients with suicidal and self-injurious behavior and borderline symptoms with a one-year follow-up. *Child and Adolescent Psychiatry and Mental Health* 5 (3).

Ford, C., English, A., and Sigman, G. (2004). Confidential health care for adolescents: position paper of the Society for Adolescent Medicine. *Journal of Adolescent Health* 35 (2): 160–167.

Fox, K.R., Franklin, J.C., Ribiero, J.D. et al. (2015). Meta-analysis of risk factors for nonsuicidal self-injury. *Clinical Psychology Review* 42: 156–167.

Fox, K.R., Hooley, J.M., Smith, D.M.Y. et al. (2018). Self-injurious thoughts and behaviors may be more common and severe among people identifying as a sexual minority. *Behavior Therapy* 49: 768–780.

Galecki, P., Mossakowska-Wojcik, J., and Talarowska, M. (2018). The anti-inflammatory mechanism of antidepressants-SSRIs, SNRIs. *Progress in Neuropsychopharmacology and Biological Psychiatry* 80: 291–294.

Gilles, D., Christou, M.A., Dixon, A.C. et al. (2018). Prevalence and characteristics of self-harm in adolescents: meta-analyses of community-based studies 1990-2015. *Journal of the American Academy of Child & Adolescent Psychiatry* 57 (8): 733–741. https://doi.org/10.1016/j.jaac.2018.06.018.

Glassman, L., Weierich, M., Hooley, J. et al. (2007). Child maltreatment, nonsuicidal self-injury, and the mediating role of self-criticism. *Behaviour Research and Therapy* 45: 2483–2490.

Glenn, C.R. and Klonsky, E.D. (eds.) (2011). One-year test-retest reliability of the Inventory of Statements about Self-Injury (ISAS). *Assessment* 18 (3): 375–378.

Gould, M., Marrocco, F., Hoagwood, K. et al. (2009). Service use by at risk youths after school-based suicide screening. *Journal of the American Academy of Child and Adolescent Psychiatry* 48 (12): 1193–1201.

Grandclerc, S., DeLabrouhe, D., Spodenkiewicz, M. et al. (2016). Relations between nonsuicidal self-injury and suicidal behavior in adolescence: a systematic review. *PLoS One* 11 (4): e0153760. https://doi.org/10.1371/journal pone. 0153760.

Gratz, K.L. (2001). Measurement of deliberate self-harm: preliminary data on the deliberate self-harm inventory. *Journal of Psychopathology and Behavioral Assessment* 23: 253–263.

Gratz, K. (2007). Targeting emotion dysregulation in the treatment of self-injury. *Journal of Clinical Psychology* 63: 1091–1103.

Gratz, K. and Roemer, L. (2004). Multidimensional assessment of emotion regulation and dysregulation: development, factor structure, and initial validation of the difficulties in emotion regulation scale. *Journal of Psychopathology and Behavioral Assessment* 26: 41–54.

Hawton, K., Witt, K.G., Taylor, S. et al. (2015). Pharmacological interventions for self-harm in adults. *Cochrane Database of Systematic Reviews* (7): CD011777. https://doi.org/10.1002/14651858. CDO11777.

Heron, M. (2018). Deaths: leading causes for 2016. *National Vital Statistics Reports* 67 (6), Centers for Disease Control and Prevention.

Hong, J.S., Espelage, D.L., and Kral, M.J. (2011). Understanding suicide among sexual minority youth in America: an ecological systems analysis. *Journal of Adolescence* 34: 885–894.

Hooley, J.M. and Germain, S.A.S. (2014). Nonsuicidal self-injury, pain, and self-criticism: Does changing self-worth change pain endurance in people who engage in self-injury? *Clinical Psychological Science* 2 (3): 297–305.

Hornor, G. (2016). Nonsuicidal self-injury. *Journal of Pediatric Health Care* 30: 261–267.

Hornor, G. (2018). Bullying: what the PNP needs to know. *Journal of Pediatric Health Care* 32: 399–408.

Joshi, S.V., Hartley, S.N., Kessler, M., and Barstead, M. (2015). School-based suicide prevention: content, process, and the role of trusted adults and peers. *Child and Adolescent Psychiatric Clinics of North America* 24 (2): 353–370.

Katz, L., Cox, B., Gunasekara, S., and Miller, A. (2004). Feasibility of dialectical behavior therapy for suicidal adolescent inpatients. *Journal of the American Academy of Child & Adolescent Psychiatry* 43 (3): 276–282.

Katz, C., Bolton, S.L., Katz, L.Y. et al. (2013). A systematic review of school-based suicide prevention programs. *Depression and Anxiety* 30 (10): 1030–1045.

Kerr, P.L., Muehlenkamp, J.J., and Turner, J.M. (2010). Non suicidal self injury: a review of current research for family medicine and primary care physicians. *Journal of the American Board of Family Physicians* 23 (2): 240–259.

Kidshealth (2015). *About teen suicide.* Available at kidshealth.org.

Kiekens, G., Hasking, P., Boyers, M. et al. (2018). The association between non-suicidal self-injury and first onset suicidal thoughts and behaviors. *Journal of Affective Disorders* 239: 171–179.

Kleinman, E.M. and Nock, M.K. (2018). Real-time assessment of suicidal thoughts and behaviors. *Current Opinion in Psychology* 22: 33–37.

Klonsky, E. (2007). The functions of deliberate self-injury, a review of the evidence. *Clinical Psychology Review* 27: 226–239.

Klonsky, E. and Glenn, C.R. (2009). Assessing the functions of non-suicidal self-injury: psychometric properties of the inventory of statements about self-injury (ISAS). *Journal of Psychopathology and Behavioral Assessment* 31 (3): 215–219.

Klonsky, E. and Muehlenkamp, J. (2007). Self-injury: a research review for the practitioner. *Journal of Clinical Psychology* 63 (11): 1045–1056.

Klonsky, E.D. and Olino, T.M. (2008). Identifying clinically distinct subgroups of self- injurers among young adults: A latent class analysis. *Journal of Consulting and Clinical Psychology* 76: 22–27.

Klonsky, E.D., Oltmanns, T.F., and Turkheimer, E. (2003). Deliberate self-harm in a nonclinical population: Prevalence and psychological correlates. *American Journal of Psychiatry* 160 (8): 1501–1508.

Klonsky, E.D., Victor, S.E., and Saffer, B.Y. (2014). Nonsuicidal self-injury: what we know, and what we need to know. *Canadian Journal of Psychiatry* 59 (11): 565–568.

Klonsky, E.D., Glenn, C.R., Styer, D.M. et al. (2015). The functions of nonsuicidal self-injury: converging evidence for a two-factor structure. *Child and Adolescent Psychiatry and Mental Health* 9: 44. https://doi.org/10.1186/s13034-015-0073-4.

Linehan, M.M. (1993a). *Cognitive Behavioral Treatment for Borderline Personality Disorder*. New York, NY: Guilford.

Linehan, M.M. (1993b). *The Skills Training Manual for Treating Borderline Personality Disorder*. New York, NY: Guilford.

Little, T.D., Roche, K.M., Chow, S.M. et al. (2016). National institutes of health pathways to prevention workshop: advancing research to prevent youth suicide. *Annals of Internal Medicine* 165: 795–799.

Macdonald, D. (1988). Substance abuse. *Pediatrics in Review* 10 (3): 89–95.

Mangnall, J. and Yurkovich, E. (2008). A literature review of deliberate self-harm. *Perspectives in Psychiatric Care* 44 (3): 175–184.

Mann, J. (2003). Neurobiology of suicidal behavior. *Nature Reviews. Neuroscience* 4 (10): 819–828.

Mann, J.J. (2013). The serotonergic system in mood disorders and suicidal behavior. *Philosophical Transactions of the Royal Society of London. Series B, Biological Sciences* 368 (1615) doi https://doi.org/10.1098/rstb.2012.0537.

Mann, J., Apter, A., Bertolote, J. et al. (2005). Suicide prevention strategies: a systematic review. *Journal of the American Medical Association* 294 (16): 2064–2074.

Marchant, A., Hawton, K., Stewart, A. et al. (2017). A systematic review of the relationship between internet use, self-harm and suicidal behavior in young people: the good, the bad and the unknown. *PLoS One* 12 (8): e0181722. https://doi.org/10.1371/journal.pone.0181722.

Marshall, A. (2016). Suicide prevention interventions for sexual & gender minority youth: an unmet need. *Yale Journal of Biology and Medicine* 89: 205–213.

McDougall, T., Armstrong, M., and Trainor, G. (2010). *Helping Children and Young People Who Self-Harm: An Introduction to Self-Harming and Suicidal Behaviours for Health Professionals*. London: Routledge.

Miller, A., Rathus, J., and Linehan, M. (2007). *Dialectical Behavior Therapy with Suicidal Adolescents*. New York, NY: Guilford.

Molina, D.K. and Farley, N.J. (2019). A 25-year reiew of pediatric suicides: distinguishing features and risk factors. *American Journal of Forensic Medicine and Pathology* 40 (3): 220–226.

Monto, M.A., McRee, N., and Frank, D. (2018). Nonsuicidal self-injury among a representative sample of US adolescents, 2015. *American Journal of Public Health* 108: 1042–1048.

Moreno, M.A., Ton, A., Selkie, E., and Evans, Y. (2016). Secret society 123: understanding the language of self-harm on Instagram. *Journal of Adolescent Health* 58: 78–84.

Muehlenkamp, J. (2006). Empirically supported treatments and general therapy guidelines for nonsuicidal self-injury. *Journal of Mental Health Counseling* 28: 166–185.

Muehlenkamp, J., Williams, K., Gutierrez, P., and Claes, L. (2009). Rates of nonsuicidal self-injury in high school students across five years. *Archives of Suicide Research* 13: 317–329.

Muehlenkamp, J.J., Claes, L., Havertape, L., and Plener, P.L. (2012). International prevalence of adolescent non-suicidl self-injury and deliberate self-harm. *Child and Adolescent Psychiatry and Mental Health* 6 (10) doi https://doi.org/10.1186/1753-2000-6-10.

Muehlenkamp, J., Brausch, A., Quigley, K., and Whitlock, J. (2013). Interpersonal features and functions of nonsuicidal self-injury. *Suicide and Life-threatening Behavior* 43 (1): 67–80.

Nafisi, N. and Stanley, B. (2007). Developing and maintaining the therapeutic alliance with self-injuring patients. *Journal of Clinical Psychology* 63: 1069–1079.

National Action Alliance for Suicide Prevention. (2015). *Fact Sheet: High risk populations*. Available from https://actionallianceforsuicideprevention.org/NSSP.

Neuroscience Education Institute (2009). *Understanding and Managing the Pieces of Major Depressive Disorder*. Carlsbad, CA: NEI.

Nock, M. (2009). Why do people hurt themselves? New insights into the nature and functions of self-injury. *Current Directions in Psychological Science* 18 (2): 78–83.

Nock, M. (2010). Self-injury. *Annual Review of Clinical Psychology* 6: 15.1–15.25.

Nock, M. and Mendes, W. (2008). Physiological arousal, distress tolerance, and social problem-solving deficits among adolescent self-injurers. *Journal of Consulting and Clinical Psychology* 76 (1): 28–38.

Nock, M.K. and Prinstein, M.J. (2004). A functional approach to the assessment of self-mutilative behavior. *Journal of Consulting and Clinical Psychology* 72 (5): 885–890.

Nock, M. and Prinstein, M. (2005). Contextual features and behavioral functions of self-mutilation among adolescents. *Journal of Abnormal Psychology* 114 (1): 140–146.

Nock, M., Holmberg, E., Photos, V., and Michel, B. (2007). Self-injurious thoughts and behaviors interview: development, reliability, and validity in an adolescent sample. *Psychological Assessment* 19 (3): 309–317.

Nock, M., Wedig, M., Holmberg, E., and Hooley, J. (2008). The emotion reactivity scale: development, evaluation, and relation to self-injurious thoughts and behaviors. *Behavior Therapy* 39: 107–116.

O'Connor, R.C. and Nock, M.K. (2014). The psychology of suicidal behavior. *Lancet Psychology* 1: 73–85.

Pfeffer, C., McBride, A., Anderson, G. et al. (1998). Peripheral serotonin measures in prepubertal psychiatric inpatients and normal children: associations with suicidal behavior and its risk factors. *Biological Psychiatry* 44 (7): 568–577.

Pfeffer, C., Jiang, H., and Kakuma, T. (2000). Child-Adolescent Suicidal Potential Index (CASPI): a screen for risk for early onset suicidal behavior. *Psychological Assessment* 12 (3): 304–318.

Plener, P.L., Brunner, R., Fegert, J.M. et al. (2016). Treating nonsuicidal self-injury (NSSI) in adolescents: consensus based German guidelines. *Child and Adolescent Psychiatry and Mental Health* 10: 46. https://doi.org/10.1186/s13034-016-0134-3.

Plener, P.L., Zohsel, K., Hohm, E. et al. (2017). *Psychoneuroendocrinology* 76: 84–87.

Rathus, J. and Miller, A. (2002). Dialectical behavior therapy adapted for suicidal adolescents. *Suicide and Life-threatening Behavior* 32 (2): 146–157.

Ream, G.L. (2019). What's unique about lesbian, gay, bisexual, and transgender (LGBT) youth and young adult suicides? Findings from the national violent death reporting system. *Journal of Adolescent Health* 64: 602–607.

Sansone, R. and Sansone, L. (2010). Measuring self-harm behavior with the self-harm inventory. *Psychiatry (Edgmont)* 7 (4): 16–20.

Shaffer, D., Scott, M., Wilcox, H. et al. (2004). The Columbia suicide screen: validity and reliability of a screen for youth suicide and depression. *Journal of the American Academy of Child and Adolescent Psychiatry* 43 (1): 71–79.

Shain, B. and AAP Committee on Adolescence (2016). Suicide and suicide attempts in adolescents. *Pediatrics* 138 (1): e20161420.

Strunk, C.M., King, K.A., Vidourek, R.A., and Sorter, M.T. (2014). Effectiveness of the surviving the Teens® suicide prevention and depression awareness program: an impact evaluation utilizing a comparison group. *Health Education & Behavior* 41 (6): 605–613.

Suyemoto, K. (1998). The functions of self-mutilation. *Clinical Psychology Review* 18 (5): 531–554.

Taliferro, L.A., Muehlenkamp, J.J., Hetler, J. et al. (2013). Nonsuicidal self-injury among adolescents: a training priority for primary care providers. *American Journal for Nurse Practitioners* 14 (5): 18–26.

Turner, M.D., Nedjai, B., Hurst, T., and Pennington, D.J. (2014a). Cytokines and chemokines: at the crossroads of cell signaling and inflammatory disease. *Biochimica et Biophysica Acta* 1843: 2563–2582.

Turner, B.J., Austin, S.B., and Chapman, A.L. (2014b). Treating non-suicidal self-injury: a systematic review of psychological and pharmacological interventions. *Canadian Journal of Psychiatry* 59 (11): 576–585.

Van Meter, A.R., Algorta, G.P., Youngstom, E.A. et al. (2018). Assessing for suicidal behavior in youth using the Achenbach system of empirically based assessment. *European Child and Adolescent Psychiatry* 27: 159–169.

Victor, S.E. and Klonsky, D. (2018). Understanding the social context of adolescent non-suicidal self-injury. *Journal of Clinical Psychology* 74 (12): 2107–2116.

Wells, J., Haines, J., and Williams, C. (1998). Severe morbid onychophagia: the classification as self-mutilation and a proposed model of maintenance. *Australian and New Zealand Journal of Psychiatry* 32: 534–545.

Whitlock, J. (2010). Self-injurious behavior in adolescents. *PLoS Medicine* 7 (5): e1000240. https://doi.org/10.1371/journal.pmed.1000240.

Whitlock, J., Powers, J., and Eckenrode, J. (2006). The virtual cutting edge: the internet and adolescent self-injury. *Developmental Psychology* 42 (3): 407–417.

Whitlock, J., Eckenrode, J., and Silverman, D. (2006). Self-injurious behaviors in a college population. *Pediatrics* 117: 1939–1948.

Whitlock, J., Lader, W., and Conterio, K. (2007). The internet and self-injury: what psychotherapists should know. *Journal of Clinical Psychology* 63 (11): 1135–1143.

Willging, C.E., Green, A.E., and Ramos, M.M. (2016). Implementing school nursing strategies to reduce LGBTQ adolescent suicide: a randomized cluster trial study protocol. *Implementation Science* 11: 145. https://doi.org/10.1186/s13012-016-0507-2.

Williams, E., Daley, M., and Iennaco, J. (2010). Assessing nonsuicidal self-injurious behaviors in adolescents. *American Journal of Nurse Practitioners* 14 (5): 18–26.

World Health Organization. (2019). *Suicide data*. Available at https://www.who.int>mental_health>prevention>suicide>suicideprevent.

You, J., Ren, Y., Zhang, X. et al. (2018). Emotional dysregulation and nonsuicidal self-injury: a meta-analytic review. *Neuropsychiatry* 8 (2): 733–748.

Zetterqvist, M., Lundh, L.G., and Svedin, C.G. (2013). A comparison of adolescents engaging in self-injurious behaviors with and without suicidal intent: self-reported experiences of adverse life events and traumatic symptoms. *Journal of Youth and Adolescence* 42 (8): 1257–1272.

14

Perceptual Alterations Disorders

Heeyoung Lee[1] and Eunjung Kim[2]

[1] University of Pittsburg, Pittsburg, PA, USA
[2] University of Washington School of Nursing, Seattle, Washington, USA

Objectives

After reading this chapter, advanced practice registered nurses (APRNs) will be able to:

1. Describe the disorders of children and adolescents that are characterized by disturbed sensory perception and altered thought processes (psychosis, not other specified and schizophrenia).
2. Identify nonspecific symptoms seen early in the prodromal phase of childhood-and adolescent-onset psychosis and schizophrenia.
3. Demonstrate knowledge of the neurodevelopmental, neurological, genetic, and environmental factors believed to be associated with disturbed sensory perception and altered thought processes.

4. Demonstrate knowledge of the use of psychotropic medications, child, adolescent, and family education, and psychosocial supports with youth diagnosed with schizophrenia.
5. Apply theoretical knowledge about individual growth and development needs and the impact on family functioning during treatment of children and adolescents with disturbed sensory perception and altered thought processes.
6. Discuss collaborative treatment strategies that APRNs in primary care and mental health can use when working with children and families affected by this disorder.

Introduction

Perceptual alterations disorders refer to conditions in which the individual experiences a change in the amount or patterning of incoming stimuli accompanied by a diminished, exaggerated, distorted, or impaired response to such stimuli (Herdman and Kamitsuru 2014). The defining characteristics are changes in the usual response to stimuli, changes in sensory acuity, visual distortions or auditory distractions, hallucinations, change in behavior pattern or in problem-solving, poor concentration, disorientation to place, and/or altered communication pattern. Disturbed thought processes are often found with disturbed sensory perceptions. The most common disorders that alter perceptions in children and adolescents include schizophrenia, unspecified schizophrenia spectrum and other psychotic disorders, bipolar disorder with psychotic features, post-traumatic stress disorder (PTSD), substance-related and addictive disorders, and organic disorders such as brain lesions (McClellan 2018; Starling et al. 2013). These disorders are severe and can be devastating to the child or adolescent and to the family.

Several of these disorders have nonspecific prodromal symptoms that are very similar. Specific

Child and Adolescent Behavioral Health: A Resource for Advanced Practice Psychiatric and Primary Care Practitioners in Nursing, Second Edition. Edited by Edilma L. Yearwood, Geraldine S. Pearson, and Jamesetta A. Newland.
© 2021 John Wiley & Sons, Inc. Published 2021 by John Wiley & Sons, Inc.
Companion website: www.wiley.com/go/Yearwood

symptoms that evolve and emerge over time include the psychotic symptoms of hallucinations or delusions. Early intervention in the management of schizophrenia and other psychotic illnesses in the child or adolescent is recognized as extremely important in preventing the transition to psychosis, shortening the duration of the psychotic episode, and effectively managing the illness to prevent further relapse episodes with resultant degenerative neurological signs (Nordentoft et al. 2014, 2015). To accomplish early intervention, it is important for primary care providers to be aware of the early signs and symptoms so that the child or adolescent can be referred to mental health professionals for immediate diagnostic workup and specialized treatment as needed (Schimmelmann et al. 2013).

This chapter describes the clinical symptoms associated with childhood- and adolescent-onset schizophrenia, the epidemiology and etiology of the disorder, assessment tools used to assist with screening, and evidence-based management strategies for use with children, adolescents, and families. A case exemplar is presented to illustrate presentation, progression, and management of the disorder.

Clinical Picture

The clinical picture in perceptual alterations disorders involves three phases. The first phase is the premorbid phase in which there may not be obvious signs or symptoms of a disorder and the child or adolescent may seem to function quite normally even though the risk factors or vulnerabilities such as genetic makeup are still present. More recently, however, premorbid developmental impairments, including language, motor, and social deficits, are being recognized as more frequent and more pronounced in children who eventually develop childhood schizophrenia (Masi and Liboni 2011; Masi et al. 2006).

The early prodromal phase includes negative and unspecific symptoms, and the late prodromal phase or psychosis phase extends from positive but attenuated psychotic symptoms or brief and limited psychosis to full psychosis. Eventually, the psychotic phase, or first psychotic episode as it is often called, occurs with the presence of such positive symptoms as hallucinations or delusions (Berger et al. 2006; Maier et al. 2003; Shioiri et al. 2007). Table 14.1 shows symptoms of the disorder in progression to the psychotic episode. It is at the point of the psychotic episode that the *Diagnostic and Statistical Manual of Mental Disorders 5* (DSM-5) diagnostic criteria can be applied and a tentative diagnosis may be made (American Psychiatric Association [APA] 2013).

Table 14.1 Symptoms in the progression to a psychotic episode

Premorbid phase
Risk factors and vulnerabilities present but no noticeable change in psychosocial functioning

Early prodromal phase
Nonspecific and general symptoms
Depression
Depressed mood
Decreased appetite
Insomnia
Anxiety
Irritation
Fear
Autonomic symptoms
Obsessive–compulsive-type symptoms
Somatoform symptoms
Eating disorder (e.g. anorexia nervosa; Kelly et al. 2004)

Late prodromal or psychosis phase
Perceptions
Hallucinations
Auditory (e.g. hearing voices that others do not hear)
Visual (e.g. seeing people or figures that others do not see)
Olfactory (e.g. smelling odors that others do not smell)
Tactile (e.g. feeling sensations others do not feel)
Thinking
Delusions (e.g. grandiose, paranoid, nihilistic)
Flight of ideas (e.g. racing thoughts, unconnected thoughts)
Cognition
Difficulty in concentrating
Difficulty in retaining memory
Difficulty in performing tasks and following instructions
Self-awareness
Loss of insight (e.g. denial of being ill or needing treatment)
Affect and emotions
Inappropriate affect
Blunted affect
Unable to express emotions or recognize emotions
Behavior
Withdrawal
Lack of socializing
Impaired functioning in all areas
Strange behaviors
Physical functioning
Change in sleep patterns
Change in eating behavior
Loss of energy
Abnormal motor activities or mannerisms

Presenting Symptoms

As seen in Table 14.1, the important phase for primary care providers as well as mental health professionals is the prodromal phase, where early recognition of the underlying disorder is the goal. The challenge in early recognition is the nonspecific nature of the signs and symptoms noted during this prodromal phase. *Prodromal* refers to the period of time from when the child or adolescent first begins to decline in baseline level of functioning to the time that the criteria for a diagnosis of the disorder are met. The prodromal phase begins with nonspecific symptoms; gradually over time, very specific symptoms of a disorder begin to manifest, including initial formation of hallucinations and/or delusions (Berger et al. 2006; David et al. 2011; McClellan et al. 1999; White et al. 2006; Woodberry et al. 2016). As the symptoms increase and become more specific, the child or adolescent's overall level of functioning declines. The specific symptoms are those symptoms that are commonly manifested for diagnosis of a disorder and are used as part of the diagnostic criteria for that disorder. Hallucinations and delusions are referred to as positive symptoms and are common in schizophrenia, especially auditory hallucinations and suspiciousness. Negative symptoms are also noted and include social withdrawal and inability to obtain pleasure from any activities. Specific symptoms noted in bipolar disorder include increased energy, elevated mood, and increased activity. In the manic stage of bipolar, psychotic symptoms such as hallucinations may be noted. Psychotic symptoms may also be noted in substance abuse in children and adolescents. Psychotic symptoms may be alleviated during abstinence, which would differentiate substance use from other disturbed sensory perception disorders. Symptoms may worsen in substance abuse with the use of cannabis and push the youth toward becoming at high risk for schizophrenia or other psychotic disorders (Gage et al. 2016, 2017).

Figure 14.1 shows the phases and the relationship between increasing symptoms and decreasing level of functioning. Emerging evidence for schizophrenia as one perceptual alterations disorder suggests that progressive deterioration occurs from neurostructural changes and that this parallels the child's or adolescent's functional decline (Koutsouleris et al. 2010; Nasrallah et al. 2009). Evidence of neurostructural changes were noted in prior studies (Jou et al. 2005; Rapoport et al. 1999; White et al. 2003; Zhang et al. 2017). Those with childhood-onset or adolescent-onset schizophrenia, or individuals at high risk for schizophrenia had progressive decrease in cortical gray matter than normal adolescents in that age group, suggesting overpruning of the cortical gray matter in those with schizophrenia. As

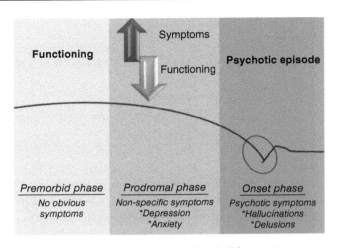

Figure 14.1 Phases, symptoms, and level of functioning leading to a psychotic episode. (*Source:* Reprinted from Kim 2010, with permission from the author.)

neurostructural changes occur, signs and symptoms of functional decline become more evident. Therefore, earlier recognition of symptoms and referral for diagnosis and treatment are the goals in order to limit or arrest developmental decline.

DSM-5 Diagnostic Criteria

Since schizophrenia is the most severe form of perceptual alterations disorder, the diagnostic criteria will be presented. The diagnostic criteria for schizophrenia in adults are also used as the diagnostic criteria for children and adolescents. According to the DSM-5 (APA 2013), the diagnosis of schizophrenia is made when the symptoms include those given in Table 14.2.

There are several challenges to diagnosing perceptual alterations disorders such as schizophrenia in children or adolescents when using adult criteria. Due to the age-related characteristics, it is often difficult to determine if the child's thinking is actually psychotic or whether the child's thinking is due to an active imagination, which would be common for this age group. The duration of 6 months, which is one of the diagnostic criteria for schizophrenia for adults, is also challenging when evaluating a child or adolescent for schizophrenia. The symptoms may resolve before 6 months, especially if medication is given, so it may be difficult to know if the psychotic symptoms would be present for that length of time. Even though normal developmental behavior may at times be difficult to differentiate from pathology, the symptoms most indicative of schizophrenia in the very early onset age group are the positive symptoms such as hallucinations and delusions. The most prominent hallucination for children and adolescents is hearing voices (David et al. 2011; Masi et al. 2006).

Table 14.2 DSM-5 criteria for schizophrenia

A. Two (or more) of the following, each present for a significant portion of time during a 1-month period (or less if successfully treated). At least one of these must be (1), (2), or (3):

1. Delusions.
2. Hallucinations.
3. Disorganized speech (e.g., frequent derailment or incoherence).
4. Grossly disorganized or catatonic behavior.
5. Negative symptoms (i.e., diminished emotional expression or avolition).

B. For a significant portion of the time since the onset of the disturbance, level of functioning in one or more major areas, such as work, interpersonal relations, or self-care, is markedly below the level achieved prior to the onset (or when the onset is in childhood or adolescence, there is failure to achieve expected level of interpersonal, academic, or occupational functioning).

C. Continuous signs of the disturbance persist for at least 6 months. This 6-month period must include at least 1 month of symptoms (or less if successfully treated) that meet Criterion A (i.e., active-phase symptoms) and may include periods of prodromal or residual symptoms. During these prodromal or residual periods, the signs of the disturbance may be manifested by only negative symptoms or by two or more symptoms listed in Criterion A present in an attenuated form (e.g., odd beliefs, unusual perceptual experiences).

D. Schizoaffective disorder and depressive or bipolar disorder with psychotic features have been ruled out because either (1) no major depressive or manic episodes have occurred concurrently with the active-phase symptoms, or (2) if mood episodes have occurred during active-phase symptoms, they have been present for a minority of the total duration of the active and residual periods of the illness.

E. The disturbance is not attributable to the physiological effects of a substance (e.g., a drug of abuse, a medication) or another medical condition.

F. If there is a history of autism spectrum disorder or a communication disorder of childhood onset, the additional diagnosis of schizophrenia is made only if prominent delusions or hallucinations, in addition to the other required symptoms of schizophrenia, are also present for at least 1 month (or less if successfully treated).

Source: American Psychiatric Association. Diagnostic and statistical manual of mental disorder, 5th edition. © 2013, American Psychiatric Association. Reprinted with permission from the American Psychiatric Association.

Because of nonspecific symptoms, it is difficult to make a definitive diagnosis and not uncommon to receive a different diagnosis over time as different specific symptom patterns become evident. Also, the stigma attached to a diagnosis of schizophrenia is a factor in many cases and psychiatrists may be hesitant to label a young person with this diagnosis at such an early age.

Differential Diagnosis

Even though symptoms may be indicative of schizophrenia, other conditions may have similar symptomatology. Bipolar disorder often has similar symptoms to those of schizophrenia. Approximately half of adolescents with bipolar disorder were originally diagnosed with schizophrenia (McClellan et al. 1993; Werry et al. 1991). Observing the symptom pattern over time may help to differentiate between the two disorders. Correll et al. (2007) and Frazier et al. (2007) differentiated between bipolar and schizophrenia and concluded that mania and schizophrenia prodromal characteristics overlapped considerably. However, social isolation, strange or unusual ideas, as well as impaired functioning in multiple domains were significantly more likely to be a part of the schizophrenia prodrome, while obsessions/compul-

sions, suicidality, difficulty thinking/communicating clearly, depressed mood, decreased concentration/memory, tiredness/lack of energy, mood lability, and physical agitation were more likely to be a part of the mania prodrome (Correll et al. 2007; Frazier et al. 2007).

Organic psychosis due to substance abuse, seizure disorders, central nervous system (CNS) lesions, or infectious diseases may present with similar symptoms to schizophrenia and also need to be ruled out. Autism is seen in children less than 5 years of age, and although extremely rare, schizophrenia can be diagnosed in children after the age of 5. Childhood disintegrative disorder and Asperger's syndrome may also resemble schizophrenia but lack the symptoms of hallucinations and delusions.

Evidence-based Data and Assessment Tools

There are two types of diagnostic assessment tools available for use with children and adolescents. Questionnaires are one type of tool that can be completed by the patient and/or caregiver, a parent, or a teacher. Questionnaires generally focus on broader domains of psychopathology and symptom occurrence. The Early Signs Scale (ESS) found in Table 14.3 is an example of a questionnaire used to measure prodromal symptoms of schizophrenia (Birchwood et al. 1989).

Table 14.3 Early signs scale

To be completed by the individual

This questionnaire describes problems and complaints that people sometimes have. Please read it carefully. After you have done so please mark the appropriate box which best describes how much each problem has bothered you during the past week, including today. Mark only one box for each of the problems listed. When you have completed the questionnaire, please return it in the stamped addressed envelope provided. Thank you very much for your help.

	Not a problem (zero times a week)	Little problem (once a week)	Moderate problem (several times a week but not daily)	Marked problem (at least once a day)
1. I talk or smile to myself.				
2. I feel unable to cope.				
3. I have aches and pains.				
4. My speech comes out jumbled or is full of odd words.				
5. I feel tired or lack energy.				
6. I feel like playing tricks or pranks.				
7. I am preoccupied with one or two things.				
8. I feel quiet and withdrawn.				
9. I feel stubborn or refuse to carry out simple requests.				
10. I do not feel like eating.				
11. My sleep has been restless or unsettled.				
12. I lose my temper easily.				
13. I feel useless or helpless.				
14. I feel violent.				
15. I feel dissatisfied with myself.				
16. I feel as if my thoughts might be controlled.				
17. Others have difficulty in following what I am saying.				
18. My movements seem slow.				
19. I feel depressed or low.				
20. I feel very excited.				
21. I feel as if I'm being laughed at or talked about.				
22. I feel as if I'm being watched.				
23. I feel confused.				
24. I feel aggressive or pushy.				
25. I think I could be someone else.				
26. I feel as if my thoughts might not be my own.				
27. I am open and explicit about sexual matters.				
28. I feel tense, afraid, or anxious.				
29. I feel forgetful or "far away."				
30. I have no interest in things.				
31. I have difficulty concentrating (e.g. on TV).				
32. I behave oddly for no reason.				
33. I am not bothered about my appearance or hygiene.				
34. I feel irritable or quick-tempered.				

Source: Reprinted from Birchwood, M., Smith, J., MacMillian, F., Hogg, B., Prasad, R., Harvey, C., & Bering, S. (1989). Predicting relapse in schizophrenia: the development and implementation of an early signs monitoring system using patients and families as observers, a preliminary investigation. Psychological Medicine, 19, 649–656. Reproduced with permission from Cambridge University Press.

The other type of assessment tool is the structured diagnostic interview, which is designed to elicit information from not only the child or adolescent but also the parent about the child's or adolescent's functioning and severity of symptoms for different psychiatric disorders. For the most part, the structured diagnostic interviews are administered by clinicians and, on completion, the diagnosis is made by the clinician. One diagnostic interview that is used often is the Schedule for Affective Disorders and Schizophrenia for School-Age Children (K-SADS) (Ambrosini 2000). The K-SADS is a semi-structured diagnostic interview designed to assess current and past psychopathology in children and adolescents. It is designed for use with children and adolescents between the ages of 6 and 18 years and takes approximately 75–90 minutes to complete (Ambrosini 2000; Calinoiu and McClellan 2004). Moreover, the K-SADS has been modified to reflect the DSM-5 criteria (APA 2013) and covers neurodevelopmental disorders, schizophrenia spectrum disorders, bipolar disorders, anxiety disorders, obsessive compulsive disorders, elimination disorders, eating and substance use disorders, and PTSD. Alternative measures include the Child and Adolescent Psychiatric Assessment (CAPA) (Angold and Costello 1995), the National Institute of Mental Health Diagnostic Interview Schedule for Children (NIMH-DISC) (Shaffer et al. 2000), and the Diagnostic Interview for Children and Adolescents (DICA) (Reich 2000).

Several scales have been developed that measure the level of functioning in children and adolescents; moreover, these scales have been used over long periods of time and feature high levels of reliability and validity. For example, the Children's Global Assessment Scale (CGAS) is a clinician rating scale (i.e. 1–100) that is used to rate the level of functioning (i.e. higher scores indicate higher functioning) (Shaffer et al. 1983). The Child and Adolescent Functional Assessment Scale (CAFAS) developed by Hodges (Hodges et al. 1999) is completed by the clinician and measures the level of functioning of the child or adolescent in domains such as behavior toward others, mood, substance use, thinking, and role performance at home, school, and community (Hodges et al. 1999).

In schizophrenia and bipolar disorder, evidence shows many adolescents experience prodromal symptoms a year or longer before the first episode. According to Bota et al. (2008), the prodromal symptoms may last as long as 4.3 years for males and as long as 6.7 years for females. With schizophrenia, as age increases, both hallucinations and delusions become more complex and elaborate. The earlier the onset and the higher the residual level of positive and negative symptoms, the poorer the functioning and prognosis. Poor functioning is also noted in social relationships and in independent living skills (Berger et al. 2006). Corcoran et al. (2007) found that narratives by family members of patients with schizophrenia were remarkably similar: patients who were previously normal but vulnerable adolescents had social withdrawal and mood symptoms. In this premorbid phase, these adolescents were particularly nonreactive to insults by others, shy, and had social awkwardness.

Epidemiology

The prevalence of schizophrenia worldwide among adults ranges from 0.5 to 1.5% of the population. Seventy-five percent of those with schizophrenia experience the onset during adolescence and early adulthood. Rates of psychosis in children show a dramatic increase in the adolescent years and especially toward late adolescence. For schizophrenia, the rate of onset increases during adolescence and reaches the adult rate of 0.1% of new cases each year (McClellan and Werry 1997). The disorder occurs more frequently in males at a ratio of 2 : 1. As age increases, more females are diagnosed with schizophrenia. The age of onset in males tends to be 5 years earlier than in females (McClellan and Werry 1997). In adolescents, both acute onset with symptoms occurring within the past year and insidious onset are noted (McClellan et al. 1993; Werry et al. 1991).

In early adolescence, which accounts for 15% of the population with schizophrenia, the onset is between ages 13 and 16. Childhood-onset schizophrenia (COS) occurs between the ages of 10–13 and comprises 4% of the population. Very early onset schizophrenia (VEOS), which occurs before the age of 10 (Mala 2008) or before age 13 (Clemmensen et al. 2012), accounts for 1% of the population with schizophrenia. VEOS is rare, with a prevalence rate estimated to be one per 10 000, and is more common among males. Eighty percent of children with VEOS report experiencing auditory hallucinations (Mala 2008). Notably, 75% of children diagnosed with schizophrenia exhibit an insidious onset; only 25% have an acute onset (Masi et al. 2006).

Etiology

No single etiology has been identified for schizophrenia in children and adolescents. Most theories include both genetic and environmental factors (Gage et al. 2017; O'Donoghue et al. 2015; Rapoport et al. 2012). With the earlier onset of schizophrenia in comparison to the adolescent or adult onset, increased genetic loading or early CNS damage due to environmental stressors may be important factors in the etiology (Howes and McCutcheon 2017).

Neurobiological/Neurophysiological Factors

Increasing evidence points to alterations in several neurotransmitters and pathways in the pathophysiological processes of schizophrenia. These include not only dopamine, glutamate, gamma-aminobutyric acid, and serotonin, but also the cholinergic and opioidergic systems. The studies that have examined the neurotransmitters and brain metabolites in children with schizophrenia report the same abnormalities as noted in adults with schizophrenia. The dopamine hypothesis maintains that hyperactivity of the dopamine system leads to an increase in positive symptoms of schizophrenia. Antipsychotics that diminish the hyperactivity of dopamine receptors decrease the positive symptoms; meanwhile, drugs that stimulate the dopamine receptors exacerbate psychotic symptoms. The other neurotransmitters also are involved in schizophrenia, and the effect of the newer psychotropic drugs on the abnormalities of these neurotransmitters is undergoing further study (Castle et al. 2013; Citrome 2016).

Neurodevelopmental hypothesis maintains that the developing brain is vulnerable to genetic and environmental insults that alter the structure and function of the brain and increase the risk of psychosis later in life. Evidence points to environmental insults such as hypoxia-associated complications during pregnancy, prenatal exposures to diseases, and famine with fetal malnutrition (Howes and McCutcheon 2017; Lukkari et al. 2012; Piper et al. 2012) as increasing the odds of developing earlier-onset schizophrenia. As noted above, excessive pruning of dopaminergic neurons in the brain during the period from birth to the age of 12–15 years also is hypothesized to lead to the development of schizophrenia (Mala 2008; Rapoport et al. 1999).

Brain imaging studies show consistent findings of brain tissue volume loss in schizophrenia. These findings provide evidence of a neurodegenerative process that occurs in the brains of people with schizophrenia. Gray matter volume loss in people with schizophrenia over time is associated with deterioration in overall clinical status (Fraguas et al. 2016; Nasrallah et al. 2009).

Genetic and Genomic Factors

Genetic and genomic factors are the best-established etiological determinants of schizophrenia (McClellan et al. 2008; Nasrallah et al. 2009). The best-established evidence comes from twin and family studies showing a strong genetic link to the development of schizophrenia. The results clearly indicate the heritability and genetic basis of schizophrenia but not specific genes. Monozygotic twins are shown to have 41–65% proband concordance rates for schizophrenia, while dizygotic twins have only 0–28% proband concordance rates (Cardno and Gottesman 2000). Future trends in searching for the etiology of schizophrenia and other perceptual alterations disorders include epigenetics, which studies changes in behavior of genes and changes in the genes as a result of our own behavior (Mala 2008).

Several chromosomal abnormalities are reported in people with schizophrenia. The 22q11.2 deletion on the maternal chromosome is of particular interest in the diagnosis of schizophrenia in children and adolescents. Children and adolescents with velocardiofacial syndrome have similar reduction in gray and white matter tissue volume, and the reduction is attributed to 22q11.2 microdeletion on the maternal chromosome (Eliez et al. 2001; Schneider et al. 2014).

Family History

Evidence of genetic etiology in schizophrenia comes from twin and family studies. Aside from genetic factors, other family history factors are not as well established as part of the etiology of schizophrenia. In the social case history, 45% of the cases of schizophrenia were found to have a history of "broken home," with most being associated with death of a parent (Mala 2008). Poor prognosis is found in cases where individuals with schizophrenia had a family history that includes psychosis and dysfunctional family behavior, but the evidence of these as determinants of schizophrenia due to environmental factors versus genetic factors is not well established (Kakela et al. 2014; Mala 2008).

Environmental and Psychosocial Factors

Previous studies reveal that certain environmental factors increase disease risk and progress. Examples of these environmental factors include advanced parental age, prenatal malnutrition and infections, obstetric complications, and cannabis use (Kuepper et al. 2011; McGrath and Susser 2009). Psychosocial factors, such as family or work settings that have highly expressed emotional atmospheres, are known to lead to an increase in symptoms and eventual relapse for some individuals with schizophrenia. However, because not all individuals exposed to such environmental and psychosocial factors develop schizophrenia, the etiological evidence is weak yet contributory.

Dysfunction of the "social brain" refers to deficits in social functioning and is present in many psychiatric disorders. This developmental disturbance affects the interconnections of the brain and leads to disorganization of thinking and perception, as well as inappropriate and flat affect and deficits in social functioning. This connectivity disturbance is hypothesized to be a factor in the etiology of schizophrenia (Mala 2008; Orban et al. 2017).

Evidence-based Nursing Intervention

Basically, treatment for children over age 12 and adolescents with schizophrenia is similar to the treatment for adults. The strongest evidence to date for effective treatment is the use of psychotropic medications (Correll et al. 2011, 2013; McClellan and Stock 2013; Pagsberg et al. 2017). Doses of medications are generally reduced for children and adolescents. Not all atypical psychotropic medications are shown to be safe and efficient for children. However, randomized clinical trials are under way to establish their efficacy with youth. Complications from the use of typical and atypical antipsychotics include marked weight gain, extrapyramidal symptoms, cardiometabolic risks, neuroleptic malignant syndrome, and other side effects. These effects become more obvious and problematic as more of these medications are used with children and adolescents (McClellan and Stock 2013; Pagsberg et al. 2017).

Medication adherence continues to be a major concern because so often even the parent who administers the medication to the child or adolescent is not aware of the importance of adhering to the medication schedule. Evidence of the effectiveness of visual feedback therapy to improve adherence to the medications by adults with schizophrenia has been noted (Kozuki and Schepp 2005). At this time, little evidence exists to show the effectiveness of visual feedback therapy when used with children and adolescents. More specific detailed information about psychotropic medications and psychopharmacology with children and adolescents is presented in Chapter 9.

Strong evidence is being established that shows the treatment effectiveness and cost effectiveness of involving the family in psychoeducational programs where all members of the family can learn about the disorder and symptoms along with skills to help the child or adolescent manage the illness (Breitborde et al. 2009; McClellan and Stock 2013; Schepp et al. 2005). Different types of psychoeducational programs are being used and more evidence is becoming available about the type of program that is most effective for each age group and cultural group (Chien and Thompson 2014; Lee and Schepp 2013; Ross 2014; Xia et al. 2011; Zhao et al. 2015). Psychoeducational programs that emphasize symptom awareness and stress management skills are reported to be effective in reducing stress for the mentally ill adolescent as well as for other family members (Lee and Schepp 2009).

The most promising advances in the treatment of early-onset schizophrenia are evidenced by the latest research supporting early treatment and aggressive use of psychotropic medications coupled with psychosocial family interventions. The less time between the onset of the first psychotic symptoms and the first adequate treatment, referred to as the duration of untreated psychosis, the better the short-term outcome is noted to be (Chang et al. 2013; Hegelstad et al. 2012; Stentebjerg-Olesen et al. 2016).

Growing evidence indicates that it may be possible to identify, treat, and potentially improve the outcome for those who are at highest risk for developing schizophrenia. Three groups found to be at highest risk are those who have experienced (i) attenuated, positive psychotic symptoms during the past year or (ii) brief intermittent episodes of frank psychotic symptoms but not lasting longer than a week and (iii) those who have a relative with a psychotic disorder or who themselves have a schizotypal personality with decreased functioning over the course of the past year (Nelson et al. 2013).

Moreover, growing evidence demonstrates cognitive behavior therapy to be effective in the treatment of schizophrenia and in psychoeducational programs for family (Hofmann et al. 2012). Likewise, appreciative inquiry, an intervention approach derived from positive psychology, has been shown to make a significant difference in the lives of young adults with schizophrenia in their perceptions of their level of happiness and hope (Buckland 2009). Moreover, rather than address *deficits*, as many interventions have done in the past, appreciative inquiry develops and emphasizes *strengths* in young adults over a period of time as part of their treatment.

Integration with Primary Care

In the context of perceptual alterations disorders among children and adolescents, the role(s) of advanced practice registered nurses (APRNs) may include (i) the early detection and referral of patients who are experiencing premorbid major delay or prodromal symptoms, (ii) monitoring and tracking patient conditions during annual well-child examinations, (iii) promoting family-centered care, (iv) educating patients and families about the relevant disorder and its management, (v) functioning as a liaison care manager among the patient, family, psychiatric specialist, and school, and (vi) helping adolescents and their families to make smooth transitions to care provided by adult primary care providers.

First, early identification of schizophrenia includes early detection and referral of patients who are experiencing premorbid major delay or prodromal symptoms. Evidence shows that 46–89% of affected children show premorbid major delay in one or all areas of motor, speech, and social development (Masi et al. 2006). Therefore, anyone who shows these early developmental delays should be monitored closely because these may be early manifestations of the disorder. Evidence shows that early identification of prodromal symptoms and intervention lead to appointments with primary care providers. Studies show that 75–90% of patients experiencing prodromal symptoms visit a physician before the onset of psychosis (Bota et al. 2008). Early prodromal symptoms are negative symptoms and include slow changes in behaviors and mood such as social isolation, decreased school functioning, anxiety/nervousness, blunted or inappropriate affect, and anhedonia.

APRNs in primary care need to distinguish whether or not these presentations are simply developmental or psychopathological. If simply developmental, the adolescents will have other symptoms. If simply psychopathological, these symptoms will not improve and may become worse to the point that they include positive symptoms. In any case, adolescents with these symptoms should be referred to a psychiatric healthcare provider for further evaluation. If adolescents who had early developmental delays show the prodromal symptoms, they need to be evaluated by a specialist.

If the primary care APRN is unsure about referral, help can be obtained by consulting with a child and adolescent psychiatric-mental health APRN in making a decision. Communications between the primary care provider and a child and adolescent psychiatric-mental health APRN may be different based on the care setting. If both providers are in the same building, direct communication can happen easily; this promotes continuity of care. In some hospitals, when the patient is referred to a specialist, the specialist sends a summary statement of the visit to the referring service provider. In this case, the primary care providers will be kept informed about the patient's condition, which allows them to stay current with the patient and schedule visits as necessary. If the specialist does not send the summary of the visit, the primary care provider should ask the patient about the visit with the specialist. If the primary care provider needs information from the specialist, then the primary care provider should contact the specialist directly to obtain the summary statement in order to provide safe care.

Second, if an adolescent is diagnosed with schizophrenia, a recommendation will be made to begin an antipsychotic medication. Side effects from antipsychotic medications are not uncommon and the adolescent and family need to be aware of these side effects. Patients with major mental illnesses also may have a greater risk of glucose intolerance diabetes and lipid abnormalities that seem to be present before treatment initiation (Chen et al. 2016) and are associated with medication effects or weight gain (Deng 2013). The use of psychotropic medication such as clozapine will require additional tests such as troponin, echocardiogram, and frequent white blood cells and granulocyte counts. The primary care provider should communicate with the specialist to verify whether or not he or she is monitoring for these risks. If not, it is recommended that the primary care provider closely monitor the patient at the annual examination along with a complete physical assessment. The child, adolescent, and/or parents should be told about potential side effects and what to do should they occur. Moreover, a full medical examination is recommended during first-episode psychosis and yearly after that includes a complete blood count, lipid panel, urea, and electrolytes, liver function, thyroid function, B12 and folate, random glucose, urinalysis, and creatinine clearance (Berger et al. 2006). Table 14.4 shows the tests that are recommended before antipsychotic medications are prescribed. Furthermore, suicidal ideation should be checked at each visit because 4 in 10 people who suffer from schizophrenia attempt suicide, and 5–13% of people who suffer from schizophrenia die by suicide (Palmer et al. 2005; Pompili et al. 2007). Those

Table 14.4 Primary care workup prior to commencement of antipsychotic medications

Timing	Tests
Before commencement of antipsychotic medications	Full blood examination
	Lipid panel (total cholesterol, triglyceride, high density lipoprotein, low density lipoprotein)
	Urea and electrolytes
	Liver function (LFTs)
	Thyroid function
	B12 and folate
	Random glucose
	Urinalysis
	Creatinine clearance glucose
	LFTs with copper, heavy metal screening
	Pregnancy test
	HIV/AIDS
	MRI to rule out organic etiology of psychosis
	Genetic testing (22q11 deletion syndrome)

who are not taking their prescribed medication as directed also are at risk for symptom resurgence, therefore medication adherence must be stressed and assessed. If adolescents stop taking prescribed medication and their symptoms return, then they are more likely to visit a primary care APRN than a psychiatric healthcare provider. When this occurs, the primary care provider should contact the specialist to obtain advice. Moreover, because consultation phone lines with psychiatric healthcare providers are present in some communities, APRNs must be familiar with all community resources available to adolescents to provide optimum care.

Third, the APRN needs to help families cope with the situation of raising an adolescent with schizophrenia, which can be very disturbing to the family. Assessing family functioning, the effect of the adolescent's illness on the family, the communication abilities of the family members, and the family member's relationship with the adolescent would be necessary. Moreover, helping the family become familiar with (i) resources in the community, such as the National Alliance on Mental Illness, (ii) websites that provide important information about schizophrenia, and (iii) the medications and treatments used and recommended for schizophrenia is extremely important. Furthermore, providing occasional respite support to both the child and family is crucial. Respite for families may occur through in-home and out-of-home settings for various lengths of time depending on the needs of the family and the available community resources. As such, primary care providers must be familiar with local government community programs that are available for funding respite support. Respite is an important part of the continuum of services for families, which helps preserve the family unit and supports family stability (Whitmore 2017).

Fourth, ongoing education of family members about schizophrenia would improve their coping skills and their ability to help the patient. including:

- knowledge about the illness and its symptoms
- advantages and disadvantages of different treatment options
- available medications and possible side effects, and signs of relapse
- better communication with the patient, other family members, healthcare providers, and school personnel
- availability of community services and supports, including respite care
- benefits and entitlements, including how to access care
- management of crises or bizarre and troubling behaviors
- importance of self-care for caregivers.

Fifth, the primary care APRN is in an ideal position to be a liaison care manager among the patient, family, other healthcare providers (e.g. the psychiatric specialist), and school. When children or adolescents develop the first psychotic episode, they may be admitted to an inpatient hospital. After a child or adolescent is discharged from the hospital, his or her school may ask for documentation from a healthcare provider to verify that the student is physically and mentally ready to manage the daily demands at school. Moreover, the primary care APRN often must function as a liaison between the family and the school to enable the child or adolescent in question to make a smooth transition to educational settings. In this event, the APRN can collaborate with the school counselor or school nurse. The APRN also can evaluate how the child or adolescent is doing at school, both academically and socially. These children or adolescents typically have trouble with declining school performance during the prodromal stage of the disorder and once they start psychotropic medications the side effects include drowsiness, which interferes with social interaction. Once the appropriate medication and dose are determined and the child or adolescent is taking the medication as prescribed, his or her functioning should improve. Nevertheless, the student may continue to struggle in school because of thought, language, perceptual, and/or motor disturbances. These children and adolescents also may be vulnerable because of decreased tolerance to normal stress. Moreover, children and adolescents may try to hide their illness from their friends, initially because of the stigma of having a mental illness. However, if the children and adolescents can be open and direct about their illness with friends, then their friends will be better positioned to understand the illness and be supportive. Peer relationships are crucially important for this developmental stage.

Last, helping the adolescent make a smooth transition to adulthood is necessary. Psychotic episodes tend to happen during stressful times when the individual feels most vulnerable, such as making transitions to living away from home, going to college or going to a new job, and trying to adjust to a new environment. Therefore, the APRN can and should help the adolescent and the family find adult care providers in the area where the adolescents will now reside.

Implications for Practice, Research, and Education

Disorders with disturbed sensory perception and thought processes are difficult to diagnose. The symptom patterns tend to be nonspecific for varying lengths of time and a clear pattern of specific symptoms may not be evident for a considerable period of time, sometimes from months to years. In the meantime, families are seeking help for their child or adolescent and many times the diagnosis is not made for at least 6 months. Often times, mental health professionals are hesitant to give a diagnosis, especially if it is schizophrenia. Diagnosing a child or adolescent as having schizophrenia can lead to labels that are difficult to get rid of and can lead to stigma toward the individual as well as to the family. The label and stigma can be devastating, especially since it can be life-long and detrimental to one's self-esteem and confidence. In recent years, efforts have been made to decrease the stigma of perceptual alterations disorders such as schizophrenia so the young person can seek treatment to lessen the persistently debilitating effects of the disorder (Asarnow et al. 2004; Lee and Schepp 2013).

As more studies yield credible evidence that can be used to guide the way for early recognition of prodromal symptoms of schizophrenia and other perception altering disorders, more interventions will become available that will be individualized to the specific needs of the child or adolescent. Genetic research will eventually lead to identification of specific genes responsible for schizophrenia and early recognition and treatment will follow. The need for early identification and early treatment prompts primary care providers to know the prodromal symptoms and refer to mental health professionals as quickly as possible so the debilitating effects of the disorder can be diminished and the disorder managed.

Research with youth with perceptual alterations disorders is challenging but the future is encouraging. More studies leading to the establishment of strong evidence-based nursing interventions for the children, adolescents, and families are being conducted. New ideas and notions that the trajectory for schizophrenia and related disorders may be altered for the good and a cure may be possible are exciting possibilities for future research. Prevention of perceptual alterations disorders is on the horizon and may one day be possible.

Because primary care providers such as pediatric nurse practitioners or family nurse practitioners often are the first healthcare providers to see the child or adolescent who is experiencing disturbed sensory perceptions and thought processes, these healthcare providers are increasingly more important as active participants of the mental health team. Their role as frontline primary care providers is crucial to early recognition and appropriate referral for those presenting with this disorder. APRNs in primary care can and should remain involved with their psychiatric APRN colleagues in collaborative management of children and adolescents presenting with these disorders. APRNs in primary care should use educational updates on psychotropic medications, management strategies for childhood psychiatric disorders, as well as new research findings in child and adolescent psychiatry to remain current in this area.

Summary

This chapter covers child and adolescent disorders with perceptual alterations such as schizophrenia or bipolar disorder or depression with psychotic features or other conditions where psychosis is present. Since depression and bipolar disorder are covered thoroughly in other chapters, this chapter specifically focused on schizophrenia as the perceptual alterations disorder. The importance of recognizing the prodromal symptoms was emphasized so that early referral for diagnostic workup can be conducted and appropriate treatment can begin. The time factor was emphasized as important because of the neurodegenerative nature of this disorder and the need to halt or reverse the debilitating effects of the disorder as quickly as possible through the use of psychotropic medications and psychosocial interventions. The symptom patterns and phases in the manifestation of schizophrenia in children and adolescents were presented. The epidemiology and current hypotheses concerning the etiology were described. Diagnostic criteria and assessment tool were discussed. Evidence-based interventions were presented and implications for practice, research, and education were addressed. The case study involved an adolescent with schizophrenia and a perceptual alterations disorder. Implications for families of children and adolescents with schizophrenia or other perceptual alterations disorders were noted throughout the chapter. Finally, resources in the form of community groups, websites, and advocacy and treatment resources were presented.

Critical Thinking Questions

1. A 15-year-old girl has visited a primary care APRN because of abdominal discomfort. The APRN notices that the girl was seen by another APRN about 2 weeks earlier for stomach discomfort and was prescribed Zantac. The girl explains, "I am very embarrassed that I have been continuously farting more than thirty times at school, and I don't to want to go school." She did not start taking the Zantac. The girl's mother explains that her daughter has been anxious and irritable, and has not been eating well. You observe that the girl's speech is incoherent and her thoughts are not well connected. As a primary care APRN, how would you approach this case?

2. A 19-year-old boy has been diagnosed with schizophrenia and treated with medications. Although he has been on medications, he smokes marijuana and cigarettes to help remain calm. The boy also has exhibited anger and irritability toward his younger sister, which results in verbal arguments. His parents are embarrassed and frustrated because they do not know what is going on with their son and do not know what to do. The boy's younger sister also worries about the possibility that the same things could happen to her. As a nurse practitioner, how would you address these issues with the family and the patient?

3. An 18-year-old girl has been on an atypical antipsychotic to manage her psychotic symptoms for 1 year. She has been stabilized with the medication and was able to go to school every day, although her academic performance was not as good as it could be. The girl does not have a close friend and does not participate in any extracurricular activities. Most of the time, she stays at home watching television or playing games. Today, she complains about the side effects of her medication: weight gain (i.e. 15 lbs over the past 3 months), which causes her stress. As a result, she does not want to take the medication, or any other medication, if it causes her to gain weight. As a psychiatric nurse practitioner, how would you approach this case?

Resources on Perceptual Alterations Disorders (Community Groups, Websites, Advocacy, and Treatment Resources)

American Psychiatric Nurses Association. www.apna.org.

American Psychiatric Association. Practice Guideline for Treatment of Patients with Schizophrenia (2004). https://psychiatryonline.org/guidelines.

American Academy of Child and Adolescent Psychiatry. www.aacap.org.

Bazelon Center for Mental Health Law. National legal advocate for people with mental illness and intellectual disability. www.bazelon.org.

Brain & Behavior Research Foundation. Research for latest advances in schizophrenia and depression. http://www.bbrfoundation.org/research.

Cochrane Database of Systematic Reviews. Excellent resource for evidence-based practice. www.cochrane.org.

Expert Consensus Guidelines. Guidelines for the treatment of schizophrenia and other disorders. www.psychguides.com.

Food and Drug Administration (FDA) Medwatch updates regarding warnings on atypical antipsychotics. http://www.fda.gov//safety/medwatch.

Health Links. an evidence-based-practice search engine at the University of Washington. http://hsl.uw.edu/toolkits/care-provider.

International Society of Psychiatric-Mental Health Nurses. http://www.ispn-psych.org.

National Alliance on Mental Health. Information, support, and advocacy. www.nami.org.

National Institute of Mental Health. Science news about children and adolescents. http://www.nimh.nih.gov/news/science-news/science-news-about-children-and-adolescents.shtml.

National Institute of Mental Health. Publication about schizophrenia. http://www.nimh.nih.gov/health/publications/schizophrenia-listing.shtml.

Open the Doors. Designed to counter the stigma and distorted facts surrounding schizophrenia. The "Families and Friends" section provides several essays useful for family members and patients newly diagnosed with schizophrenia. www.openthedoors.com.

Mental Health Consultation Outreach for Children. http://www.seattlechildrens.org/healthcare-professionals/access-services/partnership-access-line.

Psychopharmacology Algorithm Project (Harvard Medical School Department of Psychiatry). Algorithms to guide medication treatment of schizophrenia, depression, and other illnesses. http://psychopharm.mobi/algo_live.

Substance Abuse and Mental Health Services Administration (SAMHSA). Evidence-based practice resource center. http://www.samhsa.gov/ebp-resource-center.

The Reach Institute. The Resource for Advancing Children's Health. www.thereachinstitute.org.

References

Ambrosini, P.J. (2000). Historical development and present status of the schedule for affective disorders and schizophrenia for school-age children (K-SADS). *Journal of the American Academy of Child & Adolescent Psychiatry* 39: 49–58.

Angold, A. and Costello, E.J. (1995). A test-retest reliability study of child-reported psychiatric symptoms and diagnoses using the Child and Adolescent Psychiatric Assessment (CAPA-C). *Psychological Medicine* 25: 755–762.

APA (2013). *Diagnostic and Statistical Manual of Mental Disorders 5*. Washington, DC: American Psychiatric Association.

Asarnow, J.R., Tompson, M.C., and McGrath, E.P. (2004). Annotation: childhood-onset schizophrenia: clinical and treatment issues. *Journal of Child Psychology and Psychiatry* 45 (2): 180–194.

Berger, C., Fraser, R., Carbone, S., and McGorry, P. (2006). Emerging psychosis in young people, part 1: key issues for detention and assessment. *Australian Family Physician* 35 (5): 315–321.

Birchwood, M., Smith, J., MacMillian, F. et al. (1989). Predicting relapse in schizophrenia: the development and implementation of an early signs monitoring system using patients and families as observers, a preliminary investigation. *Psychological Medicine* 19: 649–656.

Bota, R.G., Sagduyu, K., Filin, E.E. et al. (2008). Toward a better identification and treatment of schizophrenia prodrome. *Bulletin of the Menninger Clinic* 72 (3): 210–227.

Breitborde, N.J., Woods, S.W., and Srihari, V.H. (2009). Multifamily psychoeducation for first-episode psychosis: a cost effectiveness analysis. *Psychiatric Services* 60 (11): 1477–1483.

Buckland, H.T. (2009). *Young adults with schizophrenia: defining happiness, building hope*. Unpublished doctoral dissertation. Seattle, WA: University of Washington.

Calinoiu, I. and McClellan, J. (2004). Diagnostic interviews. *Current Psychiatry Reports* 6: 88–95.

Cardno, A.G. and Gottesman, I.I. (2000). Twin studies of schizophrenia: from bow and arrow concordances to star wars Mx and functional genomics. *American Journal of Medical Genetics* 97 (1): 12–17.

Castle, D., Keks, N., Newton, R. et al. (2013). Pharmacological approaches to the management of schizophrenia: 10 years on.

Australasian Psychiatry 21 (4): 329–334. https://doi.org/10.1177/1039856213486211.

Chang, W.C., Hui, C.L., Tang, J.Y. et al. (2013). Impacts of duration of untreated psychosis on cognition and negative symptoms in first-episode schizophrenia: a 3-year prospective follow-up study. *Psychological Medicine* 43 (9): 1883–1893. https://doi.org/10.1017/s0033291712002838.

Chen, D.C., Du, X.D., Yin, G.Z. et al. (2016). Impaired glucose tolerance in first-episode drug-naive patients with schizophrenia: relationships with clinical phenotypes and cognitive deficits. *Psychological Medicine* 46 (15): 3219–3230. https://doi.org/10.1017/s0033291716001902.

Chien, W.T. and Thompson, D.R. (2014). Effects of a mindfulness-based psychoeducation programme for Chinese patients with schizophrenia: 2-year follow-up. *British Journal of Psychiatry* 205 (1): 52–59. https://doi.org/10.1192/bjp.bp.113.134635.

Citrome, L. (2016). Emerging pharmacological therapies in schizophrenia: what's new, what's different, what's next? *CNS Spectrums* 21 (S1): 1–12. https://doi.org/10.1017/s1092852916000729.

Clemmensen, L., Vernal, D.L., and Steinhausen, H.-C. (2012). A systematic review of the long-term outcome of early onset schizophrenia. *BMC Psychiatry* 12 (1): 150. https://doi.org/10.1186/1471-244x-12-150.

Corcoran, C., Gerson, R., Sills-Shahar, R. et al. (2007). Trajectory to a first episode of psychosis: a qualitative research study with families. *Early Intervention in Psychiatry* 1: 308–315.

Correll, C.U., Penzner, J.B., Frederickson, A.M. et al. (2007). Differentiation in the pre-onset phases of schizophrenia and mood disorders: evidence in support of a bipolar mania prodrome. *Schizophrenia Bulletin* 33 (3): 703–714.

Correll, C.U., Kratochvil, C.J., and March, J.S. (2011). Developments in pediatric psychopharmacology: focus on stimulants, antidepressants, and antipsychotics. *Journal of Clinical Psychiatry* 72 (5): 655–670. https://doi.org/10.4088/JCP.11r07064.

Correll, C.U., Zhao, J., Carson, W. et al. (2013). Early antipsychotic response to aripiprazole in adolescents with schizophrenia: predictive value for clinical outcomes. *Journal of the American Academy of Child & Adolescent Psychiatry* 52 (7): 689–698.e683. https://doi.org/10.1016/j.jaac.2013.04.018.

David, C.N., Greenstein, D., Clasen, L. et al. (2011). Childhood onset schizophrenia: high rate of visual hallucinations. *Journal of the American Academy of Child & Adolescent Psychiatry* 50 (7): 681–686.e683. https://doi.org/10.1016/j.jaac.2011.03.020.

Deng, C. (2013). Effects of antipsychotic medications on appetite, weight, and insulin resistance. *Endocrinology and Metabolism Clinics of North America* 42 (3): 545–563. https://doi.org/10.1016/j.ecl.2013.05.006.

Eliez, S., Antonarakis, S.E., Morris, M.A. et al. (2001). Parental origin of the deletion 22q11.2 and brain development in velocardiofacial syndrome: a preliminary study. *Archives of General Psychiatry* 58: 64–68.

Fraguas, D., Díaz-Caneja, C.M., Pina-Camacho, L. et al. (2016). Progressive brain changes in children and adolescents with early-onset psychosis: a meta-analysis of longitudinal MRI studies. *Schizophrenia Research* 173 (3): 132–139. https://doi.org/10.1016/j.schres.2014.12.022.

Frazier, J.A., McClellan, J., Findling, R.L. et al. (2007). Treatment of early-onset schizophrenia spectrum disorders (TEOSS): demographic and clinical characteristics. *Journal of the American Academy of Child and Adolescent Psychiatry* 46: 979–988.

Gage, S.H., Hickman, M., and Zammit, S. (2016). Association between cannabis and psychosis: epidemiologic evidence. *Biological Psychiatry* 79 (7): 549–556. https://doi.org/10.1016/j.biopsych.2015.08.001.

Gage, S.H., Jones, H.J., Burgess, S. et al. (2017). Assessing causality in associations between cannabis use and schizophrenia risk: a two-sample Mendelian randomization study. *Psychological Medicine* 47 (5): 971–980. https://doi.org/10.1017/s0033291716003172.

Hegelstad, W.T., Larsen, T.K., Auestad, B. et al. (2012). Long-term follow-up of the TIPS early detection in psychosis study: effects on 10-year outcome. *American Journal of Psychiatry* 169 (4): 374–380. https://doi.org/10.1176/appi.ajp.2011.11030459.

Herdman, T.H. and Kamitsuru, S. (eds.) (2014). *NANDA International Nursing Diagnoses: Definitions & Classification, 2015–2017.* Oxford: Wiley Blackwell.

Hodges, K., Doucette-Gates, A., and Liao, Q.L. (1999). The relationship between the child and adolescent functional assessment scale (CAFAS) and indicators of functioning. *Journal of Child and Family Studies* 8 (1): 109–122.

Hofmann, S.G., Asnaani, A., Vonk, I.J.J. et al. (2012). The efficacy of cognitive behavioral therapy: a review of meta-analyses. *Cognitive Therapy and Research* 36 (5): 427–440. https://doi.org/10.1007/s10608-012-9476-1.

Howes, O.D. and McCutcheon, R. (2017). Inflammation and the neural diathesis-stress hypothesis of schizophrenia: a reconceptualization. *Translational Psychiatry* 7 (2): e1024. https://doi.org/10.1038/tp.2016.278.

Jou, R.J., Hardan, A.Y., and Keshavan, M.S. (2005). Reduced cortical folding in individuals at high risk for schizophrenia: a pilot study. *Schizophrenia Research* 75 (2–3): 309–313. https://doi.org/10.1016/j.schres.2004.11.008.

Kakela, J., Panula, J., Oinas, E. et al. (2014). Family history of psychosis and social, occupational and global outcome in schizophrenia: a meta-analysis. *Acta Psychiatrica Scandinavica* 130 (4): 269–278. https://doi.org/10.1111/acps.12317.

Kelly, L., Moayyad, K., and Brennan, T. (2004). Anorectic symptomatology as a prodrome of schizophrenia: four case reports. *European Eating Disorders Review* 12: 230–233.

Kim, H.J. (2010). *Schizophrenia Prodrome: Phases, symptoms & level of functioning leading to psychotic episode.* University of Washington.

Koutsouleris, N., Patschurek-Kliche, K., Scheuerecker, J. et al. (2010). Neuroanatomical correlates of executive dysfunction in the at-risk mental state for psychosis. *Schizophrenia Research* 123 (2–3): 160–174. https://doi.org/10.1016/j.schres.2010.08.026.

Kozuki, Y. and Schepp, K. (2005). Visual feedback therapy to enhance medication adherence in psychosis. *Archives of Psychiatric Nursing* 19 (2): 70–80.

Kuepper, R., van Os, J., Lieb, R. et al. (2011). Continued cannabis use and risk of incidence and persistence of psychotic symptoms: 10 year follow-up cohort study. *BMJ* 342: d738. https://doi.org/10.1136/bmj.d738.

Lee, H. and Schepp, K. (2009). The relationships between symptoms and stress in adolescents with schizophrenia. *Issues in Mental Health Nursing* 30: 736–744.

Lee, H. and Schepp, K.G. (2013). Lessons learned from research with adolescents with schizophrenia and their families. *Archives of Psychiatric Nursing* 27 (4): 198–203. https://doi.org/10.1016/j.apnu.2013.03.002.

Lukkari, S., Hakko, H., Herva, A. et al. (2012). Exposure to obstetric complications in relation to subsequent psychiatric disorders of adolescent inpatients: specific focus on gender differences. *Psychopathology* 45 (5): 317–326. https://doi.org/10.1159/000336073.

Maier, W., Cornblatt, B.A., and Merikangas, K.R. (2003). Transition to schizophrenia and related disorders: toward a taxonomy of risk. *Schizophrenia Bulletin* 29 (4): 693–701.

Mala, E. (2008). Schizophrenia in childhood and adolescence. *Neuroendocrinology Letters* 29 (6): 831–836.

Masi, G. and Liboni, F. (2011). Management of schizophrenia in children and adolescents. *Drugs* 71 (2): 179–208. https://doi.org/10.2165/11585350-000000000-00000.

Masi, G., Mucci, M., and Pari, C. (2006). Children with schizophrenia: clinical picture and pharmacological treatment. *CNS Drugs* 2006 (20): 841–866.

McClellan, J. (2018). Psychosis in children and adolescents. *Journal of the American Academy of Child & Adolescent Psychiatry* 57 (5): 308–312. https://doi.org/10.1016/j.jaac.2018.01.021.

McClellan, J. and Stock, S. (2013). Practice parameter for the assessment and treatment of children and adolescents with schizophrenia. *Journal of the American Academy of Child & Adolescent Psychiatry* 52 (9): 976–990. https://doi.org/10.1016/j.jaac.2013.02.008.

McClellan, J.M. and Werry, J.S. (1997). Practice parameters for the assessment & treatment of children and adolescents with schizophrenia. *Journal of the American Academy of Child and Adolescent Psychiatry* 36 (Suppl 10): 177S–193S.

McClellan, J.M., Werry, J.S., and Ham, M. (1993). A follow-up study of early onset psychosis: comparison between outcome diagnosis of schizophrenia, mood disorders, and personality disorders. *Journal of Autism and Developmental Disorders* 23: 243–262.

McClellan, J., McCurry, C., Snell, J., and DuBose, A. (1999). Early-onset psychotic disorders: course and outcome over a 2-year period. *Journal of the American Academy of Child & Adolescent Psychiatry* 38 (11): 1380–1388.

McClellan, J., Susser, E., King, M.C. et al. (2008). Forum: the interplay of genes and environment in psychiatric disorders. *Psychiatry* 21: 322–327.

McGrath, J.J. and Susser, E.S. (2009). New directions in the epidemiology of schizophrenia. *Medical Journal of Australia* 190 (4 Suppl): S7–S9.

Nasrallah, H.A., Keshavan, M.S., Benes, F.M. et al. (2009). Proceedings and data from the schizophrenia summit: a critical appraisal to improve the management of schizophrenia. *Journal of Clinical Psychiatry* 70 (suppl 1): 4–46.

Nelson, B., Yuen, H., Wood, S.J. et al. (2013). Long-term follow-up of a group at ultra high risk ("prodromal") for psychosis: the pace 400 study. *JAMA Psychiatry* 70 (8): 793–802. https://doi.org/10.1001/jamapsychiatry.2013.1270.

Nordentoft, M., Rasmussen, J.Ø., Melau, M. et al. (2014). How successful are first episode programs? A review of the evidence for specialized assertive early intervention. *Current Opinion in Psychiatry* 27 (3): 167–172. https://doi.org/10.1097/yco.0000000000000052.

Nordentoft, M., Melau, M., Iversen, T. et al. (2015). From research to practice: how OPUS treatment was accepted and implemented throughout Denmark. *Early Intervention in Psychiatry* 9 (2): 156–162. https://doi.org/10.1111/eip.12108.

O'Donoghue, B., Lyne, J., Madigan, K. et al. (2015). Environmental factors and the age at onset in first episode psychosis. *Schizophrenia Research* 168 (1–2): 106–112. https://doi.org/10.1016/j.schres.2015.07.004.

Orban, P., Desseilles, M., Mendrek, A. et al. (2017). Altered brain connectivity in patients with schizophrenia is consistent across cognitive contexts. *Journal of Psychiatry & Neuroscience: JPN* 42 (1): 17–26. https://doi.org/10.1503/jpn.150247.

Pagsberg, A.K., Tarp, S., Glintborg, D. et al. (2017). Acute antipsychotic treatment of children and adolescents with schizophrenia-spectrum disorders: a systematic review and network meta-analysis. *Journal of the American Academy of Child & Adolescent Psychiatry* 56 (3): 191–202. https://doi.org/10.1016/j.jaac.2016.12.013.

Palmer, B.A., Pankratz, V., and Bostwick, J. (2005). The lifetime risk of suicide in schizophrenia: a reexamination. *Archives of General Psychiatry* 62 (3): 247–253. https://doi.org/10.1001/archpsyc.62.3.247.

Piper, M., Beneyto, M., Burne, T.H. et al. (2012). The neurodevelopmental hypothesis of schizophrenia: convergent clues from epidemiology and neuropathology. *The Psychiatric Clinics of North America* 35 (3): 571–584. https://doi.org/10.1016/j.psc.2012.06.002.

Pompili, M., Amador, X.F., Girardi, P. et al. (2007). Suicide risk in schizophrenia: learning from the past to change the future. *Annals of General Psychiatry* 6 (1): 10. https://doi.org/10.1186/1744-859x-6-10.

Rapoport, J.L., Giedd, J.N., Blumenthal, J. et al. (1999). Progressive cortical change during adolescence in childhood-onset schizophrenia. A longitudinal magnetic resonance imaging study. *Archives of General Psychiatry* 56 (7): 649–654.

Rapoport, J.L., Giedd, J.N., and Gogtay, N. (2012). Neurodevelopmental model of schizophrenia: update 2012. *Molecular Psychiatry* 17 (12): 1228–1238. https://doi.org/10.1038/mp.2012.23.

Reich, W. (2000). Diagnostic interview for children and adolescents (DICA). *Journal of the American Academy of Child & Adolescent Psychiatry* 39: 59–66.

Ross, R.G. (2014). Adolescents are like adults (sort of): psychosocial interventions for adolescents with or vulnerable to schizophrenia. *Journal of the American Academy of Child & Adolescent Psychiatry* 53 (8): 833–834. https://doi.org/10.1016/j.jaac.2014.04.019.

Schepp, K.G., O'Connor, F.W. & Kennedy, M. (2005). *Self-management therapy for youth with schizophrenia.* Final Report: Summary for NIMH Randomized Clinical Trial #R01-MH56580. Submitted to the National Institute of Mental Health of the National Institutes of Health, Bethesda, MD.

Schimmelmann, B.G., Walger, P., and Schultze-Lutter, F. (2013). The significance of at-risk symptoms for psychosis in children and adolescents. *Canadian Journal of Psychiatry* 58 (1): 32–40. https://doi.org/10.1177/070674371305800107.

Schneider, M., Debbane, M., Bassett, A.S. et al. (2014). Psychiatric disorders from childhood to adulthood in 22q11.2 deletion syndrome: results from the international consortium on brain and behavior in 22q11.2 deletion syndrome. *American Journal of Psychiatry* 171 (6): 627–639. https://doi.org/10.1176/appi.ajp.2013.13070864.

Shaffer, D., Gould, M.S., Brasic, J. et al. (1983). A children's global assessment scale (CGAS). *Archives of General Psychiatry* 40: 1228–1231.

Shaffer, D., Fisher, P., Lucas, C.P. et al. (2000). NIMH diagnostic interview schedule for children version IV (NIMH DISC-IV): description, differences from previous versions, and reliability of some common diagnoses. *Journal of the American Academy of Child & Adolescent Psychiatry* 39 (1): 28–38.

Shioiri, T., Shinada, K., Kuwabara, H., and Someya, T. (2007). Early prodromal symptoms and diagnoses before first psychotic episode in 219 inpatients with schizophrenia. *Psychiatry and Clinical Neurosciences* 61: 348–354.

Starling, J., Williams, L.M., Hainsworth, C., and Harris, A.W. (2013). The presentation of early-onset psychotic disorders. *Australian and New Zealand Journal of Psychiatry* 47 (1): 43–50. https://doi.org/10.1177/0004867412463615.

Stentebjerg-Olesen, M., Pagsberg, A.K., Fink-Jensen, A. et al. (2016). Clinical characteristics and predictors of outcome of schizophrenia-spectrum psychosis in children and adolescents: a systematic review. *Journal of Child and Adolescent Psychopharmacology* 26 (5): 410–427. https://doi.org/10.1089/cap.2015.0097.

Werry, J.S., McClellan, J.M., and Chard, L. (1991). Childhood and adolescent schizophrenic, bipolar and schizoaffective disorders: a clinical and outcome study. *Journal of the American Academy of Child and Adolescent Psychiatry* 30: 457–465.

White, T., Andreasen, N.C., Nopoulos, P., and Magnotta, V. (2003). Gyrification abnormalities in childhood- and adolescent-onset schizophrenia. *Biological Psychiatry* 54 (4): 418–426.

White, T., Anjum, A., and Schulz, S.C. (2006). The schizophrenia prodrome. *American Journal of Psychiatry* 163: 376–380.

Whitmore, K.E. (2017). The concept of respite care. *Nursing Forum* 52 (3): 180–187. https://doi.org/10.1111/nuf.12179.

Woodberry, K.A., Shapiro, D.I., Bryant, C., and Seidman, L.J. (2016). Progress and future directions in research on the psychosis prodrome: a review for clinicians. *Harvard Review of Psychiatry* 24 (2): 87–103. https://doi.org/10.1097/hrp.0000000000000109.

Xia, J., Merinder, L.B., and Belgamwar, M.R. (2011). Psychoeducation for schizophrenia. *The Cochrane Database of Systematic Reviews* (6): CD002831-CD002831. https://doi.org/10.1002/14651858.CD002831.pub2.

Zhang, C., Wang, Q., Ni, P. et al. (2017). Differential cortical gray matter deficits in adolescent- and adult-onset first-episode treatment-naïve patients with schizophrenia. *Scientific Reports* 7 (1): 10267. https://doi.org/10.1038/s41598-017-10688-1.

Zhao, S., Sampson, S., Xia, J., and Jayaram, M.B. (2015). Psychoeducation (brief) for people with serious mental illness. *Cochrane Database of Systematic Reviews* (4): Cd010823. https://doi.org/10.1002/14651858.CD010823.pub2.

15

Feeding and Eating Disorders in Children and Adolescents

Janiece E. DeSocio[1] and Joan B. Riley[2]

[1] Seattle University College of Nursing, Seattle, WA, USA
[2] Georgetown University School of Nursing & Health Sciences, Washington, DC, USA

Objectives

After reading this chapter, advanced practice registered nurses will be able to:

1. Identify the signs, symptoms, medical complications, psychiatric comorbidities, and developmental differences associated with anorexia nervosa, bulimia nervosa, binge eating disorder, and avoidant/restrictive food intake disorder in children and adolescents.
2. Discuss theories of etiology associated with feeding and eating disorders, including neurobiological, genetic, family dynamics, and psychosocial factors.
3. Describe evidence-based interventions for children and adolescents diagnosed with feeding and eating disorders.
4. Differentiate roles of primary care practitioners and advanced practice psychiatric mental health nurses in the diagnosis and treatment of children and adolescents with feeding and eating disorders.

Introduction

Results from the National Institute of Mental Health National Comorbidity Study Replication (NIMH-NCSR) indicate that the majority of individuals with eating disorders do not receive treatment, supporting the need for increased screening in primary care (Hudson et al. 2007). Advanced practice registered nurses (APRNs) working with children, adolescents, and young adults in any setting should (i) provide education about eating disorders to patients and families, (ii) screen for signs and symptoms of eating disorders to promote early identification, (iii) partner with patients and parents to enhance motivation and cooperation for treatment, (iv) treat medical complications, (v) restore patients to a healthy weight, (vi) correct maladaptive thoughts, attitudes, and feelings related to food and body image, (vii) improve self-esteem, (viii) enhance and utilize family support, (ix) treat associated and comorbid psychiatric conditions, and (x) prevent relapse or recurrence. An objective proposed for Healthy People 2020 is "to reduce the proportion of adolescents who engage in disordered eating in an attempt to control their weight" (US Department of Health and Human Services 2009). Reducing the health consequences of eating disorders is an essential goal for all health professionals.

Child and Adolescent Behavioral Health: A Resource for Advanced Practice Psychiatric and Primary Care Practitioners in Nursing, Second Edition. Edited by Edilma L. Yearwood, Geraldine S. Pearson, and Jamesetta A. Newland.
© 2021 John Wiley & Sons, Inc. Published 2021 by John Wiley & Sons, Inc.
Companion website: www.wiley.com/go/Yearwood

This chapter provides a framework for the recognition and treatment of four feeding and eating disorder subtypes that occur during childhood and adolescence: anorexia nervosa (AN), bulimia nervosa (BN), binge eating disorder (BED), and avoidant/restrictive food intake disorder (ARFID).

Statistics and Prevalence

Eating disorders are chronic disorders that begin in childhood or adolescence and typically continue into adulthood. The peak onset for eating disorders is between ages 16 and 20 years (Pearson et al. 2017). AN has a bimodal peak of onset at ages 13 and 18. Trends show eating disorders are increasing among younger children, males, and youth from minority populations (Campbell and Peebles 2014). There is a 13-month or longer delay in diagnosing eating disorders in children aged 7 to 10 years; twice as long as the delay in diagnosing these disorders after age 11 (Peebles et al. 2006).

The NIMH-NCSR Adolescent Supplement (NCS-A) identified the lifetime prevalence of eating disorders in adolescents as 2.7%. They occur more often in females (3.8% lifetime prevalence) than in males (1.5% lifetime prevalence) (Merikangas et al. 2010). The lifetime prevalence of AN ranges from 0.5% to 2% and the lifetime prevalence for BN ranges from 0.9% to 3% (Campbell and Peebles 2014). Subthreshold or partial syndromes, defined as falling short of meeting one or more criteria for a diagnosis of AN, have been identified in 1.3–3.7% of the population (Bulik et al. 2005). BED occurs in approximately 3% of the population and rates of binge eating increase 25% from middle to late adolescence (Hoek and van Hoeken 2003; Pearson et al. 2017).

Prevalence rates for eating disorder diagnoses do not fully represent the extent of body image concerns and patterns of disordered eating that occur during adolescence. Over 25% of middle-school and high-school age girls and 17% of boys report severe dissatisfaction with their bodies (Ackard et al. 2007). Approximately 50% of girls report dieting in the past year, 30% of girls and 15% of boys require medical attention for problems related to disordered eating, and 9% of girls report daily purging to lose weight (Campbell and Peebles 2014). At the other end of the spectrum, loss of control eating occurs in approximately 25% of adolescents and is associated with an increased risk for BED, overweight or obesity, and depression (Schlüter et al. 2016).

Historical and Cultural Perspective

The documented history of eating disorders begins in the Middle Ages with accounts of early saints and martyrs who engaged in starvation and purging as expressions of asceticism. Sir William Gull is credited with the first use of the term "anorexia nervosa" to describe a condition of starvation in adolescent girls in 1874, and Gerald Russell introduced the term "bulimia nervosa" to describe a purging variant of this condition in 1979 (Gull 1874; Halmi 2007; Madden 2004; Russell 1979).

In the 1970s and 1980s, attention was drawn to the dangers and potential deadly consequences of AN by the death of a popular singer, Karen Carpenter. This attention has continued as more athletes and celebrities disclose their personal struggles with these disorders. Unfortunately, the myth that eating disorders are trendy, media-driven conditions of white, affluent young women continues despite evidence that they are serious brain disorders with life-threatening complications affecting males and females from all racial and ethnic groups and socioeconomic backgrounds (Sonneville and Lipson 2018).

Beliefs about the rarity of eating disorders in non-Westernized countries have been dispelled by research. Keel and Klump (2003) found evidence of AN in all non-Western regions of the world, including Africa, the Middle East, India, Southeast Asia, and East Asia. Economic growth and global influences are believed to affect the recognition and reporting of eating disorders in Asian and Middle Eastern countries (Pike et al. 2014). Other factors affecting the differential reporting of eating disorders include longstanding cultural attitudes toward mental disorders in general. Stigma and lack of acceptance of mental disorders contribute to underdiagnosis and treatment avoidance in the United States and internationally. Internalization of stigma affects the self-view of individuals with eating disorders, contributing to secrecy, denial of symptoms, and feelings of alienation that reduce help-seeking behaviors (Griffiths et al. 2018). Myths about who is affected by eating disorders also impact the attitudes and practice of health providers, who may overlook symptoms in patients that do not fit the social stereotype (Sonneville and Lipson 2018). In 2015, an international effort to combat stigma was undertaken by the Academy of Eating Disorders (AED) with the publication of *Nine Truths about Eating Disorders* in 30 different languages. AED describes this publication as "a guiding document to accelerate global dissemination of accurate and evidence-informed information about eating disorders" (Schaumberg et al. 2017, p. 432). In 2018, the National Institutes of Health listed over 140 active and/or currently recruiting eating disorder research studies, an indication of the growing national and international interest in response to calls for research in this field (www.clinicaltrials.gov).

Course of Illness, Remission, and Recovery

The typical course of eating disorders is marked by periods of symptom remission and exacerbation. The cognitive symptoms (e.g. obsessions about food, distorted body perceptions, obsessive drive for exercise, and fears of weight gain) usually precede the onset of restricting, binging, and/or purging, and these cognitive symptoms are typically the last to remit. Time to remission depends on the severity of symptoms at onset of treatment and the type, duration, and degree of adherence to treatment. Milder eating disorder symptoms often first appear during childhood or early adolescence and progress to more severe symptoms over time. Symptoms that persist for 10–15 years predict a chronic, disabling course with higher rates of mortality (Treasure et al. 2015). Prevention and early intervention are essential to reduce the lifetime burden of these disorders.

With effective treatment, episodes of restricting, binging, and purging generally remit within 8–12 months (Clausen 2004; Couturier and Lock 2006; Strober et al. 1997). Research has identified the median time to full physical and cognitive/psychological remission to be shorter for patients with BN, averaging 11–26 months, while time to full remission for patients with AN can require up to 6 years (Clausen 2004).

Long-term follow-up of patients with AN reveals that approximately 50% achieve recovery, 30% improve but retain residual symptoms, and 20% persist on a chronic and disabling course. Findings for adolescents who receive treatment early in the course of illness are more optimistic, with as many as 75% achieving recovery at 10–15-year follow-up (Herzog and Eddy 2007; Yilmaz et al. 2015).

The most vulnerable time for eating disorder relapse occurs within the first 3–18 months after discharge from treatment. Relapse rates are as high as 35–50% for patients with AN (Berends et al. 2016; Khalsa et al. 2017). For AN, relapse is defined as weight loss to 85% or less of ideal body weight and return of cognitive and psychological symptoms (Khalsa et al. 2017). Relapse prevention programs that support individuals with eating disorders beyond completion of intensive treatment can reduce rates of relapse. For example, individuals with AN who were followed in a relapse prevention program for 18 months after treatment demonstrated significantly lower rates of relapse, with approximately 11% experiencing full relapse, 19% partial relapse, and 70% no relapse (Berends et al. 2016). Risk factors associated with relapse include failure to achieve symptom remission, lower body mass index (BMI) and greater caloric restriction at the onset of treatment, resistance to nutritional compliance, and persistence of self-evaluations focused on body size and shape (McFarlane et al. 2008). In a study of adolescents aged 11–19 years who achieved weight restoration, approximately 25% required readmission to the hospital within 12 months while 75% did not. Factors that increased the risk for hospital readmission included diagnosis prior to age 15, a lower rate of weight gain, and greater disturbances in eating attitudes (Castro et al. 2004). Evidence points to the importance of full weight restoration as a minimum requirement for extended periods of remission and recovery.

The mortality rate for individuals with AN is six times higher than for the general population and is among the highest mortality rates of all mental disorders (Smink et al. 2013; Yilmaz et al. 2015). Mortality rates for BN are not significantly different from rates in the general population (Berkman et al. 2007; Sokol et al. 2005). Factors associated with mortality risk include very low body weight, multiple hospital admissions, use of alcohol and substances, psychiatric comorbidities, and history of suicidal behaviors (Berkman et al. 2007). Cardiac failure and suicide are the most common causes of death, with one in five deaths attributed to suicide (Herzog and Eddy 2007; Smink et al. 2013).

Etiology

Genetic and Neurobiological Factors

Genetic and biological factors have assumed prominence in explaining the etiology of eating disorders. Twin studies estimate the heritability of these disorders to be approximately 40% for BED, 60% for BN, and 50–84% for AN (Boraska et al. 2014; Yilmaz et al. 2015). Female relatives of individuals with AN have an 11 times greater risk of developing AN than relatives of normal controls, and the risk of developing BN is four times greater among relatives of individuals with BN (Strober et al. 2000; Yilmaz et al. 2015).

Similar to large genome-wide studies of other major mental disorders, researchers have not found single genes that predispose individuals to eating disorders but rather a combination of multiple genes and polymorphisms likely to interact to increase risk (Brandys et al. 2015). The Genetic Consortium on Anorexia Nervosa (GCAN) is a large international research collaboration involved in genome-wide association studies (GWAS) of AN. GCAN has analyzed DNA samples from almost 3000 individuals across 14 countries. Variants of the SOX2OT and PPP3CA genes have shown promise in GWAS studies (Boraska et al. 2014). Other analyses have identified potential genetic variants of EBF1, a gene involved in development of adipocytes and regulation of leptin (Li et al. 2017).

Genetic studies also point to polymorphisms in serotonin (5-hydroxytryptamine, 5-HT) genes and brain-derived neurotrophic factors in individuals with eating disorders (Gamero-Villarroel et al. 2014; Klump et al. 2009). Serotonin is a major neurotransmitter involved in regulation of feeding, appetite, sleep, mood, and anxiety. Abnormalities in 5-HT receptors and a reduction in cerebrospinal fluid concentrations of 5-HT metabolites have been reported in AN. Brain-imaging studies of individuals with AN have identified reduced 5-HT2A receptor activity in the anterior cingulate, amygdala, temporal lobes, parietal lobes, and occipital region of the brain (Kaye et al. 2005).

Having one or two short alleles of the serotonin transporter gene (SLC6A4) has been described as a "vulnerable genotype" for a variety of psychiatric disorders, including major depressive disorder, bipolar disorder, panic disorder, obsessive compulsive disorder, and AN (Chen et al. 2015). Rozenblat et al. (2017) reported a significant gene-by-environment interaction in risk for eating disorders for individuals with short alleles of the promoter region (5HTTLPR) of SLC6A4 who also had histories of abuse. These authors concluded, "individuals with the risky (short-allele) genotype may be relatively resilient to low levels of environmental risk, but disproportionately affected by greater environmental adversity" (Rozenblat et al. 2017, p. 11).

Altered dopamine activity in the reward circuits of the brain has also been studied in relationship to AN (Bailer et al. 2017; Frank et al. 2005; Wagner et al. 2007). Findings implicating dopamine dysregulation include an increase in dopamine receptor binding in the striatum and a reduction in dopamine metabolites in the cerebral spinal fluid of individuals with AN. The dopamine circuits in the ventral tegmental area are associated with experiences of pleasure and reward-seeking behaviors. Modulation of pleasure seeking is achieved through top-down control exerted by the prefrontal cortex and mediated through the anterior cingulate cortex. Abnormalities in dopamine regulation and increased activation of top-down control may contribute to inhibition in pleasure seeking, increased focus on harm avoidance, and greater anxious anticipation of negative consequences in individuals with AN (Bailer et al. 2017; Frank et al. 2005; Wagner et al. 2007).

Rejection sensitivity is a trait involving attentional bias toward negative social cues and has been identified in individuals with AN and BN. In a study that exposed individuals to accepting human faces and rejecting human faces, individuals with AN and BN displayed difficulty disengaging from images of rejecting faces while disregarding accepting faces (Cardi et al. 2012).

Neuropsychological differences in individuals with AN have led to theories about brain differences that affect the processing of visual–spatial information. In response to various figure-ground tests, individuals with AN show a bias toward details and deficits in perceiving global patterns. This neurocognitive deficit is referred to as "weak central coherence" and has also been observed in individuals with obsessive compulsive disorder (OCD) and autism spectrum disorders. Additionally, individuals with AN display deficits in cognitive set shifting, which is associated with inflexibility, difficulty disengaging from tasks, and problems with transitions (Lang et al. 2016; Lopez et al. 2008; Treasure 2007).

Alexithymia is the inability to name and describe feelings and is a characteristic identified in individuals with AN (Schmelkin et al. 2017). The insula is a brain structure associated with interoceptive awareness and the ability to interpret physiological and emotional cues arising from the body. Neuroimaging studies have shown altered neuronal connections between the insula and brain regions associated with emotional expression (Strigo et al. 2013). Alexithymia has also been linked to lower levels of the neurohormone oxytocin. Oxytocin is a hormone involved in social bonding; increased oxytocin promotes social and emotional engagement with others. Lower levels of oxytocin have been identified in individuals recovered from AN compared to healthy controls (Schmelkin et al. 2017).

Biological Triggers

Estrogen plays a role in modulating serotonin activity. Serotonin receptor activity and serotonin gene transcription are influenced by estrogen. Changes in estrogen and gonadal hormones during puberty have been linked to the onset of binge eating and other eating disorder symptoms in genetically vulnerable individuals (Kaye et al. 2005; Klump and Gobrogge 2005; Klump et al. 2017).

Streptococcal infections are biological triggers that have been studied in relationship to acute onset AN and ARFID. Group A streptococcal infections are one of multiple sources of pediatric acute neuropsychiatric syndromes (PANS) that affect prepubertal age children. When the source of PANS is linked to a streptococcal infection, it is referred to as pediatric autoimmune neuropsychiatric disorder associated with streptococcal infection (PANDAS). PANDAS is characterized by sudden symptom onset within days of a strep infection or exposure, and can include obsessive fears of choking or swallowing, compulsive behaviors, motor tics, stereotypical movements, heightened sensory sensitivity, and acute food refusal. The theorized pathophysiology of PANDAS involves strep antibodies crossing the blood–brain barrier and establishing an inflammatory response in the dorsal striatum of the brain. A diagnosis of

PANDAS is based on a positive history of strep infection or positive strep culture and/or elevated anti-DNase B and antistreptolysin O (ASO) titers. Treatment includes antibiotics for active strep infections and immunomodulatory therapies such as intravenous immunoglobulin (Puxley et al. 2008; Toufexis et al. 2015).

Significant weight loss from any source, including energy-deficient exercise or weight loss secondary to acute illness, can trigger the onset of anorexia and restrictive eating. Leptin is a neuroendocrine hormone released by adipocytes that regulates energy and food intake (Blüher and Mantzoros 2004; Müller et al. 2009). Leptin signals the hypothalamus about the state of the body's fat stores. Weight loss in AN is associated with decreased levels of leptin, thyroid hormone, and gonadotropins and increased levels of adrenocorticotropic hormone and cortisol. According to Müller et al. (2009), hypoleptinemia is an important marker of the severity of AN and the extent to which an individual is progressing toward starvation. Research has linked AN to dysregulation of multiple neuroendocrine axes, including the hypothalamic–pituitary-thyroid axis, the hypothalamic–pituitary-gonadal axis, and the hypothalamic–pituitary–adrenal axis. Evidence points to leptin as a "master hormone" involved in the regulation of these neuroendocrine systems (Blüher and Mantzoros 2004, p. 2472S).

Restricting access to food and increasing access to a running wheel in laboratory animals can result in a state of activity-based anorexia. Dieting and physical exercise activate dopamine neurons in the mesolimbic pathway and noradrenergic neurons in the locus coeruleus, inducing a focused state that perpetuates the drive to exercise and suppresses food seeking (Herzog and Eddy 2007; Hillebrand et al. 2005; McCormick et al. 2008; Sodersten et al. 2003).

Psychosocial Triggers

Psychosocial factors interact with genetic and biological vulnerability to increase the risk for eating disorder onset and/or relapse. Certain personality phenotypes are associated with an increased risk for eating disorders, including American Psychiatric Association *Diagnostic and Statistical Manual of Mental Disorders*, 5th edition (DSM-5; American Psychiatric Association [APA] 2013) Cluster C personality traits of perfectionism, harm avoidance, and cognitive inflexibility (DeSocio 2013). For individuals with these personality traits, change and transitions can be stressful. Certain developmental periods are recognized as times of exceptional change, including the transition from elementary school to middle school, the onset of puberty, entry into high school, and launching into independent living during late adolescence and early adulthood. These developmental transitions coincide with peak periods for the onset and relapse of eating disorder symptoms.

Adolescence is second only to infancy in its rapid rate of physical growth and change. Body image concerns are common during adolescence, with as many as 36% of girls and 24% of boys reporting that body image is very important to their self-esteem (Ackard et al. 2007). Participation in activities such as dance, gymnastics, and competitive sports accentuates the focus on physical attributes, and may magnify body image concerns for vulnerable adolescents. Dissatisfaction with body image can result in dieting and engaging in energy-deficient exercise, both of which are potential triggers for individuals who are genetically predisposed to eating disorders (DeSocio 2013).

Being the victim of peer bullying, including cyber bullying, is distressing for all children and adolescents and increases risk for anxiety, depression, self-harm, and suicidality (Arseneault 2018). Peer bullying can be especially traumatic for children with heightened rejection sensitivity, a trait associated with eating disorder risk. For rejection-sensitive children and adolescents, peer bullying related to body size, shape or appearance can amplify the influence of body image on self-esteem and increase preoccupation with behaviors to avoid weight gain. Copeland et al. (2015) identified peer bullying as a predictor of anorexic and bulimic symptoms in adolescents.

Social stigma, victimization, and harassment have been linked to high rates of disordered eating among lesbian, gay, bisexual, transgender, and questioning (LGBTQ) youth. Watson et al. (2017) researched disordered eating among transgender youth and found almost 50% of transgender youth ages 14–18 engaged in disordered eating behaviors, including fasting and purging to control weight. Supportive relationships with parents and peers and positive connections at school are protective factors that reduce risk for eating disorder symptoms in transgender youth (Watson et al. 2017).

Analysis of data from over 36 000 adults in the National Epidemiologic Survey on Alcohol and Related Conditions (NESARC-III) revealed the significant impact of early abuse and neglect on eating disorder risk. Researchers identified gender differences, with sexual abuse and physical neglect having the strongest relationship to eating disorder risk in men, and sexual abuse and emotional abuse having the strongest relationship to eating disorder risk in women (Afifi et al. 2017).

Family Dynamics

Family adversity, including childhood exposure to trauma and maltreatment, has been cited as a factor contributing to the risk for eating disorders (Afifi et al. 2017). Family environments with low emotional connectedness, high parental expectations, and high parental discord have also been described in the eating disorder literature (Gorwood et al. 2003; Tantillo 2006).

The study of family environments in children and adolescents with eating disorders must consider the amount of stress induced by having a child or adolescent with an eating disorder and the potential impact this disorder can exert on marital, parental, and family systems. The heritability of these disorders increases the likelihood that one or both parents may be affected or partially affected by an eating disorder, an anxiety or mood disorder, or personality traits that fall within the spectrum of shared genetic risk. A no-blame approach recognizes that "parents do not cause eating disorders and children do not choose them" (Kartini Clinic n.d., para. 3). Families may be affected by the genetic transmission of these disorders, but this is not something parents or children willfully choose to inflict on each other. Anxious parents may be more likely to engage in counterproductive struggles over food with their children, just as anxious children may induce greater vigilance from their parents. Thus, the interactions between genetics, temperament, family dynamics, and eating disorder symptoms may be best understood as complex and multidirectional processes.

Other Risk Factors

Individuals identified at higher risk for developing eating disorders include LGBTQ youth (Watson et al. 2017), female college students (Barker and Galambos 2007), college athletes (Greenleaf et al. 2009), young women with type 1 diabetes mellitus (Walsh et al. 2000), and participants in activities that promote low body weight such as dance, wrestling, and crew. Sports that are evaluated by subjective scoring such as skating and gymnastics are also associated with a higher incidence of eating disorders.

Clinical Picture

Diagnostic Criteria

DSM-5 (APA 2013) includes several diagnoses within the Feeding and Eating Disorders classification. Among these diagnoses are ARFID, AN and its subtypes, BN, and BED. The diagnostic criteria for each of these diagnoses are found in Tables 15.1–15.4.

In differentiating bulimia nervosa from anorexia nervosa, it is important to determine the individual's premorbid weight. A child or adolescent who is of high body weight prior to the onset of eating disorder symptoms can present with normal or even above normal body weight, but upon further examination a history of nutritional restriction and dramatic weight loss may be detected. In these cases, a diagnosis of AN is appropriate even though current weight may not be abnormally low.

Developmental Variations in Symptom Presentations

The age of onset for eating disorder symptoms spans multiple developmental stages from school age through young adulthood. With symptoms emerging as young as age 7 years, it is not surprising to find developmental differences in symptom presentation among individuals of different ages.

Table 15.1 Avoidant/restrictive food intake disorder

Diagnostic Criteria	307.59 (F50.8)

A. An eating or feeding disturbance (e.g., apparent lack of interest in eating or food; avoidance based on the sensory characteristics of food; concern about aversive consequences of eating) as manifested by persistent failure to meet appropriate nutritional and/or energy needs associated with one (or more) of the following:

1. Significant weight loss (or failure to achieve expected weight gain or faltering growth in children).
2. Significant nutritional deficiency.
3. Dependence on enteral feeding or oral nutritional supplements.
4. Marked interference with psychosocial functioning.

B. The disturbance is not better explained by lack of available food or by an associated culturally sanctioned practice.
C. The eating disturbance does not occur exclusively during the course of anorexia nervosa or bulimia nervosa, and there is no evidence of a disturbance in the way in which one's body weight or shape is experienced.
D. The eating disturbance is not attributable to a concurrent medical condition or not better explained by another mental disorder. When the eating disturbance occurs in the context of another condition or disorder, the severity of the eating disturbance exceeds that routinely associated with the condition or disorder and warrants additional clinical attention.

Specify if:
In remission: After full criteria for avoidant/restrictive food intake disorder were previously met, the criteria have not been met for a sustained period of time.

Source: From Diagnostic and Statistical Manual of Mental Disorders, 5th edition, p. 334, by American Psychiatric Association, 2013, Arlington, VA: American Psychiatric Publishing. © 2013, American Psychiatric Association. Reprinted with permission.

Table 15.2 Anorexia nervosa

Diagnostic Criteria

A. Restriction of energy intake relative to requirements, leading to a significantly low body weight in the context of age, sex, developmental trajectory, and physical health. *Significantly low weight* is defined as a weight that is less than minimally normal or, for children and adolescents, less than that minimally expected.
B. Intense fear of gaining weight or of becoming fat, or persistent behavior that interferes with weight gain, even though at a significantly low weight.
C. Disturbance in the way in which one's body weight or shape is experienced, undue influence of body weight or shape on self-evaluation, or persistent lack of recognition of the seriousness of the current low body weight.

Coding note: The ICD-9-CM code for anorexia nervosa is 307.1, which is assigned regardless of the subtype. The ICD-10-CM code depends on the subtype (see below).

Specify whether:
   (F50.01) Restricting type: During the last 3 months, the individual has not engaged in recurrent episodes of binge eating or purging behavior (i.e., self-induced vomiting or the misuse of laxatives diuretics, or enemas). This subtype describes presentations in which weight loss is accomplished primarily through dieting, fasting, and/or excessive exercise.
   (F50.02) Binge-eating/purging type: During the last 3 months, the individual has engaged in recurrent episodes of binge eating or purging behavior (i.e., self-induced vomiting or the misuse of laxatives, diuretics, or enemas).

Specify if:
   In partial remission: After full criteria or anorexia nervosa were previously met Criterion A (low body weight) has not been met for a sustained period, but either Criterion B (intense fear of gaining weight or becoming fat or behavior that interferes with weight gain) or Criterion C (disturbances in self-perception of weight and shape) is still met.
   In full remission: After full criteria for anorexia nervosa were previously met, none of the criteria have been met for a sustained period of time.

Specify current severity:
The minimum level of severity is based, for adults, on current body mass index (BMI) (see below) or, for children and adolescents, on BMI percentile. The ranges below are derived from World Health Organization categories for thinness in adults; for children and adolescents, corresponding BMI percentiles should be used. The level of severity may be increased to reflect clinical symptoms, the degree of functional disability, and the need for supervision.
   Mild: BMI $\geq 17\,kg/m^2$
   Moderate: BMI $16–16.99\,kg/m^2$
   Severe: BMI $15–15.99\,kg/m^2$
   Extreme: BMI $< 15\,kg/m^2$

Source: From Diagnostic and Statistical Manual of Mental Disorders, 5th edition, p. 338–339, by American Psychiatric Association, 2013, Arlington, VA: American Psychiatric Publishing. © 2013, American Psychiatric Association. Reprinted with permission.

Symptoms of eating disorders in children are more likely to evade recognition or be misdiagnosed. This is particularly troubling because of the severe impact an eating disorder can have on organ development and bone growth. Prepubertal children may be less likely to verbalize fears of gaining weight or body dissatisfaction. Children and young adolescents are more likely to endorse fears of growing up or aversion to puberty, increased anxiety preceding and during mealtime, and exhibit relentless motor activity. Children and young adolescents can experience a faster rate of weight loss than older adolescents and progress more rapidly into states of medical compromise. Routine monitoring of growth curves is essential to detect early evidence of weight loss that first alters the child's weight curve and, if not interrupted, affects the child's height and can result in growth stunting (Abbate-Daga et al. 2007; Keel et al. 2004; Peebles et al. 2006).

Medical Complications

The medical complications of eating disorders affect every body system and have the greatest impact on health and quality of life when symptoms persist during normative periods of skeletal growth and organ development. All body systems are impacted, especially as the eating disorder becomes more severe and chronic (Westmoreland et al. 2016). Most medical complications arise from unhealthy weight-control behaviors and the physiologic response to malnutrition (Fairburn and Harrison 2003; Golden et al. 2016). Irreversible growth stunting is one of the most emotionally and physically devastating consequences of eating disorders (Fairburn and Harrison 2003; Katzman 2005; Rome and Ammerman 2003; Wolfe et al. 2016). A summary of medical complications can be found in Table 15.5.

Table 15.3 Bulimia nervosa

Diagnostic Criteria	307.51 (F50.2)

A. Recurrent episodes of binge eating. An episode of binge eating is characterized by both of the following:
  1. Eating, in a discrete period of time (e.g., within any 2-hour period), an amount of food that is definitely larger than what most individuals would eat in a similar period of time under similar circumstances.
  2. A sense of lack of control over eating during the episode (e.g. a feeling that one cannot stop eating or control what or how much one is eating).
B. Recurrent inappropriate compensatory behaviors in order to prevent weight gain, such as self-induced vomiting; misuse of laxatives, diuretics, or other medications; fasting; or excessive exercise.
C. The binge eating and inappropriate compensatory behaviors both occur, on average, at least once a week for 3 months.
D. Self-evaluation is unduly influenced by body shape and weight.
E. The disturbance does not occur exclusively during episodes of anorexia nervosa.

Specify if:
  In partial remission: After full criteria for bulimia nervosa were previously met, some, but not all, of the criteria have been met for a sustained period of time.
  In full remission: After full criteria for bulimia nervosa were previously met, none of the criteria have been met for a sustained period of time.

Specify current severity:
The minimum level of severity is based on the frequency of inappropriate compensatory behaviors (see below). The level of severity may be increased to reflect other symptoms and the degree of functional disability.
  Mild: An average of 1–3 episodes of inappropriate compensatory behaviors per week.
  Moderate: An average of 4–7 episodes of inappropriate compensatory behaviors per week.
  Severe: An average of 8–13 episodes of inappropriate compensatory behaviors per week.
  Extreme: An average of 14 or more episodes of inappropriate compensatory behaviors per week.

Source: From Diagnostic and Statistical Manual of Mental Disorders, 5th edition, p. 345, by American Psychiatric Association, 2013, Arlington, VA: American Psychiatric Publishing. © 2013, American Psychiatric Association. Reprinted with permission.

Ongoing medical assessment and monitoring are essential to early recognition and management of the complications of eating disorders as most are reversible with early effective treatment (Westmoreland et al. 2016). Potentially irreversible medical complications in children and adolescents include growth retardation if the disorder occurs before closure of the epiphyseal plates, loss of dental enamel due to chronic vomiting, pubertal delay or arrest, impaired acquisition of peak bone mass predisposing to osteopenia or osteoporosis (Golden et al. 2003), and myocarditis associated with chronic ipecac use (Rome 2015). Preventing these serious complications requires aggressive monitoring and treatment, and information sharing with the patient and parents to empower the family (Katzman et al. 2013).

Cardiovascular complications are among the most serious medical complications of eating disorders. These occur in up to 80% of patients with AN and account for up to 30% of mortality (Spaulding-Barclay et al. 2016). Cardiac involvement is present in the early stages of the disorder in adolescents with AN with both functional and structural cardiac abnormalities that can be reversible with early identification and treatment

(Katzman 2005). Cardiovascular complications can result from cardiac muscle wasting secondary to starvation and cardiac conduction abnormalities related to electrolyte disturbances in purging. Intractable vomiting can induce metabolic alkalosis and hypokalemia, and misuse of laxatives or water loading can result in hyponatremia and metabolic acidosis (Fairburn and Harrison 2003). Orthostatic blood pressure changes and bradycardia (daytime heart rate under 50 beats per minute or nighttime heart rate under 46 beats per minute) can be detected during physical examination in 35–95% of adolescents with AN (Katzman 2005). Orthostasis and bradycardia are the result of decreased basal metabolic rate, increased vagal tone, and reduced cardiac contractile force and output (Katzman et al.2013). Abnormal electrocardiogram (ECG) findings can include QTc prolongation, ST depression, and flattening of the T wave. QTc prolongation is commonly thought to be the primary cause of sudden death but evidence indicates that QTc prolongation is uncommon in the absence of contributing factors such as concurrent QTc prolonging medications and depletion of serum potassium and

Table 15.4 Binge-eating disorder

Diagnostic Criteria	307.51 (F50.8)

A. Recurrent episodes of binge eating. An episode of binge eating is characterized by both of the following:
   1. Eating, in a discrete period of time (e.g. within any 2-hour period), an amount of food that is definitely larger than what most people would eat in a similar period of time under similar circumstances.
   2. A sense of lack of control over eating during the episode (e.g. a feeling that one cannot stop eating or control what or how much one is eating).
B. The binge-eating episodes are associated with three (or more) of the following:
   1. Eating much more rapidly than normal.
   2. Eating until feeling uncomfortably full.
   3. Eating large amounts of food when not feeling physically hungry.
   4. Eating alone because of feeling embarrassed by how much one is eating.
   5. Feeling disgusted with oneself, depressed, or very guilty afterward.
C. Marked distress regarding binge eating is present.
D. The binge eating occurs, on average, at least once a week for 3 months.
E. The binge eating is not associated with the recurrent use of inappropriate compensatory behavior as in bulimia nervosa and does not occur exclusively during the course of bulimia nervosa or anorexia nervosa.

Specify if:
   In partial remission: After full criteria for binge-eating disorder were previously met, binge eating occurs at an average frequency of less than one episode per week for a sustained period of time.
   In full remission: After full criteria for binge-eating disorder were previously met, none of the criteria have been met for a sustained period of time.
Specify current severity:
The minimum level of severity is based on the frequency of episodes of binge eating (see below). The level of severity may be increased to reflect other symptoms and the degree of functional disability.
   Mild: 1–3 binge-eating episodes per week.
   Moderate: 4–7 binge-eating episodes per week.
   Severe: 8–13 binge-eating episodes per week.
   Extreme: 14 or more binge-eating episodes per week.

Source: From Diagnostic and Statistical Manual of Mental Disorders, 5th edition, p. 350, by American Psychiatric Association, 2013, Arlington, VA: American Psychiatric Publishing. © 2013, American Psychiatric Association. Reprinted with permission.

magnesium levels (Krantz et al. 2012; Westmoreland et al. 2016). Mitral valve prolapse has been observed in over one-third of adolescents with AN compared to 4% of controls (Casiero and Frishman 2006; Spaulding-Barclay et al. 2016). The risk for cardiac events increases during refeeding of seriously malnourished patients and is the rationale for hospitalization, gradual titration of calories, and close monitoring of electrolytes and cardiac status. Congestive heart failure can occur due to shifts in fluids and electrolytes (especially phosphate) from extracellular to intracellular spaces during refeeding (Katzman 2005). Cardiac functioning is generally restored upon return to a healthy body weight but the extent to which optimal cardiac capacity is regained varies by severity of illness and the type and duration of symptoms. Research has begun to examine presentation and complications of male patients with eating disorders. Kalla et al. (2017) examined gender and age differences, and identified

that male patients with AN had significantly more cardiac arrests, arrhythmias, and heart failure than female patients with AN. More research needs to be done to examine gender and racial differences as we better understand the epidemiological profile of patients with eating disorders.

Complications affecting the gastrointestinal (GI) system include a slowing of GI motility with delayed gastric emptying and constipation (Mehler et al. 2015). These complications are the basis for common complaints about abdominal discomfort and distention following the reintroduction of food in patients with AN. Reassurance can be given that gastric motility usually returns to normal and constipation resolves within 3 weeks of resuming a balanced diet and ordered eating. Chronic misuse of laxatives may lead to persistent problems with constipation and altered GI functioning (Fairburn and Harrison 2003; Rome and Ammerman 2003).

Table 15.5 Complications of eating disorders

Musculoskeletal	Decrease in bone density, which can result in osteopenia/osteoporosis (Golden et al. 2015; Mehler et al. 2015); stress fractures (Rome 2015)
	Growth retardation (Rosen 2010)
Dermatologic	Dry skin (Rome 2015); easy bruising (Rosen 2010)
	Lanugo hair growth; loss of hair shine, volume or thickness (Rome 2015; Westmoreland et al. 2016)
	Purging can cause petechiae around eyes (Rome 2015); dental erosions; if using finger to cause vomiting may note Russell sign (Rosen 2010); parotitis (Rome 2015)
	Brittle nails (Williams et al. 2008)
Endocrine/ reproductive	Females: oligomenorrhea or amenorrhea (primary or secondary) (Rosen 2010) with low luteinizing hormone, follicle-stimulating hormone, estradiol (Fairburn and Harrison 2003; Westmoreland et al. 2016) Males: low levels of testosterone (Golden et al. 2015)
	Male and female hypogonadism (Westmoreland et al. 2016)
	Infertility (Williams et al. 2008)
	If pregnant, greater risk for hyperemesis gravidum, spontaneous abortion, and adverse neonatal outcomes such as low birth weight (Mehler et al. 2015)
	Low T_3 and T_4 thyroid hormones (Fairburn and Harrison 2003)
Neurological	Cognitive changes (Westmoreland et al. 2016)
	Cerebral atrophy (Rome 2015; Westmoreland et al. 2016) or enlarged cerebral ventricles (Fairburn and Harrison 2003; Williams et al. 2008)
Gastrointestinal	Constipation due to decreased motility and slow gastrointestinal transit time (Mehler et al. 2015)
	Cathartic colon due to laxative abuse (Mehler et al. 2015)
	Delayed gastric emptying causing fullness, bloating, and pain (Mehler et al. 2015)
	Acid-reflux in BN (Mehler et al. 2015)
	Superior mesenteric artery syndrome is rare and due to the loss of mesenteric fat pad between the superior mesenteric artery and aorta (Mehler et al. 2015)
	Hepatitis with elevated transaminases due to starvation (Mehler et al. 2015)
	Sialadenosis (Mehler et al. 2015)
Hematologic	Anemia: 16.7–39% (as cited in Hütter et al. 2009); 16.7% (as cited in De Filippo et al. 2016)
	Leukopenia: 29–39% (as cited in Hütter et al. 2009); 7.9% (as cited in De Filippo et al. 2016)
	Thrombocytopenia: 5–11% (as cited in Hütter et al. 2009); 8.9% (as cited in De Filippo et al. 2016)
Cardiovascular	Orthostatic hypotension and bradycardia
	Cardiac conduction abnormalities (Spaulding-Barclay et al. 2016)
	Myocarditis associated with ipecac toxicity (Rome 2015)
	Structural changes: reduction in left ventricular mass (Spaulding-Barclay et al. 2016); pericardial effusions (Rosen 2010; Spaulding-Barclay et al. 2016); myocardial fibrosis; mitral valve prolapse (Mehler et al. 2015; Spaulding-Barclay et al. 2016)
	Congestive heart failure
	Transient hypercholesterolemia (Fairburn and Harrison 2003; Rome 2015)
Metabolic	Hypokalemia and metabolic alkalosis from excessive purging (Mehler et al. 2015) and laxative abuse (Fairburn and Harrison 2003; Rome 2015)
	Dehydration (Rosen 2010)
	Edema formation in BN due to purging (Rosen 2010); peripheral edema (Williams et al. 2008)
Other	Insomnia (Assad et al. 2018).

Complications of the skeletal system and bone health include failure to achieve genetic height potential, osteopenia, and osteoporosis. Catch-up growth may occur if nutritional status is restored prior to the closure of epiphyseal plates (Mehler et al. 2015). Adolescence is the peak time for bone mineralization and consolidation of bone strength. AN can result in a reduction of bone mineral density and increase the lifetime risk for fractures. In AN, deficiencies in dietary calcium and vitamin D are compounded by low levels of thyroid hormones, estradiol, and testosterone that affect growth factors necessary for bone mineralization and prevention of bone reabsorption. Restoring nutritional health, normalizing reproductive hormones, and prescription of appropriate weight-bearing exercise may reverse the osteopenia and osteoporosis associated with AN (Golden et al. 2015). Male patients with AN have more severe osteoporosis then females with AN (Mehler et al. 2008). As many as one-third of women who recover from this disorder continue to have osteopenia of the lumbar spine (Katzman 2005; Rome and Ammerman 2003).

It is important for practitioners to realize that, unlike the situation with menopausal bone loss, exogenous hormones are not useful for bone restoration in this population and should not be used (Bulik et al. 2007). Hormone replacement therapy can cause growth arrest in the adolescent who has not yet completed growth (Frank 1995). When female adolescents have monthly withdrawal bleeding, this can be confusing and inappropriately seen as adequate weight to support normal menstruation (Golden et al. 2003).

The endocrine and reproductive systems are affected by eating disorders. Malnutrition results in low levels of testosterone in males and low levels of luteinizing hormone (LH), follicle-stimulating hormone (FSH), and estradiol in females, which contributes to oligomenorrhea and amenorrhea (Golden et al. 2015; Westmoreland et al. 2016). Evidence of higher rates of infertility, low birth weight infants, and other childbearing complications have been associated with eating disorders (Fairburn and Harrison 2003; Favaro et al. 2006).

Compromised brain health and altered cognitive functioning occur in states of malnutrition. Cerebral atrophy with ventricular enlargement and loss of both gray matter and white matter have been observed on brain scans of patients with AN (Rome and Ammerman 2003; Westmoreland et al. 2016). Evidence of altered cognitive functioning can be detected during the mental status examination and includes cognitive latencies, flat affect, lack of emotional spontaneity, poor memory recall, inattention, and decreased concentration. There is some uncertainty about the extent to which these brain changes can be reversed; the evidence is more optimistic if symptoms are effectively treated in children and adolescents, and less optimistic for adults who have a prolonged symptom course (Katzman 2005).

Possible hematological complications in children and adolescents with eating disorders include anemia, leukopenia, and less frequently thrombocytopenia. Using a sample of AN postpubertal female patients ($n = 318$), the hematologic complications were related to the duration of illness ($P = 0.028$) and degree of protein energy malnutrition ($P = 0.001$) (De Filippo et al. 2016). These findings report lower incidence of hematologic impairment than previous studies (Hütter et al. 2009) and will require further evaluation to understand the hematologic risks.

As we gain knowledge of the changing demographics of children and adolescents with eating disorders more research is needed. Efforts to understand the presentation, assessment, management, complications, and evidence-based care of disordered eating should target both males and females, and should be inclusive of patients of all racial and ethnic backgrounds. Findings reported by Lipson and Sonneville (2017) identify undergraduate students, sexual minority men, and students who are overweight or obese as populations at elevated risk for eating disorders. Further research is needed to understand the racial, ethnic, and gender differences in individuals with eating disorders. Are there new complications we are not aware to assess? What treatments are effective as we come to understanding the changing landscape? Stereotypes about who develops eating disorders could contribute to disparities in eating disorder treatment and outcomes (Sonneville and Lipson 2018).

Psychiatric Comorbidities

Lifetime rates of comorbid psychiatric disorders are as high as 80% in individuals with eating disorders (Anderluh et al. 2003; Kaye et al. 2004; Keel et al. 2005; Klump et al. 2009; Wade et al. 2000). Comorbid psychiatric diagnoses associated with AN include anxiety disorders, depression, and OCD (Slof-Op't Landt et al. 2016). Maladaptive perfectionism has also been identified as a personality trait associated with restrictive eating disorders (Lavender et al. 2016). In contrast, impulsivity is a personality trait commonly identified in individuals with BN and BED (Monell et al. 2018; Slof-Op't Landt et al. 2016).

Compared to the general population, higher rates of bipolar disorder and substance use disorders have been reported for individuals with BN and BED, and to a lesser extent for individuals with AN (Campos et al. 2013). Liu et al. (2016) studied a "subphenotype" of individuals with comorbid eating disorders and bipolar disorder, and characterized these individuals as having early exposures to trauma, early onset of mood symptoms, rapid mood cycling, higher rates of suicidality, and elevated rates of co-occurring anxiety disorders and eating disorders. These psychiatric comorbidities require careful evaluation by clinicians who may focus on one or the other diagnosis without recognizing symptoms that represent co-occurring disorders. When comorbid disorders remain undetected, treatment may be ineffective or, in the worst-case scenario, treatment of one disorder can destabilize the other (Campos et al. 2013).

In evaluating individuals with weight loss from any source, including individuals with AN, it is important to consider the impact of nutritional depletion on brain functioning and neurotransmitter synthesis. Tryptophan is an amino acid present in many foods and is the precursor of serotonin synthesis. Depletion of serotonin in states of malnutrition can induce a wide variety of psychiatric symptoms, including anxiety, depression, insomnia, and inattention. Before giving an anxiety or mood disorder diagnosis, it is important to evaluate the individual's nutritional state and determine if these symptoms preceded or followed the onset of weight loss. If anxiety, insomnia, and depressed mood occur secondary to nutritional depletion, weight restoration alone may improve or resolve the symptoms (Lindseth et al. 2015; O'Toole 2015).

Continuum of Care and Treatment

The continuum of care for eating disorder patients ranges from the least intensive care at a community outpatient level to the most intensive care in hospitals and residential treatment facilities. Outpatient treatment is often provided by physicians and APRNs collaborating with therapists, nutritionists, and medical specialists. Intermediate levels of care include day treatment and partial hospitalization programs. Consultation with eating disorder specialists can assist primary care practitioners (PCPs) in making decisions about the appropriate level of care for a patient. It is important for APRNs to know the criteria for various levels of care and develop a network of referral sources so that specialized evaluations and treatment can be readily initiated. The AED provides guidelines for the medical treatment of patients with eating disorders (AED 2016). A table of the APA's Level of Care Guidelines for Eating Disorders (APA 2010) is also available online (www.psychiatryonline.com).

Life-threatening medical complications or suicidal thoughts and behaviors necessitate hospitalization. Common complications requiring hospitalization include electrolyte disturbances, life-threatening arrhythmias, orthostatic hypotension, bradycardia, hypothermia, intractable vomiting, risk of refeeding complications, and

suicidal ideations (Harrington et al. 2015). Acute food refusal can be a rationale for hospitalization, especially in children and young adolescents, who are at greater risk for irreversible effects on growth (Yager et al. 2006).

Medically compromised patients who meet hospitalization criteria (American Academy of Pediatrics 2003; Campbell and Peebles 2014) are best managed by an eating disorder specialist with experience in safely initiating and monitoring the refeeding process. For severely malnourished patients who are less than 70% of ideal body weight, rapid refeeding can cause a serious condition called *refeeding syndrome*. The goal of hospitalization is to monitor and stabilize cardiac functioning and electrolyte status while initiating refeeding. Electrolytes are monitored daily, including serum phosphorus, potassium, calcium, and magnesium. Supplements of phosphorus, magnesium, and/or potassium may be prescribed as indicated. Nasogastric feedings may be necessary to reestablish and titrate nutritional intake for patients who are unable to take sufficient nutrition by mouth. Weight gain goals during hospitalization are from 2 to 3 lbs per week. Continuous cardiac monitoring is recommended. Depending on the length and severity of illness, prolonged hospitalization may be necessary to restore cardiovascular functioning and reverse symptoms of bradycardia (especially overnight bradycardia) and orthostasis by pulse and/or blood pressure.

Outpatient goals for medical and psychiatric management of patients who do not require hospitalization (and those who return to outpatient care following hospital discharge) include continuation of weight restoration at a rate of 0.5–1 lbs per week until a healthy weight is achieved. Other goals include normalization of eating behaviors, resumption of menses in adolescent females, and an appropriate exercise and activity plan consistent with restoration of bone health. Calcium supplements of 1200–1500 mg/day in three divided doses, vitamin D 400–1000 IU/day, and zinc 30 mg/day are recommended. Menses typically resume within 6 months of achieving 90% of ideal body weight. For sexually active adolescents and young adults, the risk of pregnancy may be the rationale for continuing oral contraceptives, even though an important biological marker of health is disguised.

The Primary Care Practitioner Role in the Diagnosis and Management of Eating Disorders

PCPs and psychiatric mental health-advanced practice registered nurses (PMH-APRN) have important roles in the assessment, diagnosis, and management of children and adolescents with eating disorders. Stereotypical attitudes such as the belief that only thin, white, affluent females get eating disorders can be barriers to timely recognition of these disorders in primary care and in psychiatry. Practitioners must be aware that eating disorders affect individuals of diverse racial, ethnic, and socioeconomic backgrounds, including males and females of all body sizes and shapes. Fursland and Watson (2014) describe eating disorders as "hidden" mental health problems. Few with an eating disorder receive disease-specific care despite their higher utilization of healthcare services. Even though these individuals are reluctant to access eating disorder treatment, they do seek healthcare for medical symptoms that may be associated with their eating disorders and could be identified with informed screening (Weissman and Rosselli 2017). These disorders are the most medically serious psychiatric disorders necessitating PCPs to be knowledgeable and attentive to the possibility of an eating disorder in all patients. PCPs are in a unique position for detection at the earliest stages and to stop their progression (Rosen 2010). Knowledge of resources including eating disorder therapists, nutrition intervention, and multidisciplinary treatment teams is required to connect patients and their families to care.

Goals in primary care include prevention, health education for patients with identified risk factors, early symptom identification, and prompt referral to, or consultation with, eating disorder specialists for diagnostic clarification and management of the treatment. Identifying early signs of food and weight anxiety provides a window of opportunity to intervene before symptoms of a full-blown eating disorder develop (Rome et al. 2003; Williams et al. 2008). In order to intervene in the early stages of eating disorders, PCPs must be knowledgeable about and alert for signs and symptoms, and overcome barriers to identification. Common barriers in primary care include the infrequency of well-child visits, the busy pace of primary care practices, insufficient appointment time for in-depth exploration, and reluctance on the part of PCPs to discuss warning signs with patients and parents due to fear of inciting defensiveness (DeSocio et al. 2007).

Eating disorder treatment yields the most benefit as part of a coordinated, multidisciplinary effort, involving specialized psychological treatment, nutrition intervention, medication management, and medical monitoring (Sim et al. 2010). PCPs may be best to provide the medical monitoring and management of their outpatient adolescent with an eating disorder due to their rapport and communication with the patient and family when they have an established therapeutic relationship. PCPs must consider different levels of care based on the individual patient needs and assess for indications supporting increased levels of care up to supporting hospitalization (Golden et al. 2015).

Screening and Assessment

Most patients with eating disorders do not present to their healthcare providers with the complaint "I have an eating disorder." When patients with eating disorders seek healthcare, they typically do not voluntarily disclose their altered patterns of eating and weight control activities. The withholding of symptoms may be due to stigma, shame, or fear that discovery will interfere with their weight loss goals. Signs and symptoms in children and adolescents are often inadvertently discovered during routine health maintenance appointments or physical examinations for school and sports participation.

An alternative entry for care often comes from a parent or caretaker presenting alone with concerns about their child's eating and/or weight. This parent consultation allows the PCP or PMH-APRN to assess the child or adolescent through the lens of the parent/caretaker experiences and observations of the child using the same review of symptoms, family and social history as you would use with the patient themselves to gather information: if their child has lost weight, is restricting food, has food rules on what and when to eat, is vomiting, taking laxatives, exercising excessively, experiencing fatigue, fainting, low energy, or low mood. If these findings are present, then the child will need to be seen for follow-up. The consultation can allow the PCP or PMH-APRN to help the parent to understand the severity of an eating disorder and the significant risks and harm that need to be managed (Bould et al. 2017).

Acquiring a comprehensive health history is the most powerful tool for assessment and diagnosis of eating disorders (Pritts and Susman 2003; Rome 2015; Rosen 2010). Experienced APRNs integrate eating disorder screening questions into interviews with all patients. The interview should include a discussion of the patient's satisfaction and perceptions of his/her body size and shape. Body weight questions focus on recent changes in weight, current weight, lowest weight, highest weight, and desired weight. Individuals with eating disorders often report unrealistically low body weight goals; others report a goal weight below a given threshold (Rosen 2010).

Obtain a nutrition history and ask about eating alone and in secret, or if the patient has ever engaged in binge eating. Inquire about weight control activities including the type, frequency, and duration of exercise, restrictive patterns of eating, and any eating "rules" the patient may have. Inquire about purging behaviors, including vomiting and use of laxatives, diuretics, or diet pills. Obtain a menstrual history in female patients. Remember that primary amenorrhea may be extended beyond expected norms in nutritionally compromised adolescents, and menses may be artificially induced in females taking oral contraceptives.

Family history of eating disorders, obesity, mood disorders, anxiety disorders, OCD, and/or substance abuse should be asked. Also, a social history should be done inquiring about the use of tobacco, alcohol, or drugs such as anabolic steroids, stimulants, or other street drugs or drugs not prescribed for the patient, history of physical or sexual abuse, and involvement with pro-anorexia or pro-bulimia websites.

While it is rare for patients to self-identify the need for treatment of their eating disorders, they may seek medical advice about symptoms associated with these disorders that they have not linked to the disorder, such as constipation, heartburn, cold extremities, or thinning hair. Symptoms brought to the healthcare professional's attention may include amenorrhea, dizziness, or fainting, fatigue, palpitations, bloating, abdominal pain, regurgitation, or rumination, and/or difficulty with sleep (Fairburn and Harrison 2003; Golden et al. 2016; Rome 2015).

Asking about a history of suicidal ideation and self-injurious behaviors is an essential part of the interview. Children and adolescents with eating disorders often experience feelings of self-loathing and may participate in self-injurious behaviors such as hitting or scratching themselves, punishing themselves with strenuous exercise, or using sharp objects to carve angry words on their thighs, abdomens, or other body parts they consider unappealing.

The Physical Examination

The physical examination begins with a general survey of the patient's appearance. Children and adolescents with AN may appear lethargic and complain of feeling cold. The assessment of children and adolescents should always include identification of Tanner's stages of breast and genital development. In advanced states of malnutrition, the patient may appear cachectic, with reversal or atrophy of secondary sexual development. Adolescents with BN may have normal body weight but display signs that raise suspicions of purging. Physical signs of purging may include enlarged parotid glands, perioral dermatitis, dental erosion, or calluses at the base of fingers (Russell sign). Essential components of the physical examination include evaluation of vital signs, which can reveal compromised cardiovascular and peripheral vascular functioning with bradycardia and orthostatic changes in blood pressure and/or pulse. Physical examination of the hair, thyroid, mouth, muscle mass, extremities, abdomen, and the neurological system may reveal signs of malnutrition. During the physical examination, scan the patient's skin for signs of self-injurious behaviors (Pérez et al. 2018; Yager et al. 2006). Common physical examination findings are identified in Table 15.6 and differential diagnoses are included in Table 15.7.

Table 15.6 Physical examination findings of concern in patients with disordered eating

- *General appearance:* very thin, emaciated or cachectic, protuberant bony prominences (AN), overweight (BN), flat affect, sunken cheeks, gray/yellow coloring
- *Vital signs:* hypothermia, bradycardia, hypotension, orthostatic blood pressure and/or pulse
- *Skin/hair:* dry skin, lanugo, bruising; thinning hair, loss of hair or dry hair with loss of shine, calluses at base of fingers (Russell sign), brittle nails, acrocyanosis
- *HEENT (head, eyes, ears, nose and throat):* dry lips, inflamed gums, angular stomatitis, loss of tooth enamel, parotitis, dull, thinning scalp hair, and sunken eyes
- *Breasts:* atrophy in postmenarche women
- *Cardiac:* bradycardia, arrhythmias, hypotension, murmurs, mitral valve prolapse
- *Extremities:* cool on palpation, peripheral edema, acrocyanosis, Raynaud's phenomena
- *Abdomen:* scaphoid contour, epigastric tenderness (if purging by vomiting), palpable stool in bowel, abdominal masses
- *Neurological:* decreased deep tendon reflexes
- *Genitourinary:* delayed puberty, inability to concentrate urine

Table 15.7 Differential diagnosis for eating disorders

- Thyroid disease
- Inflammatory bowel disease, celiac disease, or other GI diseases
- Abdominal masses causing chronic vomiting
- Cancer
- Diabetes, new onset
- Adrenal insufficiency
- Psychiatric disease: primary depression, OCD, substance abuse, psychotic conditions
- Central nervous system disease that can cause vomiting, appetite suppression, and a depressed affect
- Chronic infections, e.g. HIV, TB

Calculating and Plotting Height, Weight, and BMI

Growth charts available from the Centers for Disease Control and Prevention (http://www.cdc.gov/growthcharts) should be used to plot height and weight with current data and with as many previous data points as possible (Golden et al. 2016). Routinely plotting height and weight promotes early recognition of changes in percentile patterns compared to premorbid and age-based norms. Children and adolescents with AN may fail to gain appropriate amounts of weight during periods of growth. This pattern can be visualized on the child's growth chart when the trajectory for height is not matched by a corresponding trajectory of weight gain. A weight curve that either plateaus or dips during a period of growth requires prompt evaluation.

Calculation of BMI is a measurement that compares height to weight and gives an objective indication of overweight, underweight, or a healthy weight for height. The formula for calculating BMI involves multiplying weight in pounds by 703 and dividing by height in inches squared. BMI calculations should be adjusted for age, as parameters for healthy BMI are different for children than for adolescents and adults. Age-adjusted BMI calculators are available on the Centers for Disease Control and Prevention website and the National Library of Medicine website (https://www.nhlbi.nih.gov/health/educational/lose_wt/BMI/bmi-m.htm). For adults and adolescents, BMI scores below 18.5 are considered underweight, a range of 18.5–24.5 is considered normal body weight, above 25 is overweight, and above 30 is obese. However, it is important to realize that even a high BMI does not rule out the diagnosis of an eating disorder, including AN. It is the change in BMI that is critical. The high body weight child is especially endangered by the prevailing belief that weight loss in an overweight child is always a good thing. Limitations of classifying malnutrition based on BMI is worth noting as adolescents with restrictive eating behaviors who are not underweight experience the same range of complications as adolescents with AN (Golden et al. 2015).

Laboratory Tests and Procedures

Laboratory assessment must be comprehensive when an eating disorder is suspected (Table 15.8). There is no single biomarker that definitively identifies individuals with eating disorders (Ceresa et al. 2015) so existing measures for indications of functioning must be used to recognize the effects of malnutrition. Common findings in the chemistry panel of the patient with BN include hypokalemia secondary to vomiting, decreased magnesium, and decreased chloride (Moreno and Judd 2008). Patients with AN may have hypoglycemia secondary to lack of glucose precursors in the diet or low glycogen stores. Hyponatremia reflects excess water intake or poor secretion of antidiuretic hormone. An elevated blood urea nitrogen may be due to dehydration. Hypokalemic or hypochloremic metabolic alkalosis occurs with vomiting, and acidosis may be due to laxative abuse. Minimally elevated liver function tests are associated with a malnourished state but are not as high as seen in active hepatitis. A dramatic elevation in cholesterol is consistent with states of starvation. Other abnormal laboratory findings may include low alkaline phosphatase, extremely low sedimentation rates, low levels of FSH, LH, and estradiol, and low free T_3, free T_4, and TSH. The patient may also exhibit leukopenia and thrombocytopenia (Bernstein 2008).

Table 15.8 Laboratory assessment of a patient with eating disorders

- *Chemistry:* electrolytes (K⁺, Na⁺, Cl⁻), glucose, calcium, magnesium, phosphorus, blood urea nitrogen, creatinine (BUN and Cr) important in dehydration and suspected purging), liver function (TP, ALP, AST, ALT)
- *CBC with ESR:* Hct and Hgb
- *CK:* elevated with muscle breakdown due to overexercising or severe nutrition restriction
- *Lipid profile:* elevated LDH (BN/BED), inadequate HDL
- *Thyroid function, serum prolactin, LH and FSH:* to evaluate amenorrhea and rule out prolactinoma, hyper-or hypothyroidism, or ovarian failure
- *Urinalysis:* to assess specific gravity for water loading to falsely elevate weight
- *Stool and urine for emetide* (byproduct of ipecac): if Ipecac use is suggested
- *Drug screen:* if indicated for a patient with possible drug use
- *Pregnancy test:* in amenorrheic females
- *Other laboratory tests to consider:*
  - leptin
  - pancreatice enzymes: amylase, lipase

K⁺, potassium; Na⁺, sodium; Cl⁻⁻, chloride; BUN, blood urea nitrogen; Cr, creatinine; TP, total protein; ALP, alkaline phosphatase; AST, aspartate aminotransferase; ALT, alanine transaminase; CBC, complete blood count; ESR, erythrocyte sedimentation rate; Hct, hematocrit; Hgb, hemoglobin; CK, creatine kinase; HDL, high density lipoprotein; BN, bulimia nervosa; BED, binge eating disorder; LDL, low density lipoprotein; LH, luteinizing hormone; FSH, follicle stimulating hormone.

An ECG should be considered to evaluate bradycardia, QTc prolongation, and cardiac conduction problems associated with electrolyte abnormalities. Apart from suicide, cardiovascular complications account for most of the morbidity and mortality associated with AN. A dual energy X-ray absorptiometry (DEXA) scan is indicated for males and females with 6 or more months of low body weight and secondary amenorrhea or prolonged primary amenorrhea in females. DEXA results must be interpreted with reference to age- and sex-matched populations using Z scores (not T scores). Low bone density and the associated risk for fractures can be a powerful incentive for some patients and parents to engage and commit to treatment. Conversely, normal bone density results can provide false reassurance that the problem is not medically significant.

Standardized Instruments and Assessment Tools

Most eating disorder instruments were validated prior to the publication of the revised DSM-5 criteria for AN and BN plus the DSM-5 added diagnosis of BED, which is more prevalent that AN and BN combined (APA 2013).

The generalizability of the existing instruments for the full range of DSM-5 eating disorders is unknown (Maguen 2018). In addition, application of the existing instruments to the changing demographics of eating disorders must be validated. Validated assessment instruments are crucial to diagnosis and to objective evaluation of treatment progress.

In clinical practice, unstructured clinical interviews are the most common assessment done by eating disorder professionals for diagnosis of an eating disorder (Towne et al. 2017). The Eating Disorder Examination (EDE) and Eating Disorder Examination-Questionnaire (EDE-Q) (Fairburn and Cooper 1993) are among the most commonly used instruments for clinical interviews and self-report assessment (Towne et al. 2017). The EDE is a well-established assessment instrument but requires substantial training and administrative time. The EDE-Q has been regarded as one of the most accurate self-report methods of assessing binge eating and is useful for tracking changes over time (Lydecker et al. 2016). The EDE and EDE-Q have been shown to have concordance as an assessment of BED (Lydecker et al. 2016). Further research of instrument validity with diverse populations is needed.

Instrument use is valuable as the information obtained through use of standardized tools can assist the practitioner in systematically evaluating symptoms and individualizing treatment plans. Other instrument examples include the Rating of Eating Disorder Severity for Children (REDS-C) (DeSocio et al. 2011), the Interview for Diagnosis of Eating Disorders (Kutlesic et al. 1998), the Questionnaire for Eating Disorder Diagnoses (QEDD) (Mintz et al. 1997), and the Yale-Brown-Cornell Eating Disorder Scale (Mazure et al. 1994).

Screening instruments frequently used in primary care are the Eating Disorder Screen for Primary Care (ESP) (Cotton et al. 2003) and the SCOFF (sick, control, one, fat, food) (Morgan et al. (1999). Many of these scales can be found online. The ESP and SCOFF are frequently used by PCPs and have been validated for low to normal weight university students. They have been validated to screen for the core characteristics of early stage AN and BN (Sim et al. 2010). Both are five questions in length and take only minutes to complete, allowing ease of use. Positive responses provide an opportunity for further investigation of an eating disorder. Both lack validity with diverse populations and generalizability for all DSM-5 diagnoses, inclusive of BED.

Mond et al. (2008) compared the validity of the EDE-Q and the SCOFF for use in primary care. Their results found both measures performed well in detecting cases and excluding noncases of the most common eating disorders. Advantages of the SCOFF are its brevity and ease of use in primary care settings. It has 100% sen-

sitivity but lower specificity with a 12.5% false-positive rate, thus the SCOFF is best used as a screening tool rather than for diagnostic purposes (Morgan et al. 1999).

The QEDD is a 50-item diagnostic instrument based on DSM-I criteria. Greenleaf et al. (2009) modified this instrument for use with athletes. The 36-item Bulimia Test-Revised (BULIT-R) is an instrument used to assess BN and is based on DSM-IV criteria (Thelen et al. 1996). The REDS-C is a semi-structured, clinician-administered interview to assess the severity of eating disorder symptoms in children and adolescents aged 8–18 years. This diagnostic interview allows practitioners to rate child and parent responses on 14 symptom domains and assign confidence scores to the symptom ratings (DeSocio et al. 2011).

Self-assessment instruments can be obtained online through Mental Health Screening, Inc. at http://www.mentalhealthscreening.org/screening/Default.aspx?&n=1. Self-assessments may be beneficial in raising self-awareness and encouraging individuals to seek care. They are appropriate for older adolescents and adults but are generally less useful for children and young adolescents.

Follow-up Care

After the intensive phase of medical stabilization and treatment, patients with eating disorders are often referred to their PCP for follow-up care and health maintenance. The goal of the maintenance phase of treatment is to sustain symptom remission for as long as possible in order to support healthy growth and development. The PCP establishes a relationship with the patient and his/her parents to sustain their efforts toward eating disorder recovery.

Decisions about the appropriate level of care for a patient are typically ongoing and related to the patient's symptom course, which may be marked by periods of remission and exacerbation. Parents and practitioners must remain vigilant to signs of relapse. During periods of stress and transition, more frequent appointments may be warranted to monitor the patient's status. Follow-up appointments should include evaluation of vital signs with attention to changes in cardiovascular parameters that may signal relapse. The practitioner should routinely inquire about eating patterns and remain alert to reports of skipped meals or calories shaved from the meal plan as early indications of slipping back into patterns of restricting or binge eating. Weight and weight management activities should be monitored at each appointment. Urine pH may be periodically checked for alkalinity, a common sign of purging. Assessment of mood and risk for self-harm is essential and should be ongoing. It is important to realize that the patient's mood may decline during early phases of eating disorder treatment. Physical symptoms are extinguished before psychological remission occurs; it is common for patients to remain ambivalent or even resistant to treatment until psychological remission is achieved (National Collaborating Centre for Mental Health 2004).

The Role of the PMH-APRN in the Diagnosis and Management of Eating Disorders

The PMH-APRN may be the first to identify an eating disorder in patients who present for evaluation of mood or anxiety symptoms. Thus, the role of the PMH-APRN includes aspects of the primary care role in health education, screening, and early identification. Additionally, the PMH-APRN has a role in differential psychiatric diagnosis and management of comorbid psychiatric disorders. Both the PCP and the PMH-APRN refer patients to specialized eating disorder teams for comprehensive eating disorder evaluations and the intensive phase of treatment and medical stabilization. Following the intensive phase of treatment, patients with comorbid psychiatric disorders may be referred back to the PMH-APRN for ongoing management of their psychiatric needs.

Differential Psychiatric Diagnosis

In conducting a comprehensive psychiatric evaluation, the PMH-APRN considers other psychiatric disorders that may present with changes in appetite, weight loss, and abnormal patterns of eating and screens for comorbid psychiatric disorders. In young children, a trajectory of poor growth and slow weight gain may be diagnosed as failure to thrive. Selective patterns of eating, refusal of foods because of textures or sensory sensitivities, and a narrow range of food preferences are common features in children with pervasive developmental disorders and autism spectrum disorders. ARFID can involve extreme fear of swallowing or choking and can lead to rapid weight loss in young children. Obsessive anxiety and compulsive rituals associated with order and cleanliness can make food preparation and eating a tortuous experience that contributes to weight loss in children with OCD. Major depression may be accompanied by changes in appetite and weight, including weight loss or failure to gain weight during periods of growth. Psychomotor agitation and increased goal-directed activity occur during hypomanic and manic episodes, and can result in weight loss due to forgetting to eat, having no time to prepare food, or taking in fewer calories than energy expended. Use of psychoactive drugs or opioids can induce appetite suppression and weight loss. Abnormal or bizarre eating patterns may be secondary to psychotic delusions about food, contamination, or body functions in patients with schizophrenia. In each of these conditions, an eating disorder diagnosis may be ruled out by the absence of essential features, which include fear of weight gain, an undue influence of body size and shape on self-evaluation, an obsessive focus on calories and avoidance of foods associated with weight gain, and/or a compulsive drive to exercise (Rome et al. 2003). Another important distinction is that patients with eating disorders do not experience a loss of appetite as such and may be focused to the point of obsession on food, cooking or baking for others, reading cookbooks, or watching the Food Channel.

Differentiating a diagnosis of body dysmorphic disorder (BDD) from an eating disorder diagnosis is challenging because of the overlapping focus on body appearance. BDD usually involves a more focused preoccupation with a perceived defect in a specific body part; this focal preoccupation is a distinguishing feature that differs from the obsession with overall body weight and shape, and the weight loss goals that characterize eating disorders. A diagnosis of BDD should only be given if the patient's symptoms are not better accounted for as an eating disorder (APA 2013, p. 242).

Weight loss may also be secondary to pharmacological interventions for other disorders, such as stimulants for attention deficit hyperactivity disorder and topiramate for impulse control or seizure disorders. When children and adolescents present with symptoms of poor appetite and weight loss, a variety of conditions and causes should be explored, including the potential side effects of prescribed and over-the-counter medications.

The process of differential diagnosis may be complicated by the patient's reluctance or inability to report eating disorder cognitions. Young children may not be able to articulate the basis for their anxieties about food, fat, or body size. Older children and adolescents may minimize or conceal their obsessive worries and fears about food and body image because of shame, stigma, or resistance to adult interference. Extreme malnutrition and cognitive compromise can impair the individual's insight and judgment, and make it difficult to elicit the presence or absence of eating disorder symptoms. Seeking and confirming information from parents and other sources, obtaining a nutritional history, examining trajectories of growth, and evaluating physical parameters and results of laboratory tests are necessary to corroborate the presence or absence of an eating disorder (Becker et al. 2009; Harrington et al. 2015).

Acquiring a developmental timeline of symptom onset is crucial to rule in or rule out comorbid psychiatric disorders. Malnutrition and the resulting depletion of brain neurotransmitters may contribute to or exaggerate a host of psychiatric symptoms, including depressed mood, anxiety, inattention, and hyperactivity. When these symptoms emerge subsequent to the onset of eating disorder symptoms, the effects of malnutrition on brain functioning should be suspected as the source. In such cases, psychiatric symptoms may be better accounted for as secondary to the medical condition of malnutrition.

A developmental timeline that elicits symptoms of OCD, social phobia, generalized anxiety, mood symptoms, inattention, and/or hyperactivity prior to the onset of extreme weight loss or restrictive eating provides stronger support for the existence of these psychiatric disorders. Failure to recognize and treat comorbid psychiatric disorders can complicate treatment of an eating disorder. Likewise, an undetected eating disorder can lead to inappropriate treatment that further compromises the patient's health. For example, without a thorough examination of eating patterns and growth, a child with an undetected eating disorder might be inappropriately diagnosed with an attention deficit disorder and started on a psychostimulant, which can suppress appetite and further compromise his/her nutritional state. Undetected eating disorders and malnutrition can interfere with the effectiveness of selective serotonin reuptake inhibitors (SSRIs) used to treat anxiety and depression. Inadequate nutrition, depletion of the brain's monoamine neurotransmitters, and low levels of estradiol should always be ruled out as potential factors contributing to treatment resistance when patients do not respond as expected to psychotropic medications.

Follow-up and Maintenance for Patients with Psychiatric Symptoms and Comorbidities

The maintenance phase of treatment for patients with eating disorders and comorbid psychiatric disorders is often co-managed by providers in primary care and psychiatry. The stability of a patient's eating disorder symptoms is closely linked to the effective management of his/her psychiatric symptoms, requiring ongoing communication and collaboration between providers. For example, the side effects of medications such as SSRIs may induce changes in appetite and GI symptoms that impact patient weight and meal plan compliance. Consultation between providers enables planning for more frequent medical monitoring while psychotropic medications are being initiated and adjusted. Additionally, patients managed in primary care may develop symptoms of anxiety and/or depression during the course of treatment for their eating disorders. These symptoms may represent a transitional response to coping with weight restoration and the limitations imposed by their illness. Alternatively, the symptoms may represent the emergence of a comorbid psychiatric disorder that was not previously recognized. The PCP may benefit from consultation with the PMH-APRN to determine if a psychiatric evaluation is warranted for diagnostic clarification.

Engagement in self-injurious behaviors and episodes of increased suicidality are serious mental health concerns that may accompany the symptomatic course of eating disorders. PCPs who are managing patients during these periods of crisis benefit from consultation with psychiatric colleagues in evaluating patient safety and determining the need for hospitalization.

Evidence-based Treatment for Eating Disorders

Best-practice models for treatment of children and adolescents with eating disorders are guided by research evidence, expert consensus, and exemplary programs that have achieved positive patient and family outcomes. Research evidence supports family-based treatment for children and adolescents with eating disorders and cognitive behavioral therapy (CBT) and interpersonal psychotherapy (IPT) for adults with these disorders (Hay 2013; Kass et al. 2013).

The ARFID diagnosis is new to the DSM-5, and there is limited literature on treatment specific for this disorder. This diagnosis is most often identified in young children but also occurs in older children and adolescents. There is evidence that children with ARFID and their families can receive effective treatment in the same settings as children and adolescents with other eating disorder diagnoses (Ornstein et al. 2017).

Family-based Treatment

The Maudsley method, which originated at the Maudsley Hospital in London, is an exemplary model of family-based treatment with evidence of effectiveness for adolescents with AN and possible efficacy for adolescents with BN (Kass et al. 2013). Many eating disorder programs incorporate principles of the Maudsley method. These principles include the involvement of parents in all aspects of their child's treatment, empowering parents with a blame-free approach, supporting parents to take control of meal planning and preparation during the acute phase of illness, externalizing the eating disorder as the problem rather than the child, and helping families learn how to respond to the child or adolescent with an eating disorder (Katzman et al. 2013).

There are other models of family-based treatment, but these models share the philosophy that parental involvement is essential and weight restoration is a fundamental requirement for effective treatment (Kartini Clinic, n.d.).

Parents assume responsibility for implementing their child's nutrition plan, preparing meals, supervising during and after meals, monitoring their child's activities and exercise, administering medications, and meeting regularly with the treatment team. Unity of purpose between parents and the treatment team creates an environment that supports the child in relinquishing eating disorder symptoms, developing healthier attitudes and beliefs about themselves and their bodies, and learning new coping skills. As partners in all aspects of eating disorder treatment for children and adolescents, parents and families benefit from psychoeducation and therapeutic support for their essential roles. Multifamily therapy groups have been shown to strengthen interfamilial relationships and improve patient and family outcomes. While research evidence is lacking for specific forms of family groups or family therapy in eating disorder treatment, clinical consensus indicates that providing opportunities for families to meet together for support and to learn from each other is helpful (Brockmeyer et al. 2018; Tantillo 2006).

Psychosocial Interventions and Psychotherapy

Psychological interventions are aimed toward interrupting the patient's faulty cognitions, developing stress management and distress tolerance skills, and developing new patterns in relationships. Expert consensus and research findings support the use of individual CBT and therapist-guided self-help forms of CBT for adults with BN and BED (Mitchell et al. 2007; Hay 2013). Fairburn (2008) designed a transdiagnostic model of CBT that specifically targets faulty cognitions underlying eating disorder symptoms (CBT-E), with adaptations suggested for a younger population. These cognitions include an exaggerated importance placed on control of eating, shape, and weight, perfectionistic attitudes, and over-reactivity to moods and interpersonal difficulties. CBT-E is one of the first treatment approaches to focus specifically on eating disorder symptoms that cross diagnostic categories. Empirical evidence for CBT-E is growing and will be strengthened with larger research trials involving independent teams of researchers (Groff 2015).

Cognitive remediation therapy (CRT) is a form of cognitive therapy designed to remediate problems of cognitive inflexibility, set-shifting difficulties, poor central coherence, and perfectionistic thinking. It was originally designed for individuals with traumatic brain injuries but has wide application in treatment of cognitive processing deficits associated with conditions such as OCD and eating disorders (van Passel et al. 2016). CRT has been adapted for use in treatment of AN and is identified as a promising approach that requires additional research (Brockmeyer et al. 2018; Tchanturia et al. 2017).

IPT has evidence of effectiveness in treatment of adults with AN and BED (Hay 2013). Dialectical behavior therapy (DBT) has demonstrated promising results for adolescents and young adults with BN and BED (Kass et al. 2013; Safer et al. 2009; Shapiro et al. 2007). The benefits of DBT focus on distress tolerance and emotional regulation skills, which may be especially helpful for individuals with impulsivity, self-injurious behaviors, and/or comorbid mood disorders.

The relationship of childhood adversity and trauma to risk for eating disorders highlights the importance of trauma-informed approaches for individuals with a trauma history. Trauma-focused CBT (TF-CBT) is a treatment approach for children and adolescents who have experienced trauma, physical abuse, and/or sexual abuse (Cohen et al. 2006). While the use of TF-CBT has not been specifically investigated as a treatment approach for children and adolescents with eating disorder symptoms, it has a high level of empirical evidence for treatment of children with trauma histories (Ramirez de Arellano et al. 2014).

Shame and internalized stigma contribute to emotional distress in individuals with eating disorders and can perpetuate engagement in eating disorder behaviors in an effort to alleviate this distress. An increase in self-compassion counteracts feelings of shame and guilt, and has been found to decrease eating disorder symptoms (Kelly and Tasca 2016; Stutts and Blomquist 2018). Compassion-focused therapy (CFT) encourages non-judgmental kindness toward self and the development of self-care practices to alleviate the negative spiral of shame, self-disgust, guilt, and self-harming behaviors and symptoms (Gilbert 2014). Further research is needed to determine the efficacy of CFT as a treatment approach for individuals with eating disorders.

Psychopharmacology

Fluoxetine (Prozac) is the only medication to receive US Food and Drug Administration approval for the treatment of BN. The best research evidence to date recommends the combined use of fluoxetine and CBT for remission of BN (Mitchell et al. 2013). SSRIs and the anticonvulsant medication topiramate have demonstrated positive effects in treatment of BED (Mitchell et al. 2013).

For patients with AN, nutrition is the best medicine and weight restoration is the foundation of treatment. Weight restoration alone may improve mood, reduce anxiety, and ameliorate the intensity of obsessions and compulsions. Research has shown promising results from the use of atypical antipsychotics, such as olanzapine and aripiprazole, to reduce delusional thought processes, stabilize moods, and lessen anxiety associated with refeeding (Frank and Shott 2016; Frank et al. 2017). Initiation of an SSRI following weight restoration to 90% of expected body weight has also been shown to extend periods of remission and may be helpful in treating symptoms of comorbid anxiety disorders and/or depression (Frank and Shott 2016). There is limited research evidence to guide the psychopharmacological management of eating disorders in children and adolescents. Psychotropic medications should be prescribed cautiously and in consultation with clinicians who specialize in treatment of children with these disorders.

Exemplary Models of Interdisciplinary Collaboration

Eating disorders affect all aspects of biological, psychological, and social functioning. Effective models of treatment thus exemplify the benefits of collaborative practice between primary care, psychiatry, eating disorder specialists, and a multidisciplinary team. Interdisciplinary roles within the eating disorder team include medical care provided by a physician or APRN, psychiatric evaluations and psychotropic medications provided by a psychiatrist or PMH-APRN, nutritional counseling by a nutritionist, psychotherapy provided by the psychiatric provider, a psychologist, or a clinical social worker, family education and therapy provided by a family therapist, physical therapy assessments and activity recommendations by a physical therapist, and dental care by a dentist. The APRN or physician often serves as the team leader and consults with other specialists, such as cardiologists and endocrinologists, to evaluate and manage medical complications. Communication among team members is essential to establish common goals, develop and modify the treatment plan, monitor progress, and coordinate the roles and responsibilities of team members (Yager et al. 2006). Clinicians at Stanford's Lucile Salter Packard Children's Hospital developed the first clinical pathway for the treatment of AN in adolescents. This clinical pathway can be used as a guide for the structure of the treatment plan.

Exemplary models of treatment offer a spectrum of services that support the patient and family through various phases of treatment. These services include eating disorder evaluations, inpatient hospitalization, day treatment or partial hospitalization, and outpatient treatment. Some programs also provide residential treatment for longer term and more intensive care. Table 15.9 provides a list of resources for eating disorders for providers.

Table 15.9 Resources for eating disorders

Books for patients and families	Bulik and Taylor (2005)
	Bryant-Waugh and Lask (2004)
	Collins (2014)
	Lock and LeGrange (2015)
	O'Toole (2015)
	Treasure (2013)
Self-help groups	Anorexics and Bulimics Anonymous, http://www.anorexicsandbulimicsanonymousaba.com
	FEAST (Families Empowered and Supporting Treatment of Eating Disorders – International, www.feast-ed.org
	National Eating Disorders Association's Proud2BMe Forum (United States)
	Binge Eating Disorder Association (United States)
	Overeaters Anonymous, http://www.oa.org
Patient, family, and professional internet resources	National Eating Disorder Association, www.nationaleatingdisorders.org
	Academy for Eating Disorders, https://www.aedweb.org/home
	Eating Disorder Referral and Information Center, www.edreferral.com
	International Association of Eating Disorders Professionals, www.iaedp.com
	National Association of Anorexia Nervosa and Associated Disorders, www.anad.org
Tools	SCOFF questionnaire, http://pcptoolkit.beaconhealthoptions.com/wp-content/uploads/2016/02/SCOFF-Questions.pdf

Implications for Prevention, Advocacy, Research, and Education

Prevention of eating disorders is a community-wide effort. APRNs can be involved in education and advocacy at local, state, and national levels to promote awareness of eating disorders and the disabilities these disorders cause when they remain unrecognized and untreated. Advocacy efforts are also needed to support legislation and regulations that improve mental health benefits and provide nutritional and medical support for children and their families. Outreach to parents, teachers, coaches, club leaders, and organizers of community recreation programs is necessary to raise awareness of the signs of eating disorders and the importance of healthy nutrition and balanced physical activity. Changing our culture and overcoming the stigma and myths about eating disorders are ongoing challenges and a goal for all health professionals. Current research related to treatment of children and adolescents with eating disorders is limited. APRNs are needed as research investigators and collaborators. Nursing brings a unique and valuable perspective to teams engaged in research about the etiology, symptom course, patient and family coping, and treatment of eating disorders.

Conclusion

Prevention and early detection of eating disorders should be integrated into the practice of PCPs and PMH-APRNs. Early recognition can interrupt the progression of these disorders, reduce their chronic and disabling effects, and improve patient outcomes. The prognosis for patients with eating disorders is extremely variable. When symptoms persist without recognition and treatment, the prognosis is more guarded and mortality risk is high. The PCP is in a key position to conduct health education, prevention, and routine screening for eating disorders and to support the child and family through follow-up and prevention of relapse. The PMH-APRN provides primary prevention and health education about eating disorders and considers the possibility of eating disorders in processes of differential diagnosis. Specialized eating disorder teams are essential partners in managing the intensive phase of treatment and necessitate an awareness of local and regional resources for referral. Interdisciplinary collaboration is essential given the comprehensive care needs associated with managing children and adolescents with these disorders and the typical course of treatment that extends over multiple developmental transitions.

Thought Questions

1. Name at least one distinguishing characteristic for each diagnosis: avoidant/restrictive food intake disorder, anorexia nervosa, bulimia nervosa, and binge-eating disorder.
2. How important is the involvement of significant others in the child's or adolescent's life in identifying a feeding and eating disorder and achieving a degree of success with treatment?
3. What actions should an APRN take when a patient reaches a critical point in the expression of a feeding or eating disorder?

References

Abbate-Daga, G., Piero, A., Rigardetto, R. et al. (2007). *Psychopathology* 40: 261–268.

Academy of Eating Disorders (2016). *AED Report 2016: Eating disorders: A guide to medical care*, 3rde. Reston, VA: Author Available at https://www.aedweb.org/resources/online-library/publications/medical-care-standards.

Ackard, D.M., Fulkerson, J.A., and Neumark-Sztainer, D. (2007). Prevalence and utility of DSM-IV eating disorder diagnostic criteria among youth. *International Journal of Eating Disorders* 40: 409–417.

Afifi, T.O., Sareen, J., Fortier, J. et al. (2017). Child maltreatment and eating disorders among men and women in adulthood: results from a nationally representative US sample. *International Journal of Eating Disorders* 50 (11): 1281–1296.

American Academy of Pediatrics, Committee on Adolescence. (2003).

APA (2010). *Practice guidelines for the treatment of patients with eating disorders*, 3rde. Washington, DC: Author Available at https://psychiatryonline.org/pb/assets/raw/sitewide/practice_guidelines/guidelines/eatingdisorders.pdf.

APA (2013). *Diagnostic and Statistical Manual of Mental Disorders, DSM-5*, 5e. Washington, DC: American Psychiatric Association.

Anderluh, M.B., Tchanturia, K., Rabe-Hesketh, S., and Treasure, J. (2003). Childhood obsessive compulsive personality traits in adult women with eating disorders: defining a broader eating disorder phenotype. *American Journal of Psychiatry* 160: 242–247.

Arseneault, L. (2018). Annual research review: the persistent and pervasive impact of being bullied in childhood and adolescence: implications for policy and practice. *Journal of Child Psychology & Psychiatry* 59 (4): 405–421.

Assad, A.T., Esawy, H.I., Mohamed, G.A.R. et al. (2018). Sleep profile in anorexia and bulimia nervosa female patients. *Sleep Medicine* 48: 113–116.

Bailer, U.F., Price, J.C., Meltzer, C.C. et al. (2017). Dopaminergic activity and altered reward modulation in anorexia nervosa – insight from multimodal imaging. *International Journal of Eating Disorders* 50: 593–596.

Barker, E.T. and Galambos, N.L. (2007). Body dissatisfaction, living away from parents, and poor social adjustment predict binge eating symptoms in young woman making the transition to university. *Journal of Youth and Adolescence* 36: 904–911.

Becker, E., Eddy, K.T., and Perloe, A. (2009). Clarifying criteria for cognitive signs and symptoms for eating disorders in DSM-V. *International Journal of Eating Disorders* 42: 611–619.

Berends, T., van Meijel, B., Nugteren, W. et al. (2016). Rate, timing, and predictors of relapse in patients with anorexia nervosa following a relapse prevention program: a cohort study. *BioMed Psychiatry* 16: 316.

Berkman, N.D., Lohr, K.N., and Bulik, C.M. (2007). Outcomes of eating disorders: a systematic review of the literature. *International Journal of Eating Disorders* 40: 293–309.

Bernstein, B.E. (2008). *Eating disorder: Anorexia: Differential diagnoses & workup*. Available at http://emedicine.medscape.com/article/912187-diagnosis.

Blüher, S. and Mantzoros, C.S. (2004). The role of leptin in regulating neuroendocrine function in humans. *Journal of Nutrition* 134 (Supplement): 2469S–2474S.

Boraska, V., Franklin, C.S., Floyd, J.A.B. et al. (2014). A genome-wide association study of anorexia nervosa. *Molecular Psychiatry* 19 (10): 1085–1094.

Bould, H., Newbegin, C., Fazel, M. et al. (2017). Assessment of child or young person with a possible eating disorder. *BMJ: British Medical Journal* (Online) 359 https://doi.org/10.1136/bmj.j5328.

Brandys, M.K., de Kovel, C.G.F., Kas, M.J. et al. (2015). Overview of genetic research in anorexia nervosa: the past, the present, and the future. *International Journal of Eating Disorders* 48: 814–825.

Brockmeyer, T., Friederich, H.C., and Schmidt, U. (2018). Advances in the treatment of anorexia nervosa: a review of established and emerging interventions. *Psychological Medicine* 48: 1228–1256.

Bryant-Waugh, R. and Lask, B. (2004). *Eating Disorders: A parents' guide* (Rev. edition). New York: Brunner-Rutledge.

Bulik, C.M. and Taylor, N. (2005). *Runaway Eating: The 8 Point Plan to Conquer Adult Food and Weight Obsessions*. New York, NY: Rodale Books.

Bulik, C.M., Reba, L., Siega-Riz, A.M., and Reichborn-Kjennerud, T. (2005). Anorexia nervosa: definition, epidemiology, and cycle of risk. *International Journal of Eating Disorders* 37: S2–S9.

Bulik, C.M., Berkman, N.D., Brownley, K.A. et al. (2007). Anorexia nervosa treatment: a systematic review of randomized controlled trials. *International Journal of Eating Disorders* 40: 310–320.

Campbell, K. and Peebles, R. (2014). Eating disorders in children and adolescents: state of the art review. *Pediatrics* 134: 582–592.

Campos, R.N., dos Santos, D.J.R., Cordás, T.A. et al. (2013). Occurrence of bipolar spectrum disorder and comorbidities in women with eating disorders. *International Journal of Bipolar Disorders* 1 (25): 1–6.

Cardi, V., Di Matteo, R., Corfield, F., and Treasure, J. (2012). Social reward and rejection sensitivity in eating disorders: an investigation of attentional bias and early experiences. *World Journal of Biological Psychiatry* 14 (8): 622–633.

Casiero, D. and Frishman, W.H. (2006). Cardiovascular complications of eating disorders. *Cardiology in Review* 14 (5): 227–231.

Castro, J., Gila, A., Puig, J. et al. (2004). Predictors of rehospitalization after total weight recovery in adolescents with anorexia nervosa. *International Journal of Eating Disorders* 36: 22–30.

Ceresa, A., Castiglioni, I., Salvatore, C., Funaro, A., Martino, I., Alfano, S., . . . Quattrone, A. (2015). Biomarkers of eating disorders using support vector machine analysis of structural neuroimaging data: Preliminary results. *Behavioural Neurology*. Available at https://www.ncbi.nlm.nih.gov/pmc/articles/PMC4663371.

Chen, J., Kang, Q., Jiang, W. et al. (2015). The 5-HTTLPR confers susceptibility to anorexia nervosa in Han Chinese: evidence from a case-control and family-based study. *PLoS One* 10 (3): e0119378.

Clausen, L. (2004). Time course of symptom remission in eating disorders. *International Journal of Eating Disorders* 36: 296–306.

Cohen, J.A., Mannarino, A.P., and Deblinger, E. (2006). *Treating Trauma and Traumatic Grief in Children and Adolescents*. NY: Guilford Press.

Collins, L. (2014). *Eating with your Anorexic: A mother's memoir*. Biscotti Press.

Copeland, W.E., Bulik, C.M., Zucker, N. et al. (2015). Does childhood bullying predict eating disorder symptoms? A prospective, longitudinal analysis. *International Journal of Eating Disorders* 48: 1141–1149.

Cotton, M., Ball, C., and Robinson, P. (2003). Four simple questions can help screen for eating disorders. *Journal of General Internal Medicine* 18 (1): 53–56. https://doi.org/10.1046/j.15251497.2003.20374.x.

Couturier, J. and Lock, J. (2006). What is recovery in adolescent anorexia nervosa? *International Journal of Eating Disorders* 39: 550–555.

De Filippo, E., Marra, M., Alfinito, F. et al. (2016). Hematological complications in anorexia nervosa. *European Journal of Clinical Nutrition* 70 (11): 1305.

DeSocio, J. (2013). The neurobiology of risk and pre-emptive interventions for anorexia nervosa. *Journal of Child & Adolescent Psychiatric Nursing* 26 (1): 16–22.

DeSocio, J., O'Toole, J., Nemirow, S. et al. (2007). Screening for childhood eating disorders in primary care. Primary care companion. *Journal of Clinical Psychiatry* 9: 1–20.

DeSocio, J.E., O'Toole, J.K., He, H. et al. (2011). Rating of eating disorder severity interview for children: psychometric properties and comparison with EDI-2 symptom index. *European Eating Disorders Review* 20 (1): e70–e77.

Fairburn, C.G. (2008). *Cognitive Behavior Therapy and Eating Disorders*. New York, NY: Guilford.

Fairburn, C.G. and Cooper, Z. (1993). The eating disorder examination. In: *Binge Eating: Nature, Assessment and Treatment*, 12e (eds. C. Fairburn and G. Wilson), 317–360. New York, NY: Guilford.

Fairburn, C.G. and Harrison, P.J. (2003). Eating disorders. *Lancet* 361: 407–416.

Favaro, A., Tenconi, E., and Santonastaso, P. (2006). Perinatal factors and the risk of developing anorexia nervosa and bulimia nervosa. *Archives of General Psychiatry* 63: 82–88.

Frank, G.R. (1995). The role of estrogen in pubertal skeletal physiology: epiphyseal maturation and mineralization of the skeleton. *Acta Paediatrica* 84 (6): 627–630.

Frank, G.K.W. and Shott, M.E. (2016). Role of psychotropic medication in the management of anorexia nervosa: rationale, evidence, and future prospects. *CNS Drugs* 30 (5): 419–442.

Frank, G.K., Bailer, U.F., Henry, S.E. et al. (2005). Increased dopamine D2/D3 receptor binding after recovery from anorexia nervosa measured by positron emission tomography and [11C] raclopride. *Biological Psychiatry* 58: 908–912.

Frank, G.K.W., Shott, M.E., Hagman, J.O. et al. (2017). The partial dopamine D2 receptor agonist aripiprazole is associated with weight gain in adolescent anorexia nervosa. *International Journal of Eating Disorders* 50 (4): 447–450.

Fursland, A. and Watson, H.J. (2014). Eating disorders: a hidden phenomenon in outpatient mental health? *International Journal of Eating Disorders* 47 (4): 422–425.

Gamero-Villarroel, C., Gordillo, I., Carrillo, J.A. et al. (2014). BDNF genetic variability modulates psychopathological symptoms in patients with eating disorders. *European Child & Adolescent Psychiatry* 23: 669–679.

Gilbert, P. (2014). The origin and nature of compassion focused therapy. *British Journal of Clinical Psychology* 53: 6–41.

Golden, N.H., Katzman, D.K., Kreipe, R.E. et al. (2003). Eating disorders in adolescents: position paper of the Society for Adolescent Medicine. *Journal of Adolescent Health* 33 (6): 496–503.

Golden, N.H., Katzman, D.K., Sawyer, S.M., and Ornstein, R.M. (2015). Position paper of the society for adolescent health and medicine: medical management of restrictive eating disorders in adolescents and young adults references. *Journal of Adolescent Health* 56 (1): 121–125.

Golden, N.H., Schneider, M., and Wood, C. (2016). Preventing obesity and eating disorders in adolescents. *Pediatrics* 138 (3): e20161649.

Gorwood, P., Kipmann, A., and Foulon, C. (2003). The human genetics of anorexia nervosa. *European Journal of Pharmacology* 480: 163–170.

Greenleaf, C., Petrie, T.A., Carter, J., and Reel, J.J. (2009). Female collegiate athletes: prevalence of eating disorders and disordered eating behaviors. *Journal of American College Health* 57: 489–496.

Griffiths, S., Mitchison, D., Murray, S.B. et al. (2018). How might eating disorder stigmatization worsen eating disorders symptom severity? Evaluation of a stigma internalization model. *International Journal of Eating Disorders*: 1–5. https://doi.org/10.1002/eat.22932.

Groff, S.E. (2015). Is enhanced cognitive behavioral therapy an effective intervention in eating disorders? A review. *Journal of Evidence-Informed Social Work* 12: 272–288.

Gull, S.W. (1874). Anorexia nervosa. *Transactions of the Clinical Society of London* 7: 22–28.

Halmi, K. (2007). Anorexia nervosa and bulimia nervosa. In: *Lewis's Child and Adolescent Psychiatry*, 4e (eds. A. Martin and F.R. Volmar), 592–602. Philadelphia, PA: Lippincott Williams & Wilkins.

Harrington, B.C., Jimerson, M., Haxton, C., and Jimerson, D.C. (2015). *American Family Physician* 91 (1): 46–52.

Hay, P. (2013). A systematic review of evidence for psychological treatments in eating disorders: 2005-2012. *International Journal of Eating Disorders* 46: 462–469.

Herzog, D.B. and Eddy, K.T. (2007). Diagnosis, epidemiology, and clinical course of eating disorders. In: *Clinical Manual of Eating Disorders* (eds. J. Yager and P.S. Powers), 1–30. Washington, DC: American Psychiatric Publishing.

Hillebrand, J.G., van Elburg, A.A., Kas, M.J.H. et al. (2005). Olanzapine reduces physical activity in rats exposed to activity-based anorexia: possible implications for treatment of anorexia nervosa. *Biological Psychiatry* 58: 651–657.

Hoek, H.W. and van Hoeken, D. (2003). Review of the prevalence and incidence of eating disorders. *International Journal of Eating Disorders* 29: 383–396.

Hudson, J.I., Hiripi, E., Pope, H.G., and Kessler, R.C. (2007). The prevalence and correlates of eating disorders in the National Comorbidity Survey Replication. *Biological Psychiatry* 61: 348–358.

Hütter, G., Ganepola, S., and Hofmann, W.K. (2009). The hematology of anorexia nervosa. *International Journal of Eating Disorders* 42 (4): 293–300.

Kalla, A., Krishnamoorthy, P., Gopalakrishnan, A. et al. (2017). Gender and age differences in cardiovascular complications in anorexia nervosa patients. *International Journal of Cardiology* 227: 55–57.

Kartini Clinic. (n.d.) *Kartini Clinic for Children and Families*. Available at https://kartiniclinic.com/ (accessed 29 August 2018).

Kass, A.E., Kolko, R.P., and Wilfley, D.E. (2013). Psychological treatments for eating disorders. *Current Opinions in Psychiatry* 26 (6): 549–555.

Katzman, D.K. (2005). Medical complications in adolescents with anorexia nervosa: a review of the literature. *International Journal of Eating Disorders* 37: S52–S59.

Katzman, D.K., Peebles, R., Sawyer, S.M. et al. (2013). The role of the pediatrician in family-based treatment for adolescent eating disorders: opportunities and challenges. *Journal of Adolescent Health* 53: 433–440.

Kaye, W.H., Bulik, C.M., Thornton, L. et al. (2004). Comorbidity of anxiety disorders with anorexia and bulimia nervosa. *American Journal of Psychiatry* 161: 2215–2221.

Kaye, W.H., Frank, G.K., Bailer, U.F., and Henry, S.E. (2005). Neurobiology of anorexia nervosa: clinical implications of alterations of the function of serotonin and other neuronal systems. *International Journal of Eating Disorders* 37: S15–S19. https://doi.org/10.1002/eat.20109.

Keel, P.K. and Klump, K.L. (2003). Are eating disorders culture-bound syndromes? Implications for conceptualizing their etiology. *Psychological Bulletin* 129 (5): 747–769.

Keel, P.K., Fichter, M., Quadflieg, N. et al. (2004). Application of a latent class analysis to empirically define eating disorder phenotypes. *Archives of General Psychiatry* 61: 192–200.

Keel, P.K., Klump, K.L., Miller, K.B. et al. (2005). Shared transmission of eating disorders and anxiety disorders. *International Journal of Eating Disorders* 38: 99–105.

Kelly, A.C. and Tasca, G.A. (2016). Within-persons predictors of change during eating disorders treatment: an examination of self-compassion, self-criticism, shame, and eating disorder symptoms. *International Journal of Eating Disorders* 49: 716–722.

Khalsa, S.S., Portnoff, L.C., McCurdy-McKinnon, D., and Feusner, J.D. (2017). What happens after treatment? A systematic review of relapse, remission, and recovery in anorexia nervosa. *Journal of Eating Disorders* 5: 20.

Klump, K.L. and Gobrogge, K.L. (2005). A review and primer of molecular genetic studies in anorexia nervosa. *International Journal of Eating Disorders* 37: S43–S48. https://doi.org/10.1002/eat.20116.

Klump, K.L., Bulik, C.M., Kaye, W.H. et al. (2009). Academy for eating disorders position paper: eating disorders are serious mental illnesses. *International Journal of Eating Disorders* 42: 97–103.

Klump, K.L., Culbert, K.M., O'Connor, S. et al. (2017). The significant effects of puberty on the genetic diathesis of binge eating in girls. *International Journal of Eating Disorders* 50 (8): 984–989.

Krantz, M.J., Sabel, A.L., Sagar, U. et al. (2012). Factors influencing QT prolongation in patients hospitalized with severe anorexia nervosa. *General Hospital Psychiatry* 34 (2): 173–177.

Kutlesic, V., Williamson, D.A., Gleaves, D.H. et al. (1998). The interview for the diagnosis of eating disorders – IV: Application to DSM-IV diagnostic criteria. *Psychological Assessment* 10 (1): 41–48. https://doi.org/10.1037/1040-3590.10.1.41.

Lang, K., Roberts, M., Harrison, A. et al. (2016). Central coherence in eating disorders: a synthesis of studies using the rey osterrieth complex figure test. *PLoS One* 11 (11): e0165467.

Lavender, J.M., Mason, T.B., Utzinger, L.M. et al. (2016). Examining affect and perfectionism in relation to eating disorder symptoms among women with anorexia nervosa. *Psychiatry Research* 241: 267–272.

Li, D., Connally, J.J., Tian, L. et al. (2017). A genome-wide association study of anorexia nervosa suggests a risk locus implicated in dysregulated leptin signaling. *Scientific Reports* 7: 3847.

Lindseth, G., Helland, B., and Caspers, J. (2015). The effects of dietary tryptophan on affective disorders. *Archives of Psychiatric Nursing* 29 (2): 102–107.

Lipson, S.K. and Sonneville, K.R. (2017). Eating disorder symptoms among undergraduate and graduate students at 12 US colleges and universities. *Eating Behaviors* 24: 81–88.

Liu, X., Bipolar Genome Study (BiGS), Kelsoe, J.R., and Greenwood, T.A. (2016). A genome-wide association study of bipolar disorder with co-morbid eating disorder replicates the SOX2-OT region. *Journal of Affective Disorders* 189: 141–149.

Lock, J. and LeGrange, D. (2015). *Help Your Teenager Beat an Eating Disorder*, 2e. New York, NY: Guilford.

Lopez, C., Tchanturia, K., Stahl, D., and Treasure, J. (2008). Weak central coherence in eating disorders: a step towards looking for an endophenotype of eating disorders. *Journal of Clinical and Experimental Neuropsychology* 31: 117–125.

Lydecker, J.A., White, M.A., and Grilo, C.M. (2016). Black patients with binge-eating disorder: comparison of different assessment methods. *Psychological Assessment* 28 (10): 1319.

Madden, S. (2004). Anorexia nervosa – still relevant in the twenty-first century? A review of William Gull's "Anorexia Nervosa". *Clinical Child Psychology and Psychiatry* 9: 149–154.

Maguen, S., Hebenstreit, C., Li, Y. et al. (2018). Screen for disordered eating: Improving the accuracy of eating disorder screening in primary care. *General Hospital Psychiatry* 50: 20–25. https://doi.org/10.1016/j.genhosppsych.2017.09.004.

Mazure, C.M., Halmi, K.A., Sunday, S.R. et al. (1994). The Yale-Brown-Cornell eating disorder scale: development, use, reliability and validity. *Journal of Psychiatric Research* 28: 425–445. https://doi.org/10.1016/0022-3956(94)90002-7.

McCormick, L.M., Keel, P.K., Brumm, M.C. et al. (2008). Implications of starvation induced change in right dorsal anterior cingulated volume in anorexia nervosa. *International Journal of Eating Disorders* 41: 602–610.

McFarlane, T., Olmsted, M.P., and Trottier, K. (2008). Timing and prediction of relapse in a transdiagnostic eating disorder sample. *International Journal of Eating Disorders* 41: 587–593.

Mehler, P.S., Sabel, A.L., Watson, T., and Andersen, A.E. (2008). High risk of osteoporosis in male patients with eating disorders. *International Journal of Eating Disorders* 41 (7): 666–672.

Mehler, P.S., Krantz, M.J., and Sachs, K.V. (2015). Treatments of medical complications of anorexia nervosa and bulimia nervosa. *Journal of Eating Disorders* 3 (1): 15.

Merikangas, K.R., He, J.-P., Burstein, M. et al. (2010). Lifetime prevalence of mental disorders in U. S. adolescents: results from the National Comorbidity Study- Adolescent Supplement (NCS-A). *Journal of the American Academy of Child and Adolescent Psychiatry* 49 (10): 980–989.

Mintz, L.B., O'Halloran, M.S., Mulholland, A.M., and Schneider, P.A. (1997). Questionnaire for eating disorder diagnoses: reliability and validity of operationalized DSM-IV criteria in a self-report format. *Journal of Counseling Psychology* 44: 63–79.

Mitchell, J.E., Agras, S., and Wonderlich, S. (2007). Treatment of bulimia nervosa: where are we and where are we going? *International Journal of Eating Disorders* 40: 95–101.

Mitchell, J.E., Roerig, J., and Steffen, K. (2013). Biological therapies for eating disorders. *International Journal of Eating Disorders* 46: 470–477.

Mond, J.M., Myers, T., Crosby, R. et al. (2008). Screening for eating disorders in primary care: EDE-Q versus SCOFF. *Behaviour Research and Therapy* 46 (5): 612–622.

Monell, E., Clinton, D., and Birgegård, A. (2018). Emotional dysregulation and eating disorders – Associations with diagnostic presentation and key symptoms. *International Journal of Eating Disorders*, Epub ahead of print. doi: https://doi.org/10.1002/eat.22925.

Moreno, M.A. & Judd, R. (2008). *Eating disorder: Bulimia: Differential diagnoses & workup*. Available at http://emedicine.medscape.com/article/913721-diagnosis.

Morgan, J.F., Reid, F., and Lacey, J.H. (1999). The SCOFF questionnaire: assessment of a new screening tool for eating disorders. *British Medical Journal* 319: 1467–1468.

Müller, T.D., Föcker, M., Holtcamp, K. et al. (2009). Leptin-mediated neuroendocrine alterations in anorexia nervosa: somatic and behavioral implications. *Child & Adolescent Clinics of North America* 18: 117–229.

National Collaborating Centre for Mental Health. (2004). *Eating disorders: Core interventions in the treatment and management of ano-*

rexia nervosa, bulimia nervosa and related eating disorders. Clinical guideline 9. London, UK: National Institute for Health and Clinical Excellence. Available at https://www.rcpsych.ac.uk/improving-care/nccmh.

Ornstein, R.M., Essayli, J.H., Nicely, T.A. et al. (2017). Treatment of avoidant/restrictive food intake disorder in a cohort of young patients in a partial hospitalization program for eating disorders. *International Journal of Eating Disorders* 50: 1067–1074.

O'Toole, J. (2015). *Give Food a Chance: A New View on Childhood Eating Disorders*. London, UK: Jessica Kingsley Publishers.

van Passel, B., Danner, U., Dingemans, A. et al. (2016). Cognitive remediation therapy (CRT) as a treatment enhancer of eating disorders and obsessive compulsive disorders: study protocol for a randomized controlled trial. *BioMed Psychiatry* 16: 393.

Pearson, C.M., Miller, J., Ackard, D.M. et al. (2017). Stability and change in patterns of eating disorder symptoms from adolescence to young adulthood. *International Journal of Eating Disorders* 50 (7): 748–757.

Peebles, R., Wilson, J.L., and Lock, J.D. (2006). How do children with eating disorders differ from adolescents with eating disorders at initial evaluation? *Journal of Adolescent Health* 39: 800–805.

Pérez, S., Marco, J.H., and Cañabate, M. (2018). Non-suicidal self-injury in patients with eating disorders: prevalence, forms, functions, and body image correlates. *Comprehensive Psychiatry* 84: 32–38.

Pike, K.M., Hoek, H.W., and Dunne, P.E. (2014). Cultural trends and eating disorders. *Current Opinions in Psychiatry* 27 (6): 436–442.

Pritts, S. and Susman, J. (2003). Diagnosis of eating disorders in primary care. *American Family Physician* 67 (2): 297–304.

Puxley, F., Midtsund, M., Iosif, A., and Lask, B. (2008). PANDAS anorexia nervosa – endangered, extinct or nonexistent. *International Journal of Eating Disorders* 41: 15–21.

Ramirez de Arellano, M.A., Lyman, D.R., Jobe-Shields, L. et al. (2014). Trauma focused cognitive behavioral therapy: assessing the evidence. *Psychiatric Services* 65 (5): 592–602.

Rome, E.S. (2015). Diagnosing eating disorders in children and adolescents. In: *The Wiley Handbook of Eating Disorders* (eds. L. Smolak and M.P. Levine), 157–169. Hoboken, NJ: Wiley.

Rome, E.S. and Ammerman, S. (2003). Medical complications of eating disorders: an update. *Journal of Adolescent Health* 33: 418–426.

Rome, E.S., Ammerman, S., Rosen, D.S. et al. (2003). Children and adolescents with eating disorders: the state of the art. *Pediatrics* 111: e98–e108.

Rosen, D.S. & Committee on Adolescence (2010). Clinical report: Identification and management of eating disorders in children and adolescence. *Pediatrics, 126*(6). Available at http://pediatrics.aappublications.org/content/126/6/1240.

Rozenblat, V., Ong, D., Fuller-Tyszkiewicz, M. et al. (2017). A systematic review and secondary data analysis of the interactions between the serotonin transporter 5-HTTLPR polymorphism and environmental and psychological factors in eating disorders. *Journal of Psychiatric Research* 84: 64–72.

Russell, G. (1979). Bulimia nervosa: an ominous variant of anorexia nervosa. *Psychological Medicine* 9: 429–448.

Safer, D.L., Telch, C.F., Chen, E.Y., and Linehan, M.M. (2009). *Dialectical Behavior Therapy for Binge Eating and Bulimia*. New York, NY: Guilford Press.

Schaumberg, K., Welch, E., Breithaupt, L. et al. (2017). The science behind the academy for eating Disorder's nine truths about eating disorders. *European Eating Disorders Review* 25: 432–450.

Schlüter, N., Schmidt, R., Kittel, R. et al. (2016). Loss of control eating in adolescents from the community. *International Journal of Eating Disorders* 49 (4): 413–420.

Schmelkin, C., Plessow, F., Thomas, J.J. et al. (2017). Low oxytocin levels are related to alexithymia in anorexia nervosa. *International Journal of Eating Disorders* 50: 1332–1338.

Shapiro, J.R., Berkman, N.D., Brownley, K.A. et al. (2007). Bulimia nervosa: a systematic review of randomized controlled trials. *International Journal of Eating Disorders* 40: 321–336.

Sim, L.A., McAlpine, D.E., Grothe, K.B., Himes, S.M., Cockerill, R.G., & Clark, M.M. (2010). Identification and treatment of eating disorders in the primary care setting. *Mayo Clinic Proceedings*, 85(8), 746–751.

Slof-Op't Landt, M.C., Claes, L., and van Furth, E.F. (2016). Classifying eating disorders based on "healthy" and "unhealthy" perfectionism and impulsivity. *International Journal of Eating Disorders* 49 (7): 673–680.

Smink, F.R.E., van Hoeken, D., and Hoek, H.W. (2013). Epidemiology, course, and outcome of eating disorders. *Current Opinion in Psychiatry* 26 (6): 543–548.

Sodersten, P., Bergh, C., and Ammar, A. (2003). Anorexia nervosa: towards a neurobiologically based therapy. *European Journal of Pharmacology* 480: 67–74.

Sokol, M.S., Jackson, T.K., Selser, C.T. et al. (2005). Review of clinical research in child and adolescent eating disorders. *Primary Psychiatry* 12: 52–58.

Sonneville, K.R. and Lipson, S.K. (2018). Disparities in eating disorder diagnosis and treatment according to weight status, race/ethnicity, socioeconomic background and sex among college students. *International Journal of Eating Disorders* 51: 518–526.

Spaulding-Barclay, M.A., Stern, J., and Mehler, P.S. (2016). Cardiac changes in anorexia nervosa. *Cardiology in the Young* 26 (4): 623–628.

Strigo, I.A., Matthews, S.C., Simmons, A.N. et al. (2013). Altered insula activation during pain anticipation in individuals recovered from anorexia nervosa: evidence of interoceptive dysregulation. *International Journal of Eating Disorders* 46 (1): 23–33.

Strober, M., Freeman, R., and Morrell, W. (1997). The long term course of severe anorexia nervosa in adolescents: survival analysis of recovery, relapse, and outcome predictors over 10-15 years in a prospective study. *International Journal of Eating Disorders* 22: 339–360.

Strober, M., Freeman, R., Lampert, C. et al. (2000). Controlled family study of anorexia nervosa and bulimia nervosa: evidence of shared liability and transmission of partial syndromes. *American Journal of Psychiatry* 157: 393–401.

Stutts, L.A. and Blomquist, K.K. (2018). The moderating role of self-compassion on weight and shape concerns and eating pathology: A longitudinal study. *International Journal of Eating Disorders*. [Online ahead of print]. doi: https://doi.org/10.1002/eat.22880.

Tantillo, M. (2006). A relational approach to eating disorders multifamily therapy group: moving from difference and disconnection to mutual connection. *Families, Systems and Health* 24: 82–102.

Tchanturia, K., Giombini, L., Leppanen, J., and Kinnaird, E. (2017). Evidence for cognitive remediation therapy in young people with anorexia nervosa: systematic review and meta-analysis of the literature. *European Eating Disorders Review* 25 (4): 227–236.

Thelen, M.H., Mintz, L.B., and Vander Wal, J. (1996). The bulimia test-revised: validation with DSM-IV criteria for bulimia nervosa. *Psychological Assessment* 8: 219–221.

Toufexis, M.D., Hommer, R., Gerardi, D.M. et al. (2015). Disordered eating and food restrictions in children with PANDAS/PANS. *Journal of Child & Adolescent Psychopharmacology* 25 (1): 48–56.

Towne, T.L., De Young, K.P., and Anderson, D.A. (2017). Trends in professionals' use of eating disorder assessment instruments. *Professional Psychology: Research and Practice* 48 (4): 243.

Treasure, J. (2007). Getting beneath the phenotype of anorexia nervosa: the search for viable endophenotypes and genotypes. *Canadian Journal of Psychiatry* 52: 212–219.

Treasure, J. (2013). *Anorexia Nervosa: A Survival Guide for Sufferers, Families, and Friends*. Rutledge Press.

Treasure, J., Stein, D., and Maquire, S. (2015). Has the time come for a staging model to map the course of eating disorders from high risk to severe enduring illness? An examination of evidence. *Early Intervention in Psychiatry* 9: 173–184.

US Department of Health and Human Services. (2009). *HealthyPeople. gov: Mental health and mental disorders*. Office of Disease Prevention and Health Promotion. Available at https://www. healthypeople.gov/2020/topics-objectives/topic/mental-health-and-mental-disorders/objectives.

Wade, T.D., Bulik, C.M., Neale, M., and Kendler, K.S. (2000). Anorexia and major depression: shared genetic and environmental risk factors. *American Journal of Psychiatry* 157: 469–471.

Wagner, A., Aizenstein, H., Venkatraman, V.K. et al. (2007). Altered reward processing in women recovered from anorexia nervosa. *American Journal of Psychiatry* 164: 1842–1849.

Walsh, J.M., Wheat, M., and Freund, K. (2000). Detection, evaluation, and treatment of eating disorders. *Journal of General Internal Medicine* 15: 577–590.

Watson, R.J., Adjei, J., Saewyc, E. et al. (2017). Trends and disparities in disordered eating among heterosexual and sexual minority adolescents. *International Journal of Eating Disorders* 50 (1): 22–31.

Watson, R.J., Veale, J.F., and Saewyc, E.M. (2017). Disordered eating behaviors among transgender youth: probability profiles from risk and protective factors. *International Journal of Eating Disorders* 50 (5): 515–522.

Weissman, R.S. and Rosselli, F. (2017). Reducing the burden of suffering from eating disorders: unmet treatment needs, cost of illness, and the quest for cost-effectiveness. *Behaviour Research and Therapy* 88: 49–64.

Westmoreland, P., Krantz, M.J., and Mehler, P.S. (2016). Medical complications of anorexia nervosa and bulimia. *American Journal of Medicine* 129 (1): 30–37.

Williams, P., Goodie, J., and Motsinger, C. (2008). Treating eating disorders in primary care. *American Family Physician* 77: 187–195.

Wolfe, B.E., Dunne, J.P., and Kells, M.R. (2016). Nursing care considerations for the hospitalized patient with an eating disorder. *Nursing Clinics of North America* 51 (2016): 213–235.

Yager, J., Devlin, M.J., Halmi, K.A. et al. (2006). *Practice guidelines for the treatment of patients with eating disorders*, 3rde. Washington, DC: American Psychiatric Association Available at http://www.psych.org/ psych_pract/treatg/pg/EatingDisorder-s3ePG_04-28-06.pdf.

Yilmaz, Z., Hardaway, J.A., and Bulik, C.M. (2015). Genetics and epigenetics of eating disorders. *Advances in Genomics and Genetics* 5: 131–150.

16

Autism Spectrum Disorder

Judith Coucouvanis[1] and Donna Hallas[2]

[1] University of Michigan Health System, Ann Arbor, MI, USA
[2] Rory Meyers College of Nursing, New York University, New York, NY, USA

Objectives

After reading this chapter, advanced practice registered nurses (APRNs) will be able to:

1. Define the epidemiology and etiology of autism spectrum disorder (ASD).
2. Apply the diagnostic criteria for ASD in clinical practice when children present with symptoms suggestive of the diagnosis.
3. Analyze clinical problems and evidence-based interventions for the treatment of ASD.
4. Summarize implications for the practice, research, and education of APRNs who care for children with ASD.

Introduction

It has been 75 years since child psychiatrist Leo Kanner (1943) first reported the unusual characteristics of a group of 11 children. Initially referred to as early infantile autism (Kanner 1943) and now referred to as autism spectrum disorder (ASD), the core features of this developmental disability are social communication deficits and repetitive and unusual sensory-motor behaviors (Lord et al. 2018). Prevalence estimates of ASD have consistently increased across the decades, from five cases per 10 000 persons in the 1980s to the latest Centers for Disease Control and Prevention (CDC) estimates of one in 54 (CDC 2020a). Autism is seen as a spectrum from very mild to very severe. This chapter will use the term ASD to refer to this group of syndromes.

ASD occurs in all racial, ethnic, and socioeconomic groups, yet is five times more likely to occur in boys than in girls (CDC 2020a). The majority of children with ASD receive special education services and have a documented history of concerns regarding development before 3 years of age. Cognitive impairment (i.e. intelligence quotient [IQ] of 70 or less) was reported in approximately one-third of children with ASD age 8 years in 2016 (Maenner et al. 2020).

Surrounded by confusion, intrigue, and myth, ASD is one of the most complex and controversial psychiatric disorders. Each affected individual exhibits a life-long profile of unique social-communicative, cognitive, and linguistic strengths and weaknesses, as well as sensory modulation issues. Every person with ASD is different. Individuals range from those who are nonverbal with

---

Child and Adolescent Behavioral Health: A Resource for Advanced Practice Psychiatric and Primary Care Practitioners in Nursing,
Second Edition. Edited by Edilma L. Yearwood, Geraldine S. Pearson, and Jamesetta A. Newland.
© 2021 John Wiley & Sons, Inc. Published 2021 by John Wiley & Sons, Inc.
Companion website: www.wiley.com/go/Yearwood

severe challenges to those who are extremely intelligent, yet demonstrate markedly impaired social skills and weak perspective-taking skills.

One of the core features of ASD is marked impairment in social functioning, regardless of intellectual or language ability (Carter et al. 2005). Social deficits are wide-ranging and persist through adolescence and adulthood when social demands become more complex (Tantam 2000). Developing meaningful relationships is a constant struggle for those with ASD. While typically developing children learn social skills through experience, the child with ASD must be directly taught specific skills (Bellini 2006).

Studies have shown that there is a 50- to 100-fold increase in the rate of autism in first-degree relatives of autistic children (Filipek et al. 2000). Estimates for recurrence of ASD in siblings range anywhere from 6 to 20% (Filipek et al. 2000; Ghaziuddin 2005). This represents a risk of over 100 times that of the general population (Ghaziuddin 2005). No one can predict the eventual outcome for an affected child with ASD (Koegel and LaZebnik 2004) and improvements cannot be expected to occur for all individuals even when using a specific established and evidence-based treatment.

In the past 20 years, a wealth of information has been gathered about ASD, but no one treatment meets the needs of all children (National Institute of Mental Health 2008). Each child requires an individualized, systematic, and comprehensive intervention plan (Koegel and LaZebnik 2004). Autism stories are regularly featured on internet websites, in talk and print media, and in mainstream magazines. Conflicting opinions regarding treatment, heated arguments about cause, and "evidence" of miracle cures are common, leaving parents confused and overwhelmed.

Parents face a daunting array of choices and decisions, often without guidance. Which interventions and treatments are best? Whom should parents trust? What will give parents hope? The estimated cost for each individual with ASD across the lifespan is US$3.2 million (Ganz 2007). Advanced practice registered nurses (APRNs) in pediatric settings are in prime positions to guide and support parents through the myriad of decisions parents encounter daily while parenting a child with a diagnosis of ASD.

Public awareness of ASD has increased in the last decade and is likely related to closer media coverage of studies in the scientific literature related to causation and intervention. Reasons for this increase have included heightened public awareness and consequent levels of parental concern, development of more sophisticated screening and diagnostic tools, and improved professional proficiency in identification of children at risk.

Also, changes in the DSM-IV criteria in 1994 broadened the range of disorders in the spectrum (Johnson and Myers 2007).

Etiology

ASD is a biologically based, neurobehavioral disorder, the cause of which has continued to perplex experts in the field attempting to identify causal factors. To date, the preponderance of evidence points to multifactorial transmission (i.e. genetic susceptibility exacerbated by environmental factors). Recent research has shown that genes may play a more significant role in the development of autism than previously thought. Fragile X syndrome (FXS; an inherited disorder that causes problems with intellectual capacity), tuberous sclerosis (TS; a rare condition in which benign tumors grow in the brain and other vital organs), Rett syndrome (a genetic condition primarily seen in girls, which causes slowing of head growth with a regression in intellectual disability [ID] around 2 years of age), and genetic mutations which may be inherited or a result of spontaneous mutations (Mayo Foundation for Medical Education and Research 2018) have all been implicated in the diagnosis of children with ASD. The role of genetics is discussed in more detail below. In addition, environmental factors affecting the development of ASD are under investigation by researchers. Environmental factors include but may not be limited to exposure to viruses in utero or after birth, prenatal complications, medications, and even air quality and exposure to air pollutants (Mayo Foundation for Medical Education and Research 2018). A discussion of the many factors that may contribute to the etiology of ASD are discussed below.

Disruption in Brain Structure and Function

Attempts at directly studying differences in brain structure and function in individuals with ASD has focused on the use of neuroimaging techniques such as functional magnetic resonance imaging (fMRI) and spectroscopy (Batshaw et al. 2007; Ecker et al. 2010). Macrocephaly is frequently noted during early childhood in individuals with ASD, and some neuroimaging studies have found that this finding coincides with brain growth acceleration at about 1 year of age in regions of cortical white matter, as well as abnormal growth patterns in the frontal and temporal lobes and the amygdala (Levy et al. 2009). Casanova (2004) reported an increased volume in brain white matter and linked these findings to short association fibers in the frontal and temporal lobes of the brain in children with ASD. These brain structural findings are thought to alter the entire brain networking architecture which is correlated to deficits in language, behavioral regulation, and social interactions (Li et al. 2014). The results of a meta-analysis reported by Liu et al. (2017) examined gray matter abnormalities in pediatric ASDs. The meta-regression analysis revealed that repetitive behavior scores of the Autism Diagnostic Interview – Revised demonstrated a positive association with increased gray matter volumes in the brain, specifically in the right angular gyrus. Other studies have used neuroimaging to detect neurotransmitter activity and cortical energy utilization in high-functioning adolescents with ASD. To date, these studies have identified some evidence that certain areas of the autistic brain have difficulty "networking" with other brain regions and functional abnormalities have been noted in brain areas associated with eye gaze, processing faces, and imitation (Batshaw et al. 2007). Such difficulties often translate into a range of sensory integration and processing difficulties (Levy et al. 2009).

Further analysis of electroencephalograms (EEGs) in individuals with a diagnosis of ASD has revealed changes in brain electric signals as compared to children without a diagnosis of ASD (Hashemian and Pourghassem 2014). In 2017, Reis Paula et al. (2017) published the results of their study which compared EEG results of children paired by age and gender with and without a diagnosis of ASD as the children were exposed to visual images of human faces with three expressions: neural, happy, and angry. The results revealed stronger activation in the frontal, central, parietal, and occipital regions of the brain in the ASD group. Failure in these systems may be related to the social cognitive deficits observed in children with ASD. The researchers concluded that these patterns of brain activation may correlate with developmental characteristics in children with ASD.

Genetic and Environmental Influences

A meta-analysis published by Tick et al. (2016) reported that 74–93% of ASD risk is heritable. Because of these high heritability estimates, a major focus of research has been on finding the underlying genetic causes of autism as well as potential environmental triggers. So far, no "autism gene" has been discovered, meaning that no gene is consistently mutated in every person with autism and there is no gene that causes autism every time it is mutated. Over the past decade, advances in DNA sequencing technologies along with the collection of large patient cohorts and widespread data sharing have enabled significant progress in the identification of genes implicated in ASD (Ramaswami and Geschwind 2018). Researchers have identified 65 genes they consider strongly linked to autism and more than 200 others that are weaker. Many of these genes are thought to be important for communication between neurons or control the expression of other genes.

Although researchers disagree on the relative contributions of genes and environment, some environmental factors may work with genetic factors to produce autism or intensify its features. Scientists continue to study the contribution of environmental factors and the interaction between genes. Many environmental risk factors for ASD have been suggested. Converging evidence from multiple studies indicates that advancing parental age of both the father and the mother increases risk of ASD in offspring. In a 2012 meta-analysis focused on maternal age using data from 25 687 ASD cases and 8 655 576 control subjects aggregated from 16 studies, investigators found that mothers ≥35 years of age had 1.5-fold increased odds (95% confidence interval [CI] = 1.1–1.9) of having a child with ASD compared to mothers 25–29 years old (Sandin et al. 2012). A similarly large 2010 meta-analysis of data from 11 studies found that fathers aged 40–49 had a 1.8-fold (95% CI: 1.5–2.1) increased risk of a child with ASD compared to fathers ≤29 years (Hultman et al. 2011).

Pregnancy factors such as maternal weight gain, metabolic conditions, and hypertension as well as maternal admission to hospital due to bacterial or viral infections have been associated with a mildly increased risk of ASD and developmental delay combined (Lord et al. 2018). Prenatal exposure to valproate is a recognized risk factor for ASD, especially in the first trimester of pregnancy. Children exposed in utero to valproate have 8-fold increased risk of ASD (Chaste and LeBoyer 2012; Christensen et al. 2013). A preterm birth of less than 32 weeks, low birth weight of <150 g, small for gestational age, and large for gestational age (Lampi et al. 2012: Moore et al. 2012) have all been independently associated with an increased risk. Periconceptual folic acid supplements (Schmidt et al. 2012) have been associated with a decreased risk for ASD and developmental disabilities. Associations with immunizations or vaccinations have not been found.

The Clinical Picture

ASD is a lifelong disorder that begins in early childhood and can be reliably diagnosed by an experienced professional at age 2. Nevertheless, the median age of first diagnosis is usually by 3 years of age (CDC 2020b). The American Academy of Child and Adolescent Psychiatry and the American Academy of Pediatrics recommend routine developmental screening for symptoms of ASD during well-child visits at 18 and 24 months (American Academy of Pediatrics 2019; Volkmar et al. 2014). Additional screening might be needed if a child is at high risk for ASD (e.g. has a sibling or other family member with ASD) or if signs associated with ASD are present (Zwaigenbaum et al. 2015). If any signs of a problem are noted, a comprehensive diagnostic evaluation is needed.

Clinical Features

"One of the most challenging aspects in recognizing ASD is the wide heterogeneity of features in individual children" (Johnson and Myers 2007, p. 1190). Diagnosing ASD can be challenging since there is no medical test unique to ASD and a significant number of people with ASD have co-occurring medical or psychiatric disorders. ASD shares signs and symptoms with a variety of other health and developmental problems, such as attention and adjustment disorders, obsessive–compulsive disorder (OCD), anxiety, depression, sensory and cognitive deficits, or generalized developmental delays (Ghaziuddin 2018). Identifying a child with ASD is a challenging and complex process and demands astute assessment skills. Being alert to the risk factors that raise suspicion of ASD is an essential first step in developing screening proficiency. Even if the APRN does not have any immediate suspicions about a possible diagnosis of ASD in a child, any parental concern about a child's developmental progress should be explored and serve as a compelling reason to proceed with an appropriate evaluation and screening.

Some of the early developmental red flags that indicate a child is at risk for autism and needs further evaluation are:

- By 6 months: absence of smiling or warm joyful expressions
- By 9 months: absence of reciprocal sharing of sounds, smiles or facial expressions with caregiver
- By 12 months: lack of response when a child's name is called
- By 12 months: lack of babbling or baby talk
- By 12 months: lack of gestures such as pointing, reaching, showing or waving
- By 16 months: absence of single spoken words
- By 18 months: absence of pretend play
- By 24 months: lack of spontaneous, meaningful two-word phrases
- At any age: any sudden or gradual regression in development, or a loss of speech, babbling or social skills.

(American Academy of Child and Adolescent Psychiatry 2018; Smith et al. 2018). As children age, the red flags for autism become more diverse and typically relate to impairments in social interaction, communication difficulties, and inflexible behavior.

Impairments in Social Communication and Social Interactions

The APRN should be attentive to parental reports of a child who appears disinterested in interacting with family and peers, or seems unaware of what is going on around him, or seems unaware of other people's presence in the environment. Parents may describe the child as "in his own world." They might suspect the child is deaf, as he doesn't seem to hear when others talk to him. The child may be described as one who prefers to be alone and shows little interest in making friends. He may be perfectly content engaging in solitary or parallel play, rather than the cooperative play that is typical of his/her age group. He might not engage in group or pretend games, imitate others' actions or use toys appropriately. He may have trouble identifying and understanding the feelings of others as well as talking about the interests of others. Identifying and talking about his personal feelings is frequently difficult. He may have difficulty sharing his toys or playing in a group. Depending on where a child falls on the autism spectrum, he may be described as an "easy child," who demands little attention from caregivers. Others may be very prone to tantrums that can be easily triggered by a common sound or visual cue. The APRN may find it difficult to elicit eye contact or a social smile from the child while conducting a physical assessment or screening. Recent research indicates that early difficulties with making eye contact may be one of the strongest predictors of the eventual level of social disability in a child with ASD (Jones et al. 2008).

Any unexplained lack of progression in language or social skill development is a compelling indication for screening and diagnostic referral for ASD. "Twenty-five to thirty percent of children with ASD develop some vocabulary words, but then stop speaking or using gestures" (Johnson and Myers 2007, p. 1192). Other common, classic presentations of communication difficulties include delayed or absent language and engagement in "scripted speech," such as excerpts from favorite videos, songs, or TV programs. Echolalia or "parroting" may also be observed and can give a false impression of advanced language abilities. Spontaneous "pop up" words with no connection to the social context may be exhibited, as well as giant, run-on words, such as "whatisit?" or "idontknow" (Johnson and Myers 2007, p. 1192).

Restricted, Repetitive Patterns of Behavior

These behaviors are typically represented by engagement in a narrow repertoire of activities that are repetitive, self-stimulatory, ritualistic, and nonfunctional in nature. Examples include unusual finger movements, hand flapping, head banging, rocking back and forth, spinning in a circle, bruxism, and preoccupation with an object, such as a piece of string or a wheeled toy. The child may line up toys, spin objects or wheels of toys or repeat words, sounds or phrases. The child might be preoccupied with a topic, game, celebrity, or TV show.

These fixated interests are abnormal in their intensity or focus. Often, the initial presenting problem at a health maintenance or episodic visit may be parental and family frustration with the child's inflexibility, his unusual adherence to habits, rituals, and daily routines, which significantly interfere with family functioning. This child may become distressed at small changes in the environment or schedule, or have trouble transitioning between activities or exhibit rigid thinking patterns. Some of these routines are so bizarre or entrenched that families may go to extreme lengths to adapt or acquiesce to them to avoid embarrassment in public places or to minimize continuous emotional upheaval in the home environment. Some children have very rigid patterns of eating, resulting in a very restricted diet. Finally, the child with autism may express hyper or hypo reactivity to sensory input, such as an abnormal reaction to pain, odor, sound or texture. The child may seek specific sensory input such as excessive smelling, touching, or displaying a visual fascination with lights or movement.

Once a developmental concern that may represent ASD is identified, there are several valid and reliable tools in the public domain and available for purchase that the APRN can use to screen the child. These are listed in Table 16.1.

Physical Assessment and Examination

When ASD is suspected, the child must be referred for further diagnostic testing. The APRN should compile a summary of the history, including the mother's prenatal history, the birth history, and any significant newborn problems (e.g. low Apgar scores, hyperbilirubinemia, tremors, abnormal SaO_2 levels, etc.). The child's past and current health status, including an achievement or lack of achievement of growth and developmental milestones, including speech and hearing findings prior to the suspected diagnosis of ASD, should be assessed. The family history should be reviewed with the parent and included in the referral summary. A complete physical examination should be performed and appropriate laboratory work, including complete blood count (CBC) and lead levels. The physical examination may identify findings associated with an underlying comorbid medical condition that can accompany an ASD or represent a completely different underlying disorder. The referral report should include the growth charts, including head circumference data. Excessive head growth in the first year of life has been identified as a predictor of autism diagnosed later in life (Miles et al. 2000; Ozgen et al. 2013; Sacco et al. 2007). Thus, APRNs in primary care must carefully monitor and assess head circumference in the first year of life and if excessive head circumference is observed, the APRN should perform age-appropriate screenings and refer for early evaluation. However, only a small percentage of children with autism have frank macrocephaly (Filipek et al. 2000; Lainhart et al. 1997). Children with ASD may also exhibit microcephaly, which is associated with structural brain abnormalities, lower IQ, and seizure disorders (Miles et al. 2000).

Table 16.1 Screening tools for autism spectrum disorder

Screening Tool for Autism in Toddlers and young children (STAT)	24–36 months	https://vkc.mc.vanderbilt.edu/vkc/triad/stat
Social Communication Questionnaire (SCQ)	>3 years	https://www.wpspublish.com/store/p/2954/scq-social-communication-questionnaire
Social Responsiveness Scale (SRS)	School age	https://www.wpspublish.com/srs-social-responsiveness-scale
Autism Spectrum Screening Questionnaire	7–16 years	https://psychology-tools.com/test/autism-spectrum-screening-questionnaire
Childhood Autism Spectrum Test (CAST)	5–11 years	https://psychology-tools.com/test/cast
Gilliam Autism Rating Scale–2nd Edition (GARS-2)	3–22 years	www.pearsonassessments.com
Modified Checklist for Autism in Toddlers (M-CHAT)	16–30 months	https://m-chat.org
Communication and Symbolic Behavior Scales CSBS DP™ Infant-Toddler Checklist	Infants to preschool age	https://www.brookespublishing.com/product/csbs-dp-itc
Childhood Autism Rating Scale™, second edition	6 years and older	https://www.wpspublish.com/store/p/2696/Childhood-Autism-Rating-Scale%E2%84%A2,-Second-Edition-(CARS%E2%84%A2-2)

Although no single or cluster of phenotypic features have been identified in children with an ASD, research has identified some physical findings that are more likely to be noted in the older, at-risk child, including asymmetric facial features or a prominent forehead (Wright 2012). Ozgen et al. (2013) examined the morphological features of 244 children with autism in comparison to 244 control group children without autism and reported that facial asymmetry, multiple hair whorls, and prominent forehead significantly differentiated patients with autism from the control group. Earlier work showed that dysmorphic features in a male child, such as a long face and large ears, and pubertal onset of macroorchidism, are findings that are frequently seen in FXS, a sex chromosomal disorder. The syndrome was formerly thought to be a cause of ASD, but it is now recognized that although boys with FXS often have *symptoms* of ASD, the majority do not fully meet the criteria for actual diagnosis (Batshaw et al. 2007). Recent research indicates that only about 2% of boys with ASD also have FXS (Wassink et al. 2001).

Careful examination of the skin is necessary to identify the presence of any hypopigmented areas (i.e. ash leaf spots) using a hand-held ultraviolet light (Wood's lamp). Such cutaneous findings are associated with TS, a genetic, neurocutaneous disorder (Accordina et al. 2015). A significant number of children with TS have symptoms of autism (Batshaw et al. 2007).

On neurosensory examination, the APRN should carefully evaluate for fine and gross motor delays due to hypotonia and hyporeflexia, as well as gait abnormalities and poor motor coordination, which are noted in 25% of children with an ASD. These neuromotor findings tend to be more evident in autistic children who also have cognitive impairment (Filipek et al. 1999). Those without cognitive impairment typically attain motor milestones on time. Some children in this category may even exhibit *advanced* motor skills, developed as a compensatory mechanism to obtain desired objects without using gestural or expressive language. The examiner should also observe for motor stereotypies, such as hand flapping, finger mannerisms, unusual posturing, toe walking, and rocking, which are frequently seen as motor components of ASD but do not reflect true neurological abnormalities (Filipek et al. 2000). Children with ASD usually have normal structure and function of sensory organ systems. However, they often display great difficulty in processing and integrating the sensory input, which they receive through visual, auditory, olfactory, gustatory, and proprioceptive channels. This may be manifested during physical assessment when the child is exposed to unfamiliar sights, sounds, and touch, resulting in display of unusual motor behaviors and sounds in order to cope with heightened sensitivity to sensory input (Baranek et al. 2007). Cuvo et al. (2010) have outlined a full range of behavior modification techniques that can be used during the physical examination to gain fuller cooperation of the child and to enhance the accuracy of the assessment findings.

The Healthcare Encounter

Preparation of the child and family members for the physical examination of a child with suspected ASD or known to have ASD is a critical component for a successful healthcare visit for all, including the child, parent, and healthcare providers. Children with a diagnosis of ASD often experience a high level of anxiety in a pediatric practice or clinic setting and may display this high anxiety level behaviorally through hostile, violent displays of temperament (Hall and Graff 2012). Planning for the child and parent visit is a means of averting some of these difficult behaviors. The parents may know a time of day that best suits the child's temperament and plan the visit during that time frame. The parent should be advised to bring a favorite toy with the child to the visit. The parent should be asked to inform the medical and nursing staff of successful approaches that help to calm the child at home and in out-of-home environments. These preparations may make the pediatric healthcare visit a more relaxed visit for the anxious child (Al-Sharif et al. 2017). Once the visit is complete the APRN should document the successful strategies as well as unsuccessful strategies that occurred during the physical examination. Use of electronic devices, such as smartphones and tablets, have been reported as successful ways to distract the child with ASD during an examination or office procedure and should be considered for use during the examination (Vaz 2010).

To minimize the anxiety that the child with ASD may experience in a novel and unfamiliar environment, the APRN should familiarize himself/herself with techniques and strategies to smooth this transition. To deliver appropriate and effective healthcare, "the history, approach to the child, physical evaluation and treatment options must be considered *in the context* of the patient's diagnosis of an ASD" (Myers et al. 2007, p. 1167). A variety of useful approaches cited in the literature include:

- Working closely with parents or guardians *in advance* to gather information about the child's sensory sensitivities, behavioral triggers, and preferred transitional objects that may enhance the child's level of comfort and cooperation during the visit.
- Providing the parents with a written outline of what will occur during the visit and examination before the appointment.

- Suggesting that the child and parent visit the office or clinic setting and meet staff prior to the day of the actual visit. More than one visit may be required for a child who is very easily distressed by unfamiliar experiences.
- Allowing for extra time during the visit. This provides an opportunity for the child to become familiar with the examiner and the equipment before the examiner touches the child and also allows for a slower-paced examination. A nationally representative sample found that "children with ASD spent twice as much time with the healthcare provider per visit compared with children in control groups" (Liptak et al. 2006, p. 876).
- Utilizing consistent staff whenever possible.
- Instituting procedures to lessen the child's anxiety due to the unfamiliar environment and equipment, such as:

  ◦ Using visual cues and supports, such as showing a picture of an examining tool and allowing the child to handle this equipment before attempting to use it. Providing parents with pictures or photographs ahead of time allows them to prepare at home.
  ◦ Using an examination room that is quiet, softly lit, and free of clutter and extraneous equipment.
  ◦ Using a slow, steady pace that minimizes sudden movements or activity changes.
  ◦ Talking to the child before touching him.
  ◦ Allowing the child to handle and manipulate equipment, if appropriate and safe.
  ◦ Breaking down procedures into short, simple steps using succinct, developmentally appropriate language.
  ◦ Being honest about what is going to happen and if there will be discomfort (Cuvo et al. 2010; Inglese and Elder 2009; Myers et al. 2007).

Referral

If ASD is suspected after screening and comprehensive health assessment, the APRN should refer the child and family to a professional or agency that is experienced in making this diagnosis, such as an interdisciplinary early identification program, child psychiatrist or psychologist, developmental pediatrician, speech and language pathologist, or psychiatric-mental health APRN. While a screening or assessment tool provides valuable information, it is insufficient to make a diagnostic conclusion. Accurate diagnosis requires assimilating data from a variety of sources, using methods from multiple disciplines, including psychology, speech and language therapy, education, occupational therapy, etc. The end of this chapter contains referral resources that offer the services needed to evaluate a child suspected of having ASD.

Before a referral for a comprehensive diagnostic evaluation occurs, it is vital to arrange a family meeting to review assessment findings and recommendations and to discuss parents' perceptions and reactions. Such a meeting may yield a gamut of parental reactions, ranging from relief that their concerns have been validated to denial that the child is experiencing any difficulties at all. When a parent rejects evidence of a problem with the child it may take several interpretive sessions with the family before they are able to act on recommendations for further evaluation and intervention. The APRN who is understanding of the parents' concerns and supportive of parent questions offers opportunities for the parents to reconsider their fears of a definitive diagnosis of ASD.

The APRN who remains in contact via phone or email (per patient and APRN preferences) may enable the family to make the decision to seek the referral in the best interest of helping the child to begin appropriate educational (early intervention services) in a timely fashion to best meet the child's medical, psychological, social–emotional, and behavioral needs.

Laboratory and Diagnostic Investigations

If a full diagnostic appraisal is planned, the APRN may be asked to conduct certain laboratory and diagnostic tests and forward results to the health professional that will be conducting the ASD evaluation. Although there are no specific diagnostic or laboratory procedures to definitively identify a child with ASD, certain categories of laboratory tests are generally conducted to detect disorders that may present with autism-like behaviors or are known comorbid conditions associated with ASD. Such routine, baseline evaluations include lead screening, karyotype analysis, and molecular DNA testing for FXS. The American College of Medical Genetics also recommends testing for inborn errors of metabolism when there is a history of lethargy, recurrent vomiting, dysmorphic features, developmental regression, unknown or questionable newborn screening results, intellectual disabilities, or seizures of unknown origin (Barbaresi et al. 2006; Filipek et al. 1999). Referral to a genetic laboratory for fluorescent in situ hybridization (FISH) testing is also recommended if comorbid ID is already identified in the child. FISH testing can help identify chromosomal abnormalities that have been linked to ASD, including chromosomes X, 2, 3, 7, 11, 15, 17, and 22 (Johnson and Myers 2007). An EEG should be completed if a history of seizure activity is reported. Neuroimaging studies (magnetic resonance imaging, fMRI, single-photon emission computed tomography, positron emission tomography, and computed tomography) are reserved as research tools in the study of autism or if there are asymmetrical or abnormal findings on neurological examination (Johnson and Myers 2007).

Current Diagnostic Criteria

The American Psychiatric Association's *Diagnostic and Statistical Manual of Mental Disorders*, 5th edition (DSM-5; American Psychiatric Association [APA] 2013) recognizes a single autism spectrum grounded in two domains: (i) impairments in social communication/social interaction and (ii) restricted, repetitive patterns of behavior that impair everyday functioning (APA 2013). Regardless of culture, race, ethnicity, or socioeconomic status, the child must exhibit these core features (Lord et al. 2018). Current or past pervasive and sustained deficits in three distinct social communication areas are required: (i) social–emotional reciprocity, (ii) nonverbal communication, and (iii) developing, maintaining, and understanding relationships. The diagnostic requirement for restricted, repetitive patterns of behavior, interests, or activities includes current or past evidence of at least two of four features: (i) stereotyped or repetitive motor movements, use of objects, or speech, (ii) insistence on sameness, inflexible adherence to routines, or ritualized patterns of verbal or nonverbal behavior, (iii) highly restricted, fixated interests that are abnormal in intensity or focus, or (iv) hyper or hypo reactivity to sensory input or unusual interest in sensory aspects of the environment (APA 2013).

The severity of ASD may be context specific and change over time, requiring changing levels of support. A child who requires "very substantial support" (Level 3) shows severe deficits in communication, such as unintelligible speech, and rarely initiates interaction with other people. He is extremely rigid and has great difficulty coping with change in every context. A child who requires "substantial support" (Level 2) has marked deficits in social communication, such as communication restricted to a narrow special interest, or unusual response to social initiation from others. He is inflexible and has frequent difficulty coping with change in a variety of contexts. A child who "requires support" (Level 1) engages in communication with others but has difficulty making friends and typically fails at reciprocal conversation. His inflexibility interferes with functioning in one or more contexts (APA 2013).

Associated Conditions

Children diagnosed with ASD often display one or more associated psychiatric and/or medical conditions that are not associated with the core diagnostic features of ASD. The DSM-5 recognizes that ASD can co-occur with these conditions, such as genetic syndromes and psychiatric disorders (APA 2013).

Psychiatric Comorbidities

Comorbidity in ASD is common and contributes to a child's overall level of impairment and need for services. In a population-based study of children with ASD traits in Norway, Posserud et al. (2018) found that "autism-plus" is more common than "autism-only." A study conducted by Leyfer et al. (2006) using the Autism Co-morbidity Interview identified 72% of their patient sample with at least one psychiatric disorder in addition to the primary diagnosis of autism. Clinic-based studies suggest that at least 70% of individuals with ASD also have additional psychiatric disorders. Clinical assessment for comorbid conditions should be suspected when the core features do not explain all of a child's symptoms, the child does not respond to therapeutic interventions as expected, or there is a significant change from baseline (Belardinelli et al. 2016).

1. *Intellectual disability*: ID is not an essential diagnostic feature of autism, but many individuals with ASD have intellectual and/or language impairments. As of the most recent prevalence study conducted by the Autism & Developmental Disabilities Monitoring Network at the CDC. They studied the records of 5108 children aged 8 years with ASD. Data from 2016 revealed that 33% of the children for whom IQ scores were available were classified in the range of ID (IQ <70), 24% were in the borderline range (IQ 71–85), and 42% had IQ scores in the average to above average range (i.e. IQ >85) (Maenner et al. 2020, CDC 2019).

2. *Attention deficit hyperactivity disorder (ADHD)*: It is estimated that approximately 30–80% of children with ASD have co-occurring ADHD (Belardinelli et al. 2016; Mahajan et al. 2012; van der Meer et al. 2012). As of DSM-5, children can be diagnosed with both ASD and ADHD, and therefore can be treated "on label" with regard to medications that treat ADHD (Baribeau and Anagnostou 2014a).

3. *Depressive disorders*: The reported prevalence of depression in ASD varies from 0.9% to 10%. In a study of 109 children with ASD aged 5–17 conducted by Leyfer et al. (2006), almost 25% of the sample met lifetime diagnostic criteria for a depressive episode significant enough to impair daily functioning.

4. *Anxiety disorders*: There is considerable evidence that children and adolescents with ASD are at increased risk of anxiety disorders. In a meta-analysis of 31 studies involving 2121 young people with ASD almost 40% had at least one comorbid

anxiety disorder, the most frequent being specific phobia (29.8%) followed by OCD (17.4%) and social anxiety disorder (16.6%) (van Steensel et al. 2011). Symptoms associated with anxiety can significantly interfere with the child's functioning at home, at school, and in the community and exacerbate the core deficits of ASD (Reaven 2009). Clues that an anxiety disorder may coexist with ASD include fears and worries that are out of proportion to a situation, symptoms that increase in frequency, duration, and intensity over time, and symptoms that are not responsive to normal reassurances (Reaven 2009). The development of irrational fears in children with ASD is a common finding. Specific phobias occur more frequently than social phobias, and prevalence has been estimated to range from 44% to 64% of children with autism (Leyfer et al. 2006). Fear of loud sounds is one of the most frequently noted phobias in the ASD population (Leyfer et al. 2006).

5. *OCD*: Although symptoms of generalized anxiety disorder, social phobia, and separation anxiety tend to be similar, the symptoms associated with OCD are felt to be qualitatively different. An individual with OCD has persistent, illogical, and obsessive thoughts and ideas that cannot be suppressed and are often associated with repetitive behaviors or mental acts, such as checking and rechecking, counting, hoarding, and maintaining symmetry and order within the environment. Rituals common to autism are seen as more likely to be rewarding and pleasurable for the child and are engaged in voluntarily (Belardinelli et al. 2016). Leyfer et al. (2006) note that in reviewed studies, the rate of OCD in children with ASD ranged from 1.5% to 81%.

6. *Challenging behaviors*: Challenging behaviors are not part of the diagnostic criteria of ASD but are often very common and one reason parents seek professional help. These behaviors can include self-injury, physical aggression, property destruction, defiance, tantrums, running away, extreme irritability, and inappropriate behavior in public (O'Nions et al. 2018). Children who present with one or more of these challenging behaviors negatively impact the relationship with their parents, siblings, and peers, and adversely impact their ability to attend to learning in classroom and home environments.

Medical Comorbidities

1. *Sleep Disturbances*: Sleep disturbances are a frequently reported problem in children with ASD at all levels of functioning. Prevalence estimates range from 44% to 83% and include difficulties with prolonged sleep latency, restless sleep, insistence on co-sleeping, and frequent awakenings (Wiggs and Stores 2004; Williams et al. 2004). Research evidence supports screening all children with ASD for sleep disturbances during each annual and episodic visit. Children with suspected sleep apnea warrant additional testing and should be referred to a sleep specialist for polysomnography (Ivanenko and Johnson 2008). Positive screening results should lead to a clinical diagnosis of a functional sleep disorder and formulation of an individualized treatment plan. Interventions to restore more normal sleep patterns in the child with an ASD are crucial, as sleep deprivation and disruption inevitably contribute an added stressor to already stressed families (Doo and Wing 2006).

2. *Fragile X syndrome*: FXS is an X-linked disorder that is the most common inherited cause of intellectual disabilities. The term "fragile" was assigned to this condition because of the appearance of an easily broken site at the distal end of the long arm of the X chromosome on karyotype analysis. It is estimated that FXS is a comorbidity in 5% of individuals with autism (Caglayan 2010). Caglayan (2010) further reports that it has been estimated that approximately 90% of males with FXS "exhibit one or more of the three major characteristics of autism, such as difficulties with social interaction, lack of eye contact, social anxiety and avoidance, perseverative speech, stereotypic behavior, hypersensitivity to sensory stimuli, impulsive aggression or self injurious behavior" (p. 131).

3. *Tuberous Sclerosis*: TS is an autosomal dominant, neurocutaneous disorder caused by the *TSC1* and *TSC2* genes on chromosome 16 that code for the protein tuberin. It is estimated that 1–4% of individuals with ASD have TS (Batshaw et al. 2007). Affected children display a range of features, depending on the penetrance of the gene, including adenoma sebaceum, hypopigmented skin lesions (ash leaf spots), seizures, and benign growths or tubers, which can affect the brain, skin, and major organs. Mild to moderate ID often accompanies this disorder when tuberous growths develop in the brain.

4. *Epilepsy*: The reported prevalence of seizures in children diagnosed with ASD varies widely in the literature, ranging from 11% to 39% (Barbaresi et al. 2006; Myers et al. 2007; Peacock et al. 2009). Barbaresi et al. (2006) report that onset of seizures in individuals with autism peaks in early childhood and adolescence. Although all classifications

of seizure types may be seen, complex partial seizures with a temporal lobe focus seem to be most prevalent. There is also increased likelihood of a child with ASD demonstrating an abnormal EEG pattern without the occurrence of clinical seizure activity (Batshaw et al. 2007).

5. *Tic Disorders*: Up to 9% of children with ASD also have motor or vocal tics (Ringman and Jankovic 2000). If tic behavior persists for at least 1 year, an associated diagnosis of Tourette's syndrome can be ascribed to the child. The co-occurrence of tic disorders in children with diagnosed ASD has also been linked to an increased risk of developing more complex psychiatric symptomatology (Gadow and DeVincent 2005).

Interventions and Plan

The ideal intervention for youth with ASD is individualized and treats each child's complex and unique set of communicative, behavioral, sensory, and cognitive characteristics. There is no cure, but intervention can improve quality of life and bring about substantial improvement in symptoms. Treatment must be intensive and may involve a multidisciplinary team of professionals and therapists. Most health professionals agree that the earlier the intervention, the better the prognosis. Unfortunately, the nature of the disorder has attracted many controversial and unproven treatments, and parents should use caution before adopting such approaches. APRNs are in prime positions to help parents evaluate potential treatments and develop a treatment plan.

Interventions for Social Communication Deficits

If a child is not diagnosed with ASD prior to the age of 4 or 5, the prekindergarten physical examination or the prekindergarten school screening test may be the first time that a differential diagnosis of ASD is considered by the primary care APRN. If the child received a possible diagnosis of ASD in the preschool years, the parents may have been hopeful that early intervention services would prepare the child for regular kindergarten. If the child is physically well, most often the child only has primary care visits annually beginning at the age of 3, thus the primary care APRN may suddenly be confronted with parents who are baffled with the educational system and are questioning what may happen to the child. The primary care APRN may be assessing the child for the first time in the pediatric office as the child may be a new patient or a child who has just entered the foster care system.

The primary care APRN will make referrals to the school system if the child is over 3 years old; the children then receive special services within the school system. The APRN may also refer the child for a neurodevelopmental examination with a pediatric developmental specialist and/or a psychiatrist or psychiatric APRN. Specific interventions for the child will be based on the assessment findings and the specific diagnosis.

It is imperative for parents to understand that acquisition of useful spoken language by children with a diagnosis of ASD requires intensive and lengthy educational processes that often have less than optimal outcomes (Goldstein 2002; Howlin and Rutter 1989). Children may have higher IQs and understandable language; however, the child's language skills may not "fit" normal conversation patterns and may not be socially acceptable. Speech patterns and language development for a child with a diagnosis of ASD also vary significantly as the child may use a few words or gestures or may have a severe deficit and no spoken language.

Since language proficiency and IQ have been shown to be related to the outcomes for children with ASD (Venter et al. 1992), a significant amount of research has focused on acquisition of spoken language (Rogers et al. 2006). However, results of long-term outcome studies conducted in the late 1980s and 1990s in children with a classic diagnosis of autism have estimated that between one-third and two-thirds of children with ASD never acquire spoken language (Charlop et al. 1985; Frankel et al. 1987; Weitz et al. 1997) and that 80% of children with a diagnosis of autism have no spoken language or only exhibit self-stimulatory or echolalic utterances when they enter kindergarten (Bondy and Frost 1994; Kraijer 1999). These studies are the underpinnings of the treatment for children with a diagnosis of ASD after the 1990s, when interventions for children with ASD have intensively focused on helping children acquire language skills (Rogers et al. 2006). Thus, both primary care and mental health APRNs are confronted with helping parents cope with a child who has ubiquitous speech problems. It is helpful for APRNs to understand the types of interventions that have been tested in children with a diagnosis of ASD and those that lend evidence of success; today, parents are internet savvy and may raise questions about programs that may or may not be available or applicable to their child, and the parents will need guidance from the APRN to understand the current best available evidence to help their child.

Early models for speech development focused on applying learning theory principles within a behavioral developmental context (Rogers et al. 2006). The "discrete trial teaching" described in 1964 used adult-delivered instruction in massed trials in which the children were taught to respond to simple instructions from the adult through the imitation of manual, oral motor, and vocal behavior and then to imitate speech (Wolf et al. 1964). A second developmental model described in 1968 (Hart and Risley 1968, 1980; Prizant and Wetherby 1998) used a child-initiated behavior followed by adult response of providing the child with the child-requested object, which was viewed as a "natural reinforcer." Both of these developmental approaches to speech acquisition have been found to be effective in a number of independent replications (Goldstein 2002; Koegel 2000). However, both of these approaches required a minimum of 1 year of treatment involving 25–40 hours of intervention each week in both educational and home settings.

The need to study more efficient ways to help children acquire spoken language resulted in researchers designing and testing methods that use language within the context of social interactions. An example of this approach is the Picture Exchange Communication System (PECS) (Frost and Bondy 2002). Children are taught to approach a picture of a desired item, then to give the picture to a communication partner in exchange for receiving the item. In an experimentally controlled study, Carr and Felce (2007) investigated the effect of implementing PECS as a teaching strategy. After 15 hours of PECS training over a period of 4–5 weeks, 5 of 24 children in the treatment group showed increases in speech production in either initiating communication or responding to staff or in both communicating and responding.

The Early Start Denver Model (Rogers et al. 2000), an early intervention program for children 12–60 months of age, has been shown to improve cognition, language skills, social abilities, and adaptive behavior in children with ASD.

Children have a combination of once-weekly 50-minute therapy sessions and daily home review by the parent. Teaching strategies include motivating social games, teaching imitation of actions on objects, focus on receptive understanding, object associations, increasing verbal approximations of target words, and including reinforcement at each stage of learning (Rogers et al. 2000, 2006). Dawson et al. (2010) randomly assigned 48 children diagnosed with ASD between 18 and 30 months of age to one of two groups: (i) Early Start Denver Model intervention or (ii) intervention commonly available in the community. Compared with children who received community intervention, children who received Early Start Denver Model (ESDM) showed significant improvements in IQ, adaptive behavior, and autism diagnosis. Children that receive the ESDM require fewer services in the years following intervention and thereby lowered overall health-related costs (Cidav et al. 2017).

Other researchers have suggested that part of the mechanism involving speech impairment in children with autism includes an oral motor dysfunction (Adams 1998; Page and Boucher 1998). The Prompts for Restructuring Oral Muscular Phonetic Targets (PROMPT) model was designed based on the interrelationships of developing speech motor control with integration of sensory modalities and the enhancement of social-emotional interactions.

Rogers et al. (2006) investigated the effectiveness of the Denver Model and the PROMPT model on speech acquisition in 10 nonverbal children with a diagnosis of autism that were matched in pairs and randomized to treatment. At the end of 12 weeks in which the children received 1-hour weekly sessions of therapy and daily 1-hour home interventions from the parents, 8 of the 10 children used five or more functional words spontaneously and spoke multiple times per hour by the end of the treatment program.

APRNs must relay to the parents the significance of daily parental involvement in the home environment. Research evidence suggests that parents who work closely with the classroom teachers and speech therapists by continuing the educational curriculum for speech development at home on a daily basis see greater improvements in language acquisition for their children (Rogers et al. 2000).

Interventions for Social Skill Development

In the past decade there has been a significant increase in the amount of research on social skills interventions for those with ASD (Reichow and Volkmar 2008). Comparisons of the efficacy of different training strategies are beginning (Reichow and Volkmar 2008; Wang and Spillane 2009; White et al. 2007). Several researchers have identified interventions which are best supported by scientific evidence for implementation for children with ASD to improve learning outcomes and social behaviors, as well as communication skills (Lindgren and Doobay 2011).

Applied behavior analysis (ABA) has been shown to be an effective technique for children with ASD. The interventions are led by a trained behavioral psychologist and involve prevention and correction of problem behaviors. Parents are trained to work with their child using strategies to reduce problem behaviors and build social skills (Lindgren and Doobay 2011). Social skill interventions should be individualized and focused on the unique characteristics of the specific child (Bellini and Peters 2008). Researchers at the Indiana Resource Center for Autism have published a framework to assess and intervene for social skill development in children with ASD (Bellini and Peters 2008). The five-step model includes (i) assessing for individual social functioning, which includes an evaluation of the child's current level of social functioning, (ii) distinguishing between skill acquisition and performance deficits, which distinguishes skill acquisition deficit as the absence of a particular skill or behavior as compared with performance deficit, which postulates that the child has the skill but does not perform the skill, (iii) selecting appropriate intervention strategies, which are highlighted below, (iv) implementing the intervention, and (v) evaluating and monitoring the progress toward achieving the social skills (Bellini 2006).

There is good evidence that interventions to directly train social skills can be effective. The use of peer-mediated interventions to build social skills has also been shown to be evidence-based and effective (Lindgren and Doobay 2011).

Common social skill interventions include those described in the following sections.

Direct Instruction

Individual and group instruction programs are child specific and typically focus on developing basic interpersonal skills, conversational dialogue, play and friendship skills, social problem solving, and emotion processing (Bellini 2006; Coucouvanis 2005; Krasny et al. 2003). Strategies include prompting, coaching, role modeling, role play, scripting, structured teaching, guided activities, and feedback. While promising, these strategies and programs require further study to determine treatment efficacy (Reichow and Volkmar 2008).

Video Modeling

An emerging strategy is video modeling (Bellini and Akullian 2007). Using the child or other designated models, including commercially prepared videos, the child learns by observing and imitating the social behaviors of those depicted in the video. This approach has promise as a highly effective intervention (Lindgren and Doobay 2011; Wang and Spillane 2009;

Use of a Social Story™

A social story (Gray 2000) describes a situation, skill, or concept in narrative format. It includes a clear description of the situation, the perspective of others in that same situation, and a statement of desired social response from the child. Social Stories™ require more study of treatment effectiveness (Wang and Spillane 2009).

Peer-mediated Intervention

Peer-mediated intervention strategies train nondisabled peers as buddies, mentors, and playmates. Usually

classmates, trained peers initiate interactions and respond appropriately to children with ASD in structured and natural environments (Bellini 2006). This intervention has support and should be considered a recommended practice for all individuals with autism (Reichow and Volkmar 2008).

Computer-aided Instruction

Computer-aided instruction has been shown to be an effective strategy for children with ASD to support the development of both communication and academic skills (Lindgren and Doobay 2011).

Interventions for Challenging Behaviors

In addition to social communication deficits and restrictive repetitive behaviors and interests, many children with ASD engage in challenging behavior. Such behaviors can cause harm to the child or others, result in damage to objects or disrupt the expected routines at home, at school or in the community. Managing children with problem behaviors places a considerable burden on the family (O'Nions et al. 2018). Challenging behaviors may include, but are not limited to, nonsuicidal self-injury, aggression, destruction of property, hazardous actions, sexually inappropriate behaviors, emotion dysregulation, and repetitive or compulsive acts. The increased prevalence of ASD has intensified the demand for effective treatments for autism, including challenging behaviors. Intervention science is now providing evidence about which practices and behavioral interventions are effecive (National Autism Center 2015; Wong et al. 2014).

Currently there are many behavioral interventions with sufficient evidence to demonstrate favorable outcomes. Known as effective interventions they are typically used to reduce problem behaviors and increase the likelihood of successfully teaching functional alternative behaviors. They include modifying the variables or situational events that precede a target behavior and making changes to the environment after a target behavior has occurred. Such programs may use basic principles of behavior change, such as modeling, prompting, positive reinforcement, extinction, and behavior rehearsal (National Autism Center 2015; Wong et al. 2014).

Comprehensive behavioral treatment programs for young children (ages 0–9) target essential skills and use techniques derived from ABA to increase communication, social, and pre-academic skills, and to reduce problem behaviors. Techniques might include discrete trial teaching, incidental teaching, errorless learning, shaping, and modeling. These programs of individualized instruction provide intensive services that are typically 25–40 hours a week for 2–3 years (National Autism

Center 2015). The University of California at Los Angeles Young Autism Program by Lovaas and colleagues (Lovaas 1987; Smith et al. 2000), and the Denver model designed by Rogers and colleagues (Rogers et al. 2000) are two examples of such programs. Often covered by healthcare insurance, the APRN should become familiar with the specialized behavioral treatment programs in his/her practice area.

Environmental engineering is a strategy that has shown success in altering the future likelihood of challenging behaviors (Horner et al. 2002). Strategies include changing the physical characteristics of the environment in which the child plays, learns, and interacts with others, altering schedules, reorganizing social groups at home and school, and using curricula adjustment to meet the individual needs of the child (Carr et al. 1994, 1999). Often parents modify the environment by limiting the child's exposure to aversive sensory stimuli, such as crowds, noisy events or feared stimuli. They might limit social activities and outings to reduce the risk of an outburst. Some parents stick to fixed routines to reduce the risk of problem behavior or use picture schedules or lists to inform the child about upcoming activities or changes in the schedule (O'Nions et al. 2018).

Structured teaching using the Treatment and Education of Autistic and related Communication-handicapped Children (TEACCH) method (Mesibov 1997; Mesibov et al. 2005) has shown promise as a comprehensive intervention. A meta-analysis of 13 studies demonstrated moderate to large gains in social behavior and maladaptive behavior (Virues-Ortega et al. 2013). Elements of structured teaching include organizing the physical environment, predictable sequences of activities, and visually structured activities (Myers et al. 2007).

Managing complex challenging behaviors is often stressful for families. The APRN can support parents in their efforts by connecting the family with the appropriate service providers. In addition, any acute exacerbation of challenging behaviors should be investigated by the APRN for possible medical causes such as infections and conditions that cause pain, such as otitis media, pharyngitis, dental abscesses, urinary tract infections, or onset of menstrual cycle in an adolescent (Myers et al. 2007).

Interventions for Sleep Problems

Individualized treatment plans are formulated based on the child's presenting sleep disturbance, the length of time the sleep disturbance has persisted, the pattern of the disturbance, the sleep environment, the effect on parents and all household members, previous treatments, and their impact on the problem. Treatment plans may include behavioral interventions, medication,

herbal treatments, massage therapy, or a combination of two or more of these modalities (Ivanenko and Johnson 2008; Polimeni et al. 2005). Reports of treatment success or failure are limited since the majority of the studies on treatment outcomes for sleep disturbances in children with ASD and especially autism are limited by sample size or individual case reports (Escalona et al. 2001; Ivanenko and Johnson 2008; Polimeni et al. 2005; Weiskop et al. 2001, 2005).

Behavioral interventions may focus on a gradual reduction of previously established excessive bedtime rituals, strategies to reduce and eliminate tantrums, consistent reinforcement and appropriate rewards, calming parental behaviors (i.e. speaking calmly), and a calm environment (calm background music) at least half an hour before the established bedtime (Escalona et al. 2001; Ivanenko and Johnson 2008; Polimeni et al. 2005; Weiskop et al. 2001, 2005). More recent biological research on sleep–wake cycles has the potential to contribute to affective interventions for children with ASD. Future research studies that investigate the establishment of a new pattern for sleep through activation of the suprachiasmatic nucleus (Fuller et al. 2006), for example by dimming lights prior to sleep followed by exposure to bright light immediately after awakening, may hold promise for changing the physiological mechanisms of the sleep–wake cycle in children. Medications for the treatment of insomnia may be prescribed and reevaluated 1 and 3 months after the initiation (see Chapter 9).

Psychopharmacology Interventions Specific to the ASD Population

At present there are no medications approved to treat the core symptoms of ASD, although psychopharmacology agents are used in this population. Among 33 565 commercially insured children with ASD, 64% had a filled prescription for at least one psychotropic medication while 35% had evidence of two or more classes, and 15% used medications from three or more classes concurrently (Spencer et al. 2013). Researchers studied two cohorts of 46 943 commercially insured and 46 696 Medicaid-insured subjects with ASD for the calendar year 2014. Sixty four percent of the commercially insured subjects and 69% of the Medicaid insured subjects received psychotropic medication treatment. In both cohorts, a large proportion of individuals received treatment even without a diagnosis of a second psychiatric comorbidity (commercial 31%, Medicaid 33%).

Psychiatric medications are typically used to treat severe and sustained behaviors that are negatively impacting the child's ability to participate in daily activities. Such agents may be used when other treatment approaches have failed to adequately improve symptoms. They are also used to treat coexisting psychiatric disorders, such as depression, ADHD, OCD, or Tourette's. In general, reasons for prescribing medication include irritability, aggression, temper outbursts, self-injurious behavior, hyperactivity, poor attention span, poor impulse control, anxiety, fears, obsessive phenomena, rituals, compulsions, tics, depressed mood, and sleep problems (Baribeau and Anagnostou 2014a).

The response to medications is often different than for typically developing children, requiring lower dosages and slower titration (Table 16.2). Before initiating medication treatment, the APRN should carefully identify and assess the specific problem or symptom to be treated and the degree of interference with daily functioning. If the presenting problem is within the APRN's scope of practice, the next step is to determine the frequency, intensity, and duration of the problem and any exacerbating factors, such as illness, setting, time of day, recurrent event, or coexisting condition. The response to previously tried behavioral intervention should be reviewed and a system to monitor the target behavior and adverse events at baseline and at regular intervals developed (see Chapter 20).

Atypical Antipsychotic Agents

Only two atypical antipsychotic agents (aripiprazole and risperidone) are licensed by the Food and Drug Administration (FDA) for the symptomatic treatment of irritability in children and teens with autism aged 6–17. Risperidone is the most studied second-generation antipsychotic agent in ASD and has been found to be effective in decreasing severe tantrums, aggression, and self-injurious behavior (Cauffield 2013; Scahill et al. 2007). Aripiprazole is used to treat similar behaviors.

In addition to the risk of dyskinesia, one of the principal safety concerns with atypical antipsychotic medication is increased appetite and weight gain (Baribeau and Anagnostou 2014a; McCracken 2005). Children taking these agents are at greater risk for developing later health problems. Therefore, atypical antipsychotics should only be considered if behavioral interventions have been tried and failed or if the safety concerns related to problem behaviors exceed the risk of harmful effects of medication. Prior to beginning medication management, the APRN should document family history of diabetes, dyslipidemia, and cardiac disease. The APRN should assess the child's height, weight, and body mass index (BMI) and determine the total caloric intake needed to maintain a normal growth pattern. The APRN must evaluate the child's diet and lifestyle to identify needed changes, while also monitoring height, weight, and abdominal girth at every visit. Monitoring also includes fasting plasma glucose, fasting lipid panel, blood pressure, and pulse at baseline, 3 months, and every 6 months (Correll 2008).

Dietary modifications frequently include the following: replace sugar-containing drinks with water, dilute fruit juice, replace soft drinks with sparkling water mixed with a small amount of juice, increase fresh fruits, vegetables, and fiber whenever possible, choose low-fat products, and monitor serving sizes and portions. Finally, reduce and preferably eliminate the consumption of sugared candy and treats. Lifestyle modifications include increasing exercise such as jumping on a trampoline, swimming, walking, riding bikes, or playing chase games while reducing time spent in sedentary activities.

When ongoing treatment with an atypical antipsychotic medication is indicated and there is concern for weight gain, the addition of metformin may be indicated (Handen et al. 2017).

Another side effect of risperidone is an elevated prolactin level. Hyperprolactinemia may cause gynecomastia, galactorrhea, irregular menses, amenorrhea, sexual dysfunction, and reduced fertility (Roke et al. 2009). Serum prolactin levels should be monitored every 6 months. Antipsychotic-induced hyperprolactinemia can be treated by reducing the dose or switching to a prolactin-sparing antipsychotic, such as quetiapine or ziprasidone (Roke et al. 2009).

Selective Serotonin Reuptake Inhibitors

Selective serotonin reuptake inhibitors (SSRIs) are commonly used off-label in children with ASD when a child develops symptoms of a major depression, anxiety, or OCD (Baribeau and Anagnostou 2014a), yet evidence from research has yielded mixed and often disappointing results (Cauffield 2013; Siegel and Beaulieu 2012). Open-label and retrospective studies suggest improvement in overall global functioning and in a wide range of symptoms (anxiety, aggression, repetitive behavior), but a recent analysis found no evidence that SSRIs are effective in treating autism (Williams et al. 2010).

A major concern in treating children and teens with SSRIs is the risk of activation. Activation events include irritability, anger outbursts, excitability, manic symptoms, hyperactivity, agitation, nervousness, sleep disturbance lability, and hostility. Mood must be monitored very closely and it may take up to 8–10 weeks to achieve moderate total daily doses. Mood lability, difficulty settling at night, irritability, and mild agitation may be signs of an activation syndrome (McCracken 2005). The decision to treat conditions that accompany ASD, such as OCD or depression, with an SSRI should be made on an individual basis (Baribeau and Anagnostou 2014a; Williams et al. 2010). The best responders may be those with ASD who do not have high levels of agitation or mood cycling at baseline. If activation occurs, reduce the dose and slow further titration.

Table 16.2 Psychopharmacology and ASD

Drug	Target behavior(s)	Dosing	Adverse effects
Antipsychotics			
Risperidone[a]	Irritability (aggression, agitation, temper outbursts, self-injurious behavior)	Initiation dose 0.25 mg daily Expected range 0.5–3 mg daily	Weight gain Note: Provide healthy lifestyle instruction at every visit
SSRIs			
Fluoxetine[b]	Major depression, OCD anxiety	Initiation dose Child: 2.5–5 mg daily Teen: 5 mg daily	Activation: agitation, insomnia, increased activity, increased anxiety, mood lability
		Initial target Child: 10–20 mg Teen: 10–20 mg Expected range Child: 5–40 mg Teen: 10–60 mg	To avoid activation: Initiate with very low starting doses Titrate very gradually, much slower than for a typical child/adult Nausea, vomiting sedation
Sertraline[b]	OCD anxiety	Initiation dose Child: 10–25 mg Teen: 25–50 mg Initial target Child: 50 mg Teen: 50 mg Expected range Child: 50–150 mg Teen: 50–200 mg Increase doses at 1–2 week intervals	Be aware of CAM use
Fluvoxamine[b]	OCD anxiety	Initiation dose Child: 25 mg Teen: 25–50 mg Initial target Child: 150 mg Teen: 200 mg Expected range Child: 50–200 mg Teen: 100–300 mg Divide doses >50 mg Increase by 25 mg every 1–2 weeks	
Stimulants			
Methylphenidate[c]	Hyperactivity Impulsivity Inattention		Higher than expected rate of adverse events (10% vs. <2% in typical kids) Irritability, increased aggression, insomnia, anorexia, increased stereotypic behavior

[a] FDA approved for children with autism aged 5–17.
[b] FDA approved for children with major depression/OCD.
[c] FDA approved for children with ADHD.
Source: From Gleason, M.M., Egger, H.L., Emslie, G.J., Greenhill, L.L., Kowatch, R.A., Lieberman, A.F.,. . .Zeanah, C.H. (2007). Psychopharmacological treatment for very young children: contexts and guidelines. Journal of the American Academy of Child and Adolescent Psychiatry, 46, 1532–72; and McCracken, J.T. (2005). Safety issues with drug therapies for autism spectrum disorders. The Journal of Clinical Psychiatry, 66(Suppl 10), 32–37.

Stimulants

Stimulants are used in children with ASD to treat comorbid ADHD or significantly disruptive hyperactive, inattentive, or impulsive behavior (Baribeau and Anagnostou 2014b). Clinical studies with methylphenidate suggest that 50% of children with ASD show a positive response versus 75% of typical children with ADHD. The mean improvement is 20–25% versus 50% in typical children with ADHD (Scahill and Pachler 2007). There are no data on long-term treatment with stimulants in children with ASD.

Children with ASD may have increased sensitivity to adverse effects of stimulants, and therefore short-acting formulations are sometimes recommended first in order to evaluate tolerability (Cauffield 2013). The major concerns are loss of appetite, increased agitation and irritability, tic onset, and sleep disturbance. To improve tolerance, use lower doses, longer titration periods, and extended release preparations (McCracken 2005).

Complementary and Alternative Medicine Interventions

Despite limited evidence to support use, complementary and alternative medicine (CAM) agents are widely used to treat children with ASD (DeFilippis 2018; Goel et al. 2018; Höfer et al. 2017; Levy and Hyman 2015). Special diets and dietary supplements (including vitamins) are the most frequently used treatments, likely due to easy accessibility (Höfer et al. 2017). Families who use CAM are likely to use more than one agent (Levy and Hyman 2015). Because of the pervasive use of CAM, it is prudent for the nurse practitioner to know the current evidence regarding the use of CAM treatments and to inquire about CAM use with families. Presently there is insufficient empirical data supporting or refuting claims of "cure" or even improvement and the available data are inadequate to guide treatment recommendations (Goel et al. 2018; Höfer et al. 2017; Lindly et al. 2017). In addition, the FDA specifically warns against the use of chelation therapy, hyperbaric oxygen

Table 16.3 Common CAM treatments for ASD

Biologically based treatments		
Treatment	Purpose	Method
Special diets	Treat gastrointestinal problems that are believed to cause autism	Gluten-free, casein-free, sugar-free Specific carbohydrate and yeast-free
Antifungal agents, probiotics, digestive enzymes	Reduce presumed fungal infections in the intestine	Tablet, powder
Antiviral agents, intravenous immunoglobulins	Modulate the immune system	Intravenous
Chelation therapy	Removes heavy metals from the body	Intravenous
Hyperbaric oxygen therapy	Increases oxygen levels in the brain	High-pressure chamber
Vitamin and mineral supplements: B6 (pyridoxine) and magnesium, B12, DMG (dimethylglycine), C and D, fish oil/essential fatty acids	Modulate neurotransmitter production/brain development/presumed deficiency to improve behavior, speech, learning and eye contact	Tablet, pill, powder, cream, liquid, gel, injection
Nonbiologically based treatments		
Auditory integration training	Treats sound sensitivity	Exposure to sound via earphones
Vision therapy	Affects visual scrutiny	Eye exercises, prism lens
Sensory integration therapy	Facilitates the nervous system's ability to process and modulate sensory input	Brushing, weighted vest, swinging, jumping, body sock, massage, joint compression
Animal therapy	Improves social and relationship skills	Interacting with animals

Source: From Hanson, E., Kalish, L.A., Bunce, E., Curtis, C., McDaniel, S., Ware, J., & Petry, J. (2007). Use of complementary and alternative medicine among children diagnosed with autism spectrum disorder. Journal of Autism and Development Disorders, 37, 628-36; Levy, S. & Hyman, S. (2015). Complementary and alternative medicine treatments for children with autism spectrum disorders. Child and Adolescent Psychiatric Clinics of North America, 24, 117–143; and Association for Science in Autism Treatment website: http://www.asatonline.org/intervention/treatments.desc.htm.

therapy, and detoxifying clay baths because of the improper claims about these methods of treatment and the significant health risks associated with them (US Food and Drug Administration 2017).

Common CAM treatments for children with ASD are listed in Table 16.3.

APRN best practices include the following:

- Be aware that families will use CAM.
- Inquire what treatments are being used.
- Provide unbiased information and advice.
- Identify risks and potential harmful effects.
- Monitor for interaction of therapies.
- Maintain open communication.
- Critically evaluate the scientific merits of treatments and share the information with parents (Levy and Hyman 2015; Myers et al. 2007).

Integration with Primary Care

ASDs are pervasive, chronic conditions that do not remit with the passage of time. There is no known cure. Treatment requires multimodal collaboration from numerous professionals, including those in medical, educational, mental health, and specialty-based settings.

Consumers report confidence and trust in the care provided by nurses, and nurses are cited as the most trusted health professionals (http://www.medicalnewstoday.com/articles/173627.php). Historically, APRNs are essential professionals in the management of chronic conditions. They are likely to comprehend the context within which a child and family live, thus lending an understanding of their specific needs and how to address them. A partnership between psychiatric and pediatric APRNs can offer considerable leadership and guidance to the family struggling with ASD. Such a team of APRNs is in a unique position to provide counseling, support, ongoing education, recommendations, referrals, advocacy, and case management throughout the life span of the individual with ASD.

Over the past several years, there have been numerous calls to integrate behavioral and mental health services into primary care practices (Substance Abuse and Mental Health Service Administration 2014). Children with ASD require extended care for office visits and often specialty care with a behavioral or mental health specialist. The primary care setting is an ideal place to offer these services to children, their parents, and their siblings. Primary care providers screen children at or before 18 months old using the Modified Checklist for Autism in Toddlers (M-CHAT-R/F)-Revised, with Follow-Up tool (National Institute of Health 2013). This tool detects possible signs of ASD and, when positive, the parent and child can be immediately referred for an evaluation and early onset interventions which may decrease some of the

parental stress and increase some of the communication and social skills of the child (Hallas 2019).

Implications for Practice, Research, and Education

With 1 in 59 children affected by ASD (Center for Disease Control 2018a), all APRNs need to be prepared for the unique challenges and great diversity of these children. Parents and professionals are faced with difficult decisions when choosing treatments. Clinical practice guidelines are now available for the management of individuals diagnosed within the autistic spectrum disorder of neurodevelopmental disorders (CDC 2019). Early intervention is crucial as it raises the possibility of a favorable response to highly structured behavioral programs. A growing body of empirical evidence supports the use of behavioral/psychoeducational interventions and some medications for treatment of specific symptoms (Lindgren and Doobay 2011). Many families use complementary and alternative treatments. Engaging families in open and honest discussions about the purpose, means, and desired treatment outcome(s) of any intervention option is essential for all practitioners.

Safe, effective, and personalized interventions are needed across the lifespan. Evidence-based practice has become the standard in the field of healthcare. The body of research examining the efficacy of various treatments for ASD continues to grow and has demonstrated the benefits of using cognitive behavioral therapy (CBT) for children with ASD and ABA to improve social and communication skills. Rigorous research studies need to continue to provide the evidence base for the most effective therapies available to change the outcomes for children and adults with a diagnosis of ASD. Special attention is needed to treat co-occurring medical and psychiatric conditions as well as clinical trials of widely used interventions, such as CAM.

Based on the complexities of the diagnosis and management of children with ASD and the potential for comorbid conditions, and the number of children with these diagnoses seen in primary care centers, it is time to consider changes in the educational preparation of APRNs. Pediatric advanced practice nursing students would benefit from a rotation in a behavioral management setting in which educational outcomes emphasize direct experiences in the assessment, diagnosis, and treatment of children with mental health disorders. Outcomes should also focus on the family dynamics and psychosocial support needed by parents to help their child achieve his or her potential.

Likewise, rotations in child and adolescent mental health centers should be mandatory for psychiatric mental health providers who are now being educated within a family-based framework that may not offer specific child and adolescent rotations. Psychiatric APRNs must understand the neuropsychiatric processes that influence the cognitive growth and development of children and adolescents to effectively treat children and help them become functional adults.

Summary

ASDs are life-long developmental neuropsychiatric disorders that exist on a continuum from mild to severe. Each affected individual presents with a distinct set of characteristics that include behavioral, communication, and social impairments. Comorbid psychiatric and medical conditions are common. Due to the pervasiveness, complexity, and uniqueness of these characteristics, it is essential that treatment be individualized. APRNs are in unique positions to partner with each other, family members, and other treatment providers to facilitate collaboration and optimize treatment outcomes for the child. Such working partnerships can continue to address challenges as the child transitions into adulthood.

Critical Thinking Questions

1. A 6-year-old male with a diagnosis of ASD presents to the primary care office with his mother and a note from the teacher reporting increased aggressive behaviors during all activities at school. He is hitting the other children and is refusing to complete any of the assigned work. What actions should the APRN take at this time?

2. A 12-year-old female with a diagnosis of ASD, primarily inattention, presents to the primary care office with her parents, who are very concerned about her recent behaviors, which are disruptive at home and at school. She is argumentative about completing homework assignments and in-class assignments. She seems to be more anxious about schoolwork, and often throws the book or tablet down in frustration. Her parents have always been opposed to medication as part of her therapy and have consistently supported behavior modification as the primary management strategy. What actions should the APRN take at this time?

3. A 16-year-old male with a diagnosis of ASD since 6 years old presents to the primary care office for further evaluation of failure to progress at school. He has a comorbid diagnosis of learning disability. He is now presenting with aggressive behaviors at home and at school. What actions should the APRN take at this time?

Resources

Research Journals

Journal of Autism and Developmental Disorders (JADD). Published by Springer.

FOCUS on Autism and Other Developmental Disorders. Published by Hammill Institute on Disabilities and Sage.

Autism Research. Published by Wiley InterScience.

Autism – The International Journal of Research and Practice. Published in the UK by Sage Publications.

Information and Resources

Association for Science in Autism Treatment, www.asatonline.org. The mission is to share accurate, scientifically sound information about autism and treatments for autism.

Autism Science Foundation, www.autismsciencefoundation.org. Autism Science Foundation's mission is to support autism research, provide information about autism to the general public, and increase awareness of autism spectrum disorders and the needs of individuals and families affected by autism.

Autism Society, www.autism-society.org. The Autism Society exists to improve the lives of those affected by autism, to provide public awareness about the day-to-day issues faced by people on the spectrum, to advocate for appropriate services for individuals across the lifespan, and to provide the latest information regarding treatment, education, research, and advocacy.

Autism Source, www.autismsource.org. An online referral database to find local resources, providers, services, and support.

Autism Speaks, www.autismspeaks.org: The mission of Autism Speaks is to facilitate global research into the causes, treatments, prevention, and an eventual cure for autism, to raise public awareness about autism and its effects on individuals, families, and society, and to provide information and resources to improve the outcomes of children, adolescents, and adults affected by autism.

Autism Watch, www.autism-watch.org: The purpose of Autism Watch is to provide basic information about autism, offer scientific analysis of autism therapies, discuss the merits of the many proposed causes of autism, identify reliable sources of help and information, report improper actions to regulatory agencies, and help people seek legal redress if they have been victimized.

Centers for Disease Control and Prevention, www.cdc.gov/ncbddd/autism. Information for families, people with ASD, healthcare providers, educators, and policy makers, including facts, screening and diagnosis, treatment, data and statistics, research, links, etc.

First Signs, www.firstsigns.org. First Signs is dedicated to educating parents and professionals about autism and related disorders. The First Signs website provides information on a range of issues: from monitoring development to concerns about a child, from the screening and referral process to sharing concerns.

Interactive Autism Network (IAN), www.iancommunity.org. IAN was established at the Kennedy Krieger Institute and is funded by a grant from Autism Speaks. IAN's goal is to facilitate research that will lead to advancements in understanding and treating autism spectrum disorders.

National Autism Center, www.nationalautismcenter.org. The National Autism Center is dedicated to serving children and adolescents with autism spectrum disorders by providing reliable information, promoting best practices, and offering comprehensive resources for families, practitioners, and communities.

Quackwatch, www.quackwatch.com. A nonprofit corporation whose purpose is to combat health-related frauds, myths, fads, and fallacies. Information on quackery and questionable therapies.

Treatment and Education of Autism and related Communication-handicapped CHildren (TEACCH), www.teacch.com. An evidence-based service, training, and research program for individuals of all ages and skill levels with autism spectrum disorder. https://www.autismspeaks.org/teacch-0.

100 Useful Sites, Networks, and Resources for Parents of Autistic Children,https://www.masters-in-special-education.com/50-great-websites-for-parents-of-children-with-special-needs/.

Publishers that Specialize in ASD and Related Disabilities

Autism Asperger Publishing Company, www.asperger.net.

Future Horizons, www.fhautism.com.

Woodbine Publishing House, www.woodbinehouse.com.

Brookes Publishing, www.brookespublishing.com.

Jessica Kingsley Publishers, www.jkp.com.

References

Accordina, R.E., Lucarelli, J., and Yan, A.C. (2015). Cutaneous disease in autism spectrum disorder: a review. *Wiley Online Library* https://doi.org/10.1111/pde.12582, https://onlinelibrary.wiley.com/doi/full/10.1111/pde.12582.

Adams, L. (1998). Oral-motor and motor-speech characteristics of children with autism. *Focus on Autism and Other Developmental Disabilities* 13: 108–112. https://doi.org/10.1177/108835769801300207.

Al-Sharif, S.M., Sivakumar, S., and Thiruvasahar, M. (2017). Improving quality care for children with autism spectrum disorders in doctor's office and outpatient clinics. *Journal of Pregnancy and Child Health* 2 https://doi.org/10.4172/2376-127X.1000253., https://www.omicsonline.org/open-access/improving-quality-care-for-children-with-autism-spectrum-disorders-indoctors-office-or-outpatient-clinics-2376-127X-1000253.pdf.

American Academy of Child and Adolescent Psychiatry (2018). *Autism Spectrum Disorders.* Available at https://www.aacap.org/AACAP/Families_and_Youth/Facts_for_Families/FFF-Guide/The-Child-With-Autism-011.aspx.

American Academy of Pediatrics (2019). Available at https://www.aap.org/en-us/advocacy-and-policy/aap-health-initiatives/Pages/autism-initiatives.aspx.

American Psychiatric Association (2013). *Diagnostic and Statistical Manual of Mental Disorders* 5. Washington DC: American Psychiatric Association Publishing.

Baranek, G., Boyd, B., Poe, M. et al. (2007). Hyperresponsive sensory patterns in young children with autism, developmental delay and typical development. *American Journal on Mental Retardation* 112 (4): 233–245.

Barbaresi, W., Katusic, S., and Voigt, R. (2006). Autism: a review of the state of the science for pediatric primary health care providers. *Archives of Pediatrics and Adolescent Medicine* 160: 1167–1175.

Baribeau, D.A. and Anagnostou, E. (2014a). An update on medication management of behavioral disorders and autism. *Current Psychiatry Reports* 16: 437.

Baribeau, D.A. and Anagnostou, E. (2014b). Social communication is an emerging target for pharmacotherapy in autism spectrum disorder: A review of the literature on potential agents. *Journal of the Canadian Academy of Child and Adolescent Psychiatry/Journal de l'Académie canadienne de psychiatrie de l'enfant et de l. adolescent* 23 (1): 20–30.

Batshaw, M., Pellegrino, L., and Roizen, N. (2007). *Children with Disabilities*, 6e. Baltimore, MD: Paul H. Brooks Publishing.

Belardinelli, C., Raza, M., and Taneli, T. (2016). Comorbid behavioral problems and psychiatric disorders in autism spectrum disorders. *Journal of Childhood and Developmental Disorders* 2 (2): 1–9.

Bellini, S. (2006). *Building Social Relationships: A Systematic Approach to Teaching Social Interaction Skills to Children and Adolescents with Autism Spectrum Disorders and Other Social Difficulties.* Shawnee Mission, KS: Autism Asperger Publishing Company.

Bellini, S. and Akullian, J. (2007). A meta-analysis of video modeling and video self-modeling interventions for children and adolescents with autism spectrum disorders. *Exceptional Children* 73 (3): 264–287.

Bellini, S. and Peters, J. (2008). Social skills training for youth with autism spectrum disorders. *Child and Adolescent Psychiatric Clinics of North America* 17 (4): 857–873.

Bondy, A.S. and Frost, L.A. (1994). The Delaware autistic program. In: *Preschool Education Programs for Children with Autism* (eds. S.L. Harris and J.S. Handleman), 37–54. Austin, TX: Pro-Ed.

Caglayan, A. (2010). Genetic causes of syndromic and non-syndromic autism. *Developmental Medicine and Child Neurology* 52: 130–138. https://doi.org/10.1111/j.1469-8749.2009.03523.x.

Carr, D. and Felce, J. (2007). Brief report: increase in production of spoken words in some children with autism after PECS teaching to phase III. *Journal of Autism and Developmental Disorders* 37: 780–787.

Carr, E.G., Levin, L., McConnachie, G. et al. (1994). *Communication Based Intervention for Problem Behavior: A User's Guide for Producing Positive Change.* Baltimore, MD: Paul H. Brookes.

Carr, E.G., Langdon, N.A., and Yarbrough, S. (1999). Hypothesis-based intervention for severe problem behavior. In: *Functional Analysis of Problem Behavior: From Effective Assessment to Effective Support* (eds. A.C. Repp and R.H. Horner), 9–31. Belmont, CA: Wadsworth Publishing.

Carter, A.S., Davis, N.O., Klin, A., and Volkmar, F.R. (2005). Social development in autism. In: *Handbook of Autism and Pervasive Developmental Disorders: Vol. 1, Diagnosis, Development, Neurobiology, and Behavior* (eds. F.R. Volkmar, R. Paul, A. Klin and D. Cohen), 312–334. Hoboken, NJ: Wiley.

Casanova, M.F. (2004). White matter volume increase and minicolumns in autism. *Annals of Neurology* 56: 453.

Cauffield, J.S. (2013). Medication use in autism spectrum disorders: what is the evidence? *Formulary* 48 (5): 161–162, 165–168.

CDC. (2020a). *Autism spectrum disorder: Data & statistics on autism spectrum disorder.* Available at https://www.cdc.gov/ncbddd/autism/data.html.

CDC. (2020b). *Autism spectrum disorder. What is autism spectrum disorder?* Available at https://www.cdc.gov/ncbddd/autism/facts.html.

CDC. (2019). *Autism spectrum disorder: Recommendations and guidelines.* Available at https://www.cdc.gov/ncbddd/autism/hcp-recommendations.html.

Charlop, M.H., Schreibman, L., and Thibodeau, M.G. (1985). Increasing spontaneous verbal responding in autistic children using a time delay procedure. *Journal of Applied Behavior Analysis* 18 (2): 155–166.

Chaste, P. and Leboyer, M. (2012). Autism risk factors: genes, environment, and gene-environment interactions. *Dialogues in Clinical Neuroscience* 14 (3): 281–292.

Christensen, J., Grønborg, T.K., Sørensen, M.J. et al. (2013). Prenatal valproate exposure and risk of autism spectrum disorders and childhood autism. *Journal of the American Medical Association* 309: 1696–1703.

Cidav, Z., Munson, J., Estes, A. et al. (2017). Cost offset associated with early start Denver model for children with autism. *Journal of the American Academy of Child and Adolescent Psychiatry* 56 (9): 777–783. [PMID: 28838582].

Correll, C. (2008). Antipsychotic use in children and adolescents: minimizing adverse effects to maximize outcomes. *Journal of the American Academy of Child & Adolescent Psychiatry* 47 (1): 9–20.

Coucouvanis, J. (2005). *Superskills: A Social Skills Group Program for Children with Asperger Syndrome, High Functioning Autism and Related Challenges*. Mission, KS: Autism Asperger Publishing Company.

Cuvo, A., Law-Reagan, A., Ackerlund, J. et al. (2010). Training children with autism spectrum disorders to be compliant with a physical exam. *Research in Autism Spectrum Disorders* 4: 168–185. https://doi.org/10.1016/j.rasd.2009.09.001.

Dawson, G., Rogers, S.J., Munson, J. et al. (2010). Randomized, controlled trial of an intervention for toddlers with autism: the early start Denver model. *Pediatrics* 125: 17–23. https://doi.org/10.1542/peds.2009-0958.

DeFilippis, M. (2018). The use of complementary alternative medicine in children and adolescents with autism spectrum disorder. *Psychopharmacology Bulletin* 48 (1): 40–63.

Doo, S. and Wing, Y. (2006). Sleep problems of children with pervasive developmental disorders: correlation with parental stress. *Developmental Medicine and Child Neurology* 48: 650–655. https://doi.org/10.1111/j.1469-8749.2006.tb01334.x.

Ecker, C., Marquand, A., Mourao-Miranda, J. et al. (2010). Describing the brain in autism in five dimensions: magnetic resonance imaging-assisted diagnosis of autism spectrum disorder using a multiparameter classification approach. *Journal of Neuroscience* 30 (32): 10612–10623. https://doi.org/10.1523/JNEUROSCI.5413-09.2010.

Escalona, A., Field, T., Singer-Strunk, R. et al. (2001). Brief report: improvements in the behavior of children with autism following massage therapy. *Journal of Autism and Developmental Disorders* 31: 513–516. https://doi.org/10.1023/A1012273110194.

Filipek, P.A., Accardo, P.J., Baranek, G. et al. (1999). The screening and diagnosis of autism spectrum disorders. *Journal of Autism and Developmental Disorders* 29 (6): 439–484.

Filipek, P.A., Accardo, P.J., Ashwal, S. et al. (2000). Practice parameter: screening and diagnosis of autism: report of the quality standards subcommittee of the American Academy of Neurology and the Child Neurology Society. *Neurology* 55 (4): 468–479.

Frankel, R., Leary, M., and Kilman, B. (1987). Building social skills through pragmatic analysis: assessment and treatment implications for children with autism. In: *Handbook of Autism and Pervasive Developmental Disorders* (eds. D. Cohen, O. Donellan and R. Paul), 333–359. New York: Wiley.

Frost, L.A. and Bondy, A.S. (2002). *PECS: The Picture Exchange Communication System Training Manual*, 2e. Newark, DE: Pyramid Educational Products Inc.

Fuller, P.M., Gooley, J., and Saper, C.B. (2006). Neurobiology of the sleepwake cycle: sleep architecture, circadian regulation and regulatory feedback. *Journal of Biological Rhythms* 26: 482–493. https://doi.org/10.1177/0748730406294627.

Gadow, K. and DeVincent, C. (2005). Clinical significance of tics and attention deficit hyperactivity disorder in children with pervasive developmental disorder. *Journal of Childhood Neurology* 20: 481–488.

Ganz, M.L. (2007). The lifetime distribution of the incremental societal costs of autism. *Archives of Pediatric Adolescence Medicine* 161 (4): 343–349.

Ghaziuddin, M. (2005). A family history study of Asperger syndrome. *Journal of Autism and Developmental Disorders* 35 (2): 177–182.

Ghaziuddin, M. (2018). *Medical Aspects of Autism and Asperger Syndrome*. London: Jessica Kingsley.

Gleason, M.M., Egger, H.L., Emslie, G.J. et al. (2007). Psychopharmacological treatment for very young children: contexts and guidelines. *Journal of the American Academy of Child and Adolescent Psychiatry* 46: 1532–1572.

Goel, R., Hong, J.S., Findling, R.L., and Ji, N.J. (2018). An update on pharmacotherapy of autism spectrum disorder in children and adolescents. *International Review of Psychiatry* 30 (1): 78–95.

Goldstein, H. (2002). Communication intervention for children with autism: a review of treatment efficacy. *Journal of Autism and Developmental Disorders* 32: 373–396. https://doi.org/10.1023/a:1020589821992.

Gray, C. (2000). *The New Social Story Book: Illustrated Edition*. Arlington, TX: Future Horizons.

Hall, H.R. and Graff, J.C. (2012). Maladaptive behaviors of children with autism: parent support, stress, and coping. *Contemporary Pediatric Nursing* 35: 194–214.

Hallas, D. (ed.) (2019). *Behavioral Pediatric Healthcare for Nurse Practitioners: A Growth and Developmental Approach to Intercepting Abnormal Behaviors*. New York: Springer Publishing Company.

Handen, B.L., Anagnostou, E., Aman, M.G. et al. (2017). A randomized, placebo-controlled trial of metformin for the treatment of overweight induced by antipsychotic medication in young people with autism spectrum disorder: open-label extension. *Journal of the American Academy of Child and Adolescent Psychiatry* 56 (10): 849–856.e6. [PMID: 28942807].

Hanson, E., Kalish, L.A., Bunce, E. et al. (2007). Use of complimentary and alternative medicine among children diagnosed with autism spectrum disorder. *Journal of Autism and Developmental Disorders* 37: 628–636.

Hart, B.M. and Risley, T.R. (1968). Establishing use of descriptive adjectives in the spontaneous speech of disadvantaged preschool children. *Journal of Applied Behavior Analysis* 1: 109–120.

Hart, B. and Risley, T.R. (1980). In vivo language intervention. Unanticipated general effects. *Journal of Applied Behavior Analysis* 13: 407–432. https://doi.org/10.1901/jaba.1980.13-407.

Hashemian, M. and Pourghassem, H. (2014). Diagnosis autism spectrum disorders on EEG analysis: a survey. *Neurophysiology* 46: 183–195.

Höfer, J., Hoffmann, F., and Bachmann, C. (2017). Use of complementary and alternative medicine in children and adolescents with autism spectrum disorder: a systematic review. *Autism* 21 (4): 387–402.

Horner, R.H., Carr, E.G., Strain, P.S. et al. (2002). Problem behavior interventions for young children with autism: a research synthesis. *Journal of Autism and Developmental Disorders* 32: 423–446.

Howlin, P. and Rutter, M. (1989). Mother's speech to autistic children: a preliminary causal analysis. *Journal of Child Psychology and Psychiatry* 30: 819–843.

Hultman, C.M., Sandin, S., Levine, S.Z. et al. (2011). Advancing paternal age and risk of autism: new evidence from a population-based study and a meta-analysis of epidemiological studies. *Molecular Psychiatry* 16: 1203–1212.

Inglese, M. and Elder, J. (2009). Caring for children with autism spectrum disorder, part I: prevalence, etiology and core features. *Journal of Pediatric Nursing* 24 (1): 41–48.

Ivanenko, A. and Johnson, K. (2008). Sleep disturbances in children psychiatric disorders. *Seminars in Pediatric Neurology* 15: 70–78.

Johnson, C. and Myers, S. (2007). Identification and evaluation of children with autism spectrum disorders. *Pediatrics* 120 (5): 1183–1215.

Jones, W., Carr, K., Katelin, B., and Klin, A. (2008). Absence of preferential looking to the eyes of approaching adults predicts level of social disability in 2 year old toddlers with autism spectrum disorder. *Archives of General Psychiatry* 65 (8): 946–954.

Kanner, L. (1943). Autistic disturbances of affective contact. *The Nervous Child* 2: 217–250.

Koegel, L.K. (2000). Interventions to facilitate communication in autism. *Journal of Autism and Developmental Disorders* 30: 383–391. https://doi.org/10.1023/a:1005539220932.

Koegel, L.K. and LaZebnik, C. (2004). *Overcoming Autism: Finding the Answers, Strategies and Hope that Can Transform a Child's Life*. New York, NY: Penguin Books.

Kraijer, D.W. (1999). Autism and autistic like conditions in mental retardation. *Journal of Disability Research* 43: 342–343.

Krasny, L., Williams, B.J., Provencal, S., and Ozonoff, S. (2003). Social skills interventions for the autism spectrum: essential ingredients and a model curriculum. *Child and Adolescent Psychiatric Clinics of North America* 12 (1): 107–122.

Lainhart, J., Piven, J., Wzorket, J. et al. (1997). Macrocephaly in children and adults with autism. *Journal of the American Academy of Child and Adolescent Psychiatry* 36: 282–290.

Lampi, K.M., Lehtonen, L., Tran, P.L. et al. (2012). Risk of autism spectrum disorders in low birth weight and small for gestational age infants. *Journal of Pediatrics* 161: 830–836.

Levy, S. and Hyman, S. (2015). Complementary and alternative medicine treatments for children with autism spectrum disorders. *Child and Adolescent Psychiatric Clinics of North America* 24: 117–143.

Levy, S., Mandell, D., and Schultz, R. (2009). Autism. *The Lancet* 374: 1627–1638. https://doi.org/10.1016/S01406736(09)61376-3.

Leyfer, O., Folstein, S., Bacalman, S. et al. (2006). Co-morbid psychiatric disorders in children with autism: interview development and rates of disorders. *Journal of Autism and Developmental Disorders* 36 (7): 849–861. https://doi.org/10.1007/s10803-006-0123-0.

Li, H., Xue, Z., Ellmore, T.M. et al. (2014). Network-based analysis reveals stronger local diffusion-based connectivity and different correlations with oral language skills in brains of children with high functioning autism spectrum disorders. *Human Brain Mapping* 35: 396–413. https://doi.org/10.1002/hbm.22185.

Lindgren, S. & Doobay, A (2011). *Evidence-based interventions for ASD*. Iowa Department of Human Services by the Center of Disabilities and Development of the University of Iowa's Children's Hospital. Available at http://www.interventionsunlimited.com/editoruploads/files/Iowa%20DHS%20Autism%20Interventions%206-10-11.pdf.

Lindly, O., Thorburn, S., Heisler, K. et al. (2017). Parent disclosure of complementary health approaches used for children with autism spectrum disorder: barriers and facilitators. *Complimentary and Therapeutic Medicine* 35: 47–52. https://doi.org/10.1016/j.ctim.2017.09.003.

Liptak, G., Stuart, T., and Auinger, P. (2006). Health care utilization and expenditures for children with autism: data from a US national sample. *Journal of Autism and Developmental Disorders* 36 (7): 871–879.

Liu, J., Yao, L., Zhang, W. et al. (2017). Gray matter abnormalities in pediatric autism spectrum disorder: a meta-analysis with signed differential mapping. *European Child & Adolescent Psychiatry* 26: 933–945.

Lord, C., Elsabbagh, M., Baird, G., and Veenstra-Vanderweele, J. (2018). Autism spectrum disorder. *The Lancet* 392: 508–520.

Lovaas, O.I. (1987). Behavioral treatment and normal educational and intellectual functioning in young autistic children. *Journal of Consulting and Clinical Psychology* 55: 3–9. Available at https://www.beca-aba.com/articles-and-forms/lovaas-1987.pdf doi: https://doi.org/10.1037/0022-006X.55.1.3.

Mahajan, R., Bernal, M.P., and Panzer, R. (2012). Clinical practice pathways for evaluation and medication choice for attention-deficit/hyperactivity disorder symptoms in autism spectrum disorders. *Pediatrics* 130 (Suppl. 2): S125–S138.

Maenner, M.J., Shaw, K.A., Baio, J. et al. (2020). Prevalence of autism spectrum disorder among children aged 8 years – Autism and Developmental Disabilities Monitoring Network, 11 Sites, United States. *MMWR Surveillance Summary* 69(No. SS-4): 1–12. http://dx.doi.org/10.15585/mmwr.ss6904a1.

Mayo Foundation for Medical Education and Research (2018). *Autism spectrum disorder*. Available at https://www.mayoclinic.org/diseases-conditions/autism-spectrum-disorder/symptoms-causes/syc-20352928.

McCracken, J.T. (2005). Safety issues with drug therapies for autism spectrum disorders. *Journal of Clinical Psychiatry* 66 (Suppl. 10): 32–37.

van der Meer, J.M., Oerlemans, A.M., and van Steijn, D.J. (2012). Are autism spectrum disorder and attention-deficit/hyperactivity disorder different manifestations of one overarching disorder? Cognitive and symptom evidence from a clinical and population-based sample. *Journal of the American Academy of Child and Adolescent Psychiatry* 51: 1160–1172.

Mesibov, G.B. (1997). Formal and informal measures on the effectiveness or the TEACCH programme. *Autism* 1: 25–35. https://doi.org/10.1177/1362361397011005.

Mesibov, G.B., Shea, V., and Schopler, F. (2005). *The TEACCH Approach to Autism Spectrum Disorders*. New York, NY: Kluwer Academic/Plenum.

Miles, J., Hadden, T., and Hillman, R. (2000). Head circumference is an independent clinical finding associated with autism. *American Journal of Medical Genetics* 95: 339–350. https://doi.org/10.1002/1096-8628 (20001211)954<339:AID-AJMG9>3.0CO;2-B.

Moore, G.S., Kneitel, A.W., Walker, C.K. et al. (2012). Autism risk in small- and large-for-gestational-age infants. *American Journal of Obstetrics and Gynecology* 206: 314.e1–314.e9.

Myers, S., Johnson, C., and Council on Children with Disabilities (2007). Management of children with autism spectrum disorders. *Pediatrics* 120: 1162–1182. https://doi.org/10.1542/peds.2007-2362.

National Autism Center (2015). *Findings and Conclusions: National Standards Project, Phase 2*. Randolph, MA: National Autism Center.

National Institute of Health (2013). *Revised autism screening tool offers more precise assessment [News Release]*. Washington, DC: US Department of Health and Human Services Available at https://www.nih.gov/news-events/news-releases/revised-autism-screening-tool-offers-more-precise-assessment.

National Institute of Mental Health (2008). *Autism spectrum disorder: Pervasive developmental disorders*. Washington, DC: US Department of Health and Human Services Available at http://autism-support.org/wp-content/uploads/2011/05/NIMH_Autism_Spectrum.pdf.

O'Nions, E., Happé, F., Evers, K. et al. (2018). How do parents manage irritability, challenging behaviour, non-compliance and anxiety in children with autism spectrum disorders? A meta-synthesis. *Journal of Autism and Developmental Disorders* 48: 1272–1286.

Ozgen, H., Hellemann, G.S., de Jonge, M.V. et al. (2013). Predictive values of morphological features in patients with autism versus normal controls. *Journal of Autism and Developmental Disorders* 43: 147–155. Available at https://www.ncbi.nlm.nih.gov/pmc/

articles/PMC3536966. doi: https://doi.org/10.1007/s10803-012-1554-4.

Page, J. and Boucher, J. (1998). Motor impairments in children with autistic disorder. *Child Language Teaching and Therapy* 14: 253–259. https://doi.org/10.1177/026565909801400301.

Peacock, G., Hyman, S., & Levy, S. (2009). Autism identification and management webinar. Webinar presented by the American Academy of Pediatrics and the National Center of Medical Home Initiatives for Children with Special Needs. American Academy of Pediatrics. Available at http://www.smileich.com/resources%20for%20pediatricians/autism%20ppt%20CDC%20AAP.pdf.

Polimeni, M.A., Richdale, A.L., and Francis, A.J. (2005). A survey of sleep problems in autism, Asperger's disorder and typically developing children. *Journal of Intellectual Disability Research* 49 (4): 260–268.

Posserud, M., Hysing, M., Helland, W. et al. (2018). Autism traits: the importance of "co-morbid" problems for impairment and contact with services. Data from the Bergen child study. *Research in Developmental Disabilities* 72: 275–283.

Prizant, B.M. and Wetherby, A.M. (1998). Communication intent: a framework for understanding social communicative behavior in autism. *Journal of the American Academy of Child and Adolescent Psychiatry* 26: 472–479.

Ramaswami, G. and Geschwind, D.H. (2018). Genetics of autism spectrum disorder. In: *Handbook of Clinical Neurology, Neurogenetics, Part 1*, vol. 147(3rd series) (eds. D.H. Geschwind, H.L. Paulson and C. Klein), 321–329.

Reaven, J. (2009). Children with high functioning autism spectrum disorders and co-occurring anxiety symptoms: implications for assessment and treatment. *Journal of the Society of Pediatric Nurses* 14 (3): 192–199.

Reichow, B. and Volkmar, F.R. (2008). Social skills interventions for individuals with autism: evaluation for evidence-based practices within a best evidence synthesis framework. *Journal of Autism and Developmental Disorders* 38: 1311–1318.

Reis Paula, C.A., Reategui, C., de Sousa Costa, B.K. et al. (2017). High-frequency EEG variation in children with autism spectrum disorder during human faces visualization. *BioMedical Research International*: 1–11. https://doi.org/10.1155/2017/3591914.

Ringman, J. and Jankovic, J. (2000). Occurrence of tics in Asperger syndrome and autistic disorder. *Journal of Child Neurology* 15 (6): 394–400.

Rogers, S.J., Hall, T., Osaki, D. et al. (2000). The Denver model: A comprehensive, integrated, educational approach to young children with autism and their families. In: *Preschool Education Programs for Children with Autism*, 2e (eds. S.L. Harris and J.S. Handleman), 95–134. Austin, TX: Pro-Ed.

Rogers, S.J., Hayden, D., Hepburn, S. et al. (2006). Teaching young nonverbal children with autism useful speech: a pilot study of the Denver model and PROMPT interventions. *Journal of Autism and Developmental Disorders* 3: 1007–1024. https://doi.org/10.1007/s10803-006-0142-x.

Roke, Y., van Harten, P.N., Boot, A.M., and Buitelaar, J.K. (2009). Antipsychotic medication in children and adolescents: a descriptive review of the effects on prolactin level and associated side effects. *Journal of Child and Adolescent Psychopharmacology* 19: 403–414.

Sacco, R., Militerni, R., Frolli, A. et al. (2007). Clinical, morphological, and biochemical correlates of head circumference in autism. *Biological Psychiatry* 62: 1038–1047.

Sandin, S., Hultman, C.M., Kolevzon, A. et al. (2012). Advancing maternal age is associated with increasing risk for autism: a review and meta-analysis. *Journal of the American Academy of Child and Adolescent Psychiatry* 51 (5): 477–486.

Scahill, L. and Pachler, M. (2007). Treatment of hyperactivity in children with pervasive developmental disorders. *Journal of Child and Adolescent Psychiatric Nursing* 20 (1): 59–62.

Scahill, L., Koenig, K., Carroll, D., and Pachler, M. (2007). Risperidone approved for the treatment of serious behavioral problems in children with autism. *Journal of Child and Adolescent Psychiatric Nursing* 20 (3): 188–190.

Schmidt, R.J., Tancredi, D.J., Ozonoff, S. et al. (2012). Maternal periconceptional folic acid intake and risk of autism spectrum disorders and developmental delay in the CHARGE (CHildhood Autism Risks from Genetics and Environment) case-control study. *American Journal of Clinical Nutrition* 96: 80–89.

Siegel, M. and Beaulieu, A.A. (2012). Psychotropic medications in children with autism spectrum disorders: a systematic review and synthesis for evidence-based practice. *Journal of Autism and Developmental Disorders* 42: 1592–1605.

Smith, T., Groen, A.D., and Wynn, J.W. (2000). Randomized trial of intensive early intervention for children with pervasive developmental disorder. *American Journal on Mental Retardation* 105 (4): 269–285.

Smith, M., Segal, J., & Hutman, T. (2018). *Help guide*. Available at https://www.helpguide.org/articles/autism-learning-disabilities/does-my-child-have-autism.htm.

Spencer, D., Marshall, J., Post, B. et al. (2013). Psychotropic medication use and polypharmacy in children with autism spectrum disorders. *Pediatrics* 132 (5): 833–840. https://doi.org/10.1542/peds.2012-3774.

van Steensel, F.J.A., Bögels, S.M., and Perrin, S. (2011). Anxiety disorders in children and adolescents with autistic spectrum disorders: a meta-analysis. *Clinical Child and Family Psychology Review* 14 (3): 302–317.

Substance Abuse and Mental Health Service Administration. (2014). *Behavioral health integration*. Available at https://www.samhsa.gov/sites/default/files/samhsa-behavioral-health-integration.pdf.

Tantam, D. (2000). Adolescence and adulthood of individuals with Asperger syndrome. In: *Asperger Syndrome* (eds. A. Klin, F.R. Klin and S.S. Sparrow), 367–402. New York, NY: The Guilford Press.

Tick, B., Colvert, E., McEwen, F. et al. (2016). Autism spectrum disorders and other mental health problems: exploring etiological overlaps and phenotypic causal associations. *Journal of the American Academy of Child & Adolescent Psychiatry* 55: 106–113.

US Food and Drug Administration (2017). *Autism: Beware of Potentially Dangerous Therapies and Products*. Consumer Health information. Available at https://www.fda.gov/ForConsumers/ConsumerUpdates/ucm394757.htm.

Vaz, I. (2010). Improving the management of children with learning disability and autism spectrum disorder when they attend hospital. *Child: Care, Health and Development* 36: 753–755.

Venter, A., Lord, C., and Schopler, E. (1992). A follow-up study of high-functioning autistic children. *Journal of Child Psychology and Psychiatry* 33: 489–507. Available at http://www.ncbi.nlm.nih.gov/pubmed/1577895.

Virues-Ortega, J., Julio, F.M., and Pastor-Barriuso, R. (2013). The TEACCH program for children and adults with autism: a meta-analysis of intervention studies. *Clinical Psychology Review* 33 (8): 940–949.

Volkmar, F., Siegel, M., Woorbury-Smith, M. et al. (2014). Practice parameter for the assessment and treatment of children and adolescents with autism Spectrum disorder. *Journal of the American Academy of Child and Adolescent Psychiatry* 53: 237–257.

Wang, P. and Spillane, A. (2009). Evidence-based social skills interventions for children with autism: a meta-analysis. *Education and Training in Developmental Disabilities* 44 (3): 318–342.

Wassink, T., Piven, J., and Patil, S. (2001). Chromosomal abnormalities in a clinic sample of individuals with autistic disorder. *Psychiatric Genetics* 11: 57–63.

Weiskop, S., Matthews, J., and Richdale, A. (2001). Treatment of sleep problems in a 5-year old boy with autism using behavioural principles. *Autism* 5: 209–221.

Weiskop, S., Richdale, A., and Matthews, J. (2005). Behavioural treatment to reduce sleep problems in children with autism or fragile X syndrome. *Developmental Medicine and Child Neurology* 47: 94–104. https://doi.org/10.1111/j.1469-8749.2005.tb01097.x.

Weitz, C., Dexter, M., and Moore, J. (1997). AAC and children with developmental disabilities. In: *Handbook of Augmentative and Alternative Communication* (eds. S. Glenn and D.C. Decoste). San Diego, CA: Singular Publishing.

White, S., Koenig, K., and Scahill, L. (2007). Social skills development in children with autism spectrum disorders: a review of the intervention research. *Journal of Autism and Developmental Disorders* 37: 1858–1868.

Wiggs, L. and Stores, G. (2004). Sleep patterns and sleep disorders in children with autism spectrum disorders: insights using parent report and actigraphy. *Developmental Medicine and Child Neurology* 46 (6): 372–380. https://doi.org/10.1017/S0012/62204000611.

Williams, P., Sears, L., and Allard, A. (2004). Sleep problems in children with autism. *Journal of Sleep Research* 13: 265–268.

Williams, K., Wheeler, D.M., Silove, N., and Hazell, P. (2010). Selective serotonin reuptake inhibitors (SSRIs) for autism spectrum disorders (ASD). *Cochrane Database of Systematic Reviews* (8): CD004677. https://doi.org/10.1002/14651858.CD004677.pub2.

Wolf, M., Risley, T., and Mees, H. (1964). Application of operant conditioning procedures to the behaviour problems of an autistic child. *Behaviour Research and Therapy* 1: 305–312. Available at http://www.garfield.library.upenn.edu/classics1983/A1983RG31100001.pdf.

Wong, C., Odom, S.L., Hume, K. et al. (2014). *Evidence-Based Practices for Children, Youth, and Young Adults with Autism Spectrum Disorder*. Chapel Hill: The University of North Carolina, Frank Porter Graham Child Development Institute, Autism Evidence-Based Practice Review Group. Available at http://autismpdc.fpg.unc.edu/sites/autismpdc.fpg.unc.edu/files/2014-EBP-Report.pdf.

Wright, J. (2012). Clinical research: Facial features can help diagnose autism. *Spectrum Autism Research News*, 1–2. Available at https://www.spectrumnews.org/news/clinical-research-facial-features-can-help-diagnose-autism/.

Zwaigenbaum, L., Bauman, M., Fein, D. et al. (2015). Early screening of autism spectrum disorder: recommendations for practice and research. *Pediatrics* 136: S41–S59.

17

Learning and Intellectual Disabilities

Linda M. Finke[1] and Patricia Ryan-Krause[2]

[1]Fort Wayne College of Health & Human Services, Indiana University-Purdue University, Fort Wayne, IN, USA
[2]Yale University School of Nursing, Orange, CT, USA

Objectives

After reading this chapter, advanced practice registered nurses (APRNs) will be able to:

1. Discuss assessment and identification of learning and intellectual disabilities.
2. Discuss the impact of diagnosis of learning or intellectual disability on the family and child.
3. Identify strategies to help families with a child with a learning or intellectual disability cope and navigate the complex systems of healthcare, schools, and community resources.
4. Describe how APRNs can work collaboratively to provide services to children and adolescents with learning and intellectual disabilities.

Introduction

A substantial number of school-age children are affected by intellectual disabilities or learning disabilities. These conditions often seriously impact academic ability and always require a multifaceted approach to ensure children meet their maximum potential. Learning disabilities refer to problems in the skills needed for reading, written and spoken language, and math. Children who are diagnosed with intellectual disabilities are delayed in overall development, including adaptive life skills, and may have a lower intellectual level than children of the same chronological age. Children with intellectual disabilities may have previously been labeled with the no longer used diagnoses of mental retarded, developmentally delayed, or intellectually challenged.

The total numbers of children affected by these disabilities are difficult to determine because while these conditions have variable presentations and diagnostic criteria, the terminology is not always clear. Learning disabilities refer to children with difficulties in the skills needed for reading, written and spoken language, and math. In 2018–19, the number of students aged 3–21 who received special education services under the Individuals with Disabilities Education Act (IDEA) was 7.1 million, which included 14% of all public school students. Among all students receiving special education services, 33% had specific learning disabilities (US Department of Education, 2020). Prevalence data from the Centers for Disease Control (CDC) National Survey of Children's Health in 2012 indicate that 7% of children from 3 to 17 years of age are diagnosed with learning

Child and Adolescent Behavioral Health: A Resource for Advanced Practice Psychiatric and Primary Care Practitioners in Nursing,
Second Edition. Edited by Edilma L. Yearwood, Geraldine S. Pearson, and Jamesetta A. Newland.
© 2021 John Wiley & Sons, Inc. Published 2021 by John Wiley & Sons, Inc.
Companion website: www.wiley.com/go/Yearwood

disabilities (Boyle et al. 2011). In 2016, CDC reported that 1.1% of individuals from 3 to 17 years were diagnosed with intellectual disabilities (Zablotsky et al. 2017). The prevalence figures for both learning disabilities and intellectual disabilities have remained stable, while autism spectrum disorder and attention deficit hyperactivity disorder (ADHD) have seen a statistical increase since 1997 (Boyle et al. 2011). Autism has recently been found to affect 2.76% of children between 3 and 17 years of age (Xu et al. 2019) and the CDC reports that 9.4% of children between 4 and 17 years of age have been diagnosed with ADHD (Danielson et al., 2016, 2018; Visser et al., 2016).

Although often quite dissimilar, it is important for psychiatric and primary care providers to be aware of characteristics and possible comorbidities. Important definitions from national associations are documented below. Recent changes in the Diagnostic and Statistical Manual 5 (DSM-5) are addressed in identified sections (American Psychiatric Association [APA] 2013). This chapter will describe the types of disabilities most frequently seen in primary care settings, provide screening tools, and discuss evidence-based interventions used with these populations, and present a case study highlighting the journey of a child with a learning disability to young adulthood.

Intellectual Disability

The American Association on Intellectual and Developmental Disabilities characterizes intellectual disability as "significant limitations in both intellectual functioning such as the ability to reason, learn and problem solve along with limitations in adaptive behavior including conceptual, social and practical skills beginning before the age of 18" (American Association on Intellectual and Developmental Disabilities n.d.).

It is often difficult to diagnose intellectual disabilities because there is no accurate test and symptoms, best described as behaviors, vary greatly. Intelligence testing is highly inaccurate in these children because of their delayed development and delayed ability to communicate, read, write, and perform tasks of daily living. Often their comprehension level is higher than is demonstrated by their verbal and writing skills.

While there are several identified causes of intellectual disabilities, 40% of those diagnosed cannot be connected with an identified cause. Chromosomal abnormalities are found in about 7% of children with intellectual disability (Belkady et al. 2018). These abnormalities include Down syndrome (21 chromosomes) and fragile X syndrome (changed *FMR1* gene on X chromosome). Fragile X syndrome is the most common sin-

gle-gene cause of an inherited intellectual disability (Raspa et al. 2017). The disability is two times more common in boys than in girls, with the diagnoses affecting 1 in 4000 boys. Fragile X syndrome is caused by the loss of expression of the *FMR1* gene. The *FMR1* gene is necessary for normal learning and memory development in the brain. Other identified causes of an intellectual disability include fetal alcohol syndrome, poor prenatal care or prenatal injury, and toxic environmental exposures during formative developmental periods. Readers are referred to Chapter 16 for a comprehensive description of the needs of children with an autism spectrum disorder as they, too, can present with learning and intellectual disability challenges.

To complicate matters more, the prevalence of other disabilities often co-occurs with intellectual disabilities. Physical disabilities such as cerebral palsy and other brain injuries may also be present. These children may have cardiac disorders, seizure disorders, or ADHD. They also may present with self-injurious behavior such as hand biting, hair pulling, head banging, or picking at clothing or skin. Children with intellectual disabilities are also at a high risk for psychiatric disorders (Matson et al. 2012; Tau et al. 2012). Again, the assessment of mental health problems in children with an intellectual disability is difficult because with this population, invalidated methods (i.e. methods not standardized for use with children with intellectual disabilities) are used to determine the presence of a mental health problem (Matson et al. 2012). The clinical picture may be further complicated by medications the child is taking because of physical or mental health concerns.

Intellectual Disabilities: Clinical Picture

Early diagnosis of an intellectual disability is important so children and their families can begin working towards meeting the child's potential. However, reaching an early diagnosis is complicated, as has previously been discussed. Presenting problems indicating an intellectual disability are usually as simple as the child not meeting expected developmental milestones such as sitting up, rolling over, crawling and walking, and for an older child, talking. The parent often brings this delay in developmental milestones to the healthcare provider's attention during routine well-child checks or the healthcare provider notes the lack of development. A complete physical examination might detect physical and congenital abnormalities such as large ears, an elongated face, prominent jaw line, macrocephaly, macro-orchidism, a narrow and high-arched palate, and hyperextensible joints associated with fragile X syndrome. A round face with eyes that slant upward, low muscle tone, a palm crease (simian line), and a protruding tongue may be associated with Down syndrome.

Genetic testing would be necessary to confirm the diagnosis. Various diagnostic tests may need to be conducted to rule out a variety of disorders, including neurological abnormalities, endocrine disorders, or hearing problems. Adaptive skills assessment is essential for children with a suspected intellectual disability. A commonly used tool is the Vineland Adaptive Behavior Scale or the Bayley III (Sparrow et al. 2016; Burakevych et al. 2017). APRNs can be trained to administer the Vineland scale, which is a questionnaire that can be completed while working with the child's parents and observing the child. A functional level can be determined which can serve as the baseline for interventions to improve the child's level of functioning.

Learning Disability

The American Academy of Pediatrics (AAP) uses the definition of learning disability provided in the IDEA: "a disorder in one or more of the basic psychological processes involved in understanding or in using language, spoken or written, that may manifest itself in an imperfect ability to listen, think, speak, read, write, spell, or do mathematical calculations" and "includes such conditions as perceptual disabilities, brain injury, minimal brain dysfunction, dyslexia, and developmental aphasia" (US Congress 2004). The AAP notes that the definition of learning disability "specifically excludes children who have learning problems resulting from primary visual, hearing, or motor disabilities; intellectual disability; and environmental, cultural, or economic disadvantage" (Rimrodt and Lipkin 2011, p. 316).

This chapter will describe the types of disabilities most frequently seen in primary care settings, provide screening tools, discuss evidence-based interventions used with these populations, and present a case study highlighting the journey of a child with a learning disability to young adulthood.

Specific Learning Disabilities: Clinical Picture

The recent DSM-5 manual notes that specific learning disability is a specific deficit in the individual's ability to perceive or process information. This involves below-average academic performance and can involve individuals who have strong intellectual capacities in spite of the impairment (APA 2013). The current definition of learning disability is an effort to replace the previous diagnosis of learning disability, which required only a discrepancy between a child's intellectual ability and the child's current academic performance. The goal of this

new definition is to include more information about specific aspects of the child and his/her family such as age, gender, cultural and language group, and level of education. Interventions which recognize and respond to these more comprehensive factors that are part of everyday life are more likely to be effective than those based only on IQ and performance discrepancy (APS 2013).

The newest diagnostic criteria for specific learning disabilities is very general and does not directly include the former labels of dyslexia, dysgraphia, and dyscalculia. Instead the DSM-5 criteria now require that an individual have persistent difficulties learning and using academic skills in any of the more specific areas of reading, comprehension, writing, spelling, understanding numbers and performing math calculations, and problem-solving activities to be diagnosed with learning disabilities. Additional criteria require that these difficulties cause academic performance which is much lower than expected for age and often that academics, work, and daily activities are impacted. Even though learning difficulties generally begin during the school years, sometimes the full impact of them is not felt until more complex demands are placed on an individual in more advanced educational or occupational settings (APA 203).

As noted above, the newest definition of learning disability is very general. However, when coding for a primary care visit with a child with a learning disability it is recommended that the specific area of need be identified as impairment in reading, written expression, or mathematics. Identifying differences among the characteristics of specific learning disorders provides healthcare and educational professionals with a clearer approach to assessment and interventions for the unique characteristics of the learning disability. The following describes the current descriptions for the most common severe learning disabilities.

Types of Learning Disorders

Impairment in Reading (Dyslexia)

Reading impairment is the most common specific learning disorder, affecting 5–10% of the world's population (Knight 2018). Dyslexia is often the term used to describe reading difficulties associated with poor phonological awareness, including difficulty in recognizing the unique sound patterns made by different letters and combinations of letters. This struggle makes rapid decoding of the written word very difficult and results in problems with sight word recognition, fluency, and spelling (AAP 2009). The newer DSM descriptions suggest that in addition to specific problems identifying and spelling words, comprehension is also an essential component of the diagnosis, which may not be fully recognized until high demands are placed on an individual in higher grades (Landi and Ryherd, 2017).

There are some early indicators which may be predictive of future reading difficulties. Lack of rhyming abilities in preschool children is one of these indicators. Most 4-year-olds are very aware of rhymes and can create list of three to five rhyming words (Wackerle-Hollman et al, 2015). Those without rhyming abilities may struggle with early reading. Recent research (Lim and Chew 2018) suggests that incorporating rhyming poetry and rhyming activities into the preschool curriculum facilitates development of phonological awareness and thus facilitates early reading. Most children enter kindergarten with near-adult levels of speech production but Foy and Mann (2012) discovered that children lacking near-adult speech production in early kindergarten struggled with prereading skills more than those children with near-adult speech production. They concluded that there is a link between early speech production and some aspects of phonological awareness that affect reading abilities. These early findings, which may be clearly predictive of future reading disorders, suggest that if careful assessment of language development is performed periodically in early childhood, it may be possible to identify many children at high risk for reading difficulties. This would prompt early intervention.

Impairment in Writing (Dysgraphia)

The general diagnostic criteria in the DSM-5 for this specific learning disorder include difficulties with spelling, grammar, punctuation accuracy, and organization of written expression. There are no additional characteristics described in the DSM-5. A classic article by Hamstra-Bletz and Blote in 1993 defines dysgraphia as "a disturbance or difficulty in the production of written language related to mechanics of writing. The inadequate handwriting performance is seen among children who have at least an average intelligence level and who have not been diagnosed with any apparent neurological or perceptual-motor difficulties (p. 690). Additional studies since Hamstra-Bletz and Blote have also described dysgraphia in terms of impaired motor function and many children may be referred to occupational therapists who are part of teams aimed at remediation of the disorder (Shah et al. 2019).

Dysgraphia has more recently also been attributed to difficulties in organization as a component of executive function. A very recent study (Rosenblum 2018) found that there were motor issues resulting in uneven writing, unrecognizable letters, poor spacing, and slower speed. However, of note is the finding that children with dysgraphia between 10 and 12 years had differing executive

functioning from their peers without dysgraphia. The affected children had difficulty with planning and organizing their written work on a page. Parents also report similar concerns with daily activities such as initiating and planning homework, organizing daily activities such as dressing, completing chores, and remaining on time. These children need to expend additional energy on activities that are much more easily accomplished by peers.

There are no specific early signs of disorders of written expression that may accurately identify a child at a very young age. However, individuals with dysgraphia are often found to have difficulties with sequencing information and may have fine motor difficulties, which make getting a thought onto paper a very difficult task. These individuals often have excellent verbal skills and can accurately relate information and ideas. However, they have great difficulty in combining the demands of abstract thinking with the fine motor tasks of using a writing implement and sequencing letters and words into meaningful written expression. Children with dysgraphia often produce very limited written work with little elaboration in their writing.

Although there are no clear and specific early markers for dysgraphia, parents and healthcare providers can foster motor development through a variety of activities like puzzles, drawing, and crafts. They can also engage young children in higher level thinking and executive function activities through daily age-appropriate activities like memory and guessing games and family-focused activities like sorting laundry, setting the table, and gardening.

In 2016 it was estimated that 7–15% of school-age children have a writing deficit. It was also estimated that 30–60% of an average school day is spent on writing and other fine motor tasks (Dohla and Heim 2016) so it is critical that early recognition and appropriate interventions are developed to maintain students' self-esteem, interest in learning, and therefore future academic progress

Impairments in Mathematics (Dyscalculia)

DSM-5 authors specify that a mathematics impairment involves difficulty with number sense, memorization of number facts, accurate computation, and mathematical reasoning. They caution that the term dyscalculia is not only difficulty memorizing math facts and performing calculations, but the true disorder includes additional and persistent weaknesses in reasoning or word reasoning accuracy. These weaknesses suggest that the disorder persists long after childhood. In contrast to the definition in the DSM-5, the World Health Organization suggests, in the *International Classification of Diseases*, 10th edition, that a mathematic disability "is a specific impairment in arithmetical skills that cannot be entirely explained by general mental retardation or of inadequate schooling. The deficit concerns mastery of basic computational skills of addition, subtraction, multiplication, and division. In contrast, it does not describe the more abstract mathematical skills involved in algebra, trigonometry, geometry, or calculus." (World Health Organization 2016). For the purposes of identifying young children with a mathematics impairment in this chapter, either definition is appropriate, but it should be noted that in the United States a mathematics disorder is long term and can affect many areas of an individual's personal and professional life.

Although most individuals with math impairments are typically identified in the school setting there may be indicators in early childhood of future impairments in mathematics. Preschoolers may have difficulty learning to count, sort, and understand one-to-one correspondence. A weakness in auditory memory may also be evident in a child who is unable to remember the number in his/her address or later an inability to recall the home phone number (Soares et al. 2018). Kindergarteners may have difficulty with counting sequentially to high numbers, number recognition or seeing a small number of objects and knowing how many there are without counting. Research findings since the 1970s have found a high rate of comorbidity of chronic learning disorders (Feinstein 1970). In more recent years this finding has been confirmed (Schuchardt 2013). School-age children with memory issues find it difficult to master math facts and to hold basic information in short-term memory while manipulating other information in the given problem. They may also have problems with visuospatial relationships which may contribute to math disorders. This difficulty is like that found in children with dysgraphia. These problems can interfere with the ability to learn from material presented on a white board, computer screen, or projector. Children can have difficulty organizing written math information on a page, so it then becomes impossible to correctly compute the answer. These children may also find it difficult to visualize patterns and successfully move through sequential operations.

Since some of the etiologies and risk factors for intellectual and learning disabilities are understood, it is possible to identify and intervene early with these children, making routine early pediatric screening in primary care essential. Early detection, a full assessment by a trained provider, and early interventions may ameliorate some of the actual developmental problems associated with disabilities and subsequently decrease the negative emotional effects associated with these

Table 17.1 Difficulties that may be associated with learning disabilities

- Following directions.
- Getting and staying organized at home and school.
- Understanding verbal directions.
- Learning facts and remembering information.
- Learning subjects taught in school (e.g., math, reading, or spelling) but seeming smart in other things.
- Fitting in with peers or communicating with others.
- Sounding words out and reading or spelling.
- Writing clearly (may have poor handwriting).
- Concentrating and finishing schoolwork (may daydream a lot).
- Explaining information clearly with speech or in writing.

Source: Based on American Academy of Pediatrics (AAP). Common learning disabilities. Retrieved from https://www.healthychildren.org/English/health-issues/conditions/learning-disabilities/Pages/default.aspx.

challenges (Lipkin et al. 2020). The AAP recommends that information from the child/teen and parent be gathered about intellectual and learning-related abilities during routine visits. See Table 17.1 for a list of learning abilities to screen for.

A major role for the APRN is to prepare the parents and child for any needed diagnostic testing and to explain the results of completed tests. Researchers have determined that children with intellectual disabilities suffer from pain more than their peers (Breau and Burkitt 2009). Limited communication skills and maladaptive behavior often make any kind of diagnostic testing stressful for these youngsters. Decreased comprehension by the child and an inability to express herself or himself may lead to frustration and acting out behaviors. In an advocacy role, the APRN should work with other healthcare providers to prepare for the child's procedure and to suggest changes in the normal routine that may facilitate testing and its outcomes. For example, changes in the routine such as allowing parents to stay in the room with the child, medicating the child, and breaking the procedure into smaller segments may be helpful.

Parents or caretakers may also express concerns about the impact of the intellectual disability on the child's self-concept. Donohue et al. (2010) conducted a study on 38 children, aged 7–13, classified by their school district as having mild intellectual disabilities. All children were referred to the study by their classroom teachers because of their difficulty with learning to read or with language skills. The researchers wanted to examine the appropriateness of two self-concept measures for use with this population and the multidimensionality of self-concept in children with mild intellectual disabilities, and to understand the relationship between the self-concept measures and reading achievement.

The measures used were the Harter Pictorial Scale of Perceived Competence and Social Acceptance for Children and the Self-Description Questionnaire Individual Administration, which elicited the child's response to statements read to them. The Harter Pictorial Scale proved to be the better measure to use with the children in the sample because it was a shorter tool. In addition, the findings indicated that, similar to other developing children, self-concept in children with mild intellectual disabilities matures during the elementary school years, affecting the child's academic achievement (including language and reading skills). Researchers recommended that teachers and parents focus on maximizing self-concept in this population as early as possible in order to support healthy social and emotional development and maximize academic performance (Donohue et al. 2010). Nurses can help parents focus on the child's strengths, praise accomplishments, and engage the child in activities in which they can succeed. In addition, referral to activities and groups that focus on skill development and self-concept enhancement may be helpful.

Nursing Interventions: Intellectual Disabilities

Children with an intellectual disability will have the same childhood illnesses, such as otitis media, that all children experience. The difference may be the difficulty in pinpointing the problem due to the lack of communication skills and low tolerance of pain. For the APRN, diagnosing the problem may take on an "explore and discover mission" when the child presents with an elevated temperature or pain. An assessment of the child would need to be more extensive and perhaps at a different pace than if the child could communicate symptoms in an age-appropriate fashion.

Medication management is also important for these youngsters. As mentioned earlier, a child with an intellectual disability may be on a number of medications, including anticonvulsants (for a seizure disorder or to regulate mood), stimulants (to manage symptoms of ADHD), selective serotonin reuptake inhibitors (Food and Drug Administration approved for treatment of pediatric depression), or other psychotropic medications to treat comorbid disorders. They and their parents/caregivers will need to be taught the importance of taking their medications as prescribed, the symptoms the medication targets, and the importance of reporting any worrisome side effects. For example, a stimulant medication like methylphenidate (Ritalin) may be prescribed to assist the child with tasks requiring attention.

Optimal attention skills are needed to facilitate the learning process, which may already pose a difficulty for this youngster.

Ruling out the presence of an underlying hearing deficit is a critical first step in the assessment process for children with an intellectual disability or learning disabilities. The findings from auditory screening may highlight the need for further testing and may explain the reason behind behavioral acting out by the youngster. Regardless, screening provides the APRN with information to guide appropriate supportive interventions. Although newborn screening protocols vary from state to state, it is essential that normal newborn hearing screening results be confirmed and reevaluated periodically. If timely appointments for extensive hearing evaluations are unavailable, the APRN should advocate for the child and family with the appropriate agency responsible for such evaluations. In addition, receiving results of comprehensive hearing evaluations in a timely manner is equally important. Despite a previous finding of normal newborn hearing screening, it is always important to acknowledge parental concerns about hearing difficulties at any age and to perform routine office screening. Patients should be referred to a pediatric audiologist for diagnostic evaluation following abnormal or inconclusive screening results.

In addition to hearing assessments, all children should be routinely screened for deficits in vision and referred for complete ophthalmologic evaluations if there are any issues discovered during screening procedures. Office and school screenings do not identify near-vision problems such as convergence or accommodative insufficiency and significant deficits in close vision. Any child suspected of an intellectual or learning disability should be referred to a pediatric ophthalmologist for evaluation and further treatment if needed (AAP 2009).

As noted above there may be dramatic or only subtle early signs of learning disabilities. The recommendations from the AAP about developmental surveillance, screening, and assessment are very important to follow. In addition to surveillance and screening guidelines, the AAP has published a book entitled *Guide to Learning Disabilities for Primary Care* (2011), which includes content on screening, identification, management, and advocacy.

Developmental surveillance at all well-child visits is imperative. The longitudinal process of surveillance allows the APRN to look at the child in context and gather important developmental information over time to facilitate early case-finding and engage in preventive interventions (Blows et al. 2016). Careful questioning of parents about the child's current developmental achievements at each visit provides the APRN with valuable information about the progression of milestones in each developmental domain. At regular intervals (9, 18, and 24 or 30 months), the AAP (2009) recommends the use of standardized screening tools. The AAP statement offers a variety of appropriate screening tools to use at these specific intervals. Some tools depend on parental report of developmental abilities while other tools require the child to perform a variety of developmental activities. An extensive list of recommended screening tools to be used at the recommended intervals of 9, 18, and 30 months is given in Table 17.2.

In addition to screening, it is important to discuss linguistic skills that should be emerging in the preschool years with the parents or caregivers. These include rhyming, recitation of nursery rhymes, letter recognition, auditory comprehension of multiple-step directions, and an awareness of print literacy (Marrus and Hall 2017). These activities can be easily incorporated into preschool well-child visits.

Conducting a careful history of the preschool child's participation and progress in preschool, Head Start, or structured daycare settings provides important clues about the child's overall language development and exposure to verbal and print activities. Since language

issues may impact social and emotional development, family and peer interactions are important to assess at routine primary care visits. Concerns voiced by parents or professionals in these settings merit a referral to the local school system for a complete speech and language evaluation and, if warranted by history, a complete psychoeducational and social–emotional evaluation. APRNs must be aware of community services and resources for preschool learning needs. These include services provided by the local school system, community playgroups, library literacy programs, social skills groups, or lists of professionals who provide individual services.

Although worrisome symptoms may be present in early childhood, it is often not until school age that specific concerns about learning or intellectual abilities are raised by parents and school personnel (Lipkin et al. 2020). APRNs continue to be important participants in the evaluation and referral processes since they know the family and social history as well as the child's past medical and developmental history. APRNs can identify medical conditions such as iron deficiency, lead poisoning, seizures, and asthma as well as genetic conditions such as fragile X syndrome that may impact learning

Table 17.2 Selected early developmental screening tools

Name of tool	Screening domains	Ages	Sources
Parent report tools			
Ages & Stages Questionnaires (ASQ)	Communication, fine and gross motor, problem solving, personal adaptive skills Pass /fail score for each domain	4–60 months	Squires et al. (1999)
Parents' Evaluation of Developmental Status (PEDS)	Development and behavior Useful for surveillance	Ages 0–8	Glascoe (1999)
Child Development Inventory (CDI)	Social, self-help, motor, language, and general development skills	18 months to 6 years	Ireton (1992) Doig et al. (1999)
Child performance tools			
Battelle Developmental Inventory Screening Tool, (2nd edition) (BDI-ST)	Personal-social, adaptive, motor, communication, and cognitive development Scoring is pass/fail	0–95 months	Newborg (2004)
Bayley Infant Neurodevelopmental Screen (BINS)	Neurologic functions, auditory, visual and tactile receptive function, expressive function, and cognitive processing	3–24 months	Aylward (1995) Aylward et al. (2000)
Brigance Screens-II	Articulation, expressive and receptive language, gross and fine motor skills, general knowledge, social skills, and pre-academic skills	0–90 months 0–23 months Use parent report tool	Glascoe (2005, 2002)
Denver-II Developmental Screening Test	Expressive and receptive language, gross and fine motor skills, personal–social skills Scoring: normal, questionable, and abnormal	0–6 years	Frankenburg et al. (1971, 1992) Denver Developmental Materials Inc., PO Box 371 075, Denver, CO

and academic performance. Medications for already identified chronic conditions such as seizures and asthma may impact learning potential by causing drowsiness or overactive behavior, which should be explained to the parents and school personnel as warranted.

Even in children without previously identified medical or learning problems, surveillance and screening of school progress are essential in the primary care setting and questions about school adjustment and achievements are critical components in a complete review of systems. For school-age children, the APRN can review report cards, encourage the child to read brief passages of grade-appropriate books recommended by local schools, and engage the child in memory, spelling, and math games during the health assessment visit.

Several screening tools are useful in the early assessment of school problems. These tools help to discriminate if the cause of poor school performance may be a learning issue, a mental health issue, or a behavioral issue. The Pediatric Symptom Checklist (Jellinek et al. 1999) is an easy-to-use tool that screens children from 4 through 18 years of age for cognitive, emotional,

and behavioral issues. After the general area of concern is identified, other disorder-specific tools are available to further assess concerns. Positive results on any of these tools require further assessment and management by the primary care provider, mental health specialist, and school or education personnel. Since intellectual disabilities are complex disorders often with comorbid mental health issues, a collaborative effort among all professionals is most effective. See Table 17.3 for additional behavioral, learning, and mental health screening tools.

It is not uncommon for parents of high school-age children to raise concerns about their adolescent's academic progress. Lack of motivation, failing grades, oppositional behavior, and poor self-esteem are frequently reported. Undiagnosed learning disabilities may contribute to an adolescent's downward spiral. To sort out potentially multifaceted issues, joint and separate interviews with parents and the adolescent must be conducted and a confidentiality agreement clearly established. Obtaining releases for healthcare providers to speak with school personnel is also useful since exchange of academic, behavioral, and medical information may

Table 17.3 Selected screening tools for mental health, learning, and behavioral issues

Name and authors	Age group	Number of items	Description
Center for Epidemiological Studies Depression Scale for Children (Faulstich et al. 1986)	Children, adolescents	20-item self-report	A depression inventory with possible scores ranging from 0 to 60. Higher scores indicate increasing levels of depression, with a score of 15 suggestive of depressive symptoms in children and adolescents.
Columbia DISC Depression Scale (Shaffer et al. 2003) (formerly the Diagnostic Interview Schedule for Children)	11 and older	22-question surveys for teens and parents	Completed separately by both the teen and a parent (no = 0, yes = 1). Assesses chances of depression.
Screen for Child Anxiety Related Disorders (Birmaher et al. 1995)	9- to 18-year-olds	41-item self-report	A survey to be completed by the child and parent separately. A total score of ≥25 may indicate the presence of an anxiety disorder. Scores higher than 30 are more specific to the type of anxiety disorder.
Vanderbilt Scales (Wolraich et al. 1996)	6- to 12-year-olds	55 items	A reliable, cost-effective assessment for ADHD in clinical and research settings. Evaluates for ADHD and other comorbid conditions. Takes 10 minutes or less to complete. The VADPRS has two components: symptom assessment and impairment of performance at home, in school, and in social settings. The automated feedback report provides instant scoring and item analysis.
Strengths and Difficulties Questionnaire (Goodman 1994)	4- to 16-year-olds	25 items for parents, teachers, and older children	Emotional, behavioral, and mental health screening tool
Conners' Rating Scales (Conners 1990)	3- to 17-year-olds		Screening tool for ADHD. Has both parent and teacher versions. Tool has been revised several times and the number of items is version dependent.

help define the components of school difficulties and facilitate the development of a comprehensive and transparent management plan of care.

Primary Care Screening

As with all disorders, earlier diagnosis provides more opportunities for interventions. As noted above there may be dramatic or only subtle early signs of learning disabilities. The recommendations from the AAP about developmental surveillance, screening, and assessment are very important to follow. In addition to surveillance and screening guidelines, the AAP has published a book entitled *Guide to Learning Disabilities for Primary Care* (2011), which includes content on screening, identification, management, and advocacy.

Developmental surveillance at all well-child visits is imperative. The longitudinal process of surveillance allows the APRN to look at the child in context and gather important developmental information over time to facilitate early case-finding and engage in preventive interventions (Blows et al. 2016). Careful questioning of parents about the child's current developmental achievements at each visit provides the APRN with valuable information about the progression of milestones in each developmental domain. At regular intervals (9, 18, and 24 or 30 months), the AAP (2009) recommends the use of standardized screening tools. The AAP statement offers a variety of appropriate screening tools to use at these specific intervals. Some tools depend on parental report of developmental abilities while other tools require the child to perform a variety of developmental activities. An extensive list of recommended screening tools to be used at the recommended intervals of 9, 18, and 30 months is given in Table 17.2.

In addition to screening, it is important to discuss linguistic skills that should be emerging in the preschool years with the parents or caregivers. These include rhyming, recitation of nursery rhymes, letter recognition, auditory comprehension of multiple-step directions, and an awareness of print literacy (Ozernov-Palchik et al. 2018). These activities can be easily incorporated into preschool well-child visits.

Conducting a careful history of the preschool child's participation and progress in preschool, Head Start, or structured daycare settings provides important clues about the child's overall language development and exposure to verbal and print activities. Since language issues may impact social and emotional development, family and peer interactions are important to assess at routine primary care visits. Concerns voiced by parents or professionals in these settings merit a referral to the local school system for a complete speech and language evaluation and, if warranted by history, a complete

psychoeducational and social–emotional evaluation. APRNs must be aware of community services and resources for preschool learning needs. These include services provided by the local school system, community playgroups, library literacy programs, social skills groups, or lists of professionals who provide individual services.

Although worrisome symptoms may be present in early childhood, it is often not until school age that specific concerns about learning abilities are raised by parents and school personnel (Preston et al. 2016). APRNs continue to be important participants in the evaluation and referral processes since they know the family and social history as well as the child's past medical and developmental history.

An additional tool which may illuminate mental health, social, and learning issues is the Strengths and Difficulties Questionnaire. This tool may be completed by parents and teachers in 4–17-year-olds. A self-report version is available for 11–17-year-olds. It assesses emotional problems, conduct problems, peer problems, and hyperactivity. All of these difficulties may contribute to poor school performance. The information gained from the screening is helpful in determining the next steps in evaluation and has also been found to monitor effectiveness of services received by school-age children (Goodman and Goodman 2009). It is not in the public domain and is best scored using a computer program but may also be scored manually.

Parent completion of the Vineland Adaptive Behavior Scales (3rd edition) will also add important information to a child's developmental profile if there are concerns about learning issues. DSM-5 authors suggest that information about age, gender, culture, education, and interventions be included in an evaluation for learning disorders (APA, 2013). The Vineland Adaptive Behavior Scales will provide this general information and give the evaluator a more complete profile of a child's skills and experiences (Sparrow et al. 2016). See Table 17.3 for additional behavioral, learning, and mental health screening tools.

Post Screening Assessment and Treatment Planning

After a positive screening for learning issues at any age, a specialized and focused multidisciplinary evaluation should be conducted by a birth to three program, local school system, or other professionals trained in intellectual or learning disabilities assessment. A complete list of community and professional resources with contact information is helpful to give to parents. Once a child turns 3 years of age, the local public school is responsible by federal law for the evaluation and provision of services if a disability is detected (IDEA n.d.).

A written parental request for a school evaluation is often effective in starting the evaluation process. A similar request to the school from the child's healthcare provider may hasten the scheduling of an evaluation. Individual state regulations determine the length of time allowed between request for evaluation and completion of evaluation. Assessment of school-age children and teens includes IQ testing (Wechsler 1991) to measure cognitive abilities and achievement tests such as the Woodcock-Johnson (McGrew and Woodcock 2001) or the Wide Range Achievement Test (Wilkinson and Robertson 2006) to evaluate grade-level progress in academic areas of reading, writing, and math. Additional assessments will ideally include speech and language, gross motor, visual-fine motor, auditory processing, visual and auditory acuity, and mental health evaluation. School or clinical psychologists and speech and language specialists will frequently be the healthcare providers completing most of the assessment at this level of evaluation.

Once the evaluations are completed, a joint meeting of parents and all involved professionals should be convened. The purpose of this meeting would be to review the evaluation results, determine if the child meets the diagnostic criteria of specific intellectual or learning disability, and develop an individual education plan (IEP) to meet the specific learning needs of the child. IEP meetings are held periodically or at least annually to review student progress and determine need for change in services. The IEP specifically describes goals, objectives, and the means to achieve them in measurable terms. This is a legal document to which the school is obliged to adhere (IDEA n.d.). Students with a diagnosis of a specific learning or intellectual disability may receive a variety of services to remediate the challenges the youngster faces. These services may include but are not limited to the following:

1. One-on-one tutoring or personal aide, resource room with a special education teacher, individual psychological therapy, resource support in the regular classroom, speech and language services, occupational therapy services, social work services, and assistive technology such as personal computers, tablets, and recording devices.

2. If a child is determined to have educational needs that can be met in the regular classroom a 504 plan is developed. Section 504 of the Rehabilitation Act of 1973 grants accommodations in the classroom that will eliminate barriers and enhance learning through use of reasonable accommodations.

Specific Federal Acts Protecting Those with Disabilities

Healthcare providers must be knowledgeable about federal legislation and how each state interprets and implements these regulations. The IDEA and the Americans with Disabilities Act (ADA; www.ada.gov) are both federal statutes that mandate services to ensure education services for children with disabilities to support their success. IDEA mandates that children with disabilities up to 21 years are identified, evaluated by an interdisciplinary team, and educated in the least restrictive environment and that parents have the right to due process to secure the most appropriate educational services for their youngster.

These statutes provide for accommodations to include but are not limited to preferential seating, modified assignments, human and technical assistance to support learning, extended time on assignments, and in-class and standardized tests. The IDEA requires that a written individualized IEP be developed stipulating the services needed by the child with the disability. IEPs are to be reevaluated every 3 years. It also mandates the school district to provide the revenue and or human resources to execute the plan.

Section 504 of the Rehabilitation Act of 1973 is a civil rights law that requires schools to eliminate barriers that would prevent students from participating in programs and services offered in a general curriculum. Reasonable accommodations must be made for the child with a disability. The 504 plan should be reevaluated annually to assure that accommodations are consistent with needs (National Center for Learning Disabilities n.d.).

Assisting with Family Coping

Parents are of course usually worried and anxious about the child and the identified delays or learning problems. The parents often feel guilty or responsible for the child's problems and will move through a grief cycle that begins, as for most grief, with denial and disbelief (Finke 1995). Parents may have difficulty accepting the diagnoses. Their denial is compounded by the fact that an exact cause frequently cannot be determined and a prediction of the child's future developmental level also cannot be predetermined. Families move to the next stage, which is anger followed by a searching for causes and solutions. Frequently no cause is identified so families move from searching for a cause to preoccupation with the weaknesses and disability. Families cycle through the various stages of grieving and coping over and over, and healthcare providers often only see the family when there is a crisis, illness, or behavioral issue (Finke 1995). It is important to view the process as a cycle so the APRN

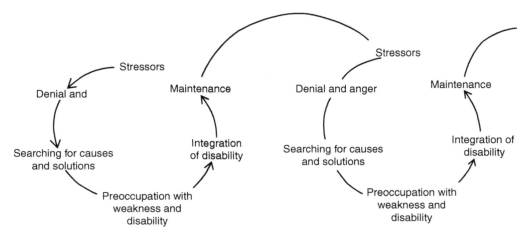

Figure 17.1 The Typology Model of Family Adjustment and Adaptation. (Reprinted from Finke, 1995, with permission from Lippincott Williams & Wilkins.)

can intervene and facilitate the move to the acceptance stage. Family members may move through the stages at different paces, which can also add to the stress on the family system (Figure 17.1).

The APRN needs to assist the family in each stage of grief by working with the child's strengths to support reaching the child's potential. Families can best assist their child if they focus on strengths and build on achievements to help the child reach her or his highest level. Families should also focus on the child's individual successes and not make comparisons to normal or appropriate milestones based on chronological age. The child's progress should be based only on his or her developmental achievements.

For adolescents with intellectual disabilities, this can be a particularly difficult time because the lack of social skills may be more noticeable to family members, peers, and the adolescent. It is also frequently at the beginning of adolescence that children with intellectual disabilities become increasingly aware of the differences between themselves and other individuals their age. Adolescence is a time for more independence and activities such as driving a car, which may not be possible for an individual who has an intellectual disability.

The APRN should also be mindful of the impact of having a brother or sister who is different than the other children in the family. Siblings are often placed in a position to watch over their brother or sister who may be chronologically older or they may find themselves defending their sibling in social situations with their own peers or others. The fact is that as the family matures, siblings will gain more responsibility for the brother or sister with an intellectual or developmental disability. Families need to plan and discuss strategies early in the process and not wait until there is a family crisis such as an illness or death of a parent.

Older children and families may be even more stressed. Co-occurring problems and difficulty in pinpointing a cause may be more frustrating, especially if mental health problems are part of the clinical picture (Faust and Scior 2007). Parents worry about the strain on their child, who does not understand what they are feeling. Parents also feel they are alone in finding answers and appropriate interventions to assist their child. It is important for the APRN to remain family focused and view the family as an essential part of the treatment team. Of course, the family knows the child best and must incorporate the child's needs and behavior into their activities and daily life. Children with an intellectual disability often have difficulty with disruptions in routines. Assessment of the family and family behavior patterns should be continuous. Behavior of family members may aggravate the child's difficult behaviors, resulting in development and maintenance of a circular pattern of negative behaviors (Skotarczak and Lee 2015).

Over the life span of the child, diagnostic labels may change. Parents and the child often struggle with labels and parents may resist a child being given a diagnosis at all. APRNs need to point out to parents and older children that without a diagnosis, the child will not qualify for any additional assistance at school or from social agencies. Funding follows diagnosis. Families who focus on the child's needs and not the title will be able to seek the most appropriate resources to help their child move forward.

Teachers and other school personnel are also important members of the treatment team. Their observations and goals need to be incorporated into the treatment plan. The APRN may also find herself or himself in the advocacy role for the family with the school and potential policy makers. Individual needs may take a backseat to larger school or classroom goals, and the APRN will need to facilitate the child's and family's needs being heard and met by the school. Parents may need coaching concerning assertiveness and advocacy so they can be more effective in navigating the healthcare system and the school system. If social services are involved, such as Medicaid, even more coordination and advocacy may be needed to combine efforts and work toward mutual goals that are in the child's best interest.

Resiliency Model

The use of the resiliency model of family stress, adjustment, and adaptation is a useful approach to assist families with children who have a disability and help them connect to community resources. The resiliency model builds on the work of McCubbin and Patterson (1983) and their Typology Model of Family Adjustment and Adaptation (McCubbin 1995). The Typology Model of Family Adjustment and Adaptation is a collaborative model that enhances the connection of the family to the community and available resources to assist them in meeting the child's needs. All families cope with stresses over time and those experiences affect the family's perceptions over time. Families with a child who has a disability face even more stresses as they interact with the healthcare system, the school system, and community systems. Stressors build up but so do the coping strategies used by the family. McCubbin and Patterson labeled the adjustment of the family to stressors as adaptation. During adaption, families try to use their usual patterns of coping and these often do not work or do not work for long due to the high level of stress. For the family to move to a more effective level of functioning, they must make changes in patterns of interaction and roles that meet the needs of the child with the disability and those of other family members (Kosciulek et al. 1993).

Families learn, with the assistance of the APRN, to use their strengths and resources within the extended family and to connect to resources in the community (Early and GlenMaye 2000). Social support and hardiness have been found to be predictors of successful adaptation by families (Weiss 2002). Using a strengths perspective, the APRN forms a collaborative partnership with the family to assist them in meeting their goals. The APRN can activate community resources such as respite care, funding sources, occupational or physical therapy, and transportation (Finke 1995). The APRN should serve as advocate for the family and as problem solver with the school system to find solutions to best meet the needs of the child and his or her family. As the child develops new problems, situations will arise that will need new interventions. Research has shown that the child, especially in adolescence, can be a reliable source to determine personal strengths and difficulties (Emerson 2005).

Tools such as genograms (pedigree) and ecomaps can provide the APRN with the information needed to assist families in reaching out to resources (Walsh 2016). A genogram is a picture of the family tree that includes genetic connections, family events such as marriages, births of children, deaths, and health conditions. The genogram is an illustration of the family resources as well as possible connections and sources of assistance such as respite relief. The genogram can also be an important diagnostic tool to identify possible genetic causes of disabilities. The ecomap is an illustration of the community systems that influence each family member and again may be turned into resources. For example, the school would be part of the ecomap as would healthcare providers and community agencies. The ecomap starts with a circle around the family with lines drawn to community systems that impact each family member. Lines can be doubled and tripled to note positive relationships, and train track lines can be drawn to demonstrate negative influences. The ecomap can be used by the APRN and family to identify possible sources for assistance such as a community agency that provides transportation or recreational activities.

The first step is always helping the family determine their own goals and not take on the goals of the APRN or other social agencies. For example, some services may push respite care away from the child's home. Some children and families may find respite care in their own home more comfortable, or the other way around. Family belief systems, finances, community resources, and extended family are just a few of the pieces that may determine what is best for the child and family.

Parents should be encouraged to pursue treatments with evidence-based parameters such as pharmacological management of ADHD symptoms (Al-Khudairi et al. 2019). APRNs must be respectful of parents' quest for a cure and seek to educate families about accepted and proven therapies and treatments for disabilities while cautioning them about the potential dangers of unproven approaches. Parents and children, when old enough, should be encouraged to reach out to others with similar issues and participate in support groups. There are many online resources such as Arc of the United States (http://TheArcLink.org), which is an organization that advocates for the rights of children and adults with developmental delays. There are state and local chapters as well. The Arc website has a wealth of information and links to resources about special education, education information about specific diagnoses, and financial resources. The National Center for Learning Disabilities (http://NCLD.org) has information about specific learning disabilities and links to other resources as well. A similar organization is the Learning

Disabilities Association of America (www.ldaamerica.org). Talking with other family members and people with similar issues can be a great comfort and provide support and a wealth of information. Another resource is Best Buddies (www.bestbuddies.org), which is a non-profit volunteer organization that offers employment, leadership development, one-to-one friendships, and inclusive living opportunities for individuals with intellectual and developmental disabilities. Best Buddies strives to decrease social isolation and stigma experienced by this population. Parents need to be referred to educational sessions early about their child's right to a "free and appropriate education" governed by federal and state regulations. The rights begin for children at birth and extend to 21 years of age, so parents need to be well informed early in the process.

Community resources vary across states and regions. Parents need to be connected to resources in their community to assist with education, health needs, social supports, financial resources, respite care, etc. APRNs can be a direct link to these resources. As children develop and progress families need to be encouraged to plan for the future. Decisions about guardianship, wills, special trusts, and living arrangements need to be discussed and put in place. Many of these children will be able to attend a job skill training program or attend post-secondary education, including pursing a college degree. It is difficult for families to plan for the future while dealing with the hurdles of daily life. APRNs need to connect families to organizations and social agencies that can help further the journey to meet the family's needs.

Conclusion

After the discovery of an intellectual or learning disability, coping is a major lifelong challenge for the child and the entire family. APRNs can provide the needed screening, interventions, and continued support to families to help their family member reach his or her potential. The APRN works with the family to progress to the highest potential for all family members. The family is assessed, connected to resources, and assisted through the continuing cycle of coping and building on strengths as the family climbs the ladder toward optimal development.

References

American Academy of Pediatrics (AAP) (2009). Learning disabilities, dyslexia, and vision. *Pediatrics* 124: 837–844.

American Academy of Pediatrics (AAP) (2010). *Common learning disabilities*. Available at http://www.healthychildren.org/English/health-issues/conditions/learning-disabilities/pages/Common-Learning-Disabilities.aspx.

Al-Khudairi, R., Perera, B., Solomou, S., and Courtenay, K. (2019). Adults with intellectual disability and attention deficit hyperactivity disorder: Clinical characteristics and medication profiles. *British Journal of Learning Disabilities* 47 (2): 145–152.

American Association on Intellectual and Developmental Disabilities. (n.d.). Definition of Intellectual Disability. Available at http://aaidd.org/intellectual-disability/definition.

American Psychiatric Association (2013). *Diagnostic and Statistical Manual of Mental Disorders*, 5e. Washington, DC: American Psychiatric Association.

Aylward, G.P. (1995). *Bayley Infant Neurodevelopmental Screener*. San Antonio, TX: Psychological Corp.

Aylward, G.P., Verhulst, S.J., and Bell, S. (2000). Predictive utility of the BSID-II infant neurodevelopmental screener (BINS) risk status classifications: clinical interpretation and application. *Developmental Medicine & Child Neurology* 42: 25–31.

Belkady, B., Elkhattabi, L., Elkarhat, Z. et al. (2018). Chromosomal abnormalities in patients with intellectual disability: A 21-year retrospective study. *Human Heredity* 83 (5): 274–282. https://doi.org/10.1159/000499710.

Birmaher, B., Khetarpal, S., Cully, M. et al. (1995). *Screen for Child Anxiety Related Disorders (SCARED)*. Pittsburgh, PA: University of Pittsburgh, Western Psychiatric Institute and Clinic.

Blows, E., Teoh, L., and Paul, S. (2016). Recognition and management of learning disabilities in early childhood by community practitioners. *Community Practitioner*, 89(5): 32–37.

Boyle, C.A., Boulet, S., Schieve, L.A., and Cohen, R.A. (2011). Trends in the prevalence of developmental disabilities in US children, 1997–2008. *Pediatrics* 127 (6): 1034–1042. https://doi.org/10.1542/peds.1010.2989.

Breau, L.M. and Burkitt, C. (2009). Assessing pain in children with intellectual disabilities. *Pain Research Management* 14: 116–120.

Burakevych, N., McKinlay, C.J.D., Alsweiler, J.M. et al. (2017). Bayley-III motor scale and neurological examination at 2 years do not predict motor skills at 4.5 years. *Developmental Medicine and Child Neurology* 59 (2): 216–223. https://doi.org/10.1111/dmcn.13232.

Conners, C.K. (1990). *Conners' Rating Scales*. North Tonawanda, NY: Multi-Health Systems, Inc.

Danielson, M.L., Bitsko, R.H., Ghandour, R.M. et al. (2016). Prevalence of parent-reported ADHD diagnosis and associated treatment among US children and adolescents, 2016. *Journal of Clinical Child and Adolescent Psychology* 47 (2): 199–212.

Danielson, M.L., Visser, S.N., Chronis-Tuscano, A., and DuPaul, G.J. (2018). A national description of treatment among US children and adolescents with ADHD. *Journal of Pediatrics*, 192 e1: 240–246.

Döhla, D. and Heim, S. (2016). Developmental dyslexia and dysgraphia: what can we learn from the one about the other? *Frontiers in Psychology* 6: 1–12.

Doig, K.B., Macias, M.M., Saylor, C.F. et al. (1999). The child development inventory: a developmental outcome measure for follow-up of the high risk infant. *Journal of Pediatrics* 135: 358–362.

Donohue, D., Wise, J., Romski, M. et al. (2010). Self-concept development and measurement in children with mild intellectual disabilities. *Developmental Neurorehabilitation* 13: 322–334.

Early, T. and GlenMaye, L. (2000). Valuing families: social work practice with families from a strengths perspective. *Social Work* 45: 118–130.

Emerson, E. (2005). Use of strengths and difficulties questionnaire to assess the mental health needs of children and adolescents with intellectual disabilities. *Journal of Intellectual and Developmental Disabilities* 30: 14–23.

Faulstich, M.E., Carey, M.P., Ruggiero, L. et al. (1986). Assessment of depression in childhood and adolescence: an evaluation of the center for epidemiological studies depression scale for children (CES-DC). *The American Journal of Psychiatry* 143: 1024–1027.

Faust, H. and Scior, K. (2007). Mental health problems in young people with intellectual disabilities: The impact on parents. *Journal of Applied Research in Intellectual Disabilities* 21 (5): 414–424. doi: 10.111/j.1468-3148.2007.00411.x.

Feinstein, A.R. (1970). The pre-therapeutic classification of co-morbidity in chronic disease. *Journal of Chronic Diseases* 3: 455–468. https://doi.org/10.1016/0021-9681(70)90054-8.

Finke, L. (1995). Mental retardation. In: *Child and Adolescent Family Psychiatric Nursing*, 174–179 (ed. B. Johnson). Philadelphia, PA: J.B. Lippincott.

Foy, J.G. and Mann, V.A. (2011). Speech production deficits in early readers: predictors of risk. *Reading and Writing* 25: 799–830.

Frankenburg, W.K., Camp, B.W., and Van Natta, P.A. (1971). Validity of the Denver developmental screening test. *Child Development* 42: 475–485.

Frankenburg, W.K., Dodds, J., Archer, P. et al. (1992). The Denver II: a major revision and restandardization of the Denver developmental screening test. *Pediatrics* 89: 91–97.

Glascoe, F.P. (1999). Toward a model for an evidenced-based approach to developmental/behavioral surveillance, promotion and patient education. *Ambulatory Child Health* 5: 197–208.

Glascoe, F.P. (2002). The Brigance infant-toddler screen (BITS): standardization and validation. *Journal of Developmental Behavioral Pediatrics* 23: 145–150.

Glascoe, F.P. (2005). *Technical Report for the Brigance Screens*. North Billerica, MA: Curriculum Associates Inc.

Goodman, R. (1994). A modified version of the Rutter parent questionnaire including items on children's strengths: a research note. *Journal of Child Psychology and Psychiatry* 35: 1483–1494.

Goodman, A. and Goodman, R. (2009). Strengths and difficulties questionnaire as a dimensional measure of child mental health. *Journal of the American Academy of Child and Adolescent Psychiatry* 48 (4): 400–403. https://doi.org/10.1097/CHI.013e3181985068.

Hamstra-Bletz, L., Blote,, A.W. (1993). A longitudinal study on dysgraphic handwriting in primary school. *Journal of Learning Disabilities* 26(10): 689–699.

IDEA. (n.d.). *Learning disabilities*. Individuals with Disability Education Improvement Act. Available at http://www2.ed.gov/policy/speced/guid/idea/idea2004.html http://www.copyright.gov/legislation/pl108-446.pdf.

Ireton, H. (1992). *Child Development Inventory Manual*. Minneapolis, MN: Behavior Science Systems Inc.

Jellinek, M., Murphy, J., and Little, M. (1999). Use of the pediatric symptom checklist (PSC) to screen for psychosocial problems in pediatric primary care: a national feasibility study. *Archives of Pediatric and Adolescent Medicine* 153: 254–260.

Knight, C. (2018). What is dyslexia? An exploration of the relationship between teachers' understandings of dyslexia and their training experiences. *Dyslexia* 24 (3): 207–219. https://doi.org/10.1002/dys.1593.

Kosiulek, J., McCubbin, M., and McCubbin, H. (1993). A theoretical framework for family adaptation to head injury. *Journal of Rehabilitation* 59: 40–45.

Landi, N. and Ryherd, K. (2017). Understanding specific reading comprehension deficit: A review. *Language and Linguistics Compass* 11 (2): e12234. Published online 22 February 2017. doi: 10.111/lnc3.12234.

Lim, C.T. & Chew, F.P. (2018). Using poems to increase phonological awareness among children. Paper presented at the *Issues and Trends in Interdisciplinary Behavior and Social Science – Proceedings of the 6th International Congress on Interdisciplinary Behavior and Social Sciences, ICIBSoS 2017*, 33–40.

Lipkin, P.H., Macias, M.M., and Council on Children with Disabilities, Section on Developmental and Behavioral Pediatrics (2020). Promoting optimal development: Identifying infants and young children with developmental disorders through developmental surveillance and screening. *Pediatrics* 145 (1): e20193449. https://doi.org/10.1542/peds.2019-3449.

Marrus, N. and Hall, L. (2017). Intellectual disability and language disorder. *Child and Adolescent Psychiatric Clinics of North America* 26 (3): 539–554. https://doi.org/10.1016/chc.2017.03.001.

Matson, J.L., Belva, B.C., Hattier, M.A., and Matson, M.L. (2012). Scaling methods to measure psychopathology in persons with intellectual disabilities. *Research in Developmental Disabilities* 33 (2): 549–562.

McCubbin, M. (1995). The typology model of adjustment and adaptation: a family stress model. *Counseling and Guidance* 10 (4): 31–37.

McCubbin, M. and Patterson, J. (1983). The family stress process: the double ABCX model of adjustment and adaptation. In: *Social Stress and the Family: Advances and Development in Family Stress Theory and Research* (eds. H. McCubbin, M. Sussman and J. Patterson), 7–37. New York, NY: Haworth Press.

McGrew, K.S. and Woodcock, R. (2001). *Woodcock-Johnson III Technical Manual*. Chicago, IL: Riverside Publishing.

National Center for Learning Disabilities. (n.d.). *Section 504 and IDEA comparison chart*. Available at http://insource.org/files/pages/0087-Section_504_vs_IEP.PDFs

Newborg, J. (2004). *Battelle developmental inventory*, 2 nde. Itasca, IL: Riverside Publishing.

Ozernov-Palchik, O., Wolf, M., and Patel, A.D. (2018). Relationships between early literacy and nonlinguistic rhythmic processes in kindergarteners. *Journal of Experimental Child Psychology* 167: 354–368. https://doi.org/10.1016/j.jecp.2017.11.009.

Preston, A., Wood, C., and Stecker, P. (2016). Response to intervention: where it came from and where it's going. *Preventing School Failure* 60 (3): 173–182.

Raspa, M., Wheeler, A., and Riley, C. (2017). Public health literature review of fragile X syndrome. *Pediatrics* 139 (suppl 3): s153–s171. https://doi.org/10.1542/peds.2016-1159C.

Rehabilitation Act of 1973, Pub. L. No. 93–112 (1973).

Rimrodt, S.L. and Lipkin, P.H. (2011). Learning disabilities and school failure. *Pediatrics in Review* 32: 315–324.

Rosenblum, S. (2018). Inter-relationships between objective handwriting features and executive control among children with developmental dysgraphia. *PLoS One* 13 (4) https://doi.org/10.1371/journal.pone.0196098.

Schuchardt, K., Bockmann, A.-K., Bornemann, G., and Maehler, C. (2013). Working memory functioning in children with learning disorders and specific language impairment. *Topics in Language Disorders* 33 (4): 298–312. https://doi.org/10.1097/01.TLD.0000437943.41140.36.

Shaffer, D., Fisher, P., and Lucas, C. (2003). The diagnostic interview schedule for children (DISC). In: *Comprehensive Handbook of Psychological Assessment*, vol. 2 (eds. M.J. Hilsenroth, D.L. Segal and M. Hersen), 256–270. New York, NY: Wiley.

Shah, H.R., Sagar, J.K.V., Somaiy, J.P., and Nagpal, J.K. (2019). Clinical practice guidelines on assessment and management of specific learning disorders. *Indian Journal of Psychiatry* 61 (suppl 2): 211–225. https://doi.org/10.4103/psychiatry.IndianJPsychiatry_564_18.

Skotarczak, L. and Lee, G.K. (2015). Effects of parent management training programs on disruptive behavior for children with a developmental disability: A meta-analyis. *Research in*

Developmental Disabilities 38: 272–287. https://doi.org/10.1016/j.ridd.2014.12.004.

Soares, N., Evans, T., and Patel, D.R. (2018). Specific learning disability in mathematics: A comprehensive review. *Translational Pediatrics* 7 (1): 48–62. https://doi.org/10.21037/tp.2017.08.03.

Sparrow, S.S., Cicchetti, D.V., and Saulnier, C.A. (2016). *Vineland Adaptive Behavior Scales*, 3e. Bloomington, MN: PsychCorp.

Squires, J., Potter, L., and Bricker, D. (1999). *The ASQ User's Guide*, 2nde. Baltimore, MD: Paul H. Brookes Publishing.

Tau, C., Hepworth, J., and Neville, C. (2012). Nurses' role in caring for people with a comorbidity of mental illness and intellectual disability: a literature review. *International Journal of Mental Health Nursing* 21 (2): 163–174.

US Department of Education. (2020). Students with disabilities. Institute of Education Sciences, National Center for Education Statistics. Available at https://nces.ed.gov/programs/coe/indicator_cgg.asp.

US Congress. (2004). *Reauthorization of the Individuals with Disabilities Education Act: Hearing of the Committee on Labor and Human Resources*. US Senate, 108th Congress, Committee on Labor and Human Resources, First Session. 3 December. Vol. 150. Washington, DC: United States Government Printing Office.

Visser, S.N., Danielson, M.L., Wolraich, M.L. et al. (2016). Vital signs: National and state-specific patterns of attention deficit/hyperactivity disorder treatment among insured children aged 2–5 years: United States, 2008–2014. *Morbidity and Mortality Weekly Report* 65: 443–450.

Wackerle-Hollman, A.K., Schmitt, B.A., Bradfield, T.A., Rodriguez, M.S., McConnell, S.R. (2015). Redefining individual growth and development indicators: Phonological awareness. *Journal of Learning Disabilities*, 48(5), 495–510.

Walsh, F. (2016). Applying a family resilience framework in training, practice, and research: Mastering the art of the possible. *Family Process* 55 (4): 616–632.

Wechsler, D. (1991). *The Wechsler Intelligence Scale for Children*, 3rde. San Antonio, TX: The Psychological Corporation.

Weiss, M.J. (2002). Hardiness and social support as predictors of stress in mothers of typical children, children with autism, and children with mental retardation. *Autism* 6: 115–130.

Wilkinson, G.S. and Robertson, G.J. (2006). *Wide Range Achievement Test*, 4 the. Lutz, FL: Psychological Assessment Resources.

Wolraich, M.L., Hannah, J.N., Pinnock, T.Y. et al. (1996). Comparison of diagnostic criteria for attention-deficit hyperactivity disorder in a county-wide sample. *Journal of the American Academy of Child and Adolescent Psychiatry* 35: 319–324.

World Health Organization. (2016). ICD-10 Version: 2016, Mental and behavioural disorders [online]. *International statistical classification of diseases and related health problems*, 10th revision. Available at http://apps.who.int/classifications/icd10/browse/2016/en#F81.2

Xu, G., Strathearn, L., Liu, B. et al. (2019). Prevalence and treatment patterns of autism spectrum disorder in the United States. *Journal of the American Medical Association Pediatrics* 173(2): 153–159. doi: 10.1001/jamapediatrics.2018.4208.

Zablotsky, B., Black, L.I., & Blumberg, S.J. (2017). *Estimated prevalence of children with diagnosed developmental disabilities in the United States, 2014-2016*. US Department of Health and Human Services, NCHS Data Brief, No. 291. Available at (https://www.cdc.gov/nchs/data/databriefs/db291_table.pdf#page=1.

18

Nonpharmacological Treatment Modalities: Play and Group Therapies

Edilma L. Yearwood[1] and Allison Grady[2]

[1]Georgetown University School of Nursing & Health Studies, Washington, DC, USA
[2]University of Wisconsin-Milwaukee, College of Nursing, Milwaukee, WI, USA

Objectives

After reading this chapter, advanced practice registered nurses (APRNs) will be able to:

1. Understand the historical, theoretical, conceptual, and treatment processes associated with play and group therapies.
2. Describe diagnostic and behavioral symptom clusters that can be addressed through use of play or group therapy techniques.
3. Critique the evidence on the effectiveness of specific play and group therapy techniques with children and adolescents.
4. Examine how APRNs can use play and group therapy techniques in their primary care and mental health practices.
5. Identify common tools and supplies needed by APRNs who use play therapy in their practice.

This chapter is posthumously dedicated to our friend and long-time colleague Judith Hirsh, who co-authored the original version of this chapter in 2012 and who we think about often.

Introduction

Nonpharmacological treatment of children with mental and behavioral health concerns includes the treatment modalities of play and group therapies. Play therapy is a complex modality and includes techniques such as child-centered, prescriptive or directive therapy, bibliotherapy, expressive play, cognitive-behavioral therapy, projective and symbolic play, filial therapy, and group therapy. Group therapy interventions with children and adolescents strive to educate, facilitate relationships, empower, and provide youngsters with corrective emotional experiences.

Therapists (psychiatric-mental health [PMH] nurse practitioners or clinical nurse specialists who are referred to as APRNs, psychologists, psychiatrists, or social workers) incorporate a variety of toys, equipment, supplies, and media during *play therapy* sessions to guide the child to better communicate with others, become self-aware, express feelings and thoughts (catharsis), and learn new or enhanced ways of relating and interacting in the world. The therapist ensures that there is safe, psychological distance from problematic issues and facilitates developmentally appropriate expression of thoughts, feelings, and behaviors (Association for Play Therapy [APT] n.d.;

Child and Adolescent Behavioral Health: A Resource for Advanced Practice Psychiatric and Primary Care Practitioners in Nursing,
Second Edition. Edited by Edilma L. Yearwood, Geraldine S. Pearson, and Jamesetta A. Newland.
© 2021 John Wiley & Sons, Inc. Published 2021 by John Wiley & Sons, Inc.
Companion website: www.wiley.com/go/Yearwood

Bonner 2004; Gil 2004; Johnson et al. 2005; Kot and Tyndall-Lind 2005; Landreth 2012; Schaefer and Reid 1986; Terr 2003). Play therapy is defined by the APT as the "systematic use of a theoretical model to establish an interpersonal process wherein trained Play Therapists use the therapeutic powers of play to help clients prevent or resolve psychosocial difficulties and achieve optimal growth and development" (APT n.d.).

Thus, play therapy conducted by trained APRN therapists has scientific underpinnings and mounting clinical evidence for support as a treatment modality. Likewise, the "art" of developmentally appropriate play is a skill set that can be taught to pediatric and family nurse practitioners for use during assessment of children and adolescents to help reduce anxiety and successfully engage young children and adolescents in a meaningful interaction during a physical examination. The art of play includes such strategies as asking the child to blow bubbles while listening to chest sounds, making a finger "become magical" by lighting up the tip of the finger with the otoscope before examining the child's ear, and role playing with school-age children and adolescents to reduce the potential for engaging in high-risk behaviors. Thus, play and play therapy are an integral part of the assessment and intervention processes in pediatric healthcare.

Group therapy involves a collection of individuals, having something in common, who meet together to work with one or more therapists or counselors toward some element of change. Change can occur at the individual, interpersonal, or group level. Group participation and effectiveness rely on dynamics and interactions within the group. A goal of group therapy is to increase knowledge, understanding, and insight while also improving social skills, promoting behavioral change and decreasing isolation (American Group Psychotherapy Association 2007; Burlingame et al. 2013).

This chapter will address the importance and evidence-based benefits of play and group therapies, highlight research on neurobiological impact from use of these modalities, and describe the significance of these interventions in promoting healthy child and adolescent growth and development. The theoretical foundations on which these modalities are based are also briefly discussed. Evidence exists for using these therapeutic modalities for specific symptom clusters, behaviors, genders, cultural, and age groups. This chapter provides an introductory overview and encourages the APRN in primary care to (i) seek further education and skills in basic play and group therapy techniques for use with common behavioral presentations, (ii) refer children and adolescents to child and adolescent PMH APRNs trained and certified in these treatment modalities, and

(iii) work collaboratively with PMH APRNs to meet both the medical and behavioral/mental health needs of the pediatric population.

Play Therapy

The Importance of Play

Play has been shown to be an essential factor in healthy cognitive, physical, and emotional development (Yogman et al. 2018). Yogman et al. further identify play as a catalyst for discovery, contributing to executive functioning and promoting school readiness. Unfortunately, studies and surveys reveal a decline in free play in children beginning in their preschool years (American Academy of Pediatrics [AAP] 2006). In a paper published in *Scientific American*, Wenner (2009) discussed the importance of free play, citing it as essential to developing healthy social skills, effectively solving problems, coping with stress, and building cognitive skills. Free play affords children the opportunity to use imagination and creativity, enhance communication skills, and master new skills. Playing with peers in unstructured ways affords the development of interpersonal skills, including sharing, learning to be fair, compromising, and taking turns. Through play, frustration tolerance develops, as well as motivation and persistence to achieve a desired goal.

In 2007, Ginsburg et al. published the AAP position paper on play, which emphasized the need for an appropriate individualized balance between scheduled organized adult-supervised activities and family/parent–child interactions related to play. The balance as related to play also included child-centered activities with peers, consideration of the child's temperament, academic needs, and environmental and family needs. This balance is believed to offer protective factors and builds resilience during stages of child development. Play recommendations included (i) the use of toys to promote childhood imagination and fantasy, (ii) education of parents on the value of being supportive and nurturing during play activities, and (iii) the need to encourage parents to involve themselves in their children's creative play while discouraging passive play. An example of passive play is time alone with computers and television. In the 2018 update on impact of play, the AAP has identified additional research that provides evidence that play in childhood is a key building block for adult problem-solving, collaboration, creativity, and overall success (Yogman et al. 2018).

Neurobiology of Play

The brain structures shown by researchers to be involved in play behaviors are the cerebellum, cortex, prefrontal cortex, and thalamus. Scientists studying human development and play conclude that play contributes to neurological growth, particularly in complex, socially skilled, and cognitively adaptable developing brains (Gaskill and Perry 2014; Henig 2008). Play has been associated with lower levels of cortisol, increased levels of norepinephrine and improved brain plasticity, all of which supports better coping with stress and challenging life events (Yogman et al. 2018, p. 5).

The brainstem has the primary function of regulating core physiology and primary sensory processing. Play activity with infants and toddlers includes peak-a-boo and tactile sensory play. Rhythmic and patterned sensory play with an attuned and responsive caregiver promotes attachment, state regulation, and resilience. Beginning in infancy through childhood, games that promote development of the midbrain also incorporate motor control and secondary sensory processing. Examples include listening to and playing music, singing, engaging in gross and fine motor games, and repeating rhymes, poems, and stories. During the period from early childhood through puberty the limbic system develops. Learning to appropriately interpret nonverbal communication, accurately reading social cues, and expressing creativity through art, music, and drama are all believed to enhance limbic system development (Gaskill 2004, 2010; Gaskill and Perry 2014). Engaging in games that facilitate social skills is thought to improve sharing, taking turns, and frustration tolerance. Participating in play groups has been attributed to improved memory, emotional regulation, attachment, affiliation, affect regulation, and primary sensory integration.

Another brain region, the (neo) cortex, develops during childhood and is believed to be responsible for reasoning, problem-solving, abstraction, socioemotional integration, and secondary sensory integration. Overall, emotional and cognitive growth in children is promoted by the use of humor, language, art, and games with rules or strategy that supports exploration, critical thinking, problem solving, and storytelling/story creation (Gaskill 2004, 2010; Gaskill and Perry 2014; Perry 2006).

Historical Development of Play Therapy
Theoretical Frameworks of Play

A concise historical overview of play therapy can be found in the *Neurobiological Power of Play* by Gaskill and Perry (2014).

There are a variety of theoretical styles that serve to inform the practitioner when conducting play therapy. One predominant framework is a child-centered play therapy (CCPT) approach, in which the child chooses the activity and paces the therapy. It is based on humanistic philosophies offered by Carl Rogers (Johnson et al. 2005; O'Connor 2000; Rogers 1951) and Axline (1978). Children control their own growth toward maturity, self-actualization, and healing. The child's perception of his reality is most important, therefore it is expressed without the therapist's interpretation or confrontation. In this method, the therapist must learn to trust the process and focus on making the experience calm, safe, and child-focused while paying attention to developing a trusting relationship with the child (Badenoch and Kestly 2015; Landreth 2012; Ritzi et al. 2017). Landreth (2012) noted that the child rather than the problem should be the focus of the treatment.

The other predominant framework is directive or prescriptive therapy. Here the therapist chooses the therapeutic activity and paces the sessions. This approach can be shorter or time-limited, attaining goals more quickly than the child-centered approach. It is flexible in that the therapist matches the technique or intervention with the presenting symptoms. The principles of prescriptive play therapy include using various play methods during a session to address identified issues or problems. Without a strict adherence to a particular technique, the treatment is customized for that particular child. It is multimodal, multicomponent, and multilayered, using scientific evidence as a guide for effectively intervening, including published practice guidelines and manuals (National Institute for Play Therapy 2009; Schaefer 2001).

In cognitive-behavioral play therapy (CBPT), Knell (1998) incorporated Beck's cognitive-behavioral therapy with therapeutic play. CBPT can be used with preschool children and relies on flexibility and a decreased need for verbalization. Therapists model improved behavior, using metaphor or other indirect expression of change via play techniques. CBPT matches the child's developmental level with an appropriate therapeutic behavioral intervention. For example, Cohen and Deblinger (2004) used dolls and puppets to cognitively reframe and gradually expose children and adolescents to trauma issues. When used, this method is directive, time-limited, structured, and problem-oriented. This intervention is considered successful if the thoughts, feelings, and beliefs of the child or adolescent are changed (Shelby and Felix 2005). For example, a sexually abused child or adolescent enters treatment feeling responsible and guilty for the abuse. The treatment process produces a change in which the child or adolescent can place responsibility and guilt with the adult or abuser for the abuse. Additional information about cognitive behavior therapy (CBT) can be found in Chapter 20.

Adlerian play therapy is based on Adler's individual psychology, which includes beliefs that humans have an inherent need to belong, feel connected to others, are goal-directed, want to feel adequate and valued, and that all behavior has a purpose (Kottman 2001). Adlerian play therapy is comprised of four phases. These include building a safe environment to promote development of trust, sharing the leadership of the experience with the child while exploring the child's experiences, directing the child to gain insight into feelings, behaviors, and thought processes, and finally allowing the child to rehearse new perceptions and behaviors (Meany-Walen et al. 2015). Filial therapy, developed in the 1960s by Louise and Bernard Guerney, is an intensive, structured, time-limited (20–24 sessions) technique in which parents are taught to be more therapeutically involved with their child. Through

weekly didactic group training, homework, role play, and supervision in the outpatient setting and then at home, parents are taught basic CCPT principles. They learn to convey empathy, acceptance, and encouragement as well as appropriate limit setting and consequences. The intervention is deemed successful when positive changes are noted in the parent–child relationship, family environment, decreased levels of parental stress, increased self-esteem in the child, child adjustment, and improved behavior (Rennie and Landreth 2000; VanFleet 2005; VanFleet et al. 2005). Table 18.1 contains a timeline illustrating the development of the science of play therapy.

Table 18.1 Historical development of play therapy

Time frame	Theorist/milestone
1900s	**S. Freud** (1909): Applied theory of instinctual drives to child psychotherapy. Bibliotherapy was used as an educational tool to provide information.
1920s	**C. Jung:** Developed analytic model of psychotherapy and interpretation (use of symbols, metaphors, and archetypes).
	M. Lowenfeld: Used sand and miniature objects to uncover unconscious issues.
	A. Freud: Developed the child psychotherapy model.
1940s	**C. Rogers:** Client-centered therapy.
	V. Axline: Developed the principles of child-centered treatment. Wrote Dibs in Search of Self.
1950s–1960s	**M. Klein:** Equated play with free association used in adult therapy.
	E. Erikson: Developed the eight stages of psychosocial development needed for emotional health.
	J. Piaget: Credited with the cognitive development model, which states that children develop intelligence by doing, imitating, observing, and interpreting. Play was viewed as a continuous organization and reorganization of experiences that begin in infancy.
	J. Bowlby: Attachment theory. Wrote about the importance of object relations (trust, protection, limits, and meeting needs) and understanding transitional objects.
	A. Jernberg: Developed the theraplay model at Head Start in Chicago.
1970s–1980s	**R. Gardner:** Created psychotherapeutic games for use with resistant children ages 4–15. Examples:
	Mutual storytelling game (1971)
	Talking, feeling and doing game (1973)
	Storytelling game (1988)
	O'Connor and Schaefer: Started the Association of Play Therapy in 1982.
	Bowlby and Ainsworth (1988): Described healthy and pathological coping styles based on the quality of parent–child attachment.
1990s	**Decade of the brain:** An increase in research led to increased knowledge and understanding of neurobiology and neurophysiology.
	Benedict (1997): Conducted research on play themes of safety, anger, loss, constancy, and nurturance. Developed thematic play therapy
2000's	**Ray, Bratton, Rhine, and Jones** (2001): Conducted meta-analysis of studies from 1940 to 2000 on the effectiveness of play therapy.
	Increased focus on evidence-based studies supporting the use of play therapy in various behavioral presentations.
2015	**APT website /resources** updated to include levels of research evidence

Source: Table developed from information on the APT website and in "A History of Play Therapy" from the British Association of Play Therapists (n.d.) (https://www.bapt.info/play-therapy/history-play-therapy).

PMH APRNs most often use child-centered and/or prescriptive models to gather assessment data and continue using these models, perhaps alternating them during the treatment process. CCPT, Adlerian play therapy, and filial therapy models require specialized training and supervision. They are also time intensive. These models reflect the basic nursing principles of care, therefore elements of these models (the need to belong, need to have value, be goal-directed, experience attachment, and a corrective experience of interaction) are used by PMH APRNs. These techniques can also be learned by APRNs who practice in pediatric primary care settings as part of brief office-based interventions to begin the process of changing unacceptable and problematic behaviors. Intradisciplinary referrals would have the advantage of APRNs using the same techniques to begin the relational and change process in children and adolescents.

Play Therapy as Evidence-based Practice

Evidence-based practice reviews of child play therapy are limited in number compared to those found in psychotherapy with adult populations. Meta-analysis of four decades of research (Bratton et al. 2005) identified 93 controlled outcome studies from 1953 to 2000, examining the efficacy of play therapy as a treatment modality. Most of the research was conducted in the 1970s ($n = 23$), 1980s ($n = 16$), and 1990s ($n = 17$).

Ray et al. (2014) conducted a meta-analysis and systematic review of 23 studies analyzing the use of CCPT in elementary schools. The analysis yielded promising to strong evidence that CCPT was effective for use with children exhibiting externalizing, internalizing, academic, self-efficacy difficulties and other challenges. Other randomized control studies conducted on the effectiveness of play therapy as an intervention with a variety of childhood behaviors have shown effective promise (Blanco and Ray 2011; Bratton et al. 2013; Ray et al. 2013). The limitations of these studies include their small sample size.

Patterson et al. (2018) conducted a pilot study on 12 school-age African-American children, half of whom had experienced three or more adverse childhood experiences (ACEs). Participants were provided with 6 weeks of individual play therapy followed by 6 weeks of group play therapy. Findings indicated that the combination of individual and group CCPT for children exposed to ACEs was successful in decreasing behavioral presentations, improving academic performance, and decreasing negative intrusive thinking. The small sample size and absence of a control group were limitations of this study.

Green and Myrick (2014) proposed the use of a phase-based integrative play therapy model with adolescents who have experienced complex trauma. The three-phase approach focuses on stabilization, trauma processing, and reconnection. During stabilization, the adolescent is guided to reduce self-destructive behaviors, understand and manage symptoms, use self-care strategies, practice self-regulation, and work on the alliance with the therapist. During the trauma processing phase, the adolescent engages in one or more strategies, including trauma-focused cognitive behavior therapy (TF-CBT), life narrative exploration, and nonverbal expressive arts including sand trays and miniatures. During the third phase, the use of music, board games, painting, and other expressive techniques can be used to improve self-esteem and relationships with others. Research is needed to establish the evidence related to use of this model with adolescents who have experienced trauma.

Symptom Clusters

Play therapy is most often used for symptoms identified as either internalizing (emotional) or externalizing (disruptive, aggressive). Internalizing symptoms reflect all the anxiety disorders, the affective or mood disorders, including suicidal ideation, psychosis, including hallucinations, and somatic disorders. The externalizing disorders include attention deficit hyperactivity disorder (ADHD), rule-breaking disorders such as conduct disorder and oppositional defiant disorder, personality disorders, Tourette's, and attachment disorders (Achenbach 1966; Achenbach and Rescorla 2001; Eisenberg et al. 2001; Tackett 2010). There is some overlap in the two clusters in behaviors, such as self-harm, eating disorders, substance use, schizophrenia, and autism spectrum disorders.

Play Techniques for Assessment and Treatment

Providing quality care involves a thorough and comprehensive assessment of the child and family. Gathering data about risk factors, mental status assessment, peer and family interactions, child and family developmental milestones, environmental factors, and social determinants of health/mental health can all contribute to successful treatment during the play therapy process. Assessment and treatment are assisted in part by using the expressive play therapies (art, stories, and sand play). A comprehensive resource on play therapy techniques can be found in Kaduson and Schaefer (2003).

Play Therapy Toolkit

Art

Using the medium of art, the PMH APRN asks a child or adolescent to draw a picture that may explain his or her feelings about an event. Likewise, during primary care visits, the primary care APRN often asks a child to draw a picture as part of a developmental assessment. Assessing artwork includes the use of colors, shading, spatial aspects, including symmetry and use of background and foreground, developmental expectations of skill, objects included or excluded, and imagery. Art is quite effective as a mode of expression for children's emotional issues (trauma, illness, and feelings). While PMH APRNs learn to assess artwork for therapeutic interventions, primary care APRNs are taught to view the artwork from a developmental perspective. However, the primary care APRN must be cognizant of "normal" versus "abnormal" drawings and make an appropriate referral for the child whose artwork is outside the norm. For example, primary care APRNs have and should continue to refer children whose drawings are suggestive of sexual or physical abuse to PMH APRNs or other mental health practitioners (Figure 18.1).

Sand play

As a therapeutic modality, the technique of sand play has evolved from its origins, which were based on Jung's theories (1968) and then incorporated Lowenfeld's concepts (1999). Jung saw play as a process in which the child's unconscious "bubbles up" with no control such as when daydreaming. He viewed toys as symbols that could be used to activate the unconscious. A central concept in Jung's work was the idea of the need for balance in order to have psychic health. Jung thought that symptoms were symbols of conflict. He

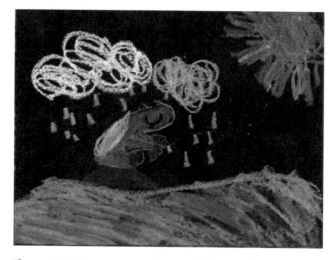

Figure 18.1 Drawing by a 7-year-old depicting bipolar experience. When given a free choice of art supplies, this youngster drew on black construction paper (mood), in appropriate crayon colors. He added a jumping frog in deep water smiling (activity level and inappropriate affect), with rain, clouds, and sun occurring simultaneously.

viewed imagination and creative fantasy as important in the therapeutic process.

The archetypes (instinctual representations and metaphor) are potentially positive or negative. Jung thought that the self was the central organizing archetype which served to heal and which sought balance by restoring equilibrium. The role of the therapist in this technique is to use knowledge of healing archetypes and symbols to validate, support, contain, and help make meanings and connections for the child or adolescent to examine (Carey 1999).

The therapist using Lowenfeld's technique has the child or adolescent use sand, landscape symbols, and animals to create a "picture." The therapist then helps the child or adolescent examine recurring themes, objects, and archetypes in order to help the youngster understand issues that were perhaps not clear when they created the "picture" (Lowenfeld 1999).

Kalff's (2003) model of sand play incorporates Jung's and Lowenfeld's models. When using Kalff's model, therapists are silent observers. Stages of psychological development are considered when evaluating a tray for how objects are placed in the sand, overall symmetry and image produced, the use of animals and vegetation, conflict between good and evil, and a balance of opposites (Carey 1999; Kalff 2003).

Puppets

Using expressive therapy techniques such as puppets to tell stories allows children to externalize their conflicts, distress, and concerns. Puppet characters effectively provide psychological distance from the issue or fantasy. Puppet shows may be used to present psychoeducational material, role play, and support cognitive change. A variety of puppet types promote symbolic expression of feelings or events (Figure 18.2). Assessment techniques have been developed that use puppets in gathering data about child and family experiences (Depa and Astramovich 2008; Knell and Beck 2000).

Bibliotherapy

Since the early 1900s, bibliotherapy has developed into a prescriptive play intervention in which the therapist selects a story that matches the client's conflict with a healthier resolution offered than the one already chosen. It may be used as part of CBPT or as an assessment technique. The process promotes growth by being centered on the guided discussions after the story is told. Hynes and Hynes-Berry (1986) defined bibliotherapy as a four-step interactive process that may take place individually or in groups. The process includes (i) recognizing the subjective value of the story (catharsis), (ii) exploring

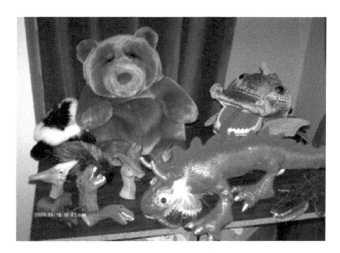

Figure 18.2 Examples of puppets used in play therapy.

the meaning of who, what, when, where, and why, (iii) examining new connections in thoughts, and (iv) applying new insights or creating new solutions. The results are evident in improved self-esteem, awareness of feelings, empathy, and assimilation of psychological or social values into the participant's behavior and personality (Hynes and Hynes-Berry).

The use of metaphor is important to mention here as it is evident not only in stories and puppet play but in other expressive modalities. A metaphor is an externalized symbolic representation of something or someone from one's own experience which allows for catharsis, insight, growth, and change. Goal-oriented metaphors have been developed into stories for therapeutic use (Lankton and Lankton 1989; Mills and Crowley 1986). Examples of metaphors include, "he was behaving like a chicken" and "the room was like a zoo."

Games

Gardner's psychotherapeutic games *Talking, Feeling and Doing* (2001) and *Storytelling* (1988) are based on his mutual storytelling technique (1975). The technique originally attempted to have uncooperative or resistant children verbalize their fantasies and, with the assistance of the therapist, analyze them. The children received chips and small prizes for their cooperation. The therapist would present stories based on the children's issues, using their characters and settings but offering healthier resolutions or adaptations. These "games" are still widely used by trained play therapists (Bellinson 2002; Gardner 2001).

"Themed" card decks were developed for the *Talking, Feeling, and Doing* game and are useful in promoting expression of feelings about issues such as anger, divorce, a range of behaviors, shyness, and teasing. Other card games that elicit data about thoughts and feelings can

also be useful during the assessment and treatment process and are most popular with adolescents (Arneson 2003; Crary and Katayama 2004). Structured games can be used as assessment tools in gathering data on social skills, self-discipline, cooperation, socioflexibility, leadership, emotional control, tolerance, and problem solving. Structured games are recognized by behaviorists as having therapeutic value in changing maladaptive behavior through the development of new skills (Bellinson 2002; Swank 2008). Assessment tools have been developed that gather data on development, potential psychiatric diagnosis, parent–child interactions, family systems, peer interactions, and projective play (Carey 1999; Gitlin-Weiner et al. 2000; Landreth 2001).

Group Therapy

The use of group therapy with adults has a long and rich history. While group work with children has been documented for over 70 years, much less research and fewer publications on the effectiveness of group therapy with children and adolescents are available. Moreno is credited with coining the term *group therapy* in 1932, and Slavson was called the Father of Group Psychotherapy in the 1940s. Early theorists who used group therapy in their work with children and adolescents included Moreno, Slavson, Fraiberg, Bettelheim, Redl, and Durkin (Kraft 1996). A good historical summary of group work can be found in a review by Barlow et al. (2000). The power of groups as a therapeutic intervention lies in its cost-effectiveness compared to individual interpersonal therapy, its ability to be both focused and time-limited, and the fact that group work as a treatment modality has the ability to promote building of relationships.

Yalom (1995) has been credited with what we know about curative group factors and functions of groups. The major strengths of groups as described by Yalom included the power of here and now interactions between group members, the opportunity for development of self-awareness secondary to repeated interactions and actions within the group, and the opportunity groups offered for corrective emotional experiences. Yalom identified 11 essential curative factors within groups that support behavioral change in group members. These included instillation of hope, universality, catharsis, imparting information, family recapitulation, altruism, socializing techniques, interpersonal learning, cohesiveness, existential factors, and imitative behaviors. Research with youth on their perceptions of the most helpful group factors included group cohesiveness (relationships), catharsis, universality, hope, interpersonal learning, and support (Mishna and Muskat 2004; Shechtman and Gluk 2005).

Group Characteristics

Most group experiences for children and adolescents occur in settings that they frequent. Schools account for approximately 79% of group activities followed by community agencies, hospitals, and clinics (Kulic et al. 2004). Most of the group work occurring in schools has a preventative focus. Group work has been conducted by a variety of individuals with various levels of training, comfort, and skills. The type and purpose of the group will often dictate who conducts the group. To be most effective, however, groups should be conducted by appropriately trained and supervised individuals.

Groups are most successful if members are motivated to participate in the process, are able to commit to attendance and appropriate group behaviors (nonaggressive, able to take turns, able to listen to others), and can maintain group confidentiality as warranted. Groups can vary in the number of times they meet (once to 10 times or more), the length of the session (i.e. 30–90 minutes), and where they meet (an office, conference room, classroom, or group room). Groups can vary in size depending on the function of the group. In order to be more effective and support member participation, counseling and therapy groups function better if size is limited to 6–10 members. Psychoeducation groups, however, can be larger but should not be so large that they overwhelm the leader, distract, or inhibit member participation.

It is generally recognized that most groups, including child and adolescent groups, go through stages in their development and work. These stages are frequently referred to as initial or beginning, working, and termination. Group members are usually unsure of what to do or say during the initial phase and will take the behavioral lead from the group leader, resist participation, or challenge and question the purpose or group process. During the working phase, the members are engaged, provide feedback, and usually do most of the work, with the leader serving as a supportive resource or catalyst to steer the group in a particular direction. In the termination phase, group members may regress to earlier behaviors due to fear about their upcoming personal capabilities in the absence of the group. Some may express anger toward the leader or fellow group members based on fear of abandonment while others may voice uncertainty about how to fill the void in time, structure, and relationships that mark the impending end of the group.

There are four common types of groups as identified by the Association for Specialists in Group Work (2001), a division of the American Counseling Association.

Each type of group requires specific training based on professional standards:

1. *Task or work groups:* Focus is on specific activities that the group develops or works to accomplish within a designated time frame. Examples include an art project, creating information manuals, or building a tree house.
2. *Psychoeducation groups:* Groups use a teaching format to impart information, skills, or knowledge about specific content area to affected and/or unaffected individuals (primary or secondary prevention). Examples include social skills development, obesity prevention, managing transitions, and learning about the effects of medications.
3. *Counseling groups:* Focus is on making positive adjustments to interpersonal or behavioral problems of group members. The process involves in-depth cognitive exploration of experiences, emotional catharsis, and ego strengthening. Development of personal competencies is often a goal of counseling groups. Examples include bereavement/loss and grief, anger management, addictions, and depression management groups.
4. *Therapy groups:* Groups use traditional psychotherapy techniques to focus on more ingrained and long-standing personality and interpersonal problems. The goal is to remediate psychological problems. Examples include groups for individuals with eating disorders, those with borderline personality, and those who self-harm.

Counseling and therapy groups have a different theoretical foundation than CBT groups, which tend to focus on cognitive changes, as discussed in Chapter 20. The framework for counseling and therapy groups is primarily humanistic, with the leader encouraging communication that fosters self-disclosure and affective exploration to support insight into personal behaviors (Shechtman 2007).

Groups are usually considered open or closed to additional members. Closed groups do not allow new members into the group once the group begins its work because of the potential to disrupt the process of the group when new members are added late. Membership in a closed group is set for the duration of the group to enhance the effectiveness of the group work. Open groups are groups that allow members to join at any point during the trajectory of the group. An example of an open group would be an Alateen support group for adolescents in the community.

Group content usually refers to what is said in the group while process refers to what happens in the group (behaviors, alliances, omissions, activities, rituals, etc.). It is important for the group leader to establish basic group norms at the beginning of any group that is formed and to invite members to add additional "rules" or behavioral expectations to the list. Common norms include getting to group on time, treating others with respect, maintaining the confidentiality of all group members (what happens in group stays in group), and refraining from aggression toward or intimidation of others. In counseling and therapy groups, leaders also discourage members from developing intimate relationships with each other as this would pose a distraction and interfere with the work of the group. This issue can be particularly problematic in adolescent and early adult aged groups where participants may also be struggling with isolation and yearning for intimate relationships.

Who is Best Suited for Groups?

The use of groups as a treatment modality is effective with most youngsters including those traumatized, learning disabled, bullying victims, substance abusers, those with low self-esteem, younger children, and older adolescents. There are differing opinions about groups for conduct disordered children. These are usually difficult groups to conduct because of the amount of resistance and testing of the leader that occur and may be more effective with the use of two group leaders. Ang and Hughes (2001) conducted a meta-analysis of social skills groups with conduct-disordered youth and concluded that homogeneous groups of conduct-disordered youth should be discouraged because they appear to result in escalation of antisocial behaviors. Gifford-Smith et al. (2005), on the other hand, thought that group characteristics could be mediated to avoid a negative outcome. Mediating factors included a skilled group therapist, groups with younger children, and group leader attention to a more heterogeneous group composition. However, the use of gender-specific groups for sensitive topics and certain developmental ages has been effective (Avinger and Jones 2007).

Shechtman (2007) reported on data that showed that among the three attachment styles of secure, anxious, and avoidant, avoidant children tended to resist self-disclosure, were less motivated to participate, and were more disruptive in groups. She recommended, however, that most children should be tried in groups and that it was the responsibility of the group leader to monitor and set limits on negative member behaviors as they occurred. Repeated negativistic and disruptive behavior should not be tolerated and would indicate that the particular group member was not ready for a group experience. It is counterproductive to maintain a disruptive member in any group.

Effective Group Leader Characteristics

It is the responsibility of the group leader to set the tone of the group experience, ensure the safety of group members, and protect the boundaries within the group and between the group and external entities. The climate or tone of the group as set by the leader and maintained by all group members can either impede or support group outcomes (Kivlighan and Tarrant 2001). It is the responsibility of the group leader to provide information, use reflection to promote communication, pose thoughtful questions, model prosocial behaviors, and gently guide the group toward its goal.

Horne et al. (2007) identified nine characteristics of group leaders that make them more effective in accomplishing the goals of the group. These included an ability to demonstrate empathy, an ability to build relationships, skills around respectful communication, an ability to maintain positive expectations for change within the group, a sense of humor, an ability to maintain structure, limits, rules, and the group focus, an ability to work with resistance from group members, good teaching skills, and skills to empower group members.

PMH APRNs receive training and supervision in this treatment modality and in their clinical practice become skilled in the dynamics and processes of group therapy. Primary care APRNs may study group therapy in their educational preparation but most have limited experiences as group therapy leaders. However, this may be an excellent opportunity for a collaborative practice model between the two APRN specialties. For example, children with diagnoses that require behavioral changes such as asthma, ADHD, and obesity in a primary care practice may be considered for their own group-specific concern with parental consent and child assent to participate. The group could be co-led by the primary care and PMH APRNs. The group could be time limited and focus on emotional adjustment to a specific condition, for example the relationship between obesity and health status and group education around safe, healthy lifestyle modifications such as exercise and healthy eating. Such office-based group strategies are an ideal forum for intradisciplinary partnerships between primary care and PMH APRNs to meet the total healthcare needs of both the child and the family.

Evidence for Group Therapy Effectiveness

D'Amico and colleagues at the University of New Mexico (2015) conducted secondary analysis of data collected from a randomized control study looking at change talk (a form of motivational interviewing) in adolescent group interventions to reduce alcohol and other drug (AOD) use in teens who were part of a Teen Court

Program. In one study, they reviewed audio recordings from 129 group sessions. Participants were engaged in weekly rolling admission group sessions. At 3-month follow-up when looking at participant AOD outcomes, group change talk was associated with decreased intent to use alcohol. Use of change talk by group facilitators trained in the strategy was found to also increase change talk in the teens (Osilla et al. 2015). Study limitations included youth who were first offenders, youth from one teen drug court program, and English speakers. Researchers recommended studying change talk in other populations with a more diverse group of adolescents and longitudinally.

In a recent abstract in the *Journal of Adolescent Health*, researchers at the University of Rochester described the use of small groups within a school environment to treat 6th and 7th graders who had experienced three or more ACEs. The group intervention used an adapted dialectic behavior therapy curriculum with 53 participants. Findings indicated that there was positive change in resilience from the baseline of students who completed the group intervention (Conn et al. 2018). Play and group therapy interventions conducted within school-based health centers are recommended as the setting is conducive to preventive efforts, early intervention, and access to a larger sample size of participants (Cossu et al. 2015).

Research indicates that CBT as a group therapy intervention with children and adolescents is effective in treating a variety of mental and behavioral challenges in children and adolescents. See Chapter 20 for additional evidence on this intervention.

Practice, Education, and Research Implications

The number of children seen today in primary care offices for routine healthcare who have a mental health diagnosis is staggering. Annually, between 13% and 20% of children and adolescents in the United States meet the criteria for a mental or behavioral disorder (Ghandour et al. 2018). In any one office day, the primary care provider may have over one-half of the children present with oppositonal defiant disorder, ADHD, an autism spectrum disorder, anxiety, or depression. As such, it is time to examine the curriculum content of advanced practice programs, in particular pediatric nurse practitioner programs, to include more content on these disorders and a clinical rotation in a pediatric psychiatric outpatient clinic to become more comfortable with assessment of these disorders in the primary care setting. The Pediatric Nursing Certification Board (PNCB; www.pncb.org) and the National Association of Pediatric Nurse Practitioners (NAPNAP; www.napnap.org) have begun to address this issue. In 2011, the PNCB began to

offer an examination for pediatric and family nurse practitioners that included content on prevention, screening, early intervention, referral to trained mental health practitioners, and collaborative follow-up of common mental and behavioral health presentations. Melnyk and Moldenhauer (2006) developed the Keep your children and yourself Safe and Secure (KySS) Guide to Child and Adolescent Mental Health Screening, Early Intervention and Health Promotion. KySS, an initiative of NAPNAP, serves as an excellent resource of assessment and screening tools for use by all APRNs working with children and adolescents with behavioral and emotional concerns.

Research on play and group therapy modalities has primarily been conducted by psychologists, social workers, and other social scientists. APRNs in child and adolescent mental health and primary care practices are in a unique position to conduct collaborative research with each other to develop a body of knowledge that is nursing specific in these areas. Topics might include conducting longitudinal inquiries on outcomes for children who participate in different treatment modalities, longitudinal outcomes of specific preventative psychoeducational groups, randomized control trials on outcomes related to group leader style or group leader discipline, the effectiveness of play or group modalities in immigrant versus nonimmigrant groups and across ages and gender, and the effectiveness of various combined modalities for specific behavioral or diagnostic disorders. Research conducted to date on play and group modalities has been criticized for not having large enough sample sizes, therefore large-scale quantitative inquiries addressing this issue would be a significant contribution to nursing science and treatment modality effectiveness.

Summary

Play and group therapies can remediate most risk factors of mental illness and behavioral difficulties, and are effective and evidenced-based psychotherapeutic interventions for a variety of emotional conditions in children and adolescents. The importance of play and the ability to function appropriately in group situations have been noted by child therapists, researchers, counselors, teachers, parents, and children themselves. The relationship-oriented, family-system, strength-based techniques characteristic of play and group therapies are synergistic to the scientific yet humanistic foundation of nursing, which also incorporates these principles in practice (Delaney 2008; Delaney et al. 2014).

APRNs without specialty education in child and adolescent mental health treatment are encouraged to seek continuing education and/or training about the specialized modalities of play and group therapies. This knowledge would enhance their practice and add additional assessment skills and interaction techniques for use with a variety of children and adolescents presenting with common diagnosable and undiagnosed behaviors in primary care (APT 2005; Saunders et al. 2004). APRNs in both specialties should keep in mind that these modalities are efficacious interventions when used with multiple child and adolescent diagnostic and behavioral presentations.

Case Exemplar

Play has been recognized in a number of fields, including nursing, medicine, child life, and psychology, as being vital to the growth and development of children. Play has been studied by giants in the developmental psychology field such as Erickson and Piaget, and they found play to be "an inseparable part of the growth and development process of the child, which assists in the building-up and consolidation of his personal identity and his effective handling of future realities" (Haiat et al. 2003, p. 210). This is particularly important for the child with illness. Illness can be acute or chronic, serious or superficial. The common denominator is that hospitalization and treatment take children out of their natural state and into a world of anxiety, pain, and unpredictability. The intersection of play and illness often involves a professional teaching about procedures or interventions that are cause for curiosity, and possibly worry and pain, and children learning how to mitigate their fears and cope with disease and the healthcare system.

Jill is a child life specialist (CLS) working in the oncology clinic. She has been working with 7-year-old Layla for the past several weeks to prepare Layla for an upcoming port placement (central venous line). During their time together, Jill shows Layla a doll named Andy that has a port "inside" of his chest just like Layla will have. Layla pushes on the port, feels the hub of the line, and even practices placing a needle inside it. Layla is curious and eager to touch the port, but when Jill directly speaks about the surgery needed to implant the port, Layla becomes withdrawn and tearful. To provide some distraction, Jill helps Layla place the port dressing over Andy's chest and "clamp" the line. Later, Jill brings out Andy and role plays the surgical planning for the port and places a mask over the face of the doll.

Layla holds the mask up to her own face and then tells Andy, "You're just going to go to sleep now: I hope that you wake up."

Jill, giggling a little to keep the mood light, asks Layla, "What do you mean that you hope that Andy wakes up?!"

Layla looks Jill directly in the eye and says, "Well, my grandma went to sleep and she didn't wake up after her surgery. And my dog went to the doctor and the doctor put him to sleep and he never woke up. So, I hope that Andy wakes up – those doctors can be tricky."

Jill considers Layla's answer before she responds. "Oh, I understand what you mean. You see all of these important people in your life going to sleep but not waking up. Layla, you should know that the doctors are going to give you a medicine so that you close your eyes and don't feel the surgery, but you will *not* be like your dog or your grandma. This surgery is to give you a port like Andy, so we can give you medicine safely and without hurting you like we do now with so many pokes."

Layla looks to Jill and then looks at Andy. "So, I'm going to wake up?"

"That's the plan. There will be lots of doctors and nurses in the room to make sure that you are safe and that when you wake up, your mom and dad will be there for you."

"Will it hurt?"

"It shouldn't hurt at all during the surgery. But when you wake up, you might be a little sore and might feel a little silly. And when we need to use the port, it might be scary the first time – just like it was for Andy. But you see the needle," Jill holds up a small port needle, "and you will have the magic cream to make it all tingly so you don't feel it very much at all." Jill squeezes a dollop of cold numbing cream onto Layla's hand. After a few minutes, Layla giggles because her hand "feels funny - like it fell asleep."

After a few minutes, Layla asks, "What will it be like to have the port dressing taken off? Will that rip my skin off? Can I have numbing cream to take *off* the dressing?"

"That's a great question," Jill responds. "No, we can't use numbing cream to take off the dressing. Taking it off is kind of like taking off a bandaid. Why don't we take off Andy's dressing?" Jill hands Layla a tube of adhesive remover and they work side-by-side to get off the tape. "Ooh, this sticker remover is kind of slimy," remarks Layla. Layla offers positive encouragement to Andy and reminds him to deep breathe while she works. "If you remember to breathe Andy, it will go much faster and it won't hurt very much at all." Layla says matter-of-factly.

"Ta-da!" Exclaims Layla when the dressing is removed.

"You did *great*, Andy!" Jill exclaims. "But Layla, you had such good ideas for keeping Andy calm and being positive. You can totally do this!"

"I CAN do this," states Layla affirmatively and gives Jill a hug.

Use of Play Therapy

This case study focuses on a child with a chronic illness. The risk for long-term anxiety and post-traumatic stress disorder is higher in this population due to ongoing negative stimuli (Secinti et al. 2017). The ability to work with a CLS can help mitigate some of Layla's fears. As

Metzger and colleagues note about the CLS working with their pediatric patients, "the CLS was able to augment... preparation for the procedure, supplement family and patient teaching, and provide one-on-one support during the procedure that reduced...stress" (Metzger et al. 2013, p. 155). The CLS accomplishes this mostly by using the principles related to preparation, sensory information, and rapport (Metzger et al. 2013, p. 155). Although these are three discrete areas, they are interconnected and depend upon each other for success.

Preparation

Preparation is key for anyone to feel comfortable in a new situation: understanding what is going to happen and how that is likely to be experienced is a major source of control. Preparation through play allows for direct and indirect "teach back" by the patient. Preparation can be performed in the actual rooms where treatment or testing will take place using actual tools or instruments, it can be performed at bedside with a doll like the one that Layla used, it can also take place in a neutral site through a video or other nontangible medium. No matter how preparation is approached, it should remain nonthreatening to the patient. By walking Andy through the steps for his anesthesia, surgical procedure, port access, and dressing change, Layla was able to verbalize her understanding, demonstrate the tone and level of engagement she perceives from her caregivers, and vocalize lingering questions and fears. These actions by Layla are effective because the reactions from an authority figure are not directed to Layla per se but rather to Andy. This provides a safe environment for Layla to learn and question, which is essential for successful preparation. Establishing comfort should be done on an age-appropriate level using accurate clinical terms whenever possible. Explanations should be simple and pseudonyms should not make children confused or scared (e.g. "going to sleep"). As demonstrated through the case study, preparation requires sustained and active listening. "Good quality communication is very powerful in identifying well-rooted concerns some may be carrying... Active listening meant I could focus on words that were shared which I then fed back to gain a deeper understanding of what was in their mind" (White 2017, p. 478). It was only by listening to Layla, questioning Layla using her own vocabulary, and answering Layla's question after seeking greater understanding did Jill have an opportunity to put some of Layla's fears at ease. This was done by calling upon Layla's previous experiences and physical play to tangibly demonstrate an idea or procedure. By learning the concerns that lurked beneath the surface, the CLS or the nurse is able to connect more intimately with the patient and empower them with the type of information and answers that they crave.

Sensory

One of the hallmarks of play is exploration. This can take place in a very tangible sense or it can be more imaginative and creative. Working hand-in-hand with preparation, sensory interventions allow a child to engage their senses – sight, touch, hearing, smell, and sometimes even taste – in an effort to make sense of their experience. Depending upon age, dolls, puppets, and stuffed animals may be used for anticipatory guidance as well as sensory stimulation. In our case study, Layla was able to hold the port needle, touch and smell the inside of the anesthesia mask, and remove the dressing when the procedure was finished. This touch and feel exercise provided a more well-rounded experience and allowed for questions that might have been missed if the tangible aspects were not included (e.g. "will it hurt?"). In addition, by using Andy and, by extension, herself, Layla can anticipate aspects of the procedures that may cause greater stress. Feeling the coldness of the "numbing cream" and the watery slickness of the adhesive remover, Layla has a deeper understanding of what is expected of her and what she might experience. In many studies, equipment like stethoscopes, blood pressure cuffs, and thermometers are allowed to be handled by a child and used either on themselves or on a doll-like proxy (Moore et al. 2015, p. 267). As Haiat and colleagues write, "play can help the hospitalized child better understand and interpret the imagery, sights, sounds, and the language of the hospital. When a child plays, he transforms himself from a passive individual into an active one because through play he creates the rules" (Haiat et al. 2003, p. 210). In our case, Layla also has a chance to be an "expert" and help Andy to cope with his treatments, which helps her to be more confident when going into her interventions.

Rapport

Overarching the subject of play therapy is rapport. The maximal benefits of preparation and sensory integration are best accomplished through a trusting and therapeutic relationship. Historically, nurses have excelled at this competency, but renewed focus on tasks, higher patient acuity, and systemic desire for speed and patient volume have diminished the importance of this role. For those able to work consistently with a CLS, their expertise in child growth and development in addition to the fact that they represent someone who will not "hurt" the child through a procedure make their contributions and presence invaluable. The CLS is able to assess "restrictions and mobility, medical stressors, emotional/coping, developmental/play/social skills, and family/community support" (Metzger et al. 2013, p. 155). When hobbies, methods of learning, preferred techniques for calming (talking, deep breathing, distraction), and appreciation for parental concerns and involvement can be gathered and synthesized into an actionable plan, the child comes to feel valued, heard, and a member of the team. Should fear or anxiety creep in due to new procedures or new caregivers, having a consistent person who has earned trust can be the difference between successful interventions and ones that ratchet up fear and anxiety. In our case study, Layla has a bond with Jill that allows her to transfer "Andy's fears" into "Layla's fears" without worry of negative judgment or minimizing of the situation by Jill. Because Jill has a rapport with Layla, Jill can ask her the more difficult questions about worries and perceptions without coming across as intrusive or inappropriate. But beyond allowing Layla to ask questions, Layla also is able to hear the answers that Jill provides and trust that they are correct. As one CLS writes, "Children need play! They need something familiar to identify with at a time when they are feeling most vulnerable. They also need to know, especially when scared, that people beside their family are there to look after them, support them and reassure them" (White 2017, p. 479).

The Role of Nursing

As noted earlier, the work of play has traditionally been left to nurses the "play ladies" who were hired to support families, provide sensory stimulation to children, and provide human touch to patients who were often alone (Metzger et al. 2013, p. 153). While the job of CLSs has brought standardized education along with research and codes of ethics and professionalism to the idea of "play ladies," it is still a relatively new profession. Many hospitals do not employ enough CLSs to cover all of the children who could use support. As a result, the job of play and preparation often falls to the nurse. While this is in part historical, as nurses have been viewed as nurturing and trusting, it is also practical. Nurses are the people who have the most regular contact with patients and are often the people who are performing the tasks that are viewed as painful and unpleasant. In our case study, it would be the nurse who would access the port as well as apply and remove the dressing. This can complicate the relationship because rapport may be established but a child may feel betrayed if they are being "hurt" by the individuals whom they identified as their allies. Various studies have demonstrated that the CLS is better at play

therapy than the nurse and the possible reasons are many, although we will offer two. First, establishing rapport and allowing for play takes time, and often nurses are running among several patients, all of whom have needs. A CLS may have more time to devote to an individual patient as this is their primary job. Next, not all nurses are trained in child development. It cannot be overstated the importance of recognizing the psychosocial and psychomotor stages that children move through. Understanding these types of development in the context of illness also allows for information to be communicated between the healthcare worker and the patient, and establishes goals and expectations that are realistic for all involved.

Resources

American Group Psychotherapy Association Practice Guidelines for Group Psychotherapy, Science to Service Task Force. www.agpa.org.

American Psychological Association (APA, Washington DC). Publishers of Magination Press, children's books on mental health issues. www.maginationpress.com.

Association for Play Therapy Inc., Clovis, CA., national and local chapter information and continuing education, regional training centers, and distance learning programs. www.a4pt.org.

Association for Specialists in Group Work. A Division of the American Counseling Association. The purpose of this association is to establish standards for professional and ethical practice, support research knowledge development and dissemination, and provide professional leadership in the field of group work. www.asgw.org

British Association of Play Therapists. https://www.bapt.info/play-therapy/history-play-therapy.

University of North Texas, Center for Play Therapy, library and education programs. http://cpt.unt.edu.

References

Achenbach, T. (1966). The classification of children's psychiatric symptoms. *Psychological Monographs* 80 (615).

Achenbach, T. and Rescorla, L. (2001). *Manual for the ASEBA School-Age Forms and Profiles.* Burlington, VT: University of Vermont Research Center for Children, Youth & Families.

AAP. (2006). *The importance of play in promoting healthy child development and maintaining strong parent-child bonds* [Clinical report]. American Academy of Pediatrics. Available at www.aap.org.

American Group Psychotherapy Association. (2007). Practice guidelines for group psychotherapy. Available at http://www.agpa.org/guidelines/AGPA%20Practice%20Guidelines%202007-PDF.pdf.

Ang, R. and Hughes, J. (2001). Differential benefits of skills training with antisocial youth based on group composition: a meta-analytic investigation. *School Psychology Review* 31: 164–185.

Arneson, L. (2003). *Thoughts and Feelings: A Sentence Completion Card Game.* Rancho Santa Fe, CA: Bright Spots Available at http://www.bright-spotsgames.com.

APT. (n.d.). *About play therapy overview.* Association for Play Therapy. Available at http://www.a4pt.org.

APT (2005). *Sample Syllabus: Introductory Graduate Play Therapy Course.* Clovis, CA: Association for Play Therapy.

APT. (2001). Why play therapy? [Video]. Association for Play Therapy. Available at www.a4pt.org.

Association for Specialists in Group Work (2001). Professional standards for the training of group workers. In: *Group Counseling and Therapy* (eds. G. Gazda, E. Ginter and A. Horne), 363–388. Boston, MA: Allyn & Bacon.

Avinger, K. and Jones, R. (2007). Group treatment of sexually abused adolescent girls: a review of outcome studies. *American Journal of Family Therapy* 35: 315–326.

Axline, V. (1978). *Play Therapy*. New York, NY: Ballantine Books, Inc.

Badendoch, B. and Kestly, T. (2015). Exploring the neuroscience of healing play at every age. In: *Play Therapy: A Comprehensive Guide to Theory and Practice* (eds. D.A. Crenshaw and A.L. Stewart), 524–538. New York, NY: Guilford Press.

Barlow, S., Burlingame, G., and Fuhriman, A. (2000). Therapeutic application of groups: from Pratt's "thought control classes" to modern group psychotherapy. *Group Dynamics: Theory, Research, and Practice* 4: 115–134.

Bellinson, J. (2002). *Children's Use of Board Games in Psychotherapy*. Northvale, NJ: Jason Aronson.

Blanco, P.J. and Ray, D.C. (2011). Play therapy in elementary schools: a best practice for improving academic achievement. *Journal of Counseling and Development* 89 (2): 235–243.

Bonner, B. (2004). Cognitive-behavioral and dynamic play therapy for children with sexual behavior problems and their caregivers. In: *Child Physical and Sexual Abuse: Guidelines for Treatment* (eds. B.E. Saunders, L. Berliner and R.F. Hanson), 34–36. Charleston, SC: National Crime Victims Research and Treatment Center.

Bratton, S., Ray, D., Rhine, T., and Jones, L. (2005). The efficacy of play therapy with children: A met-analytic review of treatment outcomes. *Professional Psychology Research and Practice* 36 (4): 376–390. https://doi.org/10.1037/0735-7028.36.4.376.

Bratton, S.C., Ceballos, P.L., Sheely-Moore, A.I. et al. (2013). Head start early mental health intervention: effects of child-centered play therapy on disruptive behaviors. *International Journal of Play Therapy* 22 (1): 28–42.

British Association of Play Therapists (n.d.). *History of play therapy*. Available at http://www.bapt.info/historyofpt.htm.

Burlingame, G.M., Strauss, B., and Joyce, A.S. (2013). Change mechanisms and effectiveness of small group treatments. In: *Handbook of Psychotherapy and Behavior Change* M.J. Lambert (ed.), 640–689. Hoboken, NJ: John Wiley & Sons.

Carey, L. (1999). *Sandplay Therapy with Children and Families*. Northvale, NJ: Jason Aronson.

Crary, E. and Katayama, M. (2004). *The Self-Calming Card Deck*. Seattle, WA: The Parenting Press. Available at http://www.ParentingPress.com.

Cohen, J. and Deblinger, E. (2004). Trauma-focused cognitive behavioral therapy. In: *Child Physical and Sexual Abuse: Guidelines for Treatment* (eds. B.E. Saunders, L. Berlinger and R.F. Hanson), 49–51. Charleston, SC: National Crime Victims Research and Treatment Center.

Conn, A.M., Urbach, K., Butler, N. et al. (2018). Building youth resilience to adverse childhood experiences: small group therapy in an urban school-based health center. *Journal of Adolescent Health* 62 (#95): S37–S140.

Cossu, G., Cantone, E., Pintus, M. et al. (2015). Integrating children with psychiatric disorders in the classroom: a systematic review. *Clinical Practice and Epidemiology in Mental Health* 11 (Suppl 1M3): 41–57.

D'Amico, E.J., Houck, J.M., Hunter, S.B. et al. (2015). Group motivational interviewing for adolescents: change talk and alcohol and marijuana outcomes. *Journal of Consulting and Clinical Psychology* 83 (1): 68–80.

Delaney, K., DeSocio, J., and Carbray, J.A. (2014). Psychotherapy with children. In: *Psychotherapy for the Advanced Practice Psychiatric Nurse*, 2nde (ed. K. Wheeler), 597–624. New York, NY: Springer.

Delaney, K. (2008). Psychotherapy with children. In: *Psychotherapy for the Advanced Practice Psychiatric Nurse* (ed. K. Wheeler), 330–352. St. Louis, MO: Mosby.

Depa, M. and Astramovich, R. (2008). Puppetwork with victims of sexual abuse. *Play Therapy* 3 (2): 10–13.

Eisenberg, N., Cumberland, T., Fabes, R. et al. (2001). The relations of regulation and emotionality to children's externalizing and internalizing problem behavior. *Child Development* 72: 1112–1134.

Erikson, E. (1980). *Identity and the Life Cycle*. New York, NY: W.W. Norton & Co., Inc.

Gardner, R. (1975). The mutual storytelling technique. In: *Psychotherapeutic Approaches to the Resistant Child* (ed. R.A. Gardner), 101–140. New York, NY: J. Aronson.

Gardner, R. (1988). *The Storytelling Card Game*. New Jersey: Creative Therapeutics.

Gardner, R. (2001). The talking, feeling and doing game. In: *Game Play* (eds. C.E. Schaefer and S.E. Reid), 78–108. New York, NY: Wiley.

Gaskill, R. (2010). Neurobiology of play therapy. *Play Therapy* 5 (4): 18–22.

Gaskill, R. (2004). Neurosequential development and experiential play therapy with traumatized children. Paper presented at the Association for Play Therapy Annual Conference. October, Denver, CO.

Gaskill, R. and Perry, B.D. (2014). The neurobiological power of play. In: *Creative Arts and Play Therapy for Attachment Problems* (eds. C.A. Malchiodi and D.A. Crenshaw), 178–194. New York, NY: Guilford Press.

Ghandour, R.M., Sherman, L.J., Vladutiu, C.J. et al. (2018). Prevalence and treatment of depression, anxiety, and conduct problems in US children. *Journal of Pediatrics.* doi https://doi.org/10.1016/j.jpeds.2018.09.021.

Gifford-Smith, M., Dodge, K., Dishion, T., and McCord, J. (2005). Peer influence in children and adolescence: crossing the bridge from development to intervention science. *Journal of Abnormal Child Psychology* 33 (3): 255–265.

Gil, E. (2004). Trauma-focused play therapy. In: *Child Physical and Sexual Abuse: Guidelines for Treatment* (eds. B.E. Saunders, L. Berlinger and R.F. Hanson), 54–55. Charleston, SC: National Crime Victims Research and Treatment Center.

Ginsburg, K.R. (2007). The importance of play in promoting healthy child development and maintaining strong parent-child bonds. *Pediatrics* 119: 182–191.the Committee on Cummunications, the Committee on Psychosocial Aspects of Child and Family Health.

Gitlin-Weiner, K., Sandgrund, A., and Schaefer, C. (eds.) (2000). *Play Diagnosis and Assessment*, 2nde. New York, NY: Wiley.

Green, E.J. and Myrick, A.C. (2014). Treating complex trauma in adolescents: a phase-based, integrative approach for play therapists. *International Journal of Play Therapy* 23 (3): 131–145.

Haiat, H., Bar-Mor, G., and Shochat, M. (2003). The world of the child: a world of play even in the hospital. *Journal of Pediatric Nursing* 18: 209–214.

Henig, R. (2008). *Taking play seriously*. Available at http://www.nytimes.com/2008/02/17/magazine/17play.html.

Horne, A., Stoddard, J., and Bell, C. (2007). Group approaches to reducing aggression and bullying in school. *Group Dynamics: Theory, Research, and Practice* 11: 262–271.

Hynes, A. and Hynes-Berry, M. (1986). *Biblio /Poetry Therapy: The Interactive Process: A Handbook*. Boulder, CO: Westview Press.

Johnson, D., Pedro-Carroll, J., and Demanchik, S. (2005). The primary mental health project: a play intervention for school-aged children. In: *Empirically Based Play Interventions for Children* (eds. L.A. Reddy, T.M. Files-Hall and C.E. Schaefer), 13–30. Washington, DC: American Psychological Association.

Jung, C. (ed.) (1968). *Man and His Symbols*. New York, NY: Dell Books.

Kaduson, H.G. and Schaefer, C.E. (eds.) (2003). *101 Favorite Play Therapy Techniques*, vol. 111. Lanham, MD: Rowman and Littlefield Publishers, Inc.

Kalff, D. (2003). *Sandplay: A Psychotherapeutic Approach to the Psyche*. Cloverdale, CA: Temenos Press.

Kivlighan, D. and Tarrant, J. (2001). Does group climate mediate the group leadership-group member outcome relationship? A test of Yalom's hypotheses about leadership priorities. *Group Dynamics: Theory, Research, and Practice* 5 (3): 220–234.

Knell, S. (1998). Cognitive-behavioral play therapy. *Journal of Clinical Child Psychology* 27: 28–34.

Knell, S. and Beck, K. (2000). The puppet sentence completion task. In: *Play Diagnosis and Assessment*, 2e (eds. K. Gitlin-Weiner, A. Sandgrund and C.E. Schaefer), 704–721. New York, NY: Wiley.

Kot, S. and Tyndall-Lind, A. (2005). Intensive play therapy with child witnesses of domestic violence. In: *Empirically Based Play Interventions for Children* (eds. L.A. Reddy, T.M. Files-Hall and C.E. Schaefer), 31–49. Washington, DC: American Psychological Association.

Kottman, T. (2001). Adlerian play therapy. *International Journal of Play Therapy* 10 (2): 1–12.

Kraft, I. (1996). History. In: *Group Therapy with Children and Adolescents* (eds. P. Kymissis and D. Halperin). Washington, DC: American Psychiatric Press.

Kulic, K., Horne, A., and Dagley, J. (2004). A comprehensive review of prevention groups for children and adolescents. *Group Dynamics: Theory, Research, and Practice* 8: 139–151.

Landreth, G. (ed.) (2001). *Innovations in Play Therapy: Issues, Process and Special Populations*. Philadelphia, PA: Brunner Routledge.

Landreth, G. (2012). *Play Therapy: The Art of the Relationship*, 3e. New York, NY: Routledge.

Lankton, C. and Lankton, S. (1989). *Tales of Enchantment: Goal Oriented Metaphors for Adults and Children in Therapy*. New York, NY: Brunner Mazel.

Lowenfeld, M. (1999). *Understanding Children's Sandplay: Lowenfeld's World Technique*. Cambridge, MA: Margaret Lowenfeld Trust.

Meany-Walen, K.K., Kottman, T., Bullis, Q., and Taylor, D.D. (2015). Effects of Adlerian play therapy on children's externalizing behavior. *Journal of Counseling and Development* 93 (4): 418–428.

Melnyk, B. and Moldenhauer, Z. (2006). *The KySS Guide to Child and Adolescent Mental Health Screening, Early Intervention and Health Promotion*. Cherry Hill, NJ: National Association of Pediatric Nurse Practitioners.

Metzger, T., Mignogna, K., and Reilly, L. (2013). Child life specialists: key members of the team in pediatric radiology. *Journal of Radiology Nursing* 32: 153–159.

Mills, J. and Crowley, R. (1986). *Therapeutic Metaphors for Children and the Child within*. New York, NY: Brunner Mazel.

Mishna, F. and Muskat, B. (2004). "I'm not the only one!" group therapy with older children and adolescents who have learning disabilities. *International Journal of Group Psychotherapy* 54: 455–476.

Moore, E.R., Bennett, K.L., Dietrich, M.S., and Wells, N. (2015). The effect of directed medical play on young children's pain and distress during burn wound care. *Journal of Pediatric Health Care* 29: 265–273.

National Institute for Play Therapy. (2009). *Play science: The seven patterns of play*. Available at http://nifplay.org.

O'Connor, K.J. (2000). *The Play Therapy Primer*, 3–58. New York, NY: Wiley.

Osilla, K.C., Ortiz, J.A., Miles, J.N. et al. (2015). How group factors affect adolescent change talk and substance use outcomes: implications for motivational interviewing training. *Journal of Counseling Psychology* 62 (1): 79–86.

Patterson, L., Stutey, D.M., and Dorsey, B. (2018). Plat therapy with African American children exposed to adverse childhood experiences. *International Journal of Play Therapy* 27 (4): 215–226.

Perry, B. (2006). Applying principles of neurodevelopment to clinical work with maltreated and traumatized children: the neurosequential model of therapeutics. In: *Working with Traumatized Youth in Child Welfare (Ch. 3)* (ed. N.B. Webb). New York, NY: Guilford Press.

Ray, D.C. & McCullough, R. (2016). *Evidence-based practice statement: Play therapy* (Research report). Association for Play Therapy. Available at http://www.a4pt.org/?page=EvidenceBased.

Ray, D.C., Armstrong, S.A., Balkin, R.S., and Jayne, K.M. (2014). Child-centered play therapy in the schools: review and meta-analysis. *Psychology in the Schools* 52 (2): 107–123.

Ray, D.C., Stulmaker, H.L., Lee, K.R., and Silverman, W.K. (2013). Child-centered play therapy and impairment: exploring relationships and constructs. *International Journal of Play Therapy* 22 (1): 13–27.

Rennie, R. and Landreth, G. (2000). Effects of filial therapy on parent and child behaviors. *International Journal of Play Therapy* 9 (2): 19–37.

Ritzi, R.M., Ray, D.C., and Schumann, B.R. (2017). Intensive short-term child-centered play therapy and externalizing behaviors in children. *International Journal of Play Therapy* 26 (1): 33–46.

Rogers, C. (1951). *Client-Centered Therapy*. Boston, MA: Houghton Mifflin.

Saunders, B.E., Berliner, L., and Hanson, R.F. (2004). *Child physical and sexual abuse: Guidelines for treatment* (Revised Report: April 26, 2004). Charleston, SC: National Crime Victims Research and Treatment Center.

Schaefer, C. (2001). Prescriptive play therapy. *International Journal of Play Therapy* 10 (2): 57–73.

Schaefer, C. and Reid, S. (1986). *Game Play: Therapeutic Use of Childhood Games*. New York, NY: Wiley.

Secinti, E., Thompson, E.J., Richards, M., and Gaysina, D. (2017). Research review: childhood chronic physical illness and adult emotional health--a systematic review and meta-analysis. *Journal of Child Psychology and Psychiatry* 58: 753–769.

Shechtman, Z. (2007). How does group process research inform leaders of counseling and psychotherapy groups? *Group Dynamics: Theory, Research, and Practice* 11 (4): 293–304.

Shechtman, Z. and Gluk, O. (2005). An investigation of therapeutic factors in children's groups. *Group Dynamics: Theory, Research, and Practice* 9 (2): 127–134.

Shelby, J. and Felix, E. (2005). Posttraumatic play therapy: the need for an integrated model of directive and non-directive approaches. In: *Empirically Based Play Interventions for Children* (eds. L. Reddy, T.M. Files-Hall and C.E. Schaefer), 79–103. Washington, DC: American Psychological Association.

Stulmaker, H.L. and Ray, D.C. (2015). Child-centered play therapy with young children who are anxious: a controlled trial. *Children and Youth Services Review* 57: 127–133.

Swank, J. (2008). The use of games: a therapeutic tool with children and families. *International Journal of Play Therapy* 17: 154–167.

Tackett, J. (2010). Toward an externalizing spectrum in DSM-V: incorporating developmental concerns. *Child Development Perspectives* 4 (3): 161–167.

Terr, L. (2003). Wild child: how three principles of healing organized 12 years of psychotherapy. *Journal of the American Academy of Child & Adolescent Psychiatry* 42: 1401–1409.

VanFleet, R. (2005). *Filial Therapy: Strengthening Parent-Child Relationships through Play*, 2e. Sarasota, FL: Professional Resource Press.

VanFleet, R., Ryan, S., and Smith, S. (2005). Filial therapy: a critical review. In: *Empirically Based Play Interventions for Children* (eds. L.A. Reddy, T.M. Files-Hall and C.E. Schaefer), 241–264.

Wenner, M. (2009). The serious need for play. *Scientific American* 20: 22–29. https://doi.org/10.1038/scientificamericanmind0209-22.

White, H.L. (2017). The working life of a play specialist. *Paediatrics and Child Health* 27: 476–480.

Yalom, I. (1995). *The Theory and Practice of Group Psychotherapy*, 4e. New York, NY: Basic Books.

Yogman, M., Garner, A., Hutchinson, J. et al. (2018). The power of play: a pediatric role in enhancing development in young children. AAP committee on psychosocial aspects of child and family health, AAP council on communication and media. *Pediatrics* 142 (3): e20182058. doi:10/1542/peds.2018-2058.

19

Individual and Family Therapies

Kathleen Scharer

University of South Carolina, Columbia, SC, USA

Objectives

After reading this chapter, advanced practice registered nurses will be able to:

1. Identify different types of therapies that would be appropriate for a particular child and/or family.
2. Discuss the evidence base for each therapy presented.
3. Determine which treatments might be provided within the APRN setting and what qualifications would be needed to provide the treatment.
4. Make an informed decision about the mental health treatment referral needs of children and adolescents.

Introduction

The purpose of this chapter is to discuss the major types of individual and family therapies useful for children and adolescents, the evidence of their effectiveness, and any particular problems for which they have been proven effective. This allows the primary care advanced practice registered nurse (APRN) to make an informed selection of treatments and providers when making referrals for their patients. Psychotherapy involves using planned interventions or counseling designed to reduce maladaptive behavior, reduce stress, or enhance adaptive behaviors. There are various forms of therapy that are developmentally appropriate for children and adolescents, and for particular types of problems; selecting the best form and type of evidence-based intervention is an important factor in the success of the therapy. Most therapies involve some type of interpersonal interactions,

that is, talk between patient and therapist or with others in the session. For children, talk is important but may be supplemented with play, rewarding certain behaviors, behavioral rehearsal, games, stories, or other activities that allow the child to express and/or practice certain emotions or behaviors. Elsewhere in this book, chapters have been devoted to important types of therapies such as play therapy, group therapy, and cognitive-behavioral therapy (CBT). This chapter will address other types of evidence-based therapies that are useful to children and their families.

Generally, the primary goal of therapy is to help individuals or families change problematic behavior. In many types of therapy, with adults and adolescents, change is believed to occur through interpretations the therapists make and share with the patients. These interpretations help patients develop a new understanding of

Child and Adolescent Behavioral Health: A Resource for Advanced Practice Psychiatric and Primary Care Practitioners in Nursing,
Second Edition. Edited by Edilma L. Yearwood, Geraldine S. Pearson, and Jamesetta A. Newland.
© 2021 John Wiley & Sons, Inc. Published 2021 by John Wiley & Sons, Inc.
Companion website: www.wiley.com/go/Yearwood

themselves and their behavior to enable them to make a change. Interpretations only work if the child can comprehend the interpretation and is cognitively mature enough to incorporate this understanding. Behavioral treatments do not rely on making interpretations but are focused on the belief that if behavior changes, the emotional and cognitive processes will also change. Some points to consider in selecting a therapy are related to the child's developmental stage. Therapies that involve mature cognition for success are not likely to be effective with young children.

Several factors about young children must be taken into account when making a choice of therapy. For example, the young child believes that the world revolves around himself or herself. As the child matures, this omnipotence diminishes and other causes for problems can be understood by the child. We know that this omnipotent stance can remain for highly emotionally charged issues into adolescence, long beyond when it disappears for routine things. Adolescents may feel responsible for their parents divorcing when the adolescent had no real responsibility for the problems of the parents. Young children have trouble linking past events and emotions to the present because their sense of time is not yet developed. An example of this undeveloped sense of time is the frequent question of young children when traveling: "Are we there yet?" Preadolescent and younger children also have difficulty understanding conscious versus unconscious motivations for behavior. Explanations that a behavior has some unconscious motivation would typically be rejected by the child in favor of a conscious explanation; this is not resistance on the child's part but an effect of normal cognitive development. Abstract reasoning does not develop until formal operations develop in adolescence so the child cannot always see the perspective of others. Selecting an intervention that relies on how a younger child's behavior affects another is not likely to be effective.

One of the most difficult decisions in psychotherapy is determining what type of therapy and which therapist are most appropriate for a particular child and family. In many cases, children and their families are referred to a mental health provider because the referring practitioner knows the mental health provider or the referral is to a mental health system or office, rather than to a specific therapist. This may not result in the best choice of therapy or therapist for the child or family. It is imperative that the therapist have experience with children. There are multiple types of therapies; some have a greater base of evidence than others and some are more suited to particular types of problems. No practitioner is an expert in all types of therapy; in reality, most practices use one or two types of therapy with perhaps some

aspects of others mixed into their practice. By understanding the various types of therapies, the primary care APRN can make the best selection for youth who need assistance. The practitioner must recognize that evidence-based means more than just the underlying research; evidence-based includes the preferences of the child and family as well as the practitioner's clinical assessment of the individual child and family. An excellent reference for the practitioner is *What works for Whom? A critical review of treatments for children and adolescents* by Fonagy, Cotrell, Phillips, Bevington, Glasser, and Allison (2nd edition, published in 2015). This book discusses the use of both medications and psychotherapies for specific disorders.

Individual Therapy

Individual therapy for children and adolescents is typically provided within a developmental framework. Some therapies, such as play therapy, which is discussed in Chapter 18, are only appropriate for younger children; the typical adolescent would be offended if offered a sand tray and puppets or other similar toys for therapy. Even within a developmental phase, what one child needs may be quite different from what another child needs.

Younger children may also have more difficulty interpreting and/or reporting events that occur, so their reporting of events must be often validated with parents and, in school-age children, with teachers. In most therapy sessions, the therapist spends at least a little time with the parents of young children. Most adolescents are very concerned about what an individual therapist might say to their parents and do not want their therapist to speak with their parents unless the teen is present. Respecting the privacy of the child of any age must be carefully balanced with the needs of the parent to understand the therapeutic process and the progress of the child in therapy. In the following material, the word "child" is used to mean individuals up to 18 years of age, unless distinctions between adolescents and children need to be specifically made.

Cognitive-Behavioral Therapy

CBT has the most extensive research base of any psychotherapy. It has been widely used with children with good effects. Because of the amount of evidence available on CBT, it is addressed on its own in Chapter 20.

Psychodynamic Psychotherapy

The term "psychodynamic psychotherapy" covers a broad spectrum of interventions that can range from child psychoanalysis to less frequent sessions with the therapist. Psychodynamic therapies are an outgrowth of the work of Sigmund Freud with modification and input from many other therapists, including Melanie Klein, Anna Freud, Heinz Kohut, Donald Winnicott, Otto Kernberg, Margaret Mahler, and John Bowlby (Fonagy 1999).

What is it?

Some psychodynamic therapies are very expressive in nature while others are more supportive. However, the commonality in these approaches is the belief that the problems that bring the child to therapy stem from the stress of a conflicting motivational states. This form of therapy is believed to be therapeutic because it helps individuals build on their own inherent capacities for understanding and emotional responsiveness. Therapists aid in this process by communicating an understanding of a child's conflicting motivations and the responses to these motivations. While there are differences in the way psychodynamic psychotherapy can be operationalized, there are some commonalities in beliefs about the treatment. The therapist sees the problem as the child's reaction to the external world as based on past representations of events. This is the notion of psychological causation. The therapist believes that there are unconscious mental processes that affect the child's reaction to the external world. The therapist also believes that the child has mental representations of events with others that form the basis of interactions with others. In the therapist's view, the child has experienced intrapsychic conflict and uses defenses to protect against these conflicts. Psychodynamic psychotherapists also believe that a child's symptoms have several layers of meaning and the job of the therapist is to interpret and explain these to the child. The therapist has the assumption that transference will occur and is the child's displacement of unresolved issues from previous relationships, usually with parents, onto the therapist. The relational aspects of the therapy relationship are also seen as beneficial to the child's functioning (Fonagy 1999).

For Whom Does it Work?

Psychodynamic psychotherapy by its nature requires that the child or adolescent have good verbal skills and the ability to think of behavior as influenced by thoughts and feelings. The child or adolescent needs to be able to tolerate some anxiety and conflicts, especially around issues previously not allowed into consciousness without experiencing increased disorganization. The parents, or caregivers in another milieu in which the child is residing, need to be able to support the child in a long-term therapeutic relationship and encourage the child's commitment to the therapeutic process. A basic assumption is that the child's problem is due to some internal conflict. Children have to be developmentally age appropriate unless the developmental deficits are the result of the internal conflict requiring therapy. Children also need to be able to sustain a long-term relationship and be able to trust the therapist. Children must have developed the understanding that they have a responsibility for their problems and behaviors (Fonagy 1999). Generally speaking, psychodynamic psychotherapy is useful for children who are considered neurotic rather than more severely disturbed children.

What Happens in Therapy?

In psychodynamic psychotherapy, the therapist attempts to understand and create a model of the child's thoughts and feelings through what the child reports, through nonverbal play, through any dreams that are reported, or through other behaviors. Additional information may be obtained from parents, teachers, and others in contact with the child. Using the model, the therapist tries to help the child understand his inappropriate or irrational feelings and beliefs. Some techniques are often used in the therapeutic process. Supportive interventions are used to reduce anxiety or increase the child's sense of mastery. This can be done through suggesting ideas to the child, reassuring the child about fears or concerns, providing information as needed, or being empathetic to the child's situation. Therapists also clarify the children's affect and verbalization to help the child understand and may make direct comments about repeated behaviors as a way of directing the child's attention to these. Sometimes summarizing or paraphrasing things the child says can help the child continue to discuss things with the therapist. Interpretations are used to describe ideas or beliefs of which the child may not be consciously aware and to which the child may not be ready to listen. It is imperative then that the therapist times interpretations carefully and selects those for which the evidence is fairly conclusive (Fonagy 1999).

What is the Evidence Base for this Therapy?

The research on psychodynamic psychotherapy has been somewhat limited because it is not a therapy that is easily manualized; it must be adapted to every child. Increasingly, research is being done on psychodynamic psychotherapy for children and adolescents. Abbass et al. (2013) completed a meta-analysis of 11 studies of short-term psychodynamic psychotherapy (STPP) of fewer than 40 sessions with children and adolescents. A total of 655 patients with varying diagnoses such as depression, anxiety disorders, anorexia nervosa, and borderline personality disorder were included in the studies. STPP was not significantly different from the comparison treatments but there were some subgroup differences. Robust within-group effect sizes (0.80–1.34) were observed, suggesting the treatment may be effective. These effects increased in follow up compared to post treatment, suggesting a tendency toward increased gains. Heterogeneity was high across most analyses, suggesting that these data need be interpreted with caution. This review suggests that STPP may be effective in children and adolescents across a range of common mental disorders (Abbass et al. 2013).

In a more recent study of psychodynamic therapy with patients 14–24 years old, Nemirovski Edlund and Carlberg (2016) used a retrospective naturalistic design to examine the ratings on the Children's Global Assessment Scale (CGAS), the Global Assessment of Functioning (GAF), and decreased symptom severity on Symptoms Checklist-90. The patients typically had internalizing disorders which have been previously shown to be more responsive to psychodynamic therapy. Unlike some previous meta-analyses, the effect sizes in the study were large. One note of caution is that often patients dropped out of therapy early because of various adversities in their lives, which may have contributed to the findings of increased duration of therapy with positive effects (Nemirovski Edlund and Carlberg 2016).

The research on psychodynamic psychotherapy's efficacy with children and adolescents is growing. The research that has been done has mixed results, but more recent research has shown greater effect sizes. Therefore, psychodynamic psychotherapy should be carefully considered for children and adolescents.

How to Become a Psychodynamic Therapist

Typically learning to be a competent psychodynamic therapist involves advanced training in psychiatry, psychology, psychiatric nursing, social work, or counseling with a focus on this method and often postgraduate training. It is important to have close supervision by a competent psychodynamic therapist to learn how to make appropriate interpretations. Sometimes individual psychodynamic therapy for the therapist is also recommended. The Psychoanalytic Association of New York, Department of Psychiatry, New York University offers postgraduate training programs. For information visit their website: https://www.pany.org.

A search did not reveal any professional organization that specifically offered training for psychodynamic therapists.

Interpersonal Psychotherapy

Interpersonal psychotherapy (IPT) is based on the interpersonal theory of Harry Stack Sullivan, who believed that personality is developed from the reflected appraisals of others. Sullivan believed that mental illnesses developed in the context of social relationships that were not effective. Sullivan met Alfred Meyer during his education in psychotherapy and was introduced to Meyer's theory that psychological disorder developed from the individual's struggle to deal with his social environment. Sullivan applied these ideas to the treatment of schizophrenia (New World Encyclopedia 2008). Later his ideas became the basis for IPT. IPT is also based on the attachment theory of John Bowlby (Mufson and Sills 2006).

What is it?

As currently practiced, IPT was developed by Gerald Klerman and Myrna Weissman (International Society for Interpersonal Psychotherapy 2018). The patient's interpersonal interactions are examined in relationship to the patient's depressive symptoms. IPT recognizes the significance of the current interpersonal world of the client in symptom development and maintenance. IPT is directive and active, with an explicit focus for the client and therapist. There are three components of depression in the IPT model of depression: (i) symptom formation, (ii) social functioning, and (iii) personality contributions.

For Whom Does it Work?

IPT was initially developed to treat major depression in short-term therapy in about 12–16 sessions. It has subsequently been modified and researched in a number of different age groups and with a wide variety of diagnoses, such as anorexia nervosa (Rieger et al. 2010), substance misuse, bulimia nervosa (Arcelus et al. 2009; Fairburn et al. 1993), dysthymia, post-traumatic stress disorder (PTSD), somatization disorder, and some anxiety disorders with adults (Cyranowski et al. 2005). It is a manualized therapy, and for each adaptation for depression the manuals are used but different components are emphasized (International Society for Interpersonal Psychotherapy 2020). A specific manual for adolescent depression, called IPT-A, has been developed and tested (Mufson and Sills 2006).

What Happens in Therapy?

There are certain theoretical assumptions underpinning IPT. First, IPT does not consider that psychological problems come only from the interpersonal realm, psychological problems all occur in an interpersonal context. This interpersonal context is interdependent with the psychological problems. IPT aims to intervene in this interpersonal context to achieve some symptom relief. The therapist presents as warm and in a collaborative relationship to the patient; however, there is strict adherence to the manual. In this short-term therapy, regression is discouraged by a focus within every session on the upcoming termination.

Sessions are usually weekly for an hour. In the first session, an assessment is done of the patient's illness and social context. The illness is explained to the patient in interpersonal terms. The process of the sessions in IPT is described to the patient. An "interpersonal inventory" is completed which depicts and categorizes the important relationships in the patient's life into the four components of depression: role transitions, grief, interpersonal disputes, and interpersonal deficits.

The remaining sessions, except the last two, deal with the problematic relationships in the patient's life; little emphasis is placed on the illness, except to ask about the severity of the symptoms. The final two sessions focus on termination, which is presented as a loss experience from which the patient can learn more about the response to loss and how well IPT has helped in modulating responses to loss. The therapist uses active listening and clarification to help demonstrate to the patient any biases. For interpersonal disputes role-playing and communication analysis can be helpful in resolving the disputes. Within the safety of the session, encouragement of affect allows the patient to experience emotions that might be considered unpleasant, such as the sadness from loss. The patient is encouraged to generate problem solutions as much on their own as possible, thus gradually phasing out the need for a therapist. It is this process of patients learning to initiate their own changes that accounts for the symptomatic improvement peaking around 3–6 months after treatment is terminated.

What is the Evidence Base for this Therapy?

Studies about IPT-A have been conducted over many years (Gunlicks-Stoessel et al. 2010; Tang et al. 2010). Young et al. (2010) evaluated the efficacy of a prevention program for depression in 57 adolescents randomized to either usual school counseling or IPT with an adolescent skills training model (IPT-AST), which was a modification of IPT-A. At the end of the intervention the adolescents in the IPT-AST group reported significantly greater improvement in symptom level and overall functioning at post intervention but during the remainder of the 18 months, rates of change slowed for the IPT-AST group while the school counseling group continued to improve so that the changes were no longer significant. However, IPT-AST has the benefit of returning the adolescents to schoolwork and other activities sooner.

Mychailyszyn and Elson (2018) conducted a meta-analysis of the effectiveness of IPT-A. A total of 10 studies yielding 766 participants were analyzed using a standardized mean gain effect size. The results indicate that IPT-A was significantly effective at reducing depressive symptoms in adolescents and significantly more effective than control or treatment-as-usual groups in treating depression in adolescents, no matter what format was used or the ethnic/racial background of the patients. IPT-A had an overall effect size (Hedges g) of 1.19, while the aggregate effect size for controls was 0.58. A significant change in symptoms of depression was found over all 10 studies with IPT-A.

How Do You Become a Therapist?

The International Society for Interpersonal Psychotherapy (ISIP) website (International Society for Interpersonal Psychotherapy 2018) describes the training for those interested in becoming IPT therapists. The first requirement is that potential trainees have a clinical background with a sound understanding of mood disorders. The trainees read the IPT manual and attend a 2–4 day training course. This is followed by supervision with a supervisor registered through the ISIP. The first case seen by the trainee must be a patient with a major depressive disorder, and the second case must be a person with dysthymia, adolescent depression, or eating disorder. The trainee must be supervised for a minimum of two cases. All sessions must be recorded. The supervisor selects a minimum of three sessions to review and rate on the IPT competency scale. After the supervisor deems the trainee has meet the competencies on two cases, the training is considered to be finished (ISIP 2018). The ISIP can be accessed online at: https://www.interpersonalpsychotherapy.org.

Multisystemic Therapy

Multisystemic therapy (MST) was developed specifically to work with children and adolescents who have demonstrated serious antisocial behavior. The program focuses on the entire world of the youth, including families, friends, schools, teachers, and even the neighborhood. It is an individual therapy integrated with family therapy and environmental therapy.

What is it?

MST is targeted for the toughest offenders, male and female, between 12 and 17 years of age. The treatment program is based on the theory of social ecology, which considers the determinants of the child's behavior to be multilayered, like an onion, with the child being the central core and family, friends, teachers, school, and neighborhood making up the additional layers. The child's behavior is influenced by the interaction among all of these groups with the child. To effectively treat the youth's antisocial behavior, MST must be able to address all of aspects of the child's life to change the youth's problem behavior. The ultimate aim of MST is to surround the youth with layers of people who promote prosocial behavior rather than antisocial behavior (Henggler et al. 2009).

For Whom Does it Work?

MST was developed specifically to treat antisocial youths. However, it has been adapted to other types of children and youth, and has been used in other countries. For example it is being tried as a treatment for youth with severe type 1 diabetes (Ellis et al. 2010), serious emotional disturbances (Rowland et al. 2005), adolescent substance abuse (Randall et al. 2001), and a history of family abuse (Brunk et al. 1987). These many adaptations of the original program speak to its strength as a treatment when a strong supportive environment is needed to encourage the youth's healthy development.

What Happens in Therapy?

MST is multifaceted treatment as its name implies. Increasing the parenting skills of the child's caregivers and changing the behavior of the antisocial youth are at the core of the treatment process, but MST is not delivered in an office on a once-a-week or once-a-month basis; rather the therapist goes to where the youth hangs out, to school, and to the home. Therapists often see the members of the youth's ecological system more than once a week since all of these individuals have affected the youth. These meetings are not conducted strictly during standard business hours. The MST team members are on call 24 hours a day and every day of the week. Naturally this requires that the therapists have quite limited caseloads. Dropouts are also reduced by this process because barriers to getting the youth to a therapy session are avoided.

Family-focused therapy is intensive; goals include increasing parenting skills, improving all relationships within the family, involving the youth with peers who do not engage in antisocial behaviors, helping the youth to achieve academically or vocationally, helping the youth find positive activities in which to engage such as sports, and creating a support network of extended family, friends, and neighbors who will aid the caregivers in maintaining change (Henggler et al. 2009). To achieve these goals, family members collaborate with MST team members to develop the treatment plan that makes sense to the family and builds on their strengths. This collaboration increases the likelihood of the success of the treatment plan.

What is the Evidence Base for this Therapy?

The evidence base for MST is extensive. The first publications began in 1986, which labeled the treatment as multisystemic and described the effects on the youth and family (Henggeler et al. 1986). Recently Henggeler and Schaeffer (2016) noted that more than 100 peer-reviewed outcome and implementation journal articles had been published as of January 2016. Many of these 100 papers were written by independent investigators. Most of the outcome research has demonstrated positive results, while implementation research has demonstrated the need for treatment fidelity to obtain the desired outcomes.

A study done by Borduin and Dopp in 2015 examined the economic impact of MST for problematic sexual behaviors (MST-PSB). They studied the cost and benefits of MST-PSB compared to the usual community services group. The total benefit was estimated to be US\$343 455 per MST-PSB participant. Another way to look at the data was every US\$1.00 spent on MST-PSB treatment resulted in a US\$48.81 saving for the taxpayers and victims.

How Do You Become a Therapist?

Four types of training are used in the MST model to maintain quality. Since MST is delivered by a team, the team trains together. First the professional attends a 5-day training session. Therapists are asked to read the MST manual prior to training, which includes both didactic and experiential learning. Therapists who are conducting MST also participate in quarterly booster training, which is an onsite, 1.5 days of training, used to enhance the team's knowledge and skills. Onsite supervision is also provided weekly and there is weekly expert consultation for the team. Supervision of MST therapists is also manualized and supervisors must also undergo training in MST. The expert consultant works with the supervisors to help them develop their supervisory skills in MST. For online information about MST go to www.mstservices.com.

Eye Movement Desensitization and Reprocessing

Eye movement desensitization and reprocessing (EMDR) is a scientifically validated, psychotherapeutic approach. The theory behind EMDR is that many psychological problems are caused by traumatic experiences or disturbing life events. These traumatic or disturbing events impair the person's processing abilities and the ability to integrate experiences in the central nervous system. EMDR seems to have a direct effect on the way that the brain processes information. Normal information processing is resumed, so following a successful EMDR session a person no longer relives the strong negative images, sounds, and feelings when the event is brought to mind.

What is it?

EMDR was developed in 1987 by Dr. Francine Shapiro, who made a chance observation that eye movements could reduce disturbing thoughts in certain situations (Shapiro 1989). The combination of remembering the traumatic event, describing the negative feelings, and the multisaccadic eye movements done in sets can desensitize the patient to the traumatic event in as little as one session. EMDR can be viewed as a physiologically based therapy that allows a person to see previously disturbing material in a new and less distressing way. EMDR has standard protocols and has helped many people since its development (Rodenburg et al. 2009).

For Whom Does it Work?

The patients most likely to benefit from EMDR are those individuals who have experienced traumatic events. These can be accidents, war trauma, rape, child abuse, domestic violence, or any other event that leaves strong negative images or feelings that recur and bother the person (Ahmad et al. 2007).

What Happens in Therapy?

The amount of time required to complete EMDR will vary according to the history of the patient. The protocol targets three areas: past memories, present disturbances, and future actions. The aim of therapy is to help patients process all of the experiences that are causing the problem, thus resolving the symptoms of the patient (Shapiro 1989).

The therapist completes a thorough history and assessment to identify the specific targets for therapy. Next, the therapist teaches the client certain skills that will be necessary for the actual treatment, including establishing a trusting relationship and calming techniques. In the third phase of treatment, the patient begins the process of selecting a particular scene from the target event that most clearly represents the target event, identifies a negative self-statement associated with the event like, "I am helpless," and develops a statement describing a more positive belief such as, "I am in control" (EMDR International Association [EMDRIA] 2018).

Reprocessing takes about three sessions in most cases but can vary for more complex problems. In the third phase the rapid eye movements or taps or tones are also used along with verbalizing the negative self-statement and recalling the target picture. Phase four involves the desensitization processes. This phase works with all of the patient's emotions as well as others that may arise during the sessions (EMDRIA 2018). In phase five, the goals are to increase the strengths of the patient's positive belief. In the sixth phase, the patient is asked to recall the disturbing event and to assess if there is any residual tension left in the body. If so, reprocessing is repeated. Calming techniques learned by the patient can be used to achieve a sense of calmness. The final phase is reevaluation, which actually occurs at the beginning of every session. In this phase, the therapist evaluates how the patient is doing, identifies any new problems that need to be resolved, and plans for this. The patient is also educated about using the techniques in the future (EMDRIA 2018).

What is the Evidence Base for this Therapy?

The clinical efficacy of EMDR in post-traumatic stress disorder treatment has been well established. Several meta-analyses and systematic reviews have been done, e.g. Rodenburg et al. (2009) and Seidler and Wagner (2006). From these reviews, EMDR could be regarded as an effective trauma therapy among other established trauma therapies for adults. Chen et al. (2018) completed a systematic review of the use of EMDR in children and adults who had experienced complex trauma, which is trauma that occurs over time, such as child abuse or war, rather than a single occurrence of trauma. Six randomized clinical trials (RCTs) with a total of 251 participants met the criteria for inclusion in the review. All six studies demonstrated favorable outcomes for both children and adults with EMDR in comparison with other therapies, treatment with fluoxetine, and other control conditions. The number of sessions per subject was also variable. The comparison groups were very heterogeneous among studies. The degree of success was not significant in every one of the studies (Chen et al. 2018). However, one of the tenets of such reviews is that when flawed or small studies achieve the same or similar outcomes, the evidence is strengthened as long as the flaws were different in the studies. It would appear from the review description of the studies that the flaws were variable among the studies.

A newer RCT compared trauma-focused CBT (TF-CBT) with EMDR (Diehle et al. 2015). The RTC examined the effectiveness and efficiency of both therapies using 48 children between 8 and 18 years of age. Children were randomly assigned to either treatment of eight sessions apiece. The researchers found that both therapies were effective and efficient in the treatment of children with PTSD. While there has been some criticism of EMRD as simply exposure therapy with some eye movements thrown in, the evidence of success with the therapy continues to grow.

How Do You Become a Therapist?

Qualifications for licensed mental health professionals vary by discipline. Physicians must have specialist training in psychiatry and be licensed. APRNs must have a master's degree in psychiatric nursing and be registered by their state board of nursing. Other mental health clinicians must have completed a masters- or doctorate-level graduate program with a focus in the mental health field *and* must be licensed or certified through their state or national credentialing board. Some limited licenses in some states, including LLP (limited liability partnership in Michigan), meet this requirement. Training can occur throughout the course of a semester for a university program or be tailored to fit the needs of the trainees if offered in some other arrangement (EMDRIA 2018). Consult the EMDRIA website for further information (http://www.emdria.org).

Family Therapy

Family therapy is often used in the treatment of a child's mental health problems because the child's problem affects the entire family unit. For many years families were believed to be the major source of childhood mental health problems; now we recognize that while families may unwittingly contribute to the child's problems, many childhood mental health problems have a neurobiological basis. Even when the problem is primarily neurobiological, the child's behavior affects the family, which in turn affects the child. Helping families sort through these issues is critical in helping the child. In some cases young children may be excluded from family therapy sessions even when they are the presenting problem for the family; this is much less true for adolescents. Sometimes this is an appropriate decision, if the child is very young or very disruptive. In some cases marital issues seem to be negatively influencing the child's behavior and sessions with just parents are needed. There is no one model that works for all families. Family therapies can be divided into two major groups: systemic therapies that are at least loosely based on systems theory and behavioral family therapies that use primarily behavioral techniques to reduce problems within the family. Behavioral therapy and CBT are described in Chapter 20 and will not be included here. The principles described in Chapter 20 are the same when applied in the context of family therapy. Evidence for specific types of family therapy other than CBT can be difficult to find. Research on therapies other than CBT decreased significantly in 1980s (Durlak and McGlinchey 1999) and sometimes the evidence available for a particular therapy is quite weak. Many of the articles about research on family therapy for children

and adolescents discuss family therapy as one method without specifying a particular type or even combining types, while other papers present case studies but clinical trials are few. Heatherington et al. (2015) noted that some systemic family therapies have had much more research and sometimes with specific disorders while others have very limited current research. For example, multidimensional family therapy (MFT) was designed for and applied to youth with externalizing behaviors, i.e. antisocial behavior, and the research supports this use. But other therapies, such as narrative family therapy and solution-focused therapy, have minimal research over the last 25 years.

Table 19.1 shows various systemic family therapies, what they are, for whom they are effective, and the extant evidence. Systems theory therapies are typically taught to mental health professionals either during their graduate education or through workshops. Supervision in the techniques is considered necessary at least until the professional becomes competent in the new techniques. Unlike many of the individual therapies, there are not websites or organizations for the various forms of family therapy. Rather, the American Association for Marriage and Family Therapy is the professional association for this group of professionals (http://www.aamft.org). There are chapters or divisions in some states that also have websites. Additionally, the International Family Therapy Association is a valuable resource (https://ifta-familytherapy.org).

Parent and Teacher Training

Directly working with parents about parenting issues is another way to influence a child's mental health. Some childhood problems do appear to be related to parenting approaches. The work of Gerald Patterson (1982) showed that different parenting styles affected the child's behavior. By helping parents learn different parenting approaches, the child's behavior can be corrected before it becomes a major problem. The parenting programs discussed here are all evidence-based, many with years of research behind them. The programs are built on social learning theory.

Triple P-Positive Parenting Program

The Triple P-Positive Parenting Program is a public health approach to parenting (Sanders 2003). It aims to prevent more serious problems in children and adolescents by delivering services to parents at five different levels, depending upon need.

Table 19.1 Comparison of different systemic family therapies

Type	What is it?	For whom does it work?	What happens in therapy?	What is the evidence base?
Attachment-based	Based on Bowlby's attachment theory, attachment-focused therapy is used to provide a secure base from which the individual can learn and grow. In this safe environment, the family can explore problems and find better ways to interact.	Depressed adolescent males (Diamond et al. 2002); young children with attachment disorders; others with attachment problems, such as abused children.	Each family member must have a solid attachment to the therapist. This is created by the therapist by being nonjudgmental and demonstrating relaxed engagement, playfulness, curiosity, and empathy. The therapist seeks to know each family member well and reflects that understanding through empathy. Information about child development, family processes, attachment, and intersubjectivity are shared to the extent needed. Within this environment, problems in the family are discussed and understood related to attachment and intersubjectivity. Family members' affect intentions and awareness are tracked, verbalized, and new meanings are co-created (Hughes 2007).	Diamond et al. (2016) report on multiple studies, including clinical trials and process studies that show that attachment-based family therapy is an empirically supported treatment specifically developed for repairing parent–child relationship that have damaged.
Experiential	In experiential family therapy, the family is involved in various activities as a family that are used to depict the family problems while encouraging family members to openly express how they are feeling. Behavior problems are believed to emanate from the smothering of emotions. The task of therapy is to unblock defenses and release people's innate vitality. This therapy stems from the work of Carl Whitaker.	This therapy has been used primarily for treating depression, based on studies in the literature.	The experience the family had is discussed and emotions are explored. A type of activity that might be used in experiential therapy is role reversal in which family members play each other during some situation. This provides the individual with an opportunity to experience the emotional reactions the other experiences during the real situation. This role reversal can be helpful in changing long-standing interaction patterns within a family. Other techniques can include family sculpting, family art therapy, family puppet interviews, and the Gestalt empty chair exercise.	Evidence for experiential therapy is fairly recent. Some studies have been testing the efficacy of the therapy (Carryer and Greenberg 2010; Ellison et al. 2009; Pos et al. 2009). Generally, the studies have shown some success with experiential therapy.
Multidimensional	Similar to multisystem therapy (MST) in that it uses an integrative, systems-oriented approach. The youth, the family, and the community are all involved in this therapy. Treatment can be provided in any number of settings, including foster care. The family develops competency in collaborating with any social systems in which the youth is involved, including school, juvenile justice system, or recreational activities.	Aimed at treating adolescents with drug use disorders and related behavior problems but has also been used for children with foster home placement behavior problems (Leve et al. 2009).	Treatment can be provided in any number of settings, including foster care. The family develops competency in collaborating with any social systems in which the youth is involved, including school, juvenile justice system, or recreational activities. Therapies are individualized to the needs of the children (Liddle 2010).	There is strong evidence of the effectiveness of this approach in various settings, including an international trial (e.g. Rigter et al. 2010). Carr (2016) in his research review noted that this therapy was much more effective than waiting-list controls and moderately more effective than usual treatment for adolescents with conduct disorders and drug use disorders.

(*continued*)

Table 19.1 *(cont'd)*

Type	What is it?	For whom does it work?	What happens in therapy?	What is the evidence base?
Narrative	In narrative therapy the focus is on using a comparison for learning. Each individual has a personal narrative, which can include different versions of the self, some of which are problematic. Families also develop narratives about themselves. Individuals and families tend to judge themselves by the narratives of the society in which they live. The therapist uses a technique for externalizing the problem story so the family can consider times when it is and is not a problem.	Narrative family therapy has been used for parent–child conflicts (Besa 1994), obsessive–compulsive disorders (McLuckie 2006), and blended families with role conflicts (Shalay and Brownlee 2007).	When a family comes into therapy, there are problem-laden narratives among the family members. These problem stories are often kept active because of their connection to others. The therapist seeks to help the family members redevelop these stories with more positive outcomes to help them look at what is stopping them from behaving in more successful ways. As a more positive account of the person develops, the problems fade into the background (White and Epston 1990). Therapists may use between-session tasks to help families re-author their narratives (Besa 1994).	Besa's study (1994) demonstrated effectiveness in changing parent–child conflicts with narrative therapy. Almost all of the current literature is of case studies or how to conduct the therapy.
Solution-focused	Brief therapy (solution-focused brief therapy) focused on developing solutions to problems the family already uses. The idea behind solution-focused therapy is to focus on the family's goals and reaching their goals. Strengths and solutions are focused on what is used when the problem is not occurring. Focus is on doing more of what is working.	Solution-focused therapy can help children with oppositional defiant disorder (Conoley et al. 2003) or with other behavior problems.	Attention is not paid to family structure or rules. The therapist, assuming an approach of curiosity, and in the role of nonexpert collaborator, helps the family construct solutions to their problems. The family sets a joint goal. The therapist poses the miracle question: "If a miracle happened tonight and removed the problem we just discussed, how would things be different?" Then family members state willingness to make it happen and confidence it could (Conoley et al. 2003). Berg and Steiner (2003) offer many suggestions on creative ways to engage children in solution-focused family therapy, e.g. puppet play. Children may feel safe discussing difficult issues through puppets when they would not feel safe talking directly about the issues. Another child-friendly activity is to ask the child to state three wishes. This allows the child to fantasize about the future and think about how life could be different.	Although much of the literature has methodological weaknesses, existing research does provide tentative support for the use of solution-focused therapy, particularly in relation to internalizing and externalizing child behavior problems. It appears particularly effective as an early intervention when presenting problems are not severe (Bond et al. 2013).

Strategic	Problems in families develop because of a lack of alternatives or an unhelpful way of linking explanations and behaviors. Emphasis is on the therapist being curious about the relationship between the beliefs and behaviors of family members. An assumption of BSFT is that if the therapist alters the family and extended family, they become a continuous positive influence on the youth (Santisteban et al. 1997).	Adolescents with substance abuse problems or conduct problems. Adolescents with anxiety disorders.	There are three major parts of the BSFT model: (i) joining, (ii) family pattern diagnosis, and (iii) restructuring. Joining with the family results in an effective collaboration and minimizes dropping out or resisting change. The therapist becomes the family leader. Family pattern diagnosis involves identifying the maladaptive family behavior patterns that are perpetuating the problem. This identification allows restructuring, which is the process of modifying the family patterns of interaction and helping the family reorganize and modify family roles. The result is to reduce the potential for drug abuse by the adolescent (Santisteban et al. 1997).	Carr (2016) noted in a review of research on family treatment that strategic family therapy was much more effective than waiting-list control comparison groups and modestly more effective than usual treatments for conduct disorders and drug use disorders. Brief strategic family therapy (BSFT) has been tested with varied populations and target problems. Experience in implementing BSFT shows an organizational-level systemic approach is necessary to ensure successful adoption of BSFT.
Structural	Problems develop from inappropriate family structure or organization. Structural family therapy focuses on reestablishing appropriate boundaries between parents and child(ren) and family and extended family (Minuchin et al. 1964). The goal of the therapy is to redesign the family structure to be more positive.	Children with conduct problems and psychosomatic problems such as intractable asthma, anorexia nervosa, and brittle diabetes	The therapist takes command of sessions, taking responsibility for moving the family in the desired direction. The therapist is very active in sessions and may redirect family members in seating arrangements or to whom each is speaking. Family may be directed to enact the problem behavior or change interactional patterns. Sometimes play activities can be used to unbalance the nonadaptive system in which the child has too much control and to reinforce the executive role of the parents.	In multiple cases, structural family therapy was effective with psychosomatic illness. Weaver et al. (2013) examined the effects of structural family therapy and results suggested it is a promising way to address both children's and mothers' mental health needs.

What is it?

Universal Triple P is delivered via media such as radio and television. The goal of Universal Triple P is to use mass media to reach many parents and provide information about common problems, such as shopping with young children (Sanders and Prinz 2008). Level two is single-session interaction with parents around a particular short-term problem. Level three is designed to be a four-session intervention delivered in the context of brief sessions, approximately 20 minutes each. One reason for the shortness of these sessions was to allow the delivery by primary healthcare providers. Parents identify a specific problematic behavior of their child, such as not following requests or being rude, and within the sessions are taught how to monitor the behavior, develop a behavioral plan, implement it, and assess the results (Sanders et al. 2003). Level four Triple P is an 8–10-session program designed to help parents manage their children's more serious problems, such as conduct disorders or attention deficit hyperactivity disorder (Bodenmann et al. 2008). Level four Triple P is more in depth and includes some parent–child sessions with the provider. Parents are taught 15 parenting behaviors, which they implement to help their child. Level five Triple P is essentially an add-on to level four and is used when more serious problems are identified (Hoath and Sanders 2002). There have been various modifications of the Triple P programs for use with different groups and problems.

For Whom Does it Work?

Because there are both preventative and treatment aspects to the interventions, Triple P is a universal approach to parenting. It has been used to decrease the amount of child abuse in a community (Prinz et al. 2009), for helping families with a disabled or autistic child (Whittingham et al. 2009), for helping teens transition to high school (Ralph and Sanders 2003; Ralph et al. 2004), for externalizing disorders such as disruptive behaviors and attention deficit hyperactivity disorder (Connell et al. 1997), for children with developmental disabilities (Plant and Sanders 2007), for preventing drug abuse (Sanders 2000), for lifestyles changes with obese children (West et al. 2010), and even for families with gifted children (Morawska and Sanders 2008). Triple P has been used in large urban areas, in rural counties, with indigenous peoples, and in many different countries. It has been delivered in person, in groups, via television or other mass media, by internet, and even self-directed. It is indeed a universal program for parents.

What Happens in Therapy?

The Triple P programs are built on a framework of self-regulation. Parents are taught self-regulations skills with the goal of building their self-regulation capacities and then modeling and teaching these to their children (Sanders 2008). Parents are helped to change their parenting strategies through increasing self-efficacy and parental self-efficacy, using self-management tools, promoting personal agency, and developing sound problem-solving skills. The program is built on five principles of positive parenting: a safe and engaging environment, a positive learning environment, assertive and consistent discipline, realistic expectations, and taking care of oneself as a parent (Sanders and Ralph 2001). Parents identify specific goals they would like to accomplish with their children based on an assessment and then in a guided participation model (Sanders and Lawton 1993) with the therapist work on a plan to accomplish the goal. Parents are taught specific skills that enhance their relationship with their child, encourage children's desirable behaviors, manage misbehaviors, anticipate and plan for risky behaviors, coach their children in learning new behaviors and skills, learn self-regulations skills, manage their own moods, and increase their coping skills and partner support skills (Sanders and Ralph 2001).

What is the Evidence Base for this Therapy?

The research base for the Triple P program is extensive, with over 100 studies completed since the early 1980s. The program has been implemented and studied internationally. It was developed in Queensland, Australia, by Dr. Mathew Sanders and has been widely implemented in Australia, Europe, Asia, and the United States (US). Triple P has been the subject of several meta-analyses, which have demonstrated effectiveness (e.g. de Graaf et al. 2008a,b; Sanders et al. 2014). Many of the previously cited articles also contribute to the evidence for this program.

How Do You Become a Therapist?

The Triple P program is tightly controlled to ensure treatment fidelity; all practitioners must undergo training for each specific type of Triple P they provide. Regular supervision or consultation is recommended and specific forms, teaching materials, and information sheets for parents must be purchased through the Triple P program. Checklists are used to help the practitioner maintain treatment fidelity. Each provider is accredited through an additional day of skills demonstration. Primary care providers or child psychiatric nurses could become trained in providing various levels of this intervention and use it in their practices. Training and certification are available through the Triple P International Website (http://www.triplep.net). Training can either be provided through open enrollment wherever Triple P is holding training or training for a group of individuals can be arranged through Triple P.

The Incredible Years

The Incredible Years (IY) Training Series is an approach to providing training for parents, teachers, and even young children with conduct problems, including oppositional defiant disorder (ODD) and conduct disorders. Many parents identify conduct problems in preschoolers that do not meet all of the criteria for a diagnosis of either conduct disorder or ODD. Children who display ODD symptoms in the preschool years have two to three times the risk of becoming violent and chronic juvenile delinquents (Loeber et al. 1993; Patterson et al. 1991). These disorders have been discussed in depth in other chapters in this book and the reader is referred to them for a more complete description of the problems.

What is It?

The IY Training Series was developed by Carolyn Webster-Stratton, a nurse and psychologist, to reduce conduct problems in young children. It was built on social learning theory. There are training programs for parents, teachers, and even for the children themselves to help learn skills to react in more socially expected ways (Webster-Stratton and Reid 2010).

For Whom Does it Work?

The underpinning of the program is that as conduct problems continue they become more entrenched and are harder to treat in older children and adolescents. By modifying family and child components of the behavior problems early, the children are able to develop healthier behaviors. Most recently, the program has been implemented and evaluated with 8–12-year-old children and has shown that children can improve their behaviors even at that age (Webster-Stratton and Reid 2010).

What Happens in Therapy?

There are three separate programs for parents, teachers, and children. The parent programs were begun in 1980 and have been recently updated to cover four age ranges: infancy, toddler, preschool, and school age up to age 12. The length of the programs varies by the age of the child, with the program for infancy lasting 8–9 weeks and increasing up to 18 weeks for the preschool and school-age parents. A series of videotaped vignettes are used by the therapist to promote discussion, problem solving, and collaborative learning (Webster-Stratton and Reid 2010, p. 196). Parents learn a series of nonviolent strategies for managing their child's behavior. Parents are taught self-control related to anger management and using positive self-talk to deal with more negative self-messages. Parents are also taught how to teach problem-solving skills to their child. The programs use a parent handbook to supplement the sessions with the therapist (Webster-Stratton and Reid 2010).

The teacher training program is a 6-day program that focuses on improving the teacher's classroom management skills, increasing the teacher's use of effective discipline strategies, helping the teacher learn to collaborate with parents, increasing the teacher's ability to foster social competence among the students, and strengthening the teacher's use of coaching for the academic, social emotional, and persistence skills of the child. Teachers are taught to monitor closely for aggressive behaviors and to intervene appropriately. There is also a book for teachers to use along with their training program (Webster-Stratton and Reid 2010).

Because children contribute to their problems of conduct, a program for children using video vignettes was developed. The training consists of 22 sessions that teach children problem-solving and social skills, with the children meeting in small groups of six. The goals of this program are to strengthen social skills and appropriate play skills, help children recognize and label their emotions, increase their empathy, boost academic skills, reduce aggression and defiance, promote compliance with others, and increase self-confidence and self-esteem.

What is the Evidence Base for this Therapy?

The IY parent programs have been well studied for effectiveness. There have been many randomized controlled trials that have shown that the program makes a significant difference in parenting behaviors, including reductions in harsh discipline compared to the waiting-list control group (Lavigne et al. 2008; Reid et al. 2007; Verardo and Cioccolanti 2017; Webster-Stratton 1998). Research has shown that the teacher and child training are also helpful, especially when combined with parent training (Webster-Stratton and Hammond 1997). The IY Child Training Program is also effective in improving children's friendship and social problem-solving skills (Baker-Henningham et al. 2012; Hutchings et al. 2012).

How Do You Become a Therapist?

To provide the IY Training Series, group leaders need to be certified through training for each component of the program either in Seattle or through onsite training within the community. Individuals seeking certification can come from a variety of disciplines, such as nursing, psychology, social work, counseling, education, or psychiatry, and should have received training in group work, behavior management, and child development. After the training, certification must be obtained by completing at least two groups and having these reviewed by a supervisor or mentor. Feedback from participants must also be obtained. These processes help ensure that the program is delivered as intended (Incredible Years 2013). When referring a family to the IY Program, it is important to know the therapist has been certified in the appropriate training needed by the family. Information about training and certification can be obtained by going to the IY website (http://www.incredibleyears.com).

Parent Management Training – Oregon Model

The Parent Management Training – Oregon Model (PMTO™) is designed to treat or prevent antisocial behavior problems in children and adolescents. It was developed at the Oregon Social Learning Center (OSLC) over more than four decades ago through research on children and their families.

What is it?

As the OSLC's name suggests, the theoretical underpinnings of PMTO are based on social learning, social interaction, and behavioral theories. Social learning and behavioral theories are used to examine how behavior patterns become entrenched, while social interaction theory is used to understand the connections among family members and friends that lead to various behavior patterns that contribute to mental health or problems (Forgatch and Patterson 2010).

For Whom Does it Work?

Antisocial behavior is seen as a continuum that begins with relatively minor problems such as temper tantrums, biting, hitting, or noncompliance in young children that parents often accidentally negatively reinforce. In some children, the behaviors stop, while in others covert antisocial behaviors such as lying, stealing, fire setting, animal cruelty, or truancy develop as the child gets older if parental discipline is harsh. These behaviors may also be reinforced through peer behaviors. Parents are seen as an important early factor in serious antisocial behavior in a child. Patterson demonstrated the cycle of coercive behavior that can develop in families in which one person starts a cycle of coercion and that is responded to with negative reciprocity; it ends when one of the players ends the cycle with a negative behavior, thus winning that round. In families with a clinical level of problem, the cycles occur quite frequently, as often as four times an hour and can begin as early as 2 years of age (Patterson 1982). Thus, children with disruptive behaviors and their families are the primary users for this program.

What Happens in Therapy?

PMTO can be delivered in single family or group sessions. Family sessions usually run 60 minutes long and 25–30 sessions are the norm; group treatment runs for 14 sessions for 90 minutes. In individual sessions, children may be involved to some degree depending upon the family's and therapist's preferences. Treatment sessions are generally highly structured and consist of a warm-up activity, then review of assigned homework, the introduction and practicing of new concepts or skills, and then end with a new assignment for homework. Midweek calls are used to promote the success of the treatment (Forgatch and Patterson 2010).

Forgatch and Patterson (2010) described the treatment as having five dimensions: scaffolding (breaking down complex behaviors into more manageable steps while using positive reinforcement to teach children more prosocial behavior), monitoring behavior by parents, limit setting, problem-solving skills, and positive involvement of parents with children. The goal of PMTO treatment is to empower parents to use positive parenting practices rather than coercive or harsh discipline. One important component is teaching parents emotional regulation though role play. Strategies used for face-to-face issues such as fighting are time-outs. For behaviors such as lying or stealing, extra chores are used or possibly fines with privilege removal being used for time-out refusal or refusing to do assigned chores.

What is the Evidence Base for this Therapy?

There is a significant body of research supporting PMTO; over 25 studies have demonstrated the efficacy of the model (e.g. DeGarmo and Forgatch 2007; Forgatch et al. 2009; Ogden et al. 2005). Many other studies are available that describe effectiveness implementations or variations on the program. A randomized experiment showed that PMTO had a positive impact on mothers' and stepfathers' parenting practices, and these improved practices in turn were associated with fewer child externalizing behavior problems (Bullard et al. 2010). An implementation of PMTO in Iceland demonstrated that the method could be transferred fully from the purveyor to the community without loss of fidelity to the method (Sigmarsdóttir and Vikar Guðmundsdóttir 2013).

How Do You Become a Therapist?

In 1997, the materials, policies, and procedures for training others to provide PMTO were developed to implement the training in Norway (Forgatch and Patterson 2010). Training was accomplished through six workshops each lasting 3 days and then coaching, which was done from videotaped therapy sessions. Trainees each had to see five families. Two of these families were seen for certification. Since then, Implementation Scientists International, Inc. has been developed at OSLC to provide training in PMTO. The group works with the community or group to ensure that the intervention will be delivered with fidelity to the core dimensions of the program. The goal is to have a sustainable implementation with a long-term commitment to PMTO and future generations of PMTO therapists trained by local PMTO coaches. Further information on resources for Parenting Inside Out, the new program grounded in the research from the PMTO program, can be obtained from the OSLC website (https://www.oslc.org/projects/parenting-inside/) or for training information from the Implementation Scientists International, Inc. website (http://www.isii.net/website.isii/NewFiles/training.html).

Parent–Child Interaction Therapy

Parent–child interaction therapy (PCIT) was developed by Shelia Eyberg et al. (2001) to treat young children with disruptive behaviors. It is designed to help parents learn to be warm and nurturing while establishing firm controls (Pincus et al. 2008).

What is it?

The goal of PCIT is to teach parents an authoritative style of parenting (Zisser and Eyberg 2010). The authoritative style of parenting has been demonstrated in various studies to be the most effective of the four identified styles of parenting: authoritative, authoritarian, neglectful, and permissive (e.g. Glasgow et al. 1997; Querido et al. 2002). In PCIT, parents are taught to interrupt the negative coercive relationship that develops between parent and child when the child has disruptive behavior problems. Parent and child are seen together in this model of parenting therapy (Zisser and Eyberg 2010).

For Whom Does it Work?

It is effective for families engaged in the coercive cycle of parenting that often evolves in families when children have a disruptive behavior problem. It is more effective for younger children since the disruptive patterns are less entrenched in younger children.

What Happens in Therapy?

In therapy, each session has a teaching component in which the therapist explains and models or role-plays certain skills, then the parent works with the child, practicing the skills while the therapist acts as coach (Zisser and Eyberg 2010). Skills include those that are child-directed interaction skills, such as letting the child lead an activity, showing approval, reflection of the child's behavior, and parent-directed interaction skills, which include making commands that are specific, age appropriate, and positively stated. Initially the child-directed interactional skills are the focus as parents learn to give positive attention and ignore negative behaviors unless they are aggressive or destructive. In this case the parent tells the child their special time has ended and to disengage until a later time when the child is calm.

During parent-directed interactions, parents learn when to give explanations, how not to argue with the child, and specific steps to follow after giving a command to the child. These steps begin with a warning and then time-out with the parent establishing the specific time-out length if the warning is insufficient. If the child leaves the time-out chair, a time-out room is used. Parents are coached about how to manage any escalation of behavior that may occur early in this process as the child learns to follow direction. Progress in therapy is measured by observation and coding of the parent's skill development and by completing the intensity scale of the Eyberg Child Behavior Inventory (Zisser and Eyberg 2010).

What is the Evidence Base for this Therapy?

The evidence base for PCIT is strong. It has been in use since the 1980s and various studies have tested PCIT with populations, in addition to families with children with disruptive behavior disorders, such as those with intellectual disability, autism spectrum disorders, or problems related to prematurity (Bagner and Eyberg 2007; Choate et al. 2005; Matos et al. 2009; Pincus et al. 2008; Solomon et al. 2008), in different ethnic, cultural, or racial groups (Leung et al. 2009; Matos et al. 2009; McCabe and Yeh 2009; Phillips et al. 2008), for families where child maltreatment has occurred (Chaffin et al. 2004; Timmer et al. 2006), or in different settings or modalities (Funderburk et al. 2008; Lyon and Budd 2010; Lyon et al. 2009; Niec et al. 2005; Timmer et al. 2010). In addition, several studies have tested the efficacy of the intervention (Bagner and Eyberg 2007; Eyberg et al. 2001; Funderburk et al. 1998). Fowles et al. (2018) studied clinic-based and in-home versions of the therapy and found both were effective in reducing child-behavior problems and increasing parenting skills. Intensive home-based treatment resulted in double the completion rate compared to clinic-based participants.

How Do You Become a Therapist?

Training to conduct PCIT requires that the therapist have a minimum of a masters degree in an appropriate discipline and complete 40 hours of face to face contact with a certified PCIT trainer that includes theoretical content, coding practice, case observations, and guided coaching with families to develop the needed skill set. This is followed in 2–6 months with advanced training with actual cases. Then the trainee must complete at least two PCIT cases and be in regular contact with their trainer for about a year. Trainees must have a skill review via some observation: live, videotape, or teleconferencing. Further information about training requirements is available on the PCIT website (www.pcit.org).

Summary

Many types of therapies are available for helping children and their families with mental health problems. Individual therapies and parent training programs have a broader evidence base than do family therapies. While other types of therapies exist, the therapies presented in this chapter have the most evidence and are among the best known for children. While most therapies need to be provided by mental healthcare providers, some parent training programs, such as Triple P level 3, could be provided by a pediatric nurse practitioner who obtained the training.

Critical Thinking Questions

1. What is the best way of determining the level of training required for an APRN to begin practicing in parent management techniques?
2. What role does psychopharmacology have in parent management training and other family modalities of care?
3. How can an APRN build in supervision and consultation into practice?

References

Abbass, A.A., Rabung, S., Leichsenring, F. et al. (2013). Psychodynamic psychotherapy for children and adolescents: a meta-analysis of short-term psychodynamic models. *Journal of the American Academy of Child and Adolescent Psychiatry* 52 (8): 863–875.

Ahmad, A., Larsson, B., and Sundelin-Wahlsten, V. (2007). EMDR treatment for children with PTSD: results of a randomized controlled trial. *Nordic Journal of Psychiatry* 61: 349–354. https://doi.org/10.1080/08039480701643464.

Arcelus, J., Whight, D., Langham, C. et al. (2009). A case series evaluation of the modified version of interpersonal psychotherapy (IPT) for the treatment of bulimic eating disorders: a pilot study. *European Eating Disorders Review* 17: 260–268. https://doi.org/10.1002/(ISSN)1099-096810.1002/erv.v17:410.1002/erv.932.

Bagner, D.M. and Eyberg, S.M. (2007). Parent-child interaction therapy for disruptive behavior in children with mental retardation: a randomized controlled trial. *Journal of Clinical Child and Adolescent Psychology* 36: 418–429.

Baker-Henningham, H., Scott, S., Jones, K., and Walker, S. (2012). Reducing child conduct problems and promoting social skills in a middle-income country: cluster randomised controlled trial. *The British Journal of Psychiatry* 201 (2): 101–108.

Berg, I.K. and Steiner, T. (2003). *Children's Solutions Work*. New York, NY: Norton.

Besa, D. (1994). Evaluating narrative family therapy using single-system research designs. *Research on Social Work Practice* 4: 309–325. https://doi.org/10.1177/104973159400400303.

Bodenmann, G., Cina, A., Ledermann, T., and Sanders, M.R. (2008). The efficacy of the triple P-positive parenting program in improving parenting and child behavior: a comparison with two other treatment conditions. *Behaviour Research and Therapy* 46: 411–427. https://doi.org/10.1016/j.brat.2008.01.001.

Bond, C., Woods, K., Humphrey, N. et al. (2013). Practitioner review: the effectiveness of solution focused brief therapy with children and families: a systematic and critical evaluation of the literature from 1990–2010. *Journal of Child Psychology and Psychiatry* 54 (7): 707–723. https://doi.org/10.1111/jcpp.12058.

Borduin, C.M. and Dopp, A.R. (2015). Economic impact of multisystemic therapy with juvenile sexual offenders. *Journal of Family* 29 (5): 687–696. Available at https://psycnet.apa.org/record/2015-25968-001.

Brunk, M., Henggeler, S.W., and Whelan, J.P. (1987). A comparison of multisystemic therapy and parent training in the brief treatment of child abuse and neglect. *Journal of Consulting and Clinical Psychology* 55: 311–318.

Bullard, L., Wachlarowicz, M., DeLeeuw, J. et al. (2010). Effects of the Oregon model of parent management training (PMTO) on marital adjustment in new stepfamilies: a randomized trial. *Journal of Family Psychology* 24 (4): 485–496. https://doi.org/10.1037/a0020267.

Carr, A. (2016). Family therapy for adolescents: a research-informed perspective. *Australian and New Zealand Journal of Family Therapy* 37: 467–479. https://doi.org/10.1002/anzf.1184.

Carryer, J.R. and Greenberg, L.S. (2010). Optimal levels of emotional arousal in experiential therapy of depression. *Journal of Consulting and Clinical Psychology* 78 (2): 190–199. https://doi.org/10.1037/a0018401.

Chaffin, M., Silovsky, J.F., Funderburk, B. et al. (2004). Parent-child interaction therapy with physically abusive parents: efficacy for reducing future abuse reports. *Journal of Consulting and Clinical Psychology* 72 (3): 500–510. https://doi.org/10.1037/0022-006x.72.3.500.

Chen, R., Gillespie, A., Zhao, Y. et al. (2018). The efficacy of eye movement desensitization and reprocessing in children and adults who have experienced complex childhood trauma: a systematic review. *Frontiers in Psychology* 9: 1–10. Available at http://journal.frontiersin.org/Journal/10.3389/fpsyg.2018.00534/abstract. https://doi.org/10.3389/fpsyg.2018.00534.

Choate, M.L., Pincus, D.B., Eyberg, S.M., and Barlow, D.H. (2005). Parent-child interaction therapy for treatment of separation anxiety disorder in young children: a pilot study. *Cognitive and Behavioral Practice* 12 (1): 126–135.

Connell, S., Sanders, M.R., and Markie-Dadds, C. (1997). Self-directed behavioral family intervention for parents of oppositional children in rural and remote areas. *Behavior Modification* 21: 379–408.

Conoley, C.W., Graham, J.M., Neu, T. et al. (2003). Solution-focused family therapy with three aggressive and oppositional-acting children: an N = 1 empirical study. *Family Process* 42 (3): 361–374.

Cyranowski, J.M., Frank, E., Shear, M.K. et al. (2005). Interpersonal psychotherapy for depression with panic spectrum symptoms: a pilot study. *Depression and Anxiety* 21: 140–142. https://doi.org/10.1002/da.20069.

DeGarmo, D.S. and Forgatch, M.S. (2007). Efficacy of parent training for stepfathers: from playful spectator and polite stranger to effective stepfathering. *Parenting-Science and Practice* 7 (4): 331–355.

Diamond, G.S., Reis, B.F., Diamond, G.M. et al. (2002). Attachment-based family therapy for depressed adolescents: a treatment development study. *Journal of the American Academy of Child and Adolescent Psychiatry* 41: 1190–1196. https://doi.org/10.1097/01.CHI.0000024836.94814.08.

Diamond, G., Russon, J., and Levy, S. (2016). Attachment-based family therapy: a review of the empirical support. *Family Process* 55: 595–610. https://doi.org/10.1111/famp.12241.

Diehle, J., Brent, C., Opmeer, B.C. et al. (2015). Trauma-focused cognitive behavioral therapy or eye movement desensitization and reprocessing: what works in children with posttraumatic stress symptoms? A randomized controlled trial. *European Child and Adolescent Psychiatry* 24: 227–236. https://doi.org/10.1007/s00787-014-0572-5.

Durlak, J.A. and McGlinchey, K.A. (1999). Child therapy outcome research. Current status and some future priorities. In: *Handbook of Psychotherapies with Children and Families* (eds. E. Russ and T.H. Ollendick), 525–539. Dordrecht: Kluwer Academic/Plenum Publishers.

Ellis, M.L., Weiss, B., Han, S., and Gallop, R. (2010). The influence of parental factors on therapist adherence in multi-systemic therapy. *Journal of Abnormal Child Psychology* 38 (6): 857–868. https://doi.org/10.1007/s10802-010-9407-0.

Ellison, J.A., Greenberg, L.S., Goldman, R.N., and Angus, L. (2009). Maintenance of gains following experiential therapies for depression. *Journal of Consulting and Clinical Psychology* 77 (1): 103–112. https://doi.org/10.1037/a0014653.

EMDR International Association. (2018). *Definition of EMDR*. Available at www.emdria.org.

Eyberg, S.M., Funderburk, B.W., Hembree-Kigin, T.L. et al. (2001). Parent-child interaction therapy with behavior problem children: one and two year maintenance of treatment effects in the family. *Child and Family Behavior Therapy* 23 (4): 1–20.

Fairburn, C.G., Jones, R., Peveler, R.C. et al. (1993). Psychotherapy and bulimia nervosa: longer-term effects of interpersonal psychotherapy, behavior therapy, and cognitive behavior therapy. *Archives of General Psychiatry* 50 (6): 419–428. https://doi.org/10.1001/archpsyc.1993.01820180009001.

Fonagy, P. (1999). Psychodynamic psychotherapy. In: *Handbook of Psychotherapies with Children and Families*, 1e (eds. S.W. Russ and T.H. Ollendick), 87–106. New York: Kluwer Academic/Plenum Publishers.

Fonagy, P., Cotrell, D., Phillips, J. et al. (2015). *What Works for Whom? A Critical Review of Treatments for Children and Adolescents*, 2e. New York: Guilford Press.

Forgatch, M.S. and Patterson, G.R. (2010). Parent management training–Oregon model. In: *Evidence-Based Psychotherapies for Children and Adolescents*, 2e (eds. J.R. Weisz and A.E. Kazdin), 159–178. New York: Guilford Press.

Forgatch, M.S., Patterson, G.R., DeGarmo, D.S., and Beldavs, Z.G. (2009). Testing the Oregon delinquency model with 9-year follow-up of the Oregon divorce study. *Development and Psychopathology* 21: 637–660. https://doi.org/10.1017/S0954579409000340.

Fowles, T.R., Masse, J.J., McGoron, L. et al. (2018). Home-based vs. clinic-based parent–child interaction therapy: comparative effectiveness in the context of dissemination and implementation. *Journal of Child and Family Studies* 27: 1115–1129. https://doi.org/10.1007/s10826-017-0958-3.

Funderburk, B.W., Eyberg, S.M., Newcomb, K. et al. (1998). Parent-child interaction therapy with behavior problem children: mainte-nance of treatment effects in the school setting. *Child and Family Behavior Therapy* 20 (2): 17–38.

Funderburk, B.W., Ware, L.M., Altshuler, E., and Chaffin, M. (2008). Use and feasibility of telemedicine technology in the dissemination of parent-child interaction therapy. *Child Maltreatment* 13 (4): 377–382. https://doi.org/10.1177/1077559508321483.

Glasgow, K.L., Dornbusch, S.M., Troyer, L. et al. (1997). Parenting styles, adolescents' attributions, and educational outcomes in nine heterogeneous high schools. *Child Development* 68 (3): 507–529.

de Graaf, I., Speetjens, P., Smit, F. et al. (2008a). Effectiveness of the triple P positive parenting program on behavioral problems in children a meta-analysis. *Behavior Modification* 32 (5): 714–735. https://doi.org/10.1177/0145445508317134.

de Graaf, I., Speetjens, P., Smit, F. et al. (2008b). Effectiveness of the triple P-positive parenting program on parenting: a meta-analysis. *Family Relations* 57: 553–566. https://doi.org/10.1111/j.1741-3729.2008.00522.x.

Gunlicks-Stoessel, M., Mufson, L., Jekal, A., and Turner, J.B. (2010). The impact of perceived interpersonal functioning on treatment for adolescent depression: IPT-A versus treatment as usual in school-based health clinics. *Journal of Consulting and Clinical Psychology* 78 (2): 260–267. https://doi.org/10.1037/a0018935.

Heatherington, L., Friedlander, M.L., Diamond, G.M. et al. (2015). 25 years of systemic therapies research: progress and promise. *Psychotherapy Research* 25 (3): 348–364. http://doi.org/10.1080/10503307.2014.983208.

Henggeler, S.W. and Schaeffer, C.M. (2016). Multisystemic therapy: clinical overview, outcomes, and implementation research. *Family Process* 55: 514–528. https://doi.org/10.1111/famp.12232.

Henggeler, S.W., Rodick, J.D., Borduin, C.A. et al. (1986). Multisystemic treatment of juvenile offenders: effects on adolescent behavior and family interactions. *Developmental Psychology* 22: 132–141.

Henggler, S.W., Schoenwald, S.K., Bourduin, C. et al. (2009). *Multisystemic Therapy for Antisocial Behavior in Children and Adolescents*, 2e. New York: Guilford Press.

Hoath, F.E. and Sanders, M.R. (2002). A feasibility study of enhanced group triple P – positive parenting program for parents of children with attention-deficit/hyperactivity disorder. *Behaviour Change* 19 (4): 191–206. Available at http://dx.doi.org.pallas2.tcl.sc.edu/10.1375/bech.19.4.191.

Hughes, D.J. (2007). *Attachment-Focused Family Therapy*. New York: W.W. Norton, Publishers.

Hutchings, J., Bywater, T., Gridley, N. et al. (2012). The incredible years therapeutic social and emotional skills programme: a pilot study. *School Psychology International* 33 (3): 285–293.

Incredible Years. (2013). *Certification in Incredible Years® Programs*. Available at http://www.incredibleyears.com/certification-gl/.

International Society for Interpersonal Psychotherapy. (2020). *Interpersonal psychotherapy: IPT manuals in English*. Available at https://interpersonalpsychotherapy.org/resources-links/books-manuals/.

Lavigne, J.V., LeBailly, S.A., Gouze, K.R. et al. (2008). Treating oppositional defiant disorder in primary care: a comparison of three models. *Journal of Pediatric Psychology* 33 (5): 449–461. https://doi.org/10.1093/jpepsy/jsm074.

Leung, C., Tsang, S., Heung, K., and Yiu, I. (2009). Effectiveness of parent-child interaction therapy (PCIT) among Chinese families. *Research on Social Work Practice* 19 (3): 304–313. https://doi.org/10.1177/1049731508321713.

Leve, L.D., Fisher, P.A., and Chamberlain, P. (2009). Multidimensional treatment foster care as a preventive intervention to promote resiliency among youth in the child welfare system. *Journal of Personality* 77 (6): 1869–1902. https://doi.org/10.1111/j.1467-6494.2009.00603.x.

Liddle, H.A. (2010). Multidimensional family therapy: a science-based treatment system. *Australian and New Zealand Journal of Family Therapy* 31 (2): 133–148.

Loeber, R., Wung, P., Keenan, K. et al. (1993). Developmental pathways in disruptive child-behavior. *Development and Psychopathology* 5 (1–2): 103–133.

Lyon, A.R. and Budd, K.S. (2010). A community mental health implementation of Parent-Child Interaction Therapy (PCIT). *Journal of Child and Family Studies* 19 (5): 654–668. https://doi.org/10.1007/s10826-010-9353-z.

Lyon, A.R., Gershenson, R.A., Farahmand, F.K. et al. (2009). Effectiveness of Teacher-Child Interaction Training (TCIT) in a preschool setting. *Behavior Modification* 33 (6): 855–884. https://doi.org/10.1177/0145445509344215.

Matos, M., Bauermeister, J.J., and Bernal, G. (2009). Parent-child interaction therapy for Puerto Rican preschool children with ADHD and behavior problems: a pilot efficacy study. *Family Process* 48 (2): 232–252. https://doi.org/10.1111/j.1545-5300.2009.01279.x.

McCabe, K. and Yeh, M. (2009). Parent-child interaction therapy for Mexican Americans: a randomized clinical trial. *Journal of Clinical Child and Adolescent Psychology* 38 (5): 753–759. https://doi.org/10.1080/15374410903103544.

McLuckie, A. (2006). Narrative family therapy for paediatric obsessive compulsive disorder. *Journal of Family Psychotherapy* 16 (4): 83–106.

Minuchin, S., Auerswald, E., King, C., and Rabinowitz, C. (1964). The study and treatment of families that produce multiple acting-out boys. *American Journal of Orthopsychiatry* 34: 125–134.

Morawska, A. and Sanders, M.R. (2008). Parenting gifted and talented children: what are the key child behaviour and parenting issues? *Australian and New Zealand Journal of Psychiatry* 42 (9): 819–827. https://doi.org/10.1080/00048670802277271.

Mufson, L. and Sills, R. (2006). Interpersonal psychotherapy for depressed adolescents (IPT-A): an overview. *Nordic Journal of Psychiatry* 60 (60): 431–437. https://doi.org/10.1080/08039480601022397.

Mychailyszyn, M.P. and Elson, D.M. (2018). Working through the blues: a meta-analysis on Interpersonal Psychotherapy for depressed adolescents (IPT-A). *Children and Youth Services Review* 87: 123–129. Available at https://psycnet.apa.org/record/2018-11316-016.

Nemirovski Edlund, J. and Carlberg, G. (2016). Psychodynamic psychotherapy with adolescents and young adults: outcome in routine practice. *Clinical Child Psychology and Psychiatry* 21 (1): 66–80. https://doi.org/10.1177/1359104514554311.

New World Encyclopedia. (2008). Harry Stack Sullivan [Electronic Version]. Available at http://www.newworldencyclopedia.org/entry/Harry_Stack_Sullivan?oldid=687861.

Niec, L.N., Hemme, J.M., Yopp, J.M., and Brestan, E.V. (2005). Parent-child interaction therapy: the rewards and challenges of a group format. *Cognitive and Behavioral Practice* 12 (1): 113–125.

Ogden, T., Forgatch, M.S., Askeland, E. et al. (2005). Implementation of parent management training at the national level: the case of Norway. *Journal of Social Work Practice* 19 (3): 317–329. https://doi.org/10.1080/02650530500291518.

Patterson, G.R. (1982). *Coercive Family Processes*. Eugene, OR: Castalia.

Patterson, G., Capaldi, D., and Bank, L. (1991). An early starter model for predicting delinquency. In: *The Development and Treatment of Childhood Aggression* (eds. D.J. Pepler and K.H. Rubun), 139–168. Hillsdale, NJ: Erlbaum.

Phillips, J., Morgan, S., Cawthorne, K., and Barnett, B. (2008). Pilot evaluation of parent-child interaction therapy delivered in an Australian community early childhood clinic setting. *Australian and New Zealand Journal of Psychiatry* 42 (8): 712–719.

Pincus, D.B., Santucci, L.C., Ehrenreich, J.T., and Eyberg, S.M. (2008). The implementation of modified parent-child interaction therapy for youth with separation anxiety disorder. *Cognitive and Behavioral Practice* 15 (2): 118–125. https://doi.org/10.1016/j.cbpra.2007.08.002.

Plant, K.M. and Sanders, M.R. (2007). Reducing problem behavior during care-giving in families of preschool-aged children with developmental disabilities. *Research in Developmental Disabilities* 28 (4): 362–385. https://doi.org/10.1016/j.ridd.2006.02.009.

Pos, A.E., Greenberg, L.S., and Warwar, S.H. (2009). Testing a model of change in the experiential treatment of depression. *Journal of Consulting and Clinical Psychology* 77 (6): 1055–1066. https://doi.org/10.1037/a0017059.

Prinz, R., Sanders, M., Shapiro, C. et al. (2009). Population-based prevention of child maltreatment: the U.S. Triple P System population trial. *Prevention Science* 10: 1–12. https://doi.org/10.1007/s11121-009-0123-3.

Querido, J.G., Warner, T.D., and Eyberg, S.M. (2002). Parenting styles and child behavior in African American families of preschool children. *Journal of Clinical Child and Adolescent Psychology* 31 (2): 272–277. https://doi.org/10.1207/S15374424JCCP3102_12.

Ralph, A. and Sanders, M.R. (2003). Preliminary evaluation of Group Ten Triple P program for parents of teenagers making the transition to high school. *Australian e-Journal for the Advancement of Mental Health* 2 (3): 1–10.

Ralph, A., Stallman, H., and Sanders, M.R. (2004). Teen Triple P: a universal approach to reducing risk factors for behavioural and emotional problems in adolescents at the transition to high school. *Australian Journal of Psychology* 56 (3 Supplement S): 217–217.

Randall, J., Henggeler, S.N., Cunningham, P.B. et al. (2001). Adapting multisystemic therapy to treat adolescent substance abuse more effectively. *Cognitive and Behavioral Practice* 8 (4): 359–366. https://doi.org/10.1016/j.addbeh.2003.08.045.

Reid, M.J., Webster-Stratton, C., and Hammond, M. (2007). Enhancing a classroom social competence and problem-solving curriculum by offering parent training to families of moderate- to high-risk elementary school children. *Journal of Clinical Child and Adolescent Psychology* 36 (4): 605–620.

Rieger, R., Van Buren, D.J., Bishop, M. et al. (2010). An eating disorder-specific model of interpersonal psychotherapy (IPT-ED): causal pathways and treatment implications. *Clinical Psychology Review* 30 (4): 400–410. https://doi.org/10.1016/j.cpr.2010.02.001.

Rigter, H., Pelc, I., Tossmann, P. et al. (2010). INCANT: a transnational randomized trial of multidimensional family therapy versus treatment as usual for adolescents with cannabis use disorder. *BMC Psychiatry* 10: 1–8. https://doi.org/10.1186/1471-244X-10-28.

Rodenburg, R., Benjamin, A., de Roos, C. et al. (2009). Efficacy of EMDR in children: a meta-analysis. *Clinical Psychology Review* 29 (7): 599–606. https://doi.org/10.1016/j.cpr.2009.06.008.

Rowland, M.D., Halliday-Boykins, C.A., Henggeler, S.W. et al. (2005). A randomized trial of multisystemic therapy with Hawaii's Felix Class Youths. *Journal of Emotional and Behavioral Disorders* 13 (1): 13–23. https://doi.org/10.1177/10634266050130010201.

Sanders, M.R. (2000). Community-based parenting and family support interventions and the preventing of drug abuse. *Addictive Behaviors* 25 (6): 929–942. https://doi.org/10.1016/S0306-4603(00)00128-3.

Sanders, M. (2003). Triple P – positive parenting program: a population approach to promoting competent parenting. *Australian e-Journal for the Advancement of Mental Health (AeJAMH)* 2 (3): 127–143. https://doi.org/10.5172/jamh.2.3.127.

Sanders, M.R. (2008). Triple P-positive parenting program as a public health approach to strengthening parenting. *Journal of Family Psychology* 22 (4): 506–517. https://doi.org/10.1037/0893-3200.22.3.506.

Sanders, M.R. and Lawton, J. (1993). Therapeutic process issues in the assessment of family problems: the guided participation model of information transfer. *Child and Family Behavior Therapy* 15 (2): 5–35.

Sanders, M.R. and Prinz, R.J. (2008). Ethical and professional issues in the implementation of population-level parenting interventions. *Clinical Psychology: Science and Practice* 15 (2): 130–136. doi: 10.1111/j.1468-2850.2008.00121.x http://org.pallas2.tcl.sc.edu.

Sanders, M.R. and Ralph, A. (2001). *Practitioner's Manual for Primary Care Teen Triple-P*. Milton, Queensland, Australia: Families International Publishing.

Sanders, M.R., Tully, L., Turner, K.M. et al. (2003). Training GPs in parent consultation skills. An evaluation of training for the Triple P-positive parenting program. *Australian Family Physician* 32 (9): 763–768.

Sanders, M.R., Kirby, J.N., Tellegen, C.L., and Day, J.J. (2014). The Triple P-positive parenting program: a systematic review and meta-analysis of a multi-level system of parenting support. *Clinical Psychology Review* 34: 337–357. https://doi.org/10.1016/j.cpr.2014.04.00.

Santisteban, D.A., Coatsworth, J.D., Perez-Vidal, A. et al. (1997). Brief structural/strategic family therapy with African American and Hispanic high-risk youth. *Journal of Community Psychology* 25 (5): 453–471. Available at doi-org.pallas2.tcl.sc.edu/10.1002/(SICI)1520-6629(199709)25:5<453::AID-JCOP6>3.0.CO;2-T.

Seidler, G.H. and Wagner, F.E. (2006). Comparing the efficacy of EMDR and trauma-focused cognitive-behavioral therapy in the treatment of PTSD: a meta-analytic study. *Psychological Medicine* 36 (11): 1515–1522. https://doi.org/10.1017/S0033291706007963.

Shalay, N. and Brownlee, K. (2007). Narrative family therapy with blended families. *Journal of Family Psychotherapy* 18 (2): 17–30.

Shapiro, F. (1989). Eye movement desensitization: a new treatment for post-traumatic stress disorder. *Journal of Behavior Therapy and Experimental Psychiatry* 20 (3): 211–217.

Sigmarsdóttir, M. and Vikar Guðmundsdóttir, E. (2013). Implementation of Parent Management Training – Oregon Model (PMTO™) in Iceland: building sustained fidelity. *Family Process* 52 (2): 216–227. https://doi.org/10.1111/j.1545-5300.2012.01421.x.

Solomon, M., Ono, M., Timmer, S., and Goodlin-Jones, B. (2008). The effectiveness of parent-child interaction therapy for families of children on the autism spectrum. *Journal of Autism and Developmental Disorders* 38 (9): 1767–1776. https://doi.org/10.1007/s10803-008-0567-5.

Tang, T.-C., Jou, S.-H., Ko, C.-H. et al. (2010). Randomized study of school-based intensive interpersonal psychotherapy for depressed adolescents with suicidal risk and parasuicide behaviors. *Psychiatry and Clinical Neurosciences* 2009 63: 463–470. https://doi.org/10.1111/j.1440-1819.2009.019.

Timmer, S.G., Urquiza, A.J., Herschell, A.D. et al. (2006). Parent-child interaction therapy: application of an empirically supported treatment to maltreated children in foster care. *Child Welfare* 85 (6): 919–939.

Timmer, S.G., Zebell, N.M., Culver, M.A., and Urquiza, A.J. (2010). Efficacy of adjunct in-home coaching to improve outcomes in parent-child interaction therapy. *Research on Social Work Practice* 20 (1): 36–45. Available at http://doi.org/10.1177/1049731509332842.

Verardo, A.R. and Cioccolanti, E. (2017). Traumatic experiences and EMDR in childhood and adolescence. A review of the scientific literature on efficacy studies. *Clinical Neuropsychiatry* 14 (5): 313–320.

Weaver, A., Greeno, C.G., Marcus, S.C. et al. (2013). Effects of structural family therapy on child and maternal mental health symptomatology. *Research on Social Work Practice* 23 (3): 294–303. https://doi.org/10.1177/1049731512470492.

Webster-Stratton, C. (1998). Preventing conduct problems in head start children: strengthening parenting competencies. *Journal of Consulting and Clinical Psychology* 66 (5): 715–730.

Webster-Stratton, C. and Hammond, M. (1997). Treating children with early-onset conduct problems: a comparison of child and parenting interventions. *Journal of Consulting and Clinical Psychology* 65 (1): 93–109.

Webster-Stratton, C. and Reid, M.J. (2010). The incredible years parent, teachers and children training series. In: *Evidenced-Based Psychotherapies for Children and Adolescents*, 2e (eds. J.R. Weisz and A.E. Kazdin), 194–210. New York: Guilford Press.

West, F., Sanders, M.R., Cleghorn, G., and Davies, P.S.W. (2010). Randomised clinical trial of a family-based lifestyle intervention for childhood obesity involving parents as the exclusive agents of change. *Behaviour Research and Therapy* 48: 1170–1179. https://doi.org/10.1016/j.brat.2010.08.008.

White, M. and Epston, D. (1990). *Narrative Means to Therapeutic Ends*. New York: Norton.

Whittingham, K., Sofronoff, K., Sheffield, J., and Sanders, M.R. (2009). Stepping stones triple P: an RCT of a parenting program with parents of a child diagnosed with an autism spectrum disorder. *Journal of Abnormal Child Psychology* 37 (4): 469–480. https://doi.org/10.1007/s10802-008-9285-x.

Young, J.F., Mufson, L., and Gallop, R. (2010). Preventing depression: a randomized trial of interpersonal psychotherapy-adolescent skills training. *Depression and Anxiety* 27 (5): 426–433. https://doi.org/10.1002/da.20664.

Zisser, A. and Eyberg, S.M. (2010). Parent-child interaction therapy and the treatment of disruptive behavior. In: *Evidence-Based Psychotherapies for Children and Adolescents*, 2e (eds. J.R. Weisz and A.E. Kazdin), 179–193. New York: The Guilford Press.

20

Cognitive Behavioral Interventions in Child and Adolescent Mental Health Treatment

Pamela Lusk[1] and Jessica Lee Kozlowski[2]

[1] Ohio State University College of Nursing, Columbus, OH, USA
[2] Brandman University, Irvine, CA, USA

Objectives

After reading this chapter, advanced practice registered nurses (APRNs) will be able to:

1. Identify cognitive behavioral models of care for children and adolescents, including individual, group and school-based interventions.
2. Describe the development of cognitive behavioral therapy (CBT) as an evidence-based psychotherapy modality.
3. Explain how the principles of CBT are adapted for children and adolescents.

4. Discuss how cognitive and behavioral approaches can be implemented in primary care/pediatric practices.
5. Describe how primary care and psychiatric-mental health APRNs can work collaboratively to provide a range of preventive, acute, and long-term behavioral healthcare to children, adolescents, and their families.

Introduction

The primary care setting has become the site for mental health treatment out of necessity (Erlich et al. 2019). Thirty-five percent of youth with a mental health disorder were only treated in the primary care setting (Platt et al. 2018). Numerous efficacious treatments exist for the mental health problems that children and adolescents experience, however the strongest evidence over the past decades has supported cognitive behavioral therapy (CBT) as the first-line intervention in primary care and specialty psychiatric/mental health settings for children and adolescents with the most common mental health concerns, anxiety and depression. If one goes to the current literature for child/adolescent treatments, there are many choices. With such a broad array of available therapies, it is critical that child/adolescent providers use techniques that are efficacious, appropriate to presentation, and consistent with the parents' and child's preference. The consumer also expects that the provider has the training to implement the intervention. In a recent meta-analysis of the past five decades of research about the effects of psychotherapy with youth, "Only youth-focused behavioral therapies, including CBT showed robust effects across youth, parent, and teacher reports" (Weisz et al. 2017, p. 81).

Child and Adolescent Behavioral Health: A Resource for Advanced Practice Psychiatric and Primary Care Practitioners in Nursing,
Second Edition. Edited by Edilma L. Yearwood, Geraldine S. Pearson, and Jamesetta A. Newland.
© 2021 John Wiley & Sons, Inc. Published 2021 by John Wiley & Sons, Inc.
Companion website: www.wiley.com/go/Yearwood

This chapter focuses on cognitive behavioral psychotherapeutic approaches that have proven effective for child/adolescent mental health disorders. The chapter begins with an explanation of cognitive and behavioral treatments and their basic mechanisms of action. Next, specific CBT techniques are explained and organized as interventions known to be efficacious for specific mental health issues of children.

In both primary care and specialty mental healthcare, nurses aim to help children and their parents change behaviors/thoughts that are causing distress or limiting functioning. Pediatric primary care is an ideal site for focused CBT or brief behavioral interventions because of the collaborative nature of the relationship between the pediatric nurse practitioner (PNP) and the patient, the use of defined goal setting and monitoring, the directive active approach, and the focus on the present rather than the past.

As a rule, intensity of services should match the intensity of the child's needs. Indicators requiring specialty mental healthcare have been discussed throughout this book. For most of this chapter, interventions are delineated for behaviors and childhood disorders without consideration of where they are used, be it primary or specialty mental healthcare. However, a set of brief interventions that will be delineated by "site" are techniques for common child behavior issues that are more likely to be addressed in primary care.

CBT as an Empirically Supported Therapy for Children and Adolescents

In the past few decades in child and adolescent mental health CBT has emerged as the evidence-based psychotherapy recommended as first-line treatment for young people with depression and anxiety. These recommendations are noted in the practice guidelines of medical disciplines such as the American Academy of Pediatrics, and the American Academy of Child and Adolescent Psychiatry (Cheung et al. 2018).

A recent meta-analysis by Weisz et al. (2017) looked at psychological treatment studies targeting (i) depression, (ii) anxiety, (iii) attention deficit/hyperactive disorders, and (iv) disruptive behaviors – the four most commons youth problems seen in primary care practice. The researchers also added a category of treatments concurrently targeting multiple problems. Clinically referred youths showed high rates of comorbidity.

Criteria for evidence-based interventions were set by the Weisz et al. study group:

> There is general agreement that for a particular psychotherapy to be considered evidence-based the intervention procedures must be well specified and documented

(e.g. in form of a treatment manual). Treatment benefit must have been shown in well controlled studies that r/o alternative explanations and beneficial effects must be robust across replication (ideally by investigators other than those who created the treatment program).

(Weisz et al. 2017, p. 81)

The team synthesized 50 years of findings reporting that across five decades, hundreds of randomized control trials (RCTs) have tested psychological therapies for youth with internalizing (anxiety depression) disorders and externalizing (disruptive behaviors and attention deficit hyperactivity disorder) disorders and problems. Meta-analysis of 447 studies, representing 30 431 youths, were included. They compared effects of therapy type and found CBT effects did not differ for Caucasian versus minority samples (Weisz et al. 2017).

Evidence-based psychotherapies in the meta-analysis were mostly administered by trained therapists using treatment manuals for regularly scheduled sessions. The most relevant and commonly prescribed evidence-based psychotherapies were behavior management therapy, behavior management training (BMT) for parents or caregivers, especially with younger children, and CBT for the school-age child or adolescent (Weisz et al. 2017).

A useful chart for clinicians and families is the *Evidence-based child and adolescent psychosocial interventions*, a printable chart that identifies the psychotherapies for each "problem area" (such as depression or anxious/avoidant behaviors), including evidence to support use. Published by Practice Wise via the American Academy of Pediatrics website, it is updated at regular intervals (http://www.aap.org/en-us/Documents/CRPsychosocialInterventions.pdf.). For clinical practice purposes the Level 1 BEST SUPPORT is most recommended. CBT has the strongest evidence to support its use in several of the "problem areas" including anxiety, depression, and trauma/stress exposure.

CBT and Psychotherapy Overview

CBT is a structured, short-term, present-oriented psychotherapy, directed toward solving current problems and modifying dysfunctional (unhelpful, inaccurate) thinking (Beck 2011). Thoughts (cognitions), whether positive or negative, affect feelings and affect behaviors/actions (see Box 20.1). Aaron T. Beck is considered the father/developer of the cognitive theory of depression and subsequent school of psychotherapy (Beck 1964). He shared his account of how CBT developed in his paper *A 60-Year Evolution of Cognitive Theory and Therapy* (Beck 2019). A psychoanalyst, he treated patients for several years and noticed that there were two different levels of thoughts expressed in treatment: the deeper free-associated thoughts and a level of automatic self-assessment thoughts that often represented a negative bias in the way the patient interpreted their experiences. An example of the automatic, here and now thinking level would be "I feel like I am boring you." When the analytic patients expressed these automatic negative thoughts, Beck challenged their accuracy and explored alternative explanations with the patient, more accurate accounts of what they experienced and believed. As he challenged negative, or unhelpful, not entirely accurate cognitions (thoughts), patients' depressive symptoms lessened. Beck's academic research during his training years in psychoanalysis initially involved dreams and anger directed inward as a component of depressive illness; he soon, along with a co-trainee, changed his research focus to the cognitive approach to psychotherapy for depression (Rush et al. 1977).

Beck developed the cognitive theory of depression and the first cognitive therapy study was published in 1970, comparing results of cognitive therapy verses treatment with a tricyclic antidepressant. Patients who received cognitive therapy generally required only up to 14 sessions before they had clinical symptom improvement in their depression and were ready to terminate therapy. This contrasted to the much longer psychoanalytic approach.

Cognitive therapy involves cognitive restructuring, problem solving, and behavioral activation. This model of psychotherapy is now referred to as CBT, with behavioral activation (increasing time spent in activities that are enjoyable to the individual) a major component of the psychotherapy. The basic principles of CBT can be adapted to the school-age child/adolescents' level of cognitive, emotional, and social understanding (see Box 20.2).

In cognitive therapy a basic premise is that one's thoughts *automatically* move to a negative assumption about presenting stimuli or events. These automatic negative thoughts are like reflexes, they are well practiced thoughts, developed from childhood experiences, interactions with others, and even interaction with media "ideals." In cognitive work, the individual challenges the "evidence" that supports these negative assumptions and formulates refuting evidence that would modify them. The client is guided to understand how the thoughts and emotions affect subsequent behavior (Beck 2011). Cognitive therapy improves anxious and depressive symptoms via challenging negative thoughts, then practicing alternative, more positive thinking (Beck 2011). Cognitive interventions with children have proven to be effective in reducing symptoms, particularly for anxiety and depressive disorders (Higa-McMillan et al. 2016; Weersing et al. 2017). In the

literature CBT is generally used for children 6 years old and older because a basic level of reading allows the child to use a CBT treatment manual or workbook and/or take-home worksheets for applications of skills learned in the CBT sessions. With the early elementary age child, flashcards can be used prior to starting CBT sessions to learn to differentiate what is a thought, what is a feeling, and what is a behavior (Melnyk 2003). Not all youth have reached cognitive maturity or have the vocabulary to distinguish rational or irrational thoughts. However, they can understand the labels of "helpful or not helpful" or "sad or coping" thoughts. They may not understand probabilities that a statement is true, but they can understand that the chances are "small or big" that a statement is entirely true, and they enjoy gathering "clues" as evidence about the possibility of an outcome (Kendall 2018, p. 4). Children enjoy assuming the role of detective in evaluating their own thoughts, behaviors, and actions, and the sense of mastery when they determine the best explanation for their situation. In CBT with youth the child's natural curiosity is leveraged. The process of CBT can be explained as the child/teen assumes the role of scientist by identifying clues, evaluating the evidence, and solving problems.

Treatment manuals are meant to be colorful, concise, and engaging. Manuals are designed to be age appropriate, developmentally sound, and interesting. CBT sessions are interactive and there are lots of opportunities for back and forth discussion as the child/teen and therapist seek to solve the dilemmas of other children/teens through short case vignettes provided in the manual using the Thinking, Feeling, Behavior model of CBT (Melnyk 2003).

Child/adolescent CBT treatment manuals with evidence to support effectiveness with children and adolescents include Coping with Depression – Adolescent (CWD-A) developed by Lewhinsoln and Clarke, COPING Cat developed by Phillip Kendall for children with anxiety (now available in a Brief 8 session COPING Cat manual (Crawley et al. 2013), and the COPE (Creating Opportunities for Personal Empowerment) manuals for children, teens, and young adults, developed by B.M. Melnyk (dually certified as a PNP and psychiatric/mental health nurse practitioner) as a seven-session cognitive behavioral skill building program (Melnyk 2003).

The COPING CAT program is considered the gold standard CBT treatment for anxiety in children and is the intervention used most in studies around the effectiveness of CBT with children. Coping Cat is one of the most researched CBT approaches for children (Kendall 1994) along with Brief Coping Cat 8 Session Manual (Kendall et al. 2013). Kendall's innovative program targets several areas of anxious behavior with slightly different interventions. Anxious feelings, thoughts, and attributions are addressed with cognitive techniques (to increase awareness and challenge unrealistic cognitions); anxious self-talk is replaced with coping self-talk and a coping plan. When the child succeeds at these new coping strategies, they are provided with a self-reward (behavioral component).

This CBT model operates on the theory that children exhibiting early signs of anxiety have developed a pattern of responding with fear to particular stimuli. This in turn affects how they pay attention to the event and the attributions they form about the cause of the event (Kendall 2006). Repeated experiences of apprehension establish a cognitive template (or filter), which then influences how the child allocates attention (i.e. they have difficulty switching attention away from anxiety-provoking events) (Muris et al. 2006; Pine 2007; Roy et al. 2008). In the CBT framework, the child learns first to recognize anxious feelings, then to examine the accompanying attributions, and to finally practice alternative ways of thinking about the situation (Kendall and Suveg 2006). Via this reappraisal of anxious thoughts, the child is building a new, more adaptive cognitive template around particular events (see Box 20.3).

Melnyk's COPE program was developed on an inpatient adolescent psychiatric unit and since has been offered in schools as an after-school group, as part of the high school health education course RCT (Melnyk et al. 2013, 2015), in individual sessions for college students (Hart et al. 2019), to children in pediatric practices (Kozlowski et al. 2015), to adolescents followed in outpatient mental health practices (Lusk and Melnyk 2011a,b), and to adolescents with depression and/or anxiety in primary care practice (Erlich et al. 2019). There have been 18 published studies supporting COPE's positive outcomes with school-age children, adolescents, and college-age young adults. COPE 7 Session manuals are available for children, teens, and young adults (in Spanish and English), and there is a 15-session COPE Healthy Lifestyles manual which includes the seven CBT sessions and additional sessions focused on health information such as exercise, diet, and healthy lifestyles (www.cope2thrive.com). Kozlowski et al. (2015) describe the implementation of COPE for children presenting with significant anxiety in a rural primary care practice where many of the children were of low socioeconomic status. Erlich et al. (2019) conducted projects with adolescents in two urban clinics in a county with predominantly high socioeconomic status. Both Kozlowski's study and Erlich's studies indicated implementation of CBT interventions in primary care by PNPs was both feasible and well accepted by the parents and children/adolescents. The cost-effectiveness of CBT in primary care has been supported by a recent study in *Pediatrics* (Dickerson et al. 2018). In the COPE program the CBT core concept is: How you think affects how you feel and how you behave. This is illustrated via the Thinking, Feeling, Behaving triangle (Figure 20.1).

McCarty and Weisz (2007) in their meta-analysis of RCTs of treatment of adolescent depression identified 12 components of CBT that were included in effective CBT interventions for depression in adolescents:

- achieving measurable goals/competency
- adolescent psycho-education
- self-monitoring
- relationship skills/social interaction
- communication training
- cognitive restructuring
- problem solving
- behavior activation
- relaxation
- emotional regulation
- parent psycho education
- improving the parent–child relationship.

The treatment manuals discussed previously include the essential therapeutic components of CBT outlined

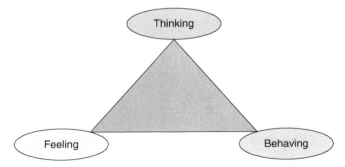

Figure 20.1 The COPE Thinking, Feeling, Behaving triangle (Melnyk 2003). *Source:* Melnyk, B. (2003). Creating Opportunities for Personal Empowerment (COPE). Retrieved from www.cope2thrive.com. Used with permission of the author.

Box 20.1   Case Example: Addressing Cognitive Distortions with a Student Using the CBT Model

Kayla and John are in English class right before lunch time. Their teacher is returning their graded book reports. Kayla looks at her returned paper and sees a lot of writing in red pen and a grade of B–. Her automatic **Thought** is I am so stupid, I can't even write a good report on a small easy book.

She **Feels**: discouraged, disappointed.
She **Behaves**: She asks to go to the school nurse because her stomach hurts and she does not want to talk to any of her classmates at lunch.

John looks at his returned paper and sees a lot of writing in red pen and a grade of B–. His automatic **Thought** is: "Oh well I got a B–, next time I will read a more interesting book, and besides I got an A on my math test this morning.

John **Feels**: OK.
John **Behaves**: John folds his paper, puts it up, and asks what his friend is having for lunch.
For both students: the trigger, or activating event, was getting their graded (B–) book report back from the teacher.
Each student's automatic **thought** affected their **feeling** and how they **behaved**.
  Employing the Beck manner of questioning (Socratic questioning) to check out or evaluate Kayla's automatic (not so helpful or completely accurate thought), what might Kayla be asked? **Thought**: Does getting a B– mean that a student is stupid? Stupid all the time? What evidence/proof can you show that you are always stupid? Is that completely true of you? That you are 100% stupid? Or just true sometimes? Have you ever written a good book report? In your many years of school?
  The clinician might then facilitate Kayla using her cognitive skills to explore solutions by asking, "What would you tell your classmate who made a B– on a book report and feels bad? What could you tell yourself? What self-statement is truer about you and your abilities to do your schoolwork? If Kayla can change/modify her initial automatic negative thought to something more accurate/truer, then she has reframed her thought – cognitive restructuring, an essential component of cognitive behavior therapy, she will **Feel** better and her subsequent **Behavior** will likely be less isolative.

Box 20.2   Beck's Principles of CBT

There are 10 principles of CBT as outlined by Beck (2011) and applied to children and adolescents in a primary care or psychiatric advanced practice registered nurse (APRN) practice:

1. Cognitive therapy is based on an ever-evolving formulation of the patient and his/her problems in cognitive terms. The initial evaluation of the child or adolescent provides a comprehensive understanding of that young person, with their strengths and interests, skills and supports, and their perceived struggles, the reason they are seeking help. Particular attention is paid to the statements the child/teen makes about themselves. The APRN formulates a diagnosis and in collaboration with the child/teen and parents develops an initial plan of treatment. As the young person and APRN work together, the plan will be updated.
2. Cognitive therapy requires a sound therapeutic alliance. Forming a therapeutic relationship with the child/teen and their parent is likely the most important factor in attaining positive outcomes from CBT. The teen and

parent need to believe that the APRN has their best interests in mind, that the goal of their work together is that the teen achieves his/her full potential.
3. Cognitive therapy emphasizes collaboration and active participation. In CBT the teen/child will be as active as the therapist in the process. Initially, the APRN will be more active in the sessions as the basic CBT model is explained, with examples. As the sessions progress the young person will provide examples from their own experiences at home, school or in social situations and will identify and evaluate their own "not so accurate thoughts" and change those thoughts to more accurate statements.
4. Cognitive therapy is goal oriented and problem focused. CBT is an active, roll up your sleeves therapy and the APRN and child/teen/parent work directly on goals and problems.
5. Cognitive therapy initially emphasizes the present. The homework assignments are stated, "In the past few days, how did you. . ." or "This past week what have you . . ." Even

though CBT is a present oriented, here and now therapy, as the therapeutic relationship develops into a safe, trusting relationship, the young person will share more of the experiences, thoughts, and feelings that have been important in their life, present and past.

6. Cognitive therapy is educative, aims to teach the patient to be his/her therapist, and emphasizes relapse prevention. In CBT the APRN is teaching the basics of how one's thinking affects feelings and behaviors. The therapist is teaching the skills that the teen can practice, master, and have at their disposal throughout their life. Coping strategies that resonate with that individual are identified and the teen outlines their own plan for catching negative or unhelpful thoughts as soon as they occur, and evaluates and restructures or dismiss the problem cognitions. Learning the process of cognitive restructuring provides relapse prevention. With children this can be presented as a fun game of Catch it, Check it, Change it (referring to the unhelpful thought).

7. Cognitive therapy aims to be time limited (4–14 sessions). In most CBT programs for youth there are seven or eight sessions.

8. Cognitive therapy sessions are structured. The structure of the sessions is clear and this structure reduces anxiety in children and adolescents – they know the focus will be on the workbook content, with a mood-monitoring check-in first (so that any acute or urgent need can be addressed as priority). Then comes a review of the homework or workbook assignments completed since the last session. The lesson, a review of the main points of the lesson, is followed with feedback (if taking medications this is a good time to review response to medications). Lastly, the new homework, a clinical skills building assignment in the manual session, is reviewed, to be done before the next session.

9. Cognitive therapy teaches patients to identify, evaluate, and respond to their dysfunctional thoughts and beliefs. Positive reappraisal, positive self-talk, and homework are all important pieces of CBT. The skills are taught and practiced and become that teen's strategies for coping with life's challenges now and in the future.

10. Cognitive therapy uses a variety of techniques to change thinking, mood, and behavior. There are many strategies taught and practiced, from relaxation techniques (deep breathing, mindfulness, visual imagery) to strategies for behavioral activation (identifying activities that are enjoyable) and change, like setting goals and moving one step at a time, adding more physical activity into the week, and cognitive techniques such as thought stopping, self-talk, and Socratic questioning of thoughts/beliefs. The teen/child selects and practices the techniques that work best for them.

All of the above CBT principles are included in the CBT manuals for children and adolescents. Even though each child/teen goes through the same content as written in the manual with the psychiatric or primary care APRN, there is individualization of the sessions, as the child/teen applies what they are learning to their own situations and experiences. For one child the regulation of strong emotions content is most applicable and interesting. For a child with social anxiety the content on coping with stress and anxiety is most applicable and challenging. This concept of the therapist/ APRN reading all of the content of the manual as printed with each child/teen (using the stories provided in the manual) and also providing the pause/ time for the child/teen to share their own examples allows for "fidelity to the treatment manual with flexibility to meet the treatment needs of the individual child/teen" (Beidas and Kendall 2014, p. 233). For the therapist, having a CBT treatment manual means the clinical notes from the previous session can be reviewed quickly, the manual homework for that session will be reviewed, and the next session is ready to begin. It has been demonstrated (Erlich et al. 2019; Kozlowski et al. 2015; Lusk and Melnyk 2011a) that the sessions in the COPE manual can be completed in 20–30-minute brief visits.

by McCarty and Weisz (2007) in developmentally appropriate language and examples. Like CBT for any age, there are homework or skills-building activities to be completed between sessions so that the young person can practice the coping strategies/skills they are learning in CBT sessions with situations that they experience at home, at school, and in social situations.

CBT Group Format

Another successful variation of CBT with children and adolescents is using a group format (Zhou et al. 2018). Based on several studies, "group format CBT for anxiety has proven efficacious for Hispanic/Latino and African American youth" (Huey and Polo 2017, p. 368).

Box 20.3 The Structure for CBT Sessions (Beck 2011)

Every CBT session, no matter the target problem or age of the participant, follows the same structure.

- Check in – mood monitoring and bridge to the previous visit.
- Setting the agenda.
- Homework (clinical skills, action plans) review.
- Work on problems.
- Summary.
- Feedback (both ways, to and from therapist and youth).
- Preview and assign homework.

This seven-step structure is built into CBT manuals. With children and teens, the agenda is already built into the sessions and assures that the CBT program addresses all essential topics/components of CBT. In most studies with youth, the CBT sessions have been 50–60 minutes. With young clients, 30-minute visits in busy primary care offices work well, both because it fits with their attention span and works well with usual scheduling of clinic patients (Erlich et al. 2019; Kozlowski et al. 2015; Lusk and Melnyk 2011a). Parents/caregivers can play important roles when their child/adolescent is being seen for a course of CBT. Parents are involved in any treatment decisions for children and teens because the young person is not yet fully independent. Roles parents can assume in cognitive behavioral interventions include:

1. Consultants – providing history of symptoms and impairment.
2. Collaborators – bringing their child to treatment, assisting with the implementation of therapy such as encouraging homework completion.
3. Co-client in the treatment program (Kendall 2018). Generally, the parents' active involvement is seen as a plus for the process. With younger anxious children, the parent being in the sessions with them is a necessity as they cannot tolerate the separation from the parent. Older teens may have their parent actively involved in the treatment plan but not attend every session. Despite variations in the roles for parents in treatment, great benefits can be gained from the parent's increased understanding of child and adolescent development, mental health, and coping strategies (Lusk and Melnyk 2011a).

Source: Based on Dorsey, S., McLaughlin, K., Kerns, S., Harrison, J., Lambert, H. & Briggs, E. (2017). Evidence base update for psychosocial treatments for children and adolescents exposed to traumatic events. Journal of Clinical Child & Adolescent Psychology, 46(3), 303–330; Weisz, J.R., Kuppens, S., Ng, M.Y., Eckshtain, D., Ugueto, A.M., Vaughn-Coaxum, R., . . .Fordwood, S.R. (2017). What five decades of research tells us about the effects of youth psychological therapy: A multilevel meta-analysis and implications for science and practice. American Psychologist, 72(2), 79–117.

Two of the previously described CBT manualized programs, the CWD-A program by Lewinsohn and Clarke (Lewinsohn et al. 1991) and the COPE (2003) CBT manualized program by Melnyk, were initially developed as group interventions.

Group sessions are typically 90 minutes long and have two therapists. Lewinsohn and Clarke and colleagues (Clarke et al. 1999) were the first to treat adolescents with depression in groups with their CWD-A course. This course proved superior to waiting-list conditions in their early studies (Bunge et al. 2017).

The COPE program was developed by Melnyk for groups on an inpatient adolescent psychiatric unit but has been offered in schools as an after-school group, as part of the high school health education course (see RCT studies) (Hoying et al. 2016; Melnyk et al. 2013, 2015). An RCT of the "No Worries!" program, a group treatment for children with generalized anxiety disorder, has also supported the efficacy of CBT delivered in groups (Holmes et al. 2015).

Advantages for delivering a CBT intervention in group format for adolescents include similarity to a classroom versus an individual psychotherapy setting; a classroom is likely more familiar to the teen/child and less stigmatizing (Creed et al. 2011; Kazdin and Weisz 2017). Teens value the feedback they receive from peers because "it comes from a peer who understands my life" (Melnyk et al. 2014, p. 4). Data suggest that "among evidence-based treatments, cognitive behavioral approaches show the strongest record of success with ethnic minority youth" (Weisz et al. 2017, p. 364). Ethnic minority youth respond best to treatments that are highly structured, time limited, pragmatic, and goal oriented (Huey and Polo 2008; Weisz et al. 2017).

The therapeutic advantages for delivering a manualized CBT program in group format lie in the power of groups as a therapeutic intervention that is cost-effective, focused, and time limited while fostering relationship building. Manuals are much like school workbooks, so are familiar to students (Creed et al. 2011; Kazdin and Weisz 2017).

Other identified advantages of group-delivered CBT include acceptability, minimized dropout rates, and increased likelihood that the teens will stay in the course and receive the full dose of treatment (Kazdin and Weisz 2017). The sessions are structured using the same structure as other CBT programs. Schools account for approximately 79% of group activities in adolescence, followed by community agencies (including after-school programs), hospitals, and clinics.

CBT in Schools

Schools are an ideal environment in which to implement intervention programs as they have unparalleled contact with youth and represent a place where the majority can be reached (Creed et al. 2011; Melnyk et al. 2013, 2015; Kazdin and Weisz 2017). Other advantages for providing a group intervention in school settings include the opportunity to teach school staff CBT principles and to learn about that community of students' stresses, cultural values, and typical home situations (Creed et al. 2011; Hoying et al. 2016). Currently, in many schools there are school-based health centers where the nursing clinical staff take an active role in providing CBT interventions (Hart et al. 2019).

Cognitive Behavioral Approaches for Children/ Adolescents with Anxiety

The interventions discussed in this section utilize a CBT approach, meaning their active elements address both thought and behavior. These interventions often combine principles of behavior therapy (e.g. reinforcement) and cognitive techniques (e.g. self-talk) to build what Kendall (2006) calls a "coping template." While many of these techniques cross over several childhood diagnoses, for clarity specific techniques will be considered under the diagnostic groups anxiety, depression, and stress-related/trauma disorders.

Anxiety in children is one of the most pervasive of childhood disorders, with a community prevalence of 15–20% in adolescents (Bennett et al. 2016; Higa-McMillan et al. 2016). Types of anxiety are as varied as underlying neurobiology. National treatment guidelines and meta-analyses of anxiety treatment research endorse CBTs as efficacious for a variety of anxiety disorders (Higa-McMillan et al. 2016). CBT programs for specific child/adolescent anxiety disorders often have additional components that address aspects of the syndrome. For example, social anxiety disorders might require a focus on social skills development.

With children who have obsessive–compulsive disorder (OCD), exposure-based CBT is the treatment of choice. The OCD intervention programs incorporate gradual exposures to the child's individual fears into the CBT framework (Franklin et al. 2017). In the cognitive model of OCD, compulsions are a response to anxious sensations (usually arising from an obsessive fear). With this theory, performing the compulsive behavior actually helps children reduce their anxious feelings and the subsequent relief reinforces their compulsions. A pattern then develops when such children encounter an anxiolytic stimulus, their response involves a focus on the related compulsions. This focus on compulsions prevents normal habituation and realistic appraisal of the fearful stimuli (Flament et al. 2007). The treatments for OCD involve CBT techniques but rely heavily on exposure and response prevention (ERP). With this intervention the youth is slowly exposed to stimuli that would normally illicit obsessive fears, but they are taught to resist engaging in compulsive behaviors (Kendall 2018).

Recent studies that inform our practice are replicated in the earlier Pediatric Obsessive–Compulsive Treatment Study (POTS) (Barrett et al. 2004; Franklin et al. 2003, 2017). These controlled studies involve several treatment conditions (family participation and medication) as well as manualized CBT with an ERP emphasis (Barrett et al. 2008). The POTS protocol also includes psychoeducation, cognitive training, mapping OCD behaviors, and ERP (Franklin et al. 2003).

The cognitive component of this intervention incorporates positive self-talk, cognitive restructuring, and cultivating a dampened response to rising anxious thoughts. The cognitive work is seen to increase a youth's sense of personal efficacy, predictability, and controllability (March et al. 2001). Nurses intervening with children struggling with OCD behaviors should familiarize themselves with these programs, particularly the accompanying explanatory models, which provide a theory for why the intervention components lead to outcomes. Such understanding is important for increasing treatment fidelity and educating the family/child on the theory of the therapy.

Neuroscience of Treatment

Many steps remain before the full potential of neuroscience to effect clinical gains in pediatrics can be realized. Clinical neuroscience has made great strides but most of the work has been done with adults, as ethical concerns are always present around research with children. Studies suggest that adults with social anxiety disorder who have a greater pretreatment response to negative facial emotions (in the dorsal and ventral occipitotemporal cortex, higher order visual processing regions of the brain) respond better to CBT (Davis 2004; Doehrmann et al. 2013). When information about structural and functional connectivity provided by diffusion tensor imaging (DTI) and functional magnetic resonance imaging (fMRI) was included in models of treatment prediction along with clinical severity data, "response to CBT treatment was predicted with 81% accuracy" (Engel et al. 2009; Whitfield-Gabrieli et al. 2016, p. 680).

As applied to children and teens, neuroscience approaches to predict treatment response have included the pretreatment viewing of fearful vs. happy faces. Greater amygdala activity was associated with higher clinician reports of symptom improvement in children receiving CBT or medication for anxiety disorders. This was also found with adolescent girls, who had greater amygdala response to threatening vs. neutral facial expressions associated with faster post-traumatic stress disorder (PTSD) symptom reduction (Cisler et al. 2015). There is much neuroscience work being done now related to children who have experienced maltreatment and adverse childhood experiences (ACEs). For instance, it has been discovered that children/teens who have experienced maltreatment require more practice and time as cognitive reappraisal requires greater cognitive resources in the prefrontal cortex (as well as increased amygdal response to negative cues). Maltreated youth also can have blunted responses to reward in the ventral striatum; behavioral activation might be a useful treatment emphasis for them. In clinical practice, these measures in the future might allow for increased ability to predict treatment response and more effective triage of cases to more effective treatments (e.g. combined CBT and medication), leading to more rapid improvement for children and adolescents and less time spent on therapies that are unlikely to be effective (Weisz 2017).

Cognitive Behavioral Approaches for Children/Adolescents with Depression

Depression in youth carries a high prevalence (11–14% of population aged 13–18) and significantly impacts important areas of functioning (Child Mind Institute 2018). CBT has proved effective for the treatment and prevention of child and adolescent depression (Cheung et al. 2018; Weisz et al. 2006).

The Guidelines for Adolescent Depression in Primary Care (GLAD-PC) Practice Guidelines for adolescent depression have recently been updated (Cheung et al. 2018; Zukerbrot et al. 2018). A recent review of 42 RCTs detailing psychosocial interventions found that the evidence for this type of child treatment is noticeably weaker than for other adolescent treatments such as CBT. No treatments achieved "well established status for school age children," but CBT for clinically depressed children is "probably efficacious." For depressed adolescents, both

CBT and interpersonal psychotherapy are "well established interventions with evidence of efficacy in multiple trials by independent investigative teams" (Weersing et al. 2017, p. 11).

Many CBT programs have success and are detailed in the literature (Erlich et al. 2019; Kozlowski et al. 2015; Lusk and Melnyk 2011a). The CBT manualized programs that have been used in most of the studies with children and adolescents include Coping with Adolescent Depression (CWDA) (Lewinsohn et al. 1991) and COPE (Clarke et al. 2006; Melnyk 2003). In studies conducted largely with adults, using neuroimaging techniques, researchers have investigated why CBT improves depression. Basically, reappraisal of negative thoughts and mood is thought to change patterns of brain activity (Dichter et al. 2008). It is believed that as individuals exercise a different (more positive) thinking pattern, growth occurs at the synaptic level and, via this neural plasticity, the circuitry supporting this new thinking pattern is strengthened (Tryon 2009).

When discussing treatment options with the youth and his/her parent, it is important to highlight the relationship between stress sensitivity, negative ruminations, and lack of involvement in pleasurable activity. Teens may resist mental health treatment because of their mistrust in mental health professionals' ability to understand their situation and the stigma that mental illness carries. When nurses encounter teens in distress, they should directly address the depression but keep in mind these developmental concerns and consider other delivery approaches, such as bibliotherapy.

Cognitive bibliotherapy has been studied for mild depression or as a preventive program for those at risk for depression. In this form of bibliotherapy a book, written for the general public that provides an overview of CBT, is given to the adolescent. The usual book assigned/given to youth in studies is *Feeling Good* by David Burns. This form of bibliotherapy may be efficacious (Rhode et al. 2015). Some early studies were promising when compared to group CBT in schools but a large RCT did not show such positive results (Moldovan et al. 2013). The long-term follow-up improvements were not as great as for students who received group CBT in schools. The advantages of bibliotherapy (over face-to-face interventions) include ease of use, low cost, low staffing demands, and greater privacy.

There are also increasing numbers of online CBT programs for children and adolescents; beginning studies indicate acceptability and success with online CBT programs (Stasiak et al. 2016).

Other Child/Adolescent Disorders Addressed with CBT Interventions

Other disorders that can be addressed with CBT include trauma and stress-related disorders (Dorsey et al. 2017; Silverman et al. 2008). Individual CBT with parent involvement and eye movement desensitization and reprocessing (EMDR) were determined to be effective among therapies studied for those children with trauma history (including expressive therapies and group CBT). When working with children and adolescents who have experienced ACEs and/or have a trauma history, it is helpful to listen for the four cognition themes of (i) powerlessness (I am helpless, powerless, not in control), (ii) safety, vulnerability (I cannot protect myself, I am not safe, I can't trust anyone), (iii) responsibility (I should have done something, I should have known better, I am inadequate/weak), and (iv) defectiveness (I am not good enough, I am not loveable, I am damaged, I am insignificant, I am worthless) (Shapiro 2018, p. 56). These four negative cognitions can be modified with a CBT approach, facilitating improvement for the child/adolescent who experiences ACEs/trauma.

Trauma-focused CBT (TF-CBT) is a well-established therapy for children and adolescents exposed to traumatic events (Cohen et al. 2017; DeArellano et al. 2014; Silverman et al. 2008). TF-CBT addresses problems specifically associated with significantly traumatic events that children experience or witness. The core target of TF-CBT is to help children overcome traumatic avoidance, shame, sadness, fear, and other traumatic specific emotional and behavioral difficulties. "TF-CBT has been highly successful in treating diverse samples of traumatized children with 80–90% remission rates of PTSD in some studies" (Cohen et al. 2017 p. 268).

Dorsey et al. (2017) described in a meta-analysis that individual CBT with parent involvement, individual CBT, and group CBT was deemed a well-established treatment for children and adolescents exposed to traumatic events. Group CBT with parental involvement and EMDR was deemed probably efficacious. TF-CBT was considered a CBT in this evidence review.

Well-established treatments for children/adolescents exposed to traumatic events include six common elements: (i) psychoeducation about trauma, prevalence, impact, and the intervention, (ii) training in emotion regulation strategies, e.g. relaxation, identification of emotion, cognitive coping, (iii) imaginal exposure, (iv) *in vivo* exposure, (v) cognitive processing, and (vi) problem solving.

The model TF-CBT program developed by Cohen and Mannarino in 1996 (TF-CBT Web) follows an intentional progression of interventions where the child is first educated on abuse and normal sexuality, and then taught relaxation techniques, coping strategies, and affect regulation, skills that gradually prepare the child to think about and discuss their trauma. It is only toward the end of the therapy, now equipped with tools to handle the accompanying emotional arousal, that the child creates a trauma narrative. TF-CBT has an accessible training protocol that is available both in live sessions and online, and can be accessed at tfcbt.org (Cohen et al. 2017).

Behavioral/Mental Health Interventions in Primary Care

The primary care setting has become the site for mental health treatment out of necessity (Erlich et al. 2019). Primary care is the preferred setting for parents and children/adolescents to receive all their healthcare (including mental healthcare) because they generally have a long-standing, trusting relationship with their primary care providers. Organizational barriers to treatment of mental and behavioral health disorders in the primary care setting include inability of the patient to pay, insurance limitations, a healthcare system which separates physical and mental/behavioral health, and functioning inadequacies within the primary care environment (Campo et al. 2018).

The pediatric practice is unique in the fact that, unlike other healthcare settings, the child is almost always seen at minimum annually across their lifespan (Campo et al. 2018; Tyler et al. 2017). The primary care provider has a distinct opportunity for education and guidance to that caregiver in a preventative, family-oriented environment (Tyler et al. 2017).

PNPs and family nurse practitioners (FNPs) frequently encounter young children and adolescents in practice who have symptoms of anxiety, depression, or disruptive behaviors. Many times, these mental health symptoms/concerns are precipitated by changes, losses, or stressful experiences. PNPs and FNPs incorporate education, anticipatory guidance, and behavioral interventions as important components of their usual practice with families.

Some cognitive behavioral techniques are already used in primary care (Box 20.4) with families. First there is an emphasis on modeling cognitive reframing for parents because it lies at the heart of many clinician–parent interactions. It has long been recognized that parents' perceptions of their children and how they see their children compared to other children may be a powerful determinant in a child's future wellbeing.

Box 20.4

Cognitive behavioral techniques useful in primary care for children with problems of mild anxiety and/or depression

Reframing (identifying and emphasizing the child/ teen's interests, strengths, efforts, contributions, vs. focus on negative behaviors)
Relaxation plans (being in the moment, guided imagery, going to one's pleasant peaceful place)
Deep breathing
Progressive relaxation
Fear hierarchies constructing anxiety ladders
Planning gradual exposures
Recognition of cognitive distortions (3Cs, Catch it, Check it, Change it [catch the automatic negative thought, check out if it is absolutely true, or maybe not totally accurate, maybe there are more realistic statements, then modify or change that automatic negative thought, to a more true thought])
ABC Model (antecedent, or activating trigger event, beliefs or thoughts about the trigger, and consequences, feelings and behaviors that follow the thought, cognition)
Use of positive self-talk
Identifying and eliminating negative self-talk
Review and encouragement of healthy sleep/ physical activity/diet
Behavior activation, ensuring pleasurable activities

(Dorsey et al. 2017, p. 324; Kazdin and Weisz 2017)

Applying Concepts

Cognitive Reframing with an Infant

Mrs. T, the mother of 2-week-old Lacy, arrived at the clinic looking exhausted. Lacy was her second baby and weighed 9 lbs at birth. She was a vigorous newborn who had already regained birth weight and more. Her mother reported that Lacy screamed loudly when she was hungry, "ate all night" and she was concerned that she was going to be "fat." Upon further questioning, the practitioner learned that her first child, Sarah, arrived 6 weeks early, weighed less than 5 lbs, slept for long periods of time, and had to be awakened to eat. At the age of 3 Sarah was a well-developed, but thin child with an easy going, quiet disposition. Further questioning revealed that Mrs. T's husband had been able to stay at home for 3 weeks when Sarah was born but now had a new job which required him to leave the house first thing in the

morning and return late at night. Mrs. T was worried about disturbing his sleep at night and wondered why Lacy was eating so often. Mrs. T also mentioned that she "used to be fat" and hoped "that Lacy wouldn't take after my side of the family."

Cognitive Reframing with a Toddler

Mr. and Mrs. J brought 4-year-old Joey in for a preschool check-up. Joey's past medical history, physical examination, and developmental assessment were normal. As part of her history taking, the practitioner asked the parents what Joey was particularly good at. Mrs. J immediately responded that he was good at putting together puzzles and working with his small cars. When they were asked, "What are the most difficult things for Joey?" she responded that Joey was shy and always found it difficult to enter new situations. The practitioner asked Mr. J if he had any ideas why this was. Mr. J responded, "No, that is just how he has always been – kind of a "scaredy cat really. He doesn't get that from me!" Further history revealed that Joey had always been slow to warm up to new people and places. Joey had one good friend with whom he played happily and at whose house he was comfortable. Mrs. J sheepishly admitted she had always wondered if he had developed this way because she had been hospitalized when he was a baby and she had had to leave him with an aunt for 2 weeks. Even though the aunt was warm and mothering, Mrs. J had always worried that Joey had been affected by her absence.

The first case example of a mother and her infant reveals many potential avenues for primary mental health interventions, including use of a screening tool for possible postpartum depression and a review of social supports available to this mother. It also illustrates how a parent may form faulty perceptions of a newborn, colored by lack of information, situational stressors, or previous experiences. As in this vignette, skilled clinicians will realize a primary consideration is the parent's need for support and, in this instance, sleep. They will also recognize the opportunity to educate new parents about the wide range of normal newborn behaviors, variations in temperament, and expected differences in term and premature infant's sleep and growth. As illustrated in this case example, the goal in primary care is to assist new parents in developing a more favorable appraisal of their infant's behaviors by helping the parent "reframe" any sense that there is something wrong with a baby displaying normal developmental behaviors.

The second case in this vignette illustrates how reframing of behaviors might occur with the parent of a toddler. In this vignette, a major task for the pediatric provider was helping the parents understand the role of temperament as an innate style of reacting; a style that is neither good nor bad. Further discussions and readings about temperament allowed Mr. and Mrs. J to form a "new cognitive appraisal" of who their son was, and what it meant (and didn't mean) to have a child with a slow-to-warm-up temperament. In this case example, over time a "goodness of fit" was achieved, and his parents were able to provide support when their child encountered normal challenges with change. Mrs. J no longer worried that she had caused him to develop this way with her absence. Mr. J was able to begin to see the strengths that often accompany a slow-to-warm-up temperament.

Evidence-Based Brief Mental Health Interventions for Primary Care (Interventions for brief visits 20–30 minutes) School-age Children and Adolescents

The American Academy of Pediatrics endorses the Screening Brief Intervention and Referral to Treatment (SBIRT) model which can be used to address mental health issues as well as substance use disorders. The APRN routinely screens for depression (Patient Health Questionnaire-9 [PhQ 9] or Center for Epidemiological Studies Depression Scale for Children [CES-DC]) and anxiety (Generalized Anxiety Disorder 7-item [GAD 7] and Screen for Child Anxiety Related Disorders [SCARED]) in primary care and now there is an emphasis on the importance of screening for ACEs. See Chapter 8 for more information about ACEs.

After the provider has screened a young child and has identified anxiety or depression as a concern, the next step is to decide if this child in need of a brief intervention in the primary care environment. Due to the lack of mental health providers, most children and adolescents will find benefit in a brief intervention even while waiting for their initial appointment with a mental health specialist. Some interventions available for primary care include bibliotherapy, Brief Coping Cat (Kendall et al. 2013) and COPE, which is useful in brief sessions for the PNP in the primary care setting (Erlich et al. 2019; Kozlowski et al. 2015; Lusk and Melnyk 2013a).

Primary care APRNs can incorporate CBT-based brief interventions into brief visits.

Brief interventions by definition:

- are time limited
- are patient driven
- are achievable
- have clear follow-up criteria that can be built upon (Lusk and Melnyk 2013a, p. 338).

Brief interventions are designed for use in busy clinical settings, are generally 5–15 minutes in duration, but no more than 30 minutes long. They are commonly used by clinicians to talk to patients about health and behavioral health issues and include behavioral approaches, supportive counseling, parent-focused interventions, motivational interviewing, and cognitive behavioral skills building (CBSB) techniques (Lusk and Melnyk 2013a, p. 338).

Handouts/worksheets based on CBT for children and adolescents have been developed to be used as stand-alone brief interventions. CBSB worksheets (see the end of this chapter) can be kept in the examination room for easy access and introduce the following topics:

- the Thinking, Feeling, Behaving triangle
- positive things about me
- healthy coping for stress and worry
- coping with strong feelings: anger, hurt, fear, sadness (Lusk and Melnyk 2013a).

The primary care APRN can review the content of the worksheets with the child and parent and then show where the child can fill in the blanks on the worksheet with their personal information/plans and bring the sheet back to their next visit (which may be scheduled the next week, or sooner if indicated).

Evidence-based brief interventions can be provided by any primary care provider in the context of brief office visits or several standard office visits. Brief interventions can be a stand-alone treatment for those children/teens at risk, as well as a vehicle for engaging those in need of more intensive specialty mental healthcare (Lusk and Melnyk 2013b). With brief interventions the clinician can begin to actively address the family's mental health concerns within the time constraints of busy primary care/pediatric practice, even if referral has been made to psychiatric specialty services.

CBT principles can also be employed with parents. As has been stated, the one evidence-based change in practice that can provide the greatest impact for children/teens and families is modifying the parents' perceptions of their child by modeling an emphasis on that child/teen's strengths and abilities (cognitive reframing). Often parents are prone to emphasize "problems" and equal emphasis on strengths/interests is a helpful reframing approach. Parents value the expertise and opinion of their primary care practitioner and the "cognitive reframing" to emphasize the child's positive traits can modify the parent's perception of their child and make a huge difference in the quality of the parent–child relationship.

Psychiatric APRNs Adding CBT to Medication Management Visits

In current practice, many parents and teens/children tell the provider they do not want to take an antidepressant as they feel the brain is still developing. When families learn of the warning that there can be increased suicidal ideation with the initiation of antidepressants in children, adolescents, and young adults (Food and Drug Administration Black Box Warning) they are more hesitant to start a trial of an antidepressant. Initiating CBT as a first-line intervention with children/teens/families that decline antidepressants can be a collaborative evidence-based treatment plan (Dickerson et al. 2018).

There have been significant studies that demonstrate adding CBT to medication (selective serotonin reuptake inhibitor, SSRI) leads to better results than those obtained with medication alone, as evidenced by the Treatment of Adolescent Depression Study (TADS) (Brent et al. 2008; March et al. 2006). The three core CBT strategies, no matter which specific program is added to the SSRI medication, are (i) cognitive restructuring, (ii) behavioral activation, and (iii) problem solving (Kendall 2018).

Clinicians can "jump start" symptom improvement in patients with CBT techniques while waiting for SSRIs produce their intended therapeutic effects (Sudak and Taormina 2018).

COPE studies have demonstrated that CBT can be delivered in 30-minute visits and the medication management interaction can be completed in these same 30 minutes (Erlich et al. 2019; Kozlowski et al. 2015; Lusk and Melnyk 2011a). Outcomes measured after APRN-delivered COPE indicated anxiety symptoms improved in children and adolescents and depressive symptoms showed significant improvement after the seven COPE CBT sessions for adolescents. Students in psychiatric and primary care APRN programs have been successfully trained in using the COPE CBT program (Lusk et al. 2018).

Most recently Dickerson et al. (2018) noted the cost-effectiveness of CBT for adolescents with depression who declined antidepressants or discontinued the medication in primary care settings and concluded "Brief primary care CBT among youth declining antidepressants is cost-effective by widely accepted standards in depression treatment. CBT becomes dominant over treatment as usual over time as revealed by a statistically significant cost offset at the end of the 2 year follow up" (Dickerson et al. 2018, p. 42). CBT sessions have been consistently reimbursed by various insurance plans and Medicaid plans of various states (Erlich et al. 2019; Kozlowski et al. 2015).

Conclusion

The future direction of behavioral and cognitive-behavioral science will likely proceed in several ways. With the increasing interest in affective neuroscience, one would anticipate that more effective regulation strategies will be included in CBT packages of treatment. CBT indirectly helps a child control affects, particularly negative and anxious emotions. But the future may hold a more concentrated effort to help children achieve regulation (Izard et al. 2008). There is a need for CBT and behavioral interventions for several serious emotional disorders of childhood, such as pediatric bipolar disorder, where only a few promising programs currently exist (Pavuluri et al. 2004). There is also a need for more evidence-based treatments for ethnic minority youth (Huey and Polo 2017).

The future will likely hold the development of additional computer-based CBT programs specifically for youth. There is also emerging evidence that computer-delivered CBT is superior to waiting-list control in helping children manage anxiety symptoms (March et al. 2009). It is likely that virtual reality applications/simulations will become available to augment CBT programs. Computer applications (apps) currently provide an opportunity for mobile CBT. Such programs hold promise for child psychiatry where the maldistribution of child mental health providers makes access to treatment a serious issue.

The near future also holds models of collaborative care where mental health specialists are co-located within the pediatric primary care home and the psychiatric APRN is an ideal mental health provider to assume that role. The concept of a healthcare home that integrates mental and physical healthcare for children is grounded in the belief that the pediatric provider recognizes the unique developmental trajectory that provides children and families with both opportunity and risk as their child grows. The pediatric primary healthcare home is also family focused and recognizes that the seeds of behavioral problems and their likely solutions lie within the family. The richness of the special relationship that can develop over time between families and a trusted APRN in pediatrics, family, or mental health sets the stage for successful behavioral intervention.

To maximize this opportunity, the pediatric APRN must take an active role in helping parents "reframe" their understanding of the well-child visit from one with a focus on physical wellbeing to one that addresses the comprehensive set of factors that are likely to threaten a child's health (Melnyk and Jensen 2013). These include a contextual approach including the child's genetic endowment, temperament, environment, early child care, the school setting, family structure, and community safety (Hagan et al. 2008).

Many APRNs are seeking additional training in addressing common child and adolescent mental health condition cognitive and behavioral skills to enhance their effectiveness in supporting families (Albury et al. 2013; Hawkins-Walsh et al. 2011). There is an online Child and Adolescent Mental Health Fellowship, KySS, at the Ohio State University College of Nursing Continuing Education Department which grants continuing education units. Many PNPs and FNPs seek an additional certification as a psychiatric mental health specialist, as granted by the Pediatric Nurse Certification Board. Some practitioners may decide to seek advanced training in specific therapy schools while other clinicians will choose a more limited role incorporating CBT and behavioral approaches within the well-child and office visits. While many pediatric providers may not identify themselves as "therapists," the American Academy of Pediatrics has endorsed active support and monitoring for symptomatic children and adolescents, and it has been noted that that active support includes psychoeducation, cognitive behavioral based brief interventions, and teaching and reviewing coping strategies such as mindfulness and regulation of strong emotions (Erlich et al. 2019; Zukerbrot et al. 2018). The question of how extensive a role the primary care provider should play in the management of common behavioral problems will continue to be addressed as changes occur within the financing and reimbursement of healthcare, the availability of mental health specialists, the changes in primary care training, and research demonstrating the effectiveness of mental health screening by pediatric primary care providers (Clarke et al. 2016).

Advanced practice nurses, and primary and psychiatric APRNs are well positioned in healthcare systems to develop and promote models of care that emphasize the importance of evidence-based therapeutic interactions. These interactions are a vital component of all visits, including screenings and brief interventions even at scheduled growth and medication check visits. APRNs serve as leaders in finding models of care that manage costs and professional time for best patient outcomes. Primary care and psychiatric-mental health APRNs can work collaboratively to provide a range of preventive, acute, and long-term behavioral healthcare to children, adolescents, and their families to improve their health, wellbeing, and functioning.

Resources

American Academy of Pediatrics Evidence-Based Child and Adolescent Psychosocial Interventions (2019). https://www.aap.org/en-us/Documents/CRPsychosocialInterventions.pdf.

KySS Online Child and Adolescent Mental Health Fellowship, The Ohio State University College of Nursing. https://nursing.osu.edu/offices-and-initiatives/office-continuing-education/kyss-mental-health-fellowship-child-and.

Pediatric Nurse Certification Board – Pediatric Mental Health Specialist eligibility and examination. https://www.pncb.org/pmhs.

CBT programs for children and adolescents can be completed online: Kendall's online program based on Coping Cat is CAMP COPE-A-LOT. https://www.copingcatparents.com/Camp_Cope_A_Lot.

The Online version of Adolescent Coping with Depression Course (CWD-A) can be accessed free at http://www.cebc4cw.org/program/adolescent-coping-with-depression-course-cwd-a/detailed. The online COPE CBT program can be accessed at www.cope2thrive.com.

Critical Thinking Questions

1. Even though CBT is not an evidence-based first-line treatment for children with oppositional defiant disorder, what components of CBT do you think would be very helpful for these children?

2. Please list the pros and cons of parents attending each CBT session with their adolescent. What is your recommendation based on what you know about CBT expected outcomes with adolescents with anxiety and depression?

3. The nurse–patient therapeutic relationship is central to CBT. What would you do in the following situations?
   - The child/adolescent comes to the session without having done his/her homework (skills building activity) for the past two sessions.
   - You have started the CBT session and the child or teen, says, "Wait, can I tell you about my problem with my friend at school?"

Brief Evidence-based CBT Worksheets for Practice

Worksheets available from Melnyk, B.M. and Jensen, P. (2013). *Practical Guide to Child and Adolescent Mental Health Screening, Early Intervention, and Health Promotion*, 2e. Cherry Hill, NJ: National Association of Pediatric Nurse Practitioners (NAPNAP).

References

Albury, R., Coehlo, D., Donohoe, M.L. et al. (2013). NAPNAP position statement on the integration of mental health care in pediatric primary care settings. *Journal of Pediatric Health Care* 27: 15A–16A.

Barrett, P.M., Healy-Farrell, L., and March, J.S. (2004). Cognitive-behavioral family treatment of child obsessive-compulsive disorder: a controlled trial. *Journal of the American Academy of Child and Adolescent Psychiatry* 32: 430–441.

Barrett, P.M., Farrell, L., Pina, A.A. et al. (2008). Evidence-based psychosocial treatments for child and adolescent obsessive-compulsive disorder. *Journal of Clinical Child and Adolescent Psychology* 37: 131–155.

Beck, A.T. (1964). Thinking and depression, II: theory and therapy. *Archives of General Psychiatry* 10: 561–571.

Beck, J. (2011). *Cognitive Behavioral Therapy: Basics and Beyond*. New York, NY: Guilford Press.

Beck, A.T. (2019). A 60-year evolution of cognitive theory and therapy. *Perspectives on Psychological Science* 14 (1): 16–20. https://doi.org/10.1177/1745691618804187.

Beidas, R.S. and Kendall, P.C. (eds.) (2014). *Dissemination and Implementation of Evidence-Based Practices in Child and Adolescent Mental Health*. New York, NY: Oxford University Press.

Bennett, K., Manassis, K., Duda, S. et al. (2016). Treating child and adolescent anxiety effectively: overview of systematic reviews. *Clinical Psychology Review* 50: 80–94. https://doi.org/10.1016/j.cpr.2016.09.006.

Brent, D., Emslie, G., Clarke, G. et al. (2008). Switching to another SSRI or to venlafaxine with or without cognitive behavioral therapy for adolescents with SSRI resistant depression: the TORDIA randomized controlled trial. *Journal of the American Medical Association* 299: 901–913.

Bunge, E., Mandil, J., Consoli, A., and Gomar, M. (2017). *CBT Strategies for Anxious and Depressed Children and Adolescents: A Clinicians' Toolkit*. New York, NY: Guilford Press.

Campo, J.V., Geist, R., and Kolko, D.J. (2018). Integration of pediatric behavioral health services in primary care: improving access and outcomes with collaborative care. *The Canadian Journal of Psychiatry* 63 (7): 432–438. https://doi.org/10.1177/0706743717751668.

Cheung, A., Zuckerbrot, R., Jensen, P. et al. (2018). Guidelines for adolescent depression in primary care (GLAD-PC): part II. Treatment and ongoing management. *Pediatrics* 141 (3): e20174082.

Child Mind Institute. (2018). *Understanding Anxiety in Children and Teens*. Available at https://childmind.org/our-impact/childrens-mental-health-report/2018report.

Cisler, J., Sigel, B., Kramer, T. et al. (2015). Amygdala response predicts trajectory of symptom reduction during trauma focused cognitive-behavioral therapy among adolescent girls with PTSD. *Journal of Psychiatric Research* 71: 33–40.

Clarke, G., Rohdi, P., Lewinsohn, P. et al. (1999). Cognitive-behavioral treatment of adolescent depression: efficacy of acute group treatment and booster sessions. *Journal of the American Academy of Child and Adolescent Psychiatry* 38 (3): 272–279.

Clarke, G., DeBar, L., Pearson, J. et al. (2016). Cognitive behavioral therapy in primary care for youth declining antidepressants: a randomized trial. *Pediatrics* 137 (5): e20151851.

Cohen, J., Mannarino, A., and Deblinger, E. (2017). Trauma-focused cognitive behavioral therapy for traumatized children. In: *Evidence-Based Psychotherapies for Children and Adolescents* (eds. J. Weisz and A. Kazdin), 253–271. New York, NY: Guilford Press.

Crawley, S.A., Kendall, P.C., Benjamin, C.L. et al. (2013). Brief cognitive-behavioral therapy for anxious youth: feasibility and initial outcomes. *Cognitive and Behavioral Practice* 20 (2) https://doi.org/10.1016/j.cbpra.2012.07.003.

Creed, T., Reisweber, J., and Beck, A. (2011). *Cognitive Therapy for Adolescents in School Settings*. New York, NY: Guilford Press.

Davis, M. (2004). Functional neuroanatomy of anxiety and fear. In: *Neurobiology of Mental Illness*, 2e (eds. D. Charney and E.J. Nestler), 584–604. New York, NY: Oxford Press.

DeArellano, M., Lyman, D., Jobe-Shields, L. et al. (2014). Trauma-focused cognitive-behavioral therapy for children and adolescents: assessing the evidence. *Psychiatric Services* 65 (5): 591–602. https://doi.org/10.1176/appi.ps.201300255.

Dichter, G.S., Felder, J.N., and Smoski, M. (2008). Treatment resistant depression: effects of psychotherapy on brain function. *Psychiatric Times* 25: 10.

Dickerson, J., Lynch, F., Leo, M. et al. (2018). Cost-effectiveness of cognitive behavioral therapy for depressed youth declining antidepressants. *Pediatrics* 141 (2): e20171969. https://doi.org/10.1542/peds.2017-1969.

Doehrmann, O., Ghosh, S., Polli, G. et al. (2013). Predicting treatment response in social anxiety disorder from functional magnetic resonance imaging. *JAMA Psychiatry* 70: 87–97.

Dorsey, S., McLaughlin, K., Kerns, S. et al. (2017). Evidence base update for psychosocial treatments for children and adolescents exposed to traumatic events. *Journal of Clinical Child & Adolescent Psychology* 46 (3): 303–330. https://doi.org/10.1080/15374416.2016.1220309.

Engel, K., Bandelow, B., and Gruber, O. (2009). Neuroimaging in anxiety disorders. *Journal of Neural Transmission* 116: 703–716.

Erlich, K.J., Li, J., Dillon, E. et al. (2019). Outcomes of a brief cognitive skills-based intervention (COPE) for adolescents in the primary care setting. *Journal of Pediatric Health Care* 00: 1–10. https://doi.org/10.1016/j.pedhc.2018.12.001.

Flament, M.F., Geller, D., Irak, M., and Blier, P. (2007). Specificities of treatment in pediatric obsessive-compulsive disorder. *CNS Spectrums* 12: 43–58.

Franklin, M., Foa, E., and March, J.S. (2003). The pediatric obsessive-compulsive disorder treatment study: rationale, design and methods. *Journal of Child and Adolescent Psychopharmacology* 13: s39–s51.

Franklin, M., Morris, S., Freeman, J., and March, J. (2017). Treating pediatric obsessive-compulsive disorder in children using exposure-based cognitive behavioral therapy. In: *Evidence-Based Psychotherapies for Children and Adolescents* (eds. J. Weisz and A. Kazdin), 35–48. New York, NY: Guilford Press.

Hagan, J.F., Shaw, J.S., and Duncan, P.M. (eds.) (2008). *Bright Futures: Guidelines for Health Supervision of Infants, Children, and Adolescents*, 3e. Elk Grove Village, IL: American Academy of Pediatrics.

Hart, B.G., Lusk, P., Hovermale, R., and Melnyk, B.M. (2019). Decreasing depression and anxiety in college youth using the creating opportunities for personal empowerment program COPE. *Journal of the American Psychiatric Nurses Association* 25 (2) https://doi.org/10.1177/1078390318779205.

Hawkins-Walsh, E., Crowley, A., Melnyk, B. et al. (2011). Improving healthcare quality through an AFPNP national nursing education collaborative to strengthen PNP curriculum in mental/behavioral health and evidence-based practice. *Journal of Professional Nursing* 27: 10–18.

Higa-McMillan, C., Francis, S., Rith-Najarian, L., and Chorpita, B. (2016). Evidence base update: 50 years of research on treatment for child and adolescent anxiety. *Journal of Clinical Child and Adolescent Psychology* 45 (2): 91–113. https://doi.org/10.1080/15374416.2015.1046177.

Holmes, M., Donovan, C., and Farrell, L. (2015). A disorder-specific, cognitively focused group treatment for childhood generalized anxiety disorder: development and case illustration for the No Worries! Program. *Journal of Cognitive Psychotherapy: An International Quarterly* 29 (4): 275–301.

Hoying, J., Melnyk, B., and Arcoleo, K. (2016). Effects of the COPE cognitive behavioral skills building TEEN program on the healthy lifestyle behaviors and mental health of Appalachian early adolescents. *Journal of Pediatric Health Care* 30 (1): 65–72. https://doi.org/10.1016/j.pedhc.2015.01.005.

Huey, S.J. and Polo, A.J. (2008). Evidence-based therapies for ethnic minority youth. *Journal of Clinical Child and Adolescent Psychology* 27: 262–301.

Huey, S. and Polo, A. (2017). Evidence-based psychotherapies with ethnic minority children and adolescents. In: *Evidence-Based*

Psychotherapies for Children and Adolescents (eds. J. Weisz and A. Kazdin), 361–378. New York, NY: Guilford Press.

Izard, C.E., King, K.A., Trentacosta, C.J. et al. (2008). Accelerating the development of emotion competence in Head Start children: effects on adaptive and maladaptive behavior. *Development and Psychopathology* 20: 369–397.

Kazdin, A.E. and Weisz, J.R. (2017). Introduction: context, background, and goals. In: *Evidence-based Psychotherapies for Children and Adolescents* (eds. J.R. Weisz and A.E. Kazdin), 3–12. New York, NY: Guilford Press.

Kendall, P.C. (1994). Treatment of anxiety disorders in children: a randomized clinical trial. *Journal of Consulting and Clinical Psychology* 62: 100–110.

Kendall, P.C. (2006). Guiding theory for therapy with children and adolescents. In: *Child and Adolescent Therapy: Cognitive-Behavioral Procedures*, 3e (ed. P.C. Kendall), 3–30. New York: Guilford Press.

Kendall, P. (ed.) (2018). *Cognitive Therapy with Children and Adolescents: A Casebook for Clinical Practice*, 3e. New York, NY: Guilford Press.

Kendall, P.C. and Suveg, C. (2006). Treating anxiety disorders in youth. In: *Child and Adolescent Therapy: Cognitive-Behavioral Procedures*, 3e (ed. P.C. Kendall), 243–294. New York, NY: Guilford Press.

Kendall, P., Beidas, R., and Mauro, C. (2013). *Brief Coping Cat: The 8 Session Coping Cat Workbook*. Ardmore, PA: Workbook Publishing, Inc.

Kozlowski, J., Lusk, P., and Melnyk, B. (2015). Pediatric nurse practitioner management of child anxiety in a rural primary care clinic with the evidence-based COPE program. *Journal of Pediatric Health Care* 29 (3): 274–282. https://doi.org/10.1016/j.pedhc.2015.01.009.

Lewinsohn, P., Rhode, P., Hops, H., & Clarke, G. (1991). Leader's manual for parent groups: Adolescent Coping with Depression Course. (The therapist and adolescent workbook may be downloaded for free at http://kpchr.org/acwd/acwd.html)

Lusk, P. and Melnyk, B.M. (2011a). The brief cognitive-behavioral COPE intervention for depressed adolescents: outcomes and feasibility of delivery in 30-minute outpatient visits. *Journal of the American Psychiatric Nurses Association* 17 (3): 226–236.

Lusk, P. and Melnyk, B.M. (2011b). COPE for the treatment of depressed adolescents: lessons learned from implementing an evidence-based practice change. *Journal of the American Psychiatric Nurses Association* 17 (4): 297–309.

Lusk, P. and Melnyk, B. (2013a). Brief evidence-based interventions for child and adolescent mental health disorders. In: *A Practical Guide to Child and Adolescent Mental Health Screening, Early Intervention, and Health Promotion*, 2e (eds. B. Melnyk and P. Jensen), 337–355. Cherry Hill, NJ: National Association of Pediatric Nurse Practitioners.

Lusk, P. and Melnyk, B.M. (2013b). COPE for depressed and anxious teens: a brief cognitive–behavioral skills building intervention to increase access to timely, evidence-based treatment. *Journal of Child and Adolescent Psychiatric Nursing* 26 (1) https://doi.org/10.1111/jcap.12017.

Lusk, P., Hart, B., and Melnyk, B.M. (2018). A successful model for clinical training in child/adolescent cognitive behavioral therapy for graduate psychiatric advanced practice nursing students. *Journal of the American Psychiatric Nurses Association* 24 (5): 457–468. https://doi.org/10.1177/1078390317723989.

March, J.S., Franklin, M., Nelson, A., and Foa, E. (2001). Cognitive-behavioral psychotherapy for pediatric obsessive-compulsive disorder. *Journal of Clinical Child Psychology* 30: 8–18.

March, J., Silva, S., and Vitiello, B. (2006). The treatment for adolescents with depression study (TADS): methods and message at 12 weeks. *Journal of the American Academy of Child and Adolescent Psychiatry* 45 (12): 1393–1403.

March, S., Spence, S., and Donovan, C.L. (2009). The efficacy of an internet-based cognitive behavioral therapy intervention for child anxiety disorders. *Journal of Pediatric Psychology* 34: 474–487.

McCarty, C. and Weisz, J. (2007). Effects of psychotherapy for depression in children and adolescents: what we can (and can't) learn from meta-analysis and component profiling. *Journal of the Academy of Child and Adolescent Psychiatry* 46 (7): 879–886.

Melnyk, B.M. (2003). *COPE: Creating opportunities for personal empowerment. A 7-session cognitive behavioral skills building program for teens/children*. Available at https://www.cope2thrive.com/.

Melnyk, B.M. and Jensen, P. (2013). *Practical Guide to Child and Adolescent Mental Health Screening, Early Intervention, and Health Promotion*, 2e. Cherry Hill, NJ: National Association of Pediatric Nurse Practitioners (NAPNAP).

Melnyk, B.M., Kelly, S., Jacobsen, D. et al. (2013). The COPE healthy lifestyles TEEN randomized controlled trial with culturally diverse high school adolescents: baseline characteristics and methods. *Contemporary Clinical Trials* 36 (1): 41–53.

Melnyk, B.M., Kelly, S., and Lusk, P. (2014). Outcomes and feasibility of a manualized cognitive-behavioral skills building intervention: group COPE for depressed and anxious adolescents in school settings. *Journal of Child and Adolescent Psychiatric Nursing* 27 (1): 3–13. https://doi.org/10.1111/jcap.12058.

Melnyk, B.M., Jacobson, D., Kelly, S.A. et al. (2015). Twelve-month effects of the COPE healthy lifestyles TEEN program on overweight and depressive symptoms in high school adolescents. *The Journal of School Health* 85 (12): 861–870.

Moldovan, R., Cobeanu, O., and David, D. (2013). Cognitive bibliotherapy for mild depression symptomatology: randomized clinical trial of efficacy and mechanisms of change. *Clinical Psychology & Psychotherapy* 20 (6): 482–493.

Muris, P., Meesters, C., and Rompelberg, L. (2006). Attention control in middle childhood: relations to psychopathological symptoms and threat perception distortions. *Behavior Research and Therapy* 45: 997–1010.

Pavuluri, M.N., Grayczyk, P., Carbray, J. et al. (2004). Child and family focused cognitive behavior therapy in pediatric bipolar disorder. *Journal of the American Academy of Child and Adolescent Psychiatry* 43: 528–537.

Pine, D.S. (2007). Research review: a neuroscience framework for pediatric anxiety disorders. *Journal of Child Psychology and Psychiatry* 48: 631–648.

Platt, R., Pustilnik, S., Connors, E. et al. (2018). Severity of mental health concerns in pediatric primary care and the role of child psychiatry access programs. *General Hospital Psychiatry* 53: 12–18. https://doi.org/10.1016/j.genhosppsych.2018.02.010.

Rhode, P., Stice, E., Shaw, H., and Gau, J. (2015). Effectiveness trial of an indicated cognitive-behavioral group adolescent depression prevention program versus bibliotherapy and brochure control at 1 and 2 year follow up. *Journal of Consulting and Clinical Psychology* 83 (4): 736–747. https://doi.org/10.1037/ccp0000022.

Roy, A.K., Vasa, R.A., Bruck, M. et al. (2008). Attention bias toward threat in pediatric anxiety disorders. *Journal of the American Academy of Child and Adolescent Psychiatry* 47: 1189–1196.

Rush, A.J., Beck, A.T., Kovacs, M., and Hollons, S. (1977). Comparative efficacy of cognitive therapy and pharmacotherapy in the treatment of depressed outpatients. *Cognitive Therapy and Research* 1: 17–37. https://doi.org/10.1007/BF01173502.

Shapiro, F. (2018). *Eye Movement Desentization and Reprocessing EMDR Therapy*. New York, NY: Guilford Press.

Silverman, W.K., Ortiz, C.D., Viswesvaran, C. et al. (2008). Evidence-based psychosocial treatments for children and adolescents exposed to traumatic events. *Journal of Clinical Child and Adolescent Psychology* 37: 156–183.

Stasiak, K., Fleming, T., Lucassen, M.F.G. et al. (2016). Computer-based and online therapy for depression and anxiety in children and adolescents. *Journal of Child and Adolescent Psychopharmacology* 26 (3): 235–245.

Sudak, D. and Taormina, S. (2018). Integrate brief CBT interventions into medication management visits. *Current Psychiatry* 17 (2): e3–e4.

Tryon, W.W. (2009). Cognitive processes in cognitive and pharmacological therapies. *Cognitive Therapy and Research* 33: 570–584.

Tyler, T., Hulkower, R., & Kaminski, J. (2017). *Behavioral health integration in pediatric primary care: Considerations and opportunities for policymakers, planners, and providers.* Available at the Milbank Memorial Fund Report website: www.milbank.org.

Weersing, V.R., Jeffreys, M., Do, M., Schwartz, K., & Bolano, C. (2017). Evidence base update of psychosocial treatments for child and adolescent depression.

Weisz, J.R., McCarty, C.A., and Valerie, S.M. (2006). Effects of psychotherapy for depression in children and adolescents: a meta-analysis. *Psychological Bulletin* 132 (1): 132–149. https://doi.org/10.1037/0033-2909.132.1.132.

Weisz, J.R., Kuppens, S., Ng, M.Y. et al. (2017). What five decades of research tells us about the effects of youth psychological therapy: a multilevel meta-analysis and implications for science and practice. *American Psychologist* 72 (2): 79–117.

Whitfield-Gabrieli, S., Ghosh, S., Nieto-Castanon, A. et al. (2016). Brain connection omics predict response to treatment in social anxiety disorder. *Molecular Psychiatry* 21: 680–685. https://doi.org/10.1038/mp.2015.109.

Zhou, X., Zhang, Y., Furukawa, T. et al. (2018). Different types and acceptability of psychotherapies for acute anxiety disorders in children and adolescents: a network meta-analysis. *JAMA Psychiatry* 76 (1): 41–50. https://doi.org/10.1001/jamapsychiatry.2018.3070.

Zukerbrot, R.A., Cheung, A., Jensen, P.S. et al. (2018). Guidelines for adolescent depression in primary care (GLAD-PC): part I. Practice preparation, identification, assessment, and initial management. *Pediatrics* 120 (5): e1299. https://doi.org/10.1542/peds.2017-4081.

21

Disorders Specific to Infants and Young Children

Joan A. Kearney[1] and Shannon Vaillancourt D'Alton[2]

[1] Yale University School of Nursing, Orange, CT, USA
[2] College of Nursing, Medical University of South Carolina, Charleston, SC, USA

Objectives

After reading this chapter, advanced practice registered nurses will be able to:

1. Identify major mental health problems experienced by infants, toddlers, and preschool children.
2. Describe varied methods for assessing the mental health problems of young children.
3. Identify psychotherapeutic approaches to intervention that consider specific symptoms, developmental issues, and family context.
4. Understand the state of the science with respect to psychopharmacological interventions and the appropriate protocols for intervention.

Introduction

Over the last 25 years, awareness has increased regarding the existence and importance of mental health problems experienced by infants, toddlers, and preschool children and a number of studies support the need for early intervention due to their long-term risk (Keenan et al. 2011; Lahey et al. 2004; Lavigne et al. 1998). Preschoolers evidence a diverse array of disorders comprising neurodevelopmental disorders, including autism spectrum disorder (ASD), attention deficit hyperactivity disorder (ADHD), mood and anxiety disorders, trauma and stressor related disorders, and sleep as well as eating and feeding disorders among others. Symptom clusters and characteristics of well-known school-age childhood disorders are similar to those seen in preschoolers (Sterba et al. 2007), and prevalence rates of preschool disorders (10–15%) show concordance with those of older children (Egger and Angold 2006). Both externalizing and internalizing disorders have shown stability in preschoolers, with evidence for a positive relationship between longer term stability and increasing age at diagnosis (Bufferd et al. 2012; Finsaas et al. 2018; Lavigne et al. 1998). The stability of disorders in younger groups of infants and toddlers has also been established (Briggs-Gowan et al. 2006). Additionally, there is growing evidence that many adult disorders have their beginnings in childhood and originate from early biological and developmental disruptions and markers of adversity (Angold and Egger 2007; Drury et al. 2012a,b; Essex et al. 2013; Lengua et al. 2015; Luby et al. 2016; Monk et al. 2012; Shonkoff et al. 2009; Zalewski et al. 2012). These recent findings articulate with evolving discussions regarding developmentally grounded continuity and discontinuity in early childhood disorders.

Child and Adolescent Behavioral Health: A Resource for Advanced Practice Psychiatric and Primary Care Practitioners in Nursing, Second Edition. Edited by Edilma L. Yearwood, Geraldine S. Pearson, and Jamesetta A. Newland.
© 2021 John Wiley & Sons, Inc. Published 2021 by John Wiley & Sons, Inc.
Companion website: www.wiley.com/go/Yearwood

These early problems are typically not transient syndromes but exhibit chronicity (Briggs-Gowan and Carter 2008; Luby et al. 2009). Due to this risk trajectory, it is essential that clinicians learn to recognize signs and symptoms associated with emotional and behavioral problems during the first few years of life. Subsequent early intervention efforts may then prevent development of more severe problems and improve the course and prognosis of existing difficulties (Carter et al. 2004, 2010; Heberle et al. 2015).

Prevalence of Mental Health Problems

A small but growing subset of studies have examined the prevalence of mental health problems in children 6 years of age or younger. Earlier work conducted in community or primary care settings with children aged 2–5 years demonstrated rates of mental illness for young children (i.e. having at least one mental disorder) ranging from 14% to 26.4% based on classifications in the past version of the Diagnostic and Statistical Manual of Mental Disorders (DSM-IV-TR) (American Psychiatric Association [APA] 2000; Carter et al. 2010; Egger and Angold 2006). Comorbidities were common in this diagnosed group, reflected in dysfunction across multiple systems. Many children also had "sub-threshold" symptoms, suggesting higher risk for later development of mental disorders.

Mental health diagnoses in children vary according to age and this is evident in infant and preschool age populations as well. A review of early research data specific to infants and toddlers referred to a community mental health clinic found that regulation disorders, developmental disorders, and adjustment difficulties were the most common diagnoses (Wright et al. 2004). Problems in the parent–child relationship were also prevalent in this group. Studies of preschoolers using both community and clinical samples demonstrated higher rates of externalizing disorders in young children when compared with internalizing disorders (Lavigne et al. 2009; Wilens et al. 2002). For instance, Wilens et al. (2002) found that 86% of children at mental health clinics were diagnosed with ADHD, and 61% with oppositional defiant disorder (ODD). Some data suggested that boys were more likely to carry an ODD diagnosis than were girls. However, despite agreement across studies, such findings may more accurately reflect difficulty in assessing emotional or internalizing symptoms in young children because of normative developmental limitations in language and cognitive capacity for abstraction and reflection. Additionally, it may be difficult for caregivers to recognize a young child's nonverbalized internal state and emotions in contrast to the child's observable behaviors.

More recent work supports these seminal studies and confirms the existence of psychiatric diagnoses in community preschoolers using standardized assessments at a rate of 26.5% for all diagnoses (Bufferd et al. 2012). As in the original studies, higher rates of externalizing disorders were found. These were followed by anxiety disorders and depression. Neurodevelopmental disorders were not included. Differentials were not made for the more recent addition of mood dysregulation disorders, i.e. disruptive mood dysregulation disorder (DMDD), which was introduced into DSM-5 (APA 2013) a year after the publication of this study and followed by the introduction of disorder of dysregulated anger and aggression of early childhood (DDAA) into DC:0–5 in 2016 (Zero to Three 2016).

Existing research also highlights the importance of ongoing mental health assessment and treatment for young children, with a focus is on early detection and prevention. Yet studies show that very few young children with mental health problems are referred for any mental health evaluation or treatment (Egger and Angold 2006; Lavigne et al. 2009). This is due to numerous issues, including the willingness to acknowledge that psychiatric problems can indeed occur in this group as well as the availability and understanding of a developmentally appropriate nosology and diagnostic systems for assessment.

The Nature of Mental Health Problems in Early Childhood

Etiology

Mental health disorders in young children are often viewed within the context of a stress diathesis model (Ingram and Luxton 2005), which operationalizes the risk/vulnerability/resilience framework. This model posits that the diathesis or constitutional (e.g. genetic, structural, neurophysiological/chemical) vulnerabilities interact with environmental stressors (e.g. biological insults/toxins, socio-emotional deprivation, trauma, loss, abuse) to precipitate mental disorders. The impact and importance of these factors vary in any given situation. For example, psychopathology (i.e. developmental psychopathology) that involves difficulty regulating sensory perception and behavior or fixed developmental impairments across systems are generally associated with neurobiological vulnerability and are impacted differentially by the child's social environment (Cicchetti 2016; Cicchetti and Curtis 2006).

Disorders such as post-traumatic stress and trauma spectrum syndromes, as well as depression, may be influenced more substantially by caregiving environments, losses, and exposure to major life stress. However, genetic predisposition or neurobiological deficits/dysfunction can render a child significantly more vulnerable to such environmental adversity (Blandon et al. 2008; Boyce and Ellis 2005), therefore increasing their psychiatric risk. Alternately, factors which contribute to resilience (constitutional strengths, positive family environment) serve as protective factors (Scorza et al. 2018). More in-depth discussion of the etiology of specific disorders can be found in relevant chapters throughout this book.

A Diagnostic Classification System for Young Children (Zero to Three)

Traditionally, concerns have been voiced about diagnostic systems for young children given rapid developmental changes and the risk of stigmatizing labels. Current views emphasize the importance of early identification of specific problems for focused treatment and the necessity of a diagnosis for services to be reimbursed. However, many mental health professionals have expressed concern about the adequacy of the DSM system for assessing young children. This concern spurred the development of alternative diagnostic frameworks such as Greenspan's DIR (developmental, individual-differences, relationship-based) model for assessment and intervention (Greenspan and Wieder 2007) and the widely used DC:0–5 system (Zero to Three 2016), which is discussed here.

For a number of years now there have been developmentally driven concerns relating to the appropriateness of assigning psychiatric diagnoses as previously defined to young children. To address these concerns, a multidisciplinary group affiliated with the National Center for

Infants, Toddlers and Families met in 1994 and developed a new diagnostic system, the Diagnostic Classification of Mental Health and Developmental Disorders of Infancy and Early Childhood (DC:0–3) (Zero to Three 1994), which has undergone two revisions (DC:0–3R: DC:0–5) (Zero to Three 2005, 2016). Although originally developed for children aged 3 years and under, it has become a useful diagnostic system for considering mental disorders of all young children, including those of preschool age. Additionally, in 2003 diagnostic criteria for preschool disorders were reviewed by the Task Force on Research Diagnostic Criteria: Infancy and Preschool (2003), further bolstering this developing clinical science.

Diagnoses using the DC:0–5 system consider a child's maturational and environmental changes over time and remain open to modification based upon these changes. It has a more significant focus on developmental and relational issues than the DSM system. Although the DSM-5 (APA 2013) no longer uses the multiaxial system of diagnosis, the DC:0–5 has retained this approach while revising and updating it to emphasize the importance of context in the diagnosis of early life disorders (Emde 2016). See Table 21.1 for comparison between these two diagnostic systems.

Earlier studies supported the validity and utility of the DC:0–3R diagnostic system (Cordeiro et al. 2003; Guedeney et al. 2003) even while early childhood psychiatric nosology was in its beginning stages. In the new version, DC:0–5, special attention has been paid to the strengthening and refinement of a specific nosology for young child disorders (Zeanah et al. 2016), rather than referring to other more general nosologies. Using specific nosologies for disorders makes assessment of

Table 21.1 Assessment within two classification systems

Axis	DC:0–5 (retains axial structure)	DSM-5 (nonaxial)
I	Clinical disorders	Primary diagnostic categories, includes former axes I, II, III
II	Relational context	Personality characteristics/disorders are assessed for all patients, a new section on emerging models has been added. Personality disorders included in the primary diagnostic considerations as outlined above
III	Physical health conditions and considerations	Medical conditions are included in the primary diagnostic considerations as outlined above
IV	Psychosocial stressors	Psychosocial and environmental stressors are considered: "Other conditions that may be a focus of concern". Z codes in the nonaxial system. Crosswalk would be to Axis II of DC:0–5
V	Developmental competence	The World Health Organization Disability Assessment Schedule is used for all to indicate impairment/functioning
Other	Cultural formulation for use with infants and toddlers	Cultural formulation

young children superior to general nosologies such as those that were used by Scheering et al. (2001). Other improvements in the newest DC:0–5 version center around extension of Axis I diagnoses through the preschool period to age 5, the use of refined diagnostic algorithms with specific descriptors and explanations, the use of distress or functional impairment criteria to distinguish actual disorders from transient conditions or behaviors, the addition of several new disorders and renaming to reflect accurate context, and extensive revision and expansion of the other axes.

For classifications shared by both systems, there has been good agreement in diagnosing young children (Frankel et al. 2004; Thomas and Guskin 2001). As DC:0–5 is the commonly used classification system for young children, a discussion of its diagnostic categories follows. DC:0–5 disorders and related diagnostic classifications from DSM-5 are shown in Table 21.2 and a full description of criteria found in the manual for DC:0–5 (Zero to Three 2016).

Neurodevelopmental Disorders

These disorders are commonly diagnosed early in life during the developmental years. Many of them were previously categorized in DSM-IV-TR as disorders typically first seen in childhood. They share additional important features, including a neurological substrate and a pattern characterized by unremitting symptoms which can be treated but are not considered curable. The disorders in this category, as outlined in Table 21.2, include ASDs, ADHD, developmental delay and disorders, and sensory processing disorders.

ASD presents with hallmark symptoms of social engagement and communication difficulties as well as

Table 21.2 DC:0–5 diagnostic classifications for mental health and developmental disorders of infancy and early childhood with crosswalk to DSM-5

DC:0–5 diagnosis	DSM-5 diagnosis
Neurodevelopmental disorders	Neurodevelopmental disorders
• Autism spectrum disorder (ASD)	• Autism spectrum disorder (ASD)
• Early atypical autism spectrum disorder (EAASD)	• Other specified neurodevelopmental disorder
• Attention deficit hyperactivity disorder (ADHD)	• Attention deficit hyperactivity disorder (ADHD)
• Overactivity disorder of toddlerhood	• ADHD, predominantly hyperactive–impulsive presentation
• Global developmental delay	• Global developmental delay
• Developmental language disorder	• Language disorder
• Developmental coordination disorder	• Developmental coordination disorder
• Other neurodevelopmental disorders of infancy/childhood	• Unspecified neurodevelopmental disorder
• Sensory processing disorders (under/over/other)	• Other specified neurodevelopmental disorder
Anxiety disorders	Anxiety disorders
• Separation anxiety disorder	• Separation anxiety disorder
• Social anxiety disorder (social phobia)	• Social anxiety disorder (social phobia)
• Generalized anxiety disorder	• Generalized anxiety disorder
• Selective mutism	• Selective mutism
• Inhibition to novelty disorder	• Other specified anxiety disorder
• Other anxiety disorder of infancy/early childhood	• Other specified anxiety disorder
Mood disorders	Depressive disorders
• Depressive disorder of early childhood	• Major depressive disorder
• Disorder of dysregulated anger and aggression of early childhood	• Disruptive mood dysregulation disorder
• Other mood disorders of early childhood	• Unspecified depressive disorder
Obsessive compulsive and related disorders	Obsessive compulsive and related disorders
• Obsessive compulsive disorder	• Obsessive compulsive disorder
• Tourettes disorder	• Tourettes disorder
• Motor or vocal tic disorder	• Persistent (chronic) motor or vocal tic disorder
• Trichotillomania	• Trichotillomania
• Skin picking disorder of infancy/early childhood	• Excoriation (skin picking) disorder
• Other obsessive compulsive and related disorders	• Unspecified obsessive compulsive and related disorder

Table 21.2 *(cont'd)*

DC:0–5 diagnosis	DSM-5 diagnosis
Sleep, eating and crying disorders Sleep disorders • Sleep onset disorder • Night waking disorder • Partial arousal sleep disorder • Nightmare disorder of early childhood	Sleep–wake disorders: feeding and eating disorders Sleep–wake disorders: • Insomnia disorder • Insomnia disorder • Nonrapid eye movement sleep arousal disorder: sleep terror type • Nightmare disorder
Eating disorders • Overeating disorder • Undereating disorder Atypical eating disorder • Hoarding • Pica • Rumination Crying disorder	Feeding and eating disorders • Unspecified feeding or eating disorder • Unspecified feeding or eating disorder • Unspecified feeding or eating disorder • Pica • Rumination disorder Unspecified, criteria not met for a specific disorder (cause not identified)
Other sleep, eating and excessive crying disorders	Other specified sleep–wake, feeding or eating disorder
Trauma, stress and deprivation disorders • Post-traumatic stress disorder • Adjustment disorder • Complicated grief disorder of infancy/early childhood • Reactive attachment disorder • Disinhibited social engagement disorder • Other trauma stress and deprivation disorder	Trauma- and stressor-related disorders • Post-traumatic stress disorder for children 6 years and younger • Adjustment disorder • Other specified trauma- and stressor-related disorders (persistent complex bereavement disorder) • Reactive attachment disorder • Disinhibited social engagement disorder • Unspecified trauma and stressor related disorder
Relationship disorders • Relationship specific disorder	Other conditions that may be a focus of clinical attention • Parent–child relational problems

restrictive repetitive behaviors. Diagnoses made after 4 years of age have shown stability over time. Prior to 36 months of age caution should be exercised and consideration given to a diagnosis of early atypical autism spectrum disorder (EAASD) as a subthreshold disorder which acknowledges the emergent trajectory of full ASD and period of risk early in life. Risk for eventual development of full ASD is high in these children. ADHD may be diagnosed as early as 3 years and symptoms of hyperactivity-impulsivity and inattention must be present for at least 6 months. Stability for ADHD diagnosis from the preschool years to early school age is high (Riddle et al. 2013). As in ASD, this diagnosis has a lower age limit for identification with consideration for a diagnosis of overactivity disorder of toddlerhood (OADT) when characteristic symptoms of hyperactivity and impulsivity exist between the ages of 24 and 36 months.

Developmental delay and specific disorders include global delay and well as disorders of language and coordination. Global developmental delay is characterized by delays across multiple developmental domains including language, verbal and nonverbal reasoning, social development, motor skills, and adaptive behaviors. Specific disorders of language and coordination indicate significant delays in these areas. Sensory processing disorders indicate difficulties in regulating sensory input and characteristically cause distress in the child. They are characterized by over- or under-responsivity or atypical responses to sensory stimuli.

Anxiety Disorders

Anxiety disorders have been established diagnostically in preschoolers, are considered leading mental health problems in this group, and are stable over time (Bufferd et al. 2012; Dougherty et al. 2013; Finsaas et al. 2018; Franz et al. 2013). They also display heterotypic continuity with adolescent depression, placing the anxious preschooler at risk for a later depressive disorder (Bufferd et al. 2012). The specific anxiety disorder symptom clusters seen in early childhood are similar to those seen in older children, but they manifest differently at various ages. The disorders most commonly seen in young children include separation anxiety disorder, social phobia, generalized anxiety disorder, and specific phobias. Central characteristics of all anxiety disorders in early childhood include distress or avoidance of anxiety-producing stimuli, occurrence during more than one daily activity or in more than one relationship, inability of the child to control symptoms, persistence for 2 weeks or more, and impairment of child and family functioning and the child's development in play, speech, sleep, relationships, and other spheres. Specific anxiety disorder symptoms in young children may include uncontrollable crying or screaming, sleeping and eating disturbances, or recklessness.

Selective mutism and inhibition to novelty disorder are also included in the anxiety disorder category. Selective mutism is an uncommon disorder in which the child fails to speak in social situations where speech is expected. Inhibition to novelty disorder is more common and a risk factor for the major anxiety disorders discussed above. It is characterized by extreme behavioral inhibition and fear of new situations, people, and/or activities.

Mood Disorders

The mood disorders category in DC:0–5 consists of depressive disorder of early childhood, DDAA, and other mood disorders of early childhood. These disorders are the early childhood correlates of major depressive disorder (MDD), DMDD, and unspecified depressive disorder of childhood in DSM-5.

Similar to those found across age groups, symptoms of mood disorders in young children include affective, behavioral, and neurovegetative symptoms (sleeping, eating, activity level). These symptoms interfere with developmentally appropriate activities and cause distress to the child and family. Affective symptoms differentiate depressive disorder of early childhood from disorder of dysregulated anger and aggression of early childhood in that children with the former often exhibit sadness and or irritability while those diagnosed with the latter often display irritability coupled with angry and aggressive outbursts reflecting characteristic dysregulation of behavior and emotion. There is evidence that this type of irritability at age 3 is associated with parental depression and anxiety, and predicts depression, ODD and functional impairments at age 6 (Dougherty et al. 2013). In the early years it is transdiagnostic and a marker of emerging mental health problems (Dougherty et al. 2017; Wiggins et al. 2018). With respect to depressive symptoms, they are also highly impairing and there is evidence for homotypic continuity into adolescence, placing these children at heightened risk throughout development (Gaffrey 2018).

To consider these diagnoses, duration and intensity of symptoms are central criteria since transient emotional, behavioral, and vegetative symptoms occur in young children, and in the absence of disorder will resolve fairly quickly as the child regulates. In depression, symptoms must be present on most days for a minimum of 2 weeks. In disorder of dysregulated anger and aggression of early childhood, symptoms must be present for at least 3 months. Neither disorder is diagnosed under the age of 2 years, the age at which depressive symptoms can be identified (Luby and Belden 2012).

Obsessive Compulsive and Related Disorders

This category includes the following diagnoses in young children: obsessive compulsive disorder (OCD), Tourette's disorder, motor or vocal tic disorder, trichotillomania, skin picking disorder of infancy/early childhood, and other obsessive compulsive and related disorders. These are the early childhood correlates of the DSM-5 diagnoses outlined for this category in Table 21.2. Although most of the research regarding these diagnoses has been conducted with older children and adults, these disorders do exist in younger children and can be diagnosed using developmentally sensitive criteria. These disorders may cause considerable distress, interfere with child and family functioning, and impede developmentally appropriate activities, leading to delays in developmental trajectories.

OCD is an established diagnosis in early childhood with an approximate mean age of onset of 5 years and criteria observed as early as 2 years (Garcia et al. 2009). Its prevalence in young children is not currently estimated. OCD is a disabling and often chronic condition characterized by repeated ritualistic thoughts and behaviors which are uncontrollable. Diagnostic criteria include the presence of obsessions (thoughts) and/or compulsions (behaviors) which occur almost every day for more than a total of an hour and are not due to another condition or traumatic experience. Symptoms must be present for at least 3 months and it is not diagnosed in children under the age of 3 years. Obsessions may include contamination fears, catastrophic thoughts, and somatic obsessions, all of which cause distress. Compulsions may include washing, checking, arranging, counting, and tapping which are linked to obsessive thoughts and are meant to reduce distress. It is important to place this disorder in developmental perspective in that rituals and repetitive behaviors often occur in young children but are transient and don't interfere with normal functioning. This differentiates them from the atypical, distressing, and chronic nature of OCD symptoms.

Tourette's disorder is more common in boys and is characterized by both motor and vocal tics which are sudden, involuntary, and repetitive. Children must evidence both types of tics and they may be in the form of simple tics (brief movements and sounds) or complex tics (a series of movements or verbal expressions (repetition of obscenities, gestures). Young children often evidence simple tics at first, later followed by complex tics. These tics may be repressed for variable periods of time in older children and are exacerbated by stress. While tics may first evidence in the second year, they are clearly identifiable between 4 and 6 years. Motor and vocal tic disorders are differentiated from Tourette's disorder in that they consist of only a motor or vocal tic per disorder and are not combined, as in the latter disorder.

Trichotillomania and skin picking disorder of infancy/early childhood have been observed in young children and are distinguished from the transient behaviors often seen in young children in their persistence, harmful physical effects (e.g. long-term wounds), and increased incidence with age.

Sleep, Eating, and Crying Disorders

These disorders indicate physiological and behavioral dysregulation which exists independent of other possible disorders or causes such as trauma. Often seen early on during the first year of life, they may be quite distressing to the child. They are differentiated from the typical range of difficulties seen in the early months in their severity and negative impact on normal developmental activities and child and family functioning. Evidence of one or more of these impairments must be present to make a diagnosis in this category. Additionally, because they occur within the context of, and are closely tied to, the regulatory functions of the attachment–caregiving relationship, it is important to assess this and determine any causal associations between both. In the absence of this association, a diagnosis can be made.

Sleep disorders include sleep onset disorder, night waking disorder, partial arousal sleep disorder, and nightmare disorder of early childhood. As in all disorders comprising the larger category, sleep disorders assume the general child and family impairment criteria discussed above. Sleep onset disorder and night waking disorder roughly correspond to insomnia disorders in DSM-5. They are characterized by difficulty falling asleep most nights beyond a 30-minute period or multiple periods of prolonged awakening. Young infants may exhibit these disorders at 6 and 8 months of age, respectively. Partial arousal sleep disorder and nightmare disorder of early childhood are parasomnias which occur at 12 months and beyond, and are characterized by sudden arousal or awakening from sleep. The former disorder includes sleep terrors which are accompanied by distress

and physiological arousal or sleep walking. The latter consists of nightmares that occur during the second half of sleep. For both of these disorders, the child may not remember any content or activities. All sleep disorders must persist for at least 1 month before diagnosis.

Eating disorders consist of overeating disorder, undereating disorder, and atypical eating disorders including hoarding, pica, and rumination disorder. Overeating and undereating disorders are characterized by excessive or inadequate food intake with differential profiles. In the former, there is overeating at or in-between meals, preoccupation with food, and distress at restriction of intake. In the latter, the child consistently eats less than the norm for their age. These disorders may result in atypical weight patterns based on height/weight norms and this would be documented on Axis III of the DC:0–5 axial schema. Overeating disorder has a lower limit of 24 months for diagnosis while undereating disorder has no diagnostic age criteria.

Atypical eating disorders include hoarding, pica, and rumination disorder. It is critical to understand certain important associations and make certain rule-outs before diagnosing these disorders. Additionally, it is important to understand the medical outcomes often associated with these disorders. For hoarding, which is indicated by hiding food in unusual places, it must be determined that the child is not chronically hungry due to food deprivation as it is often correlated with disordered caregiving and maltreatment/neglect. For pica, which is the habitual eating of nonfood substances in addition to the daily diet, it is important to rule out ADS, schizophrenia, or intellectual disability. This is particularly essential when pica is mild, requiring a primary diagnosis of these larger neurodevelopmental/psychiatric conditions. Otherwise, pica is included in the comorbidity profile. Pica is associated with medical outcomes such as iron and zinc deficiencies, intestinal obstruction and perforation as well as infections and poisoning. Rumination disorder, which is a consistent pattern of regurgitating and then reswallowing food, should not be diagnosed without first considering a number of medical conditions, including reflux, pyloric stenosis, and hiatal hernia, among others. Medical outcomes include weight loss and failure to gain weight to the point of malnutrition in more severe cases. As in hoarding, rumination disorder is often associated with disordered caregiving and maltreatment/neglect.

Hoarding and pica are not diagnosed before the age of 2 years while rumination disorder can emerge between 3 and 12 months. All eating disorders outlined here must persist for at least 1 month before a diagnosis is made.

Crying disorder of infancy/early childhood/excessive crying disorder is characterized by crying at least 3 hours a day, 3 or more days a week for at least 3 weeks (called the "rule of 3s"). As in most psychiatric diagnoses, the crying cannot be explained by medical or other causes and, as in all early childhood conditions, it impacts child and family functioning and developmental progress. It often starts in the first month, extending beyond the 3-month mark, and is associated with caregiver–child difficulties. Infants with this disorder are vulnerable due to associated attachment/caregiving problems and possible abuse, as well as related and serious medical outcomes, such as shaken baby syndrome. It can be comorbid with sensory processing and sleep disorders.

Trauma, Stress, and Deprivation Disorders

Disorders in this category include post-traumatic stress disorder (PTSD), adjustment disorder, complicated grief disorder of infancy/early childhood, reactive attachment disorder (RAD), disinhibited social engagement disorder (DSED), and other trauma, stress, and deprivation disorder. This category in DC:0–5 corresponds to the DSM-5 category of trauma- and stressor-related disorders. Unlike most other disorders in DC:0–5, these disorders have specific etiological criteria included in their diagnostic algorithms. These disorders are associated with stress, trauma of various type, and significant loss and/or deprivation, often relational in nature. Precipitants may be a single traumatic event or chronic reoccurring stress and trauma. The latter is especially pernicious to the growing child and often has long-term negative psychobiological sequelae. It is commonly referred to as complex PTSD, complex trauma, or the developmentally contextual term "toxic stress." Although significant stress, trauma, and loss may have numerous negative effects, not every child manifests symptoms of an actual disorder as defined in the DC:0–5. Although these disorders may occur within, and due to, the caregiving environment, some are temporally defined with respect to attachment relationships and are presumed to occur after these are established. These include RAD, DSED, and complicated grief disorder.

As in all early childhood disorders, each disorder in this category includes criteria which address functional impact on the child and family, including evidence of distress, relational difficulties, interference in child and family activities, and developmental progression. Duration and age limit criteria vary for each as specified. Prevalence rates for these disorders have been difficult to ascertain because of evolving diagnostic algorithms and developmentally driven limitations and nuances in symptom profiles with decreasing age. However, nosological examination of earlier (e.g. DSM-IV-R) and newer (DSM-5) developmentally sensitive criteria for

preschool PTSD disorder found prevalence rates between 44% and 49% in more than 250 traumatized young children across type of event/s and duration, showing increased sensitivity and specificity in our newer algorithm for DSM-5 (Scheeringa et al. 2012).

Symptoms of PTSD in young children generally parallel those found in the DSM-5 diagnostic rubric for PTSD in children aged 6 years and younger. The first and essential criteria for diagnosis is the direct or indirect (witnessing or learning about) exposure to a trauma-genic event. Additionally, the child will show evidence of re-experiencing the event through one or more of the following: play, preoccupation, nightmares, distress and physiological arousal, and dissociative episodes (freezing, stilling, staring, unresponsiveness) when reminded of it. Dissociation in traumatized preschoolers, although still under early study, appears to be differentially dose-related to type (e.g. sexual abuse) as well as caregiver dysfunction (Hagan Gentry et al. 2018).

The child may become avoidant of trauma-associated stimuli or show a dulling and dampening of positive affect and an increase in fearfulness and sadness, social withdrawal, and/or lack of interest in developmentally appropriate activities. They will also display two or more arousal symptoms such as sleep and concentration difficulties, hypervigilance and exaggerated startle response, and irritability, angry outbursts, and tantrums.

It is important to note that traumatic experiences in young children may have outcomes other than frank PTSD. Oppositionality is often seen in traumatized children as well as developmental regression in established skills. Moreover, the actual PTSD diagnosis is reserved for children 12 months and older due to cognitive constraints, e.g. limited representational thought in the first 12 months of life, impacting capacity for re-experiencing as currently defined. They may, however, evidence other and varied symptoms as outlined here. For a diagnosis of PTSD to be given, symptoms must persist for at least 1 month following exposure to a traumatic event.

The diagnosis of adjustment disorder is given when a child has experienced one or more stressors and develops a time-limited response with a duration of 2 weeks to 3 months. It should not be given if symptoms are explained by a more severe disorder in this category or exacerbation of a previous disorder. Conversely, it should not be given when transient symptoms are appropriate developmental reactions to environmental perturbations. Symptoms usually appear within 2 weeks of the stressor/s with disturbance of emotions or behavior (dysregulation in various domains) that clearly differ from the child's usual presentation. Age limits are not defined.

Complicated grief disorder of infancy/early childhood, another trauma/stressor disorder, is precipitated by the death or permanent loss of an attachment figure. Symptoms in infants and young children are bound by developmental stage and capacity. For example, infants often display somatic and emotional dysregulation while preschoolers may also generate idiosyncratic explanations, beliefs, and self-internalizations around the loss which may negatively impact their mental health. On the other hand, over time most children can cope, survive, and eventually thrive in the face of such loss if they are raised in healthy, loving environments and are well supported by the remaining caregivers.

Criteria for this disorder include crying and searching for the lost attachment figure, detachment, selective forgetting, extreme sensitivity regarding the lost figure or themes of loss, and preoccupation with death. Additionally, young children may display three or more of the following symptoms: neurovegetative symptoms, sadness, self-harm, lack of interest in activities, self-blaming attributions, and loss of developmental achievements. Symptoms must be present for 1 month before a diagnosis is made and given to infants and children beyond the age of 9 months when preferential attachments are considered well established.

RAD and DSED are disorders related to the lack of, or dysfunction of, early attachment/caregiving relationships. RAD is diagnosed when there is a history of inadequate care/neglect or a series of changing caregivers precluding the development of a healthy attachment to a primary caregiver. Criteria must not be met for ASD or EAASD. It is characterized by emotionally withdrawn, inhibited behavior with adult caregivers and emotional dysregulation (lack of or reduced positive affect along with periods of fearful ness/anger/irritability with strangers).

DESD is comprised of socially aberrant behavior with unfamiliar adults in children with a history of serious neglect. Children with this disorder exhibit lack of, or atypically reduced, stranger wariness, with active contact seeking of unfamiliar adults instead. They exhibit social disinhibition with adults that is culturally dystonic. The disorder may occur in children with or without established attachments. In the latter case, there is typically a history of repeated change in caregivers

Both RAD and DESD are not diagnosed until an infant is 9 months old, the age when attachments are established in typical infants. There is no minimum duration criterion for either.

Relationship Disorders

Relationship-specific disorder of infancy/early childhood comprises this category and is specifically designated apart from the general assessment of relationships for all children as outlined in Axis II of the DC:0–5 diagnostic assessment. The hallmark of this diagnosis is that the child displays symptoms related to a single caregiver only. These symptoms/behaviors do not exist with respect to other relationships. If symptoms are displayed across relationships this diagnosis is not given, but rather specific diagnoses relevant to the symptom profile.

Children may be at risk for various psychopathology due to poor attachments but they do not necessarily receive this diagnosis and, conversely, not all children who receive this diagnosis have poor attachment relationships. The category of caregiver-infant/young child adaptation on Axis II of the DC:0–5 system, which is assessed for all children, is relevant to this disorder in that only those children with seriously disturbed relationships as described on Axis II would be likely to receive a diagnosis of relationship disorder on Axis I as a primary clinical disorder. Symptoms of this disorder include persistent emotional or behavioral disturbance in a single relationship with a specific caregiver. Examples of these disturbances include aggression, oppositionality, fearfulness, and sleeping and eating problems. Additionally, as in all infant/ early childhood disorders in DC:0–5, contextual factors such as distress, functional impairment, and family difficulties must be considered. Symptoms must persist for at least 1 month and there are no age restrictions. However, it is easier to detect this disorder as the infant moves through the first year. It is thought that the disorder may be more commonly detected in infants than preschoolers because of internalization and repetition of relationship patterns as the child gets older.

Mental Health Assessment of Infants and Young Children

Practice parameters for assessment of mental disorders experienced by infants, children, and adolescents were first published by the American Academy of Child and Adolescent Psychiatry (AACAP) (1997a,b). Additional AACAP publications have addressed the assessment of specific problems that are relevant to preschool and older children with updates throughout the years. Reference to these parameters can be found in the resource section at the end of this chapter. These guidelines remain timely and recommend that assessment of young children include developmental, relational, and multidimensional perspectives. Considerations related to each follow.

Developmental Assessment

In any psychiatric evaluation of a young child, developmental assessment is essential. A valid assessment depends on knowledge of the developmental norms for this young age group (Davies 2011) as well as the nature of developmental trajectories in infancy and early childhood when rapid change is the norm. A developmental assessment provides a baseline portrait which captures deviations from the norm and often detects causative and contributory factors to early mental health problems. The assessment includes information regarding communication (including speech and language for toddlers and preschool children), motor control and coordination, adaptive behavior, regulatory and coping strategies, and social engagement/ socialization.

A number of structured developmental assessments are used for children of various ages. Multifunctional measures are widely used and may require training in administration. The Brazelton Neonatal Behavioral Assessment Scale–2 (Brazelton and Nugent 1995) is a clinician-administered developmental assessment for neonates measuring physiological reactivity and regulatory behaviors. The Bayley Scales of Infant Development (Bayley 2000) for infants and toddlers (ages 1–24 months) assess cognition, language, socioemotional, motor, and adaptive behavior domains. The Mullen Scales of Early Learning (Mullen 1995) for use with children from birth to approximately 5½ years focus on more complex processes associated with auditory, visual, and language development and are efficient in their application for a broad age range. The Infant Toddler Developmental Assessment, 2nd edition (IDA-2) (Provence et al. 2016) for children aged birth to 3 is another of these scales, as is the Brigance Inventory of Early Development (IED-II) for children aged birth through 7 years (Brigance 2006). The Battelle Developmental Inventory (BDI-II) (Newborg 2004) is also used from 5 months through 6 years to assess domains such as personal-social, motor, and communication functioning, and has a shorter parent report screening version.

In addition to these multifunction structured assessments, parent/caregiver self-report questionnaires are available to screen for developmental issues, including the typically used Ages and Stages Questionnaire (Squires and Bricker 2009), the Vineland Adaptive Behavior Scales (Sparrow et al. 2005), and earlier inventories created for infants, young children, and preschool children by Ireton (1992). These provide manuals with specific guidelines for administration and scoring and do not require extensive training for use. As a result, they are practical options for clinicians. It is important to note that since developmental capacity impacts a child's performance in an evaluation, assessment protocols and instruments must be sensitive and valid for use with respect to any limitations the child may have.

Relational Assessment

For preschool children and younger, the primary caregiver (usually the parent) is a central attachment figure and has a significant influence over the way in which the child experiences the world. Therefore, assessment of the child's interaction with this caregiver/parent is essential. However, assessment of the child's relationship with both parents or additional caregivers is the ideal when possible. Measures have been developed for assessing caregiver–child interactions. Those that have utility for clinical practice or are helpful in extended evaluations are highlighted in Table 21.3.

Table 21.3 Assessments of the parent–child relationship

Parent report assessments	Domains ASSESSED
Parenting Stress Index (PSI, PSI-SF)	Parental Distress Parent–child dysfunctional interaction Difficult child (total stress: combination of above domains)
Parental Acceptance-Rejection Questionnaire (PARQ, ECPARQ)	Acceptance Generalized rejection Aggression/hostility Neglect
Parent–Child Conflict Tactics Scales (CTSPC)	Corporal punishment Physical abuse Psychological aggression Neglect Nonviolent discipline
Observational assessments	**Domains assessed**
Parent–CHILD interaction Scale (PCI)	Parent: Sensitivity Responsiveness to distress Growth-fostering behavior: • cognitive • socioemotional Infant: Clarity of cues Responsiveness
Parent–Child Early Relational Assessment (PCERA)	Parental sensitivity/responsiveness Infant dysregulation Dyadic characteristics
Crowell procedure	Parent and child characteristics Relationship quality Child affect
Caregiver–Child Social/Emotional Relational Rating Scale (CCSERRS)	Social and emotional characteristics of relationship

Assessment of Parent–Child Interaction

Parental Report Scales

There are some well-known parent-report scales which assess important aspects and risk markers in parent–child interaction with utility in early childhood. The Parenting Stress Index (PSI and PSI/Short Form [SF]) (Abidin 2012) is a commonly used multidomain parental questionnaire assessing caregiver perceptions of stress and factors affecting the parent–child relationship.

The Parental Acceptance-Rejection Questionnaire (PARQ) (Rohner 2005) assesses general acceptance versus maltreatment of children by the caregiver based on parental report of their specific attitudes and behaviors. The PARQ Early Childhood version is used for children aged 4 to 7 years. The Parent–Child Conflict Tactics Scales (long and short versions) (CTSPC) (Straus and Mattingly 2007; Straus et al. 1998) is a parent self-report tool that also assesses child maltreatment in children 6 years and beyond. These parent report assessments often access information on parent–child interaction that otherwise may not easily be identified.

One additional consideration with respect to parent–child interaction is parental psychological status. Since infant/toddler mental health problems may occur because of, or related to, parental mental health issues, many clinicians screen for these difficulties, especially when risk factors or indicators are present. Two commonly used brief assessments of parental depression are the Edinburgh Postnatal Depression Scale (Cox et al. 1987) and the Patient Health Questionnaire (PHQ 2 or PHQ 9) (Kroenke et al. 2003; Spitzer et al. 1999).

Observational Assessments

Observational methods of parent–child interaction avoid self-report bias on the part of the parent, but often require extensive training and certification for administration. The Parent–Child Interaction Teaching and Feeding Scales (Sumner and Spietz 1994) are frequently used to assess parent–child interactions from birth to 3 years of age. Videotaped parent–child sessions facilitate validity of ratings but are not essential. Other observational measures which may require videotaping and are entailed include the Parent–Child Early Relational Assessment (PCERA) (Clark 1985) and the Crowell procedure (Crowell and Fleischman 1993). They were developed for research and may be used when a very comprehensive clinical assessment of the dyad is needed. The Caregiver–Child Social/Emotional Relational Rating Scale (CCSERRS) (McCall et al. 2010) is a more recently developed measure that has practical utility in the clinical setting.

Multidimensional Assessment

A multidimensional assessment uses varied methods to assess multiple dimensions over time rather than relying on a sole clinical encounter with the young child and family (Egger 2009). When mental health assessment of young children is based on limited information, important signs or symptoms may go unrecognized and certain behavior or input may be misconstrued or overgeneralized. Economic pressures to constrict the assessment process contribute to inaccurate or missed diagnosis, thus negatively impacting treatment.

Essential components of any psychiatric assessment with young children include an interview with, and other input from, the primary caregiver/parent, observation during the clinician's interaction with the child, and observation of the child–caregiver dyad. Additional input from other informants, such as family members or childcare providers, should be gathered whenever possible. A good example of an extended, in-depth multidimensional assessment is outlined in the Washington University School of Medicine Infant/Preschool Mental Health Clinic Assessment protocol, which has four distinct steps culminating in final integration (Navsaria and Luby 2016): (i) complete multidimensional history taking, (ii) free play observation with primary caregiver, (iii) structured observational protocols, and (iv) final integration of all assessment data with differential diagnosis and treatment planning with caregiver involvement.

Discrepant or conflicting impressions may emerge in an assessment of a young child with differences between family views and clinician observations, and data may be incongruent. For example, observation findings may be in direct opposition to parent report. When carefully considered within the integrated clinical picture, these discrepancies provide a better understanding of the child and family. It is also important to remember that observation in a clinic or hospital environment may not generalize to other times and settings.

The Psychiatric Assessment

Input from the Parents or Primary Caregiver

Parent/caregiver involvement in the assessment process is critical as they may be the only adults who can reliably comment on their child's behavior. They can also facilitate their child's comfort with aspects of the assessment that include play or developmental tests. Moreover, parent/caregiver involvement is essential to the long-term treatment process and clinical trajectory. It is important to note, however, that parents may not be completely accurate in identifying their child's emotional and behavioral problems, typically reporting fewer symptoms than children actually experience (Jensen et al. 1999). Meta-analyses of correlations between children's self-ratings of their own problems and ratings by adults raise important questions regarding the validity of parent reports in key symptom areas (Achenbach et al. 2005; Renk and Phares 2004).

In addition to the approach outlined in DC:0–5, there are a few well-established and reliable diagnostic interview protocols based on DSM criteria which have been developed for clinical research. These formal protocols can inform clinical practice as comprehensive or targeted, standardized approaches to the psychiatric assessment process. The Preschool Age Psychiatric Assessment (PAPA) (Egger and Angold 2006; Egger et al. 1999) is a well-known, reliable, and comprehensive standardized assessment protocol developed for use with children aged 2–5 years. The interview examines diagnostic criteria that are relevant to younger children, as well as other symptoms and behaviors. It also provides for assessment of family environment, family psychosocial problems, life events, and disability related to symptoms. The Diagnostic Interview Schedule for Children Version IV, modified for young children (DISC-IV-YC) (Lucas et al. 1998; Luby et al. 2009) is another structured comprehensive assessment tailored for preschoolers. The Diagnostic Infant Preschool Structured Interview (DIPA) (Scheeringa and Haslett 2010) for children 18 months to 5 years is somewhat newer than the PAPA but quite similar in reliability and its focus is on DSM criteria. It includes diagnostic guidelines. Targeted assessments include the preschool version of the Schedule for Affective Disorders and Schizophrenia for School Age Children, Present and Lifetime Version (K-SADS-PL) (Birmaher et al. 2009) and the Disruptive Behavior Diagnostic Observation Schedule (DB-DOS) (Wakschlag et al. 2008a,b), which is an observational protocol that characterizes preschool disruptive behaviors.

A number of questionnaires are also available for assessing mental health problems in young children (Table 21.4). These are usually completed by the parent(s) or primary caregiver.

The most widely used and well-tested parent self-report assessment of target behaviors is Achenbach and Rescorla's (2000) Child Behavior Checklist (CBCL) (Achenbach System of Empirically Based Assessment [ASEBS] 2012, 2018). The CBCL profiles correlate with both the PAPA and the DIPA profile findings in psychometric testing. It includes a Caregiver–Teacher Report Form, typically completed by a childcare provider or preschool teacher. The CBCL has a number of age-defined versions, including the report for ages 1½ to 5 years, which assess multiple behavioral areas and syndromal profiles. These fall into two large internalizing or externalizing categories or factors. The assessment can identify risk for major DSM-related diagnoses, including affective problems, anxiety, neurodevelopmental problems such as ADHD and ASD, and ODD. CBCL parent and teacher scales allow assessment of the child's functioning across contexts. The Early Childhood Screening Assessment (ECSA) (Gleason et al. 2010) is briefer and more limited than the CBCL for ease of use in primary care settings. This one-page parent questionnaire assesses the child's overall risk for mental health problems and asks parents to indicate their concerns regarding specific aspects of their child's behavior. A unique feature of this measure is the inclusion of four items assessing parental depression and distress.

The Infant-Toddler Social and Emotional Assessment (ITSEA), and its briefer version the (BITSEA), (Briggs-Gowan et al. 2004; Carter et al. 2003) are additional, well-studied, and reliable parent report assessments for very young children aged 1–3 years. Like the CBCL, the ITSEA examines externalizing and internalizing problems as well as dysregulation and an assessment of competencies. The brief screening version (BITSEA) provides only a general index of potential problem severity and competency. The Preschool Pediatric Symptom Checklist (PPSC) and the Baby Pediatric Symptom Checklist (BPSC) (Sheldrick et al. 2012, 2013) are used in primary care settings for children from 18 months to 5 years and birth to 18 months, respectively. They screen for internalizing and externalizing disorders, dysregulation, attention difficulties, and parenting challenges. Another general screening tool for number and frequency of problems is the Toddler Behavior Screening Inventory (TBSI) (McCain et al. 1999; Mouton-Simien et al. 1997). However, it lacks testing with ethnically and socio-economically diverse families, in contrast to the other assessments.

For children aged 2½ to 5 or 6 years, the Behavior Assessment System for Children (BASC) (Reynolds and Kamphaus 1992, 2002), the Early Childhood Symptom Inventory (ECSI) (Gadow and Sprafkin 2000; Sprafkin et al. 2002), and the older Pediatric Symptom Checklist (PSC) (Jellinek and Murphy 1990; Jellinek et al. 1988) are also available. All are easy to administer and provide cut-off scores or norms for general psychosocial impairment. Like the CBCL, the BASC and the ECSI allow for fairly comprehensive assessment of specific problems. The BASC differentiates externalizing and internalizing problems as well as adaptive skills. The ECSI identifies problems related to specific DSM diagnoses. In contrast, the PSC is a general screen for overall psychosocial impairment and when possible. The newer preschool/infant checklists (PPSC and BPSC) should be used.

Table 21.4 Assessments of mental health in early childhood

Assessment	Domains assessed	Age of child
Child Behavior Checklist (CBCL)	Clinical scales: Emotional reactivity Anxiety/depression Somatic problems Withdrawal Attention problems Aggressive behavior Sleep problems DSM scales: Affectivity Anxiety Oppositional defiant Pervasive developmental Attention-deficit/hyperactivity	1½ to 5 years
Early Childhood Screening Assessment (ECSA)	Overall problem risk	1½ to 5 years
Infant-Toddler Social and Emotional Assessment I (ITSEA/BITSEA)	ITSEA (full version): Internalizing Externalizing Dysregulation Competence BITSEA (brief version): Total problems Total competence	1 to 3 years
Toddler Behavior Screening Inventory (TBSI)	Total problems Frequency of problems	1 to 3½ years
Behavior Assessment System for Children (BASC)	Adaptive scales: Adaptability functional communication Social skills Activities of daily living Clinical scales: Aggression Anxiety Attention problems Atypicality Depression Hyperactivity Somatization Withdrawal	2 to 5 years
Pediatric Symptom Checklist (PSI)	Psychosocial impairment	3 to 6+ years

ITSEA, Infant-Toddler Social and Emotional Assessment; BITSEA, Brief Infant-Toddler Social and Emotional Assessment.

Observation and Interaction with the Child

Direct observation of young children's behavior is essential to psychiatric assessment. It is helpful to observe the child in the caregiver's presence as well as separately when possible. It is also critical to gather information about the child's behavior and functioning across contexts with caregivers and others at various time points. The assessment, while adhering to best practices and stated protocols, should be tailored to each child as much as possible to allow for the most accurate evaluation of specific functions or behaviors. Some combination of structured and unstructured formats provides a broad context for children to display strengths and limitations in a clinically meaningful way.

One integrated observational assessment developed specifically for practice purposes is the Infant and

Table 21.5 Dimensions assessed with the Infant-Toddler Mental Status Examination

---

Appearance

Reaction to the situation

Self-regulation

Motor coordination

Speech and language

Thought

Affect and mood

Structure and content of play

Cognition

Relatedness

Toddler Mental Status Examination (ITMSE) (Benham 2000). The ITMSE is useful in assessing the mental status of children from birth to 5 years and was originally published by the AACAP as part of the Practice Parameters for Assessment of Infants and Toddlers (AACAP 1997b). It provides a structure for examining traditional domains of the mental status examination but with modifications appropriate to young children while organizing observational data from a variety of sources. Instructions and guidelines for the examiner are provided. The domains examined with the ITMSE are shown in Table 21.5.

For children as young as 2 or 3 years, many play-based methods can be used to gather information. Examples include the Berkeley Puppet Interview (Measelle et al. 1998) and the story-stem technique (Gaensbauer and Kelsay 2008; Warren et al. 2000). The puppet interview helps children express their feelings by projecting them onto the puppets. In the story-stem technique, the clinician begins a story around specific toys and asks the child to complete the story. This elicits internal representations, conflicts, and impressions of caregivers and environment that a young child may not easily formulate and verbally express. Resources for assessment are referenced at the end of the chapter.

Intervention

Psychotherapy remains prominent in the treatment of young children. The Preschool Psychopharmacology Working Group (PPWG) (Gleason et al. 2007) recommended nonpharmacological treatment of young children as a first-line intervention across most diagnoses. We now have a number of evidence-based treatments for preschoolers. In addition to classic play therapy techniques which are woven into most work with young children, two general types of evidence-based interventions have currently proved effective and both include the caregivers in critical roles. These consist of parent management/behavioral models and psychodynamically based paradigms, both of which have been tested in specific preschool patient populations.

Evidence-based Techniques

The first major category of evidence-based nonpharmacological interventions address disruptive behavior disorders in young children. Two popular empirically supported treatment protocols, the Incredible Years (IY) Series (Webster-Stratton 2005) and Parent–Child Interaction Therapy (PCIT) (Eyberg and Bussing 2010; McNeil et al. 2015), are used with success in this population. This IY Series is grounded in an interactive intervention model for families of young children with early onset ODD and CD. Videotape modeling is employed for family training intervention, parental skills-training in academics, problem solving, and child social skills. Eyeberg's PCIT intervention model (Eyberg and Bussing 2010) also addresses early disruptive behavior disorders. PCIT focuses on increasing positive child behaviors through parent coaching, teaching, and skills development, thereby effecting change in both the parents and children. Other interventions include the Triple P program (triplep.org) and some address specific disorders, e.g. ADHD (Tamm et al. 2005), ASD-Triple P–Positive Parenting Program (Whittingham et al. 2009), and Helping the Noncompliant Child (McMahon and Forehand 2003), and focus on self-directed parental intervention with toddlers (Morawska and Sanders 2006).

In the psychodynamically based category of interventions, child–parent therapies build on relevant traditions, including object relations and social attachment frameworks (Bienenfeld 2006; Cassidy and Shaver 2016). Studies support the value of such interventions in improving caregiving behavior, reducing parental stress and child behavior problems, and enhancing adaptive behaviors for young children (Bakermans-Kranenburg et al. 2003; Lieberman et al. 2006). The Child Parent Psychotherapy (CPP) model for children 0–5 years (Lieberman and Van Horn 2009; Zeanah et al. 2011) focuses on unconscious processes, the parent–child relationship, internal representations of mother and child, and the relationship with the therapist. Although the evidence-based CPP model has been developed primarily with trauma populations, the conceptual underpinnings of the approach and the technique have application across preschool groups. Child–parent therapy involves dyadic psychotherapy for a young child and his/her primary caregiver with the goal of enhanced ability of the caregiver to provide responsive, therapeutic care to the young child. This type of intervention has been especially successful with young high-risk children who have been traumatized and with mothers and children who are living in violent situations (Lieberman et al. 2005).

Packaged programs in this tradition are available to assist practitioners, such as the "Circle of Security" (Marvin et al. 2002) and "Watch, Wait and Wonder" (Muir et al. 1999). Similarly, a technique called "interaction guidance" helps parents develop an understanding of their own and their infant/toddler's behavior (McDonough 2004). Additionally, the Video-based Intervention to Promote Positive Parenting (VIPP) is a home-based attachment intervention for parents of infants less than 12 months of age (Juffer et al. 2008). Each of these approaches uses discussion of videotaped interactive play sessions to highlight and reinforce a parent's positive interactions with a child and to offer suggested changes to more troublesome interactions.

Lastly, cognitive-behavioral approaches have shown promise in treating sexually abused preschool children as well as young children exposed to a variety of traumatic events (Deblinger et al. 2001; Scheeringa et al. 2007, 2011).

Play Therapy

At approximately 2 years of age a child develops the capacity for representational thought which brings with it the growing ability for imagery and symbolism. Language development occurs in synchrony with these achievements and emotional life becomes progressively sophisticated along the developmental trajectory. These capacities support increasingly complex symbolic play, enactment of situations, and storytelling throughout childhood. Play therapy for toddlers and preschool children capitalizes on these emerging capabilities using both psychodynamic and client-centered theoretical foundations (Chethik 2000; Landreth 2002a,b; Schaefer et al. 2008). This widely used therapeutic method aids in expression of emotions and experiences, and fosters the building of emotion-based skills such as coping and self-regulation. These functions comprise the expressive and formative aspects of play therapy (Benham and Slotnick 2006; Russ 2004). In the expressive component, a child explores feelings through play and verbalization. In the formative component, a child acquires new capacities for impulse control, frustration tolerance, sublimation, and other affect management strategies. Depending on a child's particular needs, clinicians can work with the child alone or, most often, in conjunction with a parent/caregiver (Landreth and Bratton 2006).

Psychopharmacological Interventions

Psychopharmacological treatment of young children is an important focus of ongoing attention. This branch of inquiry was given a formal imprimatur with the establishment of the PPWG (Gleason et al. 2007) after the AACAP Research Forum highlighted the need for focused attention to the specific issues and challenges confronting preschool psychopharmacological research (Greenhill et al. 2003). The PPWG examined a variety of issues in the psychopharmacological treatment of young children, including assessment, diagnostic, neurodevelopmental, ethical, and regulatory concerns. In addition, they looked at the place of nonpharmacological interventions in this young population. A number of recommendations followed from the efforts of the PPWG surrounding the need for careful and judicious use of medication in young children. The group reviewed the evidence for treatment of the major childhood disorders in preschoolers, including ADHD, disruptive behavior disorders, MDD, bipolar disorder, anxiety disorders including OCD, and PTSD, all of which have been treated psychopharmacologically in the preschool population. Citing the overall dearth of controlled, systematic studies for the use of the major medication classes in very young children, the group recommended nonpharmacological treatment as a first-line treatment for these disorders, with attention to the fact that it is a preferable option and should be given an adequate trial before medication is instituted. When functional impairment is mild medications are not indicated (Fanton and Gleason 2009).

Specific recommendations made by the PPWG include the following: psychopharmacological treatment should be associated only with substantial functional impairment, treatment discontinuation trials should be the norm, monotherapy should be employed, additional medications should not be used to treat side effects, and careful attention should be paid to all reports regarding medication usage in young children, including lesser level of evidence case reports (an "N of 1" approach).

Prior to these recommendations earlier large-scale studies of Medicaid as well as privately insured populations revealed a dramatic increase in the use of psychotropic medication, particularly antipsychotics, in young children during the preceding decade. This was for treatment of neurodevelopmental disorders, intellectual disability, disruptive behavior disorders, and what was designated as bipolar disorder (Olfson et al. 2009; Zito et al. 2007). Moreover, many of these children were prescribed more than one psychotropic medication and had not received complete diagnostic assessment or psychotherapy during their course of medication treatment (Olfson et al. 2009). These troubling reports dovetailed the concern regarding neurodevelopmental implications of psychopharmacological treatment in very young children. Additionally, debate continued regarding criteria for some of these diagnoses, e.g. bipolar disorder. These data also indicated that, not surprisingly, what we were treating in most cases were target symptoms. The most common of these is aggression, which is a developmentally based behavioral system and a nonspecific clinical symptom ubiquitous in young children and transdiagnostic.

Recent large-scale studies continue to show a concerning trend for some preschool prescribing without defined diagnoses and, more importantly, psychotherapeutic treatment (Ali et al. 2018). This early exposure to psychotropic medication is particularly evident in the Medicaid population (Pennap et al. 2018b). However, some states have now instituted peer review prior authorization prescribing polices as well as other regulatory practices for the use of psychotropic medication, primarily antipsychotics, in young children. These policies, for the most part, resulted in significantly decreased use in this population (Pennap et al. 2018a; Zito et al. 2018). This downward trend following the initial examination of the issue and subsequent policy changes is reflected in the finding that overall peak use of psychotropic medication in young children occurred from 2002 to 2005 and stabilized from there (Chirdkiatgumchai et al. 2013). Adding to this close scrutiny, the American Academy of Child Psychiatry has formed the Pediatric Psychopharmacology Initiative (PPI) to support research in pediatric psychopharmacology and excellence in scientific standards.

Currently only a few medications are formally approved by the Food and Drug Administration (FDA) for psychiatric treatment in children younger than 6 years. Examples are chlorpromazine, haloperidol, and risperidone for severe behavioral problems, and dextroamphetamines for ADHD. It is important to note that FDA approval does not mean that medications are necessarily preferable or used in practice. For example, despite the fact that amphetamines have FDA approval for early childhood ADHD, methylphenidate (MPH) is the preferred stimulant for use after examination in the NIMH sponsored multisite PATS trial of 300 young children (Greenhill et al. 2006; Kollins et al. 2006; Posner et al. 2007; Riddle et al. 2013). As of yet, there are no such trials for amphetamine use in young children, although it is considered a first-line treatment in older children.

There are a number of medications used "off label" in child psychiatry. The designation off-label does not imply lack of efficacy, but rather that the medication is not approved for a specific purpose in a particular age group. There are algorithms derived from research and case reports that guide clinicians in making decisions about off-label use for young children with neurodevelopmental disorders, disruptive behavior disorders, anxiety disorders,

and mood disorders (Gleason et al. 2007). Those that are most often considered in a conservative approach are MPH, alpha agonists, low dose fluoxetine (selective serotonin reuptake inhibitors [SSRIs]), and risperidone (atypical antipsychotic).

In addition to MPH, the alpha agonists clonidine and guanfacine are off-label medications that are often used for ADHD. The SSRIs fluoxetine and sertraline may be used judiciously for anxiety in preschoolers at very low starting doses and only after failure of other psychotherapeutic methods. There is little evidence for the benefits of SSRI use in preschool depression. Therefore, caution is advised and use reserved for severe impairment and failure of well-studied psychotherapeutic methods, e.g. Parent–Child Interaction Therapy – Emotion Development (PCIT-ED) (Luby et al. 2012). Atypical antipsychotics such as Risperdal have also been used for aggression or severe mood dysregulation (Biederman et al. 2005; Ercan et al. 2011) as well as ASD (Mire et al. 2015).

It bears restating that psychotropic medications must be used with caution in very young children. This is due to the still somewhat unknown neurobiological impact and post-exposure trajectory, lack of large, rigorous clinical trials, and side effect profiles. We know that younger children appear to be more sensitive to most psychotropic medications (Vitiello 2013), as seen, for example, in the age-related differential effects for SSRIs (e.g. heightened activation) and for antipsychotics (marked endocrine abnormalities, i.e. higher prolactin levels and more pronounced weight gain) (Gleason and Treverbaugh 2016). The PPWG guidelines should be adhered to as well as any protective state regulatory practices. Hopefully, future studies will move the science forward and allow for growth of the evidence base.

Environmental Intervention

Environmental interventions are those that identify and address environmental needs and problems that place children at risk or preclude the beneficial effect of other interventions. Eco-systemic models include modalities consistently used throughout child mental health practice, including family interventions. These models also address a child's immediate community and the wider culture. Interventions may target a variety of areas, including (i) the need for parent psychotherapy to target parental symptoms, (ii) family therapy to reduce conflict/violence and enhance family cohesion, adaptability, or coping, and (iii) broader social interventions to address systemic problems in foster/child care, the preschool setting, or socioeconomic constraints. These "ecological" interventions are grounded in general systems theories that recognize the impact of exposure to multiple stressors from multiple contexts on the young child's mental health (Bronfenbrenner 1989; Cowan and Cowan 2006). Environmental interventions are generally used in conjunction with other therapeutic intervention such as play therapy or child–parent therapy (Ammen and Limberg 2005; Limberg and Ammen 2008).

Environmental interventions are responsive to a "systems of care model" recommended by the Surgeon General's Commission on Mental Health of Children (US Public Health Service 2000), whereby the child and family have access to a wide range of services that address multiple needs. This approach requires collaboration between service agencies and providers to coordinate and create integrative care. Environmental approaches show good potential to improve outcomes for very young children and their families (Olds et al. 2007; Pulleyblank 2004).

Collaboration between Primary Care and Child Psychiatry

Early signs of existing or potential mental health problems are often first identified by the pediatric nurse practitioner (PNP), pediatrician, or other primary care provider (PCP) during routine well-baby/child visits. Parents or caregivers may raise specific concerns or the PCP may observe certain child behaviors during the general assessment, suggesting the need for further screening. In some agencies, the PCP may perform more focused screening of specific mental health concerns. In most agencies, the child is referred by the PCP to specialists in child mental health/psychiatry, including advanced practice child or family psychiatric nurses, child psychiatrists, social workers, or psychologists. In some cases, the PCP may use a telephone/email consultation or bring the mental health professional in for on-site consultation. A plan is then developed for intervention in the primary care setting or for more specialized assessment and treatment at a mental health clinic/agency.

In integrated practice environments, mental health professionals and pediatric practitioners may be housed in the same facility. This often reduces any stigma and fear regarding mental healthcare since the family is familiar with the environment. This practice setting and arrangement enhances service coordination and increases family awareness of the availability and importance of mental health services (Weiss et al. 2009).

Summary/Conclusions

Although empirical work in early childhood mental health has steadily increased over the past few decades, the need for more systematic study remains. Due to normative developmental constraints in language and cognition impacting the direct psychiatric assessment of very young children, extrapolating to this population from older groups is a risk. We know from current work in this area that some disorders are homotypic while others are heterotypic. The ongoing refinement of developmentally contextual nosologies and diagnostic systems like the DC:0–5 allows for greater sensitivity and specificity in this regard. In the future, we need to work on identifying within-group differences in the birth through 5-year age group and improve our understanding of symptoms in the first 2 years of life in particular. In addition, there is the need for continued development and refinement of psychometrically sound mental health assessments for children aged 6 and under, particularly those for problems during the first year of life. Refinement of screening tools for identification of specific mental disorders is also essential, especially internalizing disorders that are more difficult to assess in young children. The high incidence of diagnoses for ADHD and ODD in children under 6 years of age may be due, to some extent, to the clearly observable nature of externalizing problems combined with the wide availability of well-studied screening tools to assess these disorders. Additionally, although we have seen significant advances in this area over time, both preventive and treatment interventions for young children require further development and assessment for efficacy, including psychopharmacological interventions. Larger trials are necessary to demonstrate effectiveness and should include diverse populations of children and families.

There is also a need for improved education in the assessment and treatment of early childhood mental health problems. This includes offering specialized concentrations in child psychiatric and pediatric education that are appropriate to the scope of practice. Lack of expertise in the field and life-span training demands pose challenges to this educational gap, however. To address these issues, consideration of curricular adjustments with use of external experts and consultants may be considered. This is a clear clinical training need as we now have a scientific base to support the critical nature of these early years for psychological development, short- and long-term mental health status, and general health outcomes.

Resources

American Academy of Child and Adolescent Psychiatry. http://www.aacap.org.

American Academy of Pediatrics, Bright Futures Initiative. http://brightfutures.aap.org.

Center for Play Therapy. http://cpt.unt.edu.

Center on the Developing Child. Harvard University. https://developingchild.harvard.edu.

Head Start Programs, US Department of Health and Human Services, Administration for Children and Families. http://www.acf.hhs.gov/programs/ohs.

Center for Healthier Children, Families & Communities at UCLA. http://www.healthychild.ucla.edu.

National Child Traumatic Stress Network. https://www.nctsn.org.

National Institute of Mental Health, Medication Resource List. http://www.nimh.nih.gov/health/publications/mental-health-medications/alphabetical-list-of-medications.shtml.

Zero to Three: Center for Infants, Toddlers and Families. https://www.guidestar.org/profile/52-1105189.

Further reading

Buysse, V. and Wesley, P. (2006). *Evidence-Based Practice in the Early Childhood Field*. Washington, DC: National Center for Infants, Toddlers, and Families.

Cicchetti, D. (ed.) (2016). *Developmental Psychopathology, Maladaptation and Psychopathology*, vol. 3 of Developmental psychopathology. Wiley.

DelCarmen-Wiggins, R. and Carter, A. (eds.) (2004). *Handbook of Infant, Toddler and Preschool Mental Health Assessment*. New York, NY: Oxford University Press.

Ensher, G. and Clark, D. (2016). *The Early Years: Foundations for Best Practice with Special Children and their Families*. Washington, DC: National Center for Infants, Toddlers and Families.

Finello, K. (2005). *Handbook of Training and Practice in Infant and Preschool Mental Health*. New York, NY: Josssey Bass.

Hankin, B. and Abela, F. (2005). *Development of Psychopathology*. Thousand Oaks, CA: Sage Publications.

Keilty, B. (ed.) (2016). *The Early Intervention Guidebook for Families and Professionals: Partnering for Success*. New York, NY: Teachers College Press.

Luby, J.L. (2016). *Handbook of Preschool Mental Health: Development, Disorders and Treatment*, 2e. New York, NY: Guilford Press.

Maldonado-Duran, J.M. (2008). *Infant and Toddler Mental Health: Models of Clinical Intervention with Infants and their Families*. Washington, DC: American Psychiatric Publishing, Inc.

Papousek, M., Schieche, M., and Wurmser, H. (2007). *Disorders of Behavioral and Emotional Regulation in the First Years of Life: Early Risks and Intervention in the Developing Parent-Infant Relationship*. Washington, DC: National Center for Infants, Toddlers, and Families.

Parlakian, R. (2004). *How Culture Shapes Social–Emotional Development: Implications for Practice in Infant-Family Programs*. Washington, DC: National Center for Infants, Toddlers, and Families.

Sameroff, A.T., McDonough, S.C., and Rosenblum, K.L. (eds.) (2005). *Treating Parent–Infant Relationship Problems: Strategies for Intervention*. New York, NY: Guilford Press.

Shonkoff, J. and Meisels, S.J. (eds.) (2000). *Handbook of Early Childhood Intervention*. Cambridge, UK: Cambridge University Press.

Shonkoff, J. and Phillips, D. (2000). *From Neurons to Neighborhoods: The Science of Early Childhood Development*. Washington, DC: National Academies Press.

Zeanah, C. (2018). *Handbook of Infant Mental Health*, 4e. New York, NY: Guilford Press.

Zeanah, P., Stafford, B., and Zeanah, C. (2005). *Clinical Interventions to Enhance Infant Mental Health: A Selective Review*. Los Angeles, CA: National Center for Infant and Early Childhood Health Policy at University of California Los Angeles.

Zero to Three (2016). *Diagnostic Classification of Mental Health and Developmental Disorders of Infancy and Early Childhood. (DC:0–5)*. Washington, DC: National Center for Infants, Toddlers and Families.

References

Abidin, R.R. (2012). *Parenting Stress Index, Fourth Edition (PSI-4)*. Lutz, FL: Psychological Assessment Resources.

Achenbach, T. & Rescorla, L.A. (2000). *Manual for the ASEBA preschool forms and profiles: An integrated system of multi-informant assessment*. Available at http://www.aseba.org/aboutus/recentadvances.html.

Achenbach System of Empirically Based Assessment (2012). *The Multicultural Supplement to the Manual for the ASEBA Preschool Forms & Profiles*. Available at http://www.aseba.org/aboutus/recentadvances.html.

Achenbach System of Empirically Based Assessment. (2018) *DSM Guide for the ASEBA*. Available at http://www.aseba.org/aboutus/recentadvances.html.

Achenbach, T., Krukowski, R., Dumenci, L., and Ivanova, M. (2005). Assessment of adult psychopathology: meta-analyses and implications of cross-informant correlations. *Psychological Bulletin* 131: 361–382.

Ali, M.M., Teich, J., Lynch, S., and Mutter, R. (2018). Utilization of mental health services by preschool-aged children with private insurance coverage. *Administration & Policy in Mental Health* 45 (5): 731–740. https://doi.org/10.1007/s10488-018-0858-x.

AACAP (1997a). Practice parameters for the psychiatric assessment of children and adolescents. *Journal of the American Academy of Child and Adolescent Psychiatry* 36 (10 suppl): 4s–20s.

AACAP (1997b). Practice parameters for the psychiatric assessment of infants and toddlers (0-36 months). *Journal of the American Academy of Child and Adolescent Psychiatry* 36 (10 suppl): 21s–36s.

APA (2000). *Diagnostic and Statistical Manual of Mental Disorders* (4th edition, text revision). Washington, DC: American Psychiatric Press.

APA (2013). *Diagnostic and Statistical Manual of Mental Disorders*, 5e. Washington, DC: American Psychiatric Press.

Ammen, S. and Limberg, B. (2005). Play therapy with preschoolers using the ecosystemic model. In: *Handbook of Training and Practice in Infant and Preschool Mental Health* (ed. K. Finello), 207–232. New York, NY: Jossey Bass.

Angold, A. and Egger, H.L. (2007). Preschool psychopathology: lessons for the lifespan. *Journal of Child Psychology and Psychiatry* 48 (10): 961–966.

Bakermans-Kranenburg, M., Van IJzendoorn, M., and Juffer, F. (2003). Less is more: meta-analysis of sensitivity and attachment interventions in early childhood. *Psychological Bulletin* 129: 195–215.

Bayley, N. (2000). *Bayley Scales of Infant Development*, 3e. San Antonio, TX: Psychological Corporation.

Benham, A.L. (2000). The observation and assessment of young children including use of the infant-toddler mental status exam. In: *Handbook of Infant Mental Health*, 2e (ed. C.H. Zeanah), 249–266. New York, NY: The Guilford Press.

Benham, A.L. and Slotnick, C.F. (2006). Play therapy: integrating clinical and developmental perspectives. In: *Handbook of Preschool Mental Health* (ed. J.L. Luby), 331–371. New York, NY: Guilford Press.

Biederman, J., Mick, E., Wozniak, J. et al. (2005). An open-label trial of risperidone in children and adolescents with bipolar disorder. *Journal of Child and Adolescent Psychopharmacology* 15 (2): 311–317. https://doi.org/10.1089/cap.2005.15.311.

Bienenfeld, D. (2006). *Psychodynamic Theory for Clinicians*. Philadelphia, PA: Lippincott, Williams & Wilkins.

Birmaher, B., Ehmann, M., Axelson, D.A. et al. (2009). Schedule for Affective Disorders and Schizophrenia for School-Age Children (K-SADS-PL) for the assessment of preschool children- a preliminary psychometric study. *Journal of Psychiatric Research* 43 (7): 680–686. https://doi.org/10.1016/j.jpsychires.2008.10.003.

Blandon, A., Calkins, S., Keane, S., and O'Brien, M. (2008). Individual differences in trajectories of emotion regulation processes: the effects of maternal depressive symptomatology and children's physiological regulation. *Developmental Psychology* 44: 1110–1123.

Boyce, W.T. and Ellis, B. (2005). Biological sensitivity to context: an evolutionary developmental theory of the origins and functions of stress reactivity. *Development and Psychopathology* 17: 271–301.

Brazelton, T.B. and Nugent, K. (1995). *The Neonatal Behavioral Assessment Scale*. Cambridge, MA: MacKeith Press.

BRIGANCE® A. *Inventory of Early Development-II*. (2006) Curriculum Associates, North Billerica, MA.

Briggs-Gowan, M.J. and Carter, A.S. (2008). Social-emotional screening status in early childhood predicts elementary school outcomes. *Pediatrics* 121: 957–962.

Briggs-Gowan, M.J., Carter, A.S., Irwin, I.R. et al. (2004). The brief infant-toddler social emotional assessment: screening for social-emotional problems and delays in competence. *Journal of Pediatric Psychology* 29: 143–155.

Briggs-Gowan, M.J., Carter, A.S., Bosson-Heenan, J. et al. (2006). Are infant toddler social-emotional and behavioral problems transient? *Journal of the American Academy of Child & Adolescent Psychiatry* 45 (7): 849–858.

Bronfenbrenner, U. (1989). Ecological systems theory. In: *Annals of Child Development* (ed. R. Vasta), 187–248. Greenwich, CT: JAI.

Bufferd, S.J., Dougherty, L.R., Carlson, G.A. et al. (2012). Psychiatric disorders in preschoolers: continuity from ages 3 to 6. *American Journal of Psychiatry* 169 (11): 1157–1164. https://doi.org/10.1176/appi.ajp.2012.12020268.

Carter, A., Briggs-Gowan, M.J., Jones, S., and Little, T.D. (2003). The infant-toddler socio-emotional assessment: factor structure, reliability, and validity. *Journal of Abnormal Child Psychology* 31: 495–514.

Carter, A., Briggs-Gowan, M.J., and Davis, N. (2004). Assessment of young children's social-emotional development and psychopathology: recent advances and recommendations for practice. *Journal of Child Psychology and Psychiatry* 45: 109–134.

Carter, A.S., Wagmiller, R.J., Gray, S.A. et al. (2010). Prevalence of DSM-IV disorder in a representative, healthy birth cohort at school entry: sociodemographic risks and social adaptation. *Journal of the American Academy of Child & Adolescent Psychiatry* 49 (7): 686–698. https://doi.org/10.1016/j.jaac.2010.03.018.

Cassidy, J. and Shaver, P.R. (eds.) (2016). *Handbook of Attachment: Theory, Research and Clinical Applications*, 3e. New York, NY: Guilford Press.

Chethik, M. (2000). *Techniques of Child Therapy: Psychodynamic Strategies*, 2e. New York, NY: Guilford Press.

Chirdkiatgumchai, V., Xiao, H., Fredstrom, B.K. et al. (2013). National trends in psychotropic medication use in young children: 1994–2009. *Pediatrics* 132 (4): 615–623. https://doi.org/10.1542/peds.2013-1546.

Cicchetti, D. (2016). *Developmental Psychopathology, Maladaptation and Psychopathology*. Wiley.

Cicchetti, D. and Curtis, W.J. (2006). The developing brain and neural plasticity: implications for normality, psychopathology and resilience. In: *Developmental Psychopathology: Theory and Method*, vol. 2 (eds. D. Cicchetti and D. Cohen), 26–33. Hoboken, NJ: Wiley.

Clark, R. (1985). *The Parent-Child Early Relational Assessment: Instrument and Manual*. Madison, WI: University of Wisconsin Medical School, Department of Psychiatry.

Cordeiro, M., Caldeira da Silva, P., and Goldschmidt, T. (2003). Diagnostic classification: results from a clinical experience of three years with DC:0–3. *Infant Mental Health Journal* 24: 349–364.

Cowan, P. and Cowan, C. (2006). Developmental psychopathology from family systems and family risk factors perspectives: implications for family research, practice and policy. In: *Developmental Psychopathology: Theory and Method* (eds. D. Cicchetti and D. Cohen), 530–587. Hoboken, NJ: Wiley.

Cox, J.L., Holden, J.M., and Sagovsky, R. (1987). Detection of postnatal depression: development of the 10–item Edinburgh postnatal depression scale. *British Journal of Psychiatry* 150: 782–786.

Crowell, J.A. and Fleischman, M. (1993). Use of structured research procedures in clinical assessment of infants. In: *Handbook of Infant Mental Health* (ed. C. Zeanah), 210–221. New York: Guilford Press.

Davies, D. (2011). *Child Development: A Practitioner's Guide*, 3e. New York, NY: Guilford Press.

Deblinger, E., Stauffer, L., and Steer, R. (2001). Comparative efficacies of supportive and cognitive behavioral group therapies for young children who have been sexually abused and their non-offending mothers. *Child Maltreatment* 6: 332–343.

Dougherty, L.R., Smith, V.C., Bufferd, S.J. et al. (2013). Preschool irritability: longitudinal associations with psychiatric disorders at age 6 and parental psychopathology. *Journal of the American Academy of Child & Adolescent Psychiatry* 52 (12): 1304–1313. https://doi.org/10.1016/j.jaac.2013.09.007.

Dougherty, L.R., Barrios, C.S., Carlson, G.A., and Klein, D.N. (2017). Predictors of later psychopathology in young children with disruptive mood dysregulation disorder. *Journal of Child & Adolescent Psychopharmacology* 27 (5): 396–402. https://doi.org/10.1089/cap.2016.0144.

Drury, S.S., Gleason, M.M., Theall, K.P. et al. (2012a). Genetic sensitivity to the caregiving context: the influence of 5httlpr and BDNF val66met on indiscriminate social behavior. *Physiology & Behavior* 106 (5): 728–735. https://doi.org/10.1016/j.physbeh.2011.11.014.

Drury, S.S., Theall, K., Gleason, M.M. et al. (2012b). Telomere length and early severe social deprivation: linking early adversity and cellular aging. *Molecular Psychiatry* 17 (7): 719–727. https://doi.org/10.1038/mp.2011.53.

Egger, H. (2009). Psychiatric assessment of young children. *Child and Adolescent Psychiatric Clinics of North America* 18: 559–580.

Egger, H. and Angold, A. (2006). Common emotional and behavioral disorders in preschool children: presentation, nosology, and epidemiology. *Journal of Child Psychology and Psychiatry* 47: 313–337.

Egger, H.L., Ascher, B.H., and Angold, A. (1999). *The Preschool Age Psychiatric Assessment: Version I.I.* Unpublished interview schedule. Durham, NC: Center for Developmental Epidemiology, Department of Psychiatry and Behavior Sciences, Duke University Medical Center.

Emde, R. (2016). Building a solid platform for the diagnostic classification of mental health and developmental disorders of infancy and early childhood (DC:0–5). *Infant Mental Health Journal* 37 (5): 521–522.

Ercan, E.S., Basay, B.K., Basay, O. et al. (2011). Risperidone in the treatment of conduct disorder in preschool children without intellectual disability. *Child and Adolescent Psychiatry and Mental Health* 5: 10–10. https://doi.org/10.1186/1753-2000-5-10.

Essex, M.J., Boyce, W.T., Hertzman, C. et al. (2013). Epigenetic vestiges of early developmental adversity: childhood stress exposure and DNA methylation in adolescence. *Child Development* 84 (1): 58–75. https://doi.org/10.1111/j.1467-8624.2011.01641.x.

Eyberg, S.M. and Bussing, R. (2010). Parent-child interaction therapy for preschool children with conduct problems. In: *Clinical Handbook of Assessing and Treating Conduct Problems in Youth* (eds. R. Mullihy, A.S. Kidman and T.H. Ollendick), 139–162. New York, NY: Springer Science + Business Media.

Fanton, J.F. and Gleason, M.M. (2009). Psychopharmacology and preschoolers: a critical review of current conditions. *Child and Adolescent Psychiatric Clinics of North America* 18: 753–771.

Finsaas, M.C., Bufferd, S.J., Dougherty, L.R. et al. (2018). Preschool psychiatric disorders: homotypic and heterotypic continuity through middle childhood and early adolescence. *Psychological Medicine* 48 (13): 2159–2168. https://doi.org/10.1017/S0033291717003646.

Frankel, K.A., Boyum, L.A., and Harmon, R.J. (2004). Diagnoses and presenting symptoms in an infant psychiatry clinic: comparison of two diagnostic systems. *Journal of the American Academy of Child and Adolescent Psychiatry* 43: 578–587.

Franz, L., Angold, A., Copeland, W. et al. (2013). Preschool anxiety disorders in pediatric primary care: prevalence and comorbidity. *Journal of the American Academy of Child & Adolescent Psychiatry* 52 (12), 1294-1303.e1291. doi: https://doi.org/10.1016/j.jaac.2013.09.008.

Gadow, K.D. and Sprafkin, J. (2000). *Early Childhood Symptom Inventory–4. Screening Manual.* Stonybrook, NY: Checkmate Plus.

Gaensbauer, T.J. and Kelsay, K. (2008). Situational and story-stem scaffolding in psychodynamic play therapy with very young children. In: *Play Therapy for Very Young Children* (eds. C.E. Schaefer, S. Kelly-Zion, J. McCormick and A. Ohnogi), 173–198. Lanham, MD: Jason Aronson.

Gaffrey, M.S. (2018). Continuity and stability of preschool depression from childhood through adolescence and following the onset of puberty. *Comprehensive Psychiatry* 86: 39–46. https://doi.org/10.1016/j.comppsych.2018.07.010.

Garcia, A.M., Freeman, J.B., Himle, M.B. et al. (2009). Phenomenology of early childhood onset obsessive compulsive disorder. *Journal of Psychopathology and Behavioral Assessment* 31 (2): 104–111. https://doi.org/10.1007/s10862-008-9094-0.

Gleason, M.M. and Treverbaugh, L.A. (2016). Updates on preschool psychopahmacological treatment. In: *Handbook of Preschool Mental Health*, 2e (ed. J. Luby), 351–373. New York: Guilford Press.

Gleason, M.M., Egger, H.L., Emslie, G.J. et al. (2007). Psychopharmacological treatment for very young children: contexts and guidelines. *Journal of the American Academy of Child and Adolescent Psychiatry* 46: 1532–1572.

Gleason, M.M., Zeanah, C.H., and Dickstein, S. (2010). Recognizing young children in need of mental health assessment: development and preliminary validity of the early childhood screening assessment. *Infant Mental Health Journal* 31 (3): 335–357. https://doi.org/10.1002/imhj.20259.

Greenhill, L., Jensen, P., Abikoff, H. et al. (2003). Developing strategies for psychopharmacological studies in preschool children. *Journal of the American Academy of Child and Adolescent Psychiatry* 42: 406–414.

Greenhill, L., Kollins, S., Abikoff, H. et al. (2006). Efficacy and safety of immediate-release methylphenidate treatment for preschoolers with ADHD. *Journal of the American Academy of Child & Adolescent Psychiatry* 45 (11): 1284–1293.

Greenspan, S.I. and Wieder, S. (2007). *Infant and Early Childhood Mental Health: A Comprehensive Developmental Approach to Assessment and Intervention.* American Psychiatric Publishing.

Guedeney, N., Guedeney, A., Rabouam, C. et al. (2003). The zero to three diagnostic classification: a contribution to the validation of this classification from a sample of 85 under-threes. *Infant Mental Health Journal* 24: 313–336.

Hagan, M.J., Gentry, M., Ippen, C.G., and Lieberman, A.F. (2018). PTSD with and without dissociation in young children exposed to interpersonal trauma. *Journal of Affective Disorders* 227: 536–541. https://doi.org/10.1016/j.jad.2017.11.070.

Heberle, A.E., Krill, S.C., Briggs-Gowan, M.J., and Carter, A.S. (2015). Predicting externalizing and internalizing behavior in kindergarten: examining the buffering role of early social support. *Journal of Clinical Child & Adolescent Psychology* 44 (4): 640–654. https://doi.org/10.1080/15374416.2014.886254.

Ingram, R.E. and Luxton, D.D. (2005). Vulnerability-stress models. In: *Development of Psychopathology: A vulnerability-stress perspective* (eds. B.L. Hankin and J.R.Z. Abela), 32–46. Thousand Oaks, CA: Sage Publications.

Ireton, H.R. (1992). *Child Development Inventories.* Minneapolis, MN: Behavior Science Systems.

Jellinek, M.S. and Murphy, J.M. (1990). The recognition of psychosocial disorders in pediatric office practice: the current status of the pediatric symptom checklist. *Journal of Developmental and Behavioral Pediatrics* 11: 273–278.

Jellinek, M.S., Murphy, J.M., Robinson, J. et al. (1988). Pediatric symptom checklist: screening school-age children for psychosocial dysfunction. *Pediatrics* 112: 201–209.

Jensen, P.S., Rubio-Stipec, M., Canino, G. et al. (1999). Parent and child contributions to diagnosis of mental disorder: are both informants always necessary? *Journal of the American Academy of Child and Adolescent Psychiatry* 38: 1560–1579.

Juffer, F., Bakermans-Kranenburg, M.J., and van IJzendoorn, M.H. (eds.) (2008). Monographs in parenting series). *Promoting Positive Parenting: An Attachment-Based Intervention.* New York, NY: Taylor & Francis Group/Lawrence Erlbaum Associates.

Keenan, K., Boeldt, D., Chen, D. et al. (2011). Predictive validity of DSM-IV oppositional defiant and conduct disorders in clinically referred preschoolers. *Journal of Child Psychology & Psychiatry & Allied Disciplines* 52 (1): 47–55.

Kollins, S., Greenhill, L., Swanson, J. et al. (2006). Rationale, design, and methods of the Preschool ADHD Treatment Study (PATS). *Journal of the American Academy of Child & Adolescent Psychiatry* 45 (11): 1275–1283. https://doi.org/10.1097/01.chi.0000235074.86919.dc.

Kroenke, K., Spitzer, R.L., and Williams, J.B. (2003). The Patient Health Questionnaire-2: validity of a two-item depression screener. *Medical Care* 41 (11): 1284–1292.

Lahey, B.B., Pelham, W.E., Loney, J. et al. (2004). Three-year predictive validity of DSM-IV attention deficit hyperactivity disorder in children diagnosed at 4-6 years of age. *American Journal of Psychiatry* 161 (11): 2014–2020.

Landreth, G. (2002a). *Play Therapy: The Art of the Relationship.* New York, NY: Brunner-Routledge.

Landreth, G. (2002b). *Innovations in Play Therapy.* New York, NY: Brunner-Routledge.

Landreth, G. and Bratton, S. (2006). *Child-Parent Relationship Therapy.* New York, NY: Routledge.

Lavigne, J.V., Arend, R., Rosenbaum, D. et al. (1998). Psychiatric disorders with onset in the preschool years: I. stability of diagnoses. *Journal of the American Academy of Child and Adolescent Psychiatry* 37 (12): 1246–1254. https://doi.org/10.1097/00004583-199812000-00007.

Lavigne, J.V., LeBailly, S.A., Hopkins, J. et al. (2009). The prevalence of ADHD, ODD, depression, and anxiety in a community sample of 4 year-olds. *Journal of Clinical Child & Adolescent Psychology* 38: 315–328.

Lengua, L.J., Moran, L., Zalewski, M. et al. (2015). Relations of growth in effortful control to family income, cumulative risk, and adjustment in preschool-age children. *Journal of Abnormal Child Psychology* 43 (4): 705–720. https://doi.org/10.1007/s10802-014-9941-2.

Lieberman, A.F. and Van Horn, P. (2009). Child-parent psychotherapy: a developmental approach to mental health treatment in infancy and early childhood. In: *Handbook of Infant Mental Health*, 3e (ed. C.H. Zeanah Jr.), 439–449. New York, NY: Guilford Press.

Lieberman, A.F., Van Horn, P., and Ghosh-Ippen, C. (2005). Toward evidence-based treatment: child-parent psychotherapy with preschoolers exposed to marital violence. *Journal of the American Academy of Child and Adolescent Psychiatry* 44: 1241–1248.

Lieberman, A.F., Ghosh-Ippen, C., and Van Horn, P. (2006). Child-parent psychotherapy: 6 month follow up of a randomized controlled trial. *Journal of the American Academy of Child and Adolescent Psychiatry* 45: 913–918.

Limberg, B. and Ammen, S. (2008). Ecosystemic play therapy with infants, toddlers and their families. In: *Play Therapy for Very Young Children* (eds. C. Schaefer, P. Kelly-Zion and J. McCormick), 103–124. New York, NY: Jason Aronson.

Luby, J. and Belden, A. (2012). Depressive-symptom onset during toddlerhood in a sample of depressed preschoolers: implications for future investigations of major depressive disorder in toddlers. *Infant Mental Health Journal* 33 (2): 139–147. https://doi.org/10.1002/imhj.21314.

Luby, J., Si, X., Belden, A. et al. (2009). Preschool depression: homotypic continuity and course over 24 months. *Archives of General Psychiatry* 66 (8): 897–905.

Luby, J., Lenze, S., and Tillman, R. (2012). A novel early intervention for preschool depression: findings from a pilot randomized controlled trial. *Journal of Child Psychology and Psychiatry* 53 (3): 313–322. https://doi.org/10.1111/j.1469-7610.2011.02483.x.

Luby, J.L., Belden, A., Harms, M.P. et al. (2016). Preschool is a sensitive period for the influence of maternal support on the trajectory of hippocampal development. *Proceedings of the National Academy of Sciences* 113 (20): 5742–5747. https://doi.org/10.1073/pnas.1601443113.

Lucas, C.P., Fisher, P., and Luby, J. (1998). *Young-Child DISC-IV Research Draft: Diagnostic Interview Schedule for Children*. New York: Columbia University, Division of Child Psychiatry.

Marvin, R., Cooper, G., Hoffman, K., and Powell, B. (2002). The circle of security project: attachment-based intervention with caregiver-preschool child dyads. *Attachment and Human Development* 4: 107–124.

McCain, A., Kelley, M., and Fishbein, J. (1999). Behavioral screening in well-child care: validation of the toddler behavior screening inventory. *Journal of Pediatric Psychology* 24: 415–422.

McCall, R.B., Groark, C.J., and Fish, L. (2010). A caregiver-child social/emotional and relationship rating scale (CCSERRS). *Infant Mental Health Journal* 31: 201–219.

McDonough, S.C. (2004). Interaction guidance: promoting and guiding the caregiving relationship. In: *Treating Parent-Infant Relationship Problems: Strategies for Intervention* (eds. A. Sameroff, S. McDonough and K. Rosenblum), 79–96. New York, NY: Guilford Press.

McMahon, R.J. and Forehand, R.L. (2003). Helping the Noncompliant Child). *Family-Based treatment for Oppositional Behavior*, 2e. New York, NY: Guilford Press.

McNeil, C., Norman, C.M., and Wallace, N. (2015) Parent-child interaction therapy (PCIT). In R.L. Cautin and S.O. Lilienfeld (eds), *The Encyclopedia of Clinical Psychology*, Volume IV. Malden, MA: Wiley.

Measelle, J.R., Ablow, J.C., Cowan, P.A., and Cowan, C.P. (1998). Assessing young children's views of their academic social and emotional lives: an evaluation of the self-perception scales of the Berkeley puppet interview. *Child Development* 69: 1556–1576.

Mire, S.S., Raff, N.S., Brewton, C.M., and Goin-Kochel, R.P. (2015). Age-related trends in treatment use for children with autism spectrum disorder. *Research in Autism Spectrum Disorders* 15-16: 29–41. https://doi.org/10.1016/j.rasd.2015.03.001.

Monk, C., Spicer, J., and Champagne, F.A. (2012). Linking prenatal maternal adversity to developmental outcomes in infants: the role of epigenetic pathways. *Development & Psychopathology* 24 (4): 1361–1376. https://doi.org/10.1017/S0954579412000764.

Morawska, A. and Sanders, M.R. (2006). Self-administered behavioral family intervention for parents of toddlers: part I. Efficacy. *Journal of Consulting and Clinical Psychology* 74: 10–19.

Mouton-Simien, P., McCain, A.P., and Kelley, M.L. (1997). The development of the toddler behavior screening inventory. *Journal of the Abnormal Child Psychology* 2: 59–61.

Muir, E., Lojkasek, M., and Cohen, N. (1999). *Watch, Wait and Wonder*. Toronto, ON: Hincks-Dellcrest Institute.

Mullen, E.M. (1995). *Mullen Scales of Early Learning*. Circle Pines, MN: American Guidance Service.

Navsaria, N. and Luby, J. (2016). Assessing the preschool age child. In: *Dulcan's Textbook of Child and Adolescent Psychiatry*, 2e (ed. M. Dulcan), 37–55. Arlington, VA: American Psychiatric Publishing.

Newborg, J. (2004). *Battelle Developmental Inventory*, 2e. Itasca, IL: Riverside Publishing.

Olds, D., Sadler, L., and Kitzman, H. (2007). Programs for parents of infants and toddlers: recent evidence from randomized trials. *Journal of Child Psychology and Psychiatry* 48: 355–391.

Olfson, M., Crystal, S., Huang, C., and Gerhard, T. (2009). Trends in antipsychotic drug use by very young, privately insured children. *Journal of the American Academy of Child & Adolescent Psychiatry* 49 (1): 13–23.

Pennap, D., Burcu, M., Safer, D.J., and Zito, J.M. (2018a). The impact of a state medicaid peer-review authorization program on pediatric use of antipsychotic medications. *Psychiatric Services* 69 (3): 293–299. https://doi.org/10.1176/appi.ps.201700177.

Pennap, D., Zito, J.M., Santosh, P.J. et al. (2018b). Patterns of early mental health diagnosis and medication treatment in a medicaid-insured birth cohort. *JAMA Pediatrics* 172 (6): 576–584. https://doi.org/10.1001/jamapediatrics.2018.0240.

Posner, K., Melvin, G.A., Murray, D.W. et al. (2007). Clinical presentation of attention-deficit/hyperactivity disorder in preschool children: the Preschoolers with Attention-Deficit/Hyperactivity Treatment Study (PATS). *Journal of Child and Adolescent Psychopharmacology* 17 (5): 547–562. https://doi.org/10.1089/cap.2007.0075.

Provence, S., Erickson, J., Vater, S. et al. (2016). *Infant-Toddler Developmental Assessment Administration Manual*. Pro-Ed.

Pulleyblank, C.E. (2004). The heart of the matter: integration of ecosystemic family therapy practices with systems of care mental health services for children and families. *Family Process* 43: 161–173.

Renk, K. and Phares, V. (2004). Cross-informant ratings of social competence in children and adults. *Clinical Psychology Review* 24: 239–254.

Reynolds, C.R. and Kamphaus, R.W. (1992). *Behavior Assessment System for Children: Manual*. Circle Pines, MN: American Guidance Service.

Reynolds, C.R. and Kamphaus, R.W. (2002). *The Clinician's Guide to the Behavior Assessment System for Children*. Paris, France: Laviosier.

Riddle, M.A., Yershova, K., Lazzaretto, D. et al. (2013). The Preschool Attention-Deficit/Hyperactivity Disorder Treatment Study (PATS)

6-year follow-up. *Journal of the American Academy of Child & Adolescent Psychiatry* 52 (3), 264-278.e262. doi: https://doi.org/10.1016/j.jaac.2012.12.007.

Rohner, R. (2005). *Handbook for the Study of Parental Acceptance and Rejection: The Parental Acceptance-Rejection Test Manual.* Storrs, CT: University of Connecticut Press.

Russ, S.W. (2004). *Play in Child Development and Psychotherapy: Toward Empirically Supported Practice.* Mahwah, NJ: Erlbaum.

Schaefer, C.E., Kelly-Zion, P., McCormick, J., and Ohnogi, A. (eds.) (2008). *Play Therapy for Very Young Children.* New York, NY: Jason Aronson.

Scheeringa, M.S. and Haslett, N. (2010). The reliability and criterion validity of the diagnostic infant and preschool assessment: a new diagnostic instrument for young children. *Child Psychiatry & Human Development* 41 (3): 299–312.

Scheeringa, M.S., Peebles, C.C., Cook, C.A., and Zeanah, C.H. (2001). Toward establishing procedural, criterion, and discriminant validity for PTSD in early childhood. *Journal of the American Academy of Child and Adolescent Psychiatry* 40: 52–60.

Scheeringa, M.S., Salloum, A., Arnberger, R. et al. (2007). Feasibility and effectiveness of cognitive-behavioral therapy for PTSD in preschool children: two case reports. *Journal of Traumatic Stress* 20: 631–636.

Scheeringa, M., Weems, C., Cohen, J. et al. (2011). Trauma-focused cognitive-behavioral therapy for posttraumatic stress disorder in three-through six year-old children: a randomized clinical trial. *Journal of Child Psychology and Psychiatry* 52 (8): 853–860. https://doi.org/10.1111/j.1469-7610.2010.02354.x.

Scheeringa, M.S., Myers, L., Putnam, F.W., and Zeanah, C.H. (2012). Diagnosing PTSD in early childhood: an empirical assessment of four approaches. *Journal of Traumatic Stress* 25 (4): 359–367. https://doi.org/10.1002/jts.21723.

Scorza, P., Duarte, C.S., Hipwell, A.E. et al. (2018). Research review: intergenerational transmission of disadvantage: epigenetics and parents' childhoods as the first exposure. *Journal of Child Psychology & Psychiatry & Allied Disciplines* 23: 23. https://doi.org/10.1111/jcpp.12877.

Sheldrick, R.C., Henson, B.S., Merchant, S. et al. (2012). The Preschool Pediatric Symptom Checklist (PPSC): development and initial validation of a new social/emotional screening instrument. *Academic Pediatrics* 12 (5): 456–467.

Sheldrick, R.C., Henson, B.S., Neger, E.N. et al. (2013). The baby pediatric symptom checklist: development and initial validation of a new social/emotional screening instrument for very young children. *Academic Pediatrics* 13 (1): 72–80.

Shonkoff, J.P., Boyce, W.T., and McEwen, B.S. (2009). Neuroscience, molecular biology, and the childhood roots of health disparities: building a new framework for health promotion and disease prevention. *Journal of the American Medical Association* 301: 2252–2259.

Sparrow, S.S., Cicchetti, D.V., and Balla, D. (2005). *Vineland Adaptive Behavior Scales*, 2e. Circle Pines, MN: American Guidance Service.

Spitzer, R.L., Kroenke, K., and Williams, J.B. (1999). Validation and utility of a self-report version of the prime-MD: the PHQ primary care study. Primary care evaluation of mental disorders. Patient health questionnaire. *JAMA* 282 (18): 1737–1744.

Sprafkin, J., Volpe, R., Gadow, K. et al. (2002). A DSM-IV referenced screening instrument for preschool children: the early childhood symptom inventory. *Journal of the American Academy of Child and Adolescent Psychiatry* 41: 604–612.

Squires, J. and Bricker, D. (2009). *Ages and Stages Questionnaire: Users Guide.* Baltimore, MD: Paul H. Brookes Publishing.

Sterba, S., Egger, H.L., and Angold, A. (2007). Diagnostic specificity and nonspecificity in the dimensions of preschool psychopathology. *Journal of Child Psychology and Psychiatry* 48 (10): 1005–1013.

Straus, M. and Mattingly, M. (2007). *A Short Form and Severity Level Types for the Parent-Child Conflict Tactics Scales.* Durham, NH: Family Research Laboratory, University of New Hampshire.

Straus, M., Hamby, S., Finkelhor, D. et al. (1998). Identification of child maltreatment with the parent-child conflict tactics scales: development and psychometric data for a national sample of American parents. *Child Abuse and Neglect* 22: 249–270.

Summner, S. and Spietz, A. (1994). *NCAST: Caregiver/Parent Interaction Feeding and Teaching Scales.* Seattle, WA: University of Washington.

Tamm, L., Swanson, J., Lerner, M. et al. (2005). Intervention for preschoolers at risk for attention-deficit hyperactivity disorder (ADHD): service before diagnosis. *Clinical Neuroscience Research* 5: 247–253.

Task Force on Research Diagnostic Criteria: Infancy and Preschool (2003). Research diagnostic criteria for infants and preschool children: the process and empirical support. *Journal of the American Academy of Child & Adolescent Psychiatry* 42 (12): 1504–1512.

Thomas, J. and Guskin, K. (2001). Disruptive behavior in young children: what does it mean? *Journal of the American Academy of Child and Adolescent Psychiatry* 40: 44–51.

US Public Health Service (2000). *Report of the Surgeon general's Conference on Children's Mental Health.* Washington, DC: US Public Health Service.

Vitiello, B. (2013). Developmental aspects of pediatric psychopharmacology. In: *Clinical Manual of Child and Adolescent Psychopharmacology (Second Edition)* (eds. M. McVoy and R. Findling), 1–30. Washington, DC: American Psychiatric Publishing.

Wakschlag, L., Briggs-Gowan, M., Hill, C. et al. (2008a). Observational assessment of preschool disruptive behavior, part II: validity of the Disruptive Behavior Diagnostic Observation Schedule (DB-DOS). *Journal of the American Academy of Child & Adolescent Psychiatry* 47 (6): 632–641.

Wakschlag, L., Hill, C., Carter, A. et al. (2008b). Observational assessment of preschool disruptive behavior, part I: reliability of the Disruptive Behavior Diagnostic Observation Schedule (DB-DOS). *Journal of the American Academy of Child & Adolescent Psychiatry* 47 (6): 622–631.

Warren, S.L., Emde, R.N., and Sroufe, L.A. (2000). Internal representations: predicting anxiety from children's plan narratives. *Journal of the American Academy of Child and Adolescent Psychiatry* 39: 100–107.

Webster-Stratton, C. (2005). The incredible years: a training series for the prevention and treatment of conduct problems in young children. In: *Psychosocial Treatments for Child and Adolescent Disorders: Empirically Based Strategies for Clinical Practice*, 2e (eds. E.D. Hibbs and P.S. Jensen), 507–555. Washington, DC: American Psychological Association.

Weiss, S., Haber, J., Horowitz, J. et al. (2009). The inextricable nature of mental and physical health: implications for integrative care. *Journal of the American Psychiatric Nurses Association* 15: 371–382.

Whittingham, K., Sofronoff, K., Sheffield, J., and Sanders, M.R. (2009). Stepping stones triple P: an RCT of a parenting program with parents of a child diagnosed with an autism spectrum disorder. *Journal of Abnormal Child Psychology* 37: 469–480.

Wiggins, J.L., Briggs-Gowan, M.J., Estabrook, R. et al. (2018). Identifying clinically significant irritability in early childhood. *Journal of the American Academy of Child & Adolescent Psychiatry* 57 (3): 191–199. https://doi.org/10.1016/j.jaac.2017.12.008.

Wilens, T.E., Biederman, J., Brown, S. et al. (2002). Patterns of psychopathology and dysfunction in clinically referred preschoolers. *Journal of Developmental and Behavioral Pediatrics* 23: S31–S36.

Wright, H., Holmes, G., Stader, S. et al. (2004). Psychiatric diagnoses of infants and toddlers referred to a community mental health system. *Psychological Reports* 95: 495–503.

Zalewski, M., Lengua, L.J., Kiff, C.J., and Fisher, P.A. (2012). Understanding the relation of low income to HPA-axis functioning in preschool children: cumulative family risk and parenting as pathways to disruptions in cortisol. *Child Psychiatry & Human Development* 43 (6): 924–942. https://doi.org/10.1007/s10578-012-0304-3.

Zeanah, C.H., Berlin, L.J., and Boris, N.W. (2011). Practitioner review: clinical applications of attachment theory and research for infants and young children. *Journal of Child Psychology & Psychiatry* 52 (8): 819–833. https://doi.org/10.1111/j.1469-7610.2011.02399.x.

Zeanah, C.H., Carter, A.S., Cohen, J. et al. (2016). Diagnostic classification of mental health and developmental disorders of infancy and early childhood Dc:0–5: selective reviews from a new nosology for early childhood psychopathology. *Infant Mental Health Journal* 37 (5): 471–475. https://doi.org/10.1002/imhj.21591.

Zero to Three (1994). *Diagnostic Classification of Mental Health and Developmental Disorders of Infancy and Early Childhood (DC:0–3).* Washington, DC: National Center for Infants, Toddlers and Families.

Zero to Three (2005). *Diagnostic Classification of Mental Health and Developmental Disorders of Infancy and Early Childhood. Revised Edition (DC:0–3R).* Washington, DC: National Center for Infants, Toddlers and Families.

Zero to Three (2016). *DC: 0–5: Diagnostic Classification of Mental Health and Developmental Disorders of Infancy and Early Childhood.* Washington, DC: Zero to Three.

Zito, J.M., Safer, D.J., Valluri, S. et al. (2007). Psychotherapeutic medication prevalence in Medicaid-insured preschoolers. *Journal of Child and Adolescent Psychopharmacology* 17 (2): 195–203.

Zito, J.M., Burcu, M., McKean, S. et al. (2018). Pediatric use of antipsychotic medications before and after Medicaid peer review implementation. *JAMA Psychiatry* 75 (1): 100–103. https://doi.org/10.1001/jamapsychiatry.2017.3493.

22

Juvenile Justice Populations

Elizabeth Bonham[1] and Moriah Freeman[2]

[1] University of Southern Indiana College of Nursing, Evansville, IN, USA
[2] The New York Foundling Hospital, Astoria, NY, USA

Objectives

After reading this chapter, advanced practice registered nurses will be able to:

1. Review demographic data, risk factors, and the clinical profile for incarcerated youth.
2. Identify political and social issues affecting juvenile justice populations.
3. Discuss common comorbidities prevalent with youth in detention.
4. Review the roles and contributions of psychiatric and pediatric nurse practitioners working with juvenile offenders.

Introduction

On any day in the United States, about 60 000 youth under age 21 can be found residing in juvenile detention centers, jails, and prisons with 10 000 juveniles housed in adult prisons and jails (Sickmund et al. 2017). Youth are detained for a number of reasons, including committing a noncriminal offense (status offense), lack of an appropriate housing facility, and/or committing a criminal act. In this chapter, the authors will describe the juvenile justice population, historical information, risk factors, common physical and mental health diagnoses, special populations, nursing management of these youth, and nursing contributions to the field of juvenile justice.

During a single year, an estimated 2.1 million youth under the age of 18 are arrested in the United States. In 2016, law enforcement agencies in the United States made an estimated 856 130 arrests of persons under age 18, which is 58% less than the number of arrests in 2007. Though overall rates are declining, in 2015 courts with juvenile jurisdiction handled an estimated 884 900 delinquency cases (Office of Juvenile Justice and Delinquency Prevention [OJJDP] 2015a).

Males were involved in 72% (614 900) of the delinquency cases handled by juvenile courts in 2016. Females are the fastest growing population entering the juvenile justice system and account for more than one-fourth (29%) of the estimated 856 130 juvenile arrests in 2016 (OJJDP 2018). While the total volume of child delinquency cases handled in the juvenile courts is large, youth crime continues to decrease. The overall decline in delinquency caseloads between 2005 and 2016 was the same (49%) for both males and females.

Once incarcerated, youth are at greater risk of recidivistic behaviors. Juveniles constitute 1200 of the 1.5 million

Child and Adolescent Behavioral Health: A Resource for Advanced Practice Psychiatric and Primary Care Practitioners in Nursing,
Second Edition. Edited by Edilma L. Yearwood, Geraldine S. Pearson, and Jamesetta A. Newland.
© 2021 John Wiley & Sons, Inc. Published 2021 by John Wiley & Sons, Inc.
Companion website: www.wiley.com/go/Yearwood

people housed in federal and state prisons in this country, and nearly 200 000 youth enter the adult criminal justice system each year, most for nonviolent crimes (Campaign for Youth Justice [CFYJ] 2015). Approximately 86 900 youth under the age of 21 are detained or confined in public and private detention centers, group homes, camps, ranches, and other correctional institutions (CFYJ 2015). In addition, taxpayers may pay between $150 and $200 per day (about $58 000 annually) to detain one youth (Justice Policy Institute 2016). The physical needs of detained youth are similar to those of the general community, with increased incidences of poor dentition, untreated injuries, and sexually transmitted diseases. Mental health disorders and substance use concerns are prevalent among this group and require specific attention and treatment planning.

Significant Historical and Legal Background

History of Juvenile Justice

While juvenile delinquency has been studied for over half a century, the initial juvenile justice systems were predicated on the Society for Prevention of Cruelty to Animals (SPCA) model. By 1925, a juvenile court existed in every state except in Maine and Wyoming (Center on Juvenile and Criminal Justice [CJCJ] 2018). The notion of the court becoming the parent was termed *parens patriae*, a kind of benign community guardianship. However, in the 1970s, the legal notion of *parens patriae* gave way to due process in an attempt to assure fairness in juvenile court proceedings (Backus 2012).

Persons under the age of 18 who commit a crime will have their case heard in juvenile court (CJCJ 2018; OJJDP 2017a). This separate justice system, established approximately 100 years ago, promoted the goal of encouraging rehabilitation and protective supervision based on the individual youth's needs. In 1961, Congress enacted the Juvenile Delinquency and Youth Offenses Control Act giving authority for new methods of delinquency prevention which segued to the Juvenile Justice and Delinquency Prevention Act in 1974. This Act was reauthorized by Congress in 2018 for the first time in 16 years. Furthermore, a new requirement was added to the Act in 1988 to include a minority overrepresentation plan. The overrepresentation of people of color being incarcerated can be traced to the founding principles of America where race defined the basic structure of American society (Alexander 2012).

The 1990s in the United States brought with it a "tough on crime" attitude that made it easier to transfer youthful offenders into the criminal justice system, allowing institutional confinement to be used for even minor offenses (CJCJ 2018). Throughout the country, correctional facilities were determined to be overcrowded and conditions deteriorating, with state authorities citing widespread neglect and abuse of youth in state custody (Macallair 2010). Today, there have been major systemic reformations to improve correctional facility conditions, reduce institutional confinement, and expand community-based interventions (CJCJ 2018; OJJDP 2017c).

Criminal Responsibility

Currently there is no global consensus on the youngest age at which a child can be prosecuted for a crime. Within the United States, each individual state sets age limits for when law-violating conduct is considered "delinquent" for a child, but labeled a "crime" if the same act was committed by an adult (Juvenile Justice, Geography, Policy, Practice, and Statistics [JJGPS] 2016). According to the Child Rights International Network (CRIN), 33 states have set no minimum age of criminal responsibility, hypothetically permitting a child to be prosecuted at any age (CRIN 2018). Data collected for the National Center for Juvenile Justice provides information about the lowest age a minor's conduct can be labeled delinquent (JJGPS 2016). These numbers vary from age 6 in North Carolina, to age 10 in 10 other states. Historically, the upper age of juvenile court jurisdiction is age 18. Extended age of delinquency is up to age 21, unless otherwise determined by state law (JJGPS 2016).

Classifications of Criminality

A delinquent act is an action that is committed by a youth that an adult would be prosecuted for in criminal court, but due to the age of the child the action is within the jurisdiction of juvenile court (OJJDP 2017c). These criminal, or delinquent, acts can include crimes against persons or property, drug offenses, and crimes against public order. A criminal offense is different than a status offense, which is a nondelinquent/noncriminal offense but is illegal for underage persons (OJJDP 2017c). Examples of a status offense include underage drinking, truancy, running away from home, being ungovernable, or violating a curfew. Both delinquent/criminal offenses and status offenses are in the jurisdiction of juvenile court and charges can be brought against a juvenile. Legal terms commonly used in juvenile justice settings are listed in Appendix A for reference.

Supreme Court Rulings

Due to ongoing brain development, adolescent decision making is characterized as being susceptible to peer influence, immediate gratification, and poor forethought (Tuell et al. 2017). This evidence influenced the US Supreme Court's rationale in discerning youth culpability in significant ways. *Roper v. Simmons* in 2005 found that capital punishment for youth less than 18 years old was unconstitutional. The rationale was that a lack of maturity and underdeveloped sense of responsibility contributed to deviant behavior (Steinberg 2013). *Graham v. Florida* in 2010 ruled that life without parole for youth less than 18 years of age, and convicted of crimes other than homicide, was unconstitutional. Again, part of the rationale was based on the fact that the adolescent brain was not fully developed (Steinberg 2013). *Miller v. Alabama* in 2012 found that "states could not mandate life without parole for individuals less than 18 years old, even in the homicide cases" (Steinberg 2013).

Risk Factors for Delinquency

No single risk factor leads to delinquency (OJJDP 2015b). While some risk factors may be common among youth who commit delinquent acts, the patterns and particular combinations of risk factors are unique to that child and the context in which that child lives. It is known that the most important risks in early childhood stem from a combination of individual and family factors. At-risk youth include children who are exposed to any individual risk factor such as sexual abuse, incarcerated parents, and substance use by family members. High-risk children are determined to be "high-risk" when exposed to multiple negativistic factors, particularly when exposure is at a young age (OJJDP 2015b). An increased risk for delinquent behavior may be facilitated by individual factors, school-related factors, epigenetics, adolescent development, family, community, substance use, and homelessness.

Individual Factors

Characteristics that are directly related to, or within, a specific person may affect the likelihood of that individual engaging in violent and delinquent behavior. Such factors vary, but may originate from genetics, moral behavior, personality traits, attitudes, and negative life events. Examples of individual risk factors are antisocial behaviors and alienation, gun possession, favorable attitudes toward drug use, particularly early onset substance use, early onset of aggressive or violent tendencies, violent victimization or children exposed to violence, cognitive and neurological deficits, and mental/behavioral health disorders (Alaska Division of Behavioral Health [ADBH] 2011).

School-related Risk Factors

Academic failure and dropping out of school have been associated with the occurrence of violent behavior (le Vries et al. 2015). One theory is that exclusion from school may hinder the development of supportive social relationships, thus creating a cumulative risk for criminal

activity and behavior (Draper and Hancock 2011). Inadequate school climate, such as poorly organized instruction or negative labeling from teachers, can significantly impact the trajectory of a youth's academic pursuits and performance. Poor bonding and attachment to school may create a ripple effect, contributing to low academic aspirations, truancy, and academic failure.

Epigenetics

Epigenetics is the study of heritable changes in gene expression that do not involve changes to the underlying DNA sequence – a change in phenotype without a change in genotype – which in turn affects how cells read genes (National Institute of Health [NIH] 2019). Epigenetic change is a regular and natural occurrence, but can be influenced by factors including age, environment and lifestyle, and disease state. Childhood maltreatment and early trauma leave lasting imprints on neural mechanisms of cognition and emotion, making the study of epigenetics important as a risk factor for delinquency.

Pediatric Brain Development

Young age is associated with immature decision-making ability. The younger the youth, the less consideration is given to a decision and its consequences. Physical changes to the brain occur during development, such as synaptic pruning in neuronal connections, effecting information processing and logical reasoning (American Academy of Child and Adolescent Psychiatry [AACAP] 2016). Physiological changes, such as neurotransmitter remodeling activity, like dopamine production, may be involved with sensation-seeking activities. Myelination of prefrontal regions and subsequent prefrontal connectivity are involved with eventual higher order functions, such as planning ahead and discerning risks and consequences (AACAP 2016). These physical changes are essential in the development of coordinated thought and behavior.

Adolescent actions are more guided by the emotional and reactive amygdala and less by the thoughtful and logical frontal cortex. Exposure to drugs and alcohol during this period of development can further delay or change brain development (AACAP 2016). Based on the stage of their brain development, children and adolescents are more likely to act on impulse, get into accidents, be involved in fights, and engage in risky or dangerous behaviors. An awareness of these brain differences help parents, medical professionals, and advocates manage the behavior of adolescents.

Family

Family-based risk factors include problematic issues, such as poverty, coercive, and uninvolved parenting practices, child maltreatment and abuse, patterns of high family conflict or violence, parental mental illness, parental or sibling incarceration or criminality, and family member substance use. These issues disrupt the family environment and contribute to risk factors for delinquency (Hoeve et al. 2012; Murray and Farrington 2010). Studies have found that low parental education level and family composition (single-parent homes, youth in foster care, or the death of a parent) have a negative impact on delinquency. The absence of caring adults increases the risk for delinquent behaviors and gang involvement (OJJDP 2015b).

Community

Incarcerated youth, with a lack of familial social support, poor community monitoring, and exposure to community violence, had higher prevalence rates for high-risk sexual behaviors, suicide threats, and substance use compared to the general adolescent population (Reingle et al. 2011). Research shows that youth who have witnessed violence in their neighborhoods are more likely to engage in violent behaviors and carry weapons. The availability of alcohol, drugs, and firearms are community-level risk factors for juvenile delinquency. A community with high rates of violent crime, gang-related activity, and poor physical housing conditions increases the probability of its youth engaging in delinquent and illegal activities (OJJDP 2015b).

Substance Use

Substance use and substance use disorders are common among adolescent offenders and are associated with repeat offenses. Substance use is reported to be significantly higher among youthful offenders than for the general population. Studies of adolescent youth in the United States reveal that 56% of youth, aged 12–20, reported a lifetime use of alcohol and 40% reported using illegal drugs. These statistics are compared to 74% of youth in custody who reported a lifetime use of alcohol and 85% using illegal drugs (Sedlak and McPherson 2010).

Homelessness

Annually, over 380 000 youth in America meet the criteria for being homeless, that is, being without a home and without a parent or guardian for longer than 1 week (Pilnik 2017). Youth who experience homelessness are at risk for adverse outcomes, such as compromised health, education disruption, sexual and physical victimization, and poor nutrition and hunger (Federal Interagency Forum on Child and Family Statistics 2018). Homeless youth are often arrested or incarcerated because of their homeless status. In turn, their arrest or incarceration

may exacerbate future likelihood of being homeless. Reasons for homelessness may include parental incarceration, domestic violence, family intolerance of sexual identity, and maltreatment. More than 61% of reported runaways are females. When incarcerated for running away, these females remain in detention facilities twice as long as their male peers (Pilnik 2017).

Racial, Gender, and Ethnic Minority Groups

Historically, persons of color have been disproportionately represented in the juvenile justice system (Gase et al. 2016). The United States recognizes racial and ethnic minorities as those who identify as black, Hispanic, American Indian/Alaskan Native, Asian/Pacific Islander, and those identified as "other" (US Census Bureau 2017). Racial disparities are consistent across the various intervention points within the juvenile justice system, including arrest rates, sentencing determinations, probation or parole opportunities, and reincarceration rates (Rattan et al. 2012). The reasons for these racial and ethnic disparities remain unclear. Several studies have proposed one reason is that residential segregation in the United States increases minority contact with the juvenile and criminal justice systems (Gase et al. 2016).

These segregated areas are associated with socioeconomic disadvantage, residential instability, lack of education and economic resources, increased police presence, and higher rates of crime (Gase et al. 2016). Racial and ethnic segregation contributes to social isolation and economic disadvantages, increasing rates of neighborhood violence and decreased control over criminal activity. Whether these disparities may reflect a systematic racial and policy discrimination in criminal and juvenile justice systems or reflect disproportionate involvement of minorities in serious criminal offenses continues to be a topic of political and economic debate.

Disparities in Arrest and Incarceration

Nationwide, the ratio of the juvenile detention placement rates for minorities to that for non-Hispanic whites was 3.2 to 1, with 22 states having a ratio of more than 4 to 1 (OJJDP 2017c). In the past decade, 15 states have enacted legislation to address the over-representation of minorities in detention centers. According to the US Department of Justice and the OJJDP, between 1997 and 2015 the overall detention rate declined for all youth. Despite the overall decline, the detention rate for minority youth was more than three times that of white youth (OJJDP 2015b). The rate of detention for black youth is the highest disparity in terms of race, with black youth being detained at a rate six times that of white juveniles. Frequently, detention is an outcome of "zero-tolerance" policies in schools leading to school expulsion. This has been referred to as the "school to prison pipeline" (Cole 2019).

Meta-analysis findings from 2016 suggested that minority offenders faced greater odds of being fully prosecuted or being charged with a crime than white offenders (Wu 2016). This evidence remained constant across studies even when controlling for crime severity, criminal history, and evidentiary strength (Rattan et al. 2012). Minority disparity is stable across juvenile and adult offenders. Evidence supporting this disparity includes data collected from the 2015 National Longitudinal Surveys of Youth report, which examined juvenile justice youth from 1980 to 2000 (Stevens and Morash 2015). There was a general trend toward more punitive treatments of boys in the juvenile justice system in more recent years compared to treatment in 1980, and specifically for the treatment of racial and ethnic minority boys. These youth, once charged with a crime, were more likely to be convicted and placed in correctional institutions than non-Hispanic whites (Stevens and Morash 2015). Bias in the diagnosis and treatment of black youth has been discussed as a possible explanation for their increased involvement in juvenile justice settings.

Physical Needs of Incarcerated Youth

The health needs of youth within the correctional system are similar to those of children in the general community. Youthful offenders are considered a high-risk population and often have a history of inadequate healthcare access and unmet medical needs due to poverty, homelessness, and inconsistent healthcare services (OJJDP 2016). Experience with violence, substance abuse, sexual activity, and traumatic life events may be higher for youthful offenders than among the population of their peers.

Admission to Detention and Transfer of Care

Admission into the juvenile justice system may be the first opportunity for youth to receive comprehensive medical examinations and treatment, making continuity of care crucial upon entering detention and when transitioning back into the community. Detention center medical providers must be diligent in identifying health issues present on admission, determining if there has been, or will be, access to medical care in the community for youth. Typical primary care questions should be reviewed, including past medical/surgical/dental/family histories, medications, allergies, educational services/ learning disabilities, etc. Population-specific questioning should also be included to gather information such as prior legal involvement, offense history (including sexual and violent crimes), guardianship status, foster care history, abuse/maltreatment history, prior residential facility stays/lengths, pregnancy history, and court-mandated therapy/treatments (OJJDP 2016).

According to 2011 standards set forth by the National Commission for Correctional Health Care (NCCHC), which serves as a juvenile detention facility accreditation organization, all youth must receive a comprehensive health assessment within 7 days of admission to a detention facility, with a hands-on assessment performed by a physician, physician assistant, or nurse practitioner (NCCHC 2011). An assessment is advised to include a complete medical, dental, and mental health history, vitals, physical examination, including a genitourinary assessment, and tuberculosis screening. Laboratory diagnostic tests for sexually transmitted infections (STIs) should be determined based on risk factors, clinical judgment, and institutional guidelines.

An oral health screening is to be performed by a dentist, or a healthcare professional trained by a dentist, within 7 days of admission and a dentist-led examination within 60 days of admission. Facilities in the United States are required to provide an opportunity for the youth to request healthcare on a daily basis, and all concerns must be triaged within 24 hours of a reported complaint. Additionally, 24-hour emergency medical and dental services must be provided (NCCHC 2011). At discharge, arrangements for follow-up community care and medical management should be established prior to youth leaving the facility.

Custodial placement can make transition of medical care a challenge, particularly for youth with a history of poverty, homelessness, or limited transportation options (American Academy of Pediatrics [AAP] 2011). Continuity of care is crucial for this population and should begin at admission, with contact being made with the youth's primary care provider in the community to verify prior diagnoses, hospitalizations, medications, and ongoing treatments. In cases in which no primary care provider is found, efforts should be made to establish one in the community for the child. Federally qualified community health centers, which offer full service healthcare, might be a viable option for referral after discharge. Upon discharge, summaries of medical/dental care should be given to the outside medical provider and/or specialist. Conditions such as STIs or tuberculosis, requiring ongoing management, may need coordinated care with public health facilities (AAP 2011).

According to information provided by the Survey of Youth in Residential Placement (SYRP), collected from 7073 youth in custody in 2003, two-thirds of youth reported an unmet healthcare need, injury, concern regarding vision or hearing, dental, or other medical condition requiring intervention (Sedlak and McPherson 2010). Specific healthcare concerns for juvenile offenders include dental concerns, injuries, tuberculosis, and reproductive/sexual health.

Dental

A 30-year-old-study in a detention center in New York State identified that nearly all of the youth, 90%, required dental care (AAP 2011). A study performed in Texas between 1999 and 2003, screening 419 youth aged 12–17 years in a detention center, found that roughly half of juveniles had untreated decay and only one-fifth had preventive sealants. Asymptomatic decay and moderate gingivitis were discovered in 13.1% of the population (AAP 2011). Other research has found that approximately half of incarcerated youth have untreated tooth decay, with 6% having urgent oral health conditions including abscess, jaw fracture, or severe gum disease with bleeding (Barnert et al. 2016). It is an ongoing challenge to provide long-term dental care for this population. Numerous barriers exist prohibiting comprehensive dental treatment, as youth may be transferred to other detention facilities, records are poorly transferred, or a youth is lost to follow-up at discharge. The American Academy of Pediatric Dentistry (AAPD) recommends a routine check-up every 6 months in order to prevent cavities and other dental problems (AAPD 2013).

Medical providers should provide anticipatory guidance about practical and developmentally appropriate information for oral hygiene, dietary habits, injury prevention, substance abuse, intraoral/perioral piercings, and speech/language development (AAPD 2013). Facial trauma, resulting in fractured, displaced, or lost teeth has significant negative impact on functional, esthetic, and psychological effects on children. Age-appropriate counseling should be discussed and referrals made for necessary corrections and emergency services when required (AAPD 2013).

Injury

Incarcerated youth appear to have a higher tendency toward injury. Injuries can be traced back to various etiologies, ranging from accidental to deliberate. Approximately 25% of incarcerated US youth reported having injuries requiring medical care intervention (Barnert et al. 2016). Interpersonal violence is a significant cause of injuries for this population. In one survey, approximately 70% of incarcerated youth had been involved in a fight in the previous year, one-fourth experienced an injury requiring medical attention, and three-fourths reported fights involving a weapon (Barnert et al. 2016). The most common traumatic injury, one-third, were musculoskeletal, with one-fourth of the injuries being of a severity that the child was referred to an

outside facility for treatment. Injuries must be treated promptly by in-house detention medical providers and, when necessary, referred to specialists or emergency departments for further management.

Incarcerated populations have shown elevated rates of self-injury, including adolescents in secure facilities (Casiano et al. 2013). Self-injury is related to an increased prevalence of both psychiatric disorders and traumatic exposures. Higher rates of self-harm are found among females in numerous studies (Casiano et al. 2016). A recent review found that females were 28% more likely to report a lifetime history of self-injury, 33% more likely to report lifetime nonsuicidal cutting, and 36% more likely to report a lifetime suicide attempt (McReynolds et al. 2017). Lifetime prevalence rates for occasional and repetitive self-injury in 2018 were 21.9 and 18.4%, respectively, with 85.6% of youth endorsing a lifetime mental disorder. Due to the high prevalence of these injuries, this vulnerable population should be routinely assessed by medical personnel and detention facility staff must be trained in recognizing and handling self-harm tendencies while concurrently supporting adolescents to improve emotional regulation skills (Ludtke et al. 2018).

The high rates of traumatic brain injury (TBI) found in juvenile offenders suggests that earlier identification and intervention of brain injuries are indicated for youth. Gordon et al. (2017) found that one in four juvenile offenders met criteria for a TBI, the majority of injuries occurring prior to the adolescents' criminal offenses. History of a TBI was found to be related to youth being involved in more violent crimes and having higher levels of suicide, depression, anxiety, substance use, and maladaptive behaviors (Gordon et al. 2017).

Tuberculosis

Correctional facility residents have high rates of tuberculosis as they are housed in an environment with greater risk factors, including substance use, low socioeconomic population background, and poor access to healthcare (Centers for Disease Control and Prevention [CDC] 2017a). Luckily, few tuberculosis cases are reported in correctional facilities in children under the age of 15. The CDC) reported that from 1993 to 2017 only 19 tuberculosis cases among persons under 15 years of age were reported as residents of correctional facilities. Of the 19 cases, 13 (68%) were in a juvenile correctional facility. Between 2010 and 2017, there were four cases of tuberculosis under the age of 15, all occurring among residents of a juvenile correction facility (CDC 2017a). Detained juveniles should be screened at admission for tuberculosis with a Mantoux tuberculin skin test or blood test, according to CDC guidelines.

After admission, follow-up testing should occur at least once a year while in detention and prior to discharge (AAP 2011). The American Thoracic Society and the CDC strongly recommend direct observation therapy for the treatment of all tuberculosis patients (CDC 2017a). For further treatment instructions, the CDC and local health departments are able to facilitate early and accurate treatment recommendations.

Reproductive and Sexual Health

Incarcerated youth reported higher rates of sexual activity and reported having four or more lifetime sexual partners with significantly lower self-reported use of contraception with the most recent sexual encounter (Barnert et al. 2016).

Drug use, initiation of sexual intercourse at a young age, multiple sexual partners, and inconsistent use of condoms increases juvenile detainees' lifetime risk for developing a STI (Barnert et al. 2016). Among youth aged 12–18, a positive chlamydia infection was found in 14.8% of females from 83 juvenile detention facilities and in 6.6% of males at 123 facilities. Infections of gonorrhea were discovered at a prevalence of 3.9% of females at 71 juvenile facilities and in 1.0% of males at 118 facilities (CDC 2017b). Sexually exploited youth victims have higher incarceration rates and higher lifetime risk of contracting hepatitis C or human immunodeficiency virus (HIV). In a sample of female and male detainees aged 11–18, roughly 89% engaged in sexual activity, with the mean age of sexual initiation being 13.2 years. Females, 68.1%, were more likely than males, 31.9%, to have not used condoms in the month prior to detainment (Gowen and Aue 2011).

Approximately 1.7 million youth pass through the juvenile justice system annually, providing a unique opportunity to screen high-risk adolescents for STIs and HIV (Donaldson et al. 2013). Universal screening for chlamydia and gonorrhea for juveniles entering correctional facilities is a long-standing recommendation (CDC 2015). A major challenge to syphilis, hepatitis C, and HIV testing is that traditional methods involve blood draw and utilization of outside laboratories for analysis. Refusal of phlebotomy from youth, or transfer/ release from detention before treatment is initiated, results in poor public health outcomes for this population.

Providers working within detention centers should consider how they can improve STI and HIV treatment and prevention, including collaboration with community health and educational organizations to improve access to affordable healthcare, outpatient resources, sex education, testing services, and contraception upon release or probation from the justice system. Treatment

of STIs should be performed according to current medical guidelines, and tests for cure performed as needed (CDC 2018). While rates decrease over time, prevalence of high-risk sexual behaviors are much higher among prior juvenile delinquents than the general population (Abram et al. 2017).

Pregnancy

A study in 2003 found that 14% of incarcerated youth have a child of their own and 12% were expecting a child (Sedlak and McPherson 2010). Males, 15%, were more likely to have fathered a child compared to the 9% of females in detention who reported having a child. These statistics are significantly higher than the general population for youth of the same age group, aged 12–20, where only 2% of males and 6% of females have children.

Incarcerated female youth often have pregnancies complicated by problems such as substance abuse, posttraumatic stress disorder (PTSD), sexual abuse, and limited delivery options due to poor access to obstetric services while in detention (The American College of Obstetricians and Gynecologists [ACOG] 2012). As many as one in three girls in the juvenile justice system has been, or is currently, pregnant (National Conference of State Legislatures [NCSL] 2013; Sedlak and McPherson 2010). One recent national survey showed that only 18% of justice facilities provided pregnancy testing at admission (Saar et al. 2015).

Care for incarcerated adolescent females should be provided using the same guidelines as those who are not incarcerated, with attention to the increased risk of infectious diseases and mental health disorders common to this population. One report gathered data from 430 short- and long-term facilities and from 41 detention facility studies and evaluated obstetric services available to youth. They found that prenatal services were lacking in one-third of centers and 60% of facilities reported at least one obstetric complication (AAP 2011). Following delivery, detention centers face an additional challenge as they are not qualified, or permitted, to allow infant residency or visitation, thereby frequently forcing the placement of the youth's child into foster care (NCSL 2013). Every effort should be made for pregnant adolescents to receive routine prenatal care, access to an appropriate birthing facility, postpartum care and depression screening, and communication with foster care agencies if infants must be separated from their mothers.

Mental Health Needs of Incarcerated Youth

Research conducted over the past 10 years has expanded the understanding of the nature and prevalence of mental health disorders among the juvenile justice population.

Youth in the justice system experience substantially higher rates of mental disorders than youth in the general population (Bonham 2017; Collins et al. 2015). In one nationwide study, at least 50% of youth reported problems with anxiety, anger, and loneliness, with approximately one-fifth reporting a prior suicide attempt (Sedlak and McPherson 2010). Underwood and Washington (2016) report that 50–75% of justice-involved youth have a diagnosable mental health disorder. The National Center for Mental Health and Juvenile Justice found that approximately 80% of females in detention met the criteria for at least one mental health disorder, compared to 67% of males (Saar et al. 2015). While engaging in disruptive behavior can be a normal part of adolescent development, such behaviors are often transient. By age 28, nearly 85% of former delinquents have discontinued offending, which supports the theory that disruptive behaviors may be attributed to developmental stages (Moffitt 1993).

Youth in detention have significantly high rates of sexual and physical abuse compared with the general population, with all forms of abuse being more common in female detainees (Baglivio et al. 2014; Saar et al. 2015). Approximately 31% of females and 7% of males in juvenile detention have reported histories of being sexually abused. A National Child Traumatic Stress Network (NCTSN) literature review noted the unique link between trauma and mental health for detainees (Saar et al. 2015). At least 75% of youth in juvenile detention have experienced traumatic victimization and 93% reported exposure to adverse childhood experiences (ACEs), including child abuse, family and community violence, and serious self or family illness (Baglivio et al. 2014).

Overwhelming rates of trauma and PTSD are found among this population, more so in females, with 70% of females being exposed to some form of trauma and over 65% experiencing symptoms of PTSD (Saar et al. 2015). Females are more likely than males to have mental health diagnoses, particularly for mood and anxiety disorders, while substance use disorders have similar prevalence rates in both genders (AAP 2011). Major depression rates in detained girls was 29% and in males it was reported to be 11% (Saar et al. 2015).

Substance Use

Over 60% of youth with a mental health disorder also have a substance use disorder (National Center for Mental Health and Juvenile Justice 2014). Substance use disorders are poorly treated in the general juvenile justice population, with only 42.2% of adolescents being treated for a known substance disorder following a diagnostic interview (Mansion and Chassin 2016;

OJJDP 2017b). Mansion and Chassin (2016) conducted a study among adolescent male offenders at two detention facilities in the United States, gathering data from 1354 participants, and analyzed the ethnic and racial disparities among diagnosis and treatment for substance use and substance use disorders. This study found that minority adolescents with low to moderate levels of substance use were less likely to receive treatment services than their non-Hispanic white counterparts (Mansion and Chassin 2016). Treatment of substance abuse is relevant across all racial and ethnic backgrounds, and increased efforts must be made to address this disparity. Welty et al. (2016) concluded that gender, race, and age at detention contribute to substance use years after detention.

Substance Use Screenings

Substance use diagnoses require characterizing substance-related social consequences, dependence symptoms, and associated impairment. Diagnosing and assessing adolescent substance use can be particularly difficult for juvenile offenders as their confinement can influence false-negative results. Standardized screening methods are recommended early in the admission process to allow juveniles to be placed into community-based programs if necessary.

The National Institute on Drug Abuse (NIDA) has provided evidenced-based tools and assessment options to screen for alcohol and drug use in adolescent populations (NIDA 2018). Some of these options include self-administered or clinician-administered surveys, depending upon availability and the literacy level of the patient. The following tests can be used to screen for both drugs and alcohol and have been approved by NIDA to be administered to adolescents: Screening to Brief Intervention (S2BI), Brief Screener for Alcohol, Tobacco, and other Drugs (BSTAD), Tobacco, Alcohol, Prescription Medication, and Other Substance Use (TAPS), NIDA Drug Use Screening Tool (NMASSIST), Cut Down, Annoyed, Guilty, and Eye Opener-Adapted to Include Drug Use (CAGE-AID), and Car, Relax, Alone, Forget, Friends, Trouble (CRAFFT). Links to these resources can be found on NIDA's website for access and use (NIDA 2018).

Suicide and Suicidality

Suicide is more common among youth in juvenile detention than the general adolescent population. It is estimated that the suicide rate is 21.9 per 100 000 youth in juvenile justice facilities compared to 7 per 100 000 adolescents aged 15–19 in the general population (Teplin et al. 2015). The prevalence of lifetime suicidal ideation has been estimated to range from 16.9% to 59%, while lifetime self-injury ranges from 6.2% to 44% (Casiano et al. 2016). The average age of a first suicide attempt for juvenile delinquents is 12.7 years of age (OJJDP 2014). The most common forms of suicide are by cutting and drug overdose, similar to the general population.

In 2014, 90% of juvenile detention facilities reported that they performed suicide risk screenings on all youth, 3% evaluated "some" youth, and 7% did not evaluate any youth. Reassessment of suicide risk occurred at approximately 86% of facilities at some point during a youth's stay in detention (OJJDP 2016). Less than half of facilities used a licensed mental health professional to conduct the screening, and more than one third used neither mental health professionals nor counselors whom a mental health professional had trained to conduct suicide screenings. From the Juvenile Residential Facility Census in 2014, there were a reported five deaths from suicide, making it the leading cause of juvenile detention deaths in the United States (OJJDP 2016).

Depression is the most commonly identified predictor for both suicidal ideation and suicide attempts for this population. More than one-third of male detainees and nearly half of females felt hopeless or reported thinking a lot about death/dying in the weeks leading up to their admission to detention (OJJDP 2014). Studies have identified trauma, substance use, ACEs, particularly a history of sexual abuse, lack of parental or social support, and externalizing problems as risk factors for suicide (Teplin et al. 2015; Miller et al. 2013). This information indicates the significant need for further evaluation in the role of screening, prevention, and treatment for suicidal behavior.

Suicide Screening

Generally, detention facilities have individualized screening standards for suicide risk assessment. Providers should use their professional judgment and consult with the entire treatment team to determine if further testing or assessment interventions are indicated beyond routine screens. A suicide risk assessment test should be performed by a trained mental health professional (NCCHC 2012). Results of screenings, along with physical examination, and youth interviews help facilitate referrals to specialists needed for additional therapy and/or emergency treatment. Ongoing identification of suicide risk should be conducted throughout a youth's stay in detention as needed and on a routine periodic basis. Those with prior suicide attempts or self-harm tendencies should have special suicide precautions observed, with extra care taken to maintain a safe physical environment and increased staff monitoring (NCCHC 2012).

Mental Health Ethnic/Racial Disparities

There has been limited research performed regarding the overlap of psychiatric diagnoses and race and ethnicity among offending groups. Clinician assessment of medical compliance, patient intelligence, beliefs about the patient's likelihood of risky behavior, and beliefs about the patient's willingness to undergo treatment all influence the quality of care provided to this population. In 2012, a study was performed evaluating psychiatrists' and residents' ability to rate identical data on patients (Dana 2012). Psychiatrists saw black youth as less able to benefit from therapy based on stereotypes regarding the youth's level of introspection and sophistication. This issue of stereotyping and making racial assumptions can lead to the overdiagnosis and undertreatment of minority youth. Racial and ethnic disparities in psychiatric diagnoses do exist and must be recognized.

Baglivio et al. (2017) studied the racial and ethnic disparities in psychiatric behavioral diagnoses among serious juvenile offenders. It was determined that black males and black females were more likely to be diagnosed with conduct disorder than their white counterparts. Black and Hispanic males were less likely to be diagnosed with attention-deficit hyperactivity disorder (ADHD) than non-Hispanic white males despite controlling for behavioral indicators, prior offenses, and traumatic experiences (Baglivio et al. 2017). Research performed by the US Department of Health and Human Services (HHS) indicated that more structured clinical assessments reduce, but do not fully eliminate, racial bias (Baglivio et al. 2017). Improved cultural knowledge and elimination of racial bias involves clinician training. Untreated or undertreated psychiatric diagnoses affect the behavior of offending youth during incarceration and increase their risk for reoffense following release from detention (OJJDP 2017b).

Recommended Mental Health Assessment Instruments

There are numerous, well-known, standardized instruments to help practitioners collect information about risk factors contributing to depression, anxiety, suicidality, and substance abuse. Assessments frequently used in juvenile detention facilities include those for PTSD evaluation, neurological screenings, family relationship skills, resiliency, depression, personality, intelligence, anger, trauma, adaptive behaviors, suicidality, and recidivism risk. Two assessment instruments are presented here.

Massachusetts Youth Screening Instrument

The Massachusetts Youth Screening Instrument (MAYSI-2) has been shown to be a reliable and valid tool to identify youth with mental health needs upon entry into a detention facility (Collins et al. 2015). This 52-item standardized self-report form identifies potential mental health and substance use needs of youth at any entry or transitional point within the justice system. This assessment was designed to identify youth who report symptoms of distress, that might require immediate intervention, or who may be in need of further assessment to rule out a psychiatric disorder (Collins et al. 2015). It evaluates seven domains: alcohol/drug use, anger-irritability, depression-anxiety, somatic complaints, suicide ideation, thought disturbances for males, and trauma experiences. Criticism for this instrument includes reports that females generally scored higher on this tool than males and that the subsets may better predict severe mental illness.

Achenbach System of Empirically Based Assessment

These forms have been among checklist measures deemed useful in forensic assessments for risk of violence in juveniles (Semel 2017). These assessments utilize a multi-informant procedure with self-, teacher-, and parent-report components. Use of a multimethod, multi-informant assessment approach is essential in the assessment of juvenile delinquents, with the understanding that there are practical limitations in obtaining data from multiple sources. The Youth Self-Report of the Achenbach System of Empirically Based Assessment (ASEBA) has been associated with external correlates, including psychiatric diagnoses, antisocial cognition, family and psychosocial variables, maltreatment history, and recidivism (Semel 2017).

Mental Health Treatment and Therapy Options

Persistent disruptive behavior and child delinquency are predictors for offending later in life (AAP 2011). There is little evidence to support the notion that harsher sanctions in juvenile detention will reduce delinquency. Rather, interventions such as positive youth development and family involvement work to minimize disruptive behavior while providing a treatment-oriented and nonpunitive framework for therapy (Teplin et al. 2013). The initiation, or change of, medical treatment for psychiatric disorders while a youth is in detention is challenging. According to the Juvenile Residential Facility Census in 2014, only half of the youth in detention are placed in a facility that provides mental health evaluations of all residents and 88% of youth are in facil-

ities where mental health counselors are not licensed professionals (OJJDP 2016).

Even when youth are given a mental health diagnosis, treatment is not guaranteed. The Northwestern Juvenile Project discovered that only 15% of youth diagnosed with psychiatric disorders and functional impairment received treatment while in detention (Teplin et al. 2013). Youth with substance and mental health disorders were surveyed and a commonly cited barrier to services was that youth believed their problems would go away without getting any help. Other barriers included that youth were unsure whom to contact or where to go for help, or that it would be too difficult for them to obtain help for their problems. These barriers significantly impact whether youth pursue treatment and whether they will remain open to continuing treatment once enrolled.

Outpatient treatment is the general recommendation for first time offenders with nonviolent crime offenses and without additional psychopathology. Community-based mental health providers providing therapeutic interventions play an important role in teaching new skills, monitoring for risks of reoffense, and in managing psychological wellbeing (AAP 2011; Teplin et al. 2013). Pediatric and psychiatric medical providers involved in the care of this population should create opportunities for the youth to make healthy choices about their mental and physical health, thereby fostering a sense of independence.

Psychotropic Medication

Acute psychiatric symptoms should be treated with urgency, but medication should not be the sole means of treatment to manage behaviors. The AACAP advise that a youth's legal disposition and placement is reviewed before initiating or altering medication regimens as the length of stay in detention is often too short for most interventions to be monitored appropriately (McLaren et al. 2018). The AACAP published a document addressing mental health assessment and treatment for youth in the correctional system, advising that psychotropic medication only be used as one piece of an individual comprehensive treatment plan (McLaren et al. 2018). If medication is used, it should be in conjunction with individual, group or family therapy, along with other behavioral interventions. Initiation of new medications should be used with caution after a risk/benefit assessment is performed and alternatives for medication reviewed. Children in detention are a vulnerable population who frequently receive psychotropic medications, have high rates of polypharmacy, off-label use, and long-term medication use without adjunctive therapeutic or psychological interventions (McLaren et al. 2018).

Trauma Informed Care

Children with histories of polytrauma are found in the juvenile justice system. Trauma informed care (TIC) is an approach that recognizes trauma symptoms and the role that trauma plays in a person's life. TIC provides an effective and necessary service for children whose needs are both complex and severe. There is a growing need to train service providers in TIC and how to recognize and treat youth in a manner that does not retraumatize them but helps place them on a path toward healing (Damian et al. 2018). Service providers must set treatment goals focusing on safety and trust, recognize triggers and warning signs, manage stress, and empower youth and families (Allen et al. 2016). ACEs are stressful or traumatic events that can include abuse and neglect, having an incarcerated or mentally ill parent, or witnessing violence (Garbarino 2017). ACEs must be identified early on as they have a tremendous impact on future victimization and lifelong health consequences, making TIC a valuable therapeutic method (CDC 2016).

Cognitive Behavioral Therapy

Cognitive behavioral therapy (CBT) is one form of psychotherapy that is commonly used with youthful offenders (National Institute of Justice [NIJ] 2010). This therapy assumes that people can become conscious of their own thoughts and behaviors, and can make positive changes. This form of therapy is frequently used within the criminal justice setting, in institutions, and in community treatment centers. Research studies published between 1965 and 2005 were analyzed by Landenberger and Lipsey and they found that CBT significantly reduced recidivism, even among high-risk offenders (NIJ 2010). Characteristics addressed with this form of therapy include developmentally arrested thoughts, problem-solving abilities, egocentrism, impulsivity, and violent tendencies. This problem-focused approach helps individuals change dysfunctional beliefs, thoughts, and patterns of behavior.

Currently, CBT is the most evidence-based form of psychotherapy (David et al. 2018). Tendencies, related to the justice population, that have been particularly amenable to change through CBT include violence and criminality, substance use and abuse, teen pregnancy and risky sexual behaviors, and school failure. Combinations of CBT with family models are common for juvenile offenders. Proven successful programs include functional family therapy, multisystemic therapy, and the Michigan State Diversion Project (OJJDP 2010). These approaches attempt to integrate family and school contacts to promote change through modeling, reframing, and behavioral training.

Wraparound Therapy

Wraparound is a youth-guided, family-driven, and team process that provides individualized community-based services for youth and their families. This program emerged in the 1970s/1980s, initially as a community alternative to the institutionalization of youth with complex behavioral problems (CJCJ 2018). It is a multifaceted and coordinated intervention to keep youth at home and out of institutions when possible. As the name indicates, a "wrapping" of services and support networks around youth occurs, rather than enrollment in inflexible treatment programs (Poncin and Woolston 2016).

The National Mental Association, the US Surgeon General's Office, the National Wraparound Initiative, and the Substance Abuse and Mental Health Services Administration all have subtle differences in their definitions of what constitutes wraparound service. There is a general consensus that wraparound programs feature basic elements including a collaborative, community-based interagency team that has representatives from the justice system, public education system, and local mental health and social services agencies (CJCJ 2018). A formal interagency agreement, with care coordinators responsible for creating customized treatment programs, work with the child and their family members to ensure the child's needs are met across all domains: home, school, and in the community. A unified plan of care should be developed and updated regularly to reflect a youth's changing needs, including their progress and future goals. Enrollment may include 24/7 crisis intervention, academic tutoring, multidisciplinary therapy, after-school programs, employment training, and coordination with a wraparound team (CJCJ 2018).

Vulnerable Populations

Youth who have committed sexual offenses, female offenders, and those who self-identify as lesbian, gay, bisexual, transgender, or questioning/queer are vulnerable populations and may have additional needs while in the juvenile justice system.

Youthful Sex Offenders

A substantial portion of sex offenses against minors are committed by other minors and such perpetrators are termed juvenile sexual offenders. It was estimated that in 2014 approximately 21% of reported cases of child sexual abuse were perpetrated by juvenile sex offenders (Ryan and Otonichar 2016). Federal Bureau of Investigation (FBI) data indicate that arrest rates for sexual assault among juveniles has been declining in recent decades (FBI 2014).

Clinical Profile

There is not a single, or set, of distinguishing characteristics for juvenile sex offenders. These offenders may come from any age group or status in society. Clinical studies have identified a diversity of cultures, backgrounds, and sexual behaviors among this population (Fanniff and Kolko 2011). Social and family backgrounds can include intact family homes or those that have experienced a high burden of adversity, including abuse, poverty, maltreatment, exposure to drugs, violence, and other socioeconomic risk factors. In conjunction with a diversity in background is a diversity in motivation for criminality. Many offenders appear motivated by sexual curiosity, while others suffer from serious mental health issues or reflect impulsive, maladaptive behaviors. There are few studies on the mental illnesses prevalent among juvenile sex offenders. In a 2013 systematic review, it was estimated that 5% of juvenile sex offenders have severe mental illness, 30–40% have personality disorders, and 30% have paraphilia, abnormal sexual desires (Langstrom et al. 2013).

Rehabilitation and Recidivism

The majority of youth involved in sexual offense crimes have positive long-term outcomes, with 85–95% having no rearrests for future sexual offenses (Christiansen and Vincent 2013). According to one study of 39 248 juvenile sexual and nonsexual offenders, the reoffense rate for sexual crimes was 4.2% and the reoffense rate for nonsexual crimes, like drug use, was 40.96% (Christiansen and Vincent 2013). The major risk factors for recidivism include the selection of a stranger as a victim and deviant sexual interests (Ryan and Otonichar 2016).

Therapeutic Options for Juvenile Sex Offenders

Due to the heterogeneity of the justice population there is not a one-size-fits-all treatment plan recommended for juvenile sex offenders. Treatment that is individually tailored to the needs of the youth, via risk evaluation and psychiatric work-up, has been shown to be the best option for long-term success. Treatment must address current psychiatric disorders in addition to any deviant sexual behaviors. Due to the difficulty in obtaining accurate legal records or sexual offense histories from patients and their families, denial or minimization of

crimes is common and can lead to ineffective therapy (Craissati 2013). Particular care must be taken by clinicians involved with this population to ensure that comprehensive care is provided and treatment goals are appropriate for the individual patient.

A wide range of psychological treatments have been reported as being effective, but there is limited scientific evidence to confirm these claims. In multiple studies, multisystemic therapy was found to be the most effective, but even this option was proven to have limited evidence for reducing reoffense (Craissati 2013; Langstrom et al. 2013). CBT is a frequently used treatment for juvenile sex offenders. Criticism has arisen for this treatment method for sex offenders at a low risk for reoffense as many participants have been unresponsive to the therapy (Craissati 2013). Other treatment modalities include psychoeducation, family systems therapy, residential treatment centers, and group outpatient programs. Components of these treatment possibilities address reduction in cognitive distortions and deviant sexual arousal, attempt to resolve traumatic consequences if they themselves were victims of abuse, and enhance the management of their emotions to increase their ability to empathize with others. Problem-solving skills, age appropriate skills, and lifestyle skills are commonly taught within these therapy programs (Craissati 2013).

Female Offenders

Females tend to engage in more relational and indirect forms of aggression rather than overt physical aggression like males (Cleverley et al. 2012). Gender-specific programming for females needs to address specific risk factors, including suboptimal parenting practices, family dysfunction, maltreatment and other ACEs, and involvement with deviant peers. Females are more likely to be rejected by their prosocial peers for their behavioral problems. They are also more at risk for developing affiliations with older, deviant partners, which may increase their risk for relationship difficulties, criminality, and antisocial behaviors. Females who mature earlier have a greater risk for delinquency and mental health problems in adolescence, whereas males who are late to mature demonstrate increased disruptive behavior and substance abuse disorders in the trajectory toward adulthood (Zahn et al. 2010).

Female delinquent acts are typically less chronic and often less serious than those of males. While their offense behavior may not appear very serious, they may be fleeing victimization and illegal behavior by adults, placing them at risk for behaviors that violate the law, such as prostitution, survival sex, and drug use (Zahn et al. 2010).

Lesbian, Gay, Bisexual, Transgender, and Questioning Youth

The past decade has been instructive in naming and normalizing gender identity, gender role, and sexual orientation. The longstanding model that youth who manifest a different gender role had a psychiatric illness is being replaced with a normalizing model that includes supporting a person's identity (Olson et al. 2016). Estimates vary about numbers of lesbian, gay, bisexual, transgender, and questioning (LGBTQ) youth involved with juvenile justice systems (Development Services Group, Inc. 2014). It is estimated that 13–15% of youth in detention identify as LGBTQ compared to 5–7% in the general population (Hunt and Moodie–Mills 2012). LGBTQ youth face health disparities related to depression, suicidality, and substance use. Youth who identify as LGBTQ and are remanded to the juvenile justice system may be victimized while in detention due to deliberate or inadvertent discrimination. A 2010 survey revealed that 80% of LGBTQ youth behaved in a gender-conforming way, at least in part to avoid harassment for fear of sexual assault within the detention facility (Barnert et al. 2016). Clinicians must have a knowledge of current terminology, sensitivity to the youth's self-discovery, and awareness that this population has higher rates of depression and suicidal tendencies.

Relevant Nursing Contributions

Juvenile justice facilities offer onsite healthcare to thousands of youth annually but currently are underutilized by academic nursing institutions for educational development and instruction. Juvenile facilities in every state offer unique educational opportunities for faculty research, student learning experiences, and collaboration for the care of a vulnerable, underserved, and ethnically diverse community population. An academic partnership could enhance the progression of evidence-based practices meant to improve medical treatment for this at-risk population (Clifton and Roberts 2016).

Another nursing intervention is the community partnership nursing faculty at the University of Utah College of Nursing (UCoN) forged with juvenile justice facilities. UCoN has been serving at 10 different juvenile justice centers for the past 16 years, giving nursing students the opportunity to learn physical examination, assessment, and therapeutic techniques not frequently available in a traditional hospital or clinic setting (Clifton and Roberts 2016). UCoN established a faculty practice to care for incarcerated youths in facilities across Salt Lake

City County. Nurse practitioners hold faculty appointments with UCoN, and practice both primary and psychiatric care with patients in the detention centers. The faculty provides acute and chronic illness management and precepts undergraduate and graduate nursing students (Clifton and Roberts 2016).

Several publications demonstrate nursing influence in recent literature. One is an executive summary of a position paper (International Society of Psychiatric-Mental Health Nurses [ISPN] 2015) on the mental health needs of youth in juvenile justice (Pearson et al. 2016). The paper presents a plan to reform the juvenile justice system to aid youth with untreated mental health diagnoses.

Practice Resources for Practitioners

For psychiatric nurse practitioners who are interested in learning more about becoming effective providers for at-risk populations, the Justice Resource Institute offers an annual certificate program in Traumatic Stress Studies (Justice Resource Institute 2017). This specialized training focuses on the treatment of post-traumatic and dissociative disorders in both children and adults.

The International Association of Forensic Nursing is a nurse-founded organization that supports and complements the work of forensic nursing and practitioners throughout the world (https://www.forensicnurses.org). Nurses can access forensic nursing education, certification, and publications through membership. Another organization that nurses can be involved in for education, certification, and support is the NCCHC. Each of these organizations provides opportunities for professional nursing development, certification, and leadership.

Conclusion

Juvenile justice youth are an at-risk population with a history of unmet physical, developmental, and psychological needs. There is a current and ongoing shortage of child primary care and mental health providers throughout the United States. The limited access to healthcare funding for youth in detention, institutional variability in procedures, and lack of resources continue to be a challenge in upholding a reasonable standard of health for this population (AAP 2011). Providers must advocate for adequate medical and behavioral health services during and after incarceration.

Youth incarcerated in the juvenile corrections system are entitled to the same level and standard of medical and mental healthcare as their nonincarcerated peers.

Identifying biases, special populations, and tailoring treatment to the needs of youth promotes effective, culturally sensitive care. Ongoing support must be given to decrease the number of incarcerated youth by advocating for interventional programs in the community, addressing risk and protective factors, providing management skills for at-risk youth, and improving education for law enforcement and medical staff.

Critical Thinking Questions

1. How can nurses, nurse practitioners, and nursing educators improve the ethnic and racial disparities found in the mental and physical healthcare provided to justice-involved youth?
2. Why do you think there is such a high percentage of incarcerated youth with mental health diagnoses? Can this be changed? If so, how?
3. What are some of the main reasons children become more vulnerable to incarceration than others? What protective factors can be strengthened through preventive measures?

References

Abram, K., Stokes, M., Welty, L. et al. (2017). Disparities in HIV/AIDS risk behaviors after youth leave detention: a 14-year longitudinal study. *Pediatrics* 139 (2): 1–14. https://doi.org/10.1542/peds.2016-0360.

ADBH (2011). *Risk and Protective Factors for Adolescent Substance Use (and Other Problem Behavior)*. Anchorage, Alaska: Alaska Public Health Department, Division of Behavioral Health.

Alexander, M. (2012). *The New Jim Crow: Mass Incarceration in the Age of Colorblindness*. New York: The New Press.

Allen, O., Cocozza, J., Hill, A. et al. (2016). *Key Elements to Developing a Trauma Informed Juvenile Justice Diversion Program for Youth with Behavioral Health Conditions*. Delmar, NY: National Center for Mental Health and Juvenile Justice.

AACAP. (2016). *Teen brain: Behavior, problem solving, and decision making*. Facts for Families (95). American Academy of Child and Adolescent Psychiatry. Available at http://www.aacap.org/aacap/fffprint/article_print.aspx?dn=the-teen-brain-behavior-problem-solving-and-decision-making-095.

AAPD. (2013). *Guidelines on periodicity of examination, preventive dental services, anticipatory guidance/counseling, and oral treatments for infants, children, and adolescents*. American Academy of Pediatric Dentistry. Available at https://www.aapd.org/research/oral-health-policies--recommendations.

AAP (2011). Health care for youth in the juvenile justice system. *Pediatrics* 128 (6): 1219–1235.

ACOG (2012). Reproductive health care for incarcerated women and adolescent females. *Committee on Health Care for Underserved Women: Committee Opinion* 120: 435–429.

Backus, M. (2012). Achieving fundamental fairness for Oklahoma's juveniles: the role for competency in juvenile proceedings. *Oklahoma Law Review* 65 (1): 41–73. Available at https://digitalcommons.law.ou.edu/cgi/viewcontent.cgi?referer=https://www.google.com/&httpsredir=1&article=1086&context=olr.

Baglivio, M., Epps, N., Swartz, K. et al. (2014). The prevalence of adverse childhood experiences (ACE) in the lives of juvenile offenders. *Journal of Juvenile Justice* 3 (2): 1–23.

Baglivio, M., Wolff, K., Piquero, A. et al. (2017). Racial/ethnic disproportionality in psychiatric diagnoses and treatment in a sample of serious juvenile offenders. *Journal of Youth and Adolescence* 46 (7): 1424–1451. https://doi.org/10.1007/s10964-016-0573-4.

Barnert, E., Perry, R., and Morris, R. (2016). Juvenile incarceration and health. *Academic Pediatrics* 16 (2): 99–109. https://doi.org/10.1016/j.acap.2015.09.004.

Bonham, E. (2017). A theory of hoping for a better life grounded in youthful offender experiences. *Medical Research Archives* 5 (7): 1–16. Available at www.journals.ke-i.org/index.php/mra/article/view/1390/1136.

CFYJ. (2015). Zero tolerance: How states comply with PREA's youthful inmate standard. Campaign for Youth Justice. Available at http://cfyj.org/images/pdf/Zero_Tolerance_Report.pdf.

Casiano, H., Katz, L.Y., Globerman, D., and Sareen, J. (2013). Suicide and deliberate self-injurious behavior in juvenile correctional facilities: a review. *Journal of the Canadian Academy of Child and Adolescent Psychiatry* 22 (2): 118–124. Available at https://psycnet.apa.org/record/2013-15037-004.

Casiano, H., Bolton, S., Hildahl, K. et al. (2016). Population-based study of the prevalence and correlates of self-harm in juvenile detention. *PLoS ONE* (1): 11, e0146918. Available at https://journals.plos.org/plosone/article?id=10.1371/journal.pone.0146918.

CJCJ. (2018). *Juvenile justice history*. Center on Juvenile and Criminal Justice. Available at http://www.cjcj.org/education1/juvenile-justice-history.html.

CDC. (2015). *2015 sexually transmitted diseases treatment guidelines*. Centers for Disease Control and Prevention. Available at https://www.cdc.gov/std/tg2015/specialpops.htm.

CDC. (2016). *Adverse childhood experiences (ACEs)*. Centers for Disease Control and Prevention. Available at https://www.cdc.gov/violenceprevention/acestudy/index.html.

CDC. (2017a). *Epidemiology of tuberculosis in correctional facilities, United States, 1993–2017*. Centers for Disease Control and Prevention. Available at https://www.cdc.gov/tb/publications/slidesets/correctionalfacilities/default.htm.

CDC. (2017b). *Sexually transmitted disease surveillance 2017*. Centers for Disease Control and Prevention. Available at https://www.cdc.gov/std/stats17/2017-STD-Surveillance-Report_CDC-clearance-9.10.18.pdf.

CDC. (2018). *HIV/AIDS*. Centers for Disease Control and Prevention. Available at https://www.cdc.gov/hiv/basics/prep.html.

CRIN. (2018). *Minimum ages of criminal responsibility in the Americas*. Child Rights International Network. Available at https://www.crin.org/en/home/ages/Americas.

Christiansen, A. and Vincent, J. (2013). Characterization and prediction of sexual and nonsexual recidivism among adjudicated juvenile sex offenders. *Behavioral Sciences & the Law* 31 (4): 506–529. https://doi.org/10.1002/bsl.2070.

Cleverley, K., Szatmari, P., Vaillancourt, T. et al. (2012). Developmental trajectories of physical and indirect aggression from late childhood to adolescence: sex differences and outcomes in emerging adulthood. *Journal of the American Academy of Child & Adolescent Psychiatry* 51 (10): 1037–1051. https://doi.org/10.1016/j.jaac.2012.07.010.

Clifton, J. and Roberts, L. (2016). Innovation in faculty practice: a college of nursing and juvenile justice collaboration. *Journal of Professional Nursing* 32 (2): 94–99. https://doi.org/10.1016/j.profnurs.2015.10.007.

Cole, N.K. (2019). Understanding the school-to-prison-pipeline. Available at https://www.thoughtco.com/school-to-prison-pipeline-4136170.

Collins, O., Grisso, T., Vahl, P. et al. (2015). Standardized screening for mental health needs of detained youths from various ethnic origins: the Dutch Massachusetts Youth Screening Instrument-Second Version (MAYSI-2*). Journal of Psychopathology and Behavioral Assessment* 37 (3): 481–492.

Craissati, J. (2013). Treatment for sexual offenders against children. *British Medical Journal*: 1–2. https://doi.org/10.1136/bmj.f5397.

Damian, A., Gallo, J., and Mendelson, T. (2018). Barriers and facilitators for access to mental health services by traumatized youth. *Children and Youth Services Review* 85: 273–278. https://doi.org/10.1016/j.childyouth.2018.01.003.

Dana, R.H. (2012). Mental health services for African Americans: a cultural/racial perspective. *Journal of Human Growth & Development* 9: 63–73.

David, D., Cristea, I., and Hofmann, S. (2018). Why cognitive behavioral therapy is the current gold standard of psychotherapy. *Front Psychiatry* 9 (4).

Development Services Group, Inc (2014). *LGBTQ Youths in the Juvenile Justice System: Literature Review*. Washington, DC: OJJDP Available at https://www.ojjdp.gov/mpg/litreviews/LGBTQYouthsintheJuvenileJusticeSystem.pdf.

Donaldson, A., Burns, J., Bradshaw, C. et al. (2013). Screening juvenile justice-involved females for sexually transmitted infection: a pilot intervention for urban females in community supervision. *Journal of Correctional Health Care* 19 (4): 258–268. https://doi.org/10.1177/1078345813499310.

Draper, A. and Hancock, M. (2011). Childhood parental bereavement: the risk of vulnerability to delinquency and factors that compromise resilience. *Mortality: Promoting the Interdisciplinary Study of Death and Dying* 16 (4): 285–306.

Fanniff, A. and Kolko, D. (2011). Victim age-based subtypes of juveniles adjudicated for sexual offenses: comparisons across domains in an outpatient sample. *Sage Journals* 24 (3): 224–264. Available at https://doi.org/10.1177/1079063211416516.

Federal Bureau of Investigation. (2014). *Crime in the United States, 2010*. Available at https://ucr.fbi.gov/crime-in-the-u.s/2014/crime-in-the-u.s.-2014/persons-arrested/main.

Federal Interagency Forum on Child and Family Statistics (2018). *America's Children: Key National Indicators of Well-Being*. Washington, DC: US Government Printing Office.

Garbarino, J. (2017). ACEs in the criminal justice system. *Academic Pediatrics* 17 (7S): 32–33.

Gase, L., Glenn, B., Gomez, L. et al. (2016). Understanding racial and ethnic disparities in arrest: the role of individual, home, school, and community characteristics. *Race and Social Problems* 8 (4): 296–312.

Gordon, W., Spielman, L., Hahn-Ketter, A., and Sy, K. (2017). The relationship between traumatic brain injury and criminality in juvenile offenders. *Journal of Head Trauma Rehabilitation* 32 (6): 393–403. https://doi.org/10.1097/HTR.0000000000000274.

Gowen, L. & Aue, N. (2011). *Sexual health disparities among disenfranchised youth*. Available at https://www.pathwaysrtc.pdx.edu/pdf/pbSexualHealthDisparities.pdf.

Hoeve, M., Stams, G., van der Put, C. et al. (2012). A meta-analysis of attachment to parents and delinquency. *Journal of Abnormal Child Psychology* 40 (5): 771–785.

Hunt, J. and Moodie–Mills, A. (2012). *The Unfair Criminalization of Gay and Transgender Youth: An Overview of the Experiences of LGBT Youth in the Juvenile Justice System*. Washington, D.C.: Center for American Progress Available at http://www.americanprogress.org/wp-content/uploads/issues/2012/06/pdf/juvenile_justice.pdf.

ISPN. (2015). Meeting the mental health needs of youth in juvenile justice. International Society of Psychiatric-Mental Health Nurses. Available at https://www.ispn-psych.org/assets/docs/juvenile justicemh.pdf.

Justice Policy Institute. (2016). *Improving approaches to serving young adults in the justice system: executive summary*. Available at http://www.justicepolicy.org/uploads/justicepolicy/documents/jpi_report_summary_improving_approaches_to_serving_young_adults_in_the_justice_system.pdf.

Justice Resource Institute. (2017). *Certificate program in traumatic stress studies*. Available at http://www.traumacenter.org/training/certificate_program.php.

JJGPS. (2016). *Jurisdictional boundaries*. Juvenile Justice, Geography, Policy, Practice & Statistics. Available at http://www.jjgps.org/jurisdictional-boundaries.

Langstrom, N., Enebrink, P., Lauren, E. et al. (2013). Preventing sexual abusers of children from reoffending: systematic review of medical and psychological interventions. *British Medical Journal* 347: f4630. https://doi.org/10.1136/bmj.f4630.

Ludtke, J., In-Albon, T., Schmeck, K. et al. (2018). Nonsuicidal self-injury in adolescents placed in youth welfare and juvenile justice group homes: associations with mental health disorders and suicidality. *Journal of Abnormal Child Psychology* 46 (2): 343–354. https://doi.org/10.1007/s10802-017-0291-8.

Macallair, D. (2010). *Abuse in Youth Correctional Institutions*. Center on Juvenile and Criminal Justice. Available at http://www.cjcj.org/news/5296.

Mansion, A. and Chassin, L. (2016). The effect of race/ethnicity on the relation between substance use disorder diagnosis and substance use treatment receipt among male serious adolescent offenders. *Children and Youth Services Review* 61: 237–244. https://doi.org/10.1016/j.childyouth.2015.12.023.

McLaren, J., Barnett, E., Concepcion, Z. et al. (2018). Psychotropic medications for highly vulnerable children. *Expert Opinion on Pharmacotherapy* 19 (6): 547–560. https://doi.org/10.1080/14656566.2018.1445720.

McReynolds, L., Wasserman, G., and Ozbardakci, E. (2017). Contributors to nonsuicidal self-injury in incarcerated youth. *Health Justice* 5 (1): 13. https://doi.org/10.1186/s40352-017-0058-x.

Miller, A., Esposito-Smythers, C., Weismoore, J., and Renshaw, K. (2013). The relation between child maltreatment and adolescent suicidal behavior: a systematic review and critical examination of the literature. *Clinical Child and Family Psychology Review* 16 (2): 146–172. https://doi.org/10.1007/s10567-013-0131-5.

Moffitt, T. (1993). Adolescence-limited and life-course-persistent antisocial behavior: a developmental taxonomy. *Psychological Review* 100 (4): 674–701.

Murray, J. and Farrington, D. (2010). Risk factors for conduct disorder and delinquency: key findings from longitudinal studies. *Canadian Journal of Psychiatry* 55 (10): 633.

National Center for Mental Health and Juvenile Justice (2014). *Better solutions for youth with mental health needs in the juvenile justice system*. Available at https://www.ncmhjj.com/wp-content/uploads/2014/01/Whitepaper-Mental-Health-FINAL.pdf.

NCCHC. (2011). *Standards for health services in juvenile detention and confinement facilities*. National Commission on Correctional Health Care. Available at https://www.ncchc.org.

NCCHC. (2012). *Prevention of juvenile suicide in correctional settings*. National Commission on Correctional Health Care. Available at https://www.ncchc.org/prevention-of-juvenile-suicide-in-correctional-settings.

NCSL. (2013). *State update: Nevada: Teen pregnancy*. National Conference of State Legislatures. Available at http://www.ncsl.org/documents/health/TPinNVCWJJ1213.pdf.

NIH. (2019). *What is epigenetics?* US National Library of Medicine: Genetics Home Reference. National Institute of Health. Retrieved from https://ghr.nlm.nih.gov/primer/howgeneswork/epigenome

NIJ. (2010). *Preventing future crime with cognitive behavioral therapy*. Office of Justice Programs, National Institute of Justice. Available at https://www.nij.gov/journals/265/pages/therapy.aspx.

NIDA. (2018). *Chart of evidence-based screening tools and assessments for adults and adolescents*. National Institute on Drug Abuse. Available at https://www.drugabuse.gov/nidamed-medical-health-professionals/screening-tools-resources/chart-screening-tools.

OJJDP. (2010). *Cognitive-Behavioral Treatment*. Washington, DC: Office of Juvenile Justice and Delinquency Prevention. Available at https://www.ojjdp.gov/mpg/litreviews/Cognitive_Behavioral_Treatment.pdf.

OJJDP (2014). *Suicidal thoughts and behaviors among detained youth*. Washington, DC: Office of Juvenile Justice and Delinquency Prevention Available at https://www.ojjdp.gov/pubs/243891.pdf.

OJJDP (2015a). *Juvenile court statistics: 2015*. Washington, DC: Office of Juvenile Justice and Delinquency Prevention Available at https://www.ojjdp.gov/ojstatbb/njcda/pdf/jcs2015.pdf.

OJJDP (2015b). *Risk factors for delinquency*. Washington, DC: Office of Juvenile Justice and Delinquency Prevention Available at https://www.ojjdp.gov/mpg/litreviews/Risk%20Factors.pdf.

OJJDP (2016). *Survey of Youth in Residential Placement: Youth Characteristics and Backgrounds*. Washington, DC: Office of Juvenile Justice and Delinquency Prevention Available at https://www.ncjrs.gov/pdffiles1/ojjdp/grants/250753.pdf.

OJJDP. (2017a). *Census of juveniles in residential placement*. Washington, DC: Office of Juvenile Justice and Delinquency Prevention.

OJJDP. (2017b). *Intersection between mental health and the juvenile justice system: Literature review*. Washington, DC: Office of Juvenile Justice and Delinquency Prevention. Available at https://www.ojjdp.gov/mpg/litreviews/Intersection-Mental-Health-Juvenile-Justice.pdf.

OJJDP. (2017c). *Statistical briefing book*. Washington, DC: Office of Juvenile Justice and Delinquency Prevention. Available at https://www.ojjdp.gov/ojstatbb/crime/JAR_Display.asp?ID=qa05200.

OJJDP. (2018). *Juvenile arrests: 2016*. Washington, DC: Office of Juvenile Justice and Delinquency Prevention. Available at https://www.ojjdp.gov/pubs/251861.pdf.

Olson, K., Durwood, L., DeMeules, M., and McLaughlin, K. (2016). Mental health of transgender children who are supported in their identities. *Pediatrics* 137 (3): e20153223.

Pearson, G., Shelton, D., Shade, K. et al. (2016). Mental health needs of youth in juvenile justice: an executive summary. *Archives of Psychiatric Nursing* 31 (4): 330–331.

Pilnik, L. (2017). *Addressing the Intersections of Juvenile Justice Involvement and Youth Homelessness*. Washington, DC: Coalition for Juvenile Justice.

Poncin, Y. and Woolston, J. (2016). Systems of care, wraparound services, and home-based services. In: *Dulcan's Textbook of Child and Adolescent Psychiatry* (ed. M. Dulcan), 1007–1026. American Psychiatric Publishing Available at https://doi.org/10.1176/appi.books.9781615370306.

Rattan, A., Levine, C., Dweck, C., and Eberhardt, J. (2012). Race and the fragility of the legal distinction between juveniles and adults. *PLoS One* 7 (5) https://doi.org/10.1371/journal.pone.0036680.

Reingle, J., Jennings, W., and Maldonado-Molina, M. (2011). Generational differences in serious physical violence among Hispanic adolescents: results from a nationally representative, longitudinal study. *Race and Justice* 1: 277–291.

Ryan, E. and Otonichar, J. (2016). Juvenile sex offenders. *Current Psychiatry Reports* 18 (17): 1–10. https://doi.org/10.1007/s11920-016-0706-1.

Saar, M., Epstein, R., Rosenthal, L., & Vafa, Y. (2015). The sexual abuse to prison pipeline: The girls' story. Available at http://rights4girls.org/wp-content/uploads/r4g/2015/02/2015_COP_sexual-abuse_layout_web-1.pdf.

Sedlak, A. & McPherson K. (2010). Youth's needs and services. *OJJDP Juvenile Justice Bulletin*. Available at http://www.ncjrs.gov/pdffiles1/ojjdp/227728.pdf.

Semel, R. (2017). Utility of the ASEBA Youth Self-Report (YSR) in juvenile delinquency assessments. *EC Psychology and Psychiatry* 1 (6): 217–225.

Sickmund, M., Sladky, T.J., Kang, W., & Puzzanchera, C. (2017) *Easy access to the census of juveniles in residential placement*. Author's analysis of OJJDP's *Census of Juveniles in Residential Placement. . ..2015*. Available at http://www.ojjdp.gov/ojstatbb/ezacjrp.

Steinberg, L. (2013). The influence of neuroscience on US supreme court decisions about adolescents' criminal culpability. *Nature Reviews Neuroscience* 14: 513–518.

Stevens, T. and Morash, M. (2015). Racial/ethnic disparities in boys' probability of arrest and court actions in 1980 and 2000: the disproportionate impact of "getting tough" on crime. *Youth Violence and Juvenile Justice* 13 (1): 77–95. Available at http://dx.doi.org/10.1177/1541204013515280.

Teplin, L., Abram, K., Washburn, J. et al. (2013). *The Northwestern Juvenile Project: Overview. Juvenile Justice Bulletin*. Washington, DC: Office of Juvenile Justice and Delinquency Prevention.

Teplin, L., Stokes, M., McCoy, K. et al. (2015). Suicidal ideation and behavior in youth in the juvenile justice system: a review of the literature. *Journal of Correctional Health Care* 21 (3): 222–242.

Tuell, J., Heldman, J., & Harp, K. (2017). *Translating the science of adolescent development to sustainable best practice*. RFK National Resource Center for Juvenile Justice. Available at https://rfknrcjj.org/wp-content/uploads/2017/09/Developmental_Reform_in_Juvenile_Justice_RFKNRCJJ.pdf.

US Census Bureau. (2017). *Race & ethnicity*. Available at https://www.census.gov/mso/www/training/pdf/race-ethnicity-onepager.pdf.

Underwood, L. and Washington, A. (2016). Mental illness and juvenile offenders. *International Journal of Environmental Research and Public Health* 13 (2): 228. Available at https://doi.org/10.3390/ijerph13020228.

le Vries, S., Hoeve, M., Assink, M. et al. (2015). Practitioner review: effective ingredients of prevention programs for youth at risk of persistent juvenile delinquency–recommendations for clinical practice. *Journal of Child Psychology and Psychiatry* 56 (2): 108–121.

Welty, L., Hershfield, J., Abram, K. et al. (2016). Trajectories of substance use disorder in youth after detention: a 12-year longitudinal study. *Journal of the American Academy of Child & Adolescent Psychiatry* 56 (2): 140–148. https://doi.org/10.1016/j.jaac.2016.10.018.

Wu, J. (2016). Racial/ethnic discrimination and prosecution. *Criminal Justice and Behavior* 43 (4): 437–458. https://doi.org/10.1177/0093854815628026.

Zahn, M., Agnew, R., Fishbein, D., Miller, S., Winn, D., Dakoff, G., …Chesney-Lind, M. (2010). Causes and correlates of girls' delinquency. Office of Justice Programs. Available at https://www.ncjrs.gov/pdffiles1/ojjdp/226358.pdf.

Glossary

Adjudication	Judicial determination (judgment) that a juvenile is responsible for the delinquency or status offense that is charged in a petition or other charging document.
Age of criminal responsibility	Known as the defense of infancy: excluding a defendant from criminal liability for their actions because due to their age or developmental status they lack the capacity to appreciate the nature and wrongfulness of a crime they have committed.
Criminal offense	An act harmful not only to an individual but also to a community, society, or the state, e.g. assault, arson, robbery, theft, and drug-related crimes.
Delinquent	A young person characterized by a tendency to commit a crime, particularly minor crime.
Delinquent behavior	Something improper or criminal in nature, i.e. robbing a store.
Deviant behavior	A behavior that does not conform to social norms and values. Can also include "formal deviance," which includes acts such as robbery, theft, rape, murder, and assault.
Disruptive but nondelinquent behavior	Defiance of authority figures, angry outbursts, and other antisocial behaviors such as lying. Can include symptoms consistent with oppositional defiant disorder, conduct disorder.
Full prosecution	Holding a trial against a person and charging them with a criminal charge to the fullest extent of their suspected crimes with little to no leniency.
Judicial double standard	A set of principles that applies differently and usually more rigorously to one group of people or circumstances than to another.
Probation	The release of an offender from detention, subject to a period of good behavior under the supervision of a probation officer.
Recidivism	The tendency of a convicted criminal to reoffend.
Status offense	A noncriminal act that is considered a law violation only because of a youth's status as a minor, e.g. truancy, running away from home, violating curfew, underage use of alcohol.

23

Substance Use

Caroline R. McKinnon[1], Deborah Johnson[2], and Linda Stephan[2]

[1] Department of Biobehavioral Nursing, College of Nursing, Augusta University, Augusta, GA, USA
[2] School of Nursing, University of California San Francisco, San Francisco, CA, USA

Objectives

After reading this chapter, advanced practice registered nurses (APRNs) will be able to:

1. Identify developmental patterns and consequences of substance use, abuse, and dependence in children and adolescents.
2. Recognize evidence-based tools used to assess substance use.
3. Describe the continuum of substance use conditions.
4. Discuss evidence-based interventions and treatments for selected substance use conditions.
5. Describe implications for APRNs.

Introduction

Although substance use problems reach peak prevalence in emerging adulthood (i.e. ages 18–26), the issues also represent a significant public health concern for children and adolescents. In the United States and other high-income countries, substance use disorders (SUDs) are among the top causes of disease burden, especially among young people ages 10–24 years (Degenhardt et al. 2016; Whiteford et al. 2015). In addition, adolescence is a common age for substance use initiation, adding substantially to the extent of potential disease burden for this age group (Degenhardt et al. 2016). The Global Burden of Disease study also found that among young men aged 20–24, substance use accounted for more than 14% of the disease burden in this age group (Degenhardt et al. 2016).

This chapter will examine early use of substances including alcohol, tobacco, and illicit drugs and the misuse of prescription and over-the-counter (OTC) drugs and other psychoactive substances. A developmental lens will be used to examine patterns of adolescent alcohol and other drug (AOD) use, the trajectory of substance use conditions, and the effects of substance use on the developing adolescent. Risk and protective factors for SUDs will be examined and linked to screening, assessment, diagnosis, and treatment. These include evidence-based interventions that can be delivered by advanced practice registered nurses (APRNs) in primary care settings and criteria to use when referring for specialty treatment. This chapter concludes with implications for advanced practice nursing and a case exemplar illustrating the principles discussed in the chapter.

Child and Adolescent Behavioral Health: A Resource for Advanced Practice Psychiatric and Primary Care Practitioners in Nursing,
Second Edition. Edited by Edilma L. Yearwood, Geraldine S. Pearson, and Jamesetta A. Newland.
© 2021 John Wiley & Sons, Inc. Published 2021 by John Wiley & Sons, Inc.
Companion website: www.wiley.com/go/Yearwood

Epidemiology

Data on the overall trends in substance use among children and adolescents come from multiple annual national surveys. The *Monitoring the Future* (MTF) survey is a long-term study among US adolescents, college students, and adults through age 55 conducted with support from the National Institute of Drug Abuse (NIDA) (Johnson et al. 2018). Results have been reported separately for over four decades for 8th, 10th, and 12th graders across a range of substances and related factors. The 2017 survey included the first-ever estimate of vaping for several specific substances. Estimates for all substances on the MTF include reports for use in the past 30 days (i.e. current), past year, and lifetime. Similar to the MTF surveys, the National Survey on Drug Use and Health (NSDUH) has been compiled for several years, and includes individuals ages 12 and older (Substance Abuse and Mental Health Services Administration [SAMHSA] 2018a). Results from the NSDUH surveys are reported separately for 12–17-year-olds and include daily and past 30 days (i.e. current) use as well as data on reported substance use initiation and substance use treatment. Both surveys report on underage drinking patterns (for those aged 12–20) and binge drinking patterns, defined as five or more drinks on a single day in the past 30 days for men and four or more drinks on a single day in the past 30 days for women (Johnson et al. 2018; SAMHSA 2018a). Data on adolescent substance use patterns also come from the Youth Risk Behavior Surveillance System (YRBSS), conducted annually for the Centers for Disease Control (CDC). The YRBSS is unique in that it monitors a range of risky health behaviors commonly associated with increased morbidity and mortality, such as frequency of injury risk, risky sexual behaviors, and behaviors associated with cardiovascular health. In 2015, the YRBSS added items to allow participants a broader range of options related to gender identify, thus permitting the first opportunity to evaluate health status for sexual and gender minority students (Kann et al. 2018). Finally, the National Youth Tobacco Survey (NYTS) is a cross-sectional, voluntary, school-based survey among middle school and high school students and is analyzed by the CDC and the Food and Drug Administration (FDA). The NYTS includes questions on a range of tobacco products such as cigarettes, electronic cigarettes (e-cigarettes), smokeless tobacco, hookah, pipe tobacco, and bidis (small imported cigarettes wrapped in a leaf) (Wang et al. 2018).

Across all data sources, alcohol, marijuana, and cigarettes remain the three most commonly used substances (Johnson et al. 2018; Kann et al. 2018; SAMHSA 2018a).

In 2017 61.5% of middle school and high school aged youth reported lifetime alcohol use and 45.3% reported being drunk at least once by the time they graduated high school (Johnson et al. 2018). By comparison, these same youths endorsed a lifetime prevalence for marijuana use of 45%, for cigarette use of 26.6%, and any illicit drug other than marijuana of 14% (Johnson et al. 2018). Estimates of reported use of alcohol in the past 30 days are about 29–30% for all students and between 14% and 19% for past 30-day marijuana use, depending on the survey (Johnson et al. 2018; Kann et al. 2018).

Trends in reports of substance use by adolescents are mixed. For example, despite being among the most commonly used substances, cigarette smoking and alcohol use continue to be at historically low levels, as reported in both the 2017 MTF and the 2017 NSDUH surveys (Johnson et al. 2018; SAMHSA 2018a). In contrast, marijuana use was significantly increased in 2017, and marijuana use continues to drive trends related to the lifetime prevalence of any illicit drug use among young people. In addition, use of e-cigarettes remained the most commonly used tobacco products among middle school (3.3%) and high school students (11.7%) in 2017 (Wang et al. 2018).

Some long-standing differences in substance use patterns related to sociodemographic characteristics also appear to be changing. The historical gender gaps between male and female use of marijuana, alcohol, and cigarettes are now being reported as eliminated or significantly reduced in the 2017 MTF surveys (Johnson et al. 2018). One exception to this reduction in gender differences is the higher rate of reported misuse of prescription narcotic drugs among 12th grade males compared with female 12th graders. Gaps in reported illicit substance use by White, African American, and Hispanic students also appear to be closing, due primarily to simultaneous decreases in reported use by White students and increased use by African American and Hispanic students, especially for marijuana (Johnson et al. 2018).

Alcohol

Alcohol is the most widely used substance of abuse among youth. Although some young people begin drinking in elementary school, alcohol use typically begins in early adolescence. Rates of alcohol use increase sharply between 12 and 21 years of age. In 2017, about 2.3 million adolescents aged 12–17 used alcohol for the first time in the past year while 7.4 million people aged 12–20 reported drinking alcohol at least once in the past 30 days (SAMHSA 2018a). More specifically drinking reported in the past 30 days by 8th, 10th, and 12th graders was 8, 20, and 33% respectively (Johnson et al. 2018).

Importantly, the majority of underage alcohol use involves binge drinking (defined as having five or more drinks in a row on one or more occasions in the past 2 weeks). Reported binge drinking rates in the 2017 MTF were 4%, 10%, and 17% for grades 8, 10, and 12, respectively – reports that were all higher than the 2016 MTF (Johnson et al. 2018). Thus in 2017, one in every 20 teenagers (approximately 5.3% of adolescents) were current binge drinkers. Among 12th graders who participated in the 2017 MTF, 6% reported consuming more than 10 drinks on a single occasion at least once in the prior 2 weeks, and 3% reported consuming more than 15 drinks on a single occasion (Johnson et al. 2018).

High-risk drinking patterns such as initiation of alcohol use prior to age 15 and greater binge drinking quantity and frequency make adolescents more vulnerable to the development of alcohol dependence (Addolorato et al. 2018). Nevertheless, adolescents do not necessarily receive a diagnosis of alcohol use disorder (AUD). According to 2017 NSDUH data, the prevalence of past-year AUD was about 1.8% for individuals aged 12–17 but jumped to 10% for those aged 18–25 before dropping back to 5% for those over 26 years of age (SAMHSA 2018a). Despite these reductions in the percentage of children diagnosed with AUD, recent estimates show that less than 2% of adolescents in need of AUD treatment receive the care they need (SAMHSA 2018a). At the same time, there has been a trend for fewer and fewer treatment facilities to offer specialized adolescent AUD treatment (Mericle et al. 2015).

Nicotine/Tobacco Products

As noted above, use of conventional cigarettes by middle school and high school students has dropped steadily in recent years. In 2017, 19.6% of high school students and 5.6% of middle school students reported current use of any tobacco product in the prior 30 days (Wang et al. 2018). While these percentages represent a decreasing use trend across a range of tobacco product types, approximately one in five high school students (2.95 million) and one in 18 middle school students (0.67 million) reported current use of a tobacco product in 2017 (Wang et al. 2018). Moreover, many students who reported current tobacco product use also reported use of two or more tobacco product types (such as simultaneous use of conventional and electronic cigarettes).

In sharp contrast to conventional cigarettes, use of e-cigarettes by young people has risen sharply in recent years. From 2011 to 2015, e-cigarette use among middle and high school students increased 900% before declining slightly from 2015 to 2017 (Cullen et al. 2018). Still, since 2014, e-cigarettes have been the most commonly used tobacco product among US youth and current e-cigarette use is estimated at 3.6 million US youth in 2018 (Cullen et al. 2018).

In response to this emerging public health concern, numerous efforts are underway to restrict the sale of vaping devices, nicotine flavorings, and other paraphernalia thought to be associated with e-cigarette use for those under age 18. In 2019, the Surgeon General began a multi-media awareness campaign with information for children, parents, teachers, and health professionals on how all parties could address this public health concern (see https://e-cigarettes. surgeongeneral.gov for more details). In addition, federal regulations are also giving greater attention to marketing strategies aimed at young people, such as the language used in online and social media advertisements for e-cigarette products (Laestadius and Wang 2018).

Adolescent use of e-cigarettes poses several potential health concerns. Most importantly, nicotine exposure during adolescence is known to alter brain development in ways that can impact learning, memory, and attention (US Department of Health and Human Services [USDHHS] 2016). Adolescents using e-cigarettes may also be unaware that they are using nicotine due to specific marketing strategies that aim to conceal or minimize this kind of information (OSG 2016). Similar to the conclusions of the 2016 OSG report, a recent systematic review and meta-analysis found that e-cigarette use was associated with a greater risk of subsequent cigarette smoking initiation and past 30-day smoking (Soneji et al. 2017). Research has also shown a high correlation between e-cigarette use by 8th graders and use of other substances, especially marijuana (Westling et al. 2017). A recent small study ($n = 173$) among adolescent e-cigarette users identified factors associated with more frequent use of e-cigarettes to include receiving one's first cigarette from a family member (rather than a friend or store), using nicotine in all e-cigarettes (as compared with only some), being able to customize the device, and friends' use of e-cigarettes (Vogel et al. 2018). This same study found predictors of subsequent nicotine dependence to include younger age of e-cigarette use, friends' e-cigarette use, and recent conventional cigarette use.

Beyond the addiction potential, use of electronic nicotine delivery systems (ENDS) also has other health risks. These risks include increased exposure to toxic chemicals and/or unhealthy concentrations of nicotine; increased risk for liquid nicotine poisoning (due to the concentration of nicotine contained within a single e-cigarette cartridge), increased indoor air pollution, and increased risk of unique fire hazards (Prochnow 2017). Emerging research is also recognizing the potential health hazards of secondhand vaping exposure to youth, especially those with other respiratory illnesses such as asthma (Bayly et al. 2019). In late 2019, numerous reports began emerging of acute lung conditions related to vaping, although at this time the full association is not known. The likelihood of these health risks occurring is heightened by a combination of lack of perceived risk by adolescents and the "kid-friendly" flavors of many e-cigarettes that makes them more palatable. Several national surveys have confirmed that American teenagers do not perceive e-cigarettes as harmful, especially when compared with conventional cigarettes (Amrock et al. 2016; Johnson et al. 2018). Perception of e-cigarette risk has been associated with numerous factors, including gender, age, race, ethnicity, use of other tobacco products, and knowledge of nicotine concentration within the e-cigarette device (Amrock et al. 2016; Choi et al. 2018; Morean et al. 2016).

Marijuana

Marijuana remains the most commonly used illicit substance by adolescents. In 2017, 6.5% of adolescents aged 12–17 reported current use of marijuana, a figure representing approximately 1.6 million people (SAMHSA 2018a). The percentage of adolescents reporting current marijuana use was lower in 2017 compared with reports from 2009 to 2014, but remained similar to 2015 and 2016 reports. Reported use of synthetic marijuana by young people also continued to decline in 2017, but annual prevalence of marijuana vaping (measured separately for the first time in the 2017 MTF) was reported as 3%, 8%, and 10% for students in grades 8, 10, and 12 respectively (Johnson et al. 2018).

Changes in reported marijuana use are occurring in the context of a decline in the percentage of 12–17-year-olds who perceive marijuana as a risky substance, a phenomenon that is even more concerning as decreased risk perception has often preceded increases in substance use (SAMHSA 2018a; Volkow et al. 2014). One other factor increasing the potential for marijuana dependence among young people is the increase in the concentration of tetrahydrocannabinol (THC), the psychoactive substance in marijuana. Recent estimates suggest that the percentage of THC in illicit marijuana has increased from about 4% in 1995 to about 12% in 2014 (ElSohly et al. 2016).

As of October 2018, the majority of US states and the District of Columbia have some type of medical marijuana law (MML). Although MMLs do not specifically address adolescent use, they may still have an impact on adolescent substance use behaviors. One study of MMLs in 10 different states from 2004 to 2012 found consistent increases in marijuana use initiation among those aged 12–20, but MMLs did not have any impact on other

substance use as they did for those over age 21 (Wen et al. 2015). A more recent study analyzed data from the MTF database from 1991 to 2015 and found differences across all three grade cohorts. For eighth graders, enactment of MMLs was associated with decreases in the prevalence of several substances while 10th graders had no change in substance use prevalence, and 12th graders reported increases in nonmedical prescription opioid and cigarette use following MML enactment (Cerdá et al. 2018). These study findings are contradicted by a systematic literature review that found MML changes did not necessarily contribute to increases in adolescent marijuana use (Sarvet et al. 2018).

Other Drug Use

Illicit drugs that are recorded on the 2017 MTF included LSD, hallucinogens other than LSD, MDMA, cocaine, crack, heroin, amphetamines, sedatives, tranquilizers, methamphetamine, crystal methamphetamine, and steroids. Youth were also queried about inhalant use and nonmedical use of prescription medications (NUPM) including methylphenidate, oxycodone, and other narcotics (Johnson et al. 2018). In 2017, reported use of most illicit substances other than marijuana remained relatively low and was comparable to the prior 3 to 4 years across all three grade cohorts (Johnson et al. 2018). Among youth aged 12–17 who responded to the 2017 NSDUH survey, tranquilizers and prescription stimulants were misused by about 0.5% of the population each as compared to 0.1% or less of the population that reported use of cocaine, heroin, and/or misuse of prescription sedatives. Risk factors that increase the likelihood of NUPM include playing specific contact sports (especially ice hockey) (Veliz et al. 2017), poor school adjustment and/or lack of school attendance (Schepis et al. 2018a), and enrollment in a substance use treatment program for some other substance (Al-Tayyib et al. 2018). Gender difference related to nonmedical use of prescription opioids includes higher prevalence among male students who are also current smokers and female students who are also current smokers and/or alcohol users (Osborne et al. 2017).

Despite a public health crisis involved opioid use among adults, the extent of the problem among young people is less clear. In the 2017 MTF survey, Vicodin use dropped 51% by 8th graders, 67% by 10th graders, and 74% by 12th graders, suggesting a decrease in use. In contrast, a systematic review and meta-analysis of Americans 11–30 years of age identified a high prevalence of past-year prescription opioid misuse (Jordan et al. 2017). Likewise, analysis of national poison center data document increased accidental and/or intentional ingestion among children and adolescents, due in part to an increase in the availability of prescription opioids in the home (Chhabra and Aks 2017; Sheridan and Horowitz 2017). Analysis of NSDUH data from 2009 to 2014 showed that friends and relatives were the most common source of misused prescription opioids (Schepis et al. 2018b). Likewise, data from the 1975–2015 MTF surveys also show that medical and nonmedical use of prescription opioids are highly correlated (McCabe et al. 2017).

Neurobiology

AOD use during adolescence is associated with cognitive deficits and alterations in brain activity and structure. Specific neurobiologic changes associated with adolescent alcohol use and misuse include brain function abnormalities, decreased neurocognitive performance (primarily on tasks involving working memory and/or attention), changes in white and gray matter development, and abnormal neuronal activation in areas associated with inhibition control and sensitivity to reward/pleasure response (Bava and Tapert 2010; Jacobus and Tapert 2014; Pfefferbaum et al. 2017). Changes to specific parts of the brain anatomy related to adolescent AOD are highly relevant to subsequent adult AOD. In particular, current theories on the neurobiology of adult AOD hold that the decreased functioning of the prefrontal cortex leads to an imbalance in between desire for a drug and the ability to abstain from it (Volkow and Boyle 2018; Volkow et al. 2016). The progression from initial alcohol use in adolescence into subsequent AUDs can also be influenced by the intricate connections between brain development and environmental stress. For example, a latent class analysis study among adolescents aged 12–15 found that teens who were earlier initiators of alcohol use were also more likely to report significantly higher levels of stress and almost seven times more likely to develop an AUD by age 19 compared with late initiators (Elsayed et al. 2018).

Several of the mechanisms underlying the development of alcohol dependence are also evident in the development of nicotine dependence. Nicotine enhances dopamine release by activating nicotinic cholinergic receptors and desensitizing postsynaptic receptors on gamma aminobutyric acid (GABA) interneurons. As the receptors resensitize to their resting state, the smoker experiences craving and withdrawal (Stahl 2013). Adolescent nicotine use also has important and potentially life-long effects on brain development. Specifically, the limbic system, which controls cognition, emotion, and drug reward sensitivity, is actively maturing during adolescence (Yaun et al. 2015). Exposure to nicotine during this especially vulnerable time is associated with changes in both dopamine and serotonin receptors and

may account for an increased likelihood of nicotine being a "gateway" to other substance use and/or subsequent mood disorders in adulthood.

Etiology

The etiology of substance use and SUD is multifactorial and complex. Research has identified distinct biological and environmental factors that are correlated with initiation, use, and/or misuse of substances. In addition to the fact that no one variable or set of variables has been identified to completely explain adolescent substance use, the known biological and environmental factors also interact with each other to contribute to additional complexity.

Biological Factors

Research indicates that part of the risk of developing a SUD after adopting substance use behaviors is influenced by biological factors, such as genetics, epigenetics, and normal developmental maturation of the brain circuity and brain chemistry, all of which can be altered by adolescent AOD (Volkow and Boyle 2018; Volkow et al. 2016). Examples of genetics research related to adolescent substance use include examination of the genes associated with the enzymes responsible for nicotine metabolism (Olfson et al. 2018) as well as numerous twin and adoption studies that place the heritability of SUDs somewhere between 50 and 70% (Lynskey et al. 2010; Verhulst et al. 2015). Research on the effects of nicotine exposure shows that due to the immaturity of the adolescent brain, epigenetic changes related to nicotine are especially likely to sensitize the brain to other drugs, thus priming it for future substance abuse (Yaun et al. 2015). From a developmental perspective, once an individual's brain is exposed to a substance, brain reward systems can reinforce substance use, and repeated use can lower an individual's ability to control substance use, increasing risk for SUD (Volkow and Boyle 2018; Volkow et al. 2016). Accordingly, initiation of substance use during adolescence can place an individual at increased risk of SUD, given that the adolescent brain has not fully matured, which may predispose adolescents to more profound effects of substance on the brain's reward systems. Most research on the relationship between age of first alcohol use and subsequent adult SUD also shows that use prior to the age of 15 is a significant risk factor and is likely related to disruption of normal brain maturation (Hingson et al. 2006).

Temperament and Personality Traits

Research has identified a correlation between an individual's personality traits and risk of substance use and SUDs. In particular, research has focused on the role of impulsivity as it relates to adolescent substance use. In this context, impulsivity is defined as behaviors such sensation seeking, lack of premeditation, lack of perseverance, and the tendency to act rashly in emotional states. Notwithstanding some limitations on the research due measurement of impulsivity as a construct, meta-analyses show a relationship between impulsivity traits and increased adolescent substance use and adolescent SUD development (Bos et al. 2019; Stautz and Cooper 2013). Other personality traits associated with adolescent substance use include early childhood aggression and greater psychological dysregulation in cognitive, behavioral, and/or affective domains (Clark et al. 2012). More recently, data from the Minnesota Twin Study found that both low constraint and aggression control in teens were associated with an increased vulnerability for adult AUDs (Samek et al. 2018). Likewise, data from a twin study of adults aged 17–25 years found that those individuals with higher scores on resilience measures had a lower risk of progressing from adolescent substance use into adult SUDs (Long et al. 2017).

Environmental Risk Factors

In additional to individual personality and temperamental factors association with substance use, there are factors arising in the environment – family setting, peer group, and community – that have been found to be unique risk factors that are correlated with an individual's risk of substance use and SUD. Family factors such as poor quality of the child–parent relationship, family disruptions (e.g. divorce, acute or chronic stress), poor parenting, maternal mental health (especially depressive symptomatology), parental attitudes sympathetic to drug use, and social deprivation have been found to be associated with increased substance use (Sitnick et al. 2014). One proposed mechanism for this correlation is that through social learning, children and adolescents internalize the values and expectations of their parents and possibly acquire maladaptive coping techniques that predispose them to substance use later in life. Additionally, stress from this family setting may be a unique factor in precipitating later substance use in individuals.

Peer environment also makes a substantial contribution to adolescent substance use among adolescents, with at least some literature suggesting peer influence is the single most important factor. One way that peer environment is influential is in the extent to which teenagers tend to cluster with peers ungagged in similar behaviors. For example, longitudinal study has shown that across a range of substances, teenagers have the highest concordance of substance use with their best friend as compared with older siblings and important adult figures (Schuler et al. 2019). Other peer factors associated with increased risk of adolescent substance use include spending time with friends who are using drugs or alcohol and increased peer availability of substances.

Neighborhood, community, state, and national policies are also factors that impact an individual's substance use. Increasing restrictions on smoking in public places reinforces the norm that tobacco use is not acceptable while increasing cigarette taxes acts as a powerful economic incentive to discourage adolescent cigarette use, especially among younger adolescents (Hawkins et al. 2016). State and national tobacco policies are implemented as public health efforts to provide smoke-free environments, not only to protect nonsmokers, and promote tobacco cessation among tobacco but have resulted in a decline in tobacco use rates and delays in initiation of smoking (Been and Sheikh 2018). This is particularly relevant today for nurse practitioners in light of the currently changing local, state, and national policies in regards to vaping and marijuana policy, and the impact these policies may have on altering the general environment for adolescents and the long-term consequences these environmental changes may have on adolescent substance use.

Clinical Presentation

In 2013, with the publication of *Diagnostic and Statistical Manual of Mental Disorders 5* (DSM-5), the terminology used to categorize substance use behaviors changed. Specifically, the terms *substance abuse* and *substance dependence* were replaced with *SUD*, a condition reflecting multiple domains of problematic substance use and three levels of severity: *mild, moderate,* and *severe* (American Psychiatric Association [APA] 2013). Often used interchangeably with the term *addiction*, SUDs are defined as complex, chronic, and relapsing conditions, in which individuals compulsively and repeatedly seek substances and use them despite numerous possible negative consequences. Under DSM-5, anyone meeting at least two of 11 criteria within a 12-month period would receive a diagnosis of SUD, with the severity based on the number of criteria that were met. Other changes to the diagnostic criteria include the removal of legal problems as a criterion and the addition of cravings (APA 2013). Of note, NIDA continues to use the term *addiction* as a comparable term to the DSM-5 definition of severe SUD.

The clinical presentation of substance use, defined as a pattern of harmful use of any substance for mood-altering purposes, and SUD using the DSM-5 criteria (described below), can be challenging for healthcare providers. The reasons for this are multifactorial. While adolescent patients may present with a chief complaint of cough or arm pain or headache, they rarely present with a chief complaint of substance use or SUD, therefore the healthcare provider must evaluate subtle signs and symptoms that may be associated with substance use.

Substance Use

The observable signs and symptoms of substance use can be divided into three categories: acute intoxication, withdrawal, and the various potential clinical consequences of long-term use. Signs and symptoms of substance use are unique to the substance being used (see Table 23.1). If an adolescent presents with any of the signs and symptoms of acute intoxication, withdrawal, or the various potential clinical consequences of long-term use, then substance use and/or SUD should be considered as part of the differential diagnosis. However, the specific signs and symptoms of substance use are not pathognomonic for substance use, and the broader differential diagnosis should always be considered. Additionally, it should be noted that given the relative brief duration of adolescent substance use in comparison to adults that have used substances over years, the chronic physical manifestations of substance use are rarely noted in adolescent patients.

There is some evidence that substance use in adolescents may have unique risks that adults do not face with substance use, given that the substance use exposure occurs during a time of active development of the brain. As described earlier, nicotine exposure can be disruptive to adolescent brain development (OSG 2016). It is also known that cannabis use in adolescence is associated with reduced IQ and decreased neural connectivity (Volkow et al. 2016). It is believed that cannabis-related neurocognitive deficits in attention and memory that persist beyond abstinence suggest possible structural brain alterations (e.g. changes in gray matter tissue), changes in white matter tract integrity, and abnormalities of neural functioning (e.g. increased brain activation) (Jacobus and Tapert 2014). However, given the correlational nature of the data it is difficult to determine whether the lasting neurocognitive deficits are a product of the substance use or a risk for substance use.

Comorbid Conditions

There is a complex relationship between adolescent substance use and other mental health diagnoses. Adolescents aged 13–18 with a mental health diagnosis have been found to have a co-occurring SUD diagnosis 61–88% of the time (Couwenbergh et al. 2006). Specifically 25–50% of adolescents with conduct disorder or oppositional defiant disorder have been found to have co-occurring SUD (Bukstein 2015), 20–27% of adolescents with an SUD have comorbid attention deficit hyperactivity disorder (ADHD) (van Emmerik-van Oortmerssen et al. 2012), suicide has been found to be closely associated with substance use (Schilling et al. 2009; Wong et al. 2013), and onset of mood disorders, such as bipolar disorder, is often preceded by cannabis use (Duffy et al. 2012). A recent meta-analysis of 37 longitudinal studies found that childhood ADHD, ODD, CD, and depression all increase the risk for subsequent SUDs across a range of substances (Groenman et al. 2017). Likewise, analysis of national epidemiological survey data has also shown that mental health conditions in adolescents increases the risk of subsequent alcohol and drug use as well as the risk of transitioning into problematic use (Conway et al. 2016). Although the current evidence base is not clear on the directionality and causation of comorbid mental health and substance use conditions in adolescents, the fact remains that there is evidence that these conditions frequently coexist. Thus it is important for healthcare providers to be cognizant of the potential for the other diagnoses to be present for an individual as well. As a general rule, substance use and SUD should be considered in an adolescent patient with psychosocial problems and/or impairment.

Screening

The purpose of substance use screening is to identify individuals who have or are at risk for developing AOD-related problems, and within that group to identify individuals who need further assessment to diagnose their SUDs and develop plans to treat them (Center for Substance Abuse Treatment 1997). There is significant evidence to suggest that substance use most often begins during adolescence, increases substantially across the teenage years, and decreases during the third decade of life (Hernandez et al. 2015; Sneider et al. 2018). This can result in negative consequences including involvement with the criminal justice system, poor school performance, and health and mental health issues among substance using youth (Kelly et al. 2014). In a review of literature and meta-analytic studies of alcohol and substance use treatments, Hogue et al. (2018) conclude that prevalence rates support the importance of screening adolescents and transition age youth (TAY).

Screening, Brief Intervention, and Referral to Treatment (SBIRT) is an evidence-based approach to community-based screening for health risk behaviors, including substance use. Developed in response to a mandate by the Institute of Medicine, the SBIRT model

Table 23.1 Selected drugs of abuse, signs of intoxication and withdrawal, and potential health consequences

Substance: category and name	Examples of street names	Drug Enforcement Administration schedule/ method(s) of ingestion	Signs of intoxication/withdrawal	Potential health consequences
Cannabinoids				
Hashish	Boom, chronic, gangster, hash, hash oil, hemp	I/swallowed, smoked	Conjunctivitis, appetite stimulation, euphoria, slowed thinking and reaction time, confusion, impaired balance and coordination	Cough, frequent respiratory infections, impaired memory and learning, increased heart rate, anxiety, panic attacks, acute psychotic symptoms (auditory and visual hallucinations, paranoid delusions, confusion, and amnesia)
Marijuana (cannabis)	Grass, weed, pot, herb, dope, hash, blunt, joint, Mary Jane	I/swallowed, smoked	Withdrawal: restlessness, irritability, insomnia, loss of appetite	
Central nervous system depressants				
Alcohol	Booze, drinks, firewater, highballs, moonshine, white lightning	Not scheduled/swallowed	Disinhibition, mood lability, impaired judgment, slurred speech, incoordination, unsteady gait, nystagmus, flushed face. Withdrawal: tremors, nausea/vomiting, tachycardia, sweating, elevated blood pressure, depressed mood, irritability, transient hallucinations or illusions, headache, insomnia, seizures, delirium	Impaired memory and learning, impaired judgment, elevated liver enzymes, liver disease, disruption of hormones needed for normal organ, muscle, and bone development during puberty, peripheral neuropathy, Wernicke's encephalopathy, psychosis, cardiomyopathy, risk for fetal alcohol syndrome
Barbiturates Benzodiazepines (other than flunitrazepam)	Barbs, reds, red birds, phennies, tooies, yellows, yellow jackets Candy, downers, sleeping pills, tranks	II, II, V/injected, swallowed IV/swallowed, injected	Reduced anxiety, feeling of wellbeing, lowered inhibitions, slowed pulse and breathing, lowered blood pressure, poor concentration Barbiturates and benzodiazepines: sedation, drowsiness	Fatigue; confusion; impaired coordination, memory, and judgment Barbiturates: depression, slurred speech, irritability, dizziness, life-threatening withdrawal Benzodiazepines: dizziness
Flunitrazepam (Rohypnol)	Forget-me-pill, Mexican Valium, R2, Roche, roofies, roofinol, rope, rophies	IV/swallowed, snorted	GHB: drowsiness, nausea Methaqualone: euphoria	Flunitrazepam: visual and gastrointestinal disturbances, urinary retention, memory loss for the time of drug's effects
GHB (gamma-hydroxybutyrate)*	G, Georgia homeboy, grievous bodily harm, liquid ecstasy	I/swallowed	Withdrawal: nausea/vomiting, malaise, weakness, tachycardia, sweating, anxiety, irritability, orthostatic hypotension, tremor, insomnia, seizures	Headache, loss of consciousness, loss of reflexes, seizures, coma, death *Associated with risk of sexual assault
Methaqualone	Ludes, mandrex, quad, quay	I/injected, swallowed		Poor reflexes, slurred speech, coma
Dissociative anesthetics				
Ketamine Phencyclidine (Angel Dust) and analogs	Cat, K, Special K, vitamin K Angel dust, boat, hog, love boat, peace pill	III/injected, snorted, smoked I, II/injected, swallowed, smoked	Increased heart rate and blood pressure, impaired motor function Ketamine: delirium, depression, respiratory depression/arrest (at high doses) PCP: decreased blood pressure and heart rate, panic, aggression, violence, suicidal ideation	Memory loss, numbness, nausea/vomiting, seizures, coma, death (greatest risk at high doses and/or when used with other CNS depressants)

(continued)

Table 23.1 (cont'd)

Substance: category and name	Examples of street names	Drug Enforcement Administration schedule/method(s) of ingestion	Signs of intoxication/withdrawal	Potential health consequences
Hallucinogens				
LSD (lysergic acid diethylamide)	Acid, blotter, boomers, cubes, microdot, yellow sunshine	I/swallowed, absorbed through mouth tissues	Altered states of perception and feeling, nausea, sensitivity to light and sound LSD and mescaline: increased body temperature, heart rate, blood pressure; loss of appetite, sleeplessness, numbness, weakness, tremors	Persisting perception disorder (flashbacks)
Mescaline (Peyote)	Buttons, cactus, mesc, peyote	I/swallowed, smoked		
Psilocybin	Magic mushroom, shrooms, purple passion	I/swallowed	Psilocybin: nervousness, paranoia	
Opioids and morphine derivatives				
Codeine	Captain Cody, Cody, schoolboy, doors & fours, loads, pancakes & syrup	II, III, IV, V/injected, swallowed	Pain relief, euphoria, drowsiness, pupil constriction (or dilation due to anoxia from severe overdose), impaired attention and memory	Nausea/vomiting, confusion, sedation, respiratory depression/arrest, unconsciousness, coma, death Injectables: additional risks for HIV/AIDS, hepatitis B & C
Fentanyl and analogs	Apache, China girl, China white, dance fever, friend, goodfella, jackpot, murder 8, TNT	I, II/injected, smoked, snorted		
Heroin	Brown sugar, dope, H, horse, junk, smack, white horse	I/injected, smoked, snorted	Heroin: staggering gait Withdrawal: craving, dysphoric mood, nausea/vomiting, lacrimation or rhinorrhea, muscle aches, papillary dilation, piloerection, sweating, abdominal cramping, diarrhea, yawning, fever, insomnia	
Morphine	M, Miss Emma, monkey, white stuff	II, III/injected, swallowed, smoked		
Opium	Big O, black stuff, block, gum, hop	II, III, V/swallowed, smoked		
Oxycodone HCL	Oxy, O.C., killer	II/swallowed, snorted, injected		
Hydrocodone bitartrate, acetaminophen	Vike, Watson-387	II/swallowed		
Stimulants				
Amphetamine	Bennies, black beauties, crosses, hearts, speed, uppers	II/injected, swallowed, smoked, snorted	Increased heart rate, blood pressure, temperature, feelings of exhilaration, increased mental alertness Amphetamine: rapid breathing	Rapid/irregular heartbeat, reduced appetite, weight loss, heart failure, nervousness, insomnia, malnutrition, headaches, panic attacks, nausea, abdominal pain chest pain, respiratory failure, stroke, seizure

Cocaine	Blow, bump, C, crack, coke, rock, snow, toot	II/injected, swallowed, smoked, snorted	Cocaine: increased temperature	Amphetamine: Loss of coordination, irritability, anxiousness, delirium, panic, psychosis, impulsive behaviors, aggressiveness
Methylendioxy-methamphetamine (MDMA, nickname Ecstacy/ Molly)	Adam, clarity, ecstasy, Eve, lover's speed, peace, STP, X, XTC,	I/swallowed	MDMA: mild hallucinogenic effects, euphoria, bruxism, increased tactile sensitivity; Methamphetamine: aggression violence, psychotic behavior	Cocaine: Chest pain, respiratory failure, nausea, stroke, seizure, headache, malnutrition, panic attacks; MDMA: Impaired memory and learning, hyperthermia, cardiac toxicity, renal failure, liver toxicity
Methamphetamine	Chalk, crank, crystal, fire, glass, go fast, ice, meth, speed	II/injected, swallowed, smoked, snorted	Nicotine: Increased heart rate, blood pressure, metabolism, rapid/irregular heartbeat, heart failure, nervousness	Methamphetamine: memory loss, cardiac and neurological damage, impaired memory and learning; Nicotine: adverse pregnancy outcomes, chronic lung disease, cardiovascular disease, stroke, cancer, tolerance, addiction
Methylphenidate	JIF, MPH, R-ball, Skippy, the smart drug, vitamin R	II/injected, swallowed, snorted	Withdrawal from amphetamines and cocaine: craving, dysphoria, fatigue, vivid and unpleasant dreams, insomnia or hypersomnia, increased appetite, psychomotor retardation or agitation, severe depression, suicidal and/or paranoid ideation	
Nicotine	Cigarettes, cigars, smokeless tobacco, snuff, spit, bidis, chew	Not scheduled/smoked, snorted, taken in snuff and spit tobacco	Withdrawal from nicotine: craving, dysphoria, depressed mood, insomnia, irritability, frustration, anxiety, difficulty concentrating, decreased heart rate, increased appetite/ weight gain	
Other compounds				
Anabolic steroids	Arnolds, gym candy, juice, pumpers, shot gunning, stackers, roids	III/injected, swallowed, applied to skin	Withdrawal: mood swings, fatigue, restlessness, loss of appetite, insomnia, reduced sex drive, cravings, depression, suicidal ideation, attempts	Hostility/aggression, acne, premature growth stoppage, prostate cancer, reduced sperm production, shrunken testicles, breast enlargement, menstrual irregularities, masculine characteristics, hypertension, blood clotting, cholesterol changes, liver cysts and cancer, kidney cancer
Dextromethorphan (DMX)	Candy, dex, robotripping, Robo, skittling, Triple C	Not scheduled/swallowed	Dissociative effects, distorted visual perceptions	At higher doses, similar to dissociative anesthetic drugs
Inhalants	Laughing gas, poppers, snappers, whippets	Not scheduled/inhaled through mouth or nose	Stimulation, loss of inhibition, headache, nausea, vomiting, slurred speech, loss of motor coordination	Wheezing/unconsciousness, cramps, weight loss, muscle weakness, depression, memory impairment, damage to cardiovascular and nervous systems, sudden death, hearing loss, bone marrow damage, liver and kidney damage, increased risk of contracting and spreading infectious disease due to association with unsafe sexual practices

Source: Adapted from National Institute on Drug Abuse [NIDA] (2017). Screening Tools for Adolescent Substance Use. Retrieved from https://www.drugabuse.gov/nidamed-medical-health-professionals/screening-tools-for-adolescent-substance-use.

aims to identify, reduce, and prevent problematic use, abuse, and dependence on alcohol and illicit drugs (SAMHSA 2018b). Initially used in adult primary care, and emergency and trauma centers, SBIRT has been adapted for use with children, adolescents, and transition aged youth in primary care and university settings (SAMHSA 2018b). The President's Commission on Combating Drug Addiction and the Opioid Crisis recommended that the Department of Education collaborate with states to implement SBIRT with at-risk youth (Christie et al. 2017).

Screening for alcohol, tobacco, and drug use is recommended for youth aged 11 and older (Levy and Williams 2016). Introducing screening into primary care and other healthcare encounters can normalize discussions with adolescents about substance use, facilitating discussions that reinforce and promote healthy behaviors and choices. Among youth who are using alcohol, tobacco, or other substances and potentially at risk for a SUD, SBIRT screening guides brief interventions and referrals for treatment (NIDA 2019).

Despite evidence supporting screening youth and adolescents for substance use, there remains a significant gap in practice (Meredith et al. 2018). When developing a plan for implementing substance use screening in primary care settings, time-efficient implementation is critical to consistent and successful use (Wissow et al. 2013). In addition, screening tools should be well-validated, developmentally appropriate, and include guidelines for steps to follow subsequent to screening (Ozechowski et al. 2016). Technology-enhanced approaches are increasingly relevant to screening adolescents, given the growing appeal of digital messaging and social media (Harris et al. 2016).

Evidence-based Assessment Tools

Screening for substance use in youth begins by asking questions about use of psychoactive substances. Although the strength of the psychometric data is predominantly based on adults, a few well-validated self-report instruments are available for screening for alcohol and other substances, and these can be found in Table 23.2. Among the instruments validated with youth (NIDA 2019) the Brief Screener for Alcohol, Tobacco and other Drugs (BSTAD) and Screening to Brief Intervention (S2BI) are two brief online instruments. Recommended by NIDA (2019), both tests can be self-administered by youth and have evidence supporting validity for assess for SUD risk among adolescents 12–17 years old (Kelly et al. 2014; Levy et al. 2014). Other validated instruments include the NIDA-Modified (NM) ASSIST (APA 2018), Alcohol Screening and Brief Intervention for Youth: A Practitioner's Guide (National Institute on Alcohol Abuse and Alcoholism [NIAAA] 2015), Alcohol Abuse and Alcoholism Screening Guide (NIAAA SG), and the Personal Experience Screening Questionnaire Problem Severity Scale (PESQ-PS). Comparing psychometric performance, D'Amico et al. (2016) found that the

Table 23.2 Selected screening and assessment tools for adolescent substance use problems

Instrument	References	Items	Brief description
Screening			
Brief Screener for Alcohol, Tobacco, and other Drugs (BSTAD)	Kelly et al. (2014)	11	Endorsed by NIDA, a promising screening tool for identifying problematic tobacco, alcohol, and marijuana use in pediatric settings. Note: Consistent with the NIAAA instrument, if the respondent is aged 12–14, friends questions are asked first; if aged 15–17 (or 14-year-olds in high school), personal-use questions are asked first.
Screening to Brief Intervention (S2BI)	Boston Children's Hospital (2015)	7	Endorsed by NIDA, a frequency-based screening instrument and Quick Guide
NIDA-Modified (NM) ASSIST	American Psychiatric Association (2018)	15	For adolescents (age 11–17) and adults to self-administer the screening tool and for parents/guardians to administer with their children (age 6–17). These measures are considered by the APA as "emerging measures" and should be used to enhance clinical decision-making but not as the sole basis for making a clinical diagnosis.

(continued)

Table 23.2 (cont'd)

Instrument	References	Items	Brief description
Alcohol Screening and Brief Intervention for Youth: A Practitioner's Guide (NIAAA)	NIAAA (2015)	2–6	Endorsed by NIDA for screening and assessment. Designed for use with 9–18-year-olds. First tool to include question regarding "friends drinking." Tool and its pocket guide were designed with input from American Academy of Pediatrics to help healthcare professionals quickly identify youth at risk for alcohol-related problems.
Alcohol Abuse and Alcoholism Screening Guide (NIAAA SG)	Parast et al. (2018)	2	Brief screening identifies adults or adolescents at risk for alcohol use.
Personal Experience Screening Questionnaire Problem Severity Scale (PESQ-PS)	Shields et al. (2008)	40	Designed for a general adolescent population and assesses alcohol and drug use simultaneously. It evaluates lifetime use with special emphasis on the 12 months prior to assessment. Self-report takes about 10 minutes to complete and supports a multiscale factor structure.
Michigan Alcoholism Screening Test (MAST)	Addiction Medicine Foundation (2016); Selzer (1971); Maisto et al. (1995)	25	Recommended by Addiction Medicine Foundation for older adolescents and adults. One of the most widely used measures for assessing alcohol abuse. The measure is useful in multiple settings, designed to provide a rapid and effective screening for lifetime alcohol-related problems and alcoholism. Several briefer versions are available.
The Alcohol Use Disorders Identification Test (AUDIT)	NIAAA (n.d.); Knight et al. (2003)	10	Endorsed by NIAAA, AUDIT focuses on drinking patterns and alcohol-related behaviors in adults and adolescents aged 14–18. For youth, cut points of 2 for identifying any alcohol problem use and 3 for alcohol abuse or dependence.

Assessment

Instrument	References	Items	Brief description
Car–Relax–Alone–Forget–Family and Friends–Trouble (CRAFFT) 2.0	Harris et al. (2016)	6	Endorsed by NIDA as either self-report or clinician-interview tool for brief screen of AOD use and consequences. Designed to assess the level of alcohol and other drug problems relevant to adolescents. The name "CRAFFT" is a mnemonic to assist providers in remembering the target question.
Alcohol Screening and Brief Intervention for Youth: A Practitioner's Guide (NIAAA)	NIAAA (2015)	2–6	Endorsed by NIDA for screening and assessment. See above for description.
Drug Abuse Screening Test (DAST-20) Adolescent Version	Yudko et al. (2007)	20	Endorsed by NIDA for adolescents (DAST-10 is endorsed for adults).
Drug Abuse Screening Test (DAST-10)	Skinner (1982); Yudko et al. (2007)	10	Recommended by the Addiction Medicine Foundation for older adolescents and adults. Reduced from 28-question DAST to provide brief, self-report screening of older youth and adults. Also used for clinical case finding and treatment evaluation research.

AOD, alcohol and other drugs; NIAAA, National Institute on Alcohol Abuse and Alcoholism; NIDA, National Institute on Drug Abuse.

NIAAA SG was less sensitive for alcohol use than the CRAFFT or PESQ-PC but performed better than the Alcohol Use Disorders Identification Test (AUDIT). Sensitivity for marijuana use was similar across the instruments.

Perhaps the oldest alcohol screening test used in the United States, the 25-question Michigan Alcohol Screening Test (MAST) is validated for use with adolescents and adults (Maisto et al. 1995). Many variations are now available, including the online self-administered MAST and shorter versions (The National Center for Physician Training in Addiction Medicine 2016). Similarly, the Drug Abuse Screen Test (DAST-10) was designed as a brief, self-report instrument primarily for adults but psychometric testing has validated use in older adolescents (Skinner 1982). The DAST-10 and DAST-20 require approximately 5 minutes to administer in a self-report or interview format, and yield a quantitative index of problems associated with drug use (NIDA n.d.). The Addiction Medicine Foundation (2016) suggests that DAST-10 may be used with older adolescents, but NIDA endorses only DAST-20 for youth. DAST-20 yields a quantitative index of the degree of consequences related to drug abuse, which may serve to guide clinical intervention and the evaluation of treatment response (McCabe et al. 2006).

The CRAFFT is currently the most well-studied adolescent substance use screener available with validity among diverse populations of adolescents aged 12–18 (Harris et al. 2016) and it was updated again in 2019 to add additional items related to vaping and marijuana use (The Center for Adolescent Substance Use Research 2018). CRAFFT 2.1 has both clinician- and self-administered versions and can be accessed at http://crafft.org. Version 2.0 of the CRAFFT used three screening questions: During the past 12 months did you drink any alcohol (more than a few sips)? Smoke any marijuana or hashish? Use anything else to get high? In CRAFFT Version 2.1, the three screening questions are worded to ask more directed questions about substance use quantity over the past 12 months. Version 2.1 also includes questions about vaping administration of marijuana. If the answer to all three questions is no, only the "car" question is asked. If any of the three screening questions are endorsed, the adolescent is asked to answer the six CRAAFT questions. Positive responses to two or more questions suggest the need for further assessment by a specialist (Harris et al. 2016; Knight et al. 2003).

The Alcohol Screening and Brief Intervention for Youth: A Practitioner's Guide (NIAAA 2015) is recommended for use with children ages 9–18. The tool and related resources are available on the public domain for early detection and prevention of alcohol-related problems in youth. By incorporating a question aimed at peer alcohol use, at-risk youth can be identified at earlier stages of alcohol involvement and target advice can address the risks related to friends' drinking (NIAAA n.d.). A stepwise process is based on the patient's developmental stage, with questions for elementary (age 9–11) and middle school (age 11–14) aimed at friends' use before asking about personal use. For high school (age 14–18) patients are asked about their own use of alcohol, followed by questions about friends' use (NIAAA 2015). See Box 23.1 for the clinical decision tree.

Brief Interventions

Brief interventions are designed to be provided within the context of the primary care, school, community, or family setting. When targeting harm reduction with youth, there are multiple settings where youth may have contact with a health professional who can assess risk, advise, and assist with a plan (Das et al. 2016; NIAAA 2015). Wherever they are provided, these evidence-based practices aim to motivate behavioral change in patients at risk of substance abuse and related health problems by helping them understand the risks related to the substance use and encouraging reduction or abstinence. For serious dependence, brief interventions (BIs) focus on accepting the need for intensive treatment and referral to specialized alcohol and drug treatment (SAMHSA n.d.).

Common elements of BIs include (i) feedback on substance use and health-related harms, (ii) identification of high-risk situations for heavy drinking, (iii) simple advice about how to cut down drinking, (iv) strategies that can increase motivation to change drinking behavior, and (v) the development of a personal plan to reduce drinking (Kaner et al. 2018; Levy and Knight 2008). The counseling commonly uses brief versions of cognitive behavioral therapy (CBT) or MI within the context of the clinical visit following screening and may last from 5 minutes of brief advice to 15–30 minutes of brief counseling (SAMHSA n.d.).

In addition to the guidelines included in the SBIRT guide (NIAAA 2015), four models of BI are identified by SAMHSA (n.d.): (i) Brief Negotiated Interview (BNI) and Active Referral to Treatment: Provider Training Algorithm, (ii) BNI Steps, (iii) the Feedback on screening results, Look for change talk, Options explored (FLO) Model, and (iv) the interviewing using Feedback, Responsibility, Advice, Menu Options, Empathy, Self-Efficacy (FRAMES) Model. Each of these models provide a framework for this process, and are generally applicable to youth as well as adults. These programs and other related resources are summarized in Table 23.3.

Box 23.1 Alcohol Screening and Brief Intervention for Youth

For *all* patients

Step 1: Ask the two screening questions
For elementary and middle school patients, start with the friends' question. Choose the questions that align with the patient's school level, as opposed to age, for patients ages 11 or 14. Exclude alcohol use for religious purposes.

Elementary School (ages 9–11)
Friends: Any drinking?
"Do you have any friends who drank beer, wine, or any drink containing alcohol in the *past year*?"
ANY drinking by friends heightens concern.
Patient: Any drinking?
"How about you – have you ***ever*** had more than a few sips of any drink containing alcohol?"
ANY *drinking:* Highest risk

Middle School (ages 11–14)
Friends: Any drinking?
"Do you have any friends who drank beer, wine, or any drink containing alcohol in the *past year*?"
ANY drinking by friends heightens concern.
Patient: How many days?
"How about you – in the *past year*, on how many days have you had more than a few sips of any drink containing alcohol?"
ANY *drinking:* Moderate or highest risk (depending on age and frequency)

High school (ages 14–18)
Patient: How many days?
"In the *past year*, on how many days have you had more than a few sips of beer, wine, or any drink containing alcohol?"
Lower, moderate, or highest risk (depending on age and frequency)
Friends: How much?
"If your friends drink, *how many drinks* do they usually drink on an occasion?"
Binge drinking by friends heightens concern. (See "What counts as a drink? A binger?" on reverse.)

For patients who *do not* drink

Step 2: Guide patient

NO   Do friends drink?   **YES**

Neither patient nor patient's friends drink
• **Praise choices** of not drinking and of having nondrinking friends.

Patient does not drink, but friends do
• **Praise choice** of not drinking.
• **Consider probing a little** using a neutral tone: "When your friends were drinking, you didn't drink. Tell me more about that." If the patient admits to drinking, go to Step 2 for patients who do drink, otherwise see below.
• **Reinforce healthy choices** with praise and encouragement.
• **Elicit and affirm reasons** to stay alcohol free.
• **Educate**, if the patient is open, about drinking risks related to brain development and later alcohol dependence.
• **Rescreen next year** at the latest.
• **Explore** how your patient plans to stay alcohol free when friends drink.
• **Advise** against riding in car with driver who has been drinking or using drugs.
• **Rescreen** at next visit.

Assessment complete for patients who do not drink.

For patients who *do* drink

Step 2: Assess risk
On how many days in the *past year* did your patient drink?
Factor in friends:
• **For elementary and middle school students:** Having friends who drink heightens concern.
• **For high school students:** Having friends who binge drink heightens concern. Recent research estimates that binge drinking levels for youth start at three to five drinks, depending on age and gender (see "What Counts as a Drink? A Binge?" on reverse).

Include what you already know about the patient's physical and psychosocial development in your risk evaluation, along with other relevant factors such as the level of family support, drinking and smoking habits of parents and siblings, school functioning, or trouble with authority figures.

For moderate and highest risk patients
- **Ask about the drinking pattern:** "How much do you usually have? What's the most you've had at any one time?" If patient reports binging, ask: "How often do you drink that much?"
- **Ask about problems experienced or risks taken:** Examples include getting lower grades or missing classes; drinking and driving or riding in a car driven by someone who has been drinking; having unplanned, unsafe sex; getting into fights; getting injured having memory blackouts; and passing out.
- **Ask whether the patient has used anything else to get high in the past year**, and consider using other formal tools to help gauge risk.

Step 3: Advise and assist
- **Provide brief advice** to slop drinking.
- **Notice the good:** Reinforce strengths and healthy decisions.
- **Explore and troubleshoot** influence of friends who drink.

Moderate risk
- **Does patient have alcohol-related problems?**
  - If **no**, provide beefed-up brief advice.
  - If **yes**, conduct brief motivational interviewing (MI).
- **Ask if parents know** see Highest Risk, below, for suggestions).
- **Arrange for followup**, ideally within a month.

Highest risk
- **Conduct brief MI.**
- **Ask if parents know . . .**
  - If **no**, consider breaking confidentiality to engage parent.
  - If **yes**, ask patient permission to speak with parent.
- **Consider referral** for further evaluation or treatment.
- **If you observe signs of acute danger** (e.g. drinking and driving, binge drinking, or using alcohol with other drugs) **take immediate steps to ensure safety**.
- **Arrange for followup** within a month.

For all patients who drink
- **Collaborate on a personal goal and action plan** for your patient. Refer to page 31 in the full Guide for sample abstinence, cutting back, and contingency plans. For some patients, the goal will be accepting a referral to specialized treatment.
- **Advise your patient not to drink and drive or ride in a car with an impaired driver.**
- **Plan a full psychosocial interview** for the next visit if needed.

Step 4: At follow-up, continue support

Was patient able to meet and sustain goal(s)?
Patients may not return for an alcohol-specific follow-up, but they may do so for other reasons. In either case, **ask about alcohol use and any associated problems**. Review the patient's goal(s) and assess whether he or she was able to meet and sustain them.

No, patient was not able to meet/sustain goal(s)
- **Reassess** the risk level (see Step 2 for drinkers).
- **Acknowledge** that change is difficult, that it's normal not to be successful on the first try, and that reaching a goal is a learning process.
- **Notice the good by:**
  - **praising** honesty and efforts.
  - **reinforcing** strengths.
  - **supporting** any positive change.
- **Relate drinking to associated consequences or problems** to enhance motivation.
- **Identify and address challenges and opportunities** in reaching the goal.
- If the following measures are not already under way, **consider:**
  - **engaging** parents.
  - **referring** for further evaluation.
- **Reinforce** the importance of the goal(s) and plan and **renegotiate** specific steps, as needed.

Conduct, complete, or update the comprehensive psychosocial interview.
Yes, patient was able to meet/sustain goal(s)
- **Reinforce and support** continued adherence to recommendations.
- **Notice the good:** Praise progress and reinforce strengths and healthy decisions.
- **Elicit future goals** to build on prior ones.
- **Conduct, complete, or update** the comprehensive psychosocial interview.
- **Rescreen** at least annually.
NIH Publication No. 11-7806 NIAAA (NIH 2015).

Early intervention has particular significance when addressing substance use in children and adolescents. The impact of substance use on psychosocial and neurological development increases the urgency related to identifying use and effectively engaging the youth in a BI (Degenhardt et al. 2016; Stockings et al. 2016). Among youth who have started using (unprescribed) psychoactive substances, the goal of interventions is to motivate and support a decision to reduce use and/or harm reduction. Evidence-based methods for implementing BIs range widely in format (e.g. individual, group, family) and theory (behavioral, client-centered, cognitive-behavioral, drug counseling, family systems), providing the opportunity and challenge of selecting an approach that is applicable for the setting and population (Hogue et al. 2014).

Recent studies of BI in youth demonstrate reduction in alcohol consumption and related harms following BI with MI or motivational enhancement therapy (MET) (Jensen et al. 2011; Patton et al. 2014). The evidence suggests that even single interventions for substance use problems in youth are appropriate and have a significant effect within the context of hospital emergency departments, and primary care and mental health clinical settings (Schleider and Weisz 2017). While most significant results of MI and MET have correlated with decreased alcohol and tobacco use, MI also shows promise for reducing cannabis use when provided as a BI in a hospital emergency department, school or community settings (Hogue et al. 2014; Kaner et al. 2018).

When preparing a BI for youth, the APRN must assess the population and clinic needs and resources. Many applications are available to deliver BIs with the use of electronic devices such as computer, tablet or smart phone. Although web-based screening tools are studied and endorsed by SAMHSA and NIDA, the research is preliminary regarding e-interventions for substance use (Donoghue et al. 2014; Kaner et al. 2018; SAMHSA n.d.; Stockings et al. 2016). Nonetheless, there is evidence to support the value of integrating technology into the healthcare setting to increase the frequency and consistency of screening and BI in clinical practice (Ozechowski et al. 2016).

Within primary care and mental health settings, APRNs have the opportunity to build a trusting rapport with patients, providing a framework for effective BIs when youth screen at risk for SUDs. Whether using the CRAFFT, Alcohol Screening and Brief Intervention for Youth, or another screening tool, any youth that screens positive should be further assessed and a referral made when appropriate based on the level of severity of the adolescent's substance use and whether the adolescent meets criteria for a diagnosis of SUD or dependence.

After screening and assessing for substance use, BI with adolescents who have experimented with substance use begins with a risk reduction intervention, such as providing *advice*. Alcohol Screening and Brief Intervention for Youth takes a stepwise approach to the advice. For youth who are identified as "lower risk" brief advice includes the recommendation to stop use and positive reinforcement of strengths and healthy decisions, as well as briefly exploring potential challenges related to peer use. Adolescents at "moderate risk" warrant more rigorous advising, addressing the frequency of use and incorporating MI to elicit decision and commitment to change. In this case, follow-up is recommended within 1 month. For youth at "highest risk," advice should begin with brief MI, followed by inquiry and possible intervention regarding parental knowledge. Referral for further evaluation and treatment and follow-up are indicated (NIAAA 2015).

Within the context of a BI, if not already diagnosed, it may be appropriate to screen the adolescent for depression, anxiety, and behavioral disorders (SAMHSA 2011). Pre-existing mental disorders correlate with a significantly increased risk of transition from nonuse to first use, and from use to problematic use of either alcohol or illicit drugs (Abram 2016; Conway et al. 2016). Conway et al. (2016) found that, specifically, the rate of alcohol use correlated with anxiety disorders (17.3) and behavioral disorders (15.6%) more than phobia disorders (8.5%) or eating disorders (9.7%). Given the significant relationship between mental health and substance use, treatment of primary mental disorders is an important aspect of early intervention, with the potential to reduce

Table 23.3 Brief interventions models and resources.

Model	Developer	Number of steps	Brief description
Brief Negotiated Interview and Active Referral to Treatment: Provider Training Algorithm	Boston University School of Public Health (1996 to 2012)	5	A flowchart that includes brief screening questions health practitioners can ask during brief intervention.
Brief Negotiated Interview (BNI) Steps	Project ED Health, D'Onofrio et al. 2005)	4	Includes a listing of questions and responses that a health provider can use by during a brief intervention.
The FLO Model	Adapted from Dunn, C. and Fields, C., SBI Training for Trauma Care Providers. SAMHSA, CSAT, George Washington University (2007)	4	Includes providing feedback, listening and understanding, and exploring options.
The FRAMES Model	Miller and Sanchez (1993)	6	Involves feedback, responsibility, advice, menu of strategies, empathy, and self-efficacy.

Resources

Descriptions of Brief Intervention and Brief Therapy	Colorado Clinical Guidelines Collaborative		Details brief interventions and brief therapy.
Motivational Interviewing Network of Trainers (MINT)	Miller, W. and Rollnick, S., trainees (1997 to present)		This site offers a wealth of useful tools related to motivational interviewing to help improve clinicians' skills.
Brief Intervention: The ASSIST-Linked Brief Intervention for Hazardous and Harmful Substance Use: Manual for Use in Primary Care	Humeniuk et al. (2010)		A manual designed to explain the theoretical basis and evidence for brief intervention and to assist primary healthcare workers to conduct a simple brief intervention for risky or harmful drug use.
TIP 34 Brief Interventions and Brief Therapies for Substance Abuse	SAMHSA (2012)		Educates healthcare and social service providers on the research, results, and promise of brief interventions in the hope that they will broaden their use in clinical practice and treatment programs nationwide.
TIP 35 Enhancing Motivation for Change in Substance Abuse Treatment	SAMHSA (2013)		Describes different motivational interventions that providers can use at all stages of change, from precontemplation and preparation to action and maintenance.

Source: Adapted from SAMHSA (n.d.), https://www.integration.samhsa.gov/clinical-practice/sbirt/brief-interventions.

morbidity related to secondary SUDs in youth (Abram 2016; Conway et al. 2016).

Evidence-based Treatment

Among youth who need more than prevention or BI, treatment for SUDs may include a range of psychosocial interventions. Depending upon individual risks and needs, as well as strengths, skills, and resources, interventions can be categorized across five broad levels of care, ranging from Level 0.5 to Level 4 as defined by American Society of Addiction Medicine (ASAM) Criteria (ASAM 2018; Stallvik et al. 2015). Table 23.4 summarizes these levels of service, which may guide the APRN in referral to treatment.

Points of Contact

Most youth who enroll in treatment are linked through providers in "gateway" service systems, including juvenile justice, mental health, school clinics, emergency rooms and primary medical care, and child social services. However, a treatment gap exists between the approximately 1.7 million adolescents in the United States meeting diagnostic criteria for SUDs annually and the 7% receiving specialized alcohol or drug abuse treatment, with 25% receiving mental health services (Winters et al. 2011). This results in higher levels of entry to care and in some cases incarceration of youth who do not receive appropriate levels of evidence-based treatment (Hogue et al. 2014). A solution to this problem is for APRNs and other healthcare professionals across these "gateways" to implement screening and BI and/or referral to treatment within each of these points of contact. Rather than waiting for annual check-ups to screen, it is important to meet youth where they are at, with a plan that ensures substance use is assessed and appropriate services rendered at every encounter (Hogue et al. 2014).

Considerations When Planning Treatment and Referral to Treatment

There is movement toward integrating or pairing elements of evidence-based treatment models. Recent studies have proposed that effort be directed toward developing enhancements and population-specific adaptations for the evidence-based modalities (Goldstein et al. 2012; Hogue et al. 2014), These enhancements include using multicomponent treatment for adolescents with co-occurring disorders, such as combining CBT with medication. Another recommendation is to avoid "missed opportunity" by embedding screening questions into the check-in process for each office visit and including parents or caregivers in screening and formulation to increase sources of information and the likelihood of identifying at-risk youth (Ozechowski et al. 2016). While evidence-based BIs are effective when they are implemented, improvements are warranted to optimize the frequency and efficacy of BIs. Ozechowski et al. (2016) suggest four adaptations to optimize BIs: (i) develop and use a risk algorithm to select the BI, (ii) deliver computer-based interventions, (iii) emphasize psychoeducation, and (iv) involve caregivers. Combined with a strong commitment to improving youth access to treatment, these additional measures may increase the quality and robustness of SBIRT in practice with youth.

Family-based Therapy

Adolescent substance misuse risk has been conceptualized as a "family disease" based on genetic, epigenetic, biological, and environmental family risk factors (Kumpfer and Magalhaes 2018). While psychosocial interventions range from individual, group, and family-based treatment (FBT) models, family-based approaches have the most empirical support (Bo et al. 2018; Hogue et al. 2014, 2015, 2017; Kumpfer and Magalhaes 2018). FBT have been shown to support positive treatment engagement, treatment impact across a range of outcome domains, and durability of treatment effects across cultural settings. In a systematic review and meta-analysis, Bo et al. (2018) found that interventions aimed at both general and alcohol-specific parenting strategies had larger effect sizes than interventions that focus on alcohol-specific parenting only. They hypothesizing that targeting both general and alcohol-specific parenting strategies not only addressed alcohol contexts but also addressed parenting strategies for child wellbeing and family functioning that may indirectly affect drinking.

Family-based interventions consider the adolescent's functioning within the family, patterns of communication, and relationships with extended family members and other social systems. Given the importance of the family system and social learning in youth development, FBT for SUD in adolescents aims to break the intergenerational cycle of substance abuse by strengthening the family and parenting skills (Kumpfer and Magalhaes 2018). Several ecological models are well-established as effective interventions, including functional family therapy, (FFT) (Alexander et al. 2013), brief strategic family therapy (BSFT) (Szapocznik et al. 2013), multisystemic therapy (Fox et al. 2016), and multidimensional family therapy (MDFT) (Hoogeveen et al. 2017).

While strong evidence supports numerous ecological family therapy models, there is a need to translate these

Table 23.4 Levels of intervention

Level	Description
Early intervention (Level 0.5)	Service for individuals at risk of developing substance-related problems, or for those for whom there is not yet sufficient information to document a diagnosable substance use disorder.
Outpatient services (Level 1)	Includes less than 6 hours a week for adolescents for recovery or motivational enhancement therapies and strategies. The patient should not be at risk for withdrawal except from nicotine. Level 1 is intended for individuals who are stable and not at risk of harm to self or others.
Intensive outpatient services (Level 2.1)	Includes 6 or more hours to treat multidimensional instability in patients at high risk for relapse without close monitoring and support. These services address the complex needs of youth with addiction and co-occurring conditions, and include treatment during the day, before or after work or school, in the evening, and/or on weekends.
Partial hospitalization services (Level 2.5)	This most-structured outpatient program includes 20 or more hours of service a week for multidimensional instability that does not require 24-hour care. This encompasses an organized outpatient service that delivers treatment services usually during the day as day treatment or partial hospitalization services to meet the complex needs of adolescents with addiction and co-occurring conditions.
Clinically managed low-intensity residential services (Level 3.1)	This level of care provides 24-hour living support and structure with available trained personnel, with at least 5 hours of clinical service per week. This includes residential services that are "co-occurring capable," "co-occurring enhanced," and "complexity capable services," staffed with qualified personnel to provide addiction treatment, mental health, and general medical services.
Clinically managed population-specific high-intensity residential services (Level 3.3)	Adult-only 24-hour care with trained counselors to stabilize multidimensional imminent danger and less intense milieu and group treatment for individuals with cognitive or other impairments who are unable to use full active milieu or the therapeutic community.
Clinically managed medium-intensity residential services for adolescents (Level 3.5)	This level of care provides 24-hour care with trained counselors to stabilize multidimensional imminent danger and prepare for outpatient treatment. Patients in this level are able to tolerate and use full active milieu or therapeutic communities.
Medically monitored high-intensity inpatient services for adolescents (Level 3.7)	This level of care is for individuals at high risk of withdrawal, providing 24-hour nursing care with an available provider for acute problems and counseling access 16 hours a day. This setting is appropriate for patients with subacute biomedical and emotional, behavioral, or cognitive problems that are so severe that they require inpatient treatment and medication therapy following a recent history of withdrawal management in a less intensive level of care, and marked by past and current inability to complete withdrawal management and enter into continuing addiction treatment.
Medically managed intensive inpatient services for adolescents and adults (Level 4)	This level of care is for individuals needing 24-hour medical and nursing care perhaps due to severe risk of withdrawal or psychiatric care and addiction treatment. Counseling is available to engage patients in treatment.
Residential	Long-term treatment including psychosocial rehabilitation for those with multiple problems. Duration of 30 days to a year.
Aftercare	Ongoing support for transition to home community and family; includes relapse prevention.
Group homes	May follow a treatment program or be part of it. Transitional living with staff and consumer participation in responsibilities, governance, school, or work.
Psychosocial	Includes family treatments (multisystemic), integrated family therapy, and CBT. Individual psychoeducation for refusal skills, identification of triggers, and learning alternative options. CBT may also be included. 12-step programs include AA and NA.
Pharmacological	Withdrawal protocol from alcohol includes benzodiazepine taper, multivitamins, and seizure precautions. Medically supervised withdrawal from opiates includes clonidine, methadone, and buprenorphine (Naltrexone)

AA, Alcoholics Anonymous; CBT, cognitive behavioral therapy; NA, Narcotics Anonymous.
Source: Adapted from American Society of Addiction Medicine 2018, https://www.asamcontinuum.org/knowledgebase/what-are-the-asam-levels-of-care.

successful models into a wide range of accessible practice settings. A recent study distilled core elements of three effective family therapy models, FFT, BSFT, and MDFT, for the purpose of identifying shared elements of research-supported treatments that are more easily integrated into practice (Hogue et al. 2017). Core elements contributing to the success of these interventions include (i) family engagement, (ii) relational reframing, (iii) family behavior change, and (iv) family restructuring (Hogue et al. 2017). The APRN should consider these factors when planning family therapeutic interventions for SUD in youth.

Other Treatment Approaches

Depending upon the severity and co-occurring disorders, components of treatment may include (i) individual and group therapy, (ii) case or care management, (iii) medication, (iv) recovery support services, (v) 12-step fellowship, and (vi) peer supports (SAMHSA n.d.).

Individual Therapy

Individual therapies include behavioral treatments that teach adolescents to identify internal and external stimuli that trigger substance use, followed by providing skill training in refusal skills, relaxation techniques, and behavioral management. Behavioral interventions play an important role in relapse prevention by identifying triggers for substance use and developing alternate coping skills through reinforcement conditions. Behavioral interventions play a major role in relapse prevention. Cognitive therapies focus on distorted thoughts and maladaptive perceptions that lead to problem use behaviors. CBT explicitly aims to modify cognitive processes, beliefs, individual behaviors, and environmental reinforcers that are associated with adolescent substance use. In both MET and brief motivational interventions, the goal is to resolve ambivalence about whether the adolescent has a substance use condition and to improve his or her motivation to change (Deas 2008; Webb et al. 2007). MET's emphasis on a collaborative or proactive communication style has theoretical appeal as an intervention for adolescents (Stockings et al. 2016). MI helps build motivation toward behavior change. Brief motivational interventions consisting of one to five sessions targeted toward increasing the adolescent's motivation to decrease substance use also produced favorable outcomes in comparison studies. Numerous studies have indicated the efficacy and effectiveness of brief MI interventions (Ozechowski et al. 2016; Stockings et al. 2016).

Group Therapy

Group-based treatments are commonly implemented across the continuum of care for adolescents with substance use and co-occurring mental disorders. Groups have been studied in inpatient, residential, outpatient, school, and community settings, using interventions such as CBT and MET (Hogue et al. 2014). While their efficacy has been reported, group dynamics should be carefully considered and monitored for iatrogenic effect from exposure to peers that might reinforce negative behavior and delinquency (Dishion and Tipsord 2011; Hogue et al. 2014).

Case or Care Management

For adolescents who receive treatment for SUD, the incidence of relapse within 90 days exceeds 50% within the following year (Passetti et al. 2016). Case management may improve the outcome by providing the patient and/or parent with a single point of contact for coordinating behavioral health services with housing, employment, education, and other supports (SAMHSA 2017). The case manager can ensure that all services provided to the youth and family are efficiently coordinated and linked to continuing care. Other important roles of the case manager are to advocate for appropriate services, link individuals and families to social support, arrange transportation to pro-social activities, and support clients in securing potential employment or necessary services (Passetti et al. 2016).

Technology-enhanced Continuing Care

While substance abuse treatment may have promising results among adolescents and young adults, psychosocial pressures to use make it difficult to sustain recovery. Kaminer and Godley (2010) suggest that SUDs develop over time, and recovery requires a similar multiphasic, lengthy process. Statistically, the risk of relapse is estimated to be 60% within 3 months and 80% within 1 year once individuals discontinue treatment (Brown et al. 2001; Gonzales et al. 2014a). However, there is evidence to suggest that extending care to support sustained recovery may reduce relapse and recidivism (Passetti et al. 2016).

Post-treatment aftercare, or continuing care, aims to reduce the risk of relapse and chronic patterns that persist into adulthood (Kaminer and Godley 2010; Passetti et al. 2016). For adolescents, these interventions should utilize innovative strategies that are relevant to the population. Donoghue et al. (2014) suggest that the use of technology-enhanced screening and BI offers flexibility, anonymity, and accessibility to youth who are not otherwise engaged in traditional face-to-face treatment.

In a pilot using a mobile-based texting recovery program, Gonzales et al. (2014b) reported significant benefits of text messaging for daily self-monitoring, to provide daily wellness recovery tips with substance abuse education, and for weekend social support resources. Compared to traditional approaches, assessment and monitoring were enhanced and engagement could be personalized, targeting individual needs with minimal financial and time burden for patients or providers. The added flexibility enhanced access to this aftercare service, providing opportunity for youth to practice self-management of stressors and addiction behaviors (Gonzales et al. 2014a). Gonzales et al. (2014b) reported that most youth responded favorably to using text messaging to support recovery after treatment.

12-step Fellowship

Many programs incorporate Alcoholics Anonymous (AA) or Narcotics Anonymous (NA) into their treatment program (SAMHSA 2018a). Recent studies have shown that 12-step programs such as AA or NA strengthen and extend the benefits of typical community outpatient treatment, and may improve self-efficacy in social situations and reduce pro-drinking social networks among TAY (Bukstein 2017; Hoeppner et al. 2014; Kelly et al. 2010). There is evidence to suggest that frequency of participation in 12-step meetings is associated with more positive treatment outcomes, especially when 12-step meetings are age-matched for the participants (Passetti et al. 2016).

Pharmacological Interventions

Psychosocial interventions are the first-line treatment for adolescent SUDs (Das et al. 2016; Knudsen et al. 2011). However, recent studies have begun to evaluate complementary pharmacological interventions in youth with SUDs (Hammond and Gray 2016). Although data are limited, there is growing evidence to support a role for pharmacotherapy in youth with cannabis, alcohol, and opioid use disorders (OUDs), as well as co-occurring psychiatric disorders (Hammond and Gray 2016). When prescribing pharmacological interventions, the APRN should be aware that most medications specific for treating substance dependence and used routinely in adults lack safety and efficacy data for use in children or adolescents. Prior to off-label treatment, youth and their guardians must be thoroughly informed of the evidence supporting benefit versus risk and the reasons for the recommended treatment.

Tobacco

In a review of literature related to treatment of tobacco use disorder, Hammond and Gray (2016) report no statistically significant benefit from varenicline, nor from low dose bupropion (150 mg), nor nicotine gum or nasal spray. However, several studies suggest that bupropion sustained release 300 mg and nicotine patch may provide temporary benefit as adjunctive treatment with psychosocial and behavioral therapies (Gray et al. 2011; Hammond and Gray 2016). Long-term benefits have not been established, but further evaluation continues to explore the utility of varenicline for smoking cessation and other pharmacological approaches to long-term recovery. None of the forms of nicotine replacement therapy (NRT), varenicline, or bupropion are currently approved by the FDA for pediatric use (Miranda and Treloar 2018).

Alcohol Detoxification

Despite the prevalence of alcohol use and dependency in youth, research is lacking for psychopharmacological treatment of alcohol withdrawal syndrome and relapse prevention in the adolescent population (Hammond and Gray 2016). Neurocognitive deficits have been associated with alcohol withdrawal among adolescents, which is estimated to occur among 5–10% of adolescents with AUD (Clark 2012). Although rarely medically necessary, supervised pharmacotherapy is indicated to prevent seizure or neurocognitive damage from severe alcohol withdrawal in adolescents. As with treatment of adults, long-acting benzodiazepines such as diazepam and chlordiazepoxide are the first-line pharmacotherapy for alcohol withdrawal symptom management and seizure prevention. Other medication classes include β-adrenoceptor antagonists (beta-blockers), clonidine, baclofen, and topiramate, an anticonvulsant medication (Clark 2012).

Relapse Prevention

Small controlled studies provided preliminary support for the use of disulfiram, naltrexone, acamprosate, and topiramate with alcohol-dependent adolescents in inpatient settings following medication-assisted withdrawal/detoxification (Clark 2012; Hammond and Gray 2016). The most promising are therapies aimed at craving reduction for relapse prevention. Naltrexone, an opioidµ-receptor antagonist, has been demonstrated to reduce interest in alcohol use among adolescents more effectively than aversion therapy using disulfiram (Miranda and Treloar 2018). Similarly, the NMDA glutamate antagonist topiramate has shown promise for reducing alcohol consumption and addiction risk in adults, but has not been studied in youth to date (Clark 2012).

Ondansetron, a selective 5-HT3 (serotonin) receptor antagonist, has shown a positive effect on reduction of alcohol use in TAY and warrants further consideration in youth (Hammond and Gray 2016). In addition, the GABA agonist baclofen has shown evidence to suggest it may reduce alcohol withdrawal symptoms and alcohol use, but studies are lacking among youth to support its use (Addolorato et al. 2006; Clark 2012).

Aversion treatment warrants cautious use among adolescents who are unlikely to be committed to abstinence from alcohol use. Disulfiram is considered the prototypical aversive agent as it produces unpleasant adverse effect when taken with alcohol. A recent literature review of pharmacological treatment for SUDs identified two studies that showed an increased effectiveness for disulfiram (Yule and Wilkens 2015). As discussed in this review, both studies were limited by small sample sizes and both were conducted more than 10 years ago. Moreover, aversion therapy is considered particularly risky for unsupervised youth due to the risk of hepatotoxicity associated with disulfiram.

Cannabis

Despite recent increases in the prevalence of cannabis use among adolescents, research related to evidence-based pharmacotherapy is limited. Preliminary studies published in 2012 support the potential efficacy of gabapentin in ameliorating cannabis withdrawal symptoms (Mason et al. 2012) and the atypical antidepressant bupropion in reducing craving and withdrawal (Penetar et al. 2012). More recent study has demonstrated a possible reduction in cannabis use with the glutamatergic modulator N-acetylcysteine (NAC) (Tomko et al. 2018), however more robust evidence is needed to support the findings and to identify treatment outcomes greater than 1 month (Miranda and Treloar 2018). Another recent randomized, controlled trial found that the antiseizure medication topiramate used with and without MET was effective in quantity but not frequency of cannabis used (Miranda and Treloar 2018). To date, none of these treatments are FDA approved for adolescent use (Marshall et al. 2014).

Opioids

The increase in opioid abuse among adults has led to significant increased nonprescribed use by youth, with significant psychiatric comorbidity and psychosocial risks (Hammond and Gray 2016). Growing public awareness of the opioid crisis has increased focus on medication assisted treatment for adults using methadone, naltrexone or buprenorphine (SAMHSA 2018c). Currently, the American Academy of Pediatrics recommends medication treatment for OUD in adolescents because it effectively reduces opioid use as well as the higher rates of mortality associated with untreated OUD (Levy 2019). Two clinical trials have evaluated the efficacy of buprenorphine and naltrexone for medication-assisted treatment of OUD in youth, combined with behavioral counseling (Hammond and Gray 2016). While more studies are needed, these preliminary findings suggest that the opioid receptor antagonist naltrexone is most promising in the treatment of youth, whereas short-term opiate agonist treatment with methadone nor partial agonist buprenorphine are not generally recommended (Subramaniam et al. 2011). Hammond and Gray (2016) suggest that further studies explore the use of opioid agonists in youth with significant opioid dependence and psychiatric comorbidity.

Methamphetamine

There are no FDA approved pharmacological treatments for methamphetamine dependence, however preliminary studies in adults have suggested possible efficacy of naltrexone, mirtazapine, topiramate, bupropion, and modafinil (Courtney and Ray 2014; Miranda and Treloar 2018). As studies continue to seek effective pharmacotherapies, APRNs play an essential role in advocating for inclusion of this population in research and program funding for equitable treatment of youth with methamphetamine and other SUDs.

Co-occurring Psychiatric and Substance Use Disorders

Although large-scale epidemiological studies do not provide specific prevalence rates for adolescents, it is estimated that more than half of adolescents with a SUD also suffer from at least one psychiatric disorder (Conway et al. 2016; Hammond and Gray 2016). APRNs treating youth with depression, anxiety, ADHD, or other psychiatric conditions should be cognizant of the increased risk for early substance use and dependence as adults (Abram 2016). While the risks are significant, early identification and treatment of behavioral disorders combined with screening and substance abuse prevention are associated with decreased incidence and severity of co-occurring disorders (Hawkins 2009). Youth with anxiety and depressive disorders are at an even greater risk of substance abuse and may be more difficult to identify than youth with externalizing behavioral symptoms.

Early recognition and treatment of mood and anxiety disorders may improve prosocial skills, coping, and reduce future substance abuse (Abram 2016; Conway et al. 2016; Hulvershorn et al. 2015). Youth with co-occurring disorders are likely to experience significant barriers to treatment related to social–emotional stressors. Coordination of care is essential between primary care, behavioral health, and substance use treatment programs to provide optimal results and reduce adverse outcomes related to delayed or fragmented services. Integrated behavioral health and treatment is a favorable approach to removing barriers and stigma and increasing access to early and effective services (Hawkins 2009). While this model has gained traction in adult and family practice settings, further leadership is needed to enhance integration of services for children and adolescents (Conway et al. 2016; Hawkins 2009).

Summary

Substance use and SUDs represent a significant public health concern for children and adolescents. Across multiple national data sources, alcohol, marijuana, and cigarettes remain the three most commonly used substances. Specifically, alcohol is the most widely used substance, with the majority of underage alcohol use involving binge drinking (i.e. more than four to five drinks on a single occasion). Although the use of conventional cigarettes by middle school and high school students has dropped steadily in recent years, this trend has been replaced with a sharp increase in the use of ENDS, which represents a potential public health concern. Similar to cigarettes, marijuana use among adolescents has been declining in recent years, however the impact of newer MMLs (and associated changes in perceptions of decrease risk) is unknown. Finally, in an era of public health crisis involving opioid use among adults, children and adolescents are not necessarily misusing opioids on quite the same scale, however this trend also bears watching, especially because other substance use behaviors may be a precursor to OUDs.

The etiology of substance use and SUD is multifactorial and complex. Research has identified distinct biological, personal, and environmental factors that are correlated with initiation, use, and/or misuse of substances. In addition to research supporting each of these three factors as part of the etiology of adolescent substance use, APRNs also need to understand that these factors are highly interactive and bidirectional. More importantly, given that adolescence is a time of significant biopsychosocial development, there is even greater potential during this time to influence adult health and development outcomes by addressing substance use in young people.

APRNs should be aware of several important aspects of the clinical presentation of SUDs in children and adolescents. First of all, substance use behaviors in young people are often progressive, meaning that most children start with experimentation, and only some proceed into regular use, harmful use, and/or disordered use. While substance use is pervasive among adolescents, most teenagers who try alcohol or other drug do not

develop SUDs. Second, for those young people who do develop a SUD, the clinical presentation of the disorder is also categorized in a progressive way, ranging from mild to moderate to severe. Finally, APRNs should understand that comorbid health conditions are the norm not the exception for children with substance use behaviors and SUDs. Physical health conditions are commonly tied to the physiologic effects of the specific substance that the child is using, while common mental health conditions include depression, suicidal thinking or behaviors, and externalizing disorders (such as ADHD, conduct disorder, and oppositional defiant disorder). In addition to comorbid health conditions, adolescent substance use also commonly includes disruptions in family relationships, academic achievements, and/or legal status, all of which may impact clinical presentation.

Current practice guidelines call for providers to screen for alcohol, tobacco, and drug use for youth aged 11 and older. Numerous validated tools exist for such screening, however the strongest evidence for use specifically in young people supports use of the CRAFFT tool, a six-item mnemonic that assess risky alcohol and drug use behaviors. The CRAFFT screening tool is especially helpful in stratifying risk levels such that the APRN can respond with positive reinforcement of low-risk behaviors, provide BI for those with moderate risk, and refer high-risk patients to the necessary treatment service. Given the literature supporting the effectiveness of BI, it is important that APRNs understand how and why to apply MI skills to the care of youth engaged in risky substance use behaviors. Pediatric primary care providers may be especially well-suited for this level of care due to the greater level of patient trust associated with this more long-term patient relationship.

Among youth who need more than prevention or BI, treatment for SUDs may include a range of psychosocial and/or pharmacological interventions. Evidence-based psychosocial interventions are currently considered the first-line treatment for youth with SUDs and include individual therapy, family therapy, case management, recovery support services, 12-step groups, and peer support. There is currently much less evidence supporting the use of pharmacological therapy for adolescent SUD, due in large part to the absence of safety and efficacy data for most medications that are approved for adult use.

Regardless of the treatment modalities that are used, several common barriers exist to disrupt children receiving the services they need. Barriers to treatment include lack of adequate facilities that specialize in adolescent populations, stigma and shame issues that discourage adolescents (and their families) from seeking care, and the use of more coercive methods of entry into care such as court mandates that may discourage adolescents from being self-motivated to change behaviors. To the extent that many adolescents who use substances would try to hide or deny their use, APRNs should also understand that the nature of the behavior may discourage youth from recognizing the need for treatment.

References

Abram, K. (2016). New evidence for the role of mental disorders in the development of substance abuse. *Journal of the American Academy of Child and Adolescent Psychiatry* 55 (4): 265–266. https://doi.org/10.1016/j.jaac.2016.02.003.

Addiction Medicine Foundation (2016). Identifying and responding to substance use among adolescents and young adults: A compendium of resources for medical practice. Available at http://www.abam.net/wp-content/uploads/2016/04/MRL-Compenduim-Update-4-11-16.pdf.

Addolorato, G., Leggio, L., Agabio, R., and Colombo, G. (2006). Baclofen: A new drug for the treatment of alcohol dependence. *International Journal of Clinical Practice* 60 (8): 1003–1008. https://doi.org/10.1111/j.1742-1241.2006.01065.x.

Addolorato, G., Vassallo, G.A., Antonelli, G. et al. (2018). Binge drinking among adolescents is related to the development of alcohol use disorders: results from a cross-sectional study. *Scientific Reports* 8 (1): 12624. https://doi.org/10.1038/s41598-018-29311-y.

Alexander, J.A., Waldron, H.B., Robbins, M.S., and Neeb, A. (2013). *Functional Family Therapy for Adolescent Behavior Problems.* American Psychological Association.

Al-Tayyib, A., Riggs, P., Mikulich-Gilbertson, S., and Hopfer, C. (2018). Prevalence of nonmedical use of prescription opioids and association with co-occurring substance use disorders among adolescents in substance use treatment. *Journal of Adolescent Health* 62 (2): 241–244. https://doi.org/10.1016/j.jadohealth.2017.09.018.

APA (2013). *Diagnostic and Statistical Manual of Mental Disorders (DSM-5).* Washington, DC: American Psychiatric Association.

APA (2018). *Diagnostic and statistical manual of mental disorders (DSM-5).* Online assessment measures, Level 2 cross-cutting symptom measures. American Psychiatric Association. Available at https://www.psychiatry.org/psychiatrists/practice/dsm/educational-resources/assessment-measures#Disorder.

ASAM (2018). *ASAM Criteria.* American Society of Addiction Medicine. Available at https://www.asam.org/resources/the-asam-criteria/about.

Amrock, S.M., Lee, L., and Weitzman, M. (2016). Perceptions of e-cigarettes and noncigarette tobacco products among US youth. *Pediatrics* 138 (5): e20154306. https://doi.org/10.1542/peds.2015-4306.

Bava, S. and Tapert, S.F. (2010). Adolescent brain development and the risk for alcohol and other drug problems. *Neuropsychology Review* 20 (4): 398–413. https://doi.org/10.1007/s11065-010-9146-6.

Bayly, J.E., Bernat, D., Porter, L., and Choi, K. (2019). Secondhand exposure to aerosols from electronic nicotine delivery systems and asthma exacerbations among youth with asthma. *CHEST* 155 (1): 88–93. https://doi.org/10.1016/j.chest.2018.10.005.

Been, J.V. and Sheikh, A. (2018). Tobacco control policies in relation to child health outcomes and perinatal health outcomes. *Archives of Disease in Childhood* 103 (9): 817–819. https://doi.org/10.1136/archdischild-2017-313680.

Bo, A., Hai, A., and Jaccard, J. (2018). Parent-based interventions on adolescent alcohol use outcomes: a systematic review and meta-analysis. *Drug & Alcohol Dependence* 191: 98–109. https://doi.org/10.1016/j.drugaldep.2018.05.031.

Bos, J., Hayden, M.J., Lum, J.A., and Staiger, P.K. (2019). UPPS-P impulsive personality traits and adolescent cigarette smoking: a meta-analysis. *Drug and Alcohol Dependence* https://doi.org/10.1016/j.drugalcdep.2019.01.018.

Boston Children's Hospital (2015). Adolescent SBIRT toolkit for providers. SA3541. Available at http://massclearinghouse.ehs.state.ma.us/product/SA1099.html.

Brown, S.A., D'Amico, E.J., McCarthy, D.M., and Tapert, S.F. (2001). Four-year outcomes from adolescent alcohol and drug treatment. *Journal of Studies on Alcohol and Drugs* 62: 381–388. https://doi.org/10.15288/jsa.2001.62.381.

Bukstein, O.G. (2015). Conduct disorder and delinquency and substance use disorders. In: *Youth Substance Abuse and Co-Occurring Disorders* (ed. Y. Kaminer), 81–102. Washington, DC: American Psychiatric Association Publishing.

Bukstein, O.G. (2017). Challenges and gaps in understanding substance use problems in transitional age youth. *Child and Adolescent Psychiatric Clinics* 26 (2): 253–269. https://doi.org/10.1016/j.chc.2016.12.005.

Center for Substance Abuse Treatment (1997). *A Guide to Substance Abuse Services for Primary Care Clinicians.* Treatment Improvement Protocol (TIP) Series No. 24. Rockville (MD): Substance Abuse and Mental Health Services Administration. Available at https://www.ncbi.nlm.nih.gov/books/NBK64827/?report=reader.

Cerdá, M., Sarvet, A.L., Wall, M. et al. (2018). Medical marijuana laws and adolescent use of marijuana and other substances: alcohol, cigarettes, prescription drugs, and other illicit drugs. *Drug and Alcohol Dependence* 183: 62–68. https://doi.org/10.1016/j.drugalcdep.2017.10.021.

Chhabra, N. and Aks, S.E. (2017). Current opiate and opioid hazards in children and adolescents. *Clinical Pediatric Emergency Medicine* 18 (3): 173–180. https://doi.org/10.1016/j.cpem.2017.07.006.

Choi, H.J., Yu, M., and Sacco, P. (2018). Racial and ethnic differences in patterns of adolescent tobacco users: a latent class analysis. *Children and Youth Services Review* 84: 86–93. https://doi.org/10.1016/j.childyouth.2017.11.019.

Christie, C., Baker, C., Cooper, R., Kennedy, P., Madras, B., & Bondi, P. (2017). *The President's Commission on Combating Drug Addiction and the Opioid Crisis.* Available at https://www.whitehouse.gov/sites/whitehouse.gov/files/images/Final_Report_Draft_11-1-2017.pdf.

Clark, D. (2012). Pharmacotherapy for adolescent alcohol use disorder: therapy in practice. *CNS Drugs* 26 (7): 559–569. https://doi.org/10.2165/11634330-000000000-00000.

Clark, D.B., Chung, T., Thatcher, D.L. et al. (2012). Psychological dysregulation, white matter disorganization and substance use disorders in adolescence. *Addiction* 107 (1): 206–214. https://doi.org/10.1111/j.1360-0443.2011.03566.x.

Conway, K.P., Swendsen, J., Husky, M.M. et al. (2016). Association of lifetime mental disorders and subsequent alcohol and illicit drug use: results from the National Comorbidity Survey-Adolescent Supplement. *Journal of American Academy of Child and Adolescent Psychiatry* 55 (4): 280–288. https://doi.org/10.1016/j.jaac.2016.01.006.

Courtney, K. and Ray, L. (2014). Methamphetamine: an update on epidemiology, pharmacology, clinical phenomenology, and treatment literature. *Drug and Alcohol Dependence* 143: 11–21. https://doi.org/10.1016/j.drugalcdep.2014.08.003.

Couwenbergh, C., van den Brink, W., Zwart, K. et al. (2006). Comorbid psychopathology in adolescents and young adults treated for substance use disorders. *European Child & Adolescent Psychiatry* 15 (6): 319–328. https://doi.org/10.1007/s00787-006-0535-6.

Cullen, K.A., Ambrose, B.K., Gentzke, A.S. et al. (2018). Notes from the field: increase use of electronic cigarettes and any tobacco product among middle school and high school students – United States 2011-2018. *MMWR Morbidity and Mortality Weekly Report* 67 (45): 1276–1277. https://doi.org/10.15585/mmwr/mm6745a5.

D'Amico, E., Parast, L., Meredith, S. et al. (2016). Screening in primary care: what is the best way to identify at-risk youth for substance abuse? *Pediatrics* 138 (6): 1–11. https://doi.org/10.1542/peds. 2016-1717.

Das, J., Salam, R., Arshad, A. et al. (2016). Interventions for adolescent substance abuse: an overview of systematic reviews. *Journal of Adolescent Health* 59: S61–S75. https://doi.org/10.1016/j.jadohealth. 2016.06.021.

Deas, D. (2008). Evidence-based treatments for alcohol use disorders in adolescents. *Pediatrics* 121 (suppl 4): S348–S354.

Degenhardt, L., Stockings, E., Patton, G. et al. (2016). The increasing global health priority of substance use in young people. *The Lancet Psychiatry* 3 (3): 251–264. https://doi.org/10.1016/S2215-0366(15)00508-8.

Dishion, T.J. and Tipsord, J.M. (2011). Peer contagion in child and adolescent social and emotional development. *Annual Review of Psychology* 62: 189–214. https://doi.org/10.1146/annurev.psych. 093008.100412.

D'Onofrio, G., Pantalon, M.V., Degutis, L.C. et al. (2005). Development and implementation of an emergency practitioner–performed brief intervention for hazardous and harmful drinkers in the emergency department. *Academic Emergency Medicine* 12 (3): 249–256. https://doi.org/10.1197/j.aem.2004.10.021.

Donoghue, K., Patton, R., Phillips, T. et al. (2014). The effectiveness of electronic screening and brief intervention for reducing levels of alcohol consumption: a systematic review and meta-analysis. *Journal of Medical Internet Research* 16 (6): e142. https://doi. org/10.2196/jmir.3193.

Duffy, A., Horrocks, J., Milin, R. et al. (2012). Adolescent substance use disorder during the early stages of bipolar disorder: a prospective high-risk study. *Journal of Affective Disorders* 142 (1–3): 57–64. https://doi.org/10.1016/j.jad.2012.04.010.

Elsayed, N.M., Kim, M.J., Fields, K.M. et al. (2018). Trajectories of alcohol initiation and use during adolescence: the role of stress and amygdala reactivity. *Journal of the American Academy of Child & Adolescent Psychiatry* 57 (8): 550–560. https://doi.org/10.1016/j. jaac.2018.05.011.

ElSohly, M.A., Mehmedic, Z., Foster, S. et al. (2016). Changes in cannabis potency over the last 2 decades (1995–2014): analysis of current data in the United States. *Biological Psychiatry* 79 (7): 613–619. https://doi.org/10.1016/j.biopsych.2016.01.004.

van Emmerik-van Oortmerssen, K., van de Glind, G., van den Brink, W. et al. (2012). Prevalence of attention-deficit hyperactivity disorder in substance use disorder patients: a meta-analysis and meta-regression analysis. *Drug and Alcohol Dependence* 122 (1–2): 11–19. https://doi.org/10.1016/j.drugalcdep.2011.12.007.

Fox, S., Bibi, F., Millar, H., and Holland, A. (2016). The role of cultural factors in engagement and change in multisystemic therapy (MST). *Journal of Family Therapy.* MSTS Publication #1505. doi: https:// doi.org/10.1111/1467-6427.12134.

Goldstein, N.E., Kemp, K.A., Leff, S.S., and Lochman, J.E. (2012). Guidelines for adapting manualized interventions for new target populations: a step-wise approach using anger management as a model. *Clinical Psychology: Science and Practice* 19: 385–401.

Gonzales, R., Ang, A., Murphy, D. et al. (2014a). Substance use recovery outcomes among a cohort of youth participating in a mobile-based texting aftercare pilot program. *Journal of Substance Abuse Treatment* 47: 20–26. https://doi.org/10.1016/j. jsat.2014.01.010.

Gonzales, R., Anglin, M., and Glik, D. (2014b). Exploring the feasibility of text messaging to support substance abuse recovery among youth in treatment. *Health Education Research* 29 (1): 13–22. https://doi.org/10.1093/her/cyt094.

Gray, K.M., Carpenter, M.J., Baker, N.L. et al. (2011). Bupropion SR and contingency management for adolescent smoking cessation. *Journal of Substance Abuse Treatment* 40: 77–86. https://doi. org/10.1016/j.jsat.2010.08.010.

Groenman, A.P., Janssen, T.W., and Oosterlaan, J. (2017). Childhood psychiatric disorders as risk factor for subsequent substance abuse: a meta-analysis. *Journal of the American Academy of Child & Adolescent Psychiatry* 56 (7): 556–569. https://doi.org/10.1016/j. jaac.2017.05.004.

Hammond, C. and Gray, K. (2016). Pharmacotherapy for substance use disorders in youths. *Journal of Child and Adolescent Substance Abuse* 25 (4): 292–316. https://doi.org/10.1080/1067828X.2015.1037517.

Harris, S., Knight, J., Van Hook, S. et al. (2016). Adolescent substance use screening in primary care: validity of computer self-administered vs. clinician-administered screening. *Substance Abuse* 37 (1): 197–203. https://doi.org/10.1080/08897077.2015.1014615.

Hawkins, E.H. (2009). A tale of two systems: Co-occurring mental health and substance abuse disorders treatment for adolescents. *Annual Review of Psychology* 60: 197–227. https://doi.org/10.1146/ annurev.psych.60.110707.163456.

Hawkins, S.S., Bach, N., and Baum, C.F. (2016). Impact of tobacco control policies on adolescent smoking. *Journal of Adolescent Health* 58 (6): 679–685. https://doi.org/10.1016/j. jadohealth.2016.02.014.

Hernandez, L., Lavingne, A., Wood, M., and Weirs, R.W. (2015). Moderators and mediators of treatments for youth with substance use disorders. In: *Moderators and Mediators of Youth Treatment Outcomes* (eds. M. Maric, P.J.M. Prins and T.H. Ollendick), 174–209. New York, NY: Oxford University Press.

Hingson, R.W., Heeren, T., and Winter, M.R. (2006). Age at drinking onset and alcohol dependence: age at onset, duration, and severity. *Archives of Pediatrics & Adolescent Medicine* 160 (7): 739–746. https://doi.org/10.1001/archpedi.160.7.739.

Hoeppner, B., Hoeppner, S., and Kelly, J. (2014). Do young people benefit from AA as much, and in the same ways, as adult aged 30+? A moderated multiple mediation analysis. *Drug & Alcohol Dependence* 143: 181–188. https://doi.org/10.1016/j.drugalcdep. 2014.07.023.

Hogue, A., Henderson, C., Ozechowski, T., and Robbins, M. (2014). Evidence base on outpatient behavioral treatments for adolescent substance use: updates and recommendations 2007-2013. *Journal of Clinical Child & Adolescent Psychology* 43 (5): 695–720. https:// doi.org/10.1080/15374416.2014.915550.

Hogue, A., Dauber, S., Henderson, C. et al. (2015). Randomized trial of family therapy versus nonfamily treatment for adolescent behavior problems in usual care. *Journal of Clinical Child & Adolescent Psychology* 44 (6): 954–969. https://doi.org/10.1080/15374416.2014 .963857.

Hogue, A., Bobek, M., Dauber, S. et al. (2017). Distilling the core elements of family therapy for adolescent substance use: conceptual and empirical solutions. *Journal of Child & Adolescent Substance Abuse* 26 (6): 437–453. https://doi.org/10.1080/1067828X.2017.1322020.

Hogue, A., Henderson, C., Becker, S., and Knight, D. (2018). Evidence base on outpatient behavioral treatments for adolescent substance use, 2014–2017: outcomes, treatment delivery, and promising horizons. *Journal of Clinical Child & Adolescent Psychology* 47 (4): 499–526. https://doi.org/10.1080/15374416.2018.1466307.

Hoogeveen, C.E., Vogelvang, B., and Rigter, H. (2017). Feasibility of inpatient and outpatient multidimensional family therapy for improving behavioral outcomes in adolescents referred to residential youth care. *Residential Treatment for Children & Youth* 34: 61–82. https://doi.org/10.1080/0886571X.20161268945.

Hulvershorn, L., Quinn, P., and Scott, E. (2015). Treatment of adolescent substance use disorders and co-occurring internalizing disorders: a critical review and proposed model. *Current Drug Abuse Review* 8 (1): 41–49. https://doi.org/10.2174/1874473708666150514102745.

Humeniuk, R.E., Henry-Edwards, S., Ali, R. et al. (2010). *The ASSIST-linked brief intervention for hazardous and harmful substance use: manual for use in primary care.* Geneva, Switzerland: World Health Organization Available at https://www.who.int/substance_abuse/publications/assist_sbi/en/.

Jacobus, J. and Tapert, S.F. (2014). Effects of cannabis on the adolescent brain. *Current Pharmacological Design* 20 (13): 2186–2193. https://doi.org/10.2174/13816128113199990426.

Jensen, C., Cushing, C., Aylward, B. et al. (2011). Effectiveness of motivational interviewing interventions for adolescent substance use behavior change: a meta-analytic review. *Journal of Consulting and Clinical Psychology* 49 (4): 433–440. https://doi.org/10.1037/a0023992.

Johnson, L.D., Miech, R.A., O'Malley, P.M. et al. (2018). *Monitoring the Future National Survey Results on Drug Use: 1975–2017: Overview, Key Findings on Adolescent Drug Use.* Ann Arbor: Institute for Social Research, The University of Michigan.

Jordan, A.E., Blackburn, N.A., Des Jarlais, D.C., and Hagan, H. (2017). Past-year prevalence of prescription opioid misuse among those 11 to 30 years of age in the United States: a systematic review and meta-analysis. *Journal of Substance Abuse Treatment* 77: 31–37. https://doi.org/10.1016/j.jsat.2017.03.007.

Kaminer, Y. and Godley, M. (2010). From assessment reactivity to aftercare for adolescent substance abuse: are we there yet? *Child and Adolescent Psychiatric Clinics of North America* 19: 577–590.

Kaner, E., Beyer, F., Muirhead, C. et al. (2018). Effectiveness of brief alcohol interventions in primary care populations. *Cochrane Systematic Reviews* 2 (2) CD004148: 1–252. https://doi.org/10.1002/14651858.CD004148.pub4.

Kann, L., McManus, T., Harris, W.A. et al. (2018). Youth risk behavior surveillance – United States, 2017. *MMWR Surveillance Summaries* 67 (8): 1.

Kelly, J.F., Dow, S.J., Yeterian, J.D., and Kahler, C.W. (2010). Can 12-step group participation strengthen and extend the benefits of adolescent addiction treatment? A prospective analysis. *Drug and Alcohol Dependence* 110 (1–2): 117–125. https://doi.org/10.1016/j.drugalcdep.2010.02.019.

Kelly, S.M., Gryczynski, J., Mitchell, S.G. et al. (2014). Validity of brief screening instrument for adolescent tobacco, alcohol, and drug use. *Pediatrics* 133 (5): 819–826.

Knight, J.R., Sherritt, L., Harris, S.K. et al. (2003). Validity of brief alcohol screening tests among adolescents: a comparison of the AUDIT, POSIT, CAGE, and CRAFFT. *Alcoholism: Clinical and Experimental Research* 27: 67–73.

Knudsen, H., Abraham, A., and Oser, C. (2011). Barriers to the implementation of medication-assisted treatment for substance use disorders: the importance of funding policies and medical infrastructure. *Evaluation and Program Planning* 34: 375–381. https://doi.org/10.1016/j.evalprogplan.2011.02.004.

Kumpfer, K. and Magalhaes, C. (2018). Strengthening families program: an evidence-based family intervention for parents of high-risk children and adolescents. *Journal of Child & Adolescent Substance Abuse* 27 (3): 174–179. https://doi.org/10.1080/1067828X.2018.1443048.

Laestadius, L. and Wang, Y. (2018). Youth access to JUUL online: eBay sales of JUUL prior to and following FDA action. *Tobacco Control* https://doi.org/10.1136/tobaccocontrol-2018-054499.

Levy, S. (2019). Youth and the opioid epidemic. *Pediatrics* 143 (2): e20182752. https://doi.org/10.1542/peds.2018-2752.

Levy, S. and Knight, J.R. (2008). Screening, brief intervention and referral to treatment for adolescents. *Journal of Addiction Medicine* 2 (4): 215–221. https://doi.org/10.1097/ADM.0b013e31818a8c7a.

Levy, S.J. and Williams, J.F. (2016). Committee on substance use and prevention. Substance use screening, brief intervention, and referral to treatment. *Pediatrics* 138 (1): e20161211.

Levy, S., Weiss, R., Sherritt, L. et al. (2014). An electronic screen for triaging adolescent substance use by risk levels. *JAMA Pediatrics* 168 (9): 822–828. https://doi.org/10.1001/jamapediatrics.2014.774.

Long, E.C., Lönn, S.L., Ji, J. et al. (2017). Resilience and risk for alcohol use disorders: a Swedish twin study. *Alcoholism: Clinical and Experimental Research* 41 (1): 149–155. https://doi.org/10.1111/acer.13274.

Lynskey, M.T., Agrawal, A., and Heath, A.C. (2010). Genetically informative research on adolescent substance use: methods, findings, and challenges. *Journal of the American Academy of Child & Adolescent Psychiatry* 49 (12): 1202–1214. https://doi.org/10.1016/j.jaac.2010.09.004.

Maisto, S.A., Connors, G.J., and Allen, J.P. (1995). Contrasting self-report screens for alcohol problems: a review. *Alcoholism: Clinical and Experimental Research* 19 (6): 1510–1516.

Marshall, K., Gowing, L., Ali, R., and Le Foll, B. (2014). Pharmacotherapies for cannabis dependence. *Cochrane Database System Review* 12 (12) CD008940: 1–26. https://doi.org/10.1002/14651858.CD008940.pub2.

Mason, B.J., Crean, R., Goodell, V. et al. (2012). A proof-of-concept randomized controlled study of gabapentin: effects on cannabis use, withdrawal and executive function deficits in cannabis-dependent adults. *Neuropsychopharmacology* 37: 1689–1698. https://doi.org/10.1038/npp.2012.14.

McCabe, S., Boyd, C., Cranford, J. et al. (2006). A modified version of the drug abuse screening test among undergraduate students. *Journal of Substance Abuse Treatment* 31 (3): 297–303. https://doi.org/10.1016/j.jsat.2006.04.010.

McCabe, S.E., West, B.T., Veliz, P. et al. (2017). Trends in medical and nonmedical use of prescription opioids among US adolescents: 1976–2015. *Pediatrics* 139 (4): e20162387. https://doi.org/10.1542/peds.2016-2387.

Meredith, L.S., Ewing, B.A., Stein, B.D. et al. (2018). Influence of mental health and alcohol or other drug use risk on adolescent reported care received in primary care settings. *BioMed Central Family Practice* 19 (10): 1–9. https://doi.org/10.1186/s12875-017-0689-y.

Mericle, A.A., Arria, A.M., Meyers, K. et al. (2015). National trends in adolescent substance use disorders and treatment availability: 2003–2010. *Journal of Child & Adolescent Substance Abuse* 24 (5): 255–263. https://doi.org/10.1080/1067828X.2013.829008.

Miller, W.R. and Sanchez, V.C. (1993). Motivating young adults for treatment and lifestyle change. In: *Issues in Alcohol Use and Misuse by Young Adults* (ed. G.L. Howard), 55–82. Notre Dame, IN: University of Notre Dame Press.

Miranda, R. and Treloar, H. (2018). Pharmacotherapy for adolescent substance misuse. In: *Brief Interventions for Adolescent Alcohol and Substance Misuse* (eds. P.M. Monti, S.M. Colby and T. O'Leary Tevyaw), 318–343. New York: Guilford Press.

Morean, M.E., Kong, G., Cavallo, D.A. et al. (2016). Nicotine concentration of e-cigarettes used by adolescents. *Drug and Alcohol Dependence* 167: 224–227. https://doi.org/10.1016/j.drugalcdep.2016.06.031.

National Center for Physician Training in Addiction Medicine (2016). *Identifying and Responding to Substance Use among Adolescents and Young Adults: A Compendium of Resources for Medical Practice.* The Addiction Medicine Foundation. Available at http://www.abam.net/wp-content/uploads/2016/04/MRL-Compenduim-Update-4-11-16.pdf.

NIAAA. (n.d.). *A pocket guide for alcohol screening and brief interventions for youth.* NIH Publication No. 11–7806, National Institute on Alcohol Abuse and Alcoholism. Available at https://pubs.niaaa.nih.gov › publications › practitioner › youthguidepocket.

NIAAA (2015.) *Alcohol Screening and Brief Intervention for Youth: A Practitioner's Guide.* NIH Publication No. 11–7805, National Institute on Alcohol Abuse and Alcoholism. Available at https://pubs.niaaa.nih.gov/publications/Practitioner/YouthGuide/YouthGuide.pdf.

NIDA. (2019). *Screening tools for adolescent substance use.* Available at https://www.drugabuse.gov/nidamed-medical-health-professionals/screening-tools-resources/screening-tools-for-adolescent-substance-use.

NIDA (n.d.). *Alcohol Screening and Brief Intervention for Youth: A Practitioner's Guide.* Related Resources for Healthcare Professionals, National Institute on Drug Abuse. Available at https://www.niaaa.nih.gov/publications/clinical-guides-and-manuals/alcohol-screening-and-brief-intervention-youth/resources.

Olfson, E., Bloom, J., Bertelsen, S. et al. (2018). CYP2A6 metabolism in the development of smoking behaviors in young adults. *Addiction Biology* 23 (1): 437–447. https://doi.org/10.1111/adb.12477.

Osborne, V., Serdarevic, M., Crooke, H. et al. (2017). Non-medical opioid use in youth: gender differences in risk factors and prevalence. *Addictive Behaviors* 72: 114–119. https://doi.org/10.1016/j.addbeh.2017.03.02.

Ozechowski, T.J., Becker, S.J., and Hogue, A. (2016). SBIRT-A: adapting SBIRT to maximize developmental fit for adolescents in primary care. *Journal of Substance Abuse Treatment* 62: 28–37. https://doi.org/10.1016/j.jsat.2015.10.006.

Parast, L., Meredith, L.S., Stein, B.D. et al. (2018). Identifying adolescents with alcohol use disorder: optimal screening using the National Institute on Alcohol Abuse and Alcoholism screening guide. *Psychology of Addictive Behaviors* 32 (5): 508–516. https://doi.org/10.1037/adb0000377.

Passetti, L.L., Godley, M.D., and Kaminer, Y. (2016). Continuing care for adolescents in treatment for substance use disorders. *Child Adolescent Psychiatry Clinics in North America* 25 (4): 669–684. https://doi.org/10.1016/j.chc.2016.06.003.

Patton, R., Deluca, P., Kaner, E. et al. (2014). Alcohol screening and brief intervention for adolescents: the how, what and where of reducing alcohol consumption and related harm among young people. *Alcohol and Alcoholism* 49 (2): 207–212. https://doi.org/10.1093/alcalc/agt165.

Penetar, D.M., Looby, A.R., Ryan, E.T. et al. (2012). Bupropion reduces some of the symptoms of marihuana withdrawal in chronic marijuana users: a pilot study. *Substance Abuse: Research and Treatment* 6: 63–71. https://doi.org/10.4137/SART.S9706.

Pfefferbaum, A., Kwon, D., Brumback, T. et al. (2017). Altered brain developmental trajectories in adolescents after initiating drinking. *American Journal of Psychiatry* 175 (4): 370–380. https://doi.org/10.1176/appi.ajp.2017.17040469.

Prochnow, J.A. (2017). E-cigarettes: a practical, evidence-based guide for advanced practice nurses. *The Journal for Nurse Practitioners* 13 (7): 449–455. https://doi.org/10.1016/j.nurpra.2017.03.015.

Samek, D.R., Hicks, B.M., Durbin, E. et al. (2018). Codevelopment between key personality traits and alcohol use disorder from adolescence through young adulthood. *Journal of Personality* 86 (2): 261–282. https://doi.org/10.1111/jopy.12311.

Sarvet, A.L., Wall, M.M., Fink, D.S. et al. (2018). Medical marijuana laws and adolescent marijuana use in the United States: a systematic review and meta-analysis. *Addiction* 113 (6): 1003–1016. https://doi.org/10.1111/add.14136.

Schepis, T.S., Teter, C.J., and McCabe, S.E. (2018a). Prescription drug use, misuse and related substance use disorder symptoms vary by educational status and attainment in US adolescents and young adults. *Drug and Alcohol Dependence* 189: 172–177. https://doi.org/10.1016/j.drugalcdep.2018.05.017.

Schepis, T.S., Wilens, T.E., and McCabe, S.E. (2018b). Prescription drug misuse: sources of controlled medications in adolescents. *The Journal of the American Academy of Child & Adolescent Psychiatry* https://doi.org/10.1016/j.jaac.2018.09.438.

Schilling, E.A., Aseltine, R.H. Jr., Glanovsky, J.L. et al. (2009). Adolescent alcohol use, suicidal ideation, and suicide attempts. *Journal of Adolescent Health* 44 (4): 335–341. https://doi.org/10.1016/j.jadohealth.2008.08.006.

Schleider, J. and Weisz, J. (2017). Little treatments, promising effects? Meta-analysis of single-session interventions for youth psychiatric problems. *Journal of American Academy of Child & Adolescent Psychiatry* 56 (2): 107–115. https://doi.org/10.1016/j.jaac.2016.11.007.

Schuler, M.S., Tucker, J.S., Pedersen, E.R., and D'Amico, E.J. (2019). Relative influence of perceived peer and family substance use on adolescent alcohol, cigarette, and marijuana use across middle and high school. *Addictive Behaviors* 88: 99–105. https://doi.org/10.1016/j.addbeh.2018.08.025.

Selzer, M.L. (1971). The Michigan Alcoholism Screening Test (MAST): the quest for a new diagnostic instrument. *American Journal of Psychiatry* 127: 1653–1658.

Sheridan, D.C. and Horowitz, B.Z. (2017). Adolescent ingestions: recent national trends. *Clinical Pediatric Emergency Medicine* 18 (3): 193–196. https://doi.org/10.1016/j.cpem.2017.07.001.

Shields, A., Campfield, D., Miller, C. et al. (2008). Score reliability of adolescent alcohol screening measures: a meta-analytic inquiry. *Journal of Child & Adolescent Substance Abuse* 7 (4): 75–97. https://doi.org/10.1080/15470650802292855.

Sitnick, S.L., Shaw, D.S., and Hyde, L.W. (2014). Precursors of adolescent substance use from early childhood and early adolescence: testing a developmental cascade model. *Development and Psychopathology* 26 (1): 125–140. https://doi.org/10.1017/S0954579413000539.

Skinner, H.A. (1982). The drug abuse screening test. *Addictive Behavior* 7 (4): 363–371.

Sneider, J., Cohen-Gilbert, J., Hamilton, D. et al. (2018). Adolescent hippocampal and prefrontal brain activation during performance of the virtual Morris water task. *Frontiers in Human Neuroscience* 12 (238): 1–12. https://doi.org/10.3389/fnhum.2018.00238.

Soneji, S., Barrington-Trimis, J.L., Wills, T.A. et al. (2017). Association between initial use of e-cigarettes and subsequent cigarette smoking among adolescents and young adults: a systematic review and meta-analysis. *JAMA Pediatrics* 171 (8): 788–797. https://doi.org/10.1001/jamapediatrics.2017.1488.

Stahl, S.M. (2013). *Stahl's Essential Psychopharmacology: Neuroscientific Basis and Practical Applications.* New York: Cambridge University Press.

Stallvik, M., Gastfriend, D., and Nordah, H. (2015). Matching patients with substance use disorder to optimal level of care with the ASAM criteria software. *Journal of Substance Use* 20 (6): 389–398. https://doi.org/10.3109/14659891.2014.934305.

Stautz, K. and Cooper, A. (2013). Impulsivity-related personality traits and adolescent alcohol use: a meta-analytic review. *Clinical Psychology Review* 33 (4): 574–592. https://doi.org/10.1016/j.cpr.2013.03.003.

Stockings, E., Hall, W., Lynskey, M. et al. (2016). Prevention, early intervention, harm reduction, and treatment of substance use in young people. *Lancet Psychiatry* 3: 280–296. https://doi.org/10.1016/S2215-0366(16)00002-X.

Subramaniam, G., Warden, D., Minhajuddin, A. et al. (2011). Predictors of abstinence: NIDA multi-site buprenorphine/naloxone treatment trial in opioid dependent youth. *Journal of American Academy of Child and Adolescent Psychiatry* 50 (11): 1120–1128. https://doi.org/10.1016/j.jaac.2011.07.010.

SAMHSA. (2011). *Screening, Brief Intervention and Referral to Treatment (SBIRT) in behavioral healthcare.* SBIRT white paper, Substance Abuse and Mental Health Services Administration. Available at https://www.samhsa.gov/sites/default/files/sbirtwhite paper_0.pdf.

SAMHSA. (2012). *TIP 34 Brief Interventions and Brief Therapies for Substance Abuse.* US Department of Health and Human Services, Pub id: SMA12–3952, Substance Abuse and Mental Health Services Administration. Available at https://store.samhsa.gov/product/TIP-34-Brief-Interventions-and-Brief-Therapies-for-Substance-Abuse/SMA12-3952.

SAMHSA. (2013). *TIP 35: Enhancing Motivation for Change in Substance Abuse Treatment.* US Department of Health and Human Services, Pub id: SMA13–4212, Substance Abuse and Mental Health Services Administration. Available at https://store.samhsa.gov/product/TIP-35-Enhancing-Motivation-for-Change-in-Substance-Abuse-Treatment/SMA13-4212.

SAMHSA. (2017). *Behavioral health treatments and services.* Substance Abuse and Mental Health Services Administration. Available at https://www.samhsa.gov/treatment.

SAMHSA. (2018a). *Key substance use and mental health indicators in the United States: Results from the 2017 National Survey on Drug Use and Health.* HHS Publication No. SMA 18–5068, NSDUH Series H-53. Rockville, MD: Center for Behavioral Health Statistics and Quality, Substance Abuse and Mental Health Services Administration. Available at https://www.samhsa.gov/data.

SAMHSA. (2018b). *Treatments for substance use disorders.* Substance Abuse and Mental Health Services Administration. Available at https://www.samhsa.gov/treatment/substance-use-disorders.

SAMHSA. (2018c). *Medication-assisted treatment.* Substance Abuse and Mental Health Services Administration. Available at https://www.samhsa.gov/medication-assisted-treatment.

SAMHSA. (n.d.). *SBIRT: Screening, Brief Intervention and Referral to Treatment.* Substance Abuse and Mental Health Services Administration. Available at https://www.integration.samhsa.gov/clinical-practice/sbirt/brief-interventions.

Szapocznik, J., Zarate, M., Duff, J., and Muir, J. (2013). Brief strategic family therapy: engaging drug using/problem behavior adolescents and their families in treatment. *Social Work in Public Health* 28 (3–4): 206–223. https://doi.org/10.1080/19371918.2013.774666.

The Center for Substance Use Research. (2018). *The CRAFFT 2.1 Manual.* Available at http://crafft.org/wp-content/uploads/2018/08/FINAL-CRAFFT-2.1_provider_manual_with_CRAFFTN_2018-04-23.pdf.

Tomko, R.L., Gilmore, A.K., and Gray, K.M. (2018). The role of depressive symptoms in treatment of adolescent cannabis use disorder with N-Acetylcysteine. *Addictive Behaviors* 85: 26–30. https://doi.org/10.1016/j.addbeh.2018.05.014.

US Department of Health and Human Services. (2016). *E-Cigarette use among youth and young adults: A report of the Surgeon General.* Atlanta, GA: US Department of Health and Human Services, Centers for Disease Control and Prevention, National Center for Chronic Disease Prevention and Health Promotion, Office on Smoking and Health. Available at https://e-cigarettes.surgeongeneral.gov/documents/2016_SGR_Full_Report_508.pdf.

Veliz, P., Boyd, C.J., and McCabe, S.E. (2017). Nonmedical use of prescription opioids and heroin use among adolescents involved in competitive sports. *Journal of Adolescent Health* 60 (3): 346–349. https://doi.org/10.1016/j.jadohealth.2016.09.021.

Verhulst, B., Neale, M.C., and Kendler, K.S. (2015). The heritability of alcohol use disorders: a meta-analysis of twin and adoption studies. *Psychological Medicine* 45 (5): 1061–1072. https://doi.org/10.1017/S0033291714002165.

Vogel, E.A., Ramo, D.E., and Rubinstein, M.L. (2018). Prevalence and correlates of adolescents' e-cigarette use frequency and dependence. *Drug and Alcohol Dependence* 188: 109–112. https://doi.org/10.1016/j.drugalcdep.2018.03.051.

Volkow, N.D. and Boyle, M. (2018). Neuroscience of addiction: relevance to prevention and treatment. *American Journal of Psychiatry* 175: 729–740. https://doi.org/10.1176/appi.ajp.2018.17101174.

Volkow, N.D., Baler, R.D., Compton, W.M., and Weiss, S.R. (2014). Adverse health effects of marijuana use. *New England Journal of Medicine* 370 (23): 2219–2227. https://doi.org/10.1056/NEJMra1402309.

Volkow, N.D., Koob, G.F., and McLellan, A.T. (2016). Neurobiologic advances from the brain disease model of addiction. *New England Journal of Medicine* 374 (4): 363–371. https://doi.org/10.1056/NEJMra1511480.

Wang, T.W., Gentzke, A., Sharapova, S. et al. (2018). Tobacco product use among middle and high school students – United States, 2011–2017. *Morbidity and Mortality Weekly Report* 67 (22): 629. https://doi.org/10.15585/mmwr.mm6722a3.

Webb, C., Scudder, M., Kaminer, Y., & Kadden, R. (2007). *The Motivational Enhancement Therapy and Cognitive Behavioral Therapy Supplement: 7 Sessions of Cognitive Behavioral Therapy for Adolescent Cannabis Users,* Cannabis Youth Treatment (CYT) Series, Volume 2. DHHS Pub. No. (SMA) 07–3954. Rockville, MD: Center for Substance Abuse Treatment, SAMHSHA.

Wen, H., Hockenberry, J.M., and Cummings, J.R. (2015). The effect of medical marijuana laws on adolescent and adult use of marijuana, alcohol, and other substances. *Journal of Health Economics* 42: 64–80. https://doi.org/10.1016/j.jhealeco.2015.03.007.

Westling, E., Rusby, J.C., Crowley, R., and Light, J.M. (2017). Electronic cigarette use by youth: prevalence, correlates, and use trajectories from middle to high school. *Journal of Adolescent Health* 60 (6): 660–666. https://doi.org/10.1016/j.jadohealth.2016.12.019.

Whiteford, H.A., Ferrari, A.J., Degenhardt, L. et al. (2015). The global burden of mental, neurological and substance use disorders: an analysis from the Global Burden of Disease Study 2010. *PLoS One* 10 (2): e0116820. https://doi.org/10.1371/journal.pone.0116820.

Winters, K., Botzet, A., and Fahnhorst, T. (2011). Advances in adolescent substance abuse. *Current Psychiatry Report* 13 (5): 416–421. https://doi.org/10.1007/s11920-011-0214-2.

Wissow, L.S., Brown, J., Fothergill, K.E. et al. (2013). Universal mental health screening in pediatric primary care: a systematic review. *Journal of the American Academy of Child and Adolescent Psychiatry* 52: 1134–1147.

Wong, S.S., Zhou, B., Goebert, D., and Hishinuma, E.S. (2013). The risk of adolescent suicide across patterns of drug use: a nationally representative study of high school students in the United States from 1999 to 2009. *Social Psychiatry and Psychiatric Epidemiology* 48 (10): 1611–1620. https://doi.org/10.1007/s00127-013-0721-z.

Yaun, M., Cross, S.J., Loughlin, S.E., and Leslie, F.M. (2015). Nicotine and the adolescent brain. *Journal of Physiology* 593 (16): 3397–3412. https://doi.org/10.1113/JP270492.

Yudko, E., Lozhkina, O., and Fouts, A. (2007). A comprehensive review of the psychometric properties of the Drug Abuse Screening Test. *Journal of Substance Abuse Treatment* 32: 189–198. https://doi.org/10.1016/j.jsat.2006.08.002.

Yule, A.M. and Wilkens, T.E. (2015). Substance use disorders in adolescents with psychiatric comorbidity: when to screen and how to treat. *Current Psychiatry* 14 (4): 37–51.

24

Child and Adolescent Victims of Trauma

Dawn Bounds[1], Necole Leland[2], and Angela F. Amar[2]

[1] Rush University College of Nursing, Chicago, IL, USA
[2] University of Nevada, Las Vegas School of Nursing, Las Vegas, NV, USA

Objectives

After reading this chapter, advanced practice psychiatric nurses (APRNs) will be able to:

1. Provide an overview of childhood and adolescent trauma and the resulting health effects.
2. Outline current and emerging developments in clinical and research findings among children and adolescents who have experienced trauma.
3. Discuss clinical parameters for the identification, assessment, and psychotherapeutic intervention with children and adolescents who have experienced trauma.
4. Describe practice, research, and education implications related to an advanced practice nursing approach to the treatment of traumatized children and adolescents.

Introduction

Childhood and adolescence are times of continuous emotional, psychological, cognitive, and physical development. In this chapter, the word "child" refers to both children and adolescents unless otherwise stated. Ideally, when children face stressors or events that challenge their feelings of safety, they will have the necessary skills and support to get through these difficult times and have a positive outcome. Yet many children face stressful or traumatic situations every day that test the limits of their resilience and coping skills. Overwhelming or chronic traumatic experiences during childhood can disrupt the normal progress of development and may result in ongoing psychological and physical illness. Traumatic events can be acute, short-lived in nature, or chronic, occurring multiple times over a period of time. Examples of traumatic events or situations include violence (community, school, family/domestic, war, rape), natural/manmade disasters (earthquakes, floods, hurricanes, fire), accidents (motor vehicle, plane crashes), death of a loved one (murder, suicide, illness), child maltreatment (neglect, sexual, physical or emotional abuse), and medical trauma (illness/medical procedures). Traumatic experiences have pervasive effects on the lives of children and adolescents and profoundly affect physical, psychological, emotional, and cognitive domains.

Description of the Issue

The *Diagnostic and Statistical Manual of Mental Disorders 5* (DSM-5) defines a traumatic event as the following:

> A **traumatic event** is an incident that causes physical, emotional, spiritual, or psychological harm. The person experiencing the distressing **event** may feel threatened, anxious, or frightened as a result. In some cases, they may not know how to respond, or may be in denial about the effect such an **event** has had. (American Psychiatric Association 2013, p. 463)

By far the most common traumatic experience for children involves violence. Children can experience violence within their homes and families, such as child abuse, neglect, and sibling violence. They may also witness intimate partner violence (IPV). Outside the home, in school and community life, experience with violence is through bullying, dating violence (DV), gang membership or exposure, and as a victim and/or witness to crime. Children in many parts of the world endure oppression and traumatic experiences including being enslaved, sex trafficking, or war crimes. Many individuals immigrate to the United States following trauma in another country. Despite the variance of traumatic experiences, there is often consistency in the response to trauma. While myriad events comprise this topic, this chapter will use as an exemplar interpersonal violence, such as child maltreatment, DV, and exposure to family violence, with the understanding that the basic effects of, and responses to, interventions can apply to multiple types and forms of traumatic experiences.

The Centers for Disease Control and Prevention defines *child maltreatment* as "any act or series of acts of commission or omission by a parent or other caregiver that results in harm, potential harm or threat of harm of a child" (Leeb et al. 2008, p. 19). This includes physical abuse, neglect (emotional, physical, medical, educational), sexual abuse, emotional abuse, abandonment, and substance abuse. Not surprisingly, a large number of children who experience trauma do so at the hands of family members, including parents or caretakers (Cohen et al. 2016b). Maltreatment of children by parents and caregivers is an age-old problem; however, it was not brought to light until 1962. That year the landmark publication by Dr. C. Henry Kempe et al. titled *The Battered Child Syndrome* made child abuse a health concern (Kempe et al. 1962). The Child Abuse Prevention and Treatment Act (CAPTA), first introduced into law in 1974 and later amended and reauthorized, provided federal funding to states for prevention, identification, investigation, prosecution, and treatment. Furthermore, every state in the United States has child abuse laws that mandate that all nurses and those in advanced practice specialty areas report instances of suspected child abuse.

In recent decades, researchers have expanded their attention to focus on dating violence (DV). Dating is often viewed as a carefree time of exploration and experimentation, but the experience can also be traumatic for many adolescents. "Dating violence (DV) is defined as physical, sexual, or psychological/emotional violence between two people within a close or dating relationship" (Stonard 2019, p. 105). DV may occur as a single episode, such as date rape, or as a pattern of behavior, such as physical violence or stalking (Stonard 2019). The 2017 National Youth Risk Behavior Survey estimates that about 8% of high school students reported physical violence and about 7% reported sexual violence from a dating partner within 12 months of the survey (Kann et al. 2018).

In the DV literature, adolescent violence is accepted as bidirectional (Petering et al. 2017). Research on physical violence in adolescent intimate relationships has consistently found that the majority of female victims also report the perpetration of physical aggression against male partners (Petering et al. 2017). Despite this reciprocal nature, DV consequences are not necessarily symmetrical or mutual in that girls are more likely to be physically injured compared to boys (McNaughton Reyes et al. 2018). Younger women, aged 16–24, are more at risk for nonfatal injury from an intimate partner than are women in any other age group and their risk for murder by an intimate partner increases as these women age (Peterman et al. 2015).

Bullying, once seen as a rite of passage, is increasingly being recognized as a serious traumatic behavior that induces physical, psychological, social, and educational harm (Gillespie et al. 2018). Bullying is a form of aggression characterized by an imbalance of power that tends to peak in middle childhood. Prevalence estimates suggest that 17.9–30.9% of school-age children experience some form of bullying at school, with verbal and social bullying being most common (Flannery et al. 2016). Although all children may experience bullying, children who appear weak, insecure, sensitive, isolated, or "different" are at an increased risk of victimization from bullying. Other forms of school violence include verbal and physical assault, threats with or without a weapon, and sexual victimization (including harassment). Instances of bullying increase in frequency with age peaking in preteens to adolescents and the estimates are greater for lesbian, gay, bisexual, and transgender youth (Flannery et al. 2016). Bullying using electronic means is one of the latest forms of expression of bullying that uses technology to initiate bullying behaviors that can cause psychological and emotional abuse that traditionally happened in person (Stonard 2019). With the explosion of social media sites, cyberbullying has recently expanded to internet sex crimes that include forms of sexual exploitation including revenge porn, online solicitation, and grooming of potential victims (Citron and Franks 2014; Ehman and Gross 2019).

Sexual minority youth are at an increased risk for bullying and sexual harassment, contributing to the negative mental health consequences experienced by these youth (McGeough and Sterzing 2018). Practitioners should inquire about sexual orientation and experiences of bullying, harassment, or violence directed to sexual minority youth. If possible, provide resources and referrals that meet the unique needs of the traumatized sexual minority youth.

Runaway and/or homeless youth (RHY) include youth who have run away from home, been asked to leave or been thrown out, have contact with the juvenile justice system and/or child welfare system, and/or experience homelessness due to familial housing instability (Crosby et al. 2018). Family conflict and disintegration often precipitates their homelessness (Noh 2018). RHY often experience violence and abuse at home and on the streets. Exposure to the streets impacts RHY's physical, mental, and behavioral health with increased risks of developing depression, substance use disorders, and post-traumatic stress disorder (PTSD) (US Department of Health and Human Services [USDHHS] 2018). Prolonged exposure to life on the streets also increases the likelihood of permanent homelessness and human trafficking (USDHHS 2018). Homelessness is the number one risk factor for both sex and labor trafficking (National Research Council 2013).

US federal law considers all youth under the age of 18 who are exploited for labor or sex as human trafficking victims/survivors. The caveats for adults, "force, fraud, or coercion," need not be present. However, this component of their exploitation compounds their vulnerabilities as homeless youth (National Research Council 2013). Accurate estimates of incidence and prevalence are challenging to articulate (National Research Council 2013); however, the impact of trafficking is severe. Sexual exploitation in particular has costly sequelae that include depression, traumatic stress, substance use, and suicide attempts (Gerassi 2015). Lack of identification is a noteworthy challenge (Bounds et al. 2015, 2017). Despite high percentages of survivors reporting contact with healthcare providers while being trafficked, missed opportunities for identification and intervention within the healthcare setting abound (Lederer and Wetzel 2014). Every professional who works with youth should educate themselves on potential indicators and create policy and procedures on how to intervene (DeChesnay 2013; Ernewein and Nieves 2015; Shandro et al. 2016).

Numerous studies have established a link between traumatic experiences in childhood and negative psychological outcomes (Humphreys et al. 2018). The landmark work of Felitti and Anda in the Adverse Childhood Experiences (ACE) study identified the earliest linkages. This joint Centers for Disease Control and Prevention (CDC)–Kaiser Permanente study is the largest investigation to determine associations between child maltreatment and later life health and wellbeing (CDC 2006). Begun in 1995, the study prospectively tracks outcomes and has determined associations between ACE and alcoholism, depression, health-related quality of life, suicide attempts, risk for IPV, and illicit drug use (Felitti et al. 1998; Hughes et al. 2017). The ACE study has shifted our understanding of development toward a model that is inclusive of how social determinants of health impact development over time (Shonkoff et al. 2012). Children living in poverty are disproportionately impacted by ACES (Francis et al. 2018; Halfon et al. 2017). Please see Chapter 8 for a complete review of ACE.

Not all children display physical or psychological symptoms following a traumatic event. Following most trauma, the majority of children demonstrate resilience and have no resulting symptomatology. About half of child abuse survivors demonstrate resilience in childhood, which for nearly one-third of them persists into young adulthood (Hornor 2015). In contrast to risk factors, protective factors buffer the negative consequences from violence exposure. Protective factors include parental recognition of the problem, parental support, supportive grandparents, and accessible mental healthcare (Chen and Chan 2016).

Literature examining the physical and psychological aftermath of trauma in children reports wide variation in the prevalence of psychological and physical symptoms. Several factors, such as the type of trauma, frequency of the trauma, personality/temperament of the child, coping abilities, the relationship of the child and perpetrator, and social support, account for the differences in outcomes. Differences can exist regarding the severity of the stressor, chronicity of exposure, relationship to the offender, if appropriate, and occurrence of previous and subsequent distressful events. Multiple victimizations, five or more types in a 1-year period, can predict higher rates of trauma-related symptoms (Turner et al. 2017). Certain events, such as interpersonal violence in the form of physical and sexual abuse, are associated with more adverse effects than other events, such as natural disasters (Cohen et al. 2016b). Furthermore, evidence of psychopathology before traumatic exposure and disruptions in social networks consistently emerge as strong predictors of psychopathology after exposure to trauma. Complex trauma, or pervasive and severe traumatic events, impairs multiple domains of a child's developmental trajectory: attachment, biology, affect regulation, consciousness, behavior, cognition, and self-concept (Cook et al. 2017; van der Kolk 2005).

Epidemiology

Exposure to traumatic events during childhood is far too common. Violence is prevalent in the everyday lives of children living in the United States; children are more likely to be exposed to violence than adults are (Finkelhor et al. 2013). Several large national surveys of children and adolescents report direct and indirect exposure to violence rates as high as three of five children exposed in a year and seven out of eight children in their lifetimes, and this high exposure rate remains stable without increase (Finkelhor et al. 2013). Not surprisingly, exposure to one form of violence increases the likelihood of future victimization (Finkelhor et al. 2015).

In 2016, 3.5 million referrals were made to child protection agencies for 676 000 children who had been determined to be victims of child maltreatment (USDHHS 2018). Referrals to child protection agencies do not represent the total picture of child maltreatment, only that which is recognized, reported, responded to, and substantiated. The estimated cost for services and care to children and families of maltreatment continues to be extremely high each year (USDHHS 2018). Rates of victimization decrease with age with the youngest children, children less than 3 years of age, accounting for more than one-quarter of substantiated cases (birth to 3 years 28.5%) (USDHHS 2018). Children younger than 1 year of age account for the highest victimization (24.8%) (USDHHS 2018). Children under age 1 are at the greatest risk of death and serious injury resulting from child maltreatment, with this risk decreasing with age (McCarroll et al. 2017). Victimization is similar for both males (48.6) and females (51%), with 44.9% of victims being white, 22% Hispanic and 20.7% African American (USDHHS 2018).

According to the 2016 data, the majority of child maltreatment cases are neglect (74.8%) followed by physical abuse (18.2%) and sexual abuse (8.4%). In 2016, the rates of child fatalities were 2.36 deaths per 100 000 children (USDHHS 2018). Neglect is the failure of the offender to care for the child and to meet the basic needs of the child. Physical abuse is the use of physical force with the intention and result of hurting the child. Sexual abuse includes any attempted or completed sexual act, contact, or sexual interaction between a child and adult. Psychological abuse is any behavior that intentionally undermines the child's sense of self and self-worth. Examples include belittling, degrading, terrorizing, isolating, and rejecting.

Most often, perpetrators of child maltreatment are the people who are closest to the child, including parents (77.6%) and relatives other than a parent (6.2%), with 53.7% of offenders being women and 45.3% men (USDHHS 2018). Parents constitute the largest group of offenders (80%), with biological parents comprising nearly 90% of the parent offender group. The race and ethnicity of the perpetrators tend to mimic that of the victim.

Research has begun to explore the pervasiveness of childhood exposure to violence within communities. A nationally representative sample of children revealed that more than 67.5% were exposed to violence either directly or indirectly (Finkelhor et al. 2015). Indirect exposure occurs through witnessing or learning about a violent act. Research suggests that increased aggression is associated with witnessing community violence in young children (Fleckman et al. 2016). Emerging literature has documented the mental health consequences of exposure to IPV via one's parents. Recent studies suggest that witnessing violence impacts the child's aggression and antisocial behavior, affecting them at the cellular level (Fleckman et al. 2016). A review of published literature from 1995 to 2006 found that children and adolescents living with domestic violence had an increased risk of experiencing emotional, physical, and sexual abuse, of developing emotional and behavioral problems, and of increased exposure to other adversities in their lives (Espelage et al. 2018; Peterson et al. 2019).

Etiology

There are many possible causes of child trauma. Children across all racial, ethnic, cultural, religious, and socioeconomic groups experience interpersonal violence. As discussed, children and adolescents may be exposed to a variety of potentially traumatic situations. The risk of potential repercussions will vary greatly depending on the type of trauma. It is helpful to explore features that contribute or cause trauma from multiple perspectives on multiple levels. At the individual level, research documents risk factors that can predispose children to victimization and parents to abuse their children. In addition, individual level factors include risk factors predictive of victimization and perpetration of DV, bullying, and other forms of interpersonal violence. Factors that occur at a family level can predict exposure to violence. Finally, at a societal and community level, risk factors for violence include cultural and societal norms as well as theoretical perspectives that explain the experience of violence.

At the individual level, characteristics that make a child more likely to experience child abuse include age (younger children at greater risk of severe injury and adolescents at greater risk of sexual abuse), disabilities, chronic illness, difficult temperament, and prior maltreatment exposure (Ben-Natan et al. 2014; Fleckman et al. 2016). Risk factors for teen DV include alcohol or drug use, association with violent friends, witnessing violence at home, inability to manage anger, and poor social skills (Ludin et al. 2018).

At a family level, risk factors that identify parents at risk for violence include personality characteristics such as low self-esteem, external locus of control, and poor impulse control (Jobe-Shields et al. 2018). Parental predictors of being a perpetrator include history of child abuse, limited information about growth and development of children, lack of education, single parents, mental illness, and history of drug or alcohol use (Fluke et al. 2008). Other family attributes that increase the likelihood of child abuse are households with marital conflict, domestic violence, and lower income (Jobe-Shields et al. 2018). Several programs are available for parents and families deemed at risk of child abuse. In particular, early childhood home visitation programs and parent education programs demonstrate some success at preventing child abuse (Chen and Chan 2016).

At a community level, factors such as stress and poverty are associated with increased risk of child abuse (Jobe-Shields et al. 2018). Poverty, unemployment, and violent communities are all conditions that increase stress levels and decrease the resources and options available to families (Pascoe, Wood, Duffee, Kuo, and Committee on Psychosocial Aspects of Child and Family Health 2016). Living in communities with increased violence may create a social norm that suggests acceptance of violence (Low and Espelage 2014). Increased stress can lead to feelings of powerlessness and set a cycle of the strong preying on the weak in an effort to feel powerful. Power and control are issues at the core of violence. Children living in communities with high rates of criminal activity are at higher risk of exposure to direct or indirect forms of violence, including child maltreatment (Pascoe et al. 2016).

The US demographics continue to change, with the percentage of nonwhite individuals increasing. The change or "browning of America" also changes perceptions, attitudes, and beliefs regarding child maltreatment, child rearing, and discipline from the current Eurocentric perspective. As culture creates the lens through which an individual's experiences are interpreted, it is important to attempt to understand the unique perspectives of children, parents, caregivers, and families whose cultural and ethnic background is different from one's own. It is through the family that the individual learns about culture, and both cultural and familial features influence our definitions and perceptions of trauma, violence, and abuse. Ethnicity is a significant predictor of attitudes regarding parenting and definitions of child abuse (Merrick et al. 2017). In the

differential diagnosis of child maltreatment, the provider should consider cultural practices (Sawrikar 2016).

Theoretical perspectives commonly attributed to interpersonal violence include social cognitive theory, intergenerational transmission, feminist theory, and ecological approach. Social cognitive theory suggests that violence arises from social and contextual factors within one's world and is a learned behavior. It is a popular explanatory theory that suggests that individuals learn how to behave from exposure to and experience of violence. This leads to the intergenerational transmission of violence perspective that suggests that violence continues through generations in families as a learned behavior (Patterson et al. 2017). Feminist theory places an emphasis on power dynamics and the use of power to oppress the weak (Cannon et al. 2015). An ecological approach offers a broad contextual framework that considers individual, interpersonal, familial, community, and sociocultural factors and suggests that different levels of factors interact to cause violence (Toth and Manly 2018).

Researchers have explored the effects of trauma on the development and regulation of the neurobiological stress system and alterations in brain maturation. As childhood and adolescence are periods of neurological growth and development, any stress in this period has the potential to disrupt typical neurodevelopmental processes and contribute to long-term negative consequences. A review of existing research suggests that "the overwhelming stress of child maltreatment is associated with alterations of the biological stress systems, which, in turn, leads to adverse effects on brain development and delays in cognitive, language, and academic skills" (Teicher and Samson 2016).

Research has explored neurobiological influences of aggression and violent behavior, specifically, failures in the brain systems that modulate aggressive acts. Childhood trauma has been associated with sensitization of the stress response, glucocorticoid resistance, decreased oxytocin activity, inflammation, reduced hippocampal volume, and changes in cortical fields (Heim 2018). "Maltreated children are at higher risk for reactive aggression and deficits in emotional regulation" (Dvir et al. 2014, p. 3). Dysregulation in brain function manifests itself in anxiety, impulsivity, poor affect regulation, and motor hyperactivity (Van der Kolk 2017). For more information on neurobiology and neuropsychiatry, see Chapter 3.

Identifying the causes and risk factors associated with interpersonal violence and trauma proves to be very challenging. No specific or singular cause has been identified. Rather, the interaction of factors on multiple levels creates conditions that may be favorable for child trauma to occur. An exploration of associated risk factors that make children and families more vulnerable to abuse and neglect facilitates identification.

Profile of the Traumatized Child and Adolescent

Although not all children who experience trauma will appear to develop clinical symptoms following the event, research suggests that a significant number of children will develop immediate and long-term clinical symptoms of a stress reaction following a traumatic experience (Hodgdon et al. 2018; Hornor 2015; Spinazzola et al. 2017). Much research has documented children's behavioral, emotional, and psychological responses to trauma. Common mental health disorders include depression, PTSD, anxiety, somatization, and adjustment disorders (Cohen et al. 2016b; Kisely et al. 2018). As children often lack the cognitive ability to discuss trauma, consequences of stress are most often seen in their behavior. Adolescents also often demonstrate behavioral manifestations of trauma responses. Findings from studies suggest that even children who indirectly witness violence or traumatic events may develop symptoms of PTSD upon evaluation (Hagan et al. 2016). Children as young as 6 months who are exposed to violence or traumatic life events display clinical symptoms consistent with post-traumatic stress response and 1-year-olds have had documented trauma symptoms following hearing or witnessing IPV (Spinazzola et al. 2017).

Responses to trauma during childhood can vary depending on a number of factors, including if the events were acute or chronic, the developmental maturity of the child, the presence or absence of family/social support, the perceived threat, loss from the trauma, and prior experience with trauma. Immediately following a traumatic event, children may appear stunned, numb, or unaware of the event. As they attempt to process the trauma event and associated emotions, they may demonstrate a number of symptoms (Table 24.1). Research suggests that the greater the number of traumatic experiences or adverse childhood events, the greater the risk of developing mental health disorders (Kessler et al. 2018). In other words, the toll of traumatic experiences has a cumulative effect on mental health.

The cardinal sign that signals psychopathology and that trauma could have occurred is a change from usual behavior (Cohen et al. 2016b). This can include a change in school performance and in behavior at home or school. Common signs that could signal that a child has experienced abuse include withdrawn behavior, aggres-

Table 24.1 Symptoms seen with child abuse

Symptoms	
Emotional	Anxiety, depression, despair, hopelessness, low self-esteem, fearfulness, withdrawn, attachment difficulties, impulsivity, eating disorders
Behavioral	Aggression, anger, delinquent behaviors, self-destructive behavior, defiance, noncompliance, personality disturbances, peer conflict, sexual acting out, substance use, truancy, compulsive or obsessive behavior, suicide thoughts/attempts
Cognitive	Attention/concentration problems, attention deficit hyperactivity disorder symptoms, difficulty making decisions, memory lapses, academic difficulties
Physical	Sleep disturbances, low energy, somatic symptoms (gastrointestinal disturbances, pain, headache, etc.)

sive or angry behavior, and fearful behavior, particularly if it is attached to a person or place (Christian and Committee on Child Abuse and Neglect 2015). Children may also demonstrate regressive behavior such as bedwetting or thumb sucking in response to trauma (Joinson et al. 2016).

Health consequences to trauma can occur in multiple domains that all can potentially influence the mental health of the child. Physical injury related to abuse can be quite severe, disfiguring, and enduring. The process of obtaining the required medical treatments can be isolating, traumatic, and frightening. The psychological impact of treatment can complicate recovery from the initial traumatic event.

Recognition of the Behavioral Patterns of Abused Children

Children and adolescents who have experienced physical abuse may demonstrate behavioral signs such as extreme rage, passivity, running away from home, cheating, lying or low achievement in school, regression, and inability to form satisfactory peer relationships (Hornor 2015). Children who were sexually abused frequently present in a distinctive way, often with no external signs of child sexual abuse but with behavioral manifestations. These include unusual interest in or avoidance of all things of a sexual nature, seductiveness, statements that their bodies are dirty or damaged, and fear that there is something wrong with them in the genital area. Other signs include refusal to go to school, delinquency/conduct problems, secretiveness, aspects of sexual molestation present in drawings, games, and fantasies, and unusual aggressiveness or suicidal behavior (Hornor 2015).

Exposure to IPV can cause specific mental health symptoms in children and adolescents. Preschool children may manifest yelling, irritability, stuttering, somatic complaints, attachment behavior, sleep disturbance, and signs of terror. School-age children may respond to exposure to IPV by demonstrating a greater willingness to use violence, distractibility, feeling responsible for violence, and lability. Adolescents often act out feelings of rage, shame and betrayal, and show decreased attention span (Fusco 2017).

Implications for Clinical Practice

Assessment

A thorough assessment for past and current victimization, which includes the child, family members, and others close to the child, is essential. Gathering information from at least two sources, the child and a parent or caregiver, is necessary to obtain a complete picture (Rodriguez et al. 2018). Often, parents and children process the event and the aftermath differently and may report on different consequences. Children tend to report more internal manifestations and developmentally appropriate responses; parents tend to report the external and observable manifestations. Gathering information from multiple sources will enhance the diagnostic ability of the provider (De Los Reyes et al. 2015). While information is often gathered from parents, care must be taken when the parent is the suspected abuser to ensure that the child has a free and open place to discuss the abuse in a confidential manner.

The use of a standardized interview and diagnostic tool may aid in gathering information about the violence and the resulting symptoms (Eklund et al. 2018). It is important to inquire about experiences using questions containing specific behaviors as opposed to using labeling words. Words such as child abuse and victim can trigger societal reactions and stigma. The use of behavioral questions such as "Have you been hit or punched?" is preferred (Hornor 2015). Posing questions in a direct manner can serve to normalize the experience and lead to an assault disclosure that would not have occurred otherwise, to attenuate the patient's concern about shocking the clinician. Conversely, many children assume that their experiences must represent the norm and, therefore, will not be forthcoming about details of an assault because of a perception that the information is not relevant or important. Often, children who display behavioral or externalizing manifestations commonly

associated with traumatic events are referred for treatment. Thus, the use of screening questions with all children is necessary. Screening tools are useful in assessing a history of exposure to trauma and the impact of the event on the child or adolescent (Oh et al. 2018). The Traumatic Events Screening Instrument (TESI) is an easy-to-use screening tool for children ages 4–18 and is found in Box 24.1.

Several screening tools exist to measure traumatic events (Eklund et al. 2018). These tools have been carefully developed and tested to account for the developmental and intellectual capacity of children. They may be useful in supplementing the clinical interview. The Childhood PTSD Interview (Fletcher 1996), Childhood PTSD Inventory (Saigh et al. 2000), and University of California Los Angeles (UCLA) PTSD Reaction Index (Pynoos et al. 1998) measure both exposure to trauma and resulting PTSD symptoms. The When Bad Things Happen Scale (WBTHS) (Fletcher 1996) and the UCLA PTSD Reaction Index are both self-reported, while the others are clinician administered. All tools have been widely used with a variety of populations and are well tested. Other measures for exposure to sexual abuse include the Anatomical Doll Questionnaire (Levy et al. 1995; Saini et al. 2018). Finally, other measures screen for history of trauma. The Child Trauma Questionnaire (Bernstein and Fink 1998; Crawford-Jakubiak et al. 2017; Saini et al. 2018) can be used with adolescents aged 12 and older and assesses for emotional, physical, and sexual abuse and emotional and physical neglect. The Trauma Events Screening Inventory (Ribbe 1996) measures child maltreatment, domestic violence, community violence, disasters, and previous injuries and hospitalization in children and adolescents. For a complete discussion of trauma measures for children and adolescents, refer to Eklund et al. (2018).

Commonly used psychometric instruments, with favorable psychometric properties for the evaluation of trauma in children, can be helpful. These include the Trauma Symptom Checklist for Children (Briere 1996; Wherry and Herrington 2018), Los Angeles Symptom Checklist-Adolescent (King et al. 1995), the Child Report of Post-Traumatic Symptoms, and the Parent Report of Post-Traumatic Symptoms (Greenwald and Rubin 1999). The Child PTSD Symptom Scale (Foa et al. 2018) is a widely used measure of DSM-IV symptoms in children. Most of the above-mentioned measures are derived from the DSM-IV-TR criteria for psychiatric symptoms and disorders commonly associated with trauma. The measures are age appropriate and have been widely used so that reliability and validity have been determined.

Box 24.1   Traumatic Events Screening Instrument

Recommended use: Screening for trauma history in children or youth in clinical, educational, juvenile justice, or research settings.

Special features: Administered as a semi-structured interview to children (TESI-C) or parents (TESI-PRR), or as a staff-assisted self-report questionnaire to adolescents (ages 11–18; TESI-C-SR).

General description information:

> **Measure format**: Comes in both semi-structured interview and questionnaire formats.
>
> **Targeted age group**: Children aged 4–18.
>
> **Events assessed**: Wide range of potentially traumatic events including accidents, severe illness and hospitalization, physical or sexual abuse, separation from caregivers, neglect and emotional abuse, natural disaster, community violence, witnessing domestic violence, and traumatic losses.
>
> **Number of items; time to administer**: 15 items on TESI-C, 19 items on TESI-PRR, 26 items on TESI-C-SR; 10–30 minutes, depending on number of traumatic experiences endorsed.
>
> **Response format**: Initial response choices are "yes," "no," and "pass" (with additional choices on the Interview versions, "not sure," "refused," and "questionable validity"). "Yes" and "not sure" responses are followed up with open-ended questions about what happened and closed-ended questions to establish Criterion A from DSM-IV (See Aspects of trauma assessed below).
>
> **Training required to administer**: All versions are designed for administration by qualified mental health or juvenile services professionals or advanced trainees supervised by a qualified professional. The critical qualifications are licensure for independent practice or job classification with responsibilities for behavioral health screening and counseling with children or youth *and* supervised experience in assessment or counseling with child or youth trauma survivors.

Sample items

TESI-C-SR: Have you ever had a time in your life when *you did not have the right care*, like not having enough to eat or drink, being homeless, being left alone when you were too young to care for yourself, or being left with someone using drugs? Or have you ever been left in charge of your younger brothers or sisters for long periods of time, sometimes for several days? ☐ **Yes**   ☐ **No**   ☐ **Pass**

IF YES→ How old were you? The first time:_____ The last time:_____ The worst time:_____

Self-appraisal of fear/helplessness/horror [DSM-IV Criterion A2]:

Did you feel really bad, upset, scared, sad, or mixed up the worst time this happened? ☐ **Yes**   ☐ **No**   ☐ **Pass**

> **TESI-C**: Have you ever been in a really bad accident, like a car accident, a fall, or a fire? How old were you when this happened? Were you hurt? [What was the hurt?] Did you go to the doctor or hospital? Was someone else really hurt in the accident? [Who? What was the hurt?] Did they go to the doctor or the hospital?
>
> Clinician appraisal of objective physical threat [DSM-IV Criterion A1]: Interviewer: In your clinical judgment, was each incident life-threatening? Was or could the child or another person have been killed/severely injured?
>
> Child's appraisal of fear/helplessness/horror [DSM-IV Criterion A2]: When [event] was happening, did you feel as scared as you'd ever been, like this was one of the scariest things that EVER happened to you? [If no, ask:] When [event] happened, did you feel really confused or mixed up? [If no, ask:] Did [event] make you feel sick or disgusted?
>
> **TESI-PRR**: Has your child ever been in a serious accident like a car accident, a fall, or a fire? What happened? How old was your child when this happened? Was your child hurt? If so, what were the injuries? Was an ambulance/paramedic called? Did your child go to the doctor or hospital? Was someone else in the accident? If so, were they seriously injured or killed?
>
> Parent's appraisal of the event [DSM-IV Criterion A1]: Was or could someone have been killed or seriously physically injured in the accident?
>
> Parent's appraisal of child's fear, helplessness, or horror [DSM-IV Criterion A2]: Did your child feel extremely scared or afraid? Did your child feel sick/disgusted? Did your child appear to be really confused or mixed up?
>
> Parent's appraisal of own fear, helplessness, or horror: Did YOU feel extremely scared or afraid? Did YOU feel helpless? Did YOU feel sick/disgusted or horrified?

Scoring: Each item can be scored as a single *traumatic event* (or recurrent events, if multiple events occurred), based on the DSM-IV PTSD Criterion A for exposure to a traumatic stressor:

A1: Traumatic events must involve one of the following forms of **objective danger/harm**:

    a. **actual death** that is premature given the age of the person (*not* including death due to natural causes or expectable illness of an older adult) *or*

    b. imminent **threat of death** due to illness, accidental injury, or intentional violence *or*

    c. prolonged **separation from or loss of or failure to provide adequate basic safety and care by a primary caregiver** (including parents, other adults to whom a child's care is entrusted, or older youths including siblings) *or*

    d. **sexual acts** (witnessed or directly experienced) initiated by or involving person(s) five or more years older than the child.

and

A2: Traumatic events must include or be followed soon after by a **subjective state** *or* automatic bodily reaction of severe fear, helplessness, or horror.

Note: Children exposed to recurrent traumatic events or events that began in infancy or toddlerhood (e.g. prolonged abuse or domestic or community violence) may become sufficiently emotionally numbed or dissociated or hopeless that they do not recall ever having felt distressed and will deny these reactions or simply not be able to remember having experienced them. While it cannot be assumed that such "resilient copers" have experienced a traumatic stressor and cannot or will not acknowledge having felt emotional or bodily distress reactions when events occurred, for clinical and rehabilitative purposes these youth may be classified as having a "probable" trauma history if they (or their parents) describe:

    A. An A1 event before age 6 for which they cannot recall their emotional or bodily reaction, or

    B. A recurrent or series of A1 events that began before age 2.

Composite trauma history classifications

    A. **Physical abuse:** Item 1.8 if the perpetrator(s) were family members or caregivers

    B. **Sexual abuse:** Items 5.1 *or* 5.2

    C. **Physical assault:** Items 1.8 (if by a non-family member or non-caregiver), 2.2 (if occurred to the child/youth), *or* 2.3

    D. **Domestic violence:** Items 3.1 *or* 3.2

    E. **Community violence:** Items 2.2 (if witnessed a family member or close friend) *or* 4.1 *or* 4.2

    F. **Emotional abuse:** If by a primary caregiver or close emotional relationship, Items 2.1 or 6.1

    G. **Neglect:** Items 6.2 *or* 6.3 (the latter only if by a primary caregiver)

    H. **Interpersonal victimization trauma:** Any of A–G

    I. **Traumatic loss:** If a primary caregiver or primary emotional relationship, Items 1.4, *or* 1.6, *or* 1.7, *or* 3.3

    J. **Traumatic accident:** Items 1.1 *or* 1.2

    K. **Traumatic disaster:** Item 1.3

    L. **Traumatic illness/medical care:** Item 1.5

    M. **Non-interpersonal trauma:** J, K, L, or Item 2.4

    N. **Witnessed trauma:** If witnessed but not directly harmed/threatened, Items 1.4 *or* 1.7. *or* 2.2 *or* 3 *or* 4 *or* 5.2 *or* 6.3

    O. **Early childhood trauma:** If age of onset was 5 years old or younger

    P. **Childhood trauma:** If age(s) of occurrence was 12 years old or younger

    Q. **Adolescent trauma:** If age(s) of occurrence was 13–17 years old

    R. **Intra-familial victimization:** Any traumatic event(s) from category D (domestic violence) or (if family members were involved) A, B, C, F, or G (physical or sexual abuse or assault, emotional abuse or neglect)

Time frame assessed: Lifetime.

Correspondence with DSM: Assesses DSM-IV PTSD Criterion A-1 (experiencing or witnessing actual injury or threat of death/injury) and Criterion A-2 (subjective fear, helplessness, or horror).

Psychometric information

    Validation populations: Child psychiatry and pediatric trauma patients, juvenile justice youth.

    Reliability: TESI-C inter-rater agreement reported by Daviss et al. (2000a) and Ford et al. (2000).

    Validity: Convergent/Criterion validity reported by Daviss et al. (2000b), Ford et al. (2000, 2008).

Source: Reprinted with permission from J. D. Ford (permission granted 7 August 2019).

While empirical assessment methods are ideal, sometimes the assessment cannot proceed in this manner due to a variety of etiologies that can stem from developmental, psychological, or emotional issues. In addition, there may be other inhibiting factors such as denial or parental interference. Denial on the parent's part can occur because the parent is unaware of the trauma, because the parent is the offender, or for other reasons (AACAP 2010). Children are often unable to verbalize their symptoms in a meaningful way. Often, children have an easier time discussing somatic symptoms resulting from trauma. Assessment of the child away from the parent using age-appropriate questions is warranted. In such cases, a clinician should rely on clinical judgment and use other, less formal strategies such as the use of art and play. In analyzing the content and process of the play patterns, elements of repetition, reenactment, and developmental inappropriateness should be of concern. For example, a traumatized preschool child might display regressive behaviors such as thumb-sucking and bed-wetting; older children might present with somatic complaints and cognitive difficulties.

Only specially trained personnel should conduct interviews for the purposes of forensic evaluation and/or legal documentation; however, screening for trauma or exposure to violence should be part of a routine primary care and mental health evaluation. Practitioners need to provide children, regardless of their age, with an opportunity to talk about their trauma experiences without others, including family members, present. It is not uncommon for children to withhold details of trauma or abuse if they feel it will upset the family or parent (Alaggia et al. 2017). Furthermore, children are often reluctant to disclose abuse in an interview, especially for sexual abuse and with those who are younger and male (Azzopardi et al. 2018). Providing a private place where the practitioner and child can talk not only gives the child a chance to discuss traumatic events without a potential perpetrator present but also allows the child the opportunity to freely discuss their experiences without the child's concern for upsetting the parent.

When talking to children about their trauma experiences practitioners must be sensitive to the allegations, the child's developmental level, and the child's current mental state. The APRN can begin screening for less-threatening or traumatic experiences or begin with general statements that are not specific to the child. By also asking open-ended questions, the child is allowed to direct the conversation. It is helpful to use terms the child uses to refer to body parts or acts of violence or abuse. For example, it is helpful to begin a conversation with an adolescent patient about violence by stating, "I don't know if this is a concern for you, but many teens I see are dealing with violence or bullying issues, so I've started asking questions about violence routinely" (Alvarez et al. 2017). The provider can then follow with additional direct questions, such as, "Does anyone make you afraid? Is anyone hurting you?"

The notion of fear and being hurt can elicit responses from young children about normal daily activities. For example, a child may affirmatively respond to questions about being hit and then, through more questioning, reveal that the culprit is a classmate or sibling. In evaluating sibling abuse, the nurse also inquires further to determine if other incidences of violence occurred. Older children are capable of understanding the distinction between abusive touch as opposed to routine activities requiring touch. For example, parents routinely touch the private areas of children during bathing and toileting. The nurse may have to ask more probing questions to uncover abuse and determine inappropriate touch.

Once a child has disclosed a traumatic event, the clinician can then ask for more information such as details about onset, frequency, and duration. In screening for PTSD symptoms, it is important to use clear language about re-experiencing and avoidance items. For example, the clinician can ask the child if he or she becomes upset when in the specific place where the event occurred (AACAP 2010).

Children may display psychiatric symptoms that could indicate trauma. APRNs are encouraged to explore other psychiatric and physical conditions that may mimic PTSD, such as attention deficit hyperactivity disorder, endocrine disturbances, or seizure disorder (AACAP 2010). Children who present with symptoms suggestive of trauma but with no confirmed reports of trauma should be referred for a forensic evaluation (AACAP 2010).

Prevention

Primary prevention that can include education about the prevalence and impact of childhood trauma is imperative among all individuals in our society, particularly those who are trusted with the care of children and young people. Public awareness campaigns have continued to increase the public's awareness of traumatic stress in childhood and adolescence. Yet societal misperceptions about violence and stigma about seeking mental health treatment continue to exist. APRNs are in a position to educate the public and the healthcare system about new developments in the treatment of traumatic stress. In this time of advancing technology and knowledge explosion, education and training of APRNs to remain current are critical.

Programs designed to reduce and prevent child maltreatment have received mixed reviews over the past 20 years. However, there is growing literature to support comprehensive, evidence-based home visitation programs led by professionals, such as nurses, delivering frequent and intense interventions as cost-effective measures in preventing child maltreatment (Chaiyachati et al. 2018; Lee et al. 2018; Viswanathan et al. 2018). In addition, programs exist to prevent DV in middle and high school students. While many programs report success at changing attitudes, few programs report sustained behavior change (De La Rue et al. 2017). For a review of available programs, the reader is referred to Chaiyachati et al. (2018). An understanding of the risk factors associated with children, families, and parents enables the nurse to implement prevention programs targeted to high-risk individuals.

Bullying prevention follows three distinct approaches. First, universal prevention programs seek to reduce the risks and strengthen skills for all youth within a community or school setting. Selective preventive interventions target youth who are at risk for engaging in bullying or at risk for becoming a target for bullying. Finally, indicated preventive interventions are tailored to meet the individual needs of youths, most often those who are already demonstrating bullying behavior or being bullied. The majority of bullying prevention research focuses on universal programs. There is a need for more research on selective and indicated approaches as well as policies at the federal, state, and local level to address bullying (Rivara and LeMenestrel 2016).

Intervention

Early intervention in responding to child and adolescent trauma is essential (Hahn et al. 2016). Families that provide support and a safe, nurturing environment as soon as possible following a traumatic event effectively limit the influence of the trauma on the child or adolescent. Common mental health disorders resulting from interpersonal violence include PTSD, depression, somatization, general anxiety, and dissociative disorder. Outpatient management is appropriate for all of these symptoms; however, children and adolescents who demonstrate behavior that is harmful to self or others need inpatient hospitalization. Early treatment can alleviate symptoms of mental illness and mitigate long-term consequences. As previously stated, it is important to remember that not all who experience trauma develop mental health symptoms. The APRN who works with a child immediately after trauma can work to foster the child's resilience and help the family provide optimal support to mitigate potential health consequences.

Psychotherapy is a vital treatment modality for children's emotional, behavioral, and social problems and within the scope of the psychiatric APRN. Generally, the goal of psychotherapy following trauma is to allow the child or adolescent to talk about and integrate the event so that he or she is better able to cope with the pain or loss. Additionally, a goal of talk therapy (particularly among older patients) is to help the patient describe his or her feelings in order to recognize his or her own behaviors, symptoms, and characteristic responses to trauma. Moreover, talk therapy can help the patient gain perspective and understand the trauma within a given context.

Experiencing violence can disrupt the normal growth and development trajectory of children (Toth and Manly 2018). In therapy, the clinician can effectively use this knowledge to help children meet their developmental tasks. For example, preschool-age children are beginning to learn right from wrong, which makes them focused on punishment and rewards. When abuse occurs for children this age, it can be very confusing, causing them to feel that it is their fault. Therapists can work to restore their normal curiosity and openness while helping to repair a healthy sense of self.

Techniques used in individual psychotherapy include psychoeducational strategies, cognitive-behavioral therapy (CBT), insight-oriented therapy, and trauma-focused techniques reviws of randomized control trials consistently find strong evidence for the efficacy of CBT in treating PTSD and other psychiatric symptoms occurring after multiple traumatic experiences (Dorsey et al. 2017; Landolt and Kenardy 2015; Lewey et al. 2018). Another review of all psychosocial treatments for children exposed to traumatic events found effectiveness in trauma-focused CBT (TF-CBT) and school-based group CBT. Evidence suggests that trauma-focused therapies are more effective in treating PTSD symptoms (Wethington et al. 2008). Furthermore, treatment is essential when considering PTSD, depressive symptoms, anxiety symptoms, and externalizing behavior programs that result from traumatic experiences (Lenz and Hollenbaugh 2015).

Fundamental components of CBT include cognitive processing, exposure, and stress inoculation procedures. Cognitive processing provides opportunities to explore the child's cognitions about the event with the goal of correcting cognitive distortions. Exposure techniques help the child to disconnect thoughts and reminders of the traumatic events from overwhelming emotions using techniques such as gradual encouragement to share details of the trauma and the memories evoked. Stress inoculation techniques can include relaxation, visualization and imagery, diaphragmatic breathing, and self-talk.

TF-CBT is a highly structured program that uses an individual format that includes education on cognitive and behavioral procedures, exposure through the use of narratives, drawings, or other imaginative methods, and cognitive reprocessing of the trauma and resultant symptoms (Cohen et al. 2018). The core elements of TF-CBT provide opportunities for the child to construct a detailed trauma narrative, engage in significant cognitive processing of the event, address behavioral manifestations of PTSD, and provide a parental treatment component (Cohen et al. 2016a). The construction of a narrative is an important aspect of therapy and functions as a tool that helps the child to overcome avoidance of the traumatic memories, identify cognitive distortions, and situate the traumatic experience within the larger framework of the child's life (Knutsen and Jensen 2019). TF-CBT has demonstrated effective use with multiple traumatic experiences and has been adapted for use with children and adolescents across the age (Cohen et al. 2018). Parental involvement in TF-CBT often consists of education on the use of effective parenting skills and about incidence of trauma, common reactions to trauma, and the treatment approaches (Cohen et al. 2018). See Chapter 20 for a complete review of CBT.

Research suggests that school-based group CBT may be an effective treatment strategy for anxiety and depression in children exposed to trauma. Within this technique, emphasis centers on psychoeducation, graded exposures using writing and/or drawing, cognitive and coping skills training, and social skills training (Chafouleas et al. 2019). Another CBT technique that holds promise for resolving symptoms associated with disturbing and painful events is eye movement desensitization and reprocessing. This treatment combines exposure and cognitive psychodynamic and somatic therapies using an eight-phase approach (Dorsey et al. 2017). Effective use is reported with children as young as 6 years of age (Gutermann et al. 2016).

Play therapy is another type of psychotherapy that can be beneficial for the assessment of young children who may lack the verbal or emotional skill to access and articulate their emotions, thoughts, and fantasies regarding the traumatic event. In addition, play therapy provides a vehicle for the child to connect his or her concrete experience with abstract thought (Woodhouse 2019). For example, the child might reenact the event using dolls or via artistic expression, such as through drawing or painting. Although play therapy has been found to be beneficial to participants, insufficient evidence exists to conclude effectiveness (Dorsey et al. 2017). See Chapter 18 for further discussion of play therapy.

Children who have experienced the same trauma (e.g. surviving the same fire) can benefit from group therapy.

In addition, group therapy can be efficacious among children who have experienced similar traumas (e.g. victims of sexual abuse or domestic violence). Group therapy is particularly useful for adolescents as it complements the developmental emphasis on peers. A review of outcome studies for adolescent girls with sexual abuse histories revealed that psychodrama models decreased depressive symptoms and CBT, and group therapies using exposure were associated with PTSD reduction (Graham-Kevan and Brooks 2016). Again, the focus of the group approach can include a combination of the following treatment modalities: psychoeducation, CBT, family therapy, and problem-focused therapy. However, the most effective group treatment modality appears to be CBT (Lenz and Hollenbaugh 2015). See Chapter 18 for a complete review of group therapy.

In some instances, children benefit from the use of psychotherapy in conjunction with medication to treat symptoms of PTSD, anxiety, and depression, which are diagnoses that are associated with trauma. It is not surprising that many of these diagnoses occur in clusters since, from a neurobiological perspective, it has yet to be determined if and how the body and brain distinguish among distinct trauma responses. In particular, children with persistent symptoms that do not respond to other forms of therapy may need pharmacological treatment. Examples of commonly prescribed medications include antidepressant medications, such as fluoxetine (Prozac), sertraline (Zoloft), and citalopram (Celexa), and antianxiety medications, such as benzodiazepines and clonazepam (Klonopin), and other antianxiety agents, such as clonidine (Catapres) and guanfacine (Tenex) (Locher et al. 2017; McLaren et al. 2018). It is important to note that children are prescribed medications based on evidence and dosage recommendations that were researched with adult populations and often target adults. Selective serotonin reuptake inhibitors (SSRIs) are approved for adult use in PTSD to decrease all symptom clusters. Preliminary evidence suggests that SSRIs may be beneficial in treating children with PTSD but insufficient evidence exists to draw conclusions (Locher et al. 2017). Existing evidence has demonstrated the effectiveness of SSRIs in treating childhood depression and anxiety disorders (McClaren et al. 2018). It is important for the prescribing clinician to keep abreast of research evidence and new findings regarding psychotropic medication use with children and adolescents. Additionally, the child and adolescent brain is undergoing rather rapid development. Thus, vigilant surveillance is recommended to monitor for medication side effects and treatment response, preferably by a psychiatric APRN with expertise in pediatric psychopharmacology. See Chapter 9 for a more detailed discussion of psycho-pharmacological management for the treatment of these symptoms and diagnoses.

As children and adolescents often live with parents or caregivers, interventions are necessary at the family level. A safe and stable environment is essential for the child and adolescent to manage the trauma and resulting symptoms. Anxious parents may need assistance to be able to provide for their child's emotional and security needs. Lower levels of parental distress are associated with a more positive response to treatment by the child (Cohen et al. 2016a). When possible, emphasis should be placed on having the parents or caregivers maintain a close adherence to the usual structures and schedules of the home life so that the child can feel a sense of safety in his or her environment. Caregivers must also be taught to recognize the symptoms of escalating mental illness so they know when to bring in their child for treatment. The therapist can also ensure that the family has support systems in place to help them manage the stress associated with their child's adjustment. TF-CBT can include a parental treatment component. Inclusion of parents was found to be effective in improving the child's self-reported depressive symptoms (Cohen and Mannarino 2017). Parents can be taught strategies for coping with their own emotional difficulties resulting from their child's trauma and can learn to model coping skills. Attachment-based interventions may improve insensitive parenting and infant attachment insecurity (Landers et al. 2018; Toth and Manly 2018). Child- and parent-focused psychotherapy is indicated in families who also had exposure to domestic violence and for young children under age 7 (Sege and Amaya-Jackson 2017). Skills-based education can be helpful to increase parenting skills, and childcare and management. These relational interventions are effective in improving the parent–child relationship (Landers et al. 2018). See Chapter 19 for a complete discussion of family therapy.

Providing Specialized Care

Intervention with clients who have experienced traumatic events will be most effective when the healthcare team works together. While many health providers, including those in primary care, may recognize trauma symptoms, providing mental health treatment for children and adolescents who have experienced trauma requires a trained psychiatric practitioner. This is especially true when children require medications to manage symptoms such as depression and anxiety, as many of these medications require close follow-up and management. In routine assessments, appointments, and physical examinations, pediatric and family nurse practitioners may uncover signs of abuse and trauma. These primary care providers have the necessary skill set to document the physical findings and to testify in court if needed. However, only mental health providers have the necessary skill set for assessment and treatment of psychiatric symptoms. Further, clinicians unfamiliar with or lacking the necessary skills to assess, treat, or manage these children should refer patients and families to experts in the area of child trauma.

Forensic Implications

Psychiatric clinicians are involved in court proceedings usually by requests to confirm a diagnosis of child abuse or to assess for emotional damages to the child. Though definitions of what constitutes child abuse and neglect can vary by state, they include the minimum standards established by the federal government. The Federal CAPTA (42 U.S.C.A. §5106g), as amended by the Keeping Children and Families Safe Act of 2003, provides a seminal definition of child abuse and neglect. At minimum, a definition should include the following: Any recent act or failure to act on the part of a parent or caretaker, which results in death, serious physical or emotional harm, sexual abuse or exploitation; or an act, or failure to act which presents an imminent risk of serious harm (Christian and the Committee on Child Abuse and Neglect 2015). While definitions may vary from state to state, every state has laws that designate nurses and advanced practice nurses as mandatory reporters.

An increasing number of cases of child maltreatment and abuse are under investigation and in the courts. Accordingly, APRNs, child psychiatrists, and other qualified professionals make evaluations during legal proceedings. This can include evaluation of the competency of the child to testify, the credibility of the child's allegation, and whether it is in the child's best interest to have contact with the alleged perpetrator and under what circumstances, if any, prior to court proceedings, particularly if the perpetrator is a relative. Clinicians may also evaluate whether the child is emotionally disturbed and in need of treatment, what emotional preparation is required for court testimony, whether the child will be able to cope with the stress of giving testimony, and whether the child might experience further psychological damage by giving testimony.

Implications for Research and Education

Myriad studies document the extensive and detrimental influence of childhood trauma within social, psychological, and physical domains throughout the life span. Research is required on both diagnosis and treatment of children and adolescents who are at risk for abuse. Most of the findings on the impact of childhood trauma come from cross-sectional research. Hence, there is a need to examine and to measure the effects of the abuse over an extended period of time and within the context of a developmental framework (Ford et al. 2018). As many cases of child maltreatment are undetected, it is essential that research examine the benefits of screening and interventions.

Additionally, research within the area of neurobiology offers hope for a better understanding of childhood abuse and more effective treatment strategies that utilize advances in technology. For example, transcranial magnetic stimulation (TMS) (Trevizol et al. 2016) and virtual reality (VR) exposure therapy for the treatment of PTSD have shown promise among various populations (DiMauro 2014). TMS is a noninvasive technique that directly stimulates cortical neurons to create a therapeutic effect that, through testing with children under age18, was found to be effective (Krishnan et al. 2015). VR uses virtual reality technology to treat patients with PTSD; research suggests that it is effective in treating adults, although randomized controlled trials are not available. Well-designed studies can determine if these progressive treatments hold promise for children and adolescents.

The rapid expansion of knowledge in the basic sciences impacts research needs for practice. The increased understanding of genetics and genomics expands the need for research on familial and biological causes of mental illness and responses to trauma. The pathways between trauma and consequences such as neurostructural alterations and abnormal neuropsychological responses are important areas of study. The field could benefit from studies that examine the relationships among trauma as a form of chronic stress and the roles that neurotoxic and vulnerability effects can have on the developing brain so that early interventions can be developed (Lupien et al. 2018). In addition, there is optimism that growing research in this field will lead to a better understanding of neurobiological development of children, adolescents, and young adults. The use of more extensive neuropsychological testing will help in this area.

Research on children and adolescents and especially research on victimized children and adolescents is not without ethical and practical obstacles (see Chapter 31). It would be useful to understand the effects of participating in research with children and adolescents and if it is harmful, helpful, or neutral to the recovery process. Despite the difficulties in this research, it is important to design prospective studies that describe long- and short-term outcomes and benefits to treatment. Randomized controlled trials are needed to determine the efficacy of treatment approaches, including medication use and the effectiveness of prevention programs.

Key emerging trends include culture, treatment, and research. Cultural issues include increased use of ethnopsychology, ethnopsychiatry, ethnobiology, and ethnopharmacology, all of which entail an understanding of ethnic differences and approaches to therapy. Educational efforts must focus on readying the workforce to deal with clients of increasing diversity. Clinicians will need an understanding of the ways in which ones' ethnic and racial background can affect perceptions and treatment of mental illness. These efforts include recruitment of a more diverse workforce and cultural sensitivity training for all APRNs. Furthermore, emphasis on culture-bound syndromes and on culturally relevant and sensitive assessment, diagnosis, and treatment is important. The changing demographics of the United States necessitate that clinicians understand cultural and ethnic expression of mental health symptoms, strategies for effective relationship building, and the influence of family and community structures in diverse groups. Research that includes diverse individuals can assist in the development and testing of interventions tailored for minority populations. Research involving child trauma must also pay attention to the sociocultural impact of religion, spirituality, health disparities, socioeconomic status, and sexual orientation on child treatment.

Technological advances bring new areas of intervention, such as the use of telehealth to expand child protection services. Trends within interpersonal violence include the influence of emerging technologies used in perpetration. Internet-based crimes include child predators targeting children and adolescents in chat rooms and social networking sites. Pornography of children broadcast over the internet provides a challenge to criminal justice investigations and includes the problem of the long-term nature of pictures and videos on the web. Bullying, stalking, and harassment can also include technology in the form of text messaging, instant messaging, and social networking sites. A major problem is the intrusive, pervasive, and persistent effects of technology-assisted IPV. More research can aid in understanding prevention and intervention strategies related to technology-assisted violence.

A plethora of public policy issues exists. Due to the possibility of long-term neurological consequences, it is essential that child trauma and resulting psychiatric symptoms are identified early and intervention and treatment occur. School health nurses and school counselors can be instrumental in identifying children at risk and those who demonstrate behavioral profiles consistent with trauma. These children and their families need referrals and linkages with mental health providers, services, and resources. Programs that identify high-risk individuals and provide home visitation, education, and other social services can be helpful in preventing child abuse (Chaiyachati et al. 2018; Lee et al. 2018; Viswanathan et al. 2018). School-based programs can also be helpful in providing prevention and intervention resources around bullying, and resources and referrals for offenders and victims.

Summary

While many regard childhood and adolescence as carefree periods, this is not true for all youths. For some individuals, traumatic experiences mark childhood and adolescence. Far too many children and adolescents deal with traumatic experiences and the resulting psychiatric symptoms and distress. Often these trauma responses are misinterpreted and misdiagnosed as other psychiatric disorders and APRNs can be aided by understanding the risk factors and causes that facilitate understanding trauma experiences. Meeting the patient individually, building rapport, and gathering collateral history from parents gives context for the child's presenting symptoms. Early identification and treatment can mitigate the health consequences of trauma. A variety of therapy options exist that can aid the APRN in helping children, adolescents, and their families to manage and recover from trauma. By remaining current with research and practice trends, the APRN can provide individualized and targeted therapy to children, adolescents, and families, and develop and implement prevention and intervention strategies.

Critical Thinking Questions

1. How can a recent APRN graduate become informed about trauma in children and adolescents?
2. Identify the levels of trauma treatment that could be required by a pediatric population.
3. How do APRNs deal with their own emotional response to treating a traumatized pediatric population?

Recommended Resources

Prevent Child Abuse (PCA), America (formerly the National Committee to Prevent Child Abuse) is nationally recognized as one of the most innovative leaders in child abuse prevention. It has a nationwide network of chapters and their local affiliates in hundreds of communities. www.preventchildabuse.org.

Child Welfare League of America (CWLA) is an association of more than 1000 public and private nonprofit agencies that assist over 2.5 million abused and neglected children and their families each year with a wide range of services. http://www.cwla.org.

American Professional Society on the Abuse of Children (APSAC) works to ensure that everyone affected by child maltreatment receives the best possible professional response. http://www.apsac.org.

National Clearinghouse for Child Abuse and Neglect (NCCAN) is a national resource for professionals seeking information on the prevention, identification, and treatment of child abuse and neglect, and related child welfare issues. http://www.calib.com/nccanch, email: nccanch@calib.com.

The National Child Traumatic Stress Network works to raise the standard of care and improve access to services for traumatized children, their families, and communities throughout the United States. http://www.nctsn.org/nccts/nav.do?pid=ctr_main.

The Red Cross has a long history of helping children, families, and communities recover from disasters. http://www.redcross.org.

Cohen, J.A., Mannarino, A.P., and Deblinger, E. (2017). *Treating Trauma and Traumatic Grief in Children and Adolescents*, (2e). New York, NY: Guilford Press.

References

Alaggia, R., Collin-Vézina, D., and Lateef, R. (2017). Facilitators and barriers to child sexual abuse (CSA) disclosures: a research update (2000–2016). *Trauma, Violence & Abuse* https://doi.org/10.1177/1524838017697312.

Alvarez, C., Fedock, G., Grace, K.T., and Campbell, J. (2017). Provider screening and counseling for intimate partner violence: a systematic review of practices and influencing factors. *Trauma, Violence & Abuse* 18 (5): 479–495.

AACAP (2010). Practice parameter for the assessment and treatment of children and adolescents with posttraumatic stress disorder. *Journal of the Academy of Child and Adolescent Psychiatry* 49 (4): 414–430.

American Psychiatric Association (2013). *Diagnostic and Statistical Manual of Mental Disorders*, 5e, text revision. Washington, DC: American Psychiatric Association.

Azzopardi, C., Eirich, R., Rash, C.L. et al. (2018). A meta-analysis of the prevalence of child sexual abuse disclosure in forensic settings. *Child Abuse & Neglect*.

Ben-Natan, M., Sharon, I., Barbashov, P. et al. (2014). Risk factors for child abuse: quantitative correlational design. *Journal of Pediatric Nursing* 29 (3): 220–227.

Bernstein, D. and Fink, L. (1998). *Childhood Trauma Questionnaire: A Retrospective Self-Report*. San Antonio: The Psychological Corporation.

Bounds, D., Julion, W.A., and Delaney, K.R. (2015). Commercial sexual exploitation of children and state child welfare systems. *Policy, Politics & Nursing Practice* 16 (1–2): 17–26.

Bounds, D., Delaney, K.R., Julion, W., and Breitenstein, S. (2017). Uncovering indicators of commercial *Sexual Exploitation. Journal of Interpersonal Violence* https://doi.org/10.1177/0886260517723141.

Briere, J. (1996). *Trauma Symptom Checklist for Children (TSCC) Professional Manual*. Odessa, FL: Psychological Assessment Resources.

Cannon, C., Lauve-Moon, K., and Buttell, F. (2015). Re-theorizing intimate partner violence through post-structural feminism, queer theory, and the sociology of gender. *Social Sciences* 4 (3): 668–687.

CDC. 2006. *Adverse Childhood Experiences Study*. Centers for Disease Control and Prevention. Available from http://www.cdc.gov/nccdphp/ace/index.htm.

Chafouleas, S.M., Koriakin, T.A., Roundfield, K.D., and Overstreet, S. (2019). Addressing childhood trauma in school settings: a framework for evidence-based practice. *School Mental Health* (1): 40–53.

Chaiyachati, B.H., Gaither, J.R., Hughes, M. et al. (2018). Preventing child maltreatment: examination of an established statewide home-visiting program. *Child Abuse & Neglect* 79: 476–484.

Chen, M. and Chan, K.L. (2016). Effects of parenting programs on child maltreatment prevention. *Trauma, Violence & Abuse* 17 (1): 88–104. Available at https://doi.org/10.1177/1524838014566718.

Christian, C.W. and Committee on Child Abuse and Neglect (2015). The evaluation of suspected child physical abuse. *Pediatrics* 135 (5): e1337–e1354.

Citron, D.K. and Franks, M.A. (2014). Criminalizing revenge porn. *Wake Forest Law Review* 49: 345.

Cohen, J.A. and Mannarino, A.P. (2017). Evidence based intervention: trauma-focused cognitive behavioral therapy for children and families. In: *Parenting and Family Processes in Child Maltreatment and Intervention* (ed. D.M. Teti), 91–105. Cham: Springer.

Cohen, J.A., Mannarino, A.P., and Deblinger, E. (2016a). *Treating Trauma and Traumatic Grief in Children and Adolescents*. Guilford Publications.

Cohen, J.A., Mannarino, A.P., Jankowski, K. et al. (2016b). A randomized implementation study of trauma-focused cognitive behavioral therapy for adjudicated teens in residential treatment facilities. *Child Maltreatment* 21 (2): 156–167.

Cohen, J.A., Deblinger, E., and Mannarino, A.P. (2018). Trauma-focused cognitive behavioral therapy for children and families. *Psychotherapy Research* 28 (1): 47–57.

Cook, A., Spinazzola, J., Ford, J. et al. (2017). Complex trauma in children and adolescents. *Psychiatric Annals* 35 (5): 390–398.

Crawford-Jakubiak, J.E., Alderman, E.M., Leventhal, J.M., and Committee on Child Abuse and Neglect (2017). Care of the adolescent after an acute sexual assault. *Pediatrics* 139 (3): e20164243.

Crosby, S.D., Hsu, H.-T., Jones, K., and Rice, E. (2018). Factors that contribute to help-seeking among homeless, trauma-exposed youth: a social-ecological perspective. *Children and Youth Services Review* 93: 126–134. Available at https://doi.org/10.1016/j.childyouth.2018.07.015.

Daviss, W.B., Mooney, D., Racusin, R. et al. (2000a). Predicting posttraumatic stress after hospitalization for pediatric injury. *Journal of the American Academy of Child and Adolescent Psychiatry* 39: 576–583.

Daviss, W.B., Racusin, R., Fleischer, A. et al. (2000b). Acute stress disorder symptomatology during hospitalization for pediatric injury. *Journal of the American Academy of Child and Adolescent Psychiatry* 39: 569–575.

De La Rue, L., Polanin, J.R., Espelage, D.L., and Pigott, T.D. (2017). A meta-analysis of school-based interventions aimed to prevent or reduce violence in teen dating relationships. *Review of Educational Research* 87 (1): 7–34.

De Los Reyes, A., Augenstein, T.M., Wang, M. et al. (2015). The validity of the multi-informant approach to assessing child and adolescent mental health. *Psychological Bulletin* 141 (4): 858.

DeChesnay, M. (2013). *Sex Trafficking: A Clinical Guide for Nurses*. New York: Springer.

DiMauro, J. (2014). Exposure therapy for posttraumatic stress disorder: a meta-analysis. *Military Psychology* 26 (2): 120–130.

Dorsey, S., McLaughlin, K.A., Kerns, S.E. et al. (2017). Evidence base update for psychosocial treatments for children and adolescents exposed to traumatic events. *Journal of Clinical Child & Adolescent Psychology* 46 (3): 303–330.

Dvir, Y., Ford, J.D., Hill, M., and Frazier, J.A. (2014). Childhood maltreatment, emotional dysregulation, and psychiatric comorbidities. *Harvard Review of Psychiatry* 22 (3): 149.

Ehman, A.C. and Gross, A.M. (2019). Sexual cyberbullying: review, critique, & future directions. *Aggression and Violent Behavior* 44: 80–87. https://doi.org/10.1016/j.avb.2018.11.001.

Eklund, K., Rossen, E., Koriakin, T. et al. (2018). A systematic review of trauma screening measures for children and adolescents. *School Psychology Quarterly: The Official Journal of the Division of School Psychology, American Psychological Association* 33 (1): 30–43.

Ernewein, C. and Nieves, R. (2015). Human sex trafficking: recognition, treatment, and referral of pediatric victims. *The Journal for Nurse Practitioners* 11 (8): 797–803.

Espelage, D.L., Hong, J.S., and Valido, A. (2018). Associations among family violence, bullying, sexual harassment, and teen dating violence. In: *Adolescent Dating Violence. Theory, Research and Prevention* (eds. D.A. Wolfe and J.R. Temple), 85–102.

Felitti, V.J., Anda, R.F., Nordenberg, D. et al. (1998). Relationship of childhood abuse and household dysfunction to many of the leading causes of death in adults: the adverse childhood experiences (ACE) study. *American Journal of Preventative Medicine* 14 (4): 245–258.

Finkelhor, D., Turner, H.A., Shattuck, A., and Hamby, S.L. (2013). Violence, crime, and abuse exposure in a national sample of children and youth: an update. *JAMA Pediatrics* 167 (7): 614–621.

Finkelhor, D., Turner, H.A., Shattuck, A., and Hamby, S.L. (2015). Prevalence of childhood exposure to violence, crime, and abuse: results from the national survey of children's exposure to violence. *JAMA Pediatrics* 169 (8): 746–754. https://doi.org/10.1001/jamapediatrics.2015.0676.

Flannery, D.J., Todres, J., Bradshaw, C.P., Amar, A.F., Graham, S., Hatzenbuehler, M., & Le Menestrel, S.M. (2016). Bullying Prevention: a Summary of the Report of the National Academies of Sciences, Engineering, and Medicine. Prevention Science, 17, 1055–1053.

Fleckman, J., Drury, S., Taylor, C. et al. (2016). Role of direct and indirect violence exposure on externalizing behavior in children. *Journal of Urban Health* 93 (3): 479–492. https://doi.org/10.1007/s11524-016-0052-y.

Fletcher, K. (1996). Psychometric review of the When Bad Things Happen scale (WBTH). In: *Measurement of Stress, Trauma, and Adaptation* (ed. B.H. Stamm), 435–437. Lutherville, MD: Sidran Press.

Fluke, J.D., Shusterman, G.R., Hollinshead, D.M., and Yuan, Y.Y. (2008). Longitudinal analysis of repeated child abuse reporting and victimization: multistate analysis of associated factors. *Child Maltreatment* 13: 76–88. https://doi.org/10.1177/1077559507311517.

Foa, E.B., Asnaani, A., Zang, Y. et al. (2018). Psychometrics of the Child PTSD Symptom Scale for DSM-5 for trauma-exposed children and adolescents. *Journal of Clinical Child & Adolescent Psychology* 47 (1): 38–46.

Ford, J.D., Racusin, R., Ellis, C. et al. (2000). Child maltreatment, other trauma exposure, and posttraumatic symptomatology among children with oppositional defiant and attention deficit hyperactivity disorders. *Child Maltreatment* 5: 205–217.

Ford, J.D., Hartman, J.K., Hawke, J., and Chapman, J. (2008). Traumatic victimization, posttraumatic stress disorder, suicidal ideation, and substance abuse risk among juvenile justice-involved youths. *Journal of Child and Adolescent Trauma* 1: 75–92.

Ford, J.D., Spinazzola, J., and Grasso, D.J. (2018). Toward an empirically based developmental trauma disorder diagnosis for children: factor structure, item characteristics, reliability, and validity of the developmental trauma disorder semi-structured interview. *The Journal of Clinical Psychiatry* 79 (5) https://doi.org/10.4088/JCP.17m11675.

Francis, L., DePriest, K., Wilson, M., and Gross, D. (2018). Child poverty, toxic stress, and social determinants of health: screening and care coordination. *OJIN: The Online Journal of Issues in Nursing* 23 (3), Manuscript 2.

Fusco, R.A. (2017). Socioemotional problems in children exposed to intimate partner violence: mediating effects of attachment and family supports. *Journal of Interpersonal Violence* 32 (16): 2515–2532. https://doi.org/10.1177/0886260515593545.

Gerassi, L. (2015). From exploitation to industry: definitions, risks, and consequences of domestic sexual exploitation and sex work among women and girls. *Journal of Human Behavior in the Social Environment* 25 (6): 591–605. https://doi.org/10.1080/10911359.2014.991055.

Gillespie, G.L., Willis, D.G., and Amar, A.F. (2018). Review and application of the National Academies of Sciences, Engineering, and Medicine bullying or cyberbullying recommendations for screening and lesbian, gay, bisexual, and transgender youth. *Nursing Outlook* 66 (4): 372–378.

Graham-Kevan, N. & Brooks, M. (2016). *Effective support for victims of sexual violence: A systematic review of reviews*. Project Report, University of Central Lancashire. Available at www.uclan.ac.uk/schools/psychology.

Greenwald, R. and Rubin, A. (1999). Brief assessment of children's posttraumatic symptoms: development and preliminary validation of parent and child scales. *Research on Social Work Practice* 9: 61–75.

Gutermann, J., Schreiber, F., Matulis, S. et al. (2016). Psychological treatments for symptoms of posttraumatic stress disorder in children, adolescents, and young adults: a meta-analysis. *Clinical Child and Family Psychology Review* 19 (2): 77–93.

Hagan, M., Sulik, M., Lieberman, A. et al. (2016). Traumatic life events and psychopathology in a high risk, ethnically diverse sample of young children: a person-centered approach. *Journal of Abnormal Child Psychology* 44 (5): 833–844. https://doi.org/10.1007/s10802-015-0078-8.

Hahn, H., Oransky, M., Epstein, C. et al. (2016). Findings of an early intervention to address children's traumatic stress implemented in the child advocacy center setting following sexual abuse. *Journal of Child & Adolescent Trauma* 9 (1): 55–66.

Halfon, N., Larson, K., Son, J. et al. (2017). Income inequality and the differential effect of adverse childhood experiences in US children. *Academic Pediatrics* 17 (7): S70–S78. https://doi.org/10.1016/j.acap.2016.11.007.

Heim, C. (2018). Psychobiological consequences of child maltreatment. In: *The Biology of Early Life Stress* (ed. C. Heim), 15–30. Cham: Springer.

Hodgdon, H.B., Spinazzola, J., Briggs, E.C. et al. (2018). Maltreatment type, exposure characteristics, and mental health outcomes among clinic referred trauma-exposed youth. *Child Abuse & Neglect* 82: 12–22.

Hornor, G. (2015). Childhood trauma exposure and toxic stress: what the PNP needs to know. *Journal of Pediatric Health Care* 29 (2): 191–198.

Hughes, K., Bellis, M.A., Hardcastle, K.A. et al. (2017). The effect of multiple adverse childhood experiences on health: a systematic review and meta-analysis. *The Lancet Public Health* 2 (8): e356–e366.

Humphreys, C., Healey, L., Kirkwood, D., and Nicholson, D. (2018). Children living with domestic violence: a differential response through multi-agency collaboration. *Australian Social Work* 71 (2): 162–174. https://doi.org/10.1080/0312407X.2017.1415366.

Jobe-Shields, L., Moreland, A.D., Hanson, R.F. et al. (2018). Co-occurrence of witnessed parental violence and child physical abuse from a national sample of adolescents. *Journal of Child & Adolescent Trauma* 11 (2): 129–139. https://doi.org/10.1007/s40653-015-0057-9.

Joinson, C., Sullivan, S., von Gontard, A., and Heron, J. (2016). Stressful events in early childhood and developmental trajectories of bedwetting at school age. *Journal of Pediatric Psychology* 41 (9): 1002–1010. https://doi.org/10.1093/jpepsy/jsw025.

Kann, L., McManus, T., Harris, W.A. et al. (2018). Youth risk behavior surveillance – United States, 2017. *MMWR Surveillance Summaries* 67 (8): 1.

Kempe, C.H., Silverman, F.N., Steele, B.F. et al. (1962). The battered-child syndrome. *JAMA* 181: 17–24.

Kessler, R.C., Aguilar-Gaxiola, S., Alonso, J. et al. (2018). The associations of earlier trauma exposures and history of mental disorders with PTSD after subsequent traumas. *Molecular Psychiatry* 23 (9): 1.

King, L.A., King, D.W., Leskin, G., and Foy, D.W. (1995). The Los Angeles symptom checklist: a self-report measure of posttraumatic stress. *Assessment* 2: 1–17.

Kisely, S., Abajobir, A.A., Mills, R. et al. (2018). Child maltreatment and mental health problems in adulthood: birth cohort study. *The British Journal of Psychiatry* 213 (6): 698–703.

Knutsen, M. and Jensen, T.K. (2019). Changes in the trauma narratives of youth receiving trauma-focused cognitive behavioral therapy in relation to posttraumatic stress symptoms. *Psychotherapy Research* 29 (1): 99–111.

Krishnan, C., Santos, L., Peterson, M.D., and Ehinger, M. (2015). Safety of noninvasive brain stimulation in children and adolescents. *Brain Stimulation* 8 (1): 76–87.

Landers, A.L., McLuckie, A., Cann, R. et al. (2018). A scoping review of evidence-based interventions available to parents of maltreated children ages 0-5 involved with child welfare services. *Child Abuse & Neglect* 76: 546–560.

Landolt, M.A. and Kenardy, J.A. (2015). Evidence-based treatments for children and adolescents. In: *Evidence Based Treatments for Trauma-Related Psychological Disorders* (eds. U. Schnyder and M. Cloitre), 363–380. Cham: Springer.

Lederer, L.J. and Wetzel, C.A. (2014). The health consequences of sex trafficking and their implications for identifying victims in health-care facilities. *Annals Health Law* 23: 61.

Lee, E., Kirkland, K., Miranda-Julian, C., and Greene, R. (2018). Reducing maltreatment recurrence through home visitation: a promising intervention for child welfare involved families. *Child Abuse & Neglect* 86: 55–66.

Leeb, R.T., Paulozzi, L., Melanson, C. et al. (2008). *Child Maltreatment Surveillance: Uniform Definitions for Public Health and Recommended Data Elements, Version 1.0*. Atlanta, GA: Centers for Disease Control and Prevention, National Center for Injury Prevention and Control.

Lenz, A.S. and Hollenbaugh, K.M. (2015). Meta-analysis of trauma-focused cognitive behavioral therapy for treating PTSD and co-occurring depression among children and adolescents. *Counseling Outcome Research and Evaluation* 6 (1): 18–32.

Levy, H., Markovic, J., Kallinowski, M. et al. (1995). Child sexual abuse interviews: the use of anatomical dolls and reliability of information. *Journal of Interpersonal Violence* 10 (3): 334–353.

Lewey, J.H., Smith, C.L., Burcham, B. et al. (2018). Comparing the effectiveness of EMDR and TF-CBT for children and adolescents: a meta-analysis. *Journal of Child & Adolescent Trauma* 11 (4): 457–472.

Locher, M.C., Koechlin, M.H., Zion, M.S.R. et al. (2017). Efficacy and safety of SSRIs, SNRIs, and placebo in common psychiatric disorders: a comprehensive meta-analysis in children and adolescents. *JAMA Psychiatry* 74 (10): 1011.

Low, S. and Espelage, D. (2014). Conduits from community violence exposure to peer aggression and victimization: contributions of parental monitoring, impulsivity, and deviancy. *Journal of Counseling Psychology* 61 (2): 221–231. https://doi.org/10.1037/a0035207.

Ludin, S., Bottiani, J.H., Debnam, K. et al. (2018). A cross-national comparison of risk factors for teen dating violence in Mexico and the United States. *Journal of Youth and Adolescence* 47 (3): 547–559. https://doi.org/10.1007/s10964-017-0701-9.

Lupien, S.J., Juster, R.P., Raymond, C., and Marin, M.F. (2018). The effects of chronic stress on the human brain: from neurotoxicity, to vulnerability, to opportunity. *Frontiers in Neuroendocrinology* 49: 91–105.

McCarroll, J.E., Fisher, J.E., Cozza, S.J. et al. (2017). Characteristics, classification, and prevention of child maltreatment fatalities. *Military Medicine* 182 (1): e1551–e1557. https://doi.org/10.7205/MILMED-D-16-00039.

McGeough, B.L. and Sterzing, P.R. (2018). A systematic review of family victimization experiences among sexual minority youth. *Journal of Primary Prevention* 39 (5): 491–528. https://doi.org/10.1007/s10935-018-0523-x.

McLaren, J.L., Barnett, E.R., Concepcion Zayas, M.T. et al. (2018). Psychotropic medications for highly vulnerable children. *Expert Opinion on Pharmacotherapy* 19 (6): 547–560.

McNaughton Reyes, H.L., Foshee, V.A., Chen, M.S. et al. (2018). Consequences of involvement in distinct patterns of adolescent peer and dating violence. *Journal of Youth and Adolescence* 47 (11): 2371–2383. https://doi.org/10.1007/s10964-018-0902-x.

Merrick, M.T., Ports, K.A., Ford, D.C. et al. (2017). Unpacking the impact of adverse childhood experiences on adult mental health. *Child Abuse & Neglect* 69: 10–19.

National Research Council (2013). *Confronting Commercial Sexual Exploitation and Sex Trafficking of Minors in the United States.* National Academies Press.

Noh, D. (2018). Psychological interventions for runaway and homeless youth. *Journal of Nursing Scholarship* 50 (5): 465–472. https://doi.org/10.1111/jnu.12402.

Oh, D.L., Jerman, P., Boparai, S.K.P. et al. (2018). Review of tools for measuring exposure to adversity in children and adolescents. *Journal of Pediatric Health Care* 32 (6): 564–583.

Pascoe, J.M., Wood, D.L., Duffee, J.H. et al. (2016). Mediators and adverse effects of child poverty in the United States. *Pediatrics* 137 (4): e20160340.

Patterson, G.R., DeBaryshe, B.D., and Ramsey, E. (2017). A developmental perspective on antisocial behavior. In: *Developmental and Life-Course Criminological Theories*, 29–35. Routledge.

Petering, R., Rhoades, H., Rice, E., and Yoshioka-Maxwell, A. (2017). Bidirectional intimate partner violence and drug use among homeless youth. *Journal of Interpersonal Violence* 32 (14): 2209–2217. https://doi.org/10.1177/0886260515593298.

Peterman, A., Bleck, J., and Palermo, T. (2015). Age and intimate partner violence: an analysis of global trends among women experiencing victimization in 30 developing countries. *Journal of Adolescent Health* 57 (6): 624–630.

Peterson, C.C., Riggs, J., Guyon-Harris, K. et al. (2019). Effects of intimate partner violence and home environment on child language development in the first 3 years of life. *Journal of Developmental & Behavioral Pediatrics* 40 (2): 112–121.

Pynoos, R., Rodriguez, N., Steinberg, A. et al. (1998). *The UCLA PTSD Reaction Index for DSM IV (Revision 1).* Los Angeles: UCLA Trauma Program.

Ribbe, D. (1996). Psychometric review of Traumatic Events Screening Inventory for Children (TESI-C). In: *Measurement of Stress, Trauma, and Adaptation* (ed. B.H. Stamm), 386–387. Lutherville, MD: Sidran.

Rivara, F.P. and LeMenestrel, S.M. (eds.) (2016). *Preventing Bullying Through Science, Policy and Practice.* Washington, DC: The National Academies Press https://doi.org/10.17226/23482.

Rodriguez, C.M., Gonzalez, S., and Foiles, A.R. (2018). Maternal ADHD symptoms and physical child abuse risk: a multi-informant study. *Journal of Child and Family Studies* 27 (12): 4015–4024.

Saigh, P.A., Yasik, A., Oberfield, R. et al. (2000). The children's PTSD inventory: development and reliability. *Journal of Traumatic Stress* 13 (3): 369–380.

Saini, S.M., Hoffmann, C.R., Pantelis, C. et al. (2018). Systematic review and critical appraisal of child abuse measurement instruments. *Psychiatry Research* 272: 106–113. https://doi.org/10.1016/j.psychres.2018.12.068.

Sawrikar, P. (2016). *Working with Ethnic Minorities and Across Cultures in Western Child Protection Systems.* Routledge.

Sege, R.D., Amaya-Jackson, L., and American Academy of Pediatrics Committee on Child Abuse and Neglect (2017). Clinical considerations related to the behavioral manifestations of child maltreatment. *Pediatrics* 139 (4): e20170100.

Shandro, J., Chisolm-Straker, M., Duber, H.C. et al. (2016). Human trafficking: a guide to identification and approach for the emergency physician. *Annals of Emergency Medicine* 68 (4): 501–508.

Shonkoff, J.P., Garner, A.S., Siegel, B.S. et al. (2012). The lifelong effects of early childhood adversity and toxic stress. *Pediatrics* 129 (1): e232–e246.

Spinazzola, J., Ford, J.D., Zucker, M. et al. (2017). Survey evaluates: complex trauma exposure, outcome, and intervention among children and adolescents. *Psychiatric Annals* 35 (5): 433–439.

Stonard, K.E. (2019). Technology-assisted adolescent dating violence and abuse: a factor analysis of the nature of electronic communication technology used across twelve types of abusive and controlling behaviour. *Journal of Child and Family Studies* 28 (1): 105–115. https://doi.org/10.1007/s10826-018-1255-5.

Teicher, M.H. and Samson, J.A. (2016). Annual research review: enduring neurobiological effects of childhood abuse and neglect. *Journal of Child Psychology and Psychiatry* 57 (3): 241–266.

Toth, S.L. and Manly, J.T. (2018). Developmental consequences of child abuse and neglect: implications for intervention. *Child Development Perspectives.* Available at srcd.onlinelibrary.wiley.com. 10/1111.cdep.12317.

Trevizol, A.P., Barros, M.D., Silva, P.O. et al. (2016). Transcranial magnetic stimulation for posttraumatic stress disorder: an updated systematic review and meta-analysis. *Trends in Psychiatry and Psychotherapy* 38 (1): 50–55.

Turner, H.A., Shattuck, A., Finkelhor, D., and Hamby, S. (2017). Effects of poly-victimization on adolescent social support, self-concept, and psychological distress. *Journal of Interpersonal Violence* 32 (5): 755–780. Available at https://doi.org/10.1177/0886260515586376.

USDHHS (2018). *Child Maltreatment 2016.* US Department of Health and Human Services, Administration on Children, Youth and Families. Washington, DC: US Government Printing Office.

Van der Kolk, B.A. (2017). Developmental trauma disorder: toward a rational diagnosis for children with complex trauma histories. *Psychiatric Annals* 35 (5): 401–408.

Van der Kolk, B.A., Roth, S., Pelcovitz, D. et al. (2005). Disorders of extreme stress: The empirical foundation of a complex adaptation to trauma. *Journal of Traumatic Stress* 18: 389–399.

Viswanathan, M., Fraser, J.G., Pan, H. et al. (2018). Primary care interventions to prevent child maltreatment: updated evidence report and systematic review for the US Preventive Services Task Force. *JAMA* 320 (20): 2129–2140.

Wethington, H.R., Hahn, R.A., Fuqua-Whitley, D.S. et al. (2008). The effectiveness of interventions to reduce psychological harm from traumatic events among children and adolescents: a systematic review. *American Journal of Preventive Medicine* 35: 287–313. https://doi.org/10.1016/j.amepre.2008.06.024.

Wherry, J.N. and Herrington, S.C. (2018). Reliability and validity of the trauma symptom checklist for children and trauma symptom checklist for young children screeners in a clinical sample. *Journal of Child Sexual Abuse* 27 (8): 998–1010.

Woodhouse, T. (2019). Play therapy with children affected by sexual abuse: developing awareness of safety and trust. In: *Becoming and Being a Play Therapist: Play Therapy in Practice* (eds. P. Ayling, H. Armstrong and L.G.T. Clark), 189–203. Abington, Oxfordshire: Routledge.

25

Children in Out-of-Home Placement

Julie E. Bertram[1] and Betty Boyle-Duke[2]

[1] University of Missouri, St. Louis, MO, USA
[2] Long Island University School of Nursing, Brooklyn, NY, USA

Objectives

After reading this chapter, advanced practice registered nurses (APRNs) will be able to:

1. Describe types of formalized placements for children living out of their homes
2. Explain the potential complex physical, developmental, and mental healthcare needs of the children living in an out-of-home placement
3. Examine alternatives to out-of-home placement for children living in distressed families
4. Describe the multifaceted role of the APRN in caring for children at risk for or in an out-of-home placement

Introduction

This chapter introduces and develops the advanced practice registered nurse's (APRN) role in caring for children who are at risk for, or already live in, out-of-home placements. One of the most common reasons for out-of-home placements is court involvement due to childhood abuse and neglect, also referred to as maltreatment. The prevalence rates of maltreatment can be extrapolated from the National Child Abuse and Neglect Data System reports, which likely underestimate the true rates because not all cases are reported. It is estimated that approximately one in eight children in the United States is a victim of maltreatment (Wildeman et al. 2014). The consequences of maltreatment are a major public health issue, including high rates of health risk behaviors such as substance use, significant morbidity, substantial involvement with the criminal justice system, and early death (Campbell et al. 2016; Dube 2018; Gilbert et al. 2009; Stillerman 2018).

US children enter out-of-home placements (i.e. foster care) when unmet needs for safety, stability, and nurturance threaten their wellbeing, family functioning is severely compromised, and attempts for reunification have been unsuccessful. Childhood neglect and parental substance abuse are among the chief reasons for children being removed from their homes by the US child welfare system, with poverty being an underlying and potent contributing factor (Eckenrode et al. 2014; Kim and Drake 2018; US Department of Health and Human Services [USDHHS] 2017). Federal, state, and local funding streams support the child welfare system; however, the amount and quality of children and family needs exceed the quantity and scope of resources

Child and Adolescent Behavioral Health: A Resource for Advanced Practice Psychiatric and Primary Care Practitioners in Nursing,
Second Edition. Edited by Edilma L. Yearwood, Geraldine S. Pearson, and Jamesetta A. Newland.
© 2021 John Wiley & Sons, Inc. Published 2021 by John Wiley & Sons, Inc.
Companion website: www.wiley.com/go/Yearwood

available to meet them (Hoynes and Schanzenbach 2018; Jordan and Connelly 2016).

Children in foster care have considerably greater medical, developmental, social, behavioral, and emotional health needs when compared to their peers who are not in foster care (Turney and Wildeman 2016; Vig et al. 2005). In order to coordinate the healthcare resources necessary to meet these complex needs, children in foster care require supervision by a primary care provider (PCP) experienced in working collaboratively with other healthcare professionals and knowledgeable about the complexities of the foster care system. Thousands of children are forcibly displaced from their countries every year. Refugee and unaccompanied minor children need special protections and support (Berger Cardoso et al. 2019).

The Current State of the US Child Welfare System

The Nature of the System

The foster care system is a combination of many overlapping and interacting agencies, which include federal and state-supported agencies responsible for the protection of the foster child's welfare (Schneiderman 2005). Perhaps related to the extent and type of agency involvement, care for foster children is often fragmented, insufficient, and poorly coordinated.

Despite the availability of electronic court and medical records, databases are not shared readily or easily among the relevant entities. An inherent problem is the lack of medical records that follow a child from one setting to another, whether within a locale, within a state, or when a child moves from one state to another (Schneiderman 2008). The inability to obtain comprehensive records compromises continuity and quality of healthcare. Recent efforts to improve care coordination by establishing medical homes, integrated care models, telepsychiatry, and medical passports have been piloted but are not used consistently across the nation (Hilt et al. 2015; USDHHS 2018a).

Funding and Workforce

Child welfare services are chronically underfunded across the country (Child Trends, Inc. 2016). Child welfare workers have larger caseloads than they can adequately manage (Edwards and Wildeman 2018). Many caseworkers lack training on complex health and mental health issues. Similarly, they often do not understand medical jargon or the intricacies of the healthcare delivery system. Furthermore, approximately a 20% annual child welfare staff turnover creates additional obstacles

to the provision of timely, efficient, and appropriate healthcare (Edwards and Wildeman 2018). Due in part to inadequate human resources, the healthcare needs of foster children and adolescents are frequently unmet.

Children in Foster Care

The foster care system contained 442 995 children in 2017 in the United States (USDHHS 2019). That number accounts for children who were in care on the first day of the fiscal year (as of October 1). Foster care numbers had decreased every year from 1999 to 2012, from 567 000 to 397 000. Numbers started to rise and in 2014 were 415 000 and have steadily increased since. Trends in the number of children served over the last decade are displayed in Figure 25.1. Trend report numbers are larger because they include children who were in or entered the foster care system and who were adopted from the foster care system during a federal fiscal year. For 2017, the number of children in foster care and adoption was over 700 000 (USDHHS 2018).

Demographics

The majority of referrals to child protective services pertained to children under 4 years of age, with relatively equal gender distribution at 52% male and 48% female. Forty-four percent of children in foster care were Caucasian, 23% were African American, 21% were Hispanic, 2% were Alaska Native/American Indian, less than 1% were Asian American; the remaining 9% were multiracial or of "unknown" race/ethnicity (USDHHS 2019). While referrals to child protective services have increased over the years, the actual number of confirmed cases of abuse and neglect has decreased. However, it is estimated that 1720 children died from abuse and neglect in 2017, compared to 1750 child deaths recorded in 2016 (USDHHS 2019). Recognized predictors of maltreatment and associated childhood mortality include young mothers (less than 20 years of age), single marital status, high parenting demand, previous involvement with child protective services, previous substantiated maltreatment of the child's siblings, and criminal justice and mental health system involvement (Vaithianathan et al. 2017). Available evidence supports the benefits of home visitation to engage families at highest risk for maltreatment events and fatal outcomes (Levey et al. 2017).

Legislation

Reform movements in child welfare date back to the early 1900s, each wave occurring at approximately 10-year intervals (Murray and Gesiriech 2003). Three pieces of relevant legislation, the Adoption and Safe

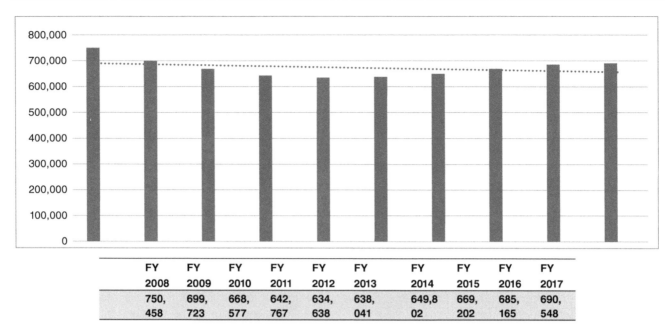

	FY 2008	FY 2009	FY 2010	FY 2011	FY 2012	FY 2013	FY 2014	FY 2015	FY 2016	FY 2017
	750, 458	699, 723	668, 577	642, 767	634, 638	638, 041	649,8 02	669, 202	685, 165	690, 548

Figure 25.1 Number of children served in US public foster care during 2008–2017. *Source:* US Department of Health and Human Services, Administration for Children and Families, Administration on Children, Youth, and Families, Children's Bureau Adoption and Foster Care Analysis and Reporting System (AFCARS) (2018). Data as of 10 August 2018.

Families Act of 1997 (ASFA-97 1997), the Fostering Connections to Success and Increasing Adoptions Act of 2008 (Fostering Connections 2008), and the Family First Preservation Services Act, are summarized below, as they represent the key policy shifts in child welfare (US Department of Justice 2009).

The ASFA-97 was passed in order to achieve several objectives to promote the adoption of children in foster care. Trends had indicated that too many children were the victims of a phenomenon called "foster care drift," whereby they were basically moved from home to home in the foster care system waiting for permanency that was never realized (Adler 2001). ASFA-97 promoted quicker adoptions via the hastening of the termination of parents' rights in certain circumstances (murder, manslaughter, and felonious assault criteria). A "fast track 15–22 months" to permanency plan was initiated, prompting state agencies to move foster children more quickly out of temporary care and into permanent living arrangements. This meant that any child who had been in foster care for 15 out of 22 months was made eligible for adoption through the termination of his/her biological parents' rights to maintain guardianship. This essentially terminated the parental rights. Permanency hearings were to be held every 12 months in order to expedite adoptions and such hearings were to be documented.

The law also allocated added health coverage funds for adoptions to states as incentives to move children out

of foster care and into adoptive homes, while also expanding healthcare coverage for adoptive children. Funding to encourage adoption was added to the budget, and greater financial resources were allocated for children with special needs. The legislation required states to document attempts to move children toward adoption. One of the barriers to adoption, interstate boundary stipulations, was removed in order to hasten the process. Additional provisions for safety were built into the legislation. For example, foster parents were specifically cited in the legislation as key informants who could testify in court cases.

In 2008, Congress passed the Fostering Connections to Success and Increasing Adoptions Act. The new law provided major reforms, including the following:

1. Supports for relatives to care for foster children in their own families and homes.
2. Educational opportunities for children transitioning from adolescence into adulthood.
3. Increased funding to foster care families living on reservations to care for Native American children within their own communities.
4. Reauthorizing the Adoption Incentives Program so that adoptive parents can receive assistance when adopting older or special needs children.
5. Requirements for states to make a concerted effort to place siblings in the same setting.

The Family First Preservation Services Act was enacted on 9 February 2018 with three main objectives, namely, (i) to prevent foster care placements by shifting funds toward families in need of mental health and substance use treatments and in-home parenting skills training, (ii) to support foster care that occurs within family-like, appropriate, and least-restrictive placements, and (iii) to fund evidence-based kinship navigator programs (H.R. 1892 2018). The enacted legislation is intended to improve the current child welfare system.

Chapter 1 of the Act stipulates who is eligible for foster care prevention activities (i.e. children at imminent risk of entering foster care) and what conditions must be met to qualify for services (i.e. services must be trauma-informed). Prevention services include mental health and substance abuse treatment, parenting skills programs, and individual and family counseling in the home setting. Services must meet evidence-based practice requirements. In particular, residential family-based treatment must be trauma-informed and service plans must include outcome measures.

Chapter 2 of the Act describes the approved placement types for foster children. Congregate care is to be avoided, and family foster homes with fewer than six children are an expected placement of children in foster care. When children require residential care, the facility should be a qualified residential treatment program. Such homes must meet specified criteria that are appropriate for the needs of the children. Kinship placements require licensing standards that are comparable to reputable model licensing standards. States must demonstrate that they are in alignment with national standards for foster family homes. Federal funds are allocated for kinship navigator programs, a set of activities that assist kinship care providers with accessing caregiver support, education, and referrals for themselves and children.

Lastly, additional investments are delineated with the intention of moving children and families toward permanency and/or reunification.

Advocacy

Socially innovative programs designated for offering services that advocate for vulnerable children are equally as important as legislation mandating services. Policy, research, and advocacy organizations drive an agenda for the reformation of the child welfare system (Children's Rights 2018). For example, The Annie E. Casey Foundation is an advocacy organization for disadvantaged children. The primary mission of the Casey Foundation is to improve the lives of the most vulnerable children by recommending public policies, advocating for human service reforms, providing community support, and identifying barriers to adequate healthcare services. The foundation provides grant funding to help states, cities, and neighborhoods develop innovative cost-effective programs to promote delivery of the best quality of care for the most disadvantaged families and children by emphasizing interdisciplinary education and practice that involves social workers, policy makers, providers, foster care families, and fragile parents. In light of the current numbers of children placed in foster care, the Casey challenge is to reduce the number of children in foster care by 50% by the year 2020 (Annie E. Casey Foundation 2009; Casey Family Programs 2017). Organizations that advocate for foster children are listed in Box 25.1.

Box 25.1 Policy, Research, and Advocacy Organizations

1. Adoption Exchange Association
2. American Bar Association
3. Annie E. Casey Foundation
4. Casey Family Programs
5. Casey Family Services
6. Center for Law and Social Policy
7. Center for the Study of Social Policy
8. Chapin Hall
9. Child Trends Databank
10. Child Welfare League of America
11. Children and Family Research Center
12. Children Awaiting Parents, Inc.
13. Children's Defense Fund
14. Court Appointed Special Advocates (CASA) for Children
15. Dave Thomas Foundation for Adoption
16. The Evan B. Donaldson Adoption Institute
17. Family Focused Treatment Association
18. The Future of Children
19. Juvenile Law Center
20. Lambda Legal
21. National Association of Counsel for Children
22. National Center for Children in Poverty
23. National Foster Care Month
24. National Foster Parent Association
25. North American Council on Adoptable Children
26. Prevent Child Abuse America
27. The Urban Institute

Source: Children's Rights (2018).

Types of Out-of-Home Placements

Although family preservation is always the goal, efforts to preserve the family fail in approximately 25% of cases (Casanueva et al. 2016). Temporary out-of-home placement is arranged in emergency or crisis settings, respite homes, traditional foster care homes, kinship care, career or behavioral foster care, therapeutic or treatment foster care, group homes, therapeutic group homes (TGHs), residential settings, transitional living, and independent living accommodations (Szilagyi et al. 2015). Permanent placement occurs through reunification, guardianship, or adoption. Placements are based on the needs of the child, guided by the principles of the least restrictive alternative and the resources of the state. The options for out-of-home placements are displayed in Figure 25.2.

Emergency or Crisis Settings

Emergency or crisis settings provide families with an opportunity to obtain parent education and support, as well as care and shelter for children when one or both caregivers are unable to adequately parent their children. Programs for parents may be offered in place (home visits) and for children at centers that are designed to support them (Casillas et al. 2016; Eddy et al. 2019).

Respite Home

Families caring for children with special needs – whether physical, emotional, or both – may access respite services under the law (Public Law 109–442 2006). Respite services can be provided in community locations other than the childhood home when indicated.

Traditional Foster Care

Placement in a traditional foster home is necessary when parents are unwilling or unable to provide adequate care for their child or children. In the case of either abuse or neglect, removal of the child from the biological family is a court-ordered intervention, which is meant to be a temporary measure rather than a long-term solution (Greater Hope Foundation for Children, Inc. 2019). Adults over the age of 21 can apply to be foster parents.

They are carefully screened for drug and alcohol use, as well as for history of child abuse and criminal behavior. Caregivers that meet the assessment criteria must be licensed or certified as a foster family upon completion of a foster parent training program, a home study conducted by the state's Department of Children & Family Services (DCFS; sometimes also called Office of Children & Family Services, depending on the state), and other licensing requirements. Foster parents are regularly supervised and are evaluated every few months, according to local and state laws, and may be dismissed upon a court order. If the birth parents' rights are not terminated, visitation rights are in place for the parents to see the child. Foster parents may act on behalf of the child for anything concerning the child's welfare, such as meeting with specialists in health or mental health services, attending individual educational planning (IEP) meetings at school, or meetings at the welfare department.

Therapeutic Foster Care

Therapeutic foster care (TFC), also referred to as treatment foster care, is a family-based home placement for foster children with serious mental and/or physical health needs. This manualized program is well-supported by the findings yielded by randomized clinical trials demonstrating efficacy and cost-effectiveness for children aged 3–18 years (Seibert et al. 2018). Recognizing the elevated needs of the children served, it is important for TFC caregivers to receive adequate support and training. TFC caregivers are supported and trained to keep systematic and descriptive daily records of the child's behavior and progress, medication administration, and all other services that the child receives in accordance with the plan of care. TFC caregivers attend the permanency placement planning meetings, where they are able to contribute their observations and predictions of how well the child may adjust to a transition to a permanent home. TFC caregivers also assist the child in maintaining an ongoing relationship with biological family members and friends.

Kinship Care

Kinship care is an out-of-home placement arrangement with relatives or other kin-like related adults (Cox 2016). The majority of kinship placements are with grandparents; approximately 2.7 million grandparents are the primary caregivers of their co-resident grandchildren under 18 years of age (Ellis and Simmons 2014). Placement with kinship providers benefits children for at least four reasons: (i) commitment of the kinship provider to the children, (ii) cultural sensitivity within the

Emergency	Respite	Traditional	Kinship	Career/Behavioral	Therapeutic	Group Home	Therapeutic	Residential	Transitional Living	Independent Living	Exit/ Re-unification or Adoption

Figure 25.2 Options for out-of-home placements.

home, (iii) continued communication with biological parents, and (iv) provision of a familiar environment. However, kinship care providers, especially when they are grandparents, tend to have high rates of health problems and often live in disadvantaged communities, while also experiencing financial hardship. Moreover, they may have conflictual relationships with foster children's parents (Cox 2016).

Despite these challenges, kinship placements are preferred over other types of foster care arrangements. Specifically, children have been found to experience a greater degree of health and placement stability when living in kinship homes (Bramlett et al. 2017; Koh et al. 2014; Winokur et al. 2014). However, grandparent kindship care providers use fewer preventative healthcare resources for themselves and experience health problems at higher rates than grandparents that do not provide this level of care (Cox 2016).

Group Homes

Group homes are intended to simulate a family environment, therefore they are frequently found in residential neighborhoods. House parents have received training in child development and behavior modification and are responsible for the residents 24 hours/day. The goals of a group home are to provide a nurturing family-type environment, integrate the residents into the school and local community, provide daily structure, coordinate all necessary community services, and prepare each resident for independence through reinforcement of daily living and self-care skills. Any facility that houses six or more children is considered a group home (USDHHS n.d.). Medicaid and other state and local funds support group homes, therefore they are subject to federal regulations and assigned a case manager from the public health department or a mental health center.

Therapeutic Group Home

A TGH houses children who are difficult to place due to complex physical and mental health problems, such as a child with diabetes who also has mental illness. The TGH is similar to TFC because of the additional training house parents receive in behavior management and child development. Training related to the specific physical needs of each child is also provided to parents. Consequently, TFC and TGH have demonstrated improved outcomes in terms of reduction in delinquent and risky behaviors exhibited by the foster child, as well as an increased number of children who are able to return to their relatives or to traditional foster care (Adopting.org n.d.).

Residential Treatment

Residential treatment settings are rarely located in the vicinity of the child's family residence and thus the child is often isolated from family and friends. Residential treatment programs are staffed by social workers, psychologists, psychiatrists, and nurses. They provide the most structure, but are also the most expensive and the most restrictive of all child protective service out-of-home placements. The residents are usually older children who are medically ill, severely mentally ill, or who may have been involved with the juvenile justice system.

Residential programs are comprehensive, providing educational and recreational activities, as well as clinical treatment programs. Treatment may include individual and group therapies, stress management, recreational therapy, and physical and occupational therapies to meet the complex needs of each child. Prior to discharge, social workers in the treatment centers work across the continuum of care to coordinate probation, court-recommended mental healthcare, medical care, and the juvenile justice system (Pearson 2006; Lister et al. 2016; American Association of Children's Residential Centers 2017).

Adoption

Approximately 2% of children grow up in adoptive families to whom they are not biologically related; foster parent adoptions account for over half of the adoptions of children from foster care. These children are more likely to be older children from minority groups or a sibling group; they are also more likely to have a history of abuse or neglect (Rushton 2010; Rushton and Dance 2006). Early childhood adoption increases the probability of positive parent–child bonding and normal child development compared with adoption in middle or late childhood (Sadock and Sadock 2009). Prolonged efforts to return children to their biological parents should be carefully examined, especially when there may be little chance of success. The longer the child remains in out-of-home placement, the more difficult the adjustment to adoption would be (Rushton and Dance 2006). All out-of-home placements are provided by the state's DCFS. States have their own laws governing out-of-home placements, but several federal laws (Child Welfare Information Gateway 2006; USDHHS n.d.) supersede individual state laws. Ultimately, it is the responsibility of each state to provide a safe and healthy environment for children in foster care (Seibert et al. 2018).

The Complex Needs of Children in Out-of-Home Placements

Many foster children suffer from physical, emotional, and sexual abuse. However, neglect is the most frequent type of maltreatment in childhood (Sadock and Sadock 2009). Unfortunately, the complex healthcare needs associated with abuse and neglect are frequently overlooked, unidentified, or untreated (Justin 2003; Kools and Kennedy 2003; Marx et al. 2003). In addition, numerous placements and frequent moves from one home to another interfere with continuity of care, contributing to high rates of poor physical and mental health outcomes among foster children.

Physical and Developmental Healthcare Needs

Maltreatment of children results in cognitive and developmental delays, as well as a wide range of complex health problems. This begins in utero if the child's developing brain is exposed to toxins such as drugs or alcohol. Alcohol causes the greatest assault on the fetal brain (Vig et al. 2005), especially when alcohol use by the mother results in fetal alcohol spectrum disorder (FASD). FASD describes a continuum of permanent birth defects that occur during pregnancy, including alcohol-related neurodevelopmental disorder and fetal alcohol syndrome. FASD is often underdiagnosed, even though alcohol exposure in utero can result in a myriad of abnormal physical findings, including prenatal and postnatal growth deficiency, microcephaly, facial and hand anomalies, heart defects, and a wide range of cognitive deficits from mild developmental delay to extreme problems with language, memory, judgment, impulse control, and aggression (Vig et al. 2005). Maternal drug and alcohol use also increases a child's risk for congenital infections such as HIV, syphilis, hepatitis, and herpes (Schneiderman 2003; Vig et al. 2005) because pregnant women using drugs and alcohol may be less likely to seek adequate prenatal care where treatments could be provided to significantly diminish disease transmission to the fetus.

Children may suffer from multiple injuries secondary to physical abuse, the most profound of which is shaken baby syndrome. This form of abuse is a result of excessive shaking of a crying infant, leading to a shearing injury to the brain, causing subdural hemorrhages. The mortality rate can be as high as 40%, but over half of surviving infants have significant neurological abnormalities and visual impairment (Vig et al. 2005).

If emotionally abused or neglected, children in foster care may regress to an earlier stage of growth and development following abuse. They may lag behind their peers in speech and language acquisition skills, and develop adaptive behavior deficits that result in bullying, lying, and disruptive behavior in social situations (Craven and Lee 2006). By the time these children attend grade school, they may be unable to meet curriculum requirements, resulting in academic failure and paving the way for teen truancy.

Other medical problems found in children in foster care include failure to thrive, malnutrition, lead toxicity, asthma, anemia, dermatological problems, vision and hearing deficits, under-immunization, and retarded growth (Schneiderman 2003; Vig et al. 2005). Despite placement in foster care with documented healthcare needs, 32% of children have at least one unmet healthcare need after placement (Vig et al. 2005). Given this alarming statistic, it is important that all children in foster care receive early childhood intervention services, such as those provided by the Early and Periodic Screening, Diagnosis, and Treatment Program (EPSDT) designed to detect and treat health problems through regular medical, dental, vision, and developmental screenings (Child Welfare Information Gateway 2006). School-age children in foster care frequently require individual tutoring and special education testing and services.

Mental Health Needs

Many foster children suffer from emotional and behavioral problems requiring mental health services. Emotional problems found in many of the children at a young age are attachment and anxiety disorders, including separation anxiety. Some foster children experience school phobias and many fear that they will be abandoned. Foster children frequently suffer from low self-esteem and feelings of personal rejection (Bruskas 2008; Kools and Kennedy 2003).

Abused and neglected children may suffer from symptoms of post-traumatic stress disorder, including hypervigilance, startle responses to noise, nightmares, and depression. Depressed children may have thoughts of suicide or exhibit self-destructive behaviors. Continuing losses due to many different out-of-home placements traumatize children, which interferes with their ability to establish positive interpersonal relationships. This is particularly difficult for children entering the teenage years because of the importance of peer relationships in this developmental period (Kools and Kennedy 2003). Adolescents in foster care often exhibit disruptive or antisocial tendencies and their attitude can be oppositional and aggressive. Many engage in risky behaviors, including drug, alcohol, and tobacco use, as well as promiscuity, resulting in an increased incidence of teen pregnancy and sexually transmitted infections (Gramkowski et al. 2009; Kools and Kennedy 2003; Sadock and Sadock 2009).

Turney and Wildeman (2016) looked at data from the 2011–2012 National Survey of Children's Health and found that children in foster care had poor mental and physical health relative to children in the general population, children across specific family types, and children in economically disadvantaged families. These findings suggest that early life circumstances might create vulnerabilities to the health of children in foster care.

Educational Needs

Owing to the poor educational achievement outcomes of children in foster care, early intervention services in childhood, special education services in the school-age years, and aftercare services are critical for youth and those aging out of foster care. In order to reduce barriers to educating children in foster care, such as lack of collaboration between child protective services and local education agencies, formal procedures need to be in place to access specialized educational programs (Weinberg et al. 2009). Agencies should initiate life skills classes as soon as the child is developmentally capable, usually in the early teen years. These classes should include education on finding employment, budgeting and managing money, going grocery shopping, finding a place to live, accessing medical and mental health services, and preventing sexually transmitted infections and pregnancy (Racusin et al. 2005). Teen parents should also be provided with parenting classes.

Transition from Out-of-Home Placement to Adulthood

As young people transition from adolescence to young adulthood, they experience numerous challenges, such as completing their education, contemplating future careers, beginning full-time employment, living independently, and choosing a partner. Few foster children have family or peer support systems for these developmental transitions and therefore they are at risk for becoming homeless, unemployed, destitute, and incarcerated (Foster and Gifford 2004). Some programs phase out young people gradually while others end services abruptly; however, transitioning to adulthood means leaving the programs children have been dependent on for many years without actually demonstrating readiness for independent living. Completion of high school or the graduation equivalency diploma (GED), availability of financial resources for further education, absence of learning problems and substance abuse, and low rates of long-standing serious emotional problems are associated with positive transitions from the foster care system to adulthood (Racusin et al. 2005).

Intensive Family Preservation

Intensive family preservation services (IFPS) is known by many names, including family-based services and family preservation, but IFPS is the most current nomenclature used in the literature. IFPS focuses on preventing

unnecessary foster care placement of minor children by providing comprehensive, short-term, in-home treatment using a family-centered approach (Berry et al. 2000). The primary goal of IFPS is to prevent out-of-home placement by adhering to key design elements and values, which involves raising children within their own family, providing services in the home, including all family members whether or not they live in the home, finding the family's strengths and weaknesses, helping parents, and empowering the family by including them in decisions (National Family Preservation Network [NFPN] 2009).

IFPS serves families with children under the age of 17 years who are considered at imminent risk of being removed from the home (Berry et al. 2000; NFPN 2009). Situations that constitute imminent risk may involve lack of effective parenting and family instability, abuse, neglect, law enforcement involvement, academic truancy, developmental disabilities, mental health issues, family violence, and health problems, especially those related to medical neglect and teen pregnancy complications. The case is then accepted based on several inclusion criteria, once willingness and ability of family members to take part in the IFPS process has been established. At least one child must be at imminent risk of removal from the home, and IFPS services will be implemented to protect the child or children from abuse or neglect in the short-term future. The child or children cannot concurrently be in the custody of any public agency.

Exclusionary criteria for IFPS may include parental substance abuse, mental illness, cognitive delay, or a history of sadistic or sexual abuse where the abuser still lives in the home (Berry et al. 2000). IFPS is not appropriate for children not at high risk for removal from the home because there are less intensive service models available for family support (NFPN 2009). Ultimately, the family preservation caseworker and supervisor make the final decision on whether IFPS intervention can safely meet the needs of the child and family.

The essential core program components of IFPS are based primarily on the HOMEBUILDERS model, the most widely used model of family preservation in the United States (NFPN 2009). The specific service components characteristic of innovative family preservation services in the child welfare system include 24-hour availability for intake, immediate response to referral, 24-hour availability to clients, intensive but time-limited services, and use of a single therapist with team back-up (NFPN 2009). Over 1000 agencies in the United States and 20 other countries use one or more of the North Carolina Family Assessment Scale (NCFAS) tools (NFPN 2015).

IFPS programs are required to provide certain interventions in order to increase the probability that a family will remain unified successfully. The interventions may vary but should include the basic fundamental elements of flexible scheduling, individually tailored services, engagement and motivation, assessment and goal setting, behavior change, skills development, personal scientist approach, concrete and advocacy services, and community coordination and interactions (NFPN 2009).

High-fidelity models such as the HOMEBUILDERS program have consistently demonstrated the success of IFPS. Empirical evidence indicates that it works equally well in a variety of circumstances, including families of color and those involved with abuse and neglect (Kirk and Griffith 2004; 2008). Although IFPS may vary considerably with respect to program characteristics, all programs seek to stabilize families, improve family functioning, use community resources for family support, and assist caregivers with developing the skills needed to nurture and protect their children.

Intensive Case Management by an Interdisciplinary Healthcare Team

In response to the daunting challenges the child welfare system faces in the twenty-first century, professionals are being asked to engage in interdisciplinary healthcare leadership teams to improve accessibility and quality of care to children in foster care (Bass et al. 2004; Magyary and Brandt 2005). Competencies required to accomplish this goal include development of collaborative relationships between multiple healthcare team providers, recognition of the significant contributions made by each member of the interdisciplinary team, and incorporation of evidence-based practices in the development of a comprehensive and culturally sensitive intensive case management program by all interdisciplinary team members.

System of Care

Implementing models of care that represent a philosophy about the way services should be delivered to children and families can provide a framework for case management services essential for ensuring the best medical and mental health outcomes for children in foster care. One model that provides this framework is the System of Care (Arbuckle and Herrick 2006). Although the organizational configuration of the System of Care may vary across communities, the system is guided by core values essential to the operations of a System of Care (Stroul 1996). The system must be child centered and family focused, community based in the most normative environment possible, and culturally competent.

Clients must be provided with comprehensive care coordination of multiple services delivered in a therapeutic manner.

The Interdisciplinary Healthcare Team

Even though the terms "multidisciplinary team" and "interdisciplinary team" are often used interchangeably, there is a distinct difference between the two concepts. Multidisciplinary teams work with clients independently of one another and share information about clients with each other. Interdisciplinary teams collaborate and are interdependent and complex, including professionals from many backgrounds who provide a variety of services. Each member of the team addresses a particular need of the child and family, and every person's role in the process is clearly identified and mutually respected (Arbuckle and Herrick 2006). The overall goal of team-based care is "to enhance communication and cooperation among the varied medical, social, and educational partners in a child's life to better meet the global needs of children and their families, helping them to achieve their best potential" (Katkin et al. 2017, p. 1).

Intensive Case Management

The purpose of all case management services provided to a child and family is to deliver a coordinated System of Care (Arbuckle and Herrick 2006). However, the case management process differs significantly from that of intensive case management. Case management focuses on provision of medical care and management of service utilization, whereas intensive case management provides attention to patients' medical and social conditions. Therefore, it is more comprehensive in its scope of services (Issel 1997).

Effective intensive case management interventions must be flexible and tailored to meet the specific needs of each family. The process is based on a core set of functions that allow adoption of a collaborative model, one of the most effective in delivering healthcare (Arbuckle and Herrick 2006). These functions should be seen as a sequential process comprising overlapping tasks that are highly personalized and family focused (Stroul 1996).

First, all agencies involved in addressing the child's and family's current healthcare needs must be identified and coordinated. Second, a plan of care must be developed in partnership with the family within the context of a multiagency team of professionals. Third, service delivery must be implemented in a timely and appropriate manner. Fourth, services must be coordinated by linking the various agencies, systems, and individuals involved with the care of the family. Finally, services must be continuously monitored and evaluated for adequacy and appropriateness. Children with complex mental health and/or medical needs require a case manager with a higher level of education. Advocacy for the individual child and family must be incorporated throughout the entire case management process (Seibert et al. 2018; Stroul 1996).

Several case management models have been developed and implemented around the country with wide variations. However, the wrap-around method of delivering coordinated and collaborative care to children requiring the services of an interdisciplinary team (Arbuckle and Herrick 2006) uses the most family-centered approach to the case management process through the development of a child and family team (CFT). The CFT is led by a parent or caregiver and is guided by specially trained individuals, such as public health nurse case managers (referred to as case coordinators among System of Care experts) who assist caregivers in partnering with relevant professionals. The wrap-around concept emphasizes extensive outreach and unconditional family-centered services, especially for those imminently at risk or already in out-of-home child placements. The wrap-around process makes it possible to combine services that match the intensity of inpatient or residential settings without actually removing a child from a foster home or an at-risk environment. Whatever services are provided to children and families, outcomes must be measured to facilitate evaluation and change.

Outcome Measures

Once the interdisciplinary care team is established and intensive case management services are coordinated, planned, and implemented, outcomes must be measured. However, developing a practical, ongoing tracking mechanism for intensive case management of children in foster care and their families has been challenging. Nonetheless, in the System of Care model, four general domains of outcome measures have been recognized as essential, namely clinical outcomes, functional outcomes, system outcomes, and family satisfaction (Stroul 1996).

The team through consensus determines which outcomes to evaluate in the quality assurance process based on what the system aims to accomplish. Synergy between individual service components within the context of the overall system and coordination leads to enhanced outcomes (Stroul 1996). Results of outcome evaluations inform future care provision. Following children in foster care and families throughout the foster care experience and into the child's adulthood, although challenging, will provide important information about the long-term implications of foster care and the benefits of strategies

designed to promote successful development for these vulnerable persons. Other challenges include model replication and sustainability, potential breakdown of agencies, financial barriers that prevent a true System of Care approach, integration of evidence-based interventions into practice, and accountability mechanisms for the system.

Specific outcomes identified by the Office of the Assistant Secretary for Planning and Evaluation (USDHHS 2008) include statewide assessments through on-site review of child and family services outcomes, program outcomes, and program improvement plans. Three outcomes are reviewed: safety, permanency, and child and family wellbeing. Seven systemic factors are considered: the statewide information, case review, and quality assurance systems, staff and provider training, service array and resource development, agency responsiveness to community, and foster and adoptive parent licensing, recruitment, and retention. The Children's Bureau works with states to achieve outcomes identified in their improvement plans and monitors progress closely. The statistics presented at the beginning of this chapter reflect outcomes from the reviews. Challenges can be overcome through a combination of education, research, policy formation, and advocacy efforts.

The Role of APRNs

Care of the foster child by a nurse practitioner (NP) should be guided by the American Academy of Pediatrics (AAP) statement on the delivery of healthcare services to children in the foster care system. These services include health information gathering at the time of removal, initial medical screen within 24 hours, ongoing health information gathering, comprehensive health assessment within 30 days of foster care placement, follow-up assessment 30 days after the comprehensive assessment, periodic preventive healthcare, and discharge encounter on final discharge from foster care. Other encounters that might warrant a health assessment can include intra-agency transfer, return to care within 90 days, return to care after 90 days, or visitation with birth parents (AAP 2005).

Initial Medical Screen

If a child is placed in the foster care system, an initial health screening must be conducted immediately before the child is placed or within 2 weeks of the most recent placement. Identification of any urgent medical needs of the child, as well as inclusion of the foster parent and caseworker in treatment planning, is essential (AAP 2002, 2005). It is imperative that the review of child's life history includes the details that led to the placement and, if possible, the past medical history. Careful measurements of height, weight, and head circumference are important to assess general nutritional status and growth. All body surfaces require an examination while unclothed to note any signs of trauma, bruises, scars, deformities, or limitations in body function. Genital and anal examinations should be conducted and, when necessary, photographic evidence should be obtained. Screening laboratory work should be carried out if clinically indicated, such as for HIV infection or other sexually transmitted diseases. Infections and communicable diseases should be noted and treated promptly (AAP 2002; 2005). The NP should discuss all findings and care instructions with the foster parent and caseworker directly and should clarify the role that the foster parent has in meeting the healthcare needs of the foster child.

Comprehensive Health Assessment

Within 1 month of placement, a comprehensive health assessment should be conducted by a PCP with whom consistent care will be established. When possible, the biological parent should provide information about the past health status of the child and should be kept informed of the child's present health status (AAP 2002, 2005; Szilagyi et al. 2015). Particular attention should be paid to assessing the child's adjustment to the foster home and any new health problems that have developed since the initial visit.

Immunization records should be reviewed. These records may have to be collated from several sources, including prior providers, schools, or vaccine registries. Many children in foster care are unimmunized or incompletely immunized, therefore they should be considered susceptible and immunized (Szilagyi et al. 2015) according to the Centers for Disease Control and Prevention immunization guidelines (Robinson et al. 2019).

As a part of the comprehensive health assessment, the PCP must also ensure that the foster child is provided with dental services. Fostered children may require an array of dental services, ranging from routine care to intensive treatment. Periodic dental screenings should be included into the ongoing process of care.

A child's growth and development should be assessed by the PCP at every well-child encounter or more frequently if indicated. This assessment may be based on a structured interview that is age-adjusted and developmentally specific, through the use of a standardized screening tool or via a review of school records (AAP 2002; 2005). All children with identified developmental delays or problems should be referred to early intervention services, local consultants, or school

resources. Some communities have established multidisciplinary programs that include professionals knowledgeable in evaluating children in foster care, who should be involved in diagnosing and treating children with developmental, mental health, and educational problems.

The prescribing provider must closely monitor any child prescribed psychotropic medication for potential adverse effects. The social worker should receive periodic updates on the child's progress, and the PCP should remain in close contact with the family to coordinate this effort.

Provision for Ongoing Care in a Medical Home Model

All children in foster care should have a medical home in which they receive ongoing primary care and assessments of their growth and development to determine if any changes in their health status require additional services or interventions. The AAP recommends that reassessments should occur monthly up to 6 months of age and semi-annually beyond 2 years through adolescence. Mental health and other primary care needs should be assessed case-by-case situation as indicated. In addition, periodic visits should be scheduled according to the AAP Recommendations for Preventive Pediatric Health Care (AAP 2017, 2019).

In order to enhance continuity of care in the primary care setting, several states have developed an abbreviated health record called a medical passport. The passport provides a brief description of the child's health, social, and family history, and is designed to enhance the transfer of essential information among health professionals. Foster parents keep the document and are required to bring it to all healthcare visits in order for the record to be updated. If the child changes foster homes, the record stays with the child to be used in a new medical home (AAP 2002, 2005).

Conclusion

APRNs, including certified family, pediatric, or psychiatric/mental health NPs, certified nurse midwives, and clinical nurse specialists face significant barriers when providing services to children in the foster care system. These barriers include lack of past medical history, social workers unable to provide details about the child's placement, foster care parents with limited training in healthcare issues, children with complicated physical and mental health conditions, lack of funding for needed services, and prior fragmentation of the child's care. To avoid some of these barriers, the APRN should provide healthcare coordination, communicate effectively with all professionals, and provide compassionate support and education to foster and birth parents. APRNs should be involved in the planning and development of a System of Care for children in foster care (AAP 2002, 2005) and recognize the important role they play in all aspects of the foster care system.

References

Adopting.org. (n.d.). *Therapeutic foster care and group homes.* Available at http://www.adopting.org/adoptions/therapeutic-foster-care-therapeutic-group-homes.html.

AAP, Committee on Early Childhood, Adoption, and Dependent Care (2002). Health care of young children in foster care. *Pediatrics* 109: 536–541.

AAP (2005). *Fostering Health: Health Care for Children and Adolescents in Foster Care*, 2e. New York, NY: American Academy of Pediatrics, Task Force on Health Care for Children in Foster Care Available at https://www.childtrends.org/publications/state-kinship-care-policies-for-children-that-come-to-the-attention-of-child-welfare-agencies.

AAP and Committee on Practice and Ambulatory Medicine and AAP Bright Futures Periodicity Schedule Workgroup (2017). 2017 Recommendations for Preventive Pediatric Health Care. *Pediatrics* 139: e20170254. https://doi.org/10.1542/peds.2017-0254.

AAP, Committee on Practice and Ambulatory Medicine, and Bright Futures Periodicity Schedule Work Group (2019). 2019 Recommendations for Preventive Pediatric Health Care. *Pediatrics* 143 (3): e20182971.

Adler, L.S. (2001). The meanings of permanence: A critical analysis of the Adoption and Safe Families Act of 1997. *Harvard Journal on Legislation* 38 (1): 1–36. Available at https://papers.ssrn.com/sol3/papers.cfm?abstract_id=2045653.

American Association of Children's Residential Centers (2017). *Redefining residential: Strategic interventions to advance youth permanency.* Milwaukee, WI: AACRC Available at https://plummeryouthpromise.org/wp-content/uploads/2017/04/AACRC-Paper-13.pdf.

Annie E. Casey Foundation. (2009). *Rebuild the national child welfare system.* Available at https://www.aecf.org/resources/rebuild-the-nations-child-welfare-system/.

Arbuckle, M. and Herrick, C. (2006). *Child and Adolescent Mental Health: Interdisciplinary Systems of Care.* Boston, MA: Jones and Bartlett Publishers.

ASFA-97. *Adoption and Safe Families Act of 1997.* P. L. 105–89, 111 Stat 2115 (1997).

Bass, S., Shields, M., and Behrman, R. (2004). Children, families, and foster care: analysis and recommendations. *The Future of Children* 14 (1): 5–29.

Berger Cardoso, J., Brabeck, K., Stinchcomb, D. et al. (2019). Integration of unaccompanied migrant youth in the United States: a call for research. *Journal of Ethnic and Migration Studies* 45: 273–292.

Berry, M., Cash, S., and Brook, J. (2000). Intensive family preservation services: an examination of critical service components. *Child and Family Social Work* 5: 191–203.

Bramlett, M.D., Radel, L.F., and Chow, K. (2017). Health and well-being of children in kinship care: findings from the National Survey of Children in Nonparental Care. *Child Welfare* 95 (3): 41–60.

Bruskas, D. (2008). Children in foster care: a vulnerable population at risk. *Journal of Child and Adolescent Psychiatric Nursing* 24: 70–77.

Campbell, J.A., Walker, R.J., and Egede, L.E. (2016). Associations between adverse childhood experiences, high-risk behaviors, and morbidity in adulthood. *American Journal of Preventive Medicine* 50: 344–352.

Casanueva, C., Burfeind, C., Tuelle, S. et al. (2016). *Patterns of Foster Care Placement and Family Reunification following Child Maltreatment Investigation.* [Research Brief]. Research Triangle, NC: RTI International Available at https://aspe.hhs.gov/system/files/pdf/258526/Reunification.pdf.

Casey Family Programs. (2017). *The evolution of hope.* Available at https://www.casey.org/hope2017.

Casillas, K.L., Fauchier, A., Derkash, B.T., and Garrido, E.F. (2016). Implementation of evidence-based home visiting programs aimed at reducing child maltreatment: a meta-analytic review. *Child Abuse & Neglect* 53: 64–80.

Child Trends, Inc. (2016). *How states fund child welfare activities.* Publication # #2016-05. Available at https://www.childtrends.org/wp-content/uploads/2016/01/2016-05HowStatesFundChild-Welfare.pdf.

Child Welfare Information Gateway (2006). *Enhancing Permanency for Older Youth in Out-of-Home Care.* Washington, DC: US Department of Health and Human Services Available at https://secure.ce-credit.com/articles/101272/enhancing.pdf.

Children's Rights. (2018). *Child welfare organizations.* Available at https://www.childrensrights.org/our-mission/our-partners/child-welfare-organizations.

Cox, C.B. (2016). *Kinship Care. Encyclopedia of Social Work.* New York, NY: Oxford University Press https://doi.org/10.1093/acrefore/9780199975839.013.966.

Craven, P.A. and Lee, R.E. (2006). Therapeutic interventions for foster children: a systematic research synthesis. *Research on Social Work Practice* 16: 287–304.

Dube, S.R. (2018). Continuing conversations about adverse childhood experiences (ACEs) screening: a public health perspective. *Child Abuse & Neglect* 85: 180–184.

Eckenrode, J., Smith, E.G., McCarthy, M.E., and Dineen, M. (2014). Income inequality and child maltreatment in the United States. *Pediatrics* 133: 454–461. https://doi.org/10.1542/peds.2013-1707.

Eddy, J.M., Shortt, J.W., Martinez, C.R. et al. (2019). Outcomes from a randomized controlled trial of the relief nursery program. *Prevention Science* 21: 36–46. https://doi.org/10.1007/s11121-019-00992-9.

Edwards, F. and Wildeman, C. (2018). Characteristics of the front-line child welfare workforce. *Children and Youth Services Review* 89: 13–26.

Ellis, R.R. and Simmons, T. (2014). *Co-resident Grandparents and Their Grandchildren: 2012.* Washington, DC: US Census Bureau Available at https://www.census.gov/library/publications/2014/demo/p20-576.html.

Foster, E.M. and Gifford, E.J. (2004). *Challenges in The Transition to Adulthood For Youth in Foster Care, Juvenile Justice and Special Education* (Policy Brief, Issue 15). Philadelphia, PA: University of Pennsylvania, Department of Sociology, MacArthur Foundation Research Network.

Fostering Connections. *Fostering Connections to Success and Increasing Adoptions Act of 2008.* P. L. 110–351 (2008).

Gilbert, R., Widom, C.S., Browne, K. et al. (2009). Burden and consequences of child maltreatment in high-income countries. *The Lancet* 373: 68–81.

Gramkowski, B., Kools, S., Paul, S. et al. (2009). High risk behavior of youth in foster care. *The Journal of Child and Adolescent Psychiatric Nursing* 22: 77–85.

Greater Hope Foundation for Children Inc. (2019). *Foster care.* Available at http://www.greaterhopefoundation.com/home.html.

Hilt, R.J., Barclay, R.P., Bush, J. et al. (2015). A statewide child telepsychiatry consult system yields desired health system changes and savings. *Telemedicine and e-Health* 21: 533–537.

Hoynes, H.W. and Schanzenbach, D.W. (2018). *Safety Net Investments in Children (No. w24594)*. Washington, DC: National Bureau of Economic Research.

Issel, L. (1997). Measuring comprehensive case management interventions: development of a tool. *Nursing Case Management* 2: 132–140.

Jordan, E. and Connelly, D.D. (2016). *An introduction to child welfare funding, and how states use it. Pub #2016-01*. Bethesda, MD: Child Trends Available at https://www.childtrends.org/wp-content/uploads/2016/01/2016-01IntroStateChildWelfareFunding.pdf.

Justin, R.G. (2003). Medical needs of foster children. *American Family Physician* 67: 474–476.

Katkin, J.P., Kressly, S.J., Edwards, A.R. et al. (2017). Guiding principles for team-based pediatric care. *Pediatrics* 140 (2): e20171489.

Kim, H. and Drake, B. (2018). Child maltreatment risk as a function of poverty and race/ethnicity in the USA. *International Journal of Epidemiology* 47: 780–787.

Kirk, R.S. and Griffith, D.P. (2004). Intensive family preservation services: demonstrating placement prevention using event history analysis. *National Association of Social Workers Inc.* 28 (1): 5–16.

Kirk, R.S. and Griffith, D.P. (2008). Impact of intensive family preservation services on disproportionality of out-of-home placement of children of color in one state's child welfare system. *Child Welfare League of America* 87 (5): 87–105.

Koh, E., Rolock, N., Cross, T.P., and Eblen-Manning, J. (2014). What explains instability in foster care? Comparison of a matched sample of children with stable and unstable placements. *Children and Youth Services* 37: 36–45.

Kools, S. and Kennedy, C. (2003). Foster child health and development. Implications for primary care. *Pediatric Nursing* 289: 39–46.

Levey, E.J., Gelaye, B., Bain, P. et al. (2017). A systematic review of randomized controlled trials of interventions designed to decrease child abuse in high-risk families. *Child Abuse & Neglect* 65: 48–57.

Lister, J., Lieberman, R.E., and Sisson, K. (2016). *Residential Treatment for Children & Youth* 33 (3-4): 177–185. Available at https://doi.org/10.1080/0886571X.2016.1240555.

Magyary, D. and Brandt, P. (2005). A leadership training model to enhance private and public service partnerships for children with special healthcare needs. *Infants and Young Children* 18 (1): 60–71.

Marx, L., Benoit, M., and Kamradt, B. (2003). Foster children in the child welfare system. In: *The Handbook of Child and Adolescent System of Care: The New Psychiatry* (eds. A.J. Pumariega and N.C. Winters), 332–350. San Francisco, CA: Jossey-Bass.

Murray, K.O. and Gesiriech, S. (2003). *A Brief Legislative History of the Child Welfare System*. Washington, DC: The Pew Commission on Children in Foster Care.

National Family Preservation Network. (2009). *IFPS ToolKit: A comprehensive guide for establishing & strengthening intensive family preservation services*. Available at https://www.nfpn.org/preservation/ifps-toolkit.

National Family Preservation Network. (2015). *Overview of assessment tools*. Available at https://www.nfpn.org/Portals/0/Documents/assessment_tools_overview.pdf.

Pearson, G. (2006). System of care with the juvenile justice population: the interface between justice and behavioral health. In: *Child and Adolescent Mental Health: Interdisciplinary Systems of Care* (eds. M. Arbuckle and C. Herrick), 221–245. Sudbury MA: Jones & Bartlett.

Racusin, R., Maerlender, A.C., Sengupta, A. et al. (2005). Psychosocial treatment of children in foster care: a review. *Community Mental Health Journal* 41: 199–221.

Robinson, C.L., Bernstein, H., Romero, J.R., and Szilagyi, P. (2019). Advisory committee on immunization practices recommended immunization schedule for children and adolescents aged 18 years or younger – United States, 2019. *Morbidity and Mortality Weekly Report* 68: 112–114. https://doi.org/10.15585/mmwr.mm6805a4.

Rushton, A. (2010). Thinking on developmental psychology in fostering and adoption. *Adoption & Fostering* 34 (3): 38–43.

Rushton, A. and Dance, C. (2006). The adoption of children from public care: a prospective study of outcomes in adolescence. *Journal of the American Academy of Child and Adolescent Psychiatry* 45: 877–883.

Sadock, B.J. and Sadock, V.A. (2009). Adoption and foster care: child maltreatment and abuse. In: *Kaplan and Sadock's Concise Book of Child and Adolescent Psychiatry* (eds. B.J. Sadock and V.A. Sadock), 214–225. Philadelphia, PA: Wolters Kluwer/Lippincott Williams & Wilkins.

Schneiderman, J.U. (2003). Health issues of children in foster care. *Contemporary Nurse* 14: 123–128.

Schneiderman, J.U. (2005). The child welfare system: through the eyes of public health nurses. *Public Health Nursing* 22: 354–359.

Schneiderman, J.U. (2008). Qualitative study on the role of nurses as health case managers of children in foster care in California. *Journal of Pediatric Nursing* 23: 241–249.

Seibert, J., Feinberg, R., Ayub, A. et al. (2018). *State Practices in Treatment/Therapeutic Foster Care*. Research Triangle Park, NC: RTI International.

Stillerman, A. (2018). Childhood adversity & lifelong health: from research to action. *The Journal of Family Practice* 67: 690–699.

Stroul, B. (1996). *Children's Mental Health: Creating Systems of Care in a Changing Society*. Baltimore, MD: Paul H. Brooks Publishing Co.

Szilagyi, M.A., Rosen, D.S., Rubin, D. et al. (2015). Health care issues for children and adolescents in foster care and kinship care. *Pediatrics* 136: e1142. https://doi.org/10.1542/peds.2015-2656.

Turney, K. and Wildeman, C. (2016). Mental and physical health of children in foster care. *Pediatrics* 138: e20161118. https://doi.org/10.1542/peds.2016-1118.

USDHHS (n.d.). *Child Welfare Information Gateway [Library Search]*. US Department of Health and Human Services, Administration for Children and Families. Washington, DC: Government Printing Office Available at https://www.childwelfare.gov.

USDHHS. (2008). *Ensuring quality in contracted child welfare services*. US Department of Health and Human Services, Office of the Assistant Secretary for Planning and Evaluation. Available at https://aspe.hhs.gov/basic-report/ensuring-quality-contracted-child-welfare-services.

USDHHS. (2017). *Child maltreatment 2017*. US Department of Health & Human Services, Administration for Children and Families, Administration on Children, Youth and Families, Children's Bureau. Available at https://www.acf.hhs.gov/sites/default/files/cb/cm2017.pdf.

USDHHS. (2018a). *AFCARS state-by-state adoption and foster care statistics*. US Department of Health and Human Services, Administration for Children and Families, Administration on Children, Youth and Families, Children's Bureau Adoption and Foster Care Analysis and Reporting System. Available at https://www.acf.hhs.gov/sites/default/files/cb/afcars_state_data_tables_08thru17.xlsx.

USDHHS (2018b). *Trends in Foster Care and Adoption: FY 2008-FY 2017*. US Department of Health and Human Services, Administration for Children and Families, Adoption and Foster Care Analysis and Reporting System. Washington, DC: Government Printing Office Available at https://www.acf.hhs.gov/sites/default/files/cb/trends_fostercare_adoption_08thru17.pdf.

USDHHS. (2019). Foster Care Statistics 2017. Washington, DC: Government Printing Office. US Department of Health and Human Services, Administration for Children and Families, Adoption and Foster Care Analysis and Reporting System. Available at https://www.acf.hhs.gov/cb/resource/afcars-report-25.

US Department of Justice (2009). *OJJDP FY 2009 Mentoring Initiative for Foster Care Youth*. Office of Justice Programs-Office of Juvenile Justice and Delinquency Prevention (OJJDP). Washington, DC: Government Printing Office Available at https://ojjdp.ojp.gov/funding/opportunities/ojjdp-2009-2214.

Vaithianathan, R., Rouland, B., and Putnam-Hornstein, E. (2017). Injury and mortality among children identified as at high risk of maltreatment. *Pediatrics* 141 (2): pii, e20172882. https://doi.org/10.1542/peds.2017-2882.

Vig, S., Chinitz, S., and Shulman, L.H. (2005). Young children in foster care: multiple vulnerabilities and complex service needs. *Infants and Young Children* 18 (2): 147–160.

Weinberg, L.A., Zetlin, A., and Shea, N.M. (2009). Removing barriers to educating children in foster care through interagency collaboration: a seven county multiple-case study. *Child Welfare* 88 (4): 77–111.

Wildeman, C., Emanuel, N., Leventhal, J.M. et al. (2014). The prevalence of confirmed maltreatment among US children, 2004 to 2011. *JAMA Pediatrics* 168: 706–713. https://doi.org/10.1001/jamapediatrics.2014.410.

Winokur, M., Holtan, A., and Batchelder, K.E. (2014). Kinship care for the safety, permanency, and well-being of children removed from the home for maltreatment [review]. *The Cochrane Library* https://doi.org/10.1002/14651858.CD006546.pub3.

26

Chronic and Palliative Care Pediatric Populations

Geraldine S. Pearson[1] and Deborah Fisher[2]

[1] University of Connecticut School of Medicine-retired, Farmington, CT, USA
[2] George Washington University, Washington, DC, USA

Objectives

After reading this chapter, advanced practice psychiatric nurses (APRNs) will be able to:

1. Define pediatric palliative care (PPC) and discuss its development.
2. Explore concepts relevant to PPC.
3. Identify and understand barriers to the provision of PPC.
4. Describe end-of-life and bereavement care for children, adolescents, and families.
5. Understand the risk factors for families of children receiving palliative and end-of-life care.
6. Explore cultural, spiritual, ethical, and legal issues unique to PPC.
7. Discuss collaborative possibilities for primary care practitioners and APRNs in the palliative care of children and families with chronic and life-shortening diseases.
8. Elucidate areas of research that will inform practice and education in PPC.

Introduction

Seldom does a topic evoke more intense emotions and feelings than the discovery that a child has a serious illness that will shorten the full, long life that he or she was expected to live. It is very likely that at some point in their practice, advanced practice psychiatric nurses (APRNs) will encounter a child who is diagnosed with a serious, life-threatening or life-limiting illness. While caring for these children, they will experience a roller coaster of emotions ranging from pure joy to profound sorrow. The goal of this chapter is to familiarize APRNs with the state of the art and science of pediatric palliative care (PPC), so that equipped with this knowledge they can meaningfully contribute to the care of a child and family facing a life-limiting or life-threatening diagnosis. Thus, this chapter will focus on the most crucial skills needed by the APRN caring for a seriously ill child: competencies in discussing the range of therapeutic and palliative options available to families, formulating realistic goals as a child's prognosis changes, and facilitating connection to the resources available to achieve the goals of care.

Child and Adolescent Behavioral Health: A Resource for Advanced Practice Psychiatric and Primary Care Practitioners in Nursing,
Second Edition. Edited by Edilma L. Yearwood, Geraldine S. Pearson, and Jamesetta A. Newland.
© 2021 John Wiley & Sons, Inc. Published 2021 by John Wiley & Sons, Inc.
Companion website: www.wiley.com/go/Yearwood

History and Evolution of PPC in the United States

From a historical perspective, palliative care for children (and adults) was often delayed until patients were very close to death, and cure-focused treatment to extend length of life was deemed no longer possible nor beneficial and discontinued. However, as the number of children who are surviving serious illness for longer periods of time has continued to increase, numerous advocacy organizations and professional groups have recognized the need to define PPC more broadly, as both a philosophy of care and an organized and structured system for delivering services. Nearly 74 million children live in the United States (Federal Interagency Forum on Child and Family Statistics and Family Statistics 2017). Of those children, approximately half a million have a life-threatening condition (Elias and Murphy 2012). Children with complex chronic conditions (CCC) represent the majority of candidates for PPC (Thrane et al. 2017). On any given day there are over 8600 children with serious or life-threatening illness who could benefit from PPC (Friebert 2009; Friebert and Williams 2015). At present, palliative care is viewed as a continuum, whose trajectory extends from the *time of diagnosis* of a serious illness to the time of cure or death and through the phase of family bereavement. Under this contemporary philosophy, the mandate for palliative care now focuses on preventing and relieving distressing symptoms experienced by the child with a serious illness, life-threatening or life-limiting condition, *regardless* of his place on the illness trajectory. Consequently, although palliative care originated from the hospice model, it is not simply a synonym for hospice (Morgan 2009). Thus, the paradigm of palliative care focuses on improving the *quality of life* of the seriously ill child and "adding life to their years, rather than years to their life" (American Academy of Pediatrics 2008, p. 353).

Although deaths in childhood are fortunately rare, the significant emotional discomfort accompanying childhood illness and death experienced by families and health professionals alike has often resulted in these children becoming "medical orphans in a health system geared to cure, and a culture where only the elderly die" (Trafford 2002, p. A7). Recommending palliative care is one of the most difficult topics for pediatric healthcare providers to broach with families of seriously ill children. This is most likely due to a variety of reasons. In addition to equating palliative care with hospice, our Western cultural heritage generally rejects the notion that children suffer and die. It is simply too difficult to conceive that a child would die before a parent, and it is uncomfortable to imagine a life of such unrealized potential coming to an early end. Society and healthcare professionals have slowly begun to recognize that such denial of suffering and death in childhood abandons the family to negotiate the perilous waters of serious childhood illness and eventual death alone. Historically, the publication of the Institute of Medicine's (IOM 2003) report *When Children Die: Improving Palliative and End-of-Life Care for Children and Their Families*, written by experts in pediatrics and palliative care, offered further support to the special needs of seriously ill children and their families.

Childhood death is a rare occurrence compared to death in adults. Approximately 50 000 infants, children, and adolescents die yearly in the United States from congenital disorders, complications of prematurity, accidental injury, cancers, and a wide variety of other life-limiting and life-threatening illnesses (Friebert and Williams 2015). More significant is the number of children who suffer from complex chronic health conditions that limit their life span. It is estimated that there are approximately 2 million children living in the United States with these serious and potentially life-limiting illnesses, who, together with their families, face a gamut of distressing symptoms and emotional upheaval (Torkildson 2010). The gradual increase in this population of seriously ill children is primarily attributed to technological and medical advances that have produced new curative and palliative therapies previously unavailable (Feudtner et al. 2015). These advances have prompted the need for a paradigm shift in care for this population, as more children who were unlikely to live past infancy now survive for months, years, or decades. It is this growing group of children who has primarily prompted the need to expand the definition of palliative care in the pediatric population just described.

The need for holistic, reimbursable care throughout the life span of seriously ill children has not kept pace with this expanded view of PPC, and the number of PPC programs that do exist is growing but is relatively small to meet the expanding needs for palliative care across the continuum. A cross-sectional survey of children's hospitals conducted in 2012 revealed that nearly 70% of the 162 responding hospitals had a PPC program. Of those, the majority were only offering inpatient palliative care (Feudtner et al. 2012). Despite this increase in available programs, many children who die in hospital do not receive palliative care consultation (Keele et al. 2013). Fiscal constraints make it difficult to create and continue palliative care programs that encompass true life span care. Obtaining insurance coverage for palliative care has proven challenging. The need to allow for a *dual focus* of care for seriously ill children was recognized by the Centers for Medicaid and Medicare Services

(CMS) as legitimate for reimbursement under the Patient Protection and Affordable Care Act of 2010. In September 2010, CMS issued a state medical director letter instructing that children receiving Medicaid or Children's Health Insurance Program health insurance coverage who have elected a hospice benefit can continue to receive all other services, *including curative therapies for which the child is eligible* (US Centers for Medicaid and Medicare Services 2010). This change will hopefully prompt more private insurers to follow suit and will make sustainability for PPC programs a more attainable goal.

Family Risk when a Child has Palliative Care Needs

Families of children requiring palliative care bear the burdens and stressors associated with this over an extended period of time. While there is a dearth of current research measuring specific changes in families receiving palliative care, several older studies looked at the impact of child death on family members (Arnold et al. 2005; Li et al. 2003; Sanders 1980). In her landmark study comparing adult bereavement after the death of a parent, spouse, and child, Sanders (1980) identified significantly higher intensities of grief among those adults surviving the death of a child. Arnold et al. (2005) explored an understanding of parental grief on the death of a child, not as episodic but as complex and ongoing. Li et al. (2003) reported an association between the death of a child and an overall increase in the mortality of mothers as well as a slightly increased early mortality in fathers. The authors posit that stress over the long term may result in pathophysiological changes, which increase susceptibility to infectious and cardiovascular disease. In addition, prolonged exposure to stress may affect changes in lifestyle, contributing to mortality (2003).

When a child dies, the impact is most profound for parents and surviving siblings (Fullerton et al. 2017). The authors describe short-term effects on these siblings as those of horror, sadness, distress, relief, and guilt, for some siblings the ill child's death may result in personal growth, increased maturation and compassion (Eilegard et al. 2013). Russell et al. (2018) note that surviving siblings, of all ages may feel emotionally abandoned as parents struggle with their own grief. Indeed, the pain of losing a brother or sister is felt deeply, and has complex effects on all the family relationships before and after the death of an ill child. There is much work to be done to better understand risk factors for families and the unique needs of siblings as health professionals provide palliative and end-of-life care for their children.

Ethical Foundations and Legal Issues

Questions and discussion about what constitutes appropriate medical and surgical treatment for children of all ages whose conditions are severe, chronic, and life threatening have become topics in the pediatric bioethics literature as well as subjects for serious consideration by bioethics committees. Not what can be done but what ought to be done is central to any ethical consideration of treatment options as rapidly exploding knowledge and advances in technology expand possibilities for intervention in the care of children with chronic illness. Juxtaposed against those expanding possibilities is the issue of quality of life, defined by the wishes, hopes, and goals for treatment established by the child, family, and caregivers. Here the developmental needs and capabilities of children, adolescents, and families converge with wishes, belief systems, and cultural values, adding richness and complexity to the decision-making process. A goal of palliative care is to mitigate conflicts that may arise as a result of failures in communication, inadequate goal setting and care planning, and inappropriate care giving (IOM 2003). Institutional efforts to identify situations posing a high risk of conflict; to develop protocols for ethics consults for patients, families, and all staff, and to draft evidence-based practice guidelines that will help clarify risks and benefits of new or experimental medical interventions are necessary to ensure a strong ethical foundation for palliative care decisions.

These are only some of the questions to be considered in the decision-making process in PPC:

1. What constitutes informed consent and/or assent by the child, adolescent, and family?
2. When and how can a child or adolescent participate in decision making?
3. Who determines what is in the best interest of a child?
4. If parent- or child-voiced wishes for care are at odds with medical recommendations, how is the conflict resolved?
5. How are risks and benefits of medical treatment determined at end of life?
6. What factors affect accessibility of palliative care?
7. What effect does the reality of limited resources have on palliative and end-of-life care?

While adults are encouraged to create advanced directives in the form of living wills and healthcare proxies, no state recognizes a formal advanced directive signed by a person under the age of 18 years (IOM 2003). In most situations, parents have the legal right to make medical treatment decisions for their children. Nonetheless, allowing children and adolescents to participate in decision making is beneficial to the child and to the parent as well. By including the child in the decision-making process and respecting their choices, dignity is promoted (Zadeh et al. 2016). Advance care planning has been associated with a decrease in suffering at end-of-life and parental decisional regret (DeCourcey et al. 2018).

The complex and difficult decisions to be made in PPC can have repercussions for caregivers. Shepard and Sheldon (2010) note that conflict between external forces (including families, institutions, and religious belief systems) and ethical principles can result in "moral distress" for the caregiver, defined as knowing the right course of action and being prevented from pursuing it. Specific bioethical principles such as beneficence, autonomy, and nonmalfeasance may be in conflict with aggressive care and may be overlooked in the effort to provide intervention. Referring conflicts to a pediatric bioethics committee or consultant may provide a context in which discrepant views can be discussed, ethical principles reviewed, "moral distress" addressed, and wishes, including the child's, heard by all involved with the child.

Basic Concepts and Quality Indicators

When investigating a referral source for PPC, the APRN should seek a provider who embraces certain philosophical principles within an organized framework for care delivery. Friebert (2015) proposes a viable and appropriate model of PPC that should encompass the following principles:

- The services are provided across a care trajectory that ideally starts at the *time of diagnosis* and in *any care setting.*
- The services should be *interdisciplinary* in order to incorporate a *holistic philosophy* and method of care delivery.
- The plan of care should be *individualized, family centered* and focused on *what matters most to the child and family.*
- The goals of care are aimed at enhancing *quality of life* and day-to-day function of the child, *minimizing suffering,* and may be concurrent with curative or life prolonging goals.

Additionally, a PPC program that supports these principles ideally implements services that are:

- sensitive to personal, cultural, and religious practices
- helpful to families as they make decisions and choices based on best practices and ethical principles
- delivered by an interdisciplinary team

- inclusive of the child's and family's community and environment
- able to offer grief counseling for bereaved families
- willing to support curative therapies concurrent with palliative treatment, if that is the family's wish
- committed to providing children and families with options and choices regarding treatment and involvement in decision making
- willing to offer effective pain and symptom management as paramount to optimizing quality of life (Friebert 2015).

Settings for Provision of PPC

Palliative care for children can be provided in a variety of models and settings and is often determined by several factors, including age at diagnosis, complexity of symptom burden, family resiliency, access to resources, location of legal residence, and, finally, insurance coverage. Corr et al. (2010), editors of the Children's Project on Palliative and Hospice Services (ChiPPS) Newsletter, have developed an overview of the range of programs, services, and pioneering collaborations that have evolved in the United States to expand and meet the unique needs of children and families requiring palliative care services (p. 6):

- *PPC waivers*: These are created to address a gap in state plan services, usually through Medicaid, aimed at specific populations prevalent in certain geographic locations.
- *Coalitions*: Statewide groups that typically focus on advocacy, education, and access to services.
- *Hospital-based services*: This is the most frequent setting for provision of palliative, hospice, and end-of-life care for children. Typically, the child remains under the care of the clinical service team that has been managing his illness, while specific palliative care recommendations and connection to resources are offered through consultation to that team and family.
- *Home-based care*: Once a child is stabilized and symptoms are under control, transition to home-based palliative care is an option that is often preferred by the child and family. Having the security and proximity of familiar surroundings and ready access to family and friends provides comfort and security to a sick child. It also offers convenience to families who must continue to meet a host of other responsibilities related to siblings, household management, work, and community. Unfortunately, the majority of palliative and hospice home care agencies provide services only for adults or have only a limited number of staff who are

competent and comfortable giving care to seriously ill children. Also, home care agencies that want to offer care to children and families who wish to receive hospice and end-of-life benefits must apply for a special license allowing them to provide these types of home-based services.

- *School as partner*: The inclusion or return of a seriously ill child to the school setting is a key factor in maintaining the quality of life of a child receiving palliative care. School can be an appropriate activity for children who have a serious, chronic, or terminal illness. Vanclooster et al. (2018) note the need for the school to have knowledge about the child's condition, education, and support requirements. Communication between parents, school, and healthcare providers can facilitate the child's transition back into the academic setting. It can be particularly stressful when a previously healthy child returns to school after diagnosis and treatment for a life-limiting or life-threatening illness. Anxiety and fear may be greater when the child's appearance has been altered because of his condition, such as weight change, hair loss, disfigurement, or the need for special devices or equipment. The child may also require special adjustments to his school routine to accommodate a diminished energy level, medication administration, or skilled nursing procedures. All of these factors may contribute to the perception of the child as "different" and increase his risk of becoming physically and socially isolated or even bullied in the school setting. Promoting a smooth transition to school is an appropriate and integral role for the APRN to assume as a child transitions back to the educational setting. The child with special needs is entitled to have an Individualized Education Plan (IEP), mandated under the Individuals with Disabilities Education Act (IDEA) and/or a 504 plan authorized under the Rehabilitation Act (American Academy of Pediatrics 2010). Although IDEA exempts schools from providing "medical services," it still stipulates that the "provision of intermittent care necessary for the student's participation cannot be used as grounds for exclusion from school" (AAP 2010, p. 1074).

Knowledge, preparation, and support are needed for a seriously ill child's transition to school. Specifically, a clear plan of communication between providers, school, parents, and the child, adapted educational programming, and support for peer relationships is recommended (Vanclooster et al. 2018).

A common source of anxiety for school staff when a seriously ill child returns to school is fear that he will experience a medical crisis while in the classroom. It will be crucial to include information about what problems

could occur, and a plan for dealing with such situations should be clearly delineated, put in writing, and made accessible to all who will interact with the child during the school day. When designing an IEP and an Individualized Health Care Plan (IHCP), it is also essential to determine what the parents' wishes are regarding resuscitation of their child, should cardiac or respiratory arrest occur in the school setting. If a "Do Not Resuscitate" (DNR) order is in place, it must be determined if the local school board will honor such a directive. [Note: In some health facilities and agencies, the acronym DNR has been replaced by AND, "Allow Natural Death" (AAP 2010).] If this is not the case, the APRN should consider acting as an advocate with the school jurisdiction to modify policies and regulations to allow the parents' and child's wishes regarding resuscitation to be honored. Advocacy efforts to achieve such a policy change should begin with systematic identification of the infrastructure needed to ensure that school personnel, the child, and the parents are supported if a DNR/AND order is in place. The National Education Association (NEA) has also published guidelines that ensure that the needs of all stakeholders will be respected when such a decision is made (NEA 2000). It is important to bear in mind, however, that "DNR" does not equate to "Do Not Care." When a DNR or AND order is in place, a clear strategy must be devised that specifies the plan for communication and comfort care for the child should cardiopulmonary arrest occur. Preparations should also be developed to support the child's classmates and teachers should a medical crisis or death occur in the school setting.

- *Free-standing hospice*: At present, the George Mark House in San Leandro, California, and Ryan House in Phoenix, Arizona are the only free-standing centers that exclusively provides palliative and hospice care for children in the United States. Exceptional Care for Children, in Newark, Delaware, initially opened in 2004 with the intent of exclusively providing end-of-life care to children. However, this agency was unable to maintain fiscal stability with this single-service focus and has now expanded its role to provide care to children requiring skilled respite, transitional, and palliative nursing care.

Assessment of Child and Family

The provision of pediatric palliative and end-of-life care is based on a complete and in-depth assessment of the family, who with the ill child are the focus of care. To develop an active partnership with the family, palliative team members gain an understanding of the family system, the factors and forces that form and impact it, and the multiple systems with which it interacts. Families are composed of the clusters of persons with whom the child lives and by whom care is given, including parents, grandparents, siblings, extended family members, godparents, and friends. Who has legal responsibility for decisions made for and about the child? Who is the custodial parent or legal guardian? Exploring with family members their ethnicity, culture, and language as well as their religious beliefs, practices, and important family rituals provides information and lends rich texture to an understanding of the family fabric (Levine et al. 2016).

In addition, information about living environment is essential in planning a context for ongoing care. Families may live in their own homes or apartments, in rooms with extended family members, or in shelters. Some families are nondomiciled. Does the child attend school? Is that school a source of normalcy, enjoyment, and socialization with peers? Are teachers aware of the child's diagnosis and plan for care so that they can support and accommodate changing needs? In addition, the team should be aware of resources in the community providing social support, including churches, community agencies, and good neighbors. Immigrant families, particularly those who are undocumented, are at risk. While they desire the utmost care for their sick children, the exposure in the hospital and community adds the risk of detention and deportation to their lives. Undocumented families may be reticent to share with the PPC team details of their precarious lives. This reticence and fear may limit the sick child's ability to communicate his needs and wishes.

Cacciatore et al. (2019) suggest that assessment should include parental observations, and the child's own physical, emotional, and social complaints. Exploration of the manifestation of the disease, documenting the history of the illness, the family's understanding of causative factors and specific pathophysiology, as well as the child's theories and notions about his disease will help the PPC team appreciate the meaning of the child's illness to the family. Wheaver and others (2015) note that youth with cancer should be introduced to palliative care concepts to reduce suffering throughout the disease process regardless of the disease status. Including the child in this exploration and eliciting his lived experience of illness and how it affects his life, his wishes, hopes, and dreams will open a pathway for discussion of symptoms and management, including traditional medical treatment, remedies tried by the patient and family, and alternative methods of care.

Barriers to PPC

Despite the growing acceptance of palliative care for children whose conditions are chronic and life threatening, there are significant barriers, both systemic and deeply personal, that limit access. These barriers exist in clinical, educational, financial, regulatory, and attitudinal forms. Cacciatore et al. (2019) note that nonhospital and human touches helped challenge the institutional constraints to care.

The relative paucity of PPC educational programs also serves as a major barrier. While nursing has taken the lead in developing teaching and training models in PPC, medicine has followed suit with the development of continuing education curriculum and a growing number of PPC fellowship sites. Despite the increase in pediatric educational programs, there are few such models that are interdisciplinary in nature. Without a designated and well-prepared PPC team to provide guidance, consultation, and education, care providers are ill-equipped to offer children and families the benefits of true palliative and end-of-life care.

Community-based PPC remains a challenge since relatively few hospices will accept pediatric patients. There are many differences between children and adult patients who qualify for hospice or palliative care. The majority of adult hospice patients have an oncologic disease, while the majority of pediatric patients have a congenital disease (Groh et al. 2014). Contrary to previous studies that have shown that children and their families' preferred location of death is in the home, DeCourcey et al. (2018) noted that more than 60% of children with life-threatening chronic conditions die within the hospital. Of those, over half died in the ICU.

Funding for PPC programs in major children's hospitals has been in short supply as the marketing of advanced lifesaving technology and care has greater public appeal than support for children with chronic illness for which there is no cure. Nonetheless, the number of PPC programs has grown in the last decade (Accreditation Council of Graduate Medical Education [ACGME] 2018). A major impediment to the provision of PPC rests in the federal Medicare model, which was used as the basis for state Medicaid hospice benefits (AAP 2000). Based on an adult patient with cancer model, hospice admission was restricted to patients with a life expectancy of 6 months or less. This stipulation has severely restricted hospice services for children because of the difficulty in predicting survival (AAP 2000). These regulations have financial implications for families who would benefit from palliative and end-of-life care services for which there is no reimbursement (Rushton 2010). Davies et al. (2010) note that cultural and linguistic differences may impede communication between families and healthcare providers. This potentially prevents family members from participating fully in decision making for their children. Without clear understanding of the nature of their child's chronic disease or condition and the options for treatment, including a full explanation of the nature of palliative care, families may misunderstand and feel demeaned, believing that such care is less valuable and less effective for their child.

When moderate to severe pain or dyspnea necessitates the use of opioids, considering their use can elicit a variety of fears and myths based on inaccurate misconceptions for both families and professionals. Uncertainty regarding respiratory depression and hastening the time of death may lead healthcare providers to delay opioid initiation or dosage increases for appropriate pain relief. Parents may interpret that a plan to use opioids signals worsening of their child's condition or imminent approach of death. Families may also worry that their child could become addicted to this type of medication, especially when opioids are referred to as "narcotics." Another common fear is that too early introduction of opioids for pain relief may lead to tolerance and ineffectiveness when the child approaches the end of life. The APRN has the opportunity to correct misconceptions, dispel myths, and calm fears through clear, honest communication and education regarding the benefits and possible side effects of medications chosen to palliate symptoms.

Facilitators of PPC

Integral to PPC is the notion of partnership between child, parents and family members, school teachers, clergy, and healthcare providers (AAP 2000). PPC, with its focus on family and child, is most effective when offered by a well-educated and -prepared multidisciplinary team engaged in open and clear communication. It is proactive, engaged care that can be introduced at the time of diagnosis of a chronic and life-threatening disease. PPC may supplement active, curative care with an ongoing focus on comfort and quality of life, or it may stand alone as aggressive care is ended. Bogetz and Friebert (2017) describe the quadruple aim of PPC as improved patient experience, better outcomes, lower costs, and improved provider experience. This includes the identification of decision makers, careful determination of the child's and family's understanding of disease and prognosis, the establishment of goals of care, and, finally, discussion of the use or not of aggressive medical interventions. Advance directives are discussed with family and, if developmentally appropriate, with children and adolescents.

Communication

Approaching children and families with a diagnosis of a chronic and life-shortening illness is a Herculean task. Finding language that conveys medical information

accurately and, understandably, assessing the parents' unique level of comprehension, and determining how much and in what way to communicate with the child and adolescent are among the greatest challenges for all pediatric caregivers. Families come with their own histories and experiences of illness and death and with their own ways of relating and communicating. Just as one considers the family system and cultural beliefs when giving difficult diagnoses, one must assess carefully the child or adolescent, considering chronological age, developmental level, and special factors contributing to cognitive and emotional status. Some of these same factors contribute to the child's and adolescent's understanding of death. The University of Rochester Medical Center offers the following developmentally based concepts of death:

Infant: Death has no real concept; rather infants react to separation and change in routine.

Toddler: Death has very little meaning; they can experiece the anxiety and emotions of those around them but death is not perceived as a permanent condition.

Preschooler: There is beginning understanding of death as something feared by adults; death may be viewed as temporary or reversible; their experience is influenced by those around them; they may blame themselves for their own illness or the illness of close family members.

School-ager: There is a more realistic understanding of death and it may be personified in a figure; death is beginning to be understood as permanent, universal, and inevitable. There is curiosity about death and fear of the unknown.

Adolescent: Influenced by past experiences and emotional development; most understand that death is permanent, universal, and inevitable; may feel immortal and exempt from death (University of Rochester Medical Center [URMC] n.d.).

Much attention in the pediatric literature has been devoted to the impact of telling versus not telling the child about diagnosis and prognosis. In the past, caregivers have colluded with parents to protect the child from knowing, believing that disclosure would cause great distress. The child's development and age, as well as relationship with parents, are factors to consider in explaining the diagnosis. The diagnosis itself marks the line dividing before from after (Arnold and Gemma 1994).

It is this heightened awareness even in very young children with chronic life-threatening disease that with cognitive and emotional developmental factors contributes to the child's understanding of illness and, in time, of impending death. Communication with children of all ages requires an understanding of normal cognitive and emotional development as well as an appreciation for the lived experience of illness. Such communication requires the use of age-appropriate language, an appreciation of bodily gestures and manner, expressive play, and drawings or writings. Frequently, children, and adolescents speak in metaphors that require acceptance without explanation. Siblings should be included in the process of telling. There may be an enormous burden of guilt carried by a child whose actions or inability to protect contributed to a sibling's injury or illness. For children whose guilt is great by virtue of their real actions or fantasies, there is a need for careful listening and discussion. This work may include parents and can be facilitated by a child therapist (Arnold and Gemma 1994).

Goals of Care

In partnership with child and family, the difficult news of diagnosis is given, and discussion shifts to formulation of goals of care. Feudtner et al. (2013) emphasize the need for an approach for involving children in decision making and goal setting. This approach focuses on understanding the abilities and vulnerabilities of children and respecting their relationship with parents.

Throughout the course of the child's illness, palliative care providers continue their responsibility of "telling," explaining changes in condition, offering new treatment options, discussing comfort measures, eliciting wishes and hopes, and renegotiating goals. Recognizing the partnership with child and family, the palliative care provider acts as an advocate strengthening the family's stance and helping their wishes and goals to remain uppermost in the medical setting and in the plan of action. In the recent past, disclosure of information to children was believed to increase fear and anxiety. However, there has been a welcome shift toward more open communication. Kreicbergs et al. (2004) discovered that in a qualitative, retrospective interview study that all parents who had discussed death and dying with their seriously ill child did not regret it. Many parents treasured those conversations and found comfort in knowing their child's wishes.

Although difficult, honest, and timely discussions regarding death facilitate healthy grieving and avoid unresolved grief, honest discussions allow for opportunities to clarify incorrect perceptions and promote assimilation of both facts and feelings. Avoidance of discussion of death contributes to the child's mistrust of adults and compounds feelings of isolation (Kubler-Ross 1983). Exclusion and dishonesty may lead to fantasies more terrible than reality. Open communication can

facilitate a child's ability to mourn in a healthy manner (Bugge et al. 2014; Ellis et al. 2013).

The adolescent and young adult (AYA) population accounts for approximately 11 000 deaths per year due to life-threatening conditions. During this developmental stage, the AYA focuses on autonomy and identity development as they prepare for a more independent life. They understand all the key concepts of death and dying, have opinions and want their goals, values, and beliefs to be heard. In order to respect their decisions and to foster a sense of control, advance care planning should be offered (Zadeh et al. 2015). In order to facilitate these discussions, the Voicing My Choices advance care planning guide has been developed and validated.

Education and Advocacy

While PPC programs are developing in major hospitals, there are few formal professional educational programs preparing healthcare providers for this work. Incorporating pediatric palliative content and experience into curricula in graduate nursing and medical programs and creating opportunities for shared learning will enhance an appreciation for team work in this area. PPC does not belong to one specialty! To counter the impression that PPC is offered when nothing more can be done, both education and information on advocacy are needed for healthcare providers and for the public. National efforts are needed to increase awareness and to improve the current healthcare professionals formal training in palliative care. By establishing workforce palliative and hospice training programs, the need for palliative care may be met by adequately trained professionals.

Case Management

As the interdisciplinary approach has become increasingly recognized as a key standard of PPC, it has also generated a need for a delivery model that can facilitate care coordination for the seriously ill child and his family. One role that is gaining increasing recognition as an effective facilitator of these services is that of *patient navigator* (PN). The PN concept was originally introduced by Freeman and colleagues in the early 1990s to improve access to healthcare for vulnerable populations whose cancer screening results indicated the need for follow-up diagnostic services (Freeman et al. 1995). As this service delivery model has grown over the years, the primary goal of the PN role evolved to simplify access to care. Thus, responsibilities typically consisted of identifying gaps in needed services and locating appropriate information, resources, and education to fill these gaps, especially with groups of patients with complex, chronic health conditions. Other crucial responsibilities frequently assumed by the PN include conducting patient needs assessments, providing education and treatment support, serving as liaison with other care providers throughout the illness trajectory, and assisting patients in navigating the healthcare system to access needed care and resources (Rollins et al. 2019). Effective PNs must have a range of core competencies and skills, including that of an expert communicator and educator who is extremely knowledgeable about the system in which the patient is seeking care. As this care delivery role has continued to expand over the years, a diverse range of individuals fulfills this function, including nurses, social workers, peer supporters, and specially trained community members (Rollins et al. 2019).

End-of-life Care

Close to the end of life, advanced care planning of the family may guide overarching decisions. However, immediate, day-to-day decisions will have to be made, which may involve withdrawal or withholding of medically provided hydration and nutrition and the stoppage of procedures causing pain and discomfort. Careful review of all medications and treatments for benefits or burdens should occur frequently and all therapies that no longer provide benefit and are burdensome should be discontinued. Within the context of the palliative care partnership with child and family, decisions are made about pain and symptom relief, presence of family members and staff, the granting of special wishes, and even preferred location of death.

Grief and Bereavement

Arnold and Gemma (2008, 1994) note that the death of a child affects all members of a family and the system itself, causing significant alterations in structures and roles. Death of a child member becomes an essential identifying piece of information about a family. It is woven into its history while affecting day-to-day functioning of the family. Parents are forever parents of their dead child. Grief for their child who has died becomes an abiding connection between parents and child (Arnold et al. 2005). While parental grief is experienced universally, the manifestations in ritual and behavior are family and culture bound (Gemma and Arnold 2002).

When a child dies, parents lose a part of themselves, leaving an empty space that can never be filled. In addition, parents lose the separate person their child was to become, their connection to the future, the embodiment

of their hopes and dreams. Parental grief is profound and lifelong regardless of the age of the child, the cause of death, and the years since death (Arnold et al. 2005). Grieving is a process through which parents learn to live without their child, and with that specific emptiness in their lives.

While the family's grief is lifelong, their acute pain lessens. Birthdays, special holidays, and anniversaries will reactivate sharp feelings of grief. For some families whose children have suffered greatly, there may be a sense of relief that the child's pain is no more. Families whose children have been cared for in hospitals and residential hospice programs may experience as well the sadness of losing a network of caregivers. Bereavement follow-up for families becomes an essential component of pediatric palliative and end-of-life care. Good bereavement care for families requires a multidisciplinary approach that guides the grieving family from hospital/hospice to home/community providing support, linkages, and referrals as necessary. A small model program developed by one of the authors in conjunction with the nursing and social work leadership staff of a large urban hospital with maternal child, neonatal, and pediatric services is described:

1. Bereavement care begins in hospital with nursing, social work, and pastoral care providing comfort, requested rituals at end of life, and information about funeral services and cremation. A designated social worker refers the bereaved family to the APRN bereavement consultant.
2. The APRN contacts family by phone at home, assessing each member of the family, providing comfort and information, and presenting resources for support and ongoing care. Phone calls are repeated at the family's request. The APRN invites parents (and grandparents) to a monthly parent support group that she leads. If the family requests additional counseling or psychiatric treatment, referral is made to a psychiatric nurse practitioner or a licensed family therapist, both of whom are experienced caring for grieving families.
3. A parent support group is held monthly in a community space in close proximity to the hospital.
4. Bereaved families are invited to attend an annual memorial service where they may share memories of their children and affix leaves with their children's names to a tree of life.
5. The bereavement committee composed of nursing and social work leadership meets quarterly to evaluate the program and plan the memorial service.

Cacciatore et al. (2019) notes that families cited the importance of compassion in healthcare providers who are with them during a child's terminal illness, from diagnosis until death. This compassion was expressed in many ways, including warmth, shared decision making, open communication, and flexibility.

For families, there is no such thing as a good child death. However, there is compassionate and informed PPC that guides the bereft family through their intense grief to a place where they can live with their loss and continue to grow. Arnold and Gemma (2008) note that bereft parents live without their dead child in a new and transformed reality.

Compassion Fatigue

Nurses caring for dying children are exposed to highly stressful and emotional situations involving children and their families. Practicing in the field of PPC requires complex knowledge, competencies, and the ability to engage in courageous advocacy (Merk 2018). These professionals must also be skilled in sustaining relationships, as the needs of children with life-limiting and life-threatening illness and their families often extend over protracted periods of time. As the longevity of some children has increased, so has the probability for health professionals experiencing protracted exposure to the distressing symptoms and suffering which threaten the identity of these children and families. These factors can generate a high level of stress and dysfunctional behavior in the professional who is not vigilant about meeting his/he needs for self-care. "Compassion fatigue" is a term first coined by Figley in 1995 to describe the inability of an individual to maintain physical and/or emotional homeostasis because of the stress resulting from helping a suffering person. During his work with trauma victims, Figley observed that health professionals who witnessed and absorbed the distressing symptoms and suffering of trauma patients sometimes experienced a type of secondary traumatic stress themselves, "resulting from helping or wanting to help a traumatized or suffering person" (p. 7). Previously, this emotional cost of caring had been described by a variety of terms, such as "burnout" and "caregiver stress." Figley (1995) also noticed that the amount of stress experienced by helping professionals was relative to the level of proximity, intensity, and duration of their exposure to the patient's distress. Health professionals who regularly witness the suffering experienced by ill children and their families are clearly at risk for experiencing compassion fatigue (Merk 2018).

The most effective tool for preventing compassion fatigue in pediatric health professionals is the ability to regularly engage in self-assessment and self-recognition of increased risk factors. It is crucial to educate providers to identify signs and symptoms of physical or emotional distress in themselves before it begins to interfere with their ability to give care. Symptoms associated with compassion fatigue include a range of physical, emotional, and spiritual warning signs, such as anxiety, sleep disturbances, irritability, anger, depression, hopelessness, anorexia, headaches, substance abuse, and feelings of general emotional and physical exhaustion. These symptoms can emerge from absorbing the problems and suffering of others (Merk 2018). Compassion fatigue can influence the health professional's personal relationships, social networks, and other aspects of their life.

Self-awareness and early recognition of the signs and symptoms of compassion fatigue are the keys to prevention or early detection of its occurrence, so that the health professional can continue to assist patients in relieving their symptom burden. Some interventions that can foster self-awareness include journaling or organizing and participating in a well-facilitated peer group where sharing personal experiences and stories is encouraged in a safe and supportive atmosphere. Identifying a mentor who is a good listener and with whom there exists an inner "connection" provides an objective observer who can serve as an early warning system when there are perceived behaviors or symptoms that may indicate compassion fatigue. Other aspects of a "self-care plan" that are recognized to prevent or alleviate compassion fatigue include arranging for regular, personal time to enjoy pleasurable activities, such as listening to preferred music, reading a favorite author, and engaging in recreational and leisure activities. Consistently meeting the body's physiologic requirements for balance in nutrition, exercise, and rest promotes both physical health and emotional wellbeing, both of which are crucial for maintaining a level of health that allows provision of compassionate, effective care to others.

Finally, the APRN should also be alert to signs that professional colleagues also may be experiencing compassion fatigue and be prepared to offer support and referral for assistance. The Resource section at the end of this chapter provides information on organizations where health professionals can find support to prevent or treat compassion fatigue.

Future Directions

Clinicians who care for children with serious illnesses need systematic processes and structures to provide quality PPC. Integration of palliative care into pediatric practice requires specific strategies focusing on clinical practice and care delivery models, professional education, research, and policy reform.

The provision of PPC has been integrated into many tertiary pediatric centers across the United States but is still insufficient to meet the needs of children and families. Similarly, there are more hospices providing care to pediatric patients and their families yet access is still limited. A recent survey conducted by the National Hospice and Palliative Care Organization (NHPCO) revealed that less than 14% of hospices accept pediatric patients (Friebert and Williams 2015).

The National Hospice and Palliative Care Coalition published Clinical Practice Guidelines for Quality Palliative Care which provide guidelines for the structure and process of providing adult and PPC (2018). Similarly, Standards for Pediatric Palliative and Hospice Care have been updated to provide guidance to those who work to improve the lives of children living with life-threatening conditions (NHPCO 2019). These standards provide the basis for designing PPC programs and care provision nationwide. Further development of standards for integrating palliative care into specific populations is ongoing (Wheaver et al. 2015).

Healthcare professionals face unique challenges when caring for dying children and their families. In particular, healthcare professionals may not have the requisite knowledge and skills to provide care in an ethically grounded and clinically competent manner (IOM 2003; Solomon et al. 2005). Although education in this area is improving, studies documenting the effectiveness of specific models and content are sparse. Innovative curricula have been developed for PPC. Two focus on essential content, while providing structure and process: (i) the Pediatric End of Life Nursing Education Consortium (ELNEC) provides extensive outlines and slide content that reflect key elements of PPC nursing and (ii) the ChiPPS offers essential resources and references for PPC. The Initiative for Pediatric Palliative Care (IPPC) is an interdisciplinary model; it provides a holistic framework for family-centered pediatric care that engages parents as co-facilitators of the process. The IPPC curriculum includes facilitation guides, videos, and educational models designed to facilitate individual and interdisciplinary learning and to serve as a vehicle for cultural transformation. A recent addition is the Education in Palliative and End-of-Life Care (EPEC) Pediatrics curriculum. Based on the adult core version of education for the physician, the EPEC-Pediatrics curriculum adaptation captures the needs of children with serious illness, their families, and their providers (Widger et al. 2018). This distance learning model is appropriate for the advance practice provider, physician, and other interdisciplinary team members.

Innovative models of teaching and learning must be evaluated and disseminated. To capture the depth of impact of these methods, novel models for evaluating the impact on healthcare professionals and their patients and families will need to be devised. Interdisciplinary research teams including parents can be instrumental in utilizing, evaluating, and disseminating family-centered, experiential palliative care curricula such as IPPC. Educational programs that offer interdisciplinary teams the opportunity to reflect on their experiences in caring for dying children and their families and to assess the effect of providing this care on their own emotional and spiritual wellbeing and quality of care are particularly promising. Collaborative research models are necessary to assess adequately the impact of these interventions on important individual and patient/family outcomes.

Similar to other areas of PPC research, interventions should be developed with preliminary data supporting their efficacy before being subjected to randomized trials. A particular challenge is to identify outcome measures that authentically reflect the lived experience of both patients and families and healthcare professionals and are able to capture the complex interplay of intellectual, emotional, and spiritual dynamics.

Anticipating the possibility of dying for children living with life-threatening conditions continues to be challenging. Researchers have begun to develop methods for earlier integration of palliative care processes and interventions and to evaluate the impact of these interventions on key areas such as earlier pain and symptom management, ongoing communication about goals of care, advance care planning, quality of life, and holistic emotional, psychosocial, and spiritual support (Zadeh et al. 2015). Researchers have evaluated the early integration of PPC in the oncology and hematopoietic stem cell transplant population (Lafond et al. 2015). Further studies examining more pediatric-specific populations, such as children with neuromuscular disorders or genetic disease, are needed. Initial findings reveal interest and satisfaction with early introduction of palliative care for families of children with CCC (Liberman et al. 2016). As children with CCC are often medically fragile and tend to be resource intensive, early integration of PPC can be beneficial in facilitating ongoing advance care planning, assessment, and reassessment of goals of care, and aggressive management of bothersome symptoms (Liberman et al. 2016).

Summary

This chapter presented PPC both as a philosophy of care and as a structured system for delivering services that focus on children and families whose conditions and diseases may not be cured and who face potentially shortened lives. There is no greater opportunity for

APRNs in primary care pediatrics and child psychiatry to collaborate than in the care of the chronically ill and dying child or adolescent. The APRNs' shared valuing of the unit of care is the child and family, and their commitment to continuing care from time of diagnosis to end of life and beyond for the family forges potential for rich and satisfying collaboration. Recognizing that each brings unique perspective to the table, APRNs are challenged to find ways to contribute to the wholeness of PPC by promoting innovative clinical practice, integration into the clinical care team, and participating in educational and research initiatives.

Resources

Family Resources

Family Voices. A national grassroots network of families and friends speaking on behalf of children with special care needs. www.familyvoices.org.

The Compassionate Friends. An international support organization for families who have experienced death of a child. www.compassionatefriends.org.

Courageous Parents Network. A national organization designed to support, guide, and strengthen parents of children with serious illness. www.courageousparentsnetwork.org.

Candlelighters' American Childhood Cancer Foundation (ACCF). This organization was formed in 1970 to provide support and information to families experiencing childhood cancer. It also advocates for children facing this disease and supports research related to childhood cancer. www.candlelighters.org.

Americans for Better Care of the Dying (ABCD). This organization is dedicated to ensuring that all Americans can count on good, end-of-life care. The mission of ABCD is to build momentum for reform, explore new methods and systems for delivering care, and shape public policy through evidence-based understanding. http://www.abcd-caring.org.

Kidsaid: 2 Kids, 4 Kids, By Kids. This is a site for children and teen grief support, including "kid-to-kid" grief support that is administered by a clinical psychologist who is a certified traumatologist. www.kidsaid.com.

Now I Lay Me Down to Sleep. This organization provides remembrance photography to parents suffering the loss of a child, with the free gift of professional portraiture. The volunteer professional photographers who participate in this program believe that these images serve as an important step in a family's healing process by honoring their child's legacy. www.nowilaymedowntosleep.org.

Make a Wish Foundation of America. The mission of this organization is to grant wishes of children with life-threatening medical conditions to enrich the human experience with hope, strength, and joy. www.wish.org.

Professional Resources

The IPPC. The goal of this organization is to enhance family-centered care for children living with life-threatening conditions through education, research, and quality improvement. www.ippcweb.org.

Education in Palliative and End-of-Life Care (EPEC). A comprehensive program to educate healthcare professionals on effective palliative care. Originally developed in 1997, a pediatric version was launched in 2013. http://www.bioethics.northwestern.edu/programs/epec.

Children's Hospice International (CHI). The mission of this organization is to ingrain the hospice concept of care into healthcare for children so it is considered an integral part of pediatric healthcare, rather than a separate specialty. www.chionline.org.

Children's Project on Palliative and Hospice Services (ChiPPS). This organization is a division of the National Hospice and Palliative Care Organization and works to enhance the science and practice of pediatric hospice and palliative care and to increase the availability of state-of-the-art services for families. www.nhpco.org.

National Coalition for Hospice and Palliative Care. *Clinical Practice Guidelines for Quality Palliative Care*, 4th edition. Richmond, VA: National Coalition for Hospice and Palliative Care 2018. https://www.nationalcoalitionhpc.org/ncp.

National Hospice and Palliative Care Organization (NHPCO). This is the largest nonprofit membership organization representing hospice and palliative care programs and professionals in the United States. The organization is committed to improving end-of-life care and expanding access to hospice care with the goal of profoundly enhancing quality of life for people dying in America and their loved ones. www.nhpco.org.

Hospice and Palliative Nurses Association (HPNA). A collaborative, professional hospice and palliative specialty nursing organization that utilizes evidence-based educational tools to assist members to deliver evidence-based care to palliative and hospice care patients. www.hpna.org.

American Society for Pain Management Nursing (ASPMN). The ASPMNs mission is to advance and promote optimal nursing care for people affected by pain by promoting best nursing practice, through education, standards, advocacy, and research. www.aspmn.org.

Association of Pediatric Hematology/Oncology Nurses (APHON). APHON provides and promotes expert practice in pediatric hematology/oncology nursing to its members and the public at large. www.aphon.org.

Center to Advance Palliative Care (CAPC). The CAPC provides healthcare professionals with the tools, training, and technical assistance necessary to start and sustain successful palliative care programs in hospitals and other healthcare settings. CAPC is a national organization dedicated to increasing the availability of quality palliative care services for people facing serious illness. http://wwww.capc.org.

Children's Hospice and Palliative Care Coalition. This advocacy organization works with hospitals and community organizations to improve PPC by promoting compassionate, all-inclusive medical treatment. www.childrenshospice.org.

International Children's Palliative Care Network. An international resource providing information about PPC services for fundraisers, professionals, caregivers, and families to raise the profile of children's palliative care while fostering an awareness of the worldwide need for children's palliative care services. www.icpcn.org.

Social Work Hospice and Palliative Care Network. www. HYPERLINK "http://swhpn.org/" http://swhpn.org

References

Accreditation Council of Graduate Medical Education. (2018). *Hospice and Palliative Medicine (Multidisciplinary) Programs Academic Year 2018–2019*. Available at https://apps.acgme.org/ads/public.

American Academy of Pediatrics. (2000). www.aap.org.

American Academy of Pediatrics. (2008). www.aap.org.

American Academy of Pediatrics Council on School Health & Committee on Bioethics (2010). Honoring do-not-attempt resuscitation requests in schools. *Pediatrics* 125 (5): 1073–1077. https://doi.org/10.1542/peds.2010-0452.

Arnold, J.H. and Gemma, P.B. (1994). *A Child Dies: A Portrait of Family Grief*. Philadelphia: Charles Press.

Arnold, J.H. and Gemma, P.B. (2008). The continuing process of parental grief. *Death Studies* 32: 658–673.

Arnold, J.H., Gemma, P.B., and Cushman, L.F. (2005). Exploring parental grief: combining quantitative and qualitative measures. *Archives of Psychiatric Nursing* 19 (6): 245–255.

Bluebond-Langner, M.B., Belasco, J.B., and Wander, M.D. (2010). "I want to live, until I don't want to live anymore": involving children with life-threatening and life-shortening illnesses in decision making about care and treatment. *Nursing Clinics of North America* 45 (3): 329–343.

Bogetz, J.F. and Friebert, S. (2017). Defining success of pediatric palliative care while tackling the the quadruple aim. *Journal of Palliative Medicine* 20: 116–119. https://doi.org/10.1089/jpm.2016.0389.

Brenneis, C. and Brown, P. (2007). International models of excellence. In: *Textbook of Palliative Nursing*, 2e (eds. B.T. Ferrell and N. Coyle). Oxford: Oxford University Press.

Bugge, K.E., Darbyshire, P., Rokholt, E.G. et al. (2014). Young children's grief: parents' understanding and coping. *Death Studies* 38: 36–43.

Cacciatore, J., Thieleman, K., Lieber, A.S. et al. (2019). The long road to farewell: the needs of families with dying children. *OMEGA-Journal of Death and Dying* 78: 404–420. https://doi.org/10.1177/0030222817697418.

Corr, C., Torkildson, C., & Horgan, M. (2010, May). Pediatric hospice and palliative care in the United States: The current state of the art. *ChiPPS E-News*. Available at http://www.nhpco.org/files/public/ChiPPS/ChiPPS_enews-19_May_2010.pdf.

Davies, B., Contro, N., Larson, J., and Widger, K. (2010). Culturally-sensitive information-sharing in pediatric palliative care. *Pediatrics* 125 (4): e859–e865.

DeCourcey, D.D., Silverman, M., Oladunjoye, A., and Wolfe, J. (2018). Advance care planning and parent-reported end-of-life outcomes in children, adolescents, and young adults with complex chronic conditions. *Critical Care Medicine* 47: 101–108. https://doi.org/10.1097/CCM.0000000000003472.

DeCourcey, D.D., Silverman, M., Oladunjoye, A. et al. (2018). Patterns of Care at the End of Life for Children and Young Adults with Life-Threatening Complex Chronic Conditions. *Journal of Pediatrics* 193: 196–203. E2. doi: https://doi.org/10.1016/j.jpeds.2017.09.078.

Eilegard, A., Steineck, G., Nybert, T., and Kreicbergs, U. (2013). Psychological health in siblings who lost a brother or sister to cancer 2 to 9 years earlier. *Psycho-Oncology* 22: 683–691. https://doi.org/10.1002/pon.3053.

Elias, E.R. and Murphy, N.A. (2012). Home care of children and youth with complex health care needs and technology dependencies. *Pediatrics* 129 (5): 996–1005. https://doi.org/10.1542/peds.2012-0606.

Ellis, J., Dowrick, C., and Lloyd-Williams, M. (2013). The long-term impact of early parental death: lessons from a narrative study. *Journal of the Royal Society of Medicine* 106: 57–67.

Federal Interagency Forum on Child and Family Statistics (2017). www.childstats.gov. (accessed 26 October 2018).

Feudtner, C., Kang, T.I., Hexem, K.R. et al. (2011). Pediatric palliative care patients: a prospective multicenter cohort study. *Pediatrics* 127: 1094–1101.

Feudtner, C., Dai, D., Hexem, K.R. et al. (2012). Prevalence of polypharmacy exposure among hospitalized children in the United States. *Archives of Pediatric and Adolescent Medicine* 166: 9–16. https://doi.org/10.1001/archpediatrics.2011.161.

Feudtner, C., Friebert, S., and Jewell, J. (2013). Pediatric palliative care and hospice care commitments, guidelines, and reommendations. *Pediatrics* 132: 966–972. https://doi.org/10.1542/peds.2013-2731.

Feudtner, C., Womer, J., Augustin, A. et al. (2013). Pediatric palliative care programs in children's hospitals: a cross-sectional national survey. *Pediatrics* 132 (6): 1063–1070. https://doi.org/10.1542/peds.2013-1286.

Feudtner, C., Walter, J.K., Faerber, J.A. et al. (2015). Good – parent beliefs of parents of seriously ill children. *JAMA Pediatr.* 169: 39–47. https://doi.org/10.1001/jamapediatrics.2014.2341.

Figley, G. (ed.) (1995). *Compassion Fatigue: Coping with Secondary Traumatic Stress Disorder in those Who Treat the Traumatized*. New York: Taylor & Francis Group.

Freeman, H., Muth, B., and Kerner, J. (1995). Expanding access to cancer screening and clinical follow-up among the medically underserved. *Cancer Practice* 3 (1): 19–30.

Friebert, S. (2009). *NHPCO Facts and Figures: Pediatric Palliative and Hospice Care in America*. Alexandria, VA: National Hospice and Palliative Care Association.

Friebert, S. and Williams, C. (2015). *NHPCO Facts and Figures: Pediatric Palliative and Hospice Care in America*. Alexandria, VA: National Hospice and Palliative Care Association.

Fullerton, J.M., Totsika, V., Hain, R., and Hastings, R.P. (2017). Siblings of children with life-limiting conditions: psychological adjustment and sibling relationships. *Child Care and Health Development* 43: 393–400. https://doi.org/10.1111/cch.12421.

Gemma, P.B. and Arnold, J.H. (2002). *Loss and Grieving in Pregnancy and the First Year of Life: A Caring Resource for Nurses*. New York, NY: March of Dimes.

Groh, G., Feddersen, B., Fuhrer, M., and Borasio, G.D. (2014). Specialized home palliative care for adults and children: differences and similarities. *Journal of Palliative Medicine* 17: 803–810.

Himelstein, B.P., Hilden, J.M., Boldt, A.M., and Weissman, D. (2004). Pediatric palliative care. *New England Journal of Medicine* 350 (17): 1752–1762.

Huff, S. (2010, September). *Standards of care for pediatric palliative and hospice care*. Paper presented at the District of Columbia Pediatric Palliative Care Collaboration, Washington, D.C.

Hutton, N., Levetown, M., and Frager, G. (2008). School and community issues. In: *The Hospice and Palliative Medicine Approach to Caring for Pediatric Patients* (ed. C.P. Storey), 27–28. Glenview, IL: American Academy of Hospice and Palliative Medicine.

Institute of Medicine (2003). *When Children Die: Improving Palliative and End-of-Life Care for Children and their Families*. Washington, D.C.: The National Academies Press.

Keele, L., Keenan, H.T., Sheetz, J., and Bratton, S.L. (2013). Differences in characteristics of dying children who receive and do not receive palliative care. *Pediatrics* 132 (72): 72–78. https://doi.org/10.1542/peds.2013-0470.

Kreicbergs, U., Valdimarsdottir, U., Onelov, E. et al. (2004). Talking about death with children who have severe malignant disease. *New England Journal of Medicine* 351: 1175–1186.

Kubler-Ross, E. (1983). *On Children and Death*. Touchstone: New York, NY.

Lafond, D.A., Kelly, K.P., Hinds, P.S. et al. (2015). Establishing feasibility of early palliative care consultation in pediatric hematopoietic stem cell transplantation. *Journal of Pediatric Oncology Nursing* 32: 265–277. https://doi.org/10.1177/1043454214563411.

Levine, D.R., Johnson, L.M., Snyder, A. et al. (2016). Integrating palliative care in pediatric oncology: evidence for an evolving paradigm for comprehensive cancer care. *Journal of the National Comprehensive Cancer Network: JNCCN* 14 (6): 741–748.

Li, J., Precht, D.H., Mortensen, P.B., and Olsen, J. (2003). Mortality in parents after death of a child in Denmark: a nationwide follow-up study. *Lancet* 361 (9355): 363–367.

Liberman, D.B., Song, E., Radbill, L.M. et al. (2016). Early integration of palliative care and advanced care planning for children with complex chronic medical conditions: a pilot study. *Child: care, health, and development* 42 (3): 439–449.

Meadors, P. and Lamson, A. (2007). Compassion fatigue and secondary traumatization: provider self care on intensive care units for children. *Journal of Pediatric Health Care* 22 (1): 24–34.

Merk, T. (2018). Compassion fatigue, compassion satisfaction & burnout among pediatric nurses: 2018 air medical transport conference scientific Assemby abstracts. *Air Medical Journal* 37: 281–298. https://doi.org/10.1016/j.amj.2018.07.020.

Morgan, D. (2009). Caring for dying children: assessing the needs of the pediatric palliative care nurse. *Pediatric Nursing* 35 (2): 86–91.

National Consensus Project for Hospice and Palliative Care (2018). *Clinical Practice Guidelines for Quality Palliative Care*, 4e. Richmond, VA: National Consensus Project for Hospice and Palliative Care Available at https://www.nationalcoalitionhpc.org/ncp.

National Education Association. (2000). *Providing safe health care: The role of educational support personnel.* Available at http://www.nea. org/home/20779.htm.

NHPCO (2019). *Updated Standards for Practice for Pediatric Palliative Care.* National Hospice and Palliative Care Organization Available at www.nhpco.org.

Rollins, M., Milone, F., Suleman, S. et al. (2019). *Paediatrics & Child Health* 24: 19–22. https://doi.org/10.1093/pch/pxy057.

Rushton, C.H. (2010). Pediatric palliative care: coming of age. *Innovations in End-of-Life Care* 2 (2) Available at http://www.edc. org/lastacts.

Russell, C.E., Widger, K., Beaune, L. et al. (2018). Siblings' voices: a prospective investigation of experiences with a dying child. *Death Studies* 42: 184–194. https://doi.org/10.1080/07481187.2017.1334009.

Sanders, C. (1980). A comparison of adult bereavement in the death of a spouse, child, and parent. *Omega* 10: 303–322.

Selekman, J. and Vessey, J. (2010). School and the child with a chronic condition. In: *Primary Care of the Child with a Chronic Condition*, 5e (eds. P. Allen, J. Vessey and N. Shapiro), 42–59. St. Louis: Mosby-Elsevier.

Shepard, A. and Sheldon, L.K. (2010). Moral distress: a consequence of caring. *Clinical J of Oncology Nursing* 14 (1): 25–27.

Solomon, M.Z., Sellers, D.E., Heller, K.S. et al. (2005). New and lingering controversies in pediatric end-of-life care. *Pediatrics* 116: 872–883.

Sourkes, B.M. (1995). *Armfuls of Time.* Pittsburgh: University of Pittsburgh Press.

Thrane, S.E., Maurer, S.H., Cohen, S.M. et al. (2017). Pediatric palliative care: A five-year retrospective chart review study. *Journal of Palliative Medicine* 20: 1104–1111. https://doi.org/10.1089/jpm.2017.0038.

Torkildson, C. (2010, May). Models of pediatric hospice and palliative care in the United States. *ChiPPS E-News* 19: 4–8. Available at http://www.nhpco.org/files/public/ChiPPS/ChiPPS_enews-19_May_2010.pdf.

Trafford, A. (2002). Second opinion: Medical orphans. *The Washington Post*, 6 August, pp. F1–7.

University of Rochester Medical Center. Health Encyclopedia. (n.d.) *A child's concept of death.* Available at https://www.urmc.rochester.edu/encyclopedia/content/aspx?ContentTypeID=90&ContentID=P03044 (accessed 3 January 2019).

US Centers for Medicaid and Medicare Services (2010). *Affordable Care Act Implementation.* Available at https://www.cms.gov/CCIIO/Resources/Fact-Sheets-and-FAQs/aca_implementation_faqs.

Van Cleave, J. and Davis, J. (2006). Bullying and peer victimization among children with special needs. *Pediatrics* 118 (4): e1212–e1219. https://doi.org/10.1542/peds.2005-3034.

Vanclooster, S., Benoot, C., Bilsen, J. et al. (2018). Stakeholders' perspectives on communication and collaboration following school reintegration of a seriously ill child: a literature review. *Child Youth Care Forum* 47: 583–612. https://doi.org/10.1007/s10566-018-9443-4.

Wheaver, M.S., Heinze, K.E., Kelly, K.P. et al. (2015). Palliative care as a standard of care in pediatric oncology. *Pediatric Blood Cancers* 62: S829–S833.

Widger, K., Wolfe, J., Friedrichsdorf, S. et al. (2018). National impact of the EPEC-pediatrics enhanced train-the-trainer model for delivering education on pediatric palliative care. *Journal of Palliative Medicine* 21 (9): 1249–1256. https://doi.org/10.1089/jpm.2017.0532.

Wright, R. (2004). Compassion fatigue: how to avoid it. *Palliative Medicine* 18: 3–4.

Zadeh, S., Pao, M., and Wiener, L. (2015). Opening end-of-life discussions: how to introduce voicing my CHOICES˜, an advance care planning guide for adolescents and young adults. *Palliative Supportive Care* 13 (3): 591–599.

27

Collaborative Treatment with Primary Care

Madeleine M. Lloyd and Jamesetta A. Newland

Rory Meyers College of Nursing, New York University, New York, NY, USA

Objectives

After reading this chapter, advanced practice registered nurses will be able to:

1. Define the concept of collaborative treatment within the context of meeting the behavioral and primary care health needs of children and adolescents.
2. Discuss evidenced-based models of collaborative care.
3. Describe roles of team members of an interprofessional team in primary care.
4. Recognize facilitators and barriers to implementing collaborative treatment models.

Introduction

The global burden of mental illness has significantly increased over the past two decades and continues to challenge health delivery systems to provide adequate mental health services across all age groups (Ion et al. 2017). Depression is the leading cause of disability worldwide, and youth suicide is the second leading cause of death for children and adolescents worldwide (World Health Organization [WHO] 2017). In 2016 alone, more than 6000 youth in the United States under the age of 25 years died by suicide, and suicide among children ages 10–14 years surpassed deaths from motor vehicle accidents (Centers for Disease Control and Prevention [CDC] 2016). Studies have found that most of the youth who died by suicide visited a healthcare provider or medical setting in the month prior to killing themselves (National Institute of Mental Health [NIMH] 2018). Mental health problems affect one in five US children

and adolescents, with 50% developing symptoms or behaviors by 14 years of age (Campo et al. 2018). Primary care providers (PCPs) play a significant role in reducing this global burden in responding to, identifying, and managing the mental health needs of children and adolescents (WHO 2017).

In the United States, challenges exist for providing high-quality mental healthcare services mainly arising from the fragmentation of medical care and mental healthcare, a shortage of mental health providers, lack of financial incentives, and a lack of access to mental health services. This shortage of mental health providers since the 1980s has resulted in the need for PCPs to manage many psychiatric disorders (American Academy of Family Physicians [AAFP] 2018; Benarous et al. 2019; Laderman and Mate 2014). Children and adolescents traditionally access medical healthcare services through a PCP, who is a pediatric nurse practitioner or family

---

Child and Adolescent Behavioral Health: A Resource for Advanced Practice Psychiatric and Primary Care Practitioners in Nursing, Second Edition. Edited by Edilma L. Yearwood, Geraldine S. Pearson, and Jamesetta A. Newland.
© 2021 John Wiley & Sons, Inc. Published 2021 by John Wiley & Sons, Inc.
Companion website: www.wiley.com/go/Yearwood

nurse practitioner (PNP/FNP), a family physician, or a pediatrician. Services for behavioral health (BH) care needs, alternatively, can be provided by the PCP but might more appropriately be delivered by a psychiatric mental health (PMH) specialist, such as a PMH advanced practice registered nurse (APRN), psychologist, social worker, psychiatrist, or other person trained to manage the BH and mental health needs of children and adolescents.

During the past 15 years, mental health emergency room visits for pediatric patients have increased 47% and the American Academy of Pediatrics (AAP) and the American Academy of Child & Adolescent Psychiatry (AACAP) reported that only 20–25% of these children received treatment (Tyler et al. 2017). This may be due to the fact that most care for children with BH disorders is referred to outside BH professionals, creating a dilemma because of the current shortage of mental health specialists, with approximately one child and adolescent psychiatrist per 15 000 US youths (Ghandour et al. 2019). To improve these statistics, collaborative care models (CCMs) with co-located primary care (PC) and BH professionals aim to reframe care as unified. In pediatrics, treatment outcomes for common BH diagnoses such as attention deficit hyperactivity disorder (ADHD), anxiety, and depression, have been shown to be effective when located under one roof with PC.

Despite the critical role of PCPs to provide more evidence-based mental healthcare, making this happen presents formidable challenges and only about one-third of adolescents with diagnosable behavioral disorders receive the appropriate care (Richardson et al. 2017). PCPs vary widely in their interests, commitment, confidence, and, most importantly, education and training in evaluating and treating mental health disorders. However, two-thirds of PCPs are unable to connect their patients to outpatient mental health services, resulting in the need for them to assume the lead in the management of mental healthcare services. In addition, PCPs serve as primary managers of psychiatric disorders in one-third of their patient panels and two-thirds of patients with depression (AAFP 2018).

Given the prevalence of BH disorders, pediatric and family clinical settings are important arenas for early identification and treatment of childhood mental and behavioral and developmental disorders, as this is often the first point of professional contact for children and their families during times of distress (Bitsko et al. 2016). Commonly, pediatric illness visits in the United States are BH related, including mental health and substance use disorders, placing a considerable demand on PCPs' ability to screen all patients for BH illness and manage them appropriately. Behavioral disorders are associated with risky sexual activity, unwanted pregnancy, higher rates of injury, and low educational and work achievement (Richardson et al. 2017). Early identification, initial management, and referral for further mental health assessment and treatment promotes healthier developmental trajectories for all children, especially those living in poverty, in rural areas, and/or who have reduced access to care. An analysis by McDermott et al. (2018) indicated that the sixth most common reason for pediatric emergency room visits was mental and BH conditions. Respiratory disorders and injury and poisoning were the two most common reasons. Therefore, collaborative models that integrate mental health into PC pediatric settings offer opportunities to provide families and children with improved coordination and delivery of BH services (Agency for Healthcare Quality and Research [AHQR] 2019; Campo et al. 2018; Olfson 2016). These approaches to PC have empirically supported models which improve access to care, improve clinical outcomes, and reduce costs (Asarnow et al. 2015; Ion et al. 2017; Vanderlip et al. 2016).

This chapter will present background information and discussion of issues in providing integrated BH and PC services through collaborative treatment models. The most common and researched collaborative and integrated practice models are presented. The team members of an interprofessional team are described. Barriers and facilitators to successful integration of BH and PC are reviewed.

Models of Collaborative Care Delivering Mental Healthcare to PC Patients

Since the passage of the Paul Wellstone and Pete Domenici Mental Health Parity and Addiction Equity Act of 2008 and the Patient Protection and Affordable Care Act (ACA) of 2010, the delivery of healthcare services to children and adolescents has changed and new opportunities for the delivery of BH within PC have been created within the US healthcare system (AACAP 2013; Institute of Medicine 2006; Tyler et al. 2017; WHO and World Organization of Family Doctors 2008). As a result of the ACA, all state Medicaid programs require basic coverage of mental healthcare as an essential service, and approximately 30 million more Americans, many with mental health disorders, gained access to insurance coverage (Olfson 2016). Of these, 8 million were children and adolescents, which expanded the demand for youth mental health services. With this increase in access to care, existing models of PC delivery systems have been challenged to expand the involvement of primary care clinicians (PCCs) in the delivery of mental healthcare. In turn, this has generated the development and dissemination of CCM for enhancing the delivery of evidence-based mental health services to children and adolescent patients who present to PC settings. (Note: In a managed care system of integrated care, a PCC is the name given to the PCP. Therefore, the term PCC is used when referring to integrated models and PCP is used when referring to general or traditional models where PC and BH are not integrated.)

Models of care that integrate BH and PC align with the Institute for Healthcare Improvement (IHI) Triple Aim: *improved quality of care* with a team-based collaborative approach, *improved health of populations*, and *reduced* per capita *costs* by improving service utilization of high-cost specialty care such as mental health (Loehrer et al. 2016). Models such as patient-centered medical homes (PCMH), accountable care organizations, and health homes enable interprofessional team-based care to address whole-person care and further encourage innovation to improve BH care (an umbrella term referring to mental health and substance abuse, health behavior change, and attention to family and other psychosocial factors) (Cohen et al. 2015) and improve provider and patient satisfaction (Asarnow et al. 2015; Cohen et al. 2015; Grazier et al. 2016; Olfson 2016; Vogt and Vogt 2017).

Patient-centered Medical Homes

Between 2009 and 2013, the number of patients enrolled in a PCMH increased from 5 million to nearly 21 million. This model of care emphasizes partnerships among patients, practitioners, and their families to help ensure patient-centered health decisions. Coordinated referrals, care transitions, multidisciplinary treatment teams, registries for chronic diseases, health information technologies such as patient portals, and integrated health records for improved communication are key elements. Fee-for-service is the dominant financial arrangement within the PCMH, based on per-member-per-month payments, and pay-for-performance bonuses are common (Olfson 2016).

Accountable Care Organizations

Under an accountable care organization, hospitals, specialists, and PCCs are encouraged to integrate care for defined Medicare beneficiary groups of patients, and financial bonuses are awarded for meeting defined quality metrics or deducted if they are not met. These financial incentives promote the integration of BH services into PC for their high-cost patients with both medical and mental healthcare needs. Reduced emergency room visits and readmissions within 30 days are key for financial rewards or penalties (Vogt and Vogt 2017).

Health Home

The health home is for Medicaid beneficiaries with complex health needs that may qualify for health home services. The ACA offers 90% federal Medicaid matching funds for health home services such as social services, health promotion, and transitional care for the first 2 years. Several states use the health home Medicaid option to enhance federal support of their efforts to integrate primary health and BH for their Medicaid beneficiaries. Although states have wide flexibility to develop an implementation strategy, many Medicaid health homes are extensions of PCMH that emphasize team-based care coordinated across different provider groups (Olfson 2016).

Defining Integrated Healthcare

Various authors and groups have defined integrated healthcare (BH and PC) and components of the concept. The descriptions are similar although the terminology varies slightly (Grazier et al. 2016). Understanding the concept of integrated care is important in designing and implementing programs. Healthcare delivery falls along a continuum from complete separation on one end to total integration on the other end. Currently consensus of terms such as "integrated behavioral health", "collaborative care", "mental health integration," and "integrated primary care," which are often used interchangeably, is important as models of collaboration are explored, created, defined, and researched. The AHQR-funded Peek and the National Integration Academy Council in 2013 published an evolving lexicon for BH and PC integration for improved communication to stakeholders, especially concerning research, practice, measurement, and development across clinical settings.

The IHI (2014) researched the core principles underlying several successful approaches to integration around the United States (including Improving Mood – Providing Access to Collaborative Treatment [IMPACT], Intermountain Healthcare, Southcentral Foundation, and Cherokee Health Systems) and determined that, although there is a perception that there are many different ways to implement integrated BH care, the commonalities among approaches are far greater than the differences, indicating that BH integration can be operationalized in a variety of ways and still be successful (Zallman et al. 2017). Additionally, integration of BH and PC has been shown to improve PCC knowledge and provider experience and improve barriers to care (Zallman et al. 2017).

The AHQR published a guidebook to assist PC and BH in identifying professional practices for developing a workforce for integrated care (Cohen et al. 2015).

Successful integrative health models within the Veterans Health Administration and Federally Qualified Health Centers have shown increased access to BH services, reduced stigma related to receiving BH services, increased patient satisfaction, and improved clinical outcomes. A Cochrane review of collaborative care trials of adult patients with depression and anxiety found significant improvements in clinical outcomes, as well as improvements in medication use and patient satisfaction across the 79 studies reviewed (Archer et al. 2012). Another meta-analysis found that collaborative chronic care models improved both medical and BH outcomes for individuals with BH disorders across different populations and settings. Quality of life for the mental health component significantly improved in a 3-year follow-up compared to standard group care (Reilly et al. 2013). Several studies of the IMPACT program have shown positive effects on integrated medical and BH outcomes and costs. Patients with comorbid diabetes and depression receiving care through IMPACT experienced 115 more depression-free days over 24 months when compared to patients in the usual care group (Archer et al. 2012; Richardson et al. 2017).

Similar to adult trials, the first systematic meta-analysis of randomized clinical trials evaluating integrated PC and behavioral care for children and adolescents found significant but modest benefits in outcomes for improved health outcomes and a greater number of treatment interventions that targeted mental health problems than usual PC (Asarnow et al. 2015). In pediatric BH integration studies that applied collaborative care interventions, integrated care demonstrated the most robust and positive effects on mental health outcomes in PC settings (Campo et al. 2018).

Models of Integrated Care Delivery

Models for structuring the PC management of mental health problems vary in complexity, required resources and barriers to integration with established clinic routines. Models of collaboration and the level of integration are multifaceted and depend on practice needs and feasibility. Three different general models of providing specialized mental health services to PC patients fall along a continuum toward fully integrated mental healthcare (Blount 2003; Collins et al. 2010; Richardson et al. 2017; Vogt and Vogt 2017).

Coordinated Care

Coordinated care models involve the least amount of collaboration but are probably the most common approach and the most researched among adolescents and young adults. When a patient in a PC practice is identified with mental health needs, a referral is made to an off-site mental health specialist for the duration of treatment. Reliance on off-site specialists to manage the patient may be inefficient, with often long wait times and transportation problems for patients. Under such coordinated care arrangements, there is variation in the extent to which PCPs and mental health specialists communicate about patients in their shared caseloads, including no record sharing (Gerrity 2014; Richardson et al. 2017).

Co-located Care

In a co-located model, patients and their families may be offered on-site mental health specialists to simplify the referral system and have easier and/or faster access to mental health services than patients served in practices that refer to off-site mental health specialists. In some practices with collocated PCCs and BH specialists, staff members share the same treatment facility, but they practice within separate cultures and develop distinct treatment plans for the same patient. In other practices, there is sharing of patient records and more direct clinical interactions between the PCCs and BH specialists. Sharing location does not necessarily mean that there will be collaboration. A mutually agreed means of communication may improve collaboration (Richardson et al. 2017; Vogt and Vogt 2017).

Integrated Care

In integrated models, there is close collaboration between PCCs and BH specialists. While providing the highest level of integration, this model involves the greatest amount of practice change for fuller collaboration. Both specialty providers develop and implement collaborative treatment plans for patients. Consultation is active and ongoing, and strong relationships exist between specialties. BH teams support PCCs in caring for identified patients. Teams are often multidisciplinary and use a defined protocol and a population-based approach. The best-studied approach to integrated care is the adult CCM. Under collaborative care, simple mental health treatment protocols are established, and patients receive mental health screenings and education. A nurse practitioner or care manager is often involved in assessing symptoms and monitoring treatment adherence over time. There is also sharing of medical records to facilitate consensus on treatment plans.

Richardson et al. (2017) identified two studies of adolescent and young adults using an "integrated care" approach, which had adapted adult CCMs for the treatment of depression. Both studies showed improved outcomes and increased treatment compliance when compared to usual care. One study from a school-based clinic showed integrated interpersonal psychotherapy, which improved depression and social dysfunction with peers. Outcomes are improved with the operational integrated care model.

Models of Collaboration

Collaborative care is a specific type of integrated behavioral and physical care derived from the chronic care model. Wayne Katon and his colleagues at the University of Washington (UoW) originally developed collaborative care as an organizing framework to improve chronic illness care. Today it is the basis for many changes in care delivery and the dominant model for PCMH. Based on the assumption that improvement in care requires an approach that incorporates patients, BH professionals working in the PC arena to help PCCs manage patients with mental health problems, and system level interventions. Collaborative care aims to improve access to evidence based mental health treatments for PC patients and has been shown to be clinically effective in randomized clinical trials globally (UoW 2018).

CCMs share five core elements: (i) patient-centered team driven, (ii) population-focused, (iii) measurement guided, (iv) evidence-based, and (v) accountable. Collaborative care relies on use of a registry to monitor treatment engagement and clinical outcomes. Collaborative care utilizes patient-reported outcomes and evidence-based clinical approaches to achieve those outcomes. Providers are accountable and reimbursed not just on the number of patients seen but for quality of care and clinical outcomes (UoW 2018). Generally, collaborative care includes measurement and monitoring by a nurse, clinical social worker, and care provider from both PC and BH using a treat to target approach for improved outcomes. A systematic review of 69 random controlled trials using the CCM for depression from 2009 found that among participants antidepressant adherence doubled and depression outcomes improved, lasting 2 to 5 years. In addition, both patient satisfaction and provider satisfaction increased with treatment of depression.

Several states have improved access to care by creating offsite BH consultation services designed to help PCPs meet the needs of children with any mental health problem. The first pilot project, in 2004, was the Massachusetts Child Psychiatry Access Project (MCPAP), a statewide system of child psychiatry consultations teams, including APRNs. The program consisted of six regional hubs, each of which had one full-time-equivalent child psychiatrist, licensed therapist, and care coordinator with a dedicated hotline as the entry point for PCPs. Services included one or more of the following: immediate clinical consultation over the telephone, expedited face-to-face psychiatric consultation, care coordination for assistance with referrals to community BH services, and continuing professional education for PCPs. Every telephone consultation increased the PCP's knowledge about child psychiatry. Outcome data reported that PCPs managed 67% of the patients that they would usually refer out to a BH specialist (Straus and Sarvet 2014).

This collaborative, scalable, and cost-effective model efficiently addresses the lack of BH access for children. Child psychiatry access programs (CPAP) now exist in over 30 states, and are based on the MCPAP, providing case-based telephone consultation, training and education, and care coordination to local mental health resources. Together, these programs have formed the National Network of CPAP. This network aims to promote the development of access programs by providing a forum for participants to learn from each other, engage in collaborative research, develop standards of practice, and maintain a website (http://nncpap.org) (Straus and Sarvet 2014).

Telemedicine, the use of electronic information and communications technologies to deliver medical care, increases access to real-time healthcare. Telepsychiatry, a subset of telemedicine for the delivery of mental health services, is of growing interest in PC and is rapidly expanding (AAFP 2018). The Extension for Community Healthcare Outcomes (ECHO) project is a model which offers both mental health and substance-use treatment via remote and telehealth training and practice support for PCP, especially in rural and underserved areas. While the research is limited on this topic, there are a growing number of studies assessing the benefits, comparative effectiveness with face-to-face visits, and cost comparisons (AACAP 2017).

The shortage of mental health resources is significantly worse in the rural communities, with 80% of all rural US counties not having a single psychiatrist or subspecialist for children. Rates of substance abuse, drug overdoses, suicide, serious mental illness, and child/adolescent/young adult deaths are in general higher than in urban settings. Additionally, families often travel hundreds of miles to visit relatives in chronic mental illness facilities (Guerrero et al. 2019). The use of several telepsychiatry models has the potential to leverage scarce specialist mental health resources to reach more patients, thereby allowing these providers to have a greater population level impact compared to traditional referral models of care. The Michigan Child Collaborative Care program provides consultation to PCPs treating youths and obtains referrals from school-based PC practices in rural areas (Marcus et al. 2019).

Team Members of Interprofessional Teams in PC

One of the most urgent global challenges is the need to strengthen primary healthcare delivery systems as human resources for health are in crisis. The WHO (2010) and National Center for Interprofessional Practice and Education [NCIPE] (2019) developed a framework providing strategies to implement interprofessional collaboration in both education and practice to strengthen this system and improve health outcomes. For healthcare workers to collaborate, interprofessional education (IPE) must be provided for the development of a collaborative practice-ready healthcare work force. IPE is defined as two or more professions learning from, about, and with each other to enable effective collaboration. Increasingly, integrated care is organized by the CCM, a service innovation emphasizing care coordination, self-management support, and use of interprofessional team-based care models in which each provider practices to the top of his or her education and training.

Collaborative practice occurs when multiple healthcare workers from different professions provide comprehensive services by working with patients, families, caregivers, and their communities to deliver high-quality evidence-based care across settings. Both clinical and nonclinical support personnel are included to provide a full range of services including diagnosis, treatment, surveillance, communication, and environmental safety (WHO 2010). Despite the level of integration that exists, education about mental health and BH disorders should be provided to PCCs to improve BH care.

The CCM is a multicomponent healthcare system level intervention that utilizes case managers to systematically follow up and coordinate the integration of PCCs, patients, and mental health specialists. All team members aim to improve routine screening and diagnosis of mental health disorders, increase use of evidence-based treatment protocols for proactive management, improve clinical and community support for active patients, engage families in goal setting, and promote self-management. Team members include the following:

- The *BH care manager* coordinates the team members and ensures effective communication. This role is typically filled by a nurse, psychologist, social worker, or licensed counselor. This role includes providing assessments, brief psychosocial interventions, education, and, if needed, medication management support.
- The *patient* is at the center of this model of care and is fully involved at all stages of care.
- The *PCC* is the clinician who takes primary responsibility for managing the patient's care. The PCC can be

the PCP if the patient's medical/physical disorder(s) are more complex and require a greater expertise for management. The PCC can be the BH specialist if the patient's mental health or BH disorder(s) are more complex conditions requiring management. Whichever specialty is the PCC, collaboration with the other specialty is expected to provide integrated care to the patient.

The Behavioral Health Specialist

Using a patient-centered, whole-person approach, PMH APRNs are educated to provide both general medical and mental healthcare across the lifespan. With this scope of practice, including an emphasis on prevention and social wellbeing, PMH APRNs are positioned well to increase the reach of the CCM and provide a critical orientation to address the mental health needs of children and adolescents, particularly within the broader socioeconomic context, such as with underserved populations and in rural areas. Each member of the CCM has a unique set of competencies which they must use to their highest scope of practice. Clear delineation of roles is essential to improve interprofessional team function and provide effective mental health services. For example, PMH APRNs are certified to provide the full scope of mental health services, including full prescription authority and therapy. These capabilities will allow them to play an important role in these teams, as state healthcare planners and health systems map out strategies to increase access to mental health services for populations and communities (Delaney 2017).

Ongoing research of outcome measures related to the patient, family, and clinician satisfaction is important. Outcomes that might be studied include the change in the quality of mental healthcare in the PC setting, reduction of emergency room visits and inpatient hospitalizations, and the dissemination of evidenced-based treatment. Individual performance might be measured by looking at the number of total encounters, psychiatric diagnoses, and treatment codes used, referrals made to mental health providers by PC, and wait time for consultations.

Interprofessional collaboration in PC is key to providing improved BH outcomes for children. Each team member from BH specialist, PCC to BH care manager needs to participate in IPE to gain an awareness of collaborative practice strategies. When interprofessional collaboration utilizes multiple healthcare workers from different professions the delivery of BH care will be strengthen and health outcomes will be improved (WHO 2010).

Facilitators and Barriers to Care

BH concerns are among the top reasons families seek care in PC medical homes. Care integration offers several advantages, including screening for BH issues and increasing access to BH care for children and adolescents in their PCMH, allowing families to work with a familiar provider and environment, promoting continuity of care. Care integration in turn reduces the risks for adverse family outcomes by the earlier identification of at-risk youth (e.g. threats to child safety, need for more intensive services or placement). With earlier identification and treatment opportunities, BH problems can be identified 2–4 years earlier, before the illness becomes more serious in the child or adolescent (Ghandour et al. 2019; Richardson et al. 2017).

Since the introduction of the Triple Aim, a fourth aim has been proposed: to improve the work life of healthcare professionals to prevent burnout and, in turn, improve population health. One way to achieve the quadruple aim is to implement CCM utilizing all team members. For example, documentation by nurses, medical assistants, and other staff has been shown to increase staff satisfaction and improve revenue (Bodenheimer and Sinsky 2014; Salyers et al. 2019).

Challenges to integrating BH and PC are similar no matter what the model: a fragmented health delivery system, cultural differences between disciplines, restrictive confidentiality laws about sharing information related to substance abuse and mental health issues, and separate payment structures. Even in areas where child psychiatry is available, access to care is limited by insurance restrictions, lack of psychological services, long delays, high cost of care, stigma, and poor communication between mental and physical health professionals (Platt et al. 2018).

Payment models for BH services are not yet available consistently across the United States for all patients. Innovative payment models are needed that address time spent in collaborative care between BH and PC professionals and other care providers, as these tasks are essential to the provision of integrated services but are often not financially incentivized in a payment system focused on face-to-face time with patients. The Medicare Physician Fee Schedule in 2017 created four new codes to allow payment to healthcare providers using the CCM (Press et al. 2017).

The findings of Ghandour et al. (2019) point toward a clear need for research and policy. First, PC settings need to consistently implement universal, standardized developmental and BH screening. Second, AAP screening guidelines should be revised to include anxiety, given the high prevalence of anxiety disorders in children and adolescents and the early onset of symptoms. Last, PCCs, in conjunction with their associated professional organizations, must advocate for increased access to BH services for their patients and for research funding to identify evidence-based alternative approaches to traditional models of care, including integrated PC models (Donohue and Aalsma 2019).

Grazier et al. (2016) identified several key categories of barriers:

1. *Vulnerable populations*: Because of the lack of culturally competent providers to treat ethnic minorities, young people with mental health disorders, in families who may not perceive a need for treatment, might wish to address the problem on their own, might be pessimistic about the effectiveness of available treatments, or might lack trust in providers of care (Campo et al. 2018). Attitudinal barriers might also exert differential effects in specific demographic, ethnic, and cultural groups and settings. For example, African American families express greater concerns about the safety of antidepressant medications than nonminority families. (Campo et al. 2018). The fear of stigma might also impede a person gaining timely access to mental health services (Mojtabai et al. 2011).

2. *Comorbidities*: Few psychiatric disorders occur singularly and many providers are faced with individuals having more than one disorder requiring intervention. Identifying the various disorders and their level of acuity while prioritizing treatment planning or referral becomes a challenge. Comorbid psychiatric and general medical illnesses commonly occur together. PCPs need to identify and assess all conditions because they may have a bidirectional adverse response to treatment and negatively impact the course of the illness. For example, the prevalence of comorbid anxiety disorders ranges from approximately 40% to 66% in youth with bipolar disorder and ADHD. Additionally, there is an increased risk of multiple medical conditions, including cardiovascular, weight concerns, neurological, and respiratory disorders, associated with the treatment of pediatric bipolar disorder (Frias et al. 2015).

3. *Provider factors*: Providers might have inadequate training and a relative discomfort in the management of pediatric mental disorders and suicidality, thus delaying early identification and intervention. Models focused on training/education of PCCs to improve their skills and capacity to care for BH problems and disorders have been developed and tested (Campo et al. 2018). A variety of approaches

have been tried, from didactic presentations and group consultations outside the specific practice site, to the application of ongoing peer consultation, and to clinical practice guidelines for the management of ADHD. Relatively large-scale efforts focused on PCC training and ongoing practice-based consultation include that of the nonprofit Resource for Advancing Children's Health (REACH) Institute (www.thereachinstitute.org) in New York City and the Ohio Minds Matter project (www.ohiomindsmatter.org), a state-sponsored program to aid PCCs in the assessment and management of pediatric mental health disorders, with the explicit goal of improving the quality and safety of psychopharmacologic practice.

4. *Financing and costs*: Challenges include the inability to pay and insurance restrictions for patients, and shortages and the misdistribution of competent, experienced care providers for healthcare systems. There is a shortage of pediatric BH specialists and access to specialty BH care is very limited, particularly for low-income, minority, and rural populations. Child and adolescent psychiatrists are especially in short supply, and this is unlikely to improve and may even become worse if existing patterns of training and support are maintained. Mental health specialists tend to cluster in more highly populated and affluent areas, contributing to an increased lack of access to services for vulnerable populations; minority youth may be at special risk (Campo et al. 2018). Families/children with low incomes or disabilities whose care is financed by the Medicaid program might be further limited in benefits. Over one-third of US counties, particularly those in rural areas and those with larger ethnic and racial minorities, do not have any outpatient mental health treatment facilities that accept Medicaid (Cummings et al. 2013). Psychiatrists are also substantially less likely than other medical specialties to accept Medicaid (43% versus 73%) or even private insurance (55% versus 89%) (Olfson 2016).

5. *Organizational issues*: Linkage with specialty mental health services is inadequate, with less than half of pediatric patients referred for off-site specialty mental health services from PC ever seeing a specialist within the ensuing 6 months (Kolko 2015; Kolko et al. 2019). The PCP's visit is often time-limited, making it challenging to effectively screen for and treat BH problems. Communication between professions is often hindered by the lack of combined medical records despite shared electronic health records, and BH notes are often not visible to other health professionals. Other organizational barriers include limited educational strategies regarding integration and a lack of support from senior management, which in turn impacts staff willingness to implement changes effectively (Chung et al. 2016; Grazier et al. 2016).

PCCs have identified several barriers to appropriate mental healthcare, such as lack of training in mental health management, insufficient time, lack of knowledge about community resources, poor referral feedback from their community mental health providers, and inadequate reimbursement. Despite these barriers, the PCC role in the PC arena includes prevention, screening, assessment, treatment, and coordination of mental health services; PCC management will depend on the level of severity and complexity of the mental health disorder.

Implications for Practice, Research, Education, and Policy

Providers can no longer be educated, trained, or work in silos. Future PCPs and PMH professionals, which include APRNs, are being asked to work within collaborative interprofessional models of care. The implications for practice, research, and education to create and maintain interprofessional relationships are compelling. Building interprofessional collaborative relationships and models of care among healthcare providers is essential to delivering mental health services in PC settings. Translating integrated models to a clinical pediatric setting from research is challenging.

Critical gaps exist in the routine assessment and management of mental health problems in PC. Without support of on-site care managers and strong consultation and referral networks to BH providers, few PC patients with mental health disorders receive evidence-based treatments for their conditions. A strong body of evidence from clinical trials and several policy opportunities within the ACA support the wisdom of placing greater emphasis on integrating mental health services into general medical settings. Emerging models of integrated care hold real promise for extending effective care to large numbers of children and adolescents who currently receive no treatment for their mental health conditions (Olfson 2016).

Compared to adults, research studies testing BH interventions with adolescents and young adults are relatively small considering the increase in mental health disorders and their impact on health outcomes (Richardson et al. 2017). Gaps in the research include evaluation of treatment strategies, especially involving technology. With the growth of telemedicine, including telepsychiatry, future research should compare satisfaction ratings within integrated settings to nonintegrated and virtual interprofessional collaborative teams and the processes they use to develop their relationships. Ultimately, understanding the characteristics of each key component of integrated care at each developmental-stage, the impact of the level of integration, and effective communication strategies will aid in evaluating outcome data required for evidence-based integrated care (Chung et al. 2016).

Tools are now available for policymakers, planners, and providers that describe the goals and strategies for implementing integrated models of care for children and young adults. A list of some of these resources are provided at the end of this chapter. Several policy issues surrounding new models of care exist, such as federal and state protections of patients' BH information as health information exchange is facilitated across electronic systems involving multiple practitioners and organizations. It is crucial for payers and policymakers to consider intermediate financial incentives to help practices support movement toward increased integration and to successfully navigate the journey of developing relationships that provide improved patient care. Innovative payment models that address time spent in collaboration with the BH and PCP team members either on site or via telecommunication and not just reimbursed solely on face-to-face time with patients is needed (Donahue and Aalsma 2019; Chung et al. 2016; Tyler et al. 2017).

To provide quality, evidence-based, and cost-effective care, health professionals must be prepared to lead and collaborate in interprofessional teams. Using IPE as a means to prepare healthcare students for collaborative practice in new models of care, the goal of improving quadruple aim can be achieved (NCIPE 2019). Just as important as equipping new nursing graduates with the basic knowledge and skills needed to be able to recognize and appropriately address mental health issues is the need to incorporate mental health content into the curricula of nonpsychiatric graduate specialties. Giving APRNs certified in PMH the opportunity and responsibility to manage the mental health needs of patients, as nurse pratitioners do in PC, would increase the numbers of accessible mental health professionals to render services to a growing population that needs such services. Other experts advocate for formal mental health competencies in practical curricula – knowledge, skills, and attitudes – training for pediatric PCCs (pediatricians) during medical school and residency programs and for physicians, nurses, social workers, and psychologists (Asarnow et al. 2015; Chung et al. 2016).

Conclusion

New models of healthcare delivery are emerging, and existing models are being adapted to accommodate behavioral and medical (primary) health within a PC setting. The particular model implemented by providers from both PC and BH will depend on many factors, including access to either professional in the community, retooling for current providers and training for new practitioners, opportunities for and willingness to collaborate, financial, and reimbursement structures, and patient acceptance. With each new report from the National Academy of Medicine, the mandate is given to change how we deliver today's healthcare services to coordinate, collaborate, and integrate these services. With a currently limited workforce, all types of providers must work better. Guidance is available through many resources offered by governmental agencies, special foundations, and professional and specialty organizations. Goals are multifaceted: (i) increased access to BH care for those in need, (ii) earlier identification and treatment of BH problems, (iii) creation of a less complex point of access to BH services for patients when they seek PC services, and vice versa, (iv) increased training among disciplines to improve interprofessional collaboration and co-management of appropriate patients, and (v) improved patient outcomes. Healthcare reform and revamping the financial/insurance health system must be priorities. These goals might be achieved by establishing integrated healthcare systems where providers from PC, BH, and other disciplines share information and decision making, including documentation, in delivering care to patients.

Providing mental health services within the PC setting can normalize and destigmatize treatment for BH disorders and offer an opportunity to blend interventions which target both physical and mental health conditions (American Psychological Association [APA] 2015). Furthermore, utilizing psychiatric providers within collaborative models of care can improve efficiencies, aid in coordinating care, enhance PC competencies, and improve use of evidence-based care (Press et al. 2017). However, implementing these models of care does not come without challenges (Emerson 2019). Making pediatrics BH integration a logical extension of team-based care coordination with PC requires healthcare integration and varies depending on which model of care exists. Regardless of whether the level of care is coordinated, colocated or integrated, the goal for seamless integration requires system level changes, effective communication and coordination as well as regulatory and payment restructuring. As policymakers, providers, and researchers across systems design models of integrated care, creating sustainable evidence-based strategies can address the mental health needs of children.

Resources

Agency for Healthcare Research and Quality (AHRQ) Academy for Integrating Behavioral Health and Primary Care. AHRQ's Lexicon for BH and PC Integration, screening, and clinical tools, and a searchable database of literature on integration. https://integrationacademy.ahrq.gov.

Advancing Integrated Mental Health Solutions (AIMS) Center. https://aims.uw.edu/collaborative-care.

American Academy of Child and Adolescent Psychiatry (AACAP). A guide to building collaborative mental health partnerships in pediatric primary care. http://www.aacap.org/App_Themes/AACAP/docs/clinical_practice_center/systems_of_care/Collaboration_Guide_FINAL_approved_6-10.pdf.

Center for American Progress Mental Health Care Services in Primary Care: Minds Matter. http://www.ohiomindsmatter.org/index.html.

Cherokee Health Systems. www.cherokeehealth.com.

Collaborative Family Healthcare Association. www.cfha.net.

Hogg Foundation for Mental Health. http://www.hogg.utexas.edu.

Improving Mood – Providing Access to Collaborative Treatment (IMPACT).http://aims.uw.edu/impact-improving-mood-promoting-access-collaborative-treatment.

Integrated Behavioral Health Partners (IBHP). http://www.ibhpartners.org/.

Integrated Primary Care, Inc. http://www.integratedprimarycare.com.

Intermountain Behavioral Health Program. http://www.intermountainhealthcare.org.

National Network of Child Psychiatric Access Programs (NNCPAP). http://www.nncpap.org.

Project TEACH. https://projectteachny.org.

SAMHSA-HRSA Center for Integration Health Solutions. Integrating behavioral health and primary care for children and youth. http://www.integration.samhsa.gov/integrated-care-models/13_June_CIHS_Integrated_Care_System_for_Children_final.pdf.

Patient Centered Primary Care Collaborative. http://pcpcc.net.

The REACH Institute. http://www.thereachinstitute.org/services/for-primary-care-practitioners/primary-pediatric-psychopharmacology-1.

University of Rochester Medical Center (URMC) Project Extension for Community Healthcare Outcomes (ECHO). Access to BH specialists through video-conferencing technology http://www.urmc.rochester.edu/project-echo.aspx.

World Health Organization (2008). Integrating Mental Health Into Primary Care: A Global Perspective. https://www.who.int/mental_health/resources/mentalhealth_PHC_2008.pdf.

References

AHQR. (2019). *Medical expenditure panel survey*. Statistical Brief #248. Agency for Healthcare Quality and Research. Available at www.http://meps.ahrq.gov/mepsweb/data_files/publications/st248/stat248.pdf.

AACAP (2017). Clinical update: telepsychiatry with children and adolescents. *Journal of American Academy of Child and Adolescent Psychiatry* 56 (10): 875–893.

AACAP. (2013). *ACOs &CAPs: Preparing for the impact of healthcare reform on child and adolescent psychiatry practice*. American Academy of Child & Adolescent Psychiatry. Available at https://www.aacap.org/App_Themes/AACAP/docs/Advocacy/policy_resources/preparing_for_healthcare_reform_201303.pdf.

AAFP. (2018). *Mental health care services by family physicians (Position paper)*. Executive Summary. American Academy of Family Physicians. Available at http://www.apa.org/about/gr/issues/cyf/child-services.aspx.

APA. (2015). *Increasing access and coordination of quality mental health services for children and adolescents*. American Psychological Association. Available at http://www.apa.org/about/gr/issues/cyf/child-services.aspx.

Archer, J., Bower, P., Gilbody, S. et al. (2012). Collaborative care for depression and anxiety problems. *Cochrane Database of Systematic Reviews* (10) Art. No. CD006525. doi: https://doi.org/10.1002/14651858.CD006525.pub2.

Asarnow, J.R., Rozenman, M., Wiblin, J., and Zeltzer, L. (2015). Integrated medical-behavioral care compared with usual primary care for child and adolescent behavioral health: a meta-analysis. *Journal of American Medical Association Pediatrics* 169: 929–937.

Benarous, X., Milhiet, V., Oppetit, A. et al. (2019). Changes in the use of emergency care for the youth with mental health problems over decades: a repeated cross sectional study. *Frontiers in Psychiatry* 10 (26): 1–8. https://doi.org/10.3389/fpsyt.2019.00026.

Bitsko, R.H., Holbrook, J.R., Kaminski, J. et al. (2016). Health-care, family and community factors associated with mental, behavioral and developmental disorders in early childhood – United States, 2011–2012. *Morbidity and Mortality Weekly Report* 65 (9): 221–226.

Blount, A. (2003). Integrated primary care: organizing the evidence. *Families, Systems & Health* 21: 121–134. Available at http://w2ww.pcpcc.net/files/organizing_the_evidence_0.pdf.

Bodenheimer, T. and Sinsky, C. (2014). From triple to quadruple aim: care of the patient requires care of the provider. *Annals of Family Medicine* 12 (6): 573–576. https://doi.org/10.1370/afm.1713.

Campo, J.V., Geist, R., and Kolko, D.J. (2018). Integration of pediatric behavioral health services in primary care: improving access and outcomes with collaborative care. *The Canadian Journal of Psychiatry* 63 (7): 432–438.

CDC. (2016). *Deaths: Final data for 2014*. National Vital Statistics Reports. National Center for Injury Prevention and Control. Available at https://www.cdc.gov/injury/wisqars/fatal.html.

Chung, H., Rostanski, N., Glassberg, H., and Pincus, H.A. (2016). *Advancing Integration of Behavioral Health into Primary Care: A Continuum-Based Framework*. New York, NY: United Hospital Fund.

Cohen, D.J., Davis, M.M., Hall, J.D. et al. (2015). *A Guidebook of Professional Practices for Behavioral Health and Primary Care Integration: Observations from Exemplary Sites*. Rockville, MD: Agency for Healthcare Research and Quality.

Collins, C., Hewson, D.L., Munger, R., and Wade, T. (2010). *Evolving Models of Behavioral Health Integration in Primary Care*. New York, NY: Milbank Memorial Fund Available at https://www.milbank.org/wp-content/uploads/2016/04/EvolvingCare.pdf.

Cummings, J.R., Wen, H., Ko, M., and Druss, B.G. (2013). Geography and the medicaid mental health care infrastructure: implications for health care reform. *Journal of American Medical Association Psychiatry* 70 (10): 1084–1090.

Delaney, K.R. (2017). Psychiatric mental health nursing advanced practice workforce: capacity to address shortages of mental health professionals. *Psychiatric Services* 68 (9): 952–954.

Donohue, K.L. and Aalsma, M.C. (2019). Identifying and managing developmental and behavioral health concerns within primary care: a push for change. *The Journal of Pediatrics* 206: 9–12.

Emerson, M.R. (2019). Implementing a hybrid-collaborative care model: practical considerations for nurse practitioners. *Mental Health Nursing* 40 (2): 112–117. https://doi.org/10.1080/01612840.2018.1524533.

Frias, A., Palma, C., and Farriols, N. (2015). Comorbidity in pediatric bipolar disorder: prevalence, clinical impact, etiology and treatment. *Journal of Affective Disorders* 174: 378–389.

Gerrity, M. (2014). *Integrating Primary Care into Behavioral Health Settings: What Works for Individuals with Serious Mental Illness*. New York, NY: Milbank Memorial Fund.

Ghandour, R.M., Sherman, L.J., Vladutiu, C.J. et al. (2019). Prevalence and treatment of depression, anxiety, and conduct problems in US children. *The Journal of Pediatrics* 206: 256–267.e3. https://doi.org/10.1016/j.peds.2018.09.021.

Grazier, K.L., Smiley, M.L., and Bondalapati, K.S. (2016). Overcoming barriers to integrating behavioral health and primary care services. *Journal of Primary Care & Community Health* 7 (4): 242–248. https://doi.org/10.1177/2150131916656455.

Guerrero, A.P.S., Balon, R., Beresin, E.V. et al. (2019). Rural mental health training: an emerging imperative to address health disparities. *Academic Psychiatry* 43 (1): 1–5.

Institute of Medicine (2006). *Adaptation to Mental Health and Addictive Disorders. Improving the Quality of Health Care for Mental and Substance Use Conditions.* Committee on Crossing the Quality Chasm. Washington, DC: National Academies Press.

Institute for Healthcare Improvement (2014). *Integrating Behavioral Health and Primary Care: IHI 90-Day r&d Project Final Summary Report.* Cambridge, MA: Institute for Healthcare Improvement Available at http://www.ihi.org/resources/Pages/Publications/BehavioralHealthIntegrationIHI90DayRDProject.aspx.

Ion, A., Sunderji, N., Jansz, G., and Ghavam-Rassoul, A. (2017). Understanding integrated mental health care in "real-world" primary care settings: what matters to health care providers and clients for evaluation and improvement? *American Psychological Association* 35: 271–282.

Kolko, D.J., Torres, E., Rumbarger, K. et al. (2019). Integrated pediatric health care in Pennsylvania: a survey of primary care and behavioral health providers. *Clinical Pediatrics* 58: 213–225.

Kolko, D.J. (2015). The effectiveness of integrated care on pediatric behavioral health: outcomes and opportunities. *Journal of American Medical Association Pediatrics* 169: 894–896.

Laderman, M. and Mate, K. (2014). Integrating behavioral health into primary care. *Health Care Executive* 29: 74–77.

Loehrer, S., Lewis, N., and Bogan, M. (2016). Improving the health of populations: a common language is key. *Healthcare Executive* 31: 82–83. Available at http://www.ihi.org/resources/Pages/Publications/Improving-the-Health-of-Populations.aspx.

McDermott, K.W., Stocks, C., & Freeman, W.J. (2018). *Overview of pediatric emergency department visits, 2015.* HCUP Statistical Brief #242. Rockville, MD: Agency for Healthcare Research and Quality. Available at http://www.hcup-us.ahrq.gov/reports/statbriefs/sb242-Pediatric-ED-Visits-2015.pdf.

Marcus, S., Malas, N., Dopp, R. et al. (2019). The Michigan child collaborative care program: building a telepsychiatry consultation service. *Psychiatric Services* 70: 849–852.

Mojtabai, R., Olfson, M., Sampson, N.A. et al. (2011). Barriers to mental health treatment: results from the National Comorbidity Survey Replication (NCS-R). *Psychological Medicine* 41: 1751–1761.

NCIPE (2019). *Guidance on Developing Quality Interprofessional Education for the Health Professions.* Chicago, IL: National Center for Interprofessional Practice and Education,: Health Professions Accreditors Collaborative.

NIMH. (2018). *New pathways for implementing universal suicide screening in healthcare settings.* National Institute of Mental Health. Available at https://www.nimh.nih.gov/news/science-news/2018/new-pathways-for-implementing-universal-suicide-risk-screening-in-healthcare-settings.shtml.

Olfson, M. (2016). The rise of primary care physicians in the provision of US mental health care. *Journal of Health Politics, Policy and Law* 41: 559–583.

Patient Protection and Affordable Care Act. *Patient Protection and Affordable Care Act of 2010*, Pub. L. No. 111–148, 124 Stat. 119 (2010).

Paul Wellstone and Pete Domenici Mental Health Parity and Addiction Equity Act. *Paul Wellstone and Pete Domenici Mental Health Parity and Addiction Equity Act of 2008*, H.R. 6983 – 110th Congress (2008).

Peek, C.J. & National Integration Academy Council. (2013). *Lexicon for behavioral health and primary care integration: Concepts and definitions developed by expert consensus.* Available at https://integrationacademy.ahrq.gov/sites/default/files/Lexicon.pdf.

Platt, R., Pustilnik, S., Connors, E. et al. (2018). Severity of mental health concerns in pediatric primary care and the role of child psychiatry access programs. *General Hospital Psychiatry* 53: 12–18.

Press, M.J., Howe, R., Schoenbaum, M. et al. (2017). Medicare payment for behavioral health integration. *The New England Journal of Medicine* 376: 405–407.

Reilly, S., Planner, C., Gask, L. et al. (2013). Collaborative care approaches for people with severe mental illness. *Cochrane Database of Systematic Reviews* (11) Art. No. CD009531. doi: https://doi.org/10.1002/14651858.CD009531.pub2.

Richardson, L.P., McCarty, C.A., Radovic, A., and Suleiman, A.B. (2017). Research in the integration of behavioral health for adolescent and young adults in primary care settings: a systematic review. *Journal of Adolescent Health* 60: 261–269.

Salyers, M.P., Garabrant, J.M., Luther, L. et al. (2019). A comparative effectiveness trial to reduce burnout and improve quality of care. *Administration and Policy in Mental Health and Mental Health Services Research* 46: 238–254. https://doi.org/10.1007/s10488-018-0908-4.

Straus, J.H. and Sarvet, B. (2014). Behavioral health care for children: the Massachusetts child psychiatry access project. *Health Affairs* 33: 2153–2161.

Tyler, E., Hulkower, R.L., & Kaminski, J.W. (2017). *Behavioral health integration in pediatric primary care: Considerations and opportunities for policymakers, planners, and providers.* Milbank Memorial Fund Report. Available at www.millbank.org.

UoW. (2018). *AIMS center: Collaborative care.* University of Washington. Available at https://aims.uw.edu/collaborative-care.

Vanderlip, E.R., Rundell, J., Avery, M. et al. (2016). *Dissemination of Integrated Care within Adult Primary Care Settings: The Collaborative Care Model.* Arlington, Virginia: American Psychiatric Association and Academy of Psychosomatic Medicine Available at https://www.psychiatry.org/psychiatrists/practice/professional-interests/integrated-care/collaborative-care-model.

Vogt, J.J. and Vogt, H. (2017). Collaboration in primary care through the integration of behavioral health professionals. *South Dakota Medicine* (Special Edition): 30–33.

WHO. (2017). *Depression fact sheet.* World Health Organization. Available at www.who.int.ezproxy.med.nyu.edu/mediacentre/factsheets/fs369/en.

WHO. (2010). *Suicide data: mental health.* World Health Organization. Available at https://www.who.int/mental_health/suicideprevention/en.

WHO & World Organization of Family Doctors. (2008). *Integrating mental health into primary care: A global perspective.* World Health Organization and World Organization of Family Doctors. Available at www.who.int.ezproxy.med.nyu.edu/mental_health/policy/services/integratingmhintoprimarycare/en.

Zallman, L., Joseph, R., O'Brien, C. et al. (2017). Does behavioral health integration improve primary care providers' perceptions of health-care system functioning and their own knowledge? *General Hospital Psychiatry* 46: 88–93. https://doi.org/10.1016/j.genhosppsych.2017.03.005.

28

Legal and Ethical Issues

Margaret Hardy[1] and Sarah B. Vittone[2]

[1] Sands Anderson PC, Richmond, VA, USA
[2] Georgetown University School of Nursing & Health Sciences, Washington, DC, USA

Objectives

After reading this chapter, advanced practice registered nurses will be able to:

1. Identify specific ethical and legal foundations in clinical practice with children and adolescents in primary care.
2. Describe basic legal obligations of advanced practice nurses in primary care and associated ethical practice implications.
3. Apply legal and ethical principles in managing child and adolescent issues in primary care.

Introduction

The delivery of healthcare to children is heavily dependent on the relationships between the providers, the children, and their parents, guardians, and caretakers. Like all relationships, each participant brings his or her own personal values, moral agency, and expectations to the interactions. An understanding of the many factors that may impact the formation and maintenance of those relationships is an important first step in caring for children, in both the pediatric and the mental health setting. In addition, advanced practice registered nurses (APRNs), as primary care providers of children, have a prevailing sensibility toward a "best interests" definition in planning care. In the ideal "shared decision-making model of care," the best interest plan for any child is the collaborative effort of the child, family, and the provider. It is with this consideration that this chapter speaks to specific issues frequently encountered in practice.

Furthermore, APRNs provide primary care adhering to professional obligations to protect individual patients and families. These obligations are at the intersection of three points of view: first, as defined by certification and licensure (*legal*), second, through professional standards of practice (SOPs) and boundaries as defined by nationally recognized authorities in evidence-based clinical practice (*clinical*), and third, as defined in professional ethics obligations (*ethical*). This chapter will introduce the legal and ethical considerations for the APRN providing care to children in primary care settings and suggest methods for resolving practical concerns that confront the APRN.

Description of the Issue

Historically speaking, society defines the scope and boundary of safe and acceptable practice in healthcare. Society changes current expectations of care and practice

---

Child and Adolescent Behavioral Health: A Resource for Advanced Practice Psychiatric and Primary Care Practitioners in Nursing,
Second Edition. Edited by Edilma L. Yearwood, Geraldine S. Pearson, and Jamesetta A. Newland.
© 2021 John Wiley & Sons, Inc. Published 2021 by John Wiley & Sons, Inc.
Companion website: www.wiley.com/go/Yearwood

through legal case precedent as well as through professional deliberation and consensus building. Professional nursing, through the American Nurses Association (ANA) Code of Ethics (Code) (2015), describes its mission as the prevention of illness, alleviation of suffering, and the protection, promotion, and optimization of health and advocacy in care of individuals, families, communities, and populations. This mission is accomplished through individuals and organizations attentive to social, ethical, and legal boundaries.

The legal status of children in the United States has undergone a major change in the last century but, in many ways, it is still poorly defined in state and federal legislation. Laws such as those restricting the use of child labor and instituting compulsory education moved society away from a mindset that children were the property of their parents, to be treated as the parents saw fit. However, the extent to which children have autonomy in making life decisions, including those related to their healthcare, is not always clear and, in many cases, varies from state to state.

Historically, mental health services for children began as institutions, then transitioned over time to community programs and integrated systems. The institutionalization of children in the United States with mental "defect," disorder, or disability has been documented since the early 1780s. Court-ordered involuntary treatment was available only in inpatient settings until the mid-1960s when the expectation of "least restrictive environment" began to prevail. In the actionable case of Willowbrook State School in Staten Island, New York, children were institutionalized for mental "defect" from 1930 to 1987 without regard to their safety or therapeutic needs (Rothman and Rothman 2005). Their deplorable care and use as research subjects stand out as an example to practitioners and consumers alike of the specific need for legislative protection of children. Through the study of the deinstitutionalization of these residents and children, we began to see the mainstreaming of children with disabilities, including those with behavioral health diagnoses, into schools as a continuing work in progress regardless of legislative requirements.

Community programs and school-based services have become a recommended standard of practice since the 1970s. Pediatric health and mental health needs are often overlapping but not addressed or met in any one program. Currently, children seen in primary care settings may be identified with acute or chronic behavioral health issues through general screening. However, poor funding, lack of adequately prepared healthcare providers, and poor or irregular utilization of services have impacted the overall health of these children. What is known is that intervention during childhood is key to limiting the growing population of emotionally, psychiatrically, and behaviorally disabled adults.

Finally, behavioral health, mental health, and mental illness are all used to identify the services described here. It is in these names that stigma may arise for the child and the family. The APRN must be aware and intervene to provide secure and private opportunities to reach children in need as well as to enhance their adherence to recommended treatment regardless of stigma.

Legal and Ethical Issues: Risks to Children

Our society views children as a vulnerable population, to be afforded the highest protection and value. Individually, children may also fall within other at-risk populations, including the poor and impoverished, the disabled, those with learning difficulties, those in foster care or in dysfunctional families, the abused, and those with chronic or serious illness.

APRNs who provide behavioral health services to children face inherent legal risks. Being cognizant of those risks, and taking steps to minimize them, can help the APRN to protect both her license and her career. Behavioral health providers have risk factors for both malpractice and licensing complaints specific to their practices, including difficult diagnoses, medication management, and suicidal and/or homicidal patients.

According to data collected by CNA, an insurer of over 26 000 nurse practitioners (NPs), malpractice claims brought against behavioral health providers are on the increase and accounted for over 15% of all claims closed in 2017, compared with 6.5% in 2012 (CNA and Nursing Service Organization 2017). In addition to civil liability for malpractice, APRNs must also be mindful of the risk of complaints filed with the Board of Nursing, the majority of which arise from office-based practices. The four most frequent complaints received by boards of nursing, comprising over 71% of all complaints, involve allegations of inappropriate prescribing, exceeding the scope of practice, inadequate treatment and care management, and unprofessional conduct. Allegations that a provider has breached a patient's confidentiality are also common and can include the unauthorized release of information, failure to provide adequate safeguards for maintaining records, and boundary violations. Although infrequent, APRNs can also face criminal liability for activities that exceed their scope of practice, including assault and excessive prescribing.

Advanced practice nurses must comply with the laws and regulations of the state in which they practice. State laws and regulations govern not only the scope of APRN practice, but also establish the criteria for licensure and the grounds for which an APRN may be disciplined. The laws and regulations vary from state to state; APRNs must familiarize themselves with those applicable to their practice. In addition, APRNs must also comply with federal laws regarding patient privacy, medical records, and prescriptive authority.

Ethical issues for children in the primary care setting cover issues related to their dependence as minors, including adherence to appointments and treatment regimens, insurance constraints and access to healthcare, quality of care, identification of safety issues related to physical, emotional, cognitive, and social abuse and neglect as well as identification of developmental delays and other behavioral concerns, and guardians being misinformed about treatment options. Furthermore, the capacity of the child or adolescent to request, assent or refuse treatment may create additional ethical challenges when paired with dissenting parents/guardians. All these issues may be influenced by the professional practice and ethical response of the healthcare providers and guardians.

Who is the Client?

When the client is a child, the APRN must consider the provider relationship within the legal relationship of the guardian. Fisher (2009) suggests that in addition to clarifying this question, another question should be posed. Due to at least two persons being in this relationship with the APRN, the APRN should consider what ethical obligations are owed to each person, a step beyond a single relational professional obligation. In behavioral health settings, where family involvement and participation may be a vital component of a child's treatment, it is important to clarify expectations and to be forthcoming regarding disclosure obligations and the confidentiality (or lack thereof) of information shared by the minor to the APRN. When providing care to a minor (in most states, an individual under the age of 18 years), the APRN must keep in mind that most states permit minors to consent to the diagnosis and treatment of specific conditions, including mental health and substance abuse treatment, but state laws vary as to the minimum age requirement and the nature and extent of treatment to which they may consent. The cognitive developmental maturity of minors with regard to capacity in decision making is discussed later in the chapter.

Who is the Guardian?

Essential to providing care to children is the identification of the person or persons with the legal right to have access to the child's health information and to make decisions on behalf of the child. In most instances, it is the parent(s) who has this right and responsibility. A provider cannot assume that is the case, however. Client intake forms should ask for the identity of the child's guardian(s). In the event that someone other than a parent is identified, the provider should request a copy of the documentation appointing the guardian and defining the parameters of the guardianship. In some instances, parental rights may have been terminated at the time a legal guardian was appointed, for example in cases of severe abuse or neglect. In cases involving divorce or custody disputes, a guardian ad litem may be appointed by the Court to protect the interests of the child while the parental rights remain intact. In those situations, the Court Order will likely give the guardian ad litem permission to obtain the child's records and communicate with the child's healthcare providers. The guardian ad litem can be a valuable resource for the providers, particularly if there is disagreement between the parents concerning the child's care. Information regarding those with legal rights regarding the child's care must be clearly documented in the treatment record and communicated to members of the treatment team. Providers should obtain clarification from the child's legal guardian regarding the person or persons authorized to act on the child's behalf. APRNs should be mindful of the fact that the person who accompanies the child to medical appointments, while perhaps not the legal guardian but a grandparent or babysitter, provides significant daily care and can be a valuable source of information for the provider. However, without the express written consent of the legal guardian, the APRN may not be able to release any information to that person.

Obligations of Children and their Guardians

In the healthcare relationship, the client is obligated to provide accurate and truthful history and pertinent information to help inform the treatment. The child and guardian are obligated to participate in clinical planning of care and to make responsible decisions. They must be honest in reporting relevant clinical symptoms and adherence to treatment. The client must also meet financial obligations as discussed with the provider. These obligations and other expectations must be shared with the client at the beginning of the relationship and reviewed as necessary thereafter. Guardians must always act in the best interests of their children. As such, a child's guardian/decision maker/surrogate must be available at all times and is required to provide consent for treatment unless an emergency exists requiring immediate treatment. Guardians as surrogates for their children are obligated to provide care that relieves suffering, preserves and restores function, as well as improves the quality and extent of the child's life. The APRN must be cognizant of the fact that guardians sometimes fail in their duties as guardians intentionally, through neglect, as a result of poor communication, or through confusion. When the provider becomes aware of such a situation there are ethical and legal duties required of the provider in order to protect the child, including a possible report to child protection services in accordance with state law and regulations.

Foundations for Practice: Legal

Duties to Patients

Each state defines the scope of practice for nurses within their state. Sometimes but not always referred to as Nurse Practice Acts, these rules are most often set out in both laws and regulations adopted by the state. The specificity of the rules varies between states but generally describes the licensure requirements, practice parameters, and means and methods of disciplinary actions within the state. Because the scopes of practice for APRNs vary widely between states, every APRN must be familiar with his or her state's rules, copies of which are available from the licensing authority of each state.

In addition to state law, some APRN activities are governed by federal law, to the extent that federal law has authority or jurisdiction over the specific activity. For example, federal law requires that APRNs register with the Drug Enforcement Administration (DEA) prior to prescribing controlled substances. Healthcare reform, changing reimbursement schedules, consumer expectations, and simple supply and demand create constant flux in the laws and regulations that apply to APRNs. Typically, APRNs and the groups that advocate for them support the expansion of the APRN role to permit more autonomy or a broader scope of practice, while other groups with conflicting interests oppose that expansion.

Duties to Others

When considering the duties of an APRN, one generally thinks of the duties owed to patients for whom the nurse is providing care. The duties of an APRN may reach beyond his or her patients, however, to third parties or to the general public. All 50 states have a law mandating the reporting of child abuse and neglect. These laws are in place to protect children but they are also required in order to qualify for funding under the Child Abuse Prevention and Treatment Act (CAPTA). Originally passed in 1974, CAPTA has been amended several times since. CAPTA establishes threshold definitions for child abuse and sexual abuse, but individual states may choose

to adopt more expansive definitions. While every state requires that certain professionals, including healthcare providers, report suspected child abuse, the extent of the knowledge that triggers the duty to report varies between states. For example, in some states, providers must report whenever they have a "reasonable cause to believe" that abuse has occurred, while other states require that providers report "known or suspected" abuse. CAPTA also requires that each state enact legislation that provides immunity from prosecution for reporting abuse. All states provide some form of immunity from criminal and civil liability for those persons who, acting in good faith, report suspected child abuse (US Department of Health and Human Services [USDHHS] 2019a,b). In a majority of states, reporters of child abuse are presumed to be acting in good faith.

In some circumstances, a provider may have a reporting duty to individuals other than his or her patients. In 1976, the Supreme Court of California recognized a health provider's duty to respond to potential danger that a patient might present to a third party. In *Tarasoff v. Regents of the University of California* et al. (1976), the parents of Tatiana Tarasoff sued, among others, a therapist named Dr. Lawrence Moore for the murder of their daughter by Prosenjit Poddar. Two months prior to the murder, Mr. Poddar had confided to Dr. Moore that he intended to kill Ms. Tarasoff, who had refused Mr. Poddar's romantic advances. Dr. Moore contacted the police and reported the threat. The police detained Mr. Poddar and questioned him but released him when he appeared to be rational and promised to stay away from Ms. Tarasoff. Neither Dr. Moore nor the police, who were also sued, notified Ms. Tarasoff or her parents of the threats made by Mr. Poddar. Despite the fact that Dr. Moore had no patient–physician relationship with Ms. Tarasoff, had never met her, and had a duty to confidentiality to Mr. Poddar, the Supreme Court of California held that Dr. Moore had a legal obligation to take steps to protect Ms. Tarasoff from being harmed by Mr. Poddar.

Since the court's ruling in Tarasoff, a majority of states have enacted laws that either require or permit providers, including APRNs in most cases, to take steps to protect third parties who may be in danger as evidenced by threats from patients. The laws define when the duty arises, for example some states require only that the healthcare provider know that a potential danger exists, while others impose a duty to act only on threats that are directly communicated to the provider. In most cases, a provider can comply with the duty in several ways, including notifying the object of the threat, contacting the police, and hospitalizing the patient. Most states provide protection from malpractice or disciplinary actions for the provider resulting from a breach of the patient's confidentiality when taking action in good faith as required by the law; failure to comply with the law can result in either or both actions being taken against the provider (Geske 1989). However, a small number of states have no law requiring or permitting a provider to warn a third party of potential danger from a patient. In those states, a provider could be subject to a claim for breaching the patient's confidentiality for warning a third party. Again, it is imperative that APRNs familiarize themselves with the laws and regulations applicable to their practices.

In addition to the duties imposed by the Tarasoff-based statutes, some states also impose statutory duties on nurses to report other healthcare providers who may have violated the rules or regulations governing their practice. Depending on the state, the duty may include reporting healthcare providers who have been hospitalized for substance abuse or psychiatric conditions or have practiced in such a way to pose a danger to patients.

Potential Liabilities for the Nurse

Like other healthcare providers, APRNs can be and are sued for malpractice, although the frequency with which APRNs are sued remains low. According to the 2018 AANP National Nurse Practitioner Sample Survey, less than 2% of NPs have been named as a primary defendant in a medical malpractice action (American Association of Nurse Practitioners [AANP] 2019). While malpractice law varies to some degree by state, all malpractice cases have four basic elements (Physicians, Surgeons, and Other Healers 2002). The first of these elements is the presence of a duty that was owed by the provider to the plaintiff. This duty may arise from common law or from statutes like those based on the Tarasoff case. For APRNs, the duty may arise from direct care provided or from the supervision of others who provided care.

The second element in a malpractice action is negligence, defined as a breach of the standard of care by the healthcare provider (Negligence 2002). Such a breach goes beyond merely what may, in hindsight, have been an error but had been justified at the time. In order to rise to the level of a breach of the standard of care, a nurse's actions or inactions must have failed to comply with what a reasonable nurse would have done under the same or similar circumstances. Generally, expert testimony from a nurse is required in a malpractice action to establish the standard of care and to testify to the defendant nurse's compliance with the statute. It is important to note that the standard is based on what a *reasonable* APRN would have learned, known, and done, not on the particular APRN being sued.

The third element in a malpractice action is harm to the patient/plaintiff that was proximately caused by the alleged negligence. Without that connection, a malpractice action cannot be established. Such a connection cannot be assumed based merely on the alleged negligence of the defendant nurse, but must be proved, usually through the use of expert testimony. For example, it may be negligent for an APRN to fail to follow up on an abnormal laboratory result, but that negligent act may bear no causal relationship to the patient's adverse outcome.

The fourth and final element of a malpractice action is damages that resulted from the harm. Such damages can include pain and suffering, medical bills, and, in some cases, emotional or mental anguish. Although this element may appear to be very straightforward, disputes often arise as to whether specific damages were caused by the harm alleged, preexisted the alleged negligence of the provider, or were caused by contributory negligence of the patient or their guardian. Psychiatric mental health practitioners may be able to defend against malpractice claims or at least apportion the damages if it is shown that the client and/or their family caused some of the harm. An example of contributory negligence occurred when a patient's family violated the contraband policy, hid cigarettes and a lighter, and gave them to a patient who suffered cognitive impairments. The patient accidentally set their clothes on fire while smoking in a wheelchair and suffered third-degree burns. Self-harm such as cutting or suicide attempts are not generally considered to be contributory negligence if the potential for self-harm is one of the reasons for treatment. The courts are reluctant to impose liability for outpatient suicide attempts unless the patient was recently discharged without appropriate documentation of risk (Yorker 1995). Psychiatric nurses who work with children and adolescents in group settings should also be aware that they may be liable for negligence if one patient harms another, e.g. sexual molestation or physical assault (Yorker 1997).

Generally speaking, an employer is responsible for the negligent acts of employees. Therefore, hospitals, medical practices, and other employers are generally liable for acts of negligence by the APRNs they employ, provided the APRN was acting within the scope of his or her employment at the time of the alleged negligence. The APRN may or may not be actually named as a defendant in the lawsuit. However, even if the APRN is not a party to the lawsuit, he or she may be required to testify in deposition or at trial regarding the care provided to the patient.

APRNs may be required by their employers to maintain malpractice insurance or the employers may provide such insurance. Insurance companies offer malpractice coverage to all levels of nurses, which includes coverage for both the cost of defending a malpractice action, as well as indemnity for any judgment that may be entered against the nurse. Adverse or unexpected outcomes are inevitable in healthcare. Fearing a malpractice suit or licensing complaint, the healthcare provider's first response to such an outcome is often avoidance, avoiding the patient and family and everyone else involved. In some situations, talking with the patient and family about the adverse outcome may diffuse the anger or mistrust that could otherwise result in a lawsuit or disciplinary action. The healthcare provider should carefully consider the information to be communicated, the method of the communication, and the individuals who should be included in the communication. Depending upon the nature and severity of the adverse event, or the patient's and family's reaction to it, it may be wise to seek the advice of a healthcare attorney.

Historically, expressions of sorrow or regret by a healthcare provider following an unanticipated outcome could be used against the provider in a subsequent malpractice action as an admission of negligence. However, a majority of states have now enacted legislation that protects healthcare providers who express sympathy to a patient or family after such an outcome (Ebert 2008). Often referred to as "I'm sorry laws," the actual protections provided by such laws vary from state to state. For example, some states protect only verbal, not written, expressions by the healthcare provider. Other states protect only statements made within a certain period of time after the unanticipated outcome. Still other states protect expressions of sympathy, but not apologies. Every healthcare provider should be aware of whether his or her own state has such a law and, if so, what protections the law offers.

Disciplinary Actions

Each state licensing board has its own rules and regulations regarding the processing of complaints and the investigatory and disciplinary process. Complaints can be filed by patients or their family members, employers, colleagues and others, and in most cases can be made anonymously. Some disciplinary actions are initiated upon receipt by the state licensing board of a report that a malpractice claim against a nurse has been settled or resulted in a judgment entered against the nurse or information that another state has disciplined the nurse. The laws and/or regulations of each state specify those actions that may result in discipline being imposed against a nurse. Often, insurance policies that provide coverage for nursing malpractice actions also provide coverage for license protection, which may cover all the legal costs and fees associated with defending oneself in a disciplinary proceeding.

Facing a disciplinary action before the state licensing board is always difficult. The possibility of having disciplinary action taken against one's license is stressful enough, but nurses who find themselves in that situation should realize that the consequences of an adverse decision by a licensing board may have far-reaching consequences. Nurses who have disciplinary actions taken against their licenses may face discipline from other states in which they are licensed, which can be imposed administratively without the opportunity to defend themselves (Porter and Mackay 2012). Depending upon the nature of the allegations, other consequences may include criminal prosecution, revocation of the provider's DEA registration number, and exclusion from participation in federal healthcare programs such as Medicare and Medicaid (Collins and Mikos 2008). Because of the potential impact that a disciplinary action may have, it is important that nurses seek the advice of an experienced attorney when faced with a licensing complaint, even though the complaint appears to be without merit.

Importance of Documentation

The medical record is one of the most important means of communication between healthcare providers. The documentation in an inpatient chart provides vital information regarding the plan of care, the implementation of that care, and the patient's response, as well as important historical information regarding the patient. In the primary care setting where multiple providers may be seeing the patient, the record is equally important. The record contains not only the documentation of the care provided in the office but also the record of communication with other providers who are involved in the patient's care.

Documentation takes on additional importance when a malpractice or disciplinary action arises. Nurses often hear the adage, "If it's not written, you didn't do it." Although in most cases a nurse would be permitted to testify during a malpractice action regarding care she provided but did not contemporaneously document, a document written at the time the care was provided, prior to any action being filed, obviously may be more persuasive and allow the nurse to avoid having to answer the question as to why if it was important enough to remember, it was not important enough to document. While the time during which a patient has to file a medical malpractice action varies by state, years may elapse from the time a nurse provided care to a patient until the time she learns she has been named as a defendant in a malpractice action. By then, the nurse may have no independent recollection of the patient or the care provided. In those situations, a well-documented record may be crucial to defending the care.

Documentation can be equally important in disciplinary actions. Typically, a copy of the patient's record is obtained during the investigation of any disciplinary action involving allegations related to patient care. Documentation that is clear, understandable, and consistent with the nurse's testimony will greatly assist the nurse in a subsequent disciplinary action. On the other hand, documentation that is missing or inaccurate may lead to additional allegations to which the nurse must respond.

It is often challenging to keep up with the documentation demands in a busy primary care setting. Providers who are overly concerned about the legal and disciplinary consequences of poor documentation may be tempted to focus more on that documentation than providing quality care. On the other hand, those who discount the importance of documentation may focus instead on providing care to the detriment of documenting that care. Neither of those extremes is appropriate. Providers must find the balance along that spectrum that fits their clinical setting, the care being provided, and the types of records being maintained.

Some general rules apply to nursing documentation, regardless of the clinical setting. Ideally, documentation should be contemporaneous with the provision of care. While that may not be realistic in every setting, it is important that care be documented as soon as possible after the care is provided. When circumstances require that late entries be added to the medical record, those entries should be clearly identified as having been added at a later time and dated and timed when actually made, while referencing the date and time of the care being documented. Entries should be patient-specific and nonjudgmental. Avoid entries in the record that reference family members or others, unless those entries are relevant to the care of the patient. Whenever possible, use direct quotes from the patient or guardian, rather than characterizing the patient using judgmental terms, such as describing the patient or family using terms such as "demanding" or "difficult."

Completeness of the record is important regardless of the patient's or parent's request to keep certain information from appearing in the record or to remove it. Sensitive information that might have long-standing implications for the child's future professional work or acceptance into areas such as the military might be included in just such a request. The APRN, while compassionate, might consider this, but should consider obligation to safety and health supported by a complete record as his/her primary obligation. Clarification of the APRN role in treatment and responsibility for documentation is key at the outset of the therapy relationship.

Electronic health records (EHRs) are increasingly common in both inpatient and outpatient settings. The EHR offer some clear advantages, including legibility, standardization, and the potential of increased availability to multiple providers. However, the EHR also presents risks. Some systems auto-populate templates with data from prior entries, creating the possibility of inaccurate or unreliable information. The EHR also presents unique risks for unauthorized access to confidential information. Federal law establishes standards for the protection of electronically maintained records.

Foundations for Practice: Ethical

Healthcare ethics is the application of bioethics principles within healthcare situations. Philosophical motivation for ethical practice may include tenets of deontology, virtue ethics, utilitarianism, or an ethics of care. These theories may guide motivation in ethical clinical practice. Ultimately, it is the applied principles, as defined here, in ethical and moral values and guidelines that produce the most successful outcomes. Moral guidance defines the motivation that produces "right or wrong" behavior. This is generally formed by individuals in society through influence of values, culture, religion, and the law. Our society has accepted a moral code of conduct for individuals to exist peacefully. The values of honesty, dignity, integrity, compassion, fairness, self-control, and duty are generally appreciated in our society (Killinger 2007).

Healthcare ethics, as a foundation, adheres to applied principles for professional guidance specifically including autonomy, beneficence, nonmaleficence, and justice (Beauchamp et al. 2019). More specifically, professional ethics are defined through codes of conduct within healthcare organizations and professional societies. Professional ethics for the APRN is most broadly defined by the ANA Code (2015), available at www.nursingworld.org. The ANA Code includes obligations to the patient's dignity through accountability, advocacy, respect, and a commitment of the nurse to the patient. Provisions in the ANA Code also articulate obligations to continue professional education, maintain professional integrity, and improve healthcare environments. In addition, APRNs practice globally and in this respect should also embrace the four-part ICN Code of Ethics for Nurses by the International Council of Nurses, available at www.icn.ch. The ICN publication identifies elements related to human rights, values, and customs and specifically identifies responsibility for supporting the health and social needs of vulnerable populations (ICN 2012).

In the United States, professional nursing specialties speak to SOPs and clinical concerns for children with behavioral health issues. These pertinent professional organizations include the American Psychiatric Nurses Association (APNA), the International Society of Psychiatric-Mental Health Nurses (ISPN), as well as the National Association of Pediatric Nurse Practitioners (NAPNAP). Yet these organizations *do not* propose separate codes of ethics for APRNs, apart from the ANA Code (2015). Furthermore, the most obvious ethical issues for APRNs that are not addressed by the ANA Code include issues related to collaboration and consultation, clearly a role for the APRN. Yet, there has been discussion of this need. In 2004, Peterson and Potter considered that the mixed role of the NP with influences from both nursing and medicine required an APRN code of ethics with mixed obligations. However, they further suggested that a standardized scope of practice must be defined prior to creating an advanced practice ethical code for nurses. Currently, the scope of practice for the APRN is still left to various state interpretations. There has been no movement for national standards for scope of practice at this time.

While ethical principles and professional codes are foundations for resolving ethical dilemmas, ethical dilemmas within healthcare are best resolved with thoughtful and careful reflection and may be best resolved through dialogue with colleagues. It is valuable to create professional relationships for reflection and discussion of common ethical concerns in practice. Ethics committees and consultants are available for conference on an individual case basis.

Moral Distress

Moral agency is generally defined as having the personal values, knowing the difference between right and wrong, and having the capacity to act based on these. The moral agent in a healthcare relationship will use personal values and the professional ethics as described previously to engage with clients. Moral distress occurs when knowing the right action, fear or other prevents the nurse from acting. Nurses and APRNs most commonly value the use of guiding principles of respect for persons (which include autonomy, individual rights and human dignity, confidentiality, privacy, veracity, and informed consent), freedom, equality, and justice. Decision making is a frequent action for an APRN and yet this can be a difficult task depending on the nature of the client and the decision involved. Laabs (2007) considered issues of moral distress in NPs, contending that at some point in a morally distressing action (even in the face of patient autonomy and strong beneficence), the moral integrity of the nurse comes at odds

with the personal self. Nurses' use of reflection and discernment may assist them in defining the limits to which their moral agency may be stretched. Laabs suggested that in the event that no successful resolution can occur, then the practitioner should be prepared to address what degree of personal moral distress would be acceptable. APRNs must be prepared to draw the line between acceptable and unacceptable actions when asked to participate in morally distressing actions. Clearly there is a risk to the relationship with the client and therefore the APRN must be clear about the role and in what situations the relationship is at risk. The American Association of Critical Care Nurses has developed a product, The 4As to Rise Above Moral Distress Toolkit (AACCN 2006), which APRNs may find helpful.

Ethical issues common to APRNs in primary care include insurance constraints, managed care policies, access to healthcare, quality of care, guardians being misinformed about treatment options, and APRNs feeling caught between managed care rules and advocacy for the patient's care. Ulrich et al. (2014) in a study of primary care NPs and physician assistants (PAs), reported 31.6% of respondents feeling overwhelmed by the needs of their patients, and 40.8% described patient relationships as becoming more adversarial than they had been. More than 40% reported that patients demand unnecessary tests and treatment. This study did find that NPs and PAs perceived quality of care was positively associated with perceived practice autonomy, ethics preparedness, ethics confidence, and physician collegiality, all factors that could be promoted through education and organizational climate.

Basic Professional Ethics Obligations

As derived from the above basic tenets of bioethical guidance, the basic professional ethics obligations for healthcare providers including APRNs are derived from a principle of respect for persons and include:

- informed consent
- privacy and confidentiality
- communication, truth telling, and disclosure
- capacity of the client (in this case the minor and the guardian).

These four areas have developed over time, historically defined by society through interpretation of the law and creation of protections through new law (Rothstein 2009). Ethical tenets through the ANA Code (2015) partner with the law to ensure that these basic obligations are upheld.

Complex Ethical Risks in Healthcare

In healthcare, there are many areas in which society, health professions, and the law have been well defined, as in confidentiality and privacy. There are other areas that are less well defined, leaving room for interpretation by stakeholders. These complex areas include:

- beginning of life concerns – reproduction, sterilization, genetic therapy, artificial reproductive technology, maternal–fetal conflicts
- end of life concerns – withholding and withdrawing life-sustaining therapy, refusal of indicated therapy, palliative sedation, euthanasia, and assisted suicide
- relational issues such as patient sovereignty and paternalism – who defines best treatment
- professional relationships related to managed care and fees
- allocation of resources.

The areas with specific implications when working with children and particularly with children in the behavioral health setting will be discussed later in the chapter.

Patient's Rights and Basic Obligations of Providers

With respect to ethical and legal foundations, all patients expect a certain degree of respect in the healthcare environment including their right to:

- privacy
- health information (medical records)
- make their own healthcare decisions
- informed consent
- refuse treatment.

These rights and obligations are founded in the ethical and legal frameworks as defined in society (Rothstein 2009). They are generally accepted and may be without written standards. In addition, the APRN as a primary healthcare provider should disclose the nature and length of the healthcare relationship and the expected outcome of the relationship. The APRN is obligated to provide honest disclosure of information received from third parties (referrals). Documentation must be timely and available as the information within is owned by the patient. The APRN who collaborates with other medical services and makes and/or receives referrals relating to this patient must be open and disclose such to the patient. Fair billing practices and information related to billing and payment should be confidential and timely. The patient seeks your care as safe, expert, and qualified in this specialty. Information about your practice should be readily available to your patient population.

Sovereignty versus Abandonment

Patient sovereignty is a model of a healthcare relationship in which the patient directs the clinical care and may request or demand therapy, medication, and treatment (Cohen and Cesta 2005). The APRN may consider withdrawal from the case for conscientious objection or refuse such demands by patients based on scientific SOPs. An APRN is not to be forced, coerced, or compelled in any way by the patient, family, colleague, or the court to provide interventions or treatment to patients that the provider considers unsafe or inappropriate. The provider should make every effort to educate the patient/family as to the standard of care. Yet, in the event of an impasse, the patient's care should be transferred to another qualified provider. The APRN must, however, take the steps necessary to transfer the care to another provider, including the transfer of treatment records. State law and/or regulations may dictate the manner in which such a transfer takes place, including the notice the patient must be given and provisions for care in the interim.

Implications for Practice

While the following concepts are based in legal and ethical foundations, the application of such in the clinical setting will be considered, including:

- confidentiality/right to information/disclosure
- decision making
  - capacity/competence
  - informed consent
  - right to refuse treatment
- involuntary treatment
- restraint
- reproductive treatment.

Confidentiality and the Right to Information

Like other healthcare providers, nurses who fall within the definition of covered entities under the Health Insurance Portability and Accountability Act (HIPAA) of 1996 (USDHHS 2013) must comply with the HIPAA Privacy Rule of 2002. The basic premise behind the HIPAA Privacy Rule – that patients have a right to privacy in their personal health information – is nothing new. The right to patient confidentiality has long been recognized in statutory and common law and is an emphasized part of nursing education at all levels. While HIPAA does not provide for private causes of action by patients for violations, meaning that a patient cannot sue a provider for a HIPAA violation, providers can face significant civil and criminal penalties for violations of the

Privacy Rule. In addition, the circumstances of a violation may also be sufficient to establish a basis for civil liability under state law.

The Office for Civil Rights (OCR) at the USDHHS (2019c) is the agency responsible for HIPAA enforcement. Between the Privacy Rule's compliance date in April 2003 and 31 August 2019, the OCR received 216 195 complaints of HIPAA violations and initiated 979 compliance reviews. The OCR has resolved 98% of those cases. As of 31 August 2019, the OCR has settled or impose a civil monetary penalty in 65 cases for a total of $102.7 million. The most commonly alleged violations are, in order of frequency, (i) the impermissible use and disclosure of protected health information, (ii) the lack of safeguards for protected health information, (iii) the lack of patient access to their protected health information, (iv) the lack of administrative safeguards for electronic protected health information, and (v) the use or disclosure of more than the minimum necessary protected health information. Hospitals and private practices are the covered entities most often alleged to have violated the Privacy Rule.

In addition to the federal Privacy Rule, most states have their own laws protecting the confidentiality of patient information. Since 2003, many of those laws have been amended to be consistent with the requirements of the HIPAA Privacy Rule. When considering confidentiality issues, it is helpful to keep in mind that a patient's health information belongs to the patient. As such, patients are entitled to access to their own information, unless there is reason to believe they could be harmed by it. The release of confidential information to anyone other than the patient or, in the case of a minor, a legal guardian must fall within the definition of a permitted or authorized disclosure. Generally speaking, healthcare providers are permitted to use and disclose information to the extent necessary for purposes of (i) treatment, including the release of information necessary for consultations and follow-up with other providers, (ii) payment, including the submission of bills to insurers, and (iii) healthcare operations, such as quality review, without the express consent of patients or their representatives. In some instances, state and federal law not only permits but requires that information be disclosed when necessary for public health or safety reasons, such as the reporting of child abuse or certain communicable diseases. Other exceptions exist for complying with court orders, such as a subpoena for medical records, protecting third parties from patients who may present a danger, and certain law enforcement purposes. In situations where the disclosure of information is not permitted or required under state or federal law, a patient or someone permitted to act on his or her behalf must authorize the release of medical information.

Generally speaking, privacy laws recognize the right of a parent to access the health information of his or her child. As described above, however, in some instances a biological parent may not be the legal guardian of the child and may no longer have the right to obtain or authorize the disclosure of the child's health information. Whenever custody and/or guardianship of a child has been transferred to someone other than the parent, healthcare providers must make sure that the treatment team is aware of the person or persons who are entitled to access the child's information and that the medical record clearly reflects that right to access.

It is important to remember that access to medical information includes more than just a copy of the medical record; it also includes verbal communications from healthcare providers. Healthcare providers must also be mindful of the risk of unintended disclosure of information, such as the potential compromise to an adolescent's confidentiality by billing a parent's health insurance for treatment sought by the adolescent without the parent's knowledge.

When working with children in the behavioral health setting, it is important to establish clear policies and procedures for maintaining the confidentiality of patient information that are both consistent with state and federal law and understood by the patient, to the extent possible. While certain protections must be in place for all private health information, healthcare providers must recognize and be able to respond to unique situations. For example, the HIPAA Privacy Rule permits a parent to agree that a minor child may obtain confidential treatment. The HIPAA Privacy Rule also permits a covered healthcare provider to choose not to provide parental access to a child's healthcare information if the provider is concerned about abuse or harm to the child. The HIPAA Privacy Rule imposes very specific requirements for written authorizations for the release of medical information. Those requirements include a description of the relationship of the person authorizing the release to the patient when signed by someone other than the patient.

Problem Solving and Decision Making

Problems within the context of healthcare require sensitivity and care. Each problem may have ethical as well as legal components in which resources may be sought to provide support and direction. The provider must weigh the outcomes from each element of an individual decision. The final decision making comes down to the provider and the guardian in a shared decision-making model seeking the best interest of the child as the outcome. The provider must collaborate with the guardian to seek the most successful outcome for the child with respect to the family as well. There must be consideration of evaluating the benefits and burdens of treating and not treating the child. The provider and guardian must consider the physical and emotional effects of treatment on the child, any pain or suffering that might be involved, any effect of the treatment on the child's life expectancy, and the potential for recovery and restorations, with and without the treatment. The indications, risks, side effects, and benefits of the treatment are included in the consent process. Finally, the decision overall should be based on family goals and values as reflected in previous healthcare decisions.

Independent providers, such as APRNs, must consider routine methods for solving problems, including using peers and mentors to voice concerns and to seek guidance. The APRN may have access to organizational ethics committees or consultants who may provide assistance in difficult matters. When in a leadership position with staff, the APRN should seek the input of all clinical parties with concerns so as to gain any pertinent or additional information necessary to formulate a solution.

General models for solving ethical problems are similar to clinical problem-solving methods such as collecting data, considering possible outcomes, and deriving a best outcome through engaging the appropriate persons for decision making. When ethical principles are at risk or have been violated outright, some of the various elements may be considered using the following method, adapted from the *Practitioner's Guide to Ethical Decision Making* (Forester-Miller and Davis 2016).

1. Identify the problem.
2. Apply the Code of Ethics.
3. Determine the nature and dimensions of the dilemma.
4. Generate potential courses of action.
5. Consider the potential consequences of all options and determine a course of action.
6. Evaluate the selected course of action.
7. Implement the course of action.

Capacity and Competence

There is a presumption of competence in the law (Physicians, Surgeons and Other Healers, *American Jurisprudence* 2002). Adult guardians and those over the age of majority are presumed competent and capable of making healthcare decisions for their children when engaged in the elements of consent and the decision-making process. The determination that an individual guardian is incompetent, and therefore incapable of giving informed consent, is a judicial one. Concurrent with a determination of incompetence is the appointment of a guardian to serve as the individual's legal representative.

When the practitioner is concerned about the soundness of a guardian's decision making or whether the guardian is acting in the best interest of the child, it may be necessary to seek the input from another guardian, if one exists, or obtain guidance from a child protective agency or a court, if the situation warrants such intervention.

When creating a sensitive professional relationship with a young child or adolescent, the provider should be motivated to allow this child some latitude in participation in decision making, based on the child's developmental age. Truthful, honest foundations are key to the therapeutic relationship. It is at this time when the APRN and guardian support the young person in their growth, playing a more active role in their care. Specifically, the adolescent has the right to a protected period in which to develop his or her decision-making skills (Mercurio 2007). The basic four elements of capacity have been established and include the ability to communicate, the ability to understand the information being presented, the ability to appreciate the decision, and the ability to reason between options, using personal values (Appelbaum 2007). Young children are capable of participating in decisions at a basic threshold, showing some evidence of choice. As the child matures, the child is more able to identify a reasonable outcome in order to base a choice. As the child matures, the child will base a choice on rational reasons and then will begin to show evidence of understanding. Finally, as an adult, the child is able to exhibit actual understanding.

When assessing the child for developmental capacity in decision making, consider a developmental assessment of cognitive and social elements. Assess the child for cognitive development, their use of preoperational versus concrete versus formal operations (Piaget and Inhelder 1969). The child must be able to form an understanding of hypothetical reasoning as in the formal operations in order to participate fully in weighing options in decisions. Furthermore, the APRN should consider elements of information processing, including attention span and memory, in the child. Capacity assessment of a child should also consider a social assessment looking for examples of conformity versus nonconformity behavior, examples of identity development, identification of personal values and resiliency, and previous experience with decisions (McCabe 1996). The child may be involved at different levels: being informed, voicing a view, influencing the decision, and then finally being the final decision maker (Alderson 2007). Children over 14 years of age but under the age of majority who are developmentally capable should be engaged in all disclosure elements. The guardian and APRN should consider an individualized threshold for participation in decision making. Children aged 7–14 years should be engaged in disclosure to their level of capacity for participation but should strictly use an assent/dissent model with regard to plan of care. If the plan is not to be disclosed to the child, the provider should document the nature of the decision. Finally, children as they approach the age of majority may be engaged by the practitioner and guardian to enact a psychiatric advanced directive (PAD) to specify their wishes for therapy should their ability to participate in the decision making be impaired related to their mental health or other reasons.

Informed Consent

One of the first and most fundamental steps in providing care to any patient is obtaining the informed consent of the patient, or someone authorized to act on behalf of the patient. In the case of a minor child, we usually assume it is the parent who must provide that consent, and in most instances that is true. In fact, the Fourteenth Amendment of the US Constitution protects the fundamental right of parents to make decisions concerning the care, custody, and control of their children. That right is not absolute, however, and it may be waived or supplanted by circumstance or government action.

As a general rule, parents must provide consent for the treatment of a child until the child reaches the age of majority. One exception to that rule is created by a change in the legal status of the child. Most, but not all, states have laws in place that permit a minor to become emancipated, thereby separating the minor from the control of his or her parents and relieving the parents from responsibility for the minor. An emancipated minor has the legal right to consent to treatment, regardless of the parents' wishes (Parent and Child, *American Jurisprudence* 2002). The procedure and requirements for becoming emancipated vary between the states that permit it but can result in documentary evidence of emancipation. A healthcare provider should not act on the belief that a child is emancipated without a copy of that evidence. In addition to legal emancipation, some states recognize the rights of homeless minors and/or those fitting the statutory definition of mature to consent to medical treatment.

State and federal law creates other exceptions to the rule of parental consent. For example, a minor has the right to obtain HIV testing in every state without having parental consent. Depending on the state, minors may also have the right to seek testing, counseling, and treatment for other conditions, such as pregnancy, sexually transmitted disease, sexual assault, substance abuse, and mental health issues. A healthcare provider offering any of these services to minors should know the laws of his or her state regarding parental consent and have clear policies and procedures in place for when these issues arise.

Another exception to the need for parental consent arises in the case of an emergency. If a minor presents to a healthcare provider in need of emergency treatment, the parents are deemed to have given "implied consent" for that treatment (Parent and Child, *American Jurisprudence* 2002). It is the same concept that allows healthcare providers to render treatment to patients who are unconscious; there is an assumption that the patient or parent of the patient would consent to the treatment if he or she were able to do so. Obviously, there can be disagreements over what constitutes an emergency. Generally speaking, if the patient is at risk for serious harm or death without immediate treatment, the implied consent rule applies. If, however, treatment can be delayed until someone with the authority to provide consent can be contacted, without harm to the patient, efforts should be made to obtain consent.

Even in the absence of any of the exceptions described above, the issue of parental consent is not always simple. In the case of divorced or unmarried parents, the parent with legal custody is authorized to provide consent. Healthcare providers cannot assume that the parent with physical custody also has legal custody. Therefore, before consent to treatment is obtained, the parent with the legal right to provide that consent must be identified. For some children, there may be a guardian or governmental entity, such as a department of social services, that has the right to consent to treatment, not the biological parents. In those instances, the healthcare provider must obtain documentation describing the parameters of the parental rights that have been transferred to the guardian or entity and what, if any, rights the biological parents continue to have.

Once the person authorized to provide consent is identified, the next step is to provide the information necessary to allow an informed decision. Such information generally includes the indications for, the risks and benefits of, and the alternatives to the proposed therapy. The depth of the information to be provided is dependent, in large part, on the nature of the proposed therapy. Various standards for disclosure are described in practice, but the "reasonable person standard" is most widely accepted. Significant risks, likely side effects, and those therapies that require invasive procedures also require that more information be given to the guardian in advance. It is important that children and their guardians be given the opportunity to ask questions and obtain clarity regarding the proposed therapy. Consent for more complex or invasive procedures should be written, along with documentation of the information provided. Finally, the consent must be voluntary without undue influence based on the decision maker's value system.

Right to Refuse Treatment

Inherent in the concept of informed consent is the right to withhold consent. The right to refuse treatment is based upon more than just the doctrine of informed consent, however. The right of a patient, or in the case of a minor, a guardian, to refuse treatment is also rooted in the constitutionally protected right to privacy (*Cruzan v. Missouri Department of Health* 1990). In most instances, declining to consent to treatment is, in essence, a refusal of treatment and absent an emergency of some sort, the matter is closed. Situations do arise, however, where public policy or safety override one's right to refuse certain treatment. In the behavioral health setting, situations most often involve patients who are deemed to be a danger to themselves or others and in need of involuntary detention and treatment by means of a civil commitment. The standards for involuntary commitment are established by state law, but most require some degree of immediacy of the threat of self-harm or harm to others. The more difficult situations often involve the refusal of treatment that may be vital, even lifesaving, in the absence of immediate danger or any suicidal or homicidal threat. News stories have detailed the accounts of parents who have refused treatment for their children on religious or other grounds. In some instances, providers have petitioned the courts for the right to treat without the patient's or parents' consent; in other instances, the state has assumed legal custody of the child to ensure that treatment was given. Some courts have upheld the patients' and/or parents' rights to refuse treatment, regardless of the likely outcome of that refusal. Each of these situations is fact-specific and the options available to the healthcare providers dependent on state law. It is important in each of these situations, however, that the treatment team work together, with input from an ethics committee, if available, and legal counsel to determine the best course to take.

Medication Management

Prescribing medication always presents potential risks. That is particularly true when prescribing psychotropic medication for children and adolescents. It is important that the APRN takes steps to minimize those risks when ordering or monitoring medications. As with any healthcare decision, the APRN should consider the risks and benefits of the medication. An analysis of the risks should include not only a review of the potential side effects and contraindications, but also any history of allergy or adverse reaction to medication and potential interaction with other medication the child may be taking. A thorough history should be obtained and documented in the child's record, along with an ongoing review of the child's response to the medication and rationale for its continued use. Patient education is vital, not only for the child, but for the parent/guardian as well.

Involuntary Patients

In the case of court-mandated outpatient therapy or inpatient treatment, the APRN must provide the assessment and therapy as defined by the involuntary commitment and the provisions of the state Nurse Practice Act. Much of the recent trend in involuntary therapy is in the outpatient environment. Guardians and children must be informed with full disclosure of the nature of this order and the consequences. Nonadherence to therapy recommendations is common in clinical settings but in the case of children in involuntary therapy, nonadherence must be documented and reported to the legal authorities. Clearly, adherence to the appointment schedule and medication therapy are crucial, as would be attendance in a school setting and group sessions outside the provider's supervision.

Chemical or Physical Restraint

In the event that a child must be restrained or put into seclusion, there must be clear documentation of the danger to self, and the provider must assess and agree with the need. It is preferable that therapeutic holding be used should the situation require it. Yet, the provider must follow state law and organizational policies governing the restraint of minors, including any disclosure to the guardians and to the patient. Restraints should be limited and appropriate with respect to the escalation and danger, and removed as soon as the child has regained control and the provider's assessment deems it so. Emergency restraint may be applied if necessary to protect the child while the appropriate medical care or provider is en route. This must be time-limited and the child must be informed of the safety and concerns requiring the restraint throughout (Baren et al. 2008). Documentation in the narrative is valuable to the review of the care during a restraint or seclusion episode.

Reproductive Issues

Providing reproductive care and advice to minors presents a special challenge for healthcare providers. Although the days of forced sterilization are long past, the pendulum has not swung so far as to permit minors full autonomy in making decisions regarding reproductive issues. Most states have laws concerning a minor's rights to birth control, but the specifics of those laws vary between states. Fewer than half of the states permit minors to obtain contraceptive services without restrictions, although some of those states permit the healthcare provider to notify the parents without the consent of the minor. A few states permit only married minors to obtain contraceptive services without parental consent, while others require only a determination that the minor is mature. As with many aspects of healthcare governed in whole or in part by state law, it is essential that providers who prescribe contraceptive services to minors familiarize themselves with the laws of their state.

Implications for Research

Historically, research with children has had some unfortunate outcomes, as exemplified by the Willowbrook Hepatitis Experiments 1956–1970 (Rothman and Rothman 2005). In 1979 the Belmont Report established the key principles for research ethics as respect for persons, beneficence and justice (National Commission for the Protection of Human Subjects of Biomedical and Behavioral Research). These principles influenced further the protections and regulations begun from the 1974 National Research Act, including the establishment of local institutional review boards for research oversight. In 1983, 45 Code of Federal Regulations Part 46 added research with children as a specifically protected population in their protection of human subjects, which was further revised in 2009 (Protection of Human Subjects 2009). Emmanuel et al. (2000) provided a comprehensive grouping of requirements that ethical research must satisfy, which continues to present and include:

1. value – for the knowledge from the work itself
2. scientific validity
3. fair subject selection
4. favorable risk–benefit ratio
5. independent review
6. informed consent
7. respect for the enrolled subjects.

Furthermore, with the enrollment of children in studies, specifically within the behavioral health context and with respect to informed consent (proxy consent), researchers need to include the child in a process of "informed assent." Assent has been recognized historically within clinical and research areas for adults and children. The American Academy of Pediatrics (AAP) published their findings and recommendations for assent in 1995 (which were reaffirmed in 2006); these recommendations have been widely referred to since. Securing assent for the child's participation in a research study, especially when the study outcome has a low benefit impact for the child, is in the general sense securing an agreement by the child to participate.

The information shared with the child should include age-specific language and a brief explanation of the child's role as a subject. The child must be informed that she/he can stop participation whenever she/he needs to and that any questions she/he has will be answered. The child should also understand that there is no penalty for not participating. Furthermore, a lack of disagreement by the child does not indicate an agreement or assent to participate AAP. The child's assent should be in conjunction with the guardians' consent. Guardians must be confident that participation is consistent with the child's interests and values. In relation to proxy consent, caution should be used when the actual individual benefit is low and the risks or uncertainty of risks/benefits are unknown. Guardian consent as proxy for the child should also be scrutinized for obvious power influences, that is, persuasion by the guardian (Coyne 2010). APRNs who serve as primary investigators should not enroll their own clients for obvious influential persuasion. The research team and process should include many checks and balances to ensure that respect for subjects includes options for subjects to opt out, for subjects to gain information as gleaned from the study, and for subjects to be given information about harms or benefits during the course of the study (which may influence their willingness to continue).

Implications for Education and Continuing Education

Continuing education of practitioners is a professional obligation as stated in the ANA Code (2015) as well as being legally required by many state boards of nursing. It is recommended that an official review of licensure, scope of practice, and change in state statute occur annually as part of routine continuing education. Ethical issues that arise from legal precedent and various other avenues should be reviewed annually as well. Historically, a core competency in *The Essentials of Master's Education for Advanced Practice Nurses*, originally stated by Shugars, O'Neil, and Bader, was the ability for all health profession graduates to "provide counseling for patients in situations where ethical issues arise, as well as participate in discussions of ethical issues in healthcare as they affect communities, society and the health professions" (as cited in American Association of Colleges of Nursing [AACN] 1996, p. 9). Ethical decision making may be enhanced through the networking with peers and colleagues, and should be encouraged especially where APRNs are in solo practice or are further isolated in rural and remote areas.

Accreditation of Educational Programs

Several nursing organizations recommend content for undergraduate and graduate curricula related to ethical and legal knowledge and application. Content at the baccalaureate level should include professional values, including altruism, autonomy, human dignity, and integrity, as well as social justice (AACN 2008). Additional material should include ethical and legal frameworks, professional accountability, and the ANA Code (2015). Legal information at the undergraduate level should include Nurse Practice Acts and scope of practice. Ethical content for the undergraduate should also include moral agency, privacy, confidentiality, self-reflection, and professional accountability. Content for graduate programs specific to ethics should include identification and analysis of ethical dilemmas, decision-making process, personal, organizational, and research perspectives, conflict of interest, dilemma resolution, and professional accountability (AACN 2006, 2011). Surprisingly, there has been no mention of legal content or education recommendations. This seems to be an oversight on the part of the graduate recommendations where scope of practice and liability issues are accentuated due to the independent role of the APRN.

Implications for Primary Care: Ethical Situations

Primary care has in its nature the true basic relationship of provider to client and client to provider in a total trusting relationship based on integrity, altruism, and loyalty by both parties. The provider is required both ethically and legally to document an accurate reflection of the assessment, diagnosis, plan, therapy intervention, and an evaluation of such. The relationship in most instances is ongoing and this continuity is a basic foundation for both. In part due to the private nature of this relationship, ethical concerns are generated. Jeremy Sugarman in 2000 published *Twenty Common Problems: Ethics in Primary Care*, which provided an important early foundation. In this section we will consider other additional primary care issues, including:

- requests for nonindicated therapy and tests
- requests for medical exemptions and privileges
- adherence to therapeutic regimen
- managed care
- conflicts of interest and obligations
- consultation and referral
- requests for therapy outside of the client relationship.

Requests for Nonindicated Therapy and Tests

The concept of patient sovereignty as expressed previously lends itself to the issues for providers in which the client and/or family requests therapy or tests that are not indicated. While the provider is obligated to engage the client and guardian in a collaborative plan of care, the APRN should not shirk professional liability and acquiesce to the requests of clients that are not clinically indicated. Should the issues of power be so forceful, the provider with support of beneficence and nonmaleficience must insist on following clinically sound judgment, decline to prescribe the requested therapy, and, if necessary, assist the client in obtaining a second opinion and/or transfer the care to another provider.

Requests for Medical Exemptions and Privileges

Similarly, with regard to clients and guardians requesting medical exemptions and privileges, the APRN is supported through sound clinical judgment and ethical tenets of beneficence and nonmaleficience in a decision to decline from providing exemptions or privileges to patients upon their request. This is common in caring for children who must frequently miss school or sports activities for health reasons, and yet in missing those activities the APRN is accountable for the health of the child. The APRN should use sound judgment when considering such requests and work collaboratively with the family as a unit.

Adherence to Therapeutic Regimen

Adherence to medical recommendations can be complicated when working with clients who are children. Many times, the lack of adherence to therapy may be a result of the child's inability to cooperate, the guardian's inability to follow therapy based on finances, or perhaps even a misunderstanding of instructions or the like. Nonadherence can have significant implications: (i) it can be dangerous for the client not to take prescribed medications, (ii) it can cause the provider to misinterpret clinical assessment, and (iii) it can perhaps cause the provider even to make further unnecessary recommendations based on misinformation. Interventions for children who are not adhering to therapy includes an evaluation of the home setting and the guardian's ability to provide the care required, including making appropriate follow-up appointments and being at the appointments on time.

Managed Care

Managed care and the role of primary providers have led to various issues for clinicians in maintaining access to patients balanced with sound clinical practice.

Previously, it was a common practice to provide care as available without regard for cost. It is the accountable professional who will provide beneficent clinical sound care, while taking into account the cost to the society as a whole. For example, diagnostic procedures that will provide information that will not be used in treatment planning need not be performed. Information for the sake of information is not necessary. Sabin in 1994 addressed four rules for primary providers that were particularly valuable and have been extrapolated now for use within the APRN's practice. First, the APRN should view her dual duty as advocating for both the individual patient and other patients in the group by resource decisions. Second, always use the least expensive treatment unless there is substantial evidence that a more expensive treatment will be more effective. Third, spend some time reviewing the rules and practices of the managed care plan to assure the practices are fair. Finally, if the plan does not provide reimbursement for a therapy the provider believes would be beneficial, the provider should discuss the therapy, including the clinical indications, benefits, and costs, with the guardian to allow the guardian to make an informed decision on how to proceed.

Conflicts of Interest and Obligation

Clinicians have a primary duty to their clients; in the case where a provider's own interests conflict with such, an ethical conflict exists. Conflicts of interest as identified by Goold (2000) include investment in medical facilities, reimbursements for services, gifts from commercial or industry (pharmaceuticals), industry sponsorship of research, pursuit of nonmonetary goods (power, reputation), and peer pressure. Goold also identified conflicts of obligations as in clinical research, educating clinicians in training, needs of other patients for more time, and family needs. In considering the implications of these conflicts, the APRN should consider the following questions: Is the conflict avoidable or unavoidable? Is the conflict reasonable or unreasonable? What is the strength or intrusiveness of the conflict on the relationship and client trust?

Consultation and Referral

APRNs as primary providers may have opportunity to refer or consult with other APRNs, physicians, or other specialists related to the care of their clients. This stems from an ethical responsiveness to nonmaleficence. If the APRN deems that she or he is not the best suited to diagnose or treat the client, then the APRN must in an intention of "do no harm" engage another, more qualified clinician for the client. Employment concerns over self-referral or fee splitting are valid in these times where

healthcare organizations are often large and can be an obvious referral empire. The client must be aware of financial relationships that the APRN or the organization may have. Clients should be offered a choice where possible related to referrals.

Request for Therapy Outside of the Client Relationship

This is a common request known as the "curb side" consult or "neighbor" friendly advice. In this relationship, the APRN is not engaged in a professional relationship and should therefore be cautious about providing treatment or opinion for persons and children for whom there is no assessment or history taken or implications for relational veracity between this person and the APRN. Furthermore, documentation of this type of interaction would be unlikely and may cause further moral, ethical, or legal conflict for the APRN. An obvious exception to this would be in the event of urgent or emergency care for a person's life and safety.

Application

It is the hope of these authors that the material presented here is applicable to your practice and will be beneficial to your client base in a successful practice. The following two cases are presented along with the various actual and potential risks and violations or legal and ethical foundations. The resolution to each case is obviously dependent on many variables. Outcomes should be based on best interest standards with the balance of burdensome outcomes in the negative. Furthermore, it should be noted that legal and/or ethical consultation may be warranted. Table 28.1 contains definitions of terms used in the chapter.

Concept Illustration 1

This example involves a conflict with respect to a plan of care decision between the guardian and the APRN. While shared decision making is best practice, at times the interpretation of safety or protection of the patient by each may create moral distress or an ethical challenge for the APRN. The role of family may be key to successful treatment of the child and the APRN may be hesitant to create a division in this family unit even if there is identifiable risk. Yet, the primary legal obligation is to the patient. Interrupting the decision making of a guardian may lead to a sense of mistrust or overt confrontation. Furthermore, in all cases, while the child may not have legal standing, their voice being heard in these situations is foundational to respect. First, when the clinical recommendation is less certain, the guardian and/or child's wishes may be ultimately respected based on a principle of respect for persons. This ethical

Table 28.1 Glossary of ethical and legal terms

Term	Definition
Assent	In the case of categorical or functional incapacity, this is the general agreement to understanding and agreement to cooperation with treatment by the minor child. Informed consent is required from the guardian.
Autonomy	An ethical principle that is derived from a principle of respect for persons. Persons have the right to self-determination and choice about actions that impact their life and livelihood.
Benefits/ burdens balance	Desired outcome in ethically challenging decisions, with benefits outweighing burdens for the identified client as well as others with ethical standing.
Beneficence	An ethical principle that intends that actions will promote good.
Best interest	An ethical standard for decision making used with clients who have not reached mature adult capacity or competence. Best interest is generally thought to be best defined by the family and gradually by the child as he/she matures. In healthcare, the primary provider has considerable influence in defining this through the collaborative nature of the relationship with the child and family.
Capacity	A clinical assessment for capability to make independent decisions. Adults achieve a categorical definition of capacity by age of majority. Childhood as a category is defined as incapacitated. Elements of capacity include an ability to understand, communicate, reason, and appreciate the information/decision being considered with a set of personal values. Threshold for capacity required for certain decisions may be flexible depending on the significance of the decision.
Confidentiality/ privacy	Derived from a principle of respect for persons in which personal information shared in any form with any person representing the healthcare relationship may not be repeated or disclosed except by the client who owns all personal health information in any form.
Conflict of interest	A situation in which a provider's interests, whether professional, personal, economic, or otherwise, conflict with that of the patient.
Deontology	A moral philosophy credited to Immanuel Kant in which the moral actions are based on specific moral duties or obligations. More recent use of this philosophy incorporates use of a variety of duties and with these an evaluative nature of consequences in order to achieve a balance or right over wrong.
Disclosure	An element of informed consent in which information pertinent to the decision is shared with those involved with the decision. The content of the disclosure may be based on various standards, including the professional standard and the reasonable person standard. Disclosure should include nature of the therapy, purpose, risks, benefits, and alternatives.
Dissent	In the case of categorical or functional incapacity, this is the general agreement to understanding and disagreement to cooperation with treatment. Informed consent is required from the guardian.
Ethic of care	While similar in foundations to feminist ethic, this ethical theory is based on relationships and engages communication and cooperation as strategies for problem solving. This theory does emphasize sensitivity and emotion, and while this is a valid motivator for clinical practice, its use in challenging decision making is limited.
Ethical dilemma	A potential or actual violation of an ethical principle with regard to an individual client in a healthcare relationship, whether intentional or unintentional, with actual or potential for burdensome outcome.
Ethical standing	Also referred to as moral standing or ethical right, this is the claim by someone other than the legal guardian that their perspective or information is valuable to the care of the patient. This may be a consistent caregiver in the case of a child.
Feminist ethic	A contextual theory that highlights the relationship of the provider and the client with regard to actions from a sense of justice and care. Decision making itself in the healthcare arena is embedded in this relationship, and for this reason this theory does not provide specific guidance in decision making, more in the context of the relationship usually specific to power and vulnerable groups.
Fidelity	An ethical value in a trusting relationship from which loyalty and accountability are derived.

(continued)

Table 28.1 (*cont'd*)

Term	Definition
Informed consent	Derived from the principle of respect for persons; an ethical ideal with intended outcome to engage the person to make efficient and effective decisions with regard to beneficial outcomes as defined by the person. Elements generally include a voluntary and capable decision maker (capacity), as well as the adequate disclosure and comprehension of information.
Integrity	A self-actualized set of values, including accuracy, honesty, and truthfulness, as a professional in clinical practice and professional relationships.
Justice	A general ethical principle that intends that actions are fair with equal impact and outcome. In healthcare, specifically, distributive justice as a principle considers the allocation of scarce resources such as access to providers and outpatient therapy.
Least restrictive environment	One of six principles included in the protection of students with disabilities as defined by the Individuals with Disabilities Education Act (2004), which is interpreted that children with disabilities should be included in classrooms with nondisabled students to the extent possible.
Malpractice	Professional misconduct; the failure to exercise the degree of skill and education that would be expected of a reasonable professional in the same situation.
Moral distress	With respect to healthcare professionals, this anguish may not only be professional but also personal and may violate one or more various personal values of self-defined moral agency. This distress may not be an ethical dilemma for the client but rests solely as dilemma for the professional.
Negligence	The failure to act as a reasonable person would act under given circumstances, or the taking of action that a reasonable and prudent person would not.
Nonmaleficence	An ethical principle that intends that actions will not cause harm.
Paternalism	An ethical principle for which the practitioner makes independent clinical treatment decisions without the input of the client or with disregard of the client's input.
Patient sovereignty	Power demanded by the patient to make clinical requests for care regardless of the practitioner's judgment in the healthcare context.
Professional ethics	In healthcare professions certain societal obligations of a caregiver are paramount, including a duty to help; that actions will promote health and palliate illness and distress.
Power	A dynamic force at work in relationships, as a result of individual perception and conflict of authority. This force may be overt or discrete. In the case of an imbalance, the individuals may choose to address this and resolve it or not. The choice to address the imbalance is dependent on the obligation of the individual to advocate for an outcome.
Respect for persons	A principle highly valued in Western society in which human beings are highly valued as individuals and in that various principles and values are derived including self-determination, autonomy, privacy, and veracity.
Shared decision-making model of care	This blends respect for autonomy and clinical expertise as defined by both clinicians and other persons. The success of treatment plans depends on the adherence and motivation of the client as well as the expertise and flexibility of the provider.
Truth-telling/ veracity	Derived from a principle of respect for persons. Disclosure with fundamental intent on sharing information as well as meaning and recommendation; this differs from "telling the truth," which may be described as sharing only the most comfortable knowledge with a trend toward paternalism. This may be to individual clients or in professional relationships.
Utilitarianism	A moral theory credited to Jeremy Bentham and John Stuart Mill in which the morality of an action is based on its consequences, moreover that the balance of good outweighs any costs.
Virtue ethics	An ethical theory that is based in the character of the person and their actions based in this character. Virtuous behavior is motivated by such values as honesty, kindness, fairness, and loyalty. Decision making is not from principles or obligations but from the person's sense of value in personal virtues. This theory, while providing motivation in clinical practice, is difficult to apply to an ethical dilemma.

Definitions developed by authors. Refer to *The Stanford Encyclopedia of Philosophy* (Zalta 2019).

outcome commonly results as the guardian, using their parental authority, makes a best interest decision for the child/adolescent. Documentation of this decision is vital. In some cases, a second clinical opinion may be sought. Second, when the clinical recommendation is clear, such as intervention for acute depression, the provider has actionable legal responsibilities to protect and treat, including notifying authorities if the guardian intends to remove the child from protective treatment. APRN confidence in duty to protect and ethical obligations to intervene regardless of the risk to the family unit is key to addressing a conflict between guardian and APRN which puts the child at risk. Documentation must include the specific risks and indication for legal protection.

Concept Illustration 2

This example involves the explicit request by the guardian for specific treatment interventions, such as medication or hospitalization, which the APRN does not recommend. The intense relationship of guardian to child may be expressed in many ways. Advocacy behaviors of the guardian may be expressed not only as a request, but as an insistence for specific treatment. Guardian stress or angst with a child's behavior may incite these requests for medication, a quick fix. Further, guardians may intentionally or unintentionally use the threat of these potential clinical interventions for their own parenting/behavior management with the child. The APRN is legally and professionally obligated to adhere to standard of care and professional guidelines in diagnostic and treatment decisions regardless of guardian persistence. Ethically the consideration of the guardian's understanding, reasoning, and appreciation of these requests is key. Documentation of the requests should be included in the assessment and outcome of these requests in the treatment plan of care notes.

Summary

The APRN providing care to children in the pediatric or mental health setting has a unique relationship to his or her patients, one that presents both great opportunity and great responsibility. While it is essential for the APRN to always consider the best interests of the child, he or she is often confronted with diverse, and sometimes competing, interests. The APRN must understand the potential legal and ethical challenges that may arise, and be cognizant of the way in which his or her own personal values and ethical code of practice may impact decision making and interactions with patients, families, and colleagues. Establishing procedures and protocols that are based on sound clinical practice and compliant with state and federal law and regulations is a critical

first step. Knowledge of what, when, and where to document information is not only important clinically but also necessary for sound risk management. While unexpected outcomes are inevitable in healthcare, a practice that incorporates sound clinical decisions, respect for patients and their families and guardians, and an awareness of one's ethical and legal obligations provides a solid foundation to enable one to respond appropriately when dealing with those outcomes. When a provider is confronted with a situation that presents ethical or legal challenges that are unusual or beyond the experience of the provider, it is important that the provider reach out for guidance. Depending upon the situation, colleagues, ethical advisors, and/or a healthcare attorney may be able to provide valuable support to assist in protecting the interests of both the patient and the provider.

References

Alderson, P. (2007). Competent children? Minors' consent to health care treatment and research. *Social Science and Medicine* 65: 2272–2283.

AAP (1995). Informed consent, parental permission, and assent in pediatric practice. *Pediatrics* 95: 314–317.

AACN (1996). *The Essentials of Master's Education for Advanced Practice Nurses.* Washington, DC: American Association of Colleges of Nursing.

AACN (2006). *The Essentials of Doctoral Education for Advanced Nursing Practice.* Washington, DC: American Association of Colleges of Nursing Available at https://www.aacnnursing.org/Portals/42/Publications/DNPEssentials.pdf.

AACN (2008). *The Essentials of Baccalaureate Education for Professional Nursing Practice.* Washington, DC: American Association of Colleges of Nursing. Available at https://www.aacnnursing.org/Portals/42/Publications/BaccEssentials08.pdf.

AACN (2011). *The Essentials of Master's Education in Nursing.* Washington, DC: American Association of Colleges of Nursing Available at https://www.aacnnursing.org/Portals/42/Publications/MastersEssentials11.pdf.

AACCN (2006). *The 4As to Rise Above Moral Distress Toolkit.* Aliso Viejo, CA: American Association of Critical Care Nurses, Ethics Work Group.

AANP (2019). *NP Fact Sheet.* Austin, TX: American Association of Nurse Practitioners Available at https://www.aanp.org/about/all-about-nps/np-fact-sheet.

ANA (2015). *Code of Ethics for Nurses with Interpretive Statements.* Silver Spring, MD: American Nurses Association Available at https://www.nursingworld.org/practice-policy/nursing-excellence/ethics/code-of-ethics-for-nurses/.

Appelbaum, P. (2007). Assessment of patient's competence to consent to treatment. *The New England Journal of Medicine* 357: 1834–1840.

Baren, J., Mace, S., Hendry, P. et al. (2008). Children's mental health emergencies: part 2. *Emergency Department Evaluation and Treatment of Children with Mental Health Disorders. Pediatric Emergency Care* 24: 485–498.

Beauchamp, T.L. and Childress, J.F. (2019). *Principles of Biomedical Ethics.* New York: Oxford University Press.

Child Abuse Prevention and Treatment Act of 1974 (CAPTA), 42 U.S.C. §5101 et seq. (1974).

CNA & National Service Organization. (2017). *A Guide to Identifying and Addressing Professional Liability Exposures, Nurse Practitioner Claim Report*, 4th Edition. Available at https://aonaffinity.blob.core. windows.net/affinitytemplate-prod/media/nso/images/documents/cna_cls_np_exec_101617_cf_prod_asize_online_sec.pdf.

Cohen, E. and Cesta, T. (2005). *Nursing Case Management: From Essentials to Advanced Practice Applications*, 4e. St. Louis, MO: Mosby.

Collins, S. and Mikos, C. (2008). Evolving taxonomy of nurse practice act violators. *Journal of Nursing Law* 12: 85–91.

Coyne, I. (2010). Research with children and young people: the issue of parental (proxy) consent. *Children & Society* 24: 227–237.

Cruzan v. Missouri Department of Health. 492 U.S. 261, 271 (1990).

Ebert, R.E. (2008). Attorneys, tell your clients to say they're sorry: apologies in the health care industry. *Indiana Health Law Review* 5: 337.

Emmanuel, E., Wendler, D., and Grady, C. (2000). What makes clinical research ethical. *Journal of the American Medical Association* 283: 2701–2711.

Fisher, M. (2009). Replacing "who is the client" with a different ethical question. *Professional Psychology: Research and Practice* 40: 1–7.

Forester-Miller, H. & Davis, T.E. (2016). *Practitioner's guide to ethical decision making*, revised edition. Available at https://www.counseling.org/docs/default-source/ethics/practioner-39-s-guide-to-ethical-decision-making.pdf?sfvrsn=10.

Geske, M.R. (1989). Statutes limiting mental health professionals' liability for the violent acts of their patients. *Indiana Law Journal* 64: 391–399.

Goold, S. (2000). Conflicts of interest and obligation. In: *Twenty Common Problems: Ethics in Primary Care* (ed. J. Sugarman), 93–102. New York, NY: McGraw-Hill.

International Council for Nurses (2012). *The ICN Code of Ethics for Nurses*. Geneva, Switzerland: International Council for Nurses.

Killinger, B. (2007). *Integrity: Doing the Right Thing for the Right Reason*. Montreal, Quebec: University Press.

Laabs, C.A. (2007). Primary care nurse practitioners' integrity when faced with moral conflict. *Nursing Ethics* 14: 795–809. https://doi.org/10.1177/0969733007082120.

McCabe, M.A. (1996). Involving children and adolescents in medical decision making: developmental and clinical considerations. *Journal of Pediatric Psychology* 21: 505–516.

Mercurio, M.R. (2007). An adolescent's refusal of medical treatment: implications of the Abraham Cheerix case. *Pediatrics* 120: 1357–1358.

National Commission for the Protection of Human Subjects of Biomedical and Behavioral Research. (1979). *The Belmont report: Ethical principles and guidelines for the protection of human subjects of research*. Available at https://www.hhs.gov/ohrp/regulations-and-policy/belmont-report/index.html.

Negligence. In *American Jurisprudence*, 2nd edn. 57B, §1106. Eagan, MN: West Publishing (2002).

Parent and Child. In *American Jurisprudence*, 2nd edn. 59, §792. Eagan, MN: West Publishing (2002).

Peterson, M. and Potter, R. (2004). A proposal for a code of ethics for nurse practitioners. *Journal of the American Academy of Nurse Practitioners* 16: 116–124.

Physicians, Surgeons, and Other Healers. In *American Jurisprudence*, 2nd edn. 61, §§158, 167, 287. Eagan, MN: West Publishing (2002).

Piaget, J. and Inhelder, B. (1969). *The Psychology of the Child*, 2nde. New York, NY: Basic Books.

Porter, J. and Mackay, T. (2012). The collateral damage to nursing licenses caused by nursing board disciplinary actions. *Journal of Nursing Law* 15: 1–6.

Protection of Human Subjects, 45 C.F.R. §46.101 (2009).

Rothman, D. and Rothman, S. (2005). *The Willowbrook Wars: Bringing the Disabled into the Community*. New Brunswick, NJ: Transaction Publishers.

Rothstein, M. (2009). The role of law in the development of American bioethics. *The International Journal of Bioethics* 20: 73–84, 110–111.

Sabin, J. (1994). A credo for ethical managed care in mental health practice. *Hospital Community Psychiatry* 45: 859–860.

Sugarman, J. (2000). *Twenty Common Problems: Ethics in Primary Care*. New York, NY: McGraw-Hill.

Tarasoff v. Pregents of the University of California, et al., 551 P, 2d 334 (1976).

USDHHS. (2013). *Summary of the HIPAA Privacy Rule*. US Department of Health and Human Services Available at http://www.hhs.gov/ocr/privacy/hipaa/understanding/summary/index.html.

USDHHS. (2019a). *About CAPTA: A legislative history*. US Department of Health and Human Services, Child Welfare Information Gateway. Available at https://www.childwelfare.gov/pubPDFs/about.pdf.

USDHHS. (2019b). *Immunity for reporters of child abuse and neglect: Summary of state laws*. US Department of Health and Human Services, Child Welfare Information Gateway. Available at https://www.childwelfare.gov/pubPDFs/immunity.pdf.

USDHHS. (2019c). *Enforcement highlights: Enforcement results as of August 31, 2019*. US Department of Health and Human Services, Office for Civil Rights. Available at https://www.hhs.gov/hipaa/for-professionals/compliance-enforcement/data/enforcement-highlights/index.html.

Ulrich, C.M., Zhou, Q.P., Hanlon, A. et al. (2014). The impact of ethics and work-related factors on nurse practitioners' and physician assistants' views on quality of primary healthcare in the United States. *Applied Nursing Research: ANR* 27 (3): 152–156. https://doi.org/10.1016/j.apnr.2014.01.001.

Yorker, B. (1995). Liability issues for nurses who work with psychiatric mental health patients. *Journal of Nursing Law* 2: 7–20.

Yorker, B. (1997). Institutional liability for children who molest other children. *American Professional Society on the Abuse of Children-Advisor* 10: 9–15.

Zalta, E.N. (ed.) (2019). *The Stanford Encyclopedia of Philosophy*. Stanford, CA: The Metaphysics Research Lab, Center for the Study of Language and Information, Stanford University. Available at https://plato.stanford.edu.

29

Evidence-based Nursing Practice

Donna Hallas[1] and Pamela Lusk[2]

[1]Rory Meyers College of Nursing, New York University, New York City, NY, USA
[2]Ohio State University College of Nursing, Columbus, OH, USA

Objectives

After reading this chapter, advanced prctice registered nurses (APRNs) will be able to:

1. Describe the process for implementation of evidence-based practice (EBP) in pediatric and adolescent primary care and mental health practice settings.
2. Describe the significance of using EBP in clinical settings.
3. Apply the evidence-based format for use in clinical practice settings:
   a. Identify a practice problem.
   b. Formulate clinically relevant PICO questions.
   c. Describe strategies to search for the best available evidence.
   d. Discuss the use of critical appraisal tools in the evidence-based process.
4. Identify national and international EBP resources that are available to improve care for children/adolescents and their families using the best available evidence.

Introduction

Evidence-based medicine (EBM) was first described by Sackett, Rosenberg, Muir Gray, Haynes, and Richardson in 1996: "Evidence-based medicine is the conscientious, explicit, and judicious use of current best evidence in making decisions about the care of individual patients. The practice of evidence-based medicine means integrating individual clinical expertise with the best available external clinical evidence from systematic research" (p. 71). The underpinnings of this work have been the analysis of the results of research studies conducted to examine the efficacy of interventions and treatments using an experimental treatment and control group design. Included in the description of evidence-based

practice (EBP) was the concept of considering patient preferences in the decision-making process (Sackett et al. 2000).

EBM has evolved into an EBP framework that has been embraced by nursing, the social sciences, including psychology, and other allied health professions. Evidence-based nursing has adopted Sackett et al.'s definition of EBM. Thus, nurses make clinical decisions based on the best available current research evidence with use of critical appraisal tools, his or her own clinical expertise, and the needs and preferences of the patient (Melynk and Fineout-Overholt 2019).

Implementation of EBP requires a commitment from each healthcare provider to search for and use the best

---

Child and Adolescent Behavioral Health: A Resource for Advanced Practice Psychiatric and Primary Care Practitioners in Nursing,
Second Edition. Edited by Edilma L. Yearwood, Geraldine S. Pearson, and Jamesetta A. Newland.
© 2021 John Wiley & Sons, Inc. Published 2021 by John Wiley & Sons, Inc.
Companion website: www.wiley.com/go/Yearwood

available evidence to establish the diagnosis and care management plans for each patient encountered in every practice settings. Prior to implementation of a practice guideline or the evidence-based work, a critical appraisal of the literature must be performed to determine if the guideline or evidence is relevant for the patient population to which it will be applied. For each pediatric patient, implementation also includes assessing the preferences of the child and family members and incorporating these preferences into care management plans to achieve optimum healthcare for each individual and family.

Analysis of the interrelatedness of primary healthcare, including the behavioral, mental and emotional healthcare for each patient encountered in primary care and mental health settings, represents major practice changes by pediatric nurse practitioners (PNPs), family nurse practitioners (FNPs), psychiatric nurse practitioners (PMHNPs), or psychiatric clinical nurse specialists (PMHCNSs). Collaborative practice between these providers has been shown to improve the care provided to each child, adolescent, and family with a focus on both the physical and emotional health of the child/adolescent and the family unit. Pediatric, family, and psychiatric practitioners (referred to as advanced practice registered nurses [APRNs] throughout this chapter) who understand the significance of these interrelationships are able to enhance their care management plans through critical analysis of the best available evidence for both primary care management and the mental healthcare management of patients.

This chapter describes current issues related to the implementation of EBP for APRNs in their individual and collaborative practices. Over the past several years, a call for integration of primary care and mental health services has continued to change the delivery of care, thus primary care providers interact and apply EBP within one clinical setting, so serving the needs of the children and families under one roof (Substance Abuse and Mental Health Service Administration n.d.)

The steps for implementing EBP in practice settings are (Melynk and Fineout-Overholt 2019, p. 17):

Step 0: Cultivate a spirit of inquiry within an EBP culture and environment.

Step 1: Ask the burning question in PICOT (population, intervention, comparison, outcome) format.

Step 2: Search for and collect the most relevant best evidence.

Step 3: Critically appraise the evidence (i.e. rapid critical appraisal, evaluation, and synthesis)

Step 4: Integrate the best evidence with one's clinical expertise and patient preferences and values in making a practice decision or change.

Step 5: Evaluate outcomes of the practice decision or change based on evidence.

Step 6: Disseminate the outcomes of the EBP decision or change.

National and international resources for using EBP in primary and mental health practice settings are highlighted in Table 29.1.

Significance of Implementing Evidence-based Practice

The standard of practice is for APRNs to continuously raise relevant evidence-based formatted questions, critically appraise and analyze each phase of the evidence-based care management process, and use the best available evidence for each clinical decision to provide care that is scientifically based. EBP is based on the use of interventions for which there is consistent

Table 29.1 Evidence-based resources

Agency for Healthcare Research and Quality, http://www.ahrq.gov

AGREE Tools, https://www.agreetrust.org/2011/06/new-agree-ii-training-tools

American Academy of Child and Adolescent Psychiatry (AACAP), http://www.aacap.org

American Academy of Pediatrics (AAP), http://www.aap.org

American Psychiatric Association (APA), https://www.psychiatry.org

Clinical trials, http://clinicaltrials.gov

Cochrane Collaboration, http://www.cochrane.org

Joanna Briggs Institute, http://joannabriggs.org

Agency for Healthcare Research Quality (AHRQ), https://www.ahrq.gov/gam/index.html

Critical Appraisal Skills Programme (CASP), http://www.casp-uk.net

PubMed, https://www.ncbi.nlm.nih.gov/pubmed

scientific evidence showing that the interventions improve healthcare outcomes (Black et al. 2015; Drake et al. 2001). When patient preferences are integrated within the clinical decision-making process, patients achieve improved healthcare outcomes (Ganz 2002; Siminoff 2013). Thus, APRNs who incorporate EBP for each patient encounter have the potential to significantly improve patient outcomes, patient and family satisfaction with their care, and the overall physical and emotional health of their patients and their family members.

Evidence-based Practice in Classroom and Clinical Settings

Practicing in an evidence-based classroom and clinical environment has evolved over the past 20 years to one in which students learn by examining cases and applying the evidence-based literature and clinical practice guidelines (CPGs) in both classroom and clinical environments. Faculty, preceptor, and clinical mentors are facilitators of learning and are expected to embrace student and clinician inquiries, offering students and clinicians opportunities to explore all diagnostic and treatment possibilities for each individual patient presentation. Students and clinicians are expected to be active lifelong learners who critically question everything and search for the best available evidence to diagnose and treat the pediatric and adolescent patient and family. Textbooks are resources but database searches for the best available evidence are daily occurrences in an EBP environment. In clinical EBP environments, new and experienced clinicians who have embraced the EBP practice model explore established and intentional inquisitive processes to design treatment plans for patients that include implementation of a CPG, individual patient preferences as well as expert opinion, in the absence of CPGs or individual high-quality studies.

Hospital-based clinical practices are also driven by EBP guidelines with the goal of improving healthcare outcomes for each individual patient and the populations that they serve. Hospitals that have attained Magnet status from the American Nurses Credentialing Center (ANCC) and those that desire to attain Magnet status must demonstrate the use of EBP as well as quality improvement (QI) projects to achieve the best outcomes for their patients. Thus, EBP has become the standard of care for all inpatient and outpatient centers and providers at all levels of care, e.g. nurses, nurse practitioners, physicians and physician assistants, must be familiar with the implementation and evaluation of EBP.

The Evidence-based Process

The evidence-based process for clinical practice includes using the following strategies:

1. Cultivate a spirit of inquiry within an EBP culture and environment.
2. Critically analyze problems at the patient level and the systems level to develop relevant clinical questions in PICO format.
3. Search the databases for systematic reviews of the literature, meta-analyses, CPGs, and randomized controlled studies or case studies that address the clinical questions.
4. Appraise the literature using Critical Appraisal Skills Program (CASP) tools or the Appraisal of Guidelines Research & Evaluation (AGREE) tool (for CPGs) (Advancing the Science of Practice Guidelines n.d.).
5. Combine the best available evidence, the APRN's clinical expertise, and patient preferences and values to make and implement practice decisions.
6. Evaluate the clinical decisions.
7. Disseminate the outcomes of the EBP decision or change (Melynk and Fineout-Overholt 2019).

As outlined in the EBP steps above, the APRN who has searched and appraised the best evidence from research also considers his/her own level of clinical expertise in delivering interventions with the strongest support from the literature. Just as APRN clinical competence with specific interventions informs the clinical action plan, the patient and family preferences and values are a significant consideration in treatment planning. As an example, parents may bring in their 7-year-old child with a copy of the recent psychological evaluation completed by the school psychologist and psychiatrist. The diagnosis is attention deficit hyperactive disorder (ADHD) and the recommendation is for stimulant medication. The APRN reviews the literature using the EBP process. Systematic reviews are found that support stimulant medication and behavioral interventions. Clinical guidelines accessed also recommend stimulant medication and behavioral interventions. In the pediatric visit, the parents inform the APRN of their belief that children should never take medications that might affect their growing brain. This is a belief that has been held in their family for generations. The APRN will incorporate the parent's strong preferences and values about not using medication into the practice decision. In this case the behavioral interventions identified in the literature as having strong support for being effective with children diagnosed with ADHD are part of the APRN's usual practice and these interventions are acceptable and welcomed by the parents. The evidence-based behavioral interventions will be implemented. EBP always considers the best evidence from the literature, the clinician's expertise with recommended interventions, and the child/adolescent/family's preferences and values (Melynk and Fineout-Overholt 2019).

Formulating Relevant Clinical (PICO) Questions

Successful implementation of the evidence-based process in clinical practice is dependent on formulating relevant clinical questions, using a format commonly referred to as PICO questions. The PICO mnemonic refers to the following: Population (P), Intervention (I), Comparison (C) intervention, and Outcome (O) (Melynk and Fineout-Overholt 2005). PICO questions emerge directly from clinical practice during daily encounters with patients and their presenting problems. Raising relevant PICO questions is an integral component of clinical practice in the EBP process and requires APRNs to develop an inquiring mind where everything is questioned, researched, and evaluated throughout the clinical decision-making process. As stated in Melynk and Fineout-Overholt (2019), "The PICO question guides the systematic search of healthcare databases to find the best available evidence to answer the clinical question" (p. 40). The outcome is rendering care based on the best available clinically based research evidence.

Identifying the population of interest (P) is an essential first step in formulating a relevant clinical question. By defining the specific population, the database search will be narrowed and more precise. An example of a population is children with a diagnosis of ADHD. Once the population is identified, the APRN questions which interventions (I) are based on the best available evidence for treatment, i.e. medications versus play therapy for management of children with ADHD, thus comparing (C) the two interventions to determine the best management outcome (O) for the child with a particular presenting problem.

To summarize, the final PICO question is, "In children with a diagnosis of ADHD (P), is medication management (I) more effective than play therapy (C) in improving the child's focus in school (O)?"

Searching for the Best Available Evidence

To find the best available evidence, two skills are essential: (i) the ability to conduct database searches based on the PICO question and (ii) the ability to understand and use techniques for critical appraisal of the research evidence identified in the database searches. Ideally, practicing APRNs and all clinicians should have access to a health science librarian to help with the database searches. However, lack of access to librarians and or university libraries is not a barrier to implementing EBP. APRNs can perform searches in some databases that are free to the public and readily available on the internet.

The Cochrane Collaboration (www.cochrane.org) has established standards for reviews of medical, health, and mental health treatments. The Cochrane Collaboration also provides systematic reviews of the research literature. Systematic reviews of the literature represent the highest level of evidence that can be considered for decision making in clinical practice.

An excellent free internet resource is PubMed (https://www.ncbi.nlm.nih.gov/pubmed). PubMed contains more than 19 million articles from MEDLINE and other science journals, making it an invaluable resource for all clinicians using an EBP model to deliver high-quality care to each client and their families.

The American Psychiatric Association (APA) (https://psychiatryonline.org/guidelines) provides a number of practice guidelines for use by clinicians. Their website address can be found in Table 29.1 along with other evidence-based resources. Part A of each APA practice guideline is first published in a supplement to the *American Journal of Psychiatry*. The APA website is an excellent resource to search for practice guidelines and current practice parameters, including excerpts from the *Diagnostic and Statistical Manual of Mental Disorders 5* (DSM-5) (APA 2013).

The American Academy of Pediatrics (AAP) website (https://www.aap.org) provides an excellent resource for the assessment, treatment, and management of children's physical and mental health problems. The AAP requires membership to access many of their resources; however, some of the practice guidelines are available free of charge in their journal publication. The AAP has an Evidence-based Child and Adolescent Psychosocial Interventions chart that is updated regularly. The American Academy of Child and Adolescent Psychiatry (AACAP) website (https://www.aacap.org) also provides exemplary mental health resources for providers and families, such as the AACAP Practice Parameters (now called Clinical Updates/Clinical Practice Guidelines). Practice-wise also offers EBP related to mental health problems in children (https://www.aap.org/en-us/Documents/CRPsychosocialInterventions.pdf). It is best to begin a search with the databases that contain CPGs since an answer for the clinical PICO question often can be found within a few seconds of beginning the search, a significant advantage for an APRN in a busy practice environment.

The best available evidence can be found in the literature as critically appraised synopses, systematic reviews and meta-analyses of randomized controlled trials (RCTs), and CPGs (DiCenso et al. 2005; Melynk and Fineout-Overholt 2019). If a systematic review cannot be located for the PICO question under investigation, then the next best available evidence is from at least one RCT. If an RCT is not available, then the best evidence may be case or cohort studies and/or reports based on expert clinical opinions, both of which are considered lower levels of evidence.

APRNs with access to a health science university library can search multiple databases simultaneously. Efficient, refined searches can also yield results in these databases in just a few minutes. Two commonly used databases are CINAHL and MEDLINE. Searches on these databases can be refined using Boolean search strategies in which "AND" and "OR" are used between the keywords that are being searched. Mileham (2009) provides a helpful discussion on how to do a literature search as well as a list of commonly used databases. Most university libraries now have an extensive list of suggested databases with direct links to the specific site. Hospitals and outpatient centers that have their own medical libraries or are linked to university libraries provide an excellent resource for APRNs and all healthcare professionals.

Searching for an Answer to the PICO Question

The PICO question exemplar is, "In children with a diagnosis of ADHD, is medication management more effective than play therapy in improving the child's focus in school?"

When this chapter was first written in 2012, a search of PubMed using the keywords "ADHD AND medication treatment" found 24 relevant articles in less than 1 minute. Searching PubMed today using the keywords "ADHD AND children AND medication treatment" located 2975 articles within 1 second. Refining the search in Pubmed using the keywords "ADHD AND children AND medication AND/OR ADHD AND play therapy" revealed a list of 300 articles in less than 1 second. Searching the Cochrane Library using the keywords "ADHD AND medication treatment" provided 13 Cochrane Reviews in contrast to the six relevant articles found when searching the same keywords for the first edition. Searching the Cochrane Library using the keywords "ADHD AND children AND medication AND/OR ADHD AND play therapy" revealed one registered clinical trial in 2018. Searching CINHAL Plus using the keywords "ADHD AND children AND medication treatment" revealed 239 articles while changing the keywords to "ADHD AND play therapy" provided 15 articles in 1 second.

It is ideal for APRNs to collaborate with reference librarians to formalize the keyword searches to assure a comprehensive search that provides the best available evidence for the PICO question. Thus, several options are available to APRNs to search for the best available evidence. However, once this evidence is identified, the APRN must critically appraise the evidence to determine if the particular practice guideline or specific evidence "fits" the PICO question that is under investigation and the population in the APRN's practice setting.

Understanding the Evidence

Systematic reviews of the literature were initially defined by Evans and Kowanko (2000) as "scientific tools which are used to summarize and communicate the results and implications of otherwise unmanageable quantities of research" (p. 35). Systematic reviews of the literature examine the best available evidence for a specific clinical question and the particular methods used. A systematic review of the literature provides a thorough search of the primary studies that pertain to the question. Furthermore, systematic reviews communicate and summarize study results and make recommendations based on the findings. Cochrane further defines a systematic review as "summarises [of] the results of available carefully designed healthcare studies (controlled trials) and provides a high level of evidence on the effectiveness of healthcare interventions. Judgments may be made about the evidence and inform recommendations for healthcare" (https://consumers.cochrane.org/what-systematic-review). Systematic reviews are considered to be the highest level of evidence.

If a systematic review of the literature is not available, a search for a meta-analysis should be conducted.

A meta-analysis is a powerful research methodology that uses statistical techniques to combine results from different studies that have addressed the same clinical question. A meta-analysis provides a quantitative estimate of the overall effect of the intervention under study for the desired outcome (Gurevitch et al. 2018; McGraw-Hill 2002). A meta-analysis provides a more powerful estimate and conclusion of the effects of the proposed interventions since several studies are included in the meta-analysis rather than just one study (Cannon and Boswell 2007; Mileham 2009). The role of the practicing APRN is to read the meta-analysis, interpret the findings, and analyze the findings to determine whether they are relevant for application in the APRN's practice (Haber and Krainovich-MIller 2019).

Melynk and Fineout-Overholt (2019) rate evidence from systematic reviews and meta-analyses as Level I, or the most reliable evidence, on the hierarchy of evidence. This rating indicates that these reviews have examined

Table 29.2 Rating system for hierarchy of evidence

Level of evidence	Type of evidence
Level I	A systematic review or meta-analysis of all relevant RCTs or evidence-based clinical practice guidelines based on systematic reviews
Level II	At least one well-designed RCT
Level III	Well-designed controlled trials without randomization
Level IV	Well-designed case control or cohort study
Level V	Systematic reviews of descriptive and qualitative studies
Level VI	A single descriptive or qualitative study
Level VII	Opinion of authorities and/or reports of expert committees

Source: Reprinted from Melynk, B.M. & Fineout-Overholt, E. Evidence-based practice in nursing and healthcare: A guide to best practice (4th ed.). © 2019, Wolters Kluwer.

relevant RCTs, long considered the gold standard of empirical evidence. Table 29.2 contains the hierarchy of evidence for all seven levels of evidence. Table 29.3 provides a summary of filtered and unfiltered evidence. Filtered evidence is evidence that has been critically appraised by researchers and includes systematic reviews of the literature, authors who evaluate and synthesize multiple research studies, or authors who have evaluated an individual research study. Unfiltered evidence has not been critically appraised and includes RCTs, cohort studies, case reports, and expert opinions. Other reviews include integrative reviews and narrative reviews. Integrative reviews synthesize and generalize a set of studies, while narrative reviews are more subjective and describe study results written in trade or lay publications.

The United States Preventive Services Task Force (USPSTF) has developed a system to grade evidence to determine whether preventive recommendations should be offered in practice. The definitions apply to their prevention suggestions (2018). In the past clinicians relied

Table 29.3 Summary of filtered and unfiltered evidence

Type of evidence	Description	Filtered information[a]	Unfiltered information[b]	Evaluation
Systematic review	Authors raise a specific question, perform a comprehensive search of all available literature, review the materials from the search, set particular criteria for acceptance or elimination of the studies from the systematic review, determine the levels of evidence in the study, and often make recommendations for practice based on the outcomes of the analysis	Yes	NO	CASP tools
Critically appraised evidence (referred to as synthesized evidence)	Authors evaluate and synthesize multiple research studies based on a particular topic	Yes	No	CASP tools
Critically appraised individual articles	Authors evaluate and provide a synopsis of one article	Yes	No	CASP tools
Randomized controlled trial (RCT)	An experimental test for a new treatment or intervention that includes random assignment to treatment or control group, and a large and diverse sample	No	Yes	"The gold standard" Evaluates for rigor in research design CASP tool
Cohort study	A study that focuses on a particular subpopulation	No	Yes	Evaluates for rigor in design
Case-controlled study	A study of one individual case	No	Yes	Evidence is not sufficient to make recommendations for practice
Expert opinion	No formal studies are available Recommendations are based on the opinions of experts The opinion may be made by one individual or a group of experts	No	Yes	Evidence is not sufficient to make recommendations for practice

[a] Filtered information has been appraised formally.
[b] Unfiltered information has not been formally appraised.

on the National Guideline Clearinghouse (NGC) to assess CPGs that included both prevention and management; the NGC, however, has been defunct since 2015. The revised 2012 grade definitions identify five levels: A, B, C, D, and I. For A and B levels, the net benefit of a service can be rated sufficient to moderate, respectively, and the service should be offered. For level D, the use of the service is discouraged; harms might outweigh benefits. For level I, current evidence is insufficient to assess the balance of benefits and harms of the service, therefore the use of the service cannot be determined. The USPSTF recommends offering the service to selected patients depending on individual circumstances; evidence demonstrates at least a small net benefit.

Evidence-based experts from Canada rate critically appraised evidence referred to as synthesized evidence or synopses rather systematic reviews. Synthesized evidence is a critical appraisal of multiple research studies based on a particular topic that has been evaluated and synthesized by a group of expert authors/researchers (DiCenso et al. 2009).

Finally, CPGs are a mechanism to transform knowledge, that is, results from individual studies are used in the development of clinical protocols and standards for care from the systematic research reviews (Brown 2009). Practice guidelines may be institution specific, which by definition limits generalization to other populations and contexts but works well for the facility. CPGs are also developed by organizations with expert clinicians who review the evidence for the topic and develop guidelines for the professional organizations and for practitioners. These are accessible to the public and other practitioners. CPGs are used at the point of care for decision making by individual APRNs for diagnosis and treatment planning options as these guidelines are based on the best available evidence.

To summarize, using the PICO question, "In children with a diagnosis of ADHD (P), is medication management (I) more effective than play therapy (C) in improving the child's focus in school (O)?" as an exemplar, the literature search revealed a practice guideline from the AAP that was originally developed from a systematic review of the literature (level I evidence) and then updated in 2011 (AAP 2001; Subcommittee on Attention-Deficit/Hyperactive Disorders, Steering Committee on Quality Improvement and Management, Wolraich et al. 2011). Thus, the systematic review, level 1 evidence, specifically addresses the PICO question on ADHD.

Evaluating the Evidence through Critical Appraisals

A critical appraisal of a research article (i.e. systematic review, RCT, or CPG) that the APRN is considering implementing in practice assures that the evidence is not flawed and may be appropriate for implementation in her or his practice. Several questions are considered during the critical appraisal, including whether the research population is consistent with the populations in my practice? Was the research methodologically sound and rigorous by design? What were the study results? Were the results valid? Will the results benefit my patients? (DiCenso et al. 2005; LoBionde-Wood et al. 2019; Melynk and Fineout-Overholt 2019).

The National Health Services Critical Appraisal Skills Program provides tools that can be used for appraising a variety of studies including systematic reviews, qualitative studies, randomized controlled studies, case controlled studies, diagnostic checklists, cohort studies, economic checklists, and clinical predictions (CASP-UK, https://casp-uk.net/casp-tools-checklists). Using the CASP tools (see Table 29.3), the research evidence is judged for credibility, clinical significance, and applicability (Brown 2009). Study results are reviewed for credibility. For example, are the results from one study similar to another? If not, a knowledge gap may be identified or flawed methodology may be determined.

Reviewing a study that uses a quantitative methodology requires a different appraisal than reviewing a study that uses a qualitative methodological approach. In addition, CPGs and integrative research reviews result in evidence that impacts a clinical population with the appropriate intervention. When results demonstrate clinical significance, the results are sizable enough to make practical differences and demonstrate validity (Brown 2009; CASP-UK, https://casp-uk.net/casp-tools-checklists; Salmond 2007).

Finally, applicability is determined by implementing the study findings in the practitioner's own setting. The study recommendation or intervention works well for the APRN when the evidence from the study being implemented "fits" the APRN's setting, the client population, and institution (LoBionde-Wood et al. 2019; Stetler 1994). Other components that are in place for applicability include feasibility (the setting result is similar to the study result), safety (few risks are identified for the patient), and expected benefits for improved patient outcomes.

Practice Guidelines

Practice guidelines are developed as mechanisms to ensure that a certain intervention for a particular population will have the desired outcome, which, in turn, will result in better care as well as best practice. Brown (2009) describes a 22-step method for producing evidence-based CPGs. After a comprehensive search of the literature, the best available evidence for the research (PICO) question under investigation is systematically examined, categorized by the levels of evidence (see Table 29.2 for hierarchy of evidence), analyzed, and then recommendations for practice are presented in the guideline based on the review of the best available evidence and expert opinions.

Evaluation and Implementation of Clinical Practice Guidelines

AGREE is an international collaboration of researchers and policy makers whose goal was to improve the quality and effectiveness of CPGs. Countries that participate in this collaboration include Denmark, Finland, Germany, Italy, the Netherlands, Spain, Switzerland, the United Kingdom, Canada, New Zealand, and the United States. The AGREE collaboration produced and validated an instrument that is used to evaluate the quality of CPGs. Categories of the instrument include scope and purpose, stakeholder involvement, rigor of development, clarity, applicability, and editorial independence (Brown 2009; Brouwers et al. 2010) The Cochrane Collaboration (cochrane.org) and the Joanna Briggs Institute (Joannabriggs.org) are two organizations that offer standards and methods that can be developed into evaluation measures of CPGs.

For the PICO question, "In children with a diagnosis of ADHD (P), is medication management (I) more effective than play therapy (C) in improving the child's focus in school (O)?", the AGREE II tool (Brouwers et al. 2010) remains a leading tool to critically appraise all practice guidelines, as well as the AAP practice guideline for the diagnosis and treatment of school-age children with ADHD (AAP 2001). Analysis of the CPG with the critical appraisal tool revealed that the practice guideline met the criteria for an EBP guideline for implementation in clinical practice for the child/adolescent population.

Today, QI projects in hospital and outpatient settings are designed to determine the effectiveness of the EBP guidelines and standards that are in place at the institution with the overall goal of improving healthcare outcomes for individuals, families, and communities.

Barriers to Implementing Evidence-based Practice

Barriers previously encountered by APRNs and all clinicians to the implementation of CPGs have changed over the years as accrediting bodies now require the use of EBP and QI as part of routine care and practice implementation. One barrier to implementation of EBP and QI measures is the time and commitment of all providers to implement and evaluate the process in various settings. Teams of clinicians in hospital settings are now responsible for identifying best practice guidelines, determining the desired outcomes after implementation, and then

conducting QI projects to determine the effectiveness of the practice change. Primary care settings, whether private or public care centers, with multiple healthcare providers experience time commitment challenges. Practice improvement outcomes for individuals and system-level changes are dependent upon all APRNs and providers having a foundation in evidence-based knowledge and QI projects to assure quality care and attainment of quality measures for reimbursement related to the delivered healthcare services (Djukic and Gilmaratin (2019).

Implications for Future Directions

All clinical educational programs need to provide experiences for students to acquire EBP competencies and to implement care based on the best available clinical evidence. In addition, programs must educate students on ways to evaluate the evidence to improve healthcare outcomes. Thus, the newest charge for educational programs and for continuing education programs is a focus on student exposure to QI projects to improve healthcare outcomes for all individuals, families, and the community/population as a whole. APRNs, and especially those prepared at the doctorate in nursing practice level (DNP), are now participating or leading QI studies in all healthcare settings. APRNs educated before the implementation of QI projects or studies need continuing education opportunities to learn the principles of QI followed by mentoring opportunities at practice sites to develop the new skills of QI implementation and evaluation.

Summary

EBP requires the use of a systematic method to raise relevant PICO (clinical) questions, search for the best available evidence relevant to the question, and identify the best available evidence and/or CPGs for treatment of all individuals, families, and populations. Systematic reviews, RCTs, CPGs, quantitative studies, case-controlled studies, and cohort studies are appraised by the APRN using standardized critical appraisal tools (Brouwers et al. 2010) to determine the goodness of fit for implementation in the APRN's practice. APRNs who implement the tenets of EBP in their clinical practice settings are using the best available evidence for the assessment, diagnosis, and clinical decision making for the treatment of their patients. Research studies examining the implementation of EBP in practice settings have demonstrated an improvement in patient healthcare outcomes in practices that consistently use an evidence-based approach in their practice settings. Today, QI projects are evaluating the results of EBP initiatives to determine the effectiveness of the healthcare and to improve practice outcomes.

Critical Thinking Questions

1. Consider your personal practice experiences (students, your clinical placement experiences). Describe a problem that you encountered. Develop a question using the PICO format.
2. Identify the methods used to conduct a literature search that you can use to locate the best available evidence for your PICO question.

References

Advancing the Science of Practice Guidelines (n.d.). *AGREE II*. Available at https://www.agreetrust.org/resource-centre/agree-ii.

AAP, Committee on Quality Improvement, Subcommittee on Attention Deficit/Hyperactivity Disorder (2001). Clinical practice guideline: treatment of the school-age child with attention-deficit/hyperactive disorder. *Pediatrics* 108: 1033–1044.

APA (2013). *Diagnostic and Statistical Manual of Mental Disorders V*, 5e. Washington, DC: American Psychiatric Association.

Association of Child and Adolescent Psychiatric Nursing (ACAPN). *ACAPN Guidelines for Care and Practice*. Retrieved from http://www.ispn-psych.org/html/acapn.html [membership required].

Black, A.T., Balneaves, L.G., Garossino, C. et al. (2015). Promoting evidence-based practice through a research training program for point-of-care clinicians. *Journal of Nursing Administration* 45 (1): 14–20. https://doi.org/10.1097/NNA.0000000000000151, https://www.ncbi.nlm.nih.gov/pubmed/25390076.

Brouwers, M.C., Kho, M.E., Browman, G.P. et al. (2010). AGREE II: advancing guideline development, reporting and evaluation in health care. *Canadian Medical Association Journal* 182 (18): E839–E842.

Brown, S.J. (2009). *Evidence-Based Nursing: The Research-Practice Connection*. Sudbury, MA: Jones and Bartlett Publishers.

Cannon, S. and Boswell, C. (2007). Application of evidence-based nursing practice with research. In: *Introduction to Nursing Research: Incorporating Evidence-Based Practice* (eds. C. Boswell and S. Cannon), 317–332. Sudbury, MA: Jones and Bartlett Publishers.

DiCenso, A., Guyatt, G., and Ciliska, D. (2005). *Evidence-Based Nursing: A Guide to Clinical Practice*. St. Louis, MO: Elsevier.

DiCenso, A., Bayley, L., and Haynes, R.B. (2009). Editorial: Accessing preappraised evidence: fine-tuning the 5S model into a 6S model. *Annals of Internal Medicine* 151 (6): JC3–JC2. JC3-3. doi: https://doi.org/10.7326/0003-4819-151-6-200909150-02002.

Djukic, M. and Gilmaratin, M.J. (2019). Evidence-based approaches for improving healthcare quality. Chapter 11. In: *Evidence-Based Practice for Nursing and Healthcare Quality Improvement* (eds. G. LoBiondo-Wood, J. Haber and M.G. Titler), 156–182. St. Louis, MO: Elsevier.

Drake, R.E., Goldman, H.H., Leff, H.S. et al. (2001). Implementing evidence-based practices in routine mental health service settings. *Psychiatric Services* 52: 179–182.

Evans, D. and Kowanko, I. (2000). Literature reviews: evolution of a research methodology. *The Australian Journal of Advanced Nursing* 18 (2): 33–38. Available at http://www.ncbi.nlm.nih.gov/pubmed/11878498.

Ganz, P.A. (2002). What outcomes matter to patients: a physician-researcher point of view. *Medical Care* 40 (6) Suppl: III-11-III-19. Available at http://www.jstor.org/pss/3767708.

Gurevitch, J., Koricheva, J., Nakagawa, S., and Stewart, G. (2018). Meta-analysis and the science of research synthesis. *Nature* 555: 175–182. Available at https://www.nature.com/articles/nature25753.

Haber, J. and Krainovich-MIller, B. (2019). Systematic reviews and clinical practice guidelines. In: *Evidence-Based Practice for Nursing and Healthcare Quality Improvement* (eds. G. LoBiondo-Wood, J. Haber and M.G. Titler), 94–116. St. Louis, MO: Elsevier.

LoBionde-Wood, G., Haber, J., and Titler, M.G. (2019). *Evidence-Based Practice for Nursing and Healthcare Quality Improvement*. St. Louis, MO: Elsevier.

Melnyk, B.M. and Fineout-Overholt, E. (2005). *Evidence-based practice in nursing & healthcare*, 6–10. Philadelphia, PA: Lippincott Williams & Wilkins.

Melynk, B.M. and Fineout-Overholt, E. (2019). *Evidence-Based Practice in Nursing and Healthcare: A Guide to Best Practice*, 4e. Philadelphia, PA: Wolters Kluwer.

Mileham, P. (2009). Finding sources of evidence. In: *Evidence-Based Practice for Nurses: Appraisal and Application of Research* (eds. N.A. Schmidt and J.M. Brown), 75–104. Sudbury, MA: Jones & Bartlett Publishers.

Sackett, D., Rosenberg, W., Muir Gray, J. et al. (1996). Evidence based medicine: what it is and what it isn't. *British Medical Journal* 312: 71–72.

Sackett, D.L., Straus, S.E., Richardson, W.S. et al. (2000). *Evidence-Based Medicine: How to Practice and Teach EBM*. London, UK: Churchill Livingstone.

Salmond, S. (2007). Advancing evidence-based practice: a primer. *Orthopaedic Nursing* 26 (2): 114–123. Available at http://www.ncbi.nlm.nih.gov/pubmed/17414381.

Segan, J.C. (2002). *McGraw-Hill Concise Dictionary of Modern Medicine*. New York, NY: The McGraw-Hill Companies Available at http://medical-dictionary.thefreedictionary.com/meta-analysis.

Siminoff, L.A. (2013). Incorporating patient and family preferences into evidence-based medicine. *BMC Medical Informatics and Decision Making* 13 (Suppl 3): s.6. https://doi.org/10.1186/1472-6947-13-S3-S6, https://www.ncbi.nlm.nih.gov/pmc/articles/PMC4029304.

Stetler, C.B. (1994). Refinement of the Stetler/Marram model for application of research findings to practice. *Nursing Outlook* 42: 15–25. https://doi.org/10.1016/0029-6554(94)90067-1.

Subcommittee on Attention-Deficit/Hyperactive Disorder, Steering Committee on Quality Improvement and Management, Wolraich et al (2011). ADHD: clinical practice guideline for the diagnosis and treatment of ADHD disorder in children and adolescents. *Pediatrics* 128: 1007–1022. doi: https://doi.org/10.1542/peds.2011-2654. Epub 16 October 2011. Available at https://www.ncbi.nlm.nih.gov/pubmed/22003063.

Substance Abuse and Mental Health Services (2017). *What Is Integrated Health Care*. Rockville, MD: Substance Abuse and Mental Health Services, HRSA Center for Integrated Health Solutions Available at https://www.integration.samhsa.gov/about-us/what-is-integrated-care.

US Preventive Services Task Force. (2018). *Grade definitions*. Available at https://www.uspreventiveservicestaskforce.org/Page/Name/grade-definitions.

30

Cultural Influences on Child and Adolescent Mental Health: Needs of Immigrant, Refugee, Displaced, and Culturally Vulnerable Youth

Edilma L. Yearwood[1] and Mikki Meadows-Oliver[2]

[1] Georgetown University School of Nursing & Health Studies, Washington, DC, USA
[2] Quinnipiac University School of Nursing, Hamden, CT, USA

Objectives

After reading this chapter, advanced practice registered nurses (APRNs) will be able to:

1. Define culture and understand the cultural context of mental health.
2. Explain the unique psychosocial experiences and needs of immigrant, refugee, and culturally vulnerable youth.
3. Describe common behavioral and psychiatric disorders seen in immigrant, refugee, displaced, and culturally vulnerable youth and their parents/caretakers.

4. Identify ways that primary care and psychiatric-mental health APRNs can collaborate to deliver seamless, comprehensive, and quality care to this population.
5. Develop personal learning strategies aimed at developing knowledge supporting culturally informed and sensitive nursing care.

Introduction

Discussion of culture is complex and, within a mental health context, may prove to be complicated and controversial. Some prefer not to engage in the conversation, professing that everyone is the same, others minimize the role and impact of culture on presenting behaviors, while others embrace and value their own culture but disrespect or marginalize the culture of others. Lastly, some are eager to learn more about culture and how it works within different contexts in order to maximize care rendered. This chapter will define culture,

acculturation, and marginalization, explore cultural factors that advanced practice registered nurses (APRNs) must understand. It will address the complex needs of immigrant, refugee, displaced, and culturally vulnerable youth living in challenging in country environments or who are crossing numerous global geographic boundaries. Cultural factors have an impact on the mental/behavioral health of immigrant and refugee children and the children of immigrant parents. Practitioners must be aware of and assess for specific cultural factors across their diverse patient caseload and formulate

Child and Adolescent Behavioral Health: A Resource for Advanced Practice Psychiatric and Primary Care Practitioners in Nursing,
Second Edition. Edited by Edilma L. Yearwood, Geraldine S. Pearson, and Jamesetta A. Newland.
© 2021 John Wiley & Sons, Inc. Published 2021 by John Wiley & Sons, Inc.
Companion website: www.wiley.com/go/Yearwood

culturally informed and patient-centered treatment strategies to enhance the mental health of children and adolescents with whom they work. Practitioners should never assume that cultural experiences or values fit everyone within a specific cultural group but instead need to embrace the uniqueness within and across groups. The chapter will also include practice, education, and research implications along with recommendations for APRNs working with immigrant, refugee, displaced, and culturally vulnerable populations, and will conclude with a case exemplar to illustrate key considerations.

Culture

There are many definitions of culture. The authors of this chapter are in support of the notion that healthcare is a cultural construct that influences provider–patient interactions and relationships and, as such, influences treatment engagement, adherence, empowerment, valuing, and inclusion. We have chosen the following adapted definition to guide the content presented here.

Culture refers to the thoughts, communications, actions, customs, beliefs, values, and institutions of racial, ethnic, religious, or social groups. Culture is complex, multidimensional, involves intersectionality, defines how we receive and understand health, illness, and healthcare information, how symptoms are manifested, how and who treats the symptoms, and how we perceive and accept treatment support (Cross et al. 1989; Kleinman 1988; Kagawa-Singer, M., Dressler, W., & George, S. (2015).

Foundational Relevant Concepts

Keesing and Strathern (1998) and Helman (2007; cited in Andrews et al. 2010) viewed culture as a contextual system of shared ideas and learned guidelines that affect how the individual or group views the world and behaves in response to that world view. Hall (1984; cited in Andrews et al. 2010) stated that there are three levels of culture: *primary* (made up of rules followed by group members but which are rarely stated), *secondary* (foundational rules known by members but rarely shared with nonmembers), and *tertiary* (explicit rules and behaviors of the group or individuals seen by others). Primary and secondary levels of culture are more intrinsic and difficult to change.

An understanding of culture matters because culture influences how individuals understand health and illness and the contextual practices used to manage their illness (Anderson et al. 2010; Bronfenbrenner 1994, 2005; Campinha-Bacote 1998; Kleinman 1988). Members of some cultures believe that physical or mental illnesses are caused by bad spirits visiting the individual or family, while others believe that illness occurs when the body is not in harmony or as a punishment for wrong doing (Andrews et al. 2010). Adolescents in the study conducted by Du Pont et al. expressed different views about mental illnesses across racial, gender, and ethnic identity groups (2019). An understanding of cultural experiences, including those specific to mental health, along with context, must be acknowledged and factored into health encounters and co-created interventions (agreed upon by the patient and clinician), as these actions are foundational for positive health outcomes and improved wellbeing (Gopalkrishnan 2018; Greene et al. 2017; Kirmayer and Bhugra 2009).

Changing Demographics

There are approximately 19.6 million immigrant children in the United States and that number is expected to rise to 33 million by 2050 (Child Trends n.d.; Passel 2011). First-generation US immigrant children are children born in another country who then migrate to the United States; their parents are foreign born. There are three million first-generation children in the United States (Childtrends n.d.). Generation 1.5 immigrant children refers to youth with the following characteristics: (i) not born in the United States, (ii) migrated to the United States at an early age, (iii) have resided in the United States for a long period of time, (iv) have foreign-born parents, and (v) are sociologically closer in behaviors to second-generation youth (Portes and Rivas 2011). Second-generation immigrant children are children born in the United States who have at least one immigrant parent (Perreira and Ornelas 2011). Children who reside in mixed legal status households (with one or both parent[s] an undocumented immigrant) are more at risk for accessing healthcare later, not having a primary care health provider, experiencing stress, anxiety, and depression related to documentation status, and not having health insurance (Perreira and Ornelas 2011). Third-generation status refers to children born to US-born parents (Passel 2011). Globally, the United Nations High Commissioner for Refugees (UNHCR) identified that in 2017, of the 68.5 million displaced individuals, 52% were children under the age of 18 years (2018). See Table 30.1 for a summary of definitions.

Cultural Factors

Cultural Vulnerability

Culturally vulnerable youth have been described as youngsters who are at risk for poor outcomes due to a variety of factors, including poverty, living in poor or

Table 30.1 Definitions

Migrant children	Individuals under the age of 18 who are living in a country/area other than where they were born They may or may not be accompanied by a parent or guardian
Planned migration	An intentional and nonreactive move
Refugee Asylum seeker Displaced person	An individual who leaves his/her country due to war, ethnic cleansing, religious violence, persecution, natural disaster, gang violence, or gang recruitment attempts
Unaccompanied immigrant minor (UIM)	An individual under the age of 18 who travels to another location without a parent or guardian
Internally displaced	Individuals who are removed from or flee their original place of birth/residence within a country

From International Society for Social Pediatrics and Child Health (2018) and the United Nations High Commissioner for Refugees (2018).

low resource environments, violence exposure, and poor academic achievement (Fernandes-Alcantara 2018). Additional factors that can impact vulnerability include race, gender, ethnicity, homelessness, runaway behaviors, residing in the juvenile justice system, limited English proficiency, geographic residence (rural versus city dweller), special education designation, emancipated minor status, being a school dropout, experiencing social exclusion, and having symptoms of or a mental health diagnosis. As can be seen from this list of factors, the APRN needs to be aware of a wide variety of factors and experiences that may play a role in symptom generation, maintenance, and treatment outcomes.

Intersectionality

Crenshaw (1989) first coined the term intersectionality to refer to the connection and intersection of social constructs such as age, race, gender, ethnicity, sexual orientation, religion, and class. Intersectionality as a critical theory concept can be used to explain and understand issues of difference, power, advantage/disadvantage, and privilege across multiple environments (Atewologun 2018). By understanding issues of compounded intersectionality and marginalization, APRN awareness can be enhanced about treatment challenges, healthcare outcomes, and struggles with sustainability of health promotion behaviors. This knowledge can further inform priority setting and treatment actions. Two current research studies on intersectionality in adolescence points to inequality based on immigration and socio-economic status and the

imperative for designing diverse educational strategies for racial, ethnic, and gender minority youth (DuPont-Reyes et al. 2019; Evans and Erickson 2019). Intersectionality is a dynamic concept that is ripe for collaborative and interprofessional research by APRNs.

Acculturation

APRNs working with immigrant youth and their families must understand the concept of acculturation and be able to determine where the child, adolescent, and/or family is on the acculturation trajectory. This knowledge helps the APRN fully grasp the social, cultural, emotional, and interactional experiences and stressors that the youngster is dealing with in their status as an immigrant. The place where the child, adolescent, and/or family is on the acculturation trajectory has been implicated in health, health practices, and health inequities (Campinha-Bacote 1998; Lopez-Class et al. 2011).

Berry described the acculturation process as two cultures coming into contact, resulting in conflict within the individual who comes from the nondominant (nonhost) culture. As a result of this interaction and over time, the individual adopts one of four behaviors: *integration* (embraces behaviors and values from both cultures), *assimilation* (embraces behaviors and values of the dominant culture and rejects own culture of origin), *separation* (immerses self in own culture of origin, rejecting behaviors and values of the dominant culture), or *marginalization* (rejects both cultures) (Berry 1997, 2015). McDermott-Levy's concept analysis of acculturation emphasized that the process is bidirectional but uneven, occurs over time (can occur over several generations), and is a phenomenon that is, "interactive, multifactorial, developmental and multidimensional" (2009, p. 283).

Kim (2004) conducted a grounded theory study on the experiences of young Korean immigrants in the United States looking at negotiation of social, cultural, and generational boundaries. Qualitative interview data were obtained from 19 youths with a mean age of 21.5 years who had been in the United States between 4 and 19 years. A major theme identified was negotiating boundaries. Participants spoke of conflicts they encountered that made them painfully aware of the cultural differences between their culture and the dominant culture, the difficulties they had with parents and peers, difficulties at home and school, navigating both the Korean and English languages, and, because of the length of time in the United States, feeling that they were neither first-generation nor second-generation immigrants. Participants also reported feeling that they were a visible minority when not living in or going to school in Korean cultural enclaves. Participants who were less than

10 years of age when they migrated to the United States reported having less difficulty with social, cultural, and generational boundaries than participants who migrated when they were 15 years or older.

In other research conducted with youth, researchers found that positive acculturation experiences promote resilience and that resilience was correlated with wellbeing (Wu et al. 2018), and an increase in acculturation stress increased anxiety and depression symptoms (Perreira et al. 2018).

As described previously by McDermott-Levy (2009) and Kim (2004), acculturation is an ecologically dynamic process that affects cultural identity and the psychological state of individuals and groups (Berry 2005). Researchers and clinicians have moved away from a simplistic and unidimensional view of acculturation that focuses on language or generational factors. Current acculturation research, which is a good fit with nursing research, focuses on attitudes, values, behaviors, environmental factors, identity, discrimination, economics, family relationships, and cultural and psychological changes (Berry 2015). Similar to Bronfenbrenner's ecological system to explain child development, Liboro (2018) encourages researchers to examine society of origin factors, host society factors, and community level acculturation factors when working with racial minority immigrants to better understand what drives and maintains behaviors and symptoms. In their study on 189 high school newcomers, Patel et al. (2016) found that the combination of multiple life events and separation from extended family/social support increased stress and resulted in unhealthy behavioral adjustments. A review by Abraido-Lanza et al. (2016) provides guidance on additional acculturation research pathways.

Marginalization

Marginalization is described by Phinney et al. (2006) as having little interest in cultural maintenance and little interest in having relations with other groups as a result of being excluded or discriminated against. Individuals who are marginalized do not feel embraced by others and are not integrated into the fiber of the culture, the group, or the environment. They experience isolation and are made to feel inconsequential or powerless. Ultimately, these individuals are at risk for poor self-esteem, depression, self-harm, and physical illnesses (Barber and Vega 2011; Park 2017). Park collected data following an ethnographic and classroom observation methodology on African refugees in an American urban high school. Several participants experienced social and linguistic marginalization in the form of verbal and non-verbal derogatory actions and comments by peers as a result of their race, religion, and distinct language

presentation. The researcher pointed out the importance of creating a tolerant and inclusive learning environment for all students to minimize and eliminate biases and marginalization and promote learning.

Immigrant Paradox

The immigrant paradox (healthy immigrant phenomenon) refers to a frequently observed trend that, compared to children from native-born families, first-generation "immigrant children present with better physical health, less involvement in risky behaviors and similar or greater academic achievement and psychological well-being" (Fuligni 1998, p. 100; Kwak and Rudmin 2014; Linton et al. 2016). Cultural foods, complementary and alternative health practices, being raised in more supportive community environments, and a more physically active lifestyle in the country of origin are reasons offered for these findings (Mendoza 2009).

However, data indicate that the longer immigrants are in the United States (shift from first generation to second), the further they navigate away from high academic aspirations and good physical and emotional health (Suarez-Orozco et al. 2009) and experience lower self-esteem and poorer health outcomes (Smokowski et al. 2010). Findings from a Canadian study of 4069 students in three generations of immigrant youth from grades 7 through 12 revealed that drug use, harmful drinking, and delinquency increased with second- and third-generation immigrant status; however, psychological distress was higher in the first-generation youth, possibly due to migration stress and uncertainty associated with relocation (Hamilton et al. 2009). This shift toward poorer outcomes with longer residence is believed to occur as a result of acculturation and adoption of the behaviors, values, and lifestyles of the host or dominant culture. APRNs need to know the medical and psychosocial history of the child or adolescent but also understand the community environment where the child lives, specifically issues of tolerance or intolerance that the child and family may experience.

Child Fostering

APRNs working with immigrant populations may encounter a rare phenomenon known as "child fostering" that might impact the parent–child relationship. The child's sense of belonging within the family may be affected and can result in behavioral and psychological symptoms such as anger, isolation, anxiety, and depression. Child fostering, or what Leinaweaver refers to as "outsourcing care" (2010), refers to the "informal care and placement of children in a household where their biological parent does not reside" (Miller 1998, p. 36). This practice appears to have originated during the time when African slaves were brought to the United States and their children were given to other adults to be cared for. It continues as a practice in Latin America and the Caribbean when primarily single parents migrate to another country for employment and to establish a home prior to sending for their children. In the current child fostering process, parents working in the United States, Canada, or other resource-rich or high-income environments send money back to the country of origin to the adult raising their children for the care being rendered (Leinaweaver 2010; Yearwood 1998).

While there are clear economic advantages to this practice, the length of separation from the child can extend from weeks to years, causing a disruption in the parent–child bond and establishing a level of uncertainty for the child as to when and whether they will see their parent again. Compounding this practice might be the undocumented status of the parent who cannot return to the country of origin to visit the child for fear of not being allowed back into the country where they are now working and living. In addition, the child left behind in the care of a friend or acquaintance might be at risk for sexual, physical, or emotional abuse and/or abandonment. When reunification with the biological parent does occur, the child then experiences the loss of the person who was caring for them while their parent was away, anger toward the biological parent over the delay in reunification, new rules and behavioral expectations that may be imposed, and worry that she/he may be separated from the parent again. This adds increased risk to disturbances in psychological wellness and adjustment to their new environment (Yearwood 1998).

Transnationals

Transnationals are individuals who maintain contact and ties with their country of origin through frequent visits (cyclical migration), frequent communication via technology, and by sending goods and money to friends and relatives who remain in the country of origin. There may be confusion as to where these individuals "fit" and challenges to their experience of acculturation. Transnationals may be at risk for relational stress secondary to frequent separations and reunions, and to generational stress secondary to contact with several generations each having beliefs and values that may challenge those held by the transnational (Falicov 2007).

Discrimination

Discrimination, racism, and various levels of aggression are other experiences immigrant youth report as newcomers to the United States. Adair (2015) reported on the personal and structural discriminatory experiences of immigrants in schools. Personal experiences include negative interaction with both peers and staff, narrow learning experiences that focuses on teaching to the test rather than exploring, embracing, and exposing immigrant children to a variety of learning strategies, offering low educational experiences, and devaluing the primary language of the immigrant. Structural discriminatory indicators included less access to educational resources, school segregation, fewer attempts to engage parents in the school and child learning process, and higher diagnosing and misdiagnosing of special education needs.

Implicit Bias

Implicit bias is the unconscious view toward individuals within one or more social groups. Social conditioning and learned associations propel the bias and impact reaction to and behavior toward the individual or group. Implicit biases are held by all individuals and APRNs are encouraged to assess and become aware of their personal biases which can serve as barriers to authentic care. Hall et al. (2015) conducted a systematic review of the literature looking at implicit bias in healthcare providers and found that implicit bias impacts provider–patient interactions, decision making, treatment adherence, and, ultimately, healthcare outcomes. The APRN is encouraged to access and review the recent American Nurses Association Standard 8 on Culturally Congruent Practice (Marion et al. 2016) as part of the self-assessment process aimed at minimizing biases and practicing from a more culturally inclusive perspective.

Poverty

As stated previously, many immigrant children and families live in poverty. With poverty status comes the lack of health insurance, inability to access a variety of resources, worse health outcomes, poorer living situations, risk for not completing school, future job insecurity, and lower wages (Tienda and Haskins 2011). Poorer community environments have little or no resources to meet the complex needs of individuals and families residing in those environments. For example, schools may lack human and material resources to have smaller classroom sizes staffed with bilingual or English as a second language (ESOL) proficient teachers. A 5-year mixed method longitudinal study of 408 immigrant children from Central America, China, Haiti, the Dominican Republic, and Mexico was conducted to identify academic trajectories across the study population. Researchers found that high-achieving and academically successful immigrant children were from families that had structure and family capital to support the child's school success, were in less segregated schools, and had stronger English skills (Suarez-Orozco et al. 2010). However, at year four of the study, most of the participants displayed a significant decline in their academic grades, with the exception of the children from China, who consistently maintained good academic achievement (Suarez-Orozco et al. 2009).

Children and adolescents raised in poverty are more at risk for anxiety and depression, violence, gang involvement, substance abuse, food insecurity, and sleep difficulties (Suarez-Orozco and Carhill 2008; Suarez-Orozco et al. 2009). Having knowledge of the socioeconomic status of the child will help the APRN understand potential risk for poor physical and mental health outcomes. However, it should also prompt the APRN to assess further for the presence of any protective factors or strengths (which are often overlooked) that can mitigate a negative outcome.

Protective Cultural Factors

Suarez-Orozco et al. (2009) identified several protective factors that promote success, social self-efficacy, and resilience in immigrant youth. These factors include academic self-sufficiency, English language proficiency, residing in a two-parent household, having a positive relationship with parent(s) with clear and respectful communication, being female, positive relationships with teachers at school, and social supports (peers, non-parental supportive adult(s), extended and supportive family members). The International Society for Social Pediatrics and Child Health (ISSOP 2018) supports the protective factors described by Suarez-Orozco and their research findings identified social inclusion, supportive family environment, good caregiver mental health, and positive school experiences as factors contributing to resilience in immigrant youth. From interviews conducted with clinicians who work with immigrant and refugee populations, Whitfield (2017) identified themes that support positive immigrant and refugee outcomes. These included existence of protective factors, family involvement, use of expressive arts as an engagement strategy, mindfulness-based strategies such as guided imagery, working in multidisciplinary teams, use of group work and cultural brokers, and culturally responsive clinicians. Concerns identified included paucity of culturally responsive clinicians, family use of physical discipline, parental misunderstanding of mental health provider role, and use of mindfulness interventions.

In addition to gaining an understanding of cultural factors impacting mental health, part of a good comprehensive mental health assessment of immigrant, refugee, displaced, and culturally vulnerable youth includes screening for the type and experiences encountered during migration.

Migration

Planned Migration

The process and characteristics of *planned migration* differ from the process involved in resettlement as a refugee. Refugees are concerned with personal or family safety and protection from people in the country being fled. Having to emigrate quickly and inconspicuously from a country poses physical and psychological challenges for refugees, who experience multiple losses during resettlement (i.e. place, family and friends, and culture), uncertainty (i.e. where to live, how to earn a living, and fear about the safety and status of those left behind), and change in personal status (i.e. socioeconomic, professional, and possible change from majority to minority status).

Specific to child and adolescent refugees, children are increasingly victims of torture and sexual exploitation or are witnesses to mass tragedy associated with wars or persecution. They can become refugees by virtue of these experiences. As a result, they may have had to live in refugee camps, endure multiple moves, or be separated from parents or caretakers in order to remain safe. Food, warmth, clothing, stability, ability to attend school, and unconditional and predictable parental "presence" may be lacking or compromised (Birman and Chan 2008; Llabre and Hadi 2009). Over time, post-traumatic stress, depression, anxiety, sleep disturbance, substance abuse, and suicidality are some of the mental health consequences of these traumatic experiences (Downes and Graham 2011).

The events in the United States at the southern border with Mexico have been at the forefront of one of the significant global immigrant/refugee crises in recent years. Other similar crises involve Syrians fleeing to Turkey and Europe, and the internal conflict in Myanmar (formerly Burma) between Rohingya Muslims and Rakhine Buddhists. With the announcement in 2012 of the Deferred Action for Childhood Arrivals (DACA) policy (US Department of Homeland Security), and the subsequent increase in individuals and families fleeing violence from Nicaragua, El Salvador, Honduras, and Guatemala (Martinez 2018), traveling through Mexico to the United States has been controversial and challenging. Advocates have called for humanitarian treatment of these refugees based on social justice principles (equity, human rights, access, and participation) (Kagan et al. 2014) and researchers point to the need for interdisciplinary and transdisciplinary research efforts to better understand clinical practice needs, influence a more caring and protective set of policies, and propel immigration reform (Gomez and Castaneda 2019; Zayas et al. 2017).

Multiple organizations have voiced their concern and strongly urged the US government to rethink its harsh treatment and detention of refugees in camps, and separation of children from their parents at the border. A sample of these communications is given in Table 30.2.

Forced Migration

Forced migration, also referred to as involuntary or displacement, is when an individual or group is made to move, by force, from their place of origin or residence. It occurs secondary to violence, danger, persecution or a

Table 30.2 Communications from organizations regarding migration

Organization	Date	Type of communication	Web link
American Association of Colleges of Nursing (AACN)	19 June 2018	Press release announcing AACN joins 32 national nursing groups to voice concern in a joint letter to the US Secretary of the Department of Homeland Security about US immigration policies	https://www.magnetmail.net/actions/email_web_version.cfm?ep=6xX3RWT_y-Zgujfys_wwVkRGGCsKXlDaepEmTtUbLpt DKLu3Ttt1eYpB-vas2C2h7aqlonSWtTH3Uk UNao2TEpWs86W4Vj14RWvuVMkfF5p1sZ QZM_N2fxlRUMC1ms9j
American Academy of Nursing	19 June 2018	Press release: American Academy of Nursing Releases Statement on Separation of Families at the US Border	https://higherlogicdownload.s3. amazonaws.com/AANNET/c8a8da9e-918c-4dae-b0c6-6d630c46007f/UploadedImages/docs/Press%20Releases/2018/2018-Acadeny_Statement_on_Separation_of_Children-Parents_at_Border-B.pdf
American Academy of Pediatrics	15 June 2018	AAP statement opposing the Border Security and Immigration Reform Act	https://www.aap.org/en-us/about-the-aap/aap-press-room/Pages/AAPStatementOppos ingBorderSecurityandImmigrationReform Act.aspx
American Psychiatric Nurses Association (APNA)	19 June 2018	APNA calls for an end to the policy that separates families	https://www.apna.org/m/pages. cfm?pageID=6455
International Council of Nurses	2018	Position statement: Health of migrants, refugees and displaced persons	https://www.icn.ch/sites/default/files/inline-files/PS_A_Health_migrants_refugees_displaced%20persons.pdf
International Family Nursing Association (IFNA)		IFNA response to the global refugee crisis: Caring for Refugee Families.	https://internationalfamilynursing. org/2016/02/18/caring-for-refugee-families
United Nations Health Commission on Refugees	18 June 2018	UNHCR urges family unity at southern US border	http://www.unhcr.org/news/press/2018/6/5b27fea84/unhcr-urges-family-unity-southern-border.html
National Association for Mental Illness (NAMI)		NAMI statement on family separations at US border.	https://www.nami.org/About-NAMI/NAMI-News/2018/Statement-about-Border-Separation-from-NAMI

directive from an individual or group in a position of power (International Organization for Migration 2019).

Stages of Migration

There are three distinct stages involved with planned migration or the move from one country to another. *Premigration*, or the period before the move, involves making the decision to move, planning, discussion with family and friends, and leave taking. Premigration can be stressful because of uncertainty about the new place of residence, economic hardship, or if significant people, things, or status is being left behind (Perreira and Ornelas 2011). *Intramigration*, or the period during travel to the new country, can evoke anxiety if the travel is difficult, long, circuitous, fraught with unexpected danger, or if family members are separated during the process. *Postmigration* involves settling in the new country, maneuvering a new environment without the usual source of social support, acculturation stress, adjusting to a different educational system, and possibly dealing with changes in language, roles, downward mobility, and/or undocumented status (Perreira and Ornelas 2011; Suarez-Orozco and Todorova 2003). Many refugees and immigrants spend time in other countries before immigrating to the United States, which may prolong the uncertainty and disruption experienced.

Crea et al. (2017) conducted a study on unaccompanied youth in long-term foster care in the United States between 2012 and 2015, looking at placement stability. These youth (N = 256) were in placements in Massachusetts, Michigan, Pennsylvania, and Oregon through the Lutheran Immigration and Refugee Service. Study participants were from Mexico, Central and South America, Haiti, Ethiopia, China, Russia, Saudi Arabia, Somalia, India, and Nigeria. Study measures included obtaining data on demographics, placement changes, and child behaviors during stages of migration. Researchers found that migration-related trauma was not significant in this sample; however, fear of returning to the country of origin and trauma unrelated to migration were associated with lower levels of placement changes. In addition, violence experience in the country of origin along with higher levels of acting out while in care were associated with more frequent changes in placement.

During the assessment process, APRNs in primary care or psychiatric-mental health practice should include questions about health status and experiences before, during, and post migration, being alert to possible exposure to traumatic events (ISSOP 2018). Children and adolescents may fear deportation and forced separation from parents, siblings, and other family members (Ciaccia and John 2016; Siemons et al. 2017).

Behavioral and Psychiatric Presentations of Immigrant Youth

Globally, what is known about behavioral and psychiatric disorders in children and adolescents is limited due to a lack of age and culturally appropriate screening tools, inconsistent epidemiological data-gathering methods across countries, lack of adequately trained mental health practitioners in low- and middle-income countries, and myopic priorities of medical and communicable diseases despite evidence that psychiatric disorders are a significant component of the noncommunicable disorders seen worldwide (Patel et al. 2007; Yearwood and DeLeon Siantz 2010) and a driver of overall wellbeing. Research conducted with immigrant youth in the United States has focused on youth behaviors in the school, parent–child behaviors, the protective role of healthy parenting, behaviors associated with the level of acculturation the youth is navigating, common behavioral or psychiatric presentations, and the youth's perception of host country discrimination/racism.

Mood disorders are expected to be the second largest contributor to global burden of disease by 2030, with a significant increase of mood symptoms and diagnoses expected in adolescence (Lewinsohn et al. and WHO as cited in Yearwood et al. 2007; WHO 2004). Immigrant youth must be carefully assessed for pre-, intra-, and postmigration stressors, untreated premigration psychopathology, behavioral and psychological responses to perceived losses, cultural stigma surrounding mental illness, academic competence, self-concept, and parent–child relationship (ISSOP 2018). All of these issues have the potential to affect the emotional, social, relational, and psychological development of the child or adolescent. In clinical practice, presentations will include isolation, anger, irritability, self-harm, poor self-esteem, depression, and anxiety. Additional information about mood disorders and recommended management approaches can be found in Chapter 12.

Post-traumatic stress disorder (PTSD) is another significant finding in migrant, refugee, and US-born youth exposed to violence and other traumas (natural disasters). Betancourt et al. (2017), Hodes and Vostanis (2019), and Yayan (2018) provide reviews of PTSD stressing the importance of assessing and intervening early to prevent long-term and potentially significant effects of untreated associated symptoms. Physical health, relationships, trust, self-concept, anxiety, depression, self-medication, school performance, and overall quality of life are potential consequences of untreated PTSD.

Assessment and Screening Tools

Explanatory models are tools that can be used to obtain the perspective of an interviewee about their experience and beliefs about his/her illness (Kirmayer and Bhugra 2009; Kleinman 1988). A frequently used tool is Kleinman's explanatory model. The questions posed try to elicit what the person believes causes the illness, how the illness is explained in the culture, how the illness affects the social world of the individual or group, and how the illness is usually managed. The illness can be either physical or psychological. Specific questions include (Anderson et al. 2010; Kleinman 1988; Kleinman and Benson 2006):

1. What do you call the problem?
2. What do you think is wrong?
3. What do you want the healthcare practitioner to do?
4. Why do you think you are experiencing these symptoms at this time?
5. How has the illness affected your life?
6. What about this illness worries you the most?
7. What do you think needs to be done to treat the illness?
8. How do people in your culture talk about and understand the illness?
9. How long do you think the illness will last?
10. Does the illness serve a purpose?

The APRN must be aware that in some cultures, direct conversation with the child or adolescent about the illness experience is not endorsed by adults because of the low status children may have within the culture. The explanatory model questions can be modified by the healthcare practitioner to facilitate age-appropriate interaction, or if there is a need to gather additional data or a need to better translate the questions to ensure understanding. The questions, however, are expected to facilitate communication between the care provider and the individual seeking care, broaden the provider's understanding of the cultural world of the patient/client, and deter the usual provider-dominant or top-down conversation style. As can be seen by the questions, the model is quite conducive to understanding how older children and adolescents understand their behavioral and/or psychological difficulties within their cultural context.

The *Diagnostic and Statistical Manual of Mental Disorders 5* (DSM-5) (American Psychiatric Association 2013) includes the cultural formulation interview (CFI), which focuses on four domains containing a total of 16 questions. The domains are the definition of the problem, perception of the cause(s), context and support, cultural factors such as past coping and help seeking, and current self-coping/help seeking such as preferences and provider–patient relationship. The CFI should be incorporated into the assessment of all patients seen regardless of immigrant status and should not be a static assessment but revisited and updated periodically.

The Achenbach system of empirically based assessment (ASEBA) is an evidence-based culturally informed assessment tool that is available in over 100 languages. The tool includes self and other report measures of behavioral, emotional, social, and thought problems along with strengths (Achenbach 2015).

Table 30.3 provides a brief overview of additional recommended screening tools for use with immigrant children and adolescents. Caballero et al. (2017) reviewed Spanish-language mental health screening tools and models of care for Latino children and concluded that providers need to be aware of risk factors for mental health symptoms, need to integrate evidence-based screening tools in their assessment, and serve as strong advocates for additional culturally appropriate tools, treatment services, and expansion of available workforce providers with the skills to work with this population. The development of additional evidence-based and comprehensive cultural screening tools is an area ripe for further research by nurse scientists.

Care Delivery

The information discussed in this chapter clarifies that work with immigrant, refugee, and culturally vulnerable children and adolescents is complex and informed by multiple factors. As the number of immigrant, refugee, displaced, and vulnerable families in the United States increases, pediatric, family, and psychiatric-mental health APRNs will be caring for many of these families in inpatient, primary care, schools, and other community settings. Often, the needs of these families are insufficiently met by existing treatment settings. The timely identification and treatment of mental health disorders in immigrant, refugee, displaced, and culturally vulnerable youth may be compromised by limited healthcare access, lack of knowledge about the complex needs of this population, variability in the comfort level of the provider, as well as failure to use evidence-based and culturally appropriate mental health screening tools. To address such situations, the American Academy of Pediatrics (AAP) released a Position Statement on Providing Care for Immigrant, Migrant, and Border Children (2013). This statement provides guidance to primary care clinicians who work with these families in their practice. Pediatric, family, and psychiatric-mental health APRNs have a professional responsibility to be aware of and address the distinct medical, mental health, cultural, and social needs of immigrant, refugee, displaced, and culturally vulnerable children and adolescents (Walden 2017).

Conducting routine medical care and obtaining a comprehensive medical, developmental, family, cultural,

Table 30.3 Recommended screening tools

Name of tool	Developed by	Targeted age	Characteristics
Strengths and Difficulties Questionnaire (SDQ)	Goodman (1999)	3- to 16-year-olds	25-item brief behavioral screening tool for positive and negative behaviors. Screens for emotional, conduct, hyperactivity, peer relationship, and prosocial behaviors. Translated into 66 languages.
Child Self-Rating Scale (CSRS)	Hightower et al. (1987)	5- to 13-year-olds	40-item self-report measure. Screens for rule compliance (adherence) and acting out, anxiety and withdrawal, friend and peer relationships, and school interest.
Pediatric Symptom Checklist (PSC)	Jellinek et al. 1988	6- to 16-year-olds	35-item screening tool that parents respond to. Available in several languages and takes approximately 10 minutes to complete.
Behavioral Assessment System for Children (BASC)	Reynolds and Kamphaus (1992)	2- to 21-year-olds	Screens for both adaptive and maladaptive thought and behaviors. Available for teachers, parents, and the child to complete. Version 2 of the scale is more comprehensive. Parent and teacher scales take 1 to 20 minutes to complete and child self-report takes 30 minutes to complete.
Child Behavior Checklist (CBCL)	Achenbach (1991, 2015)	1.5 to 18-year-olds	Multiple versions of the scale in many languages. Can be used by parent, teacher, and child. Measures internalizing and externalizing behaviors.
War Trauma Questionnaire	Macksoud (1992)	3- to 16-year-olds	45-item scale that is grouped into the following: exposure to shelling or combat, separation from parents, bereavement, witnessing violence, suffering injuries, victim of violence, emigration, displacement, involvement in violence, and deprivation.
PTSD Reaction Index	Pynoos et al. (1998)	7- to 18-year-olds	22-item self-report scale that takes approximately 30 minutes to complete. Translated into many languages. Assesses symptoms of PTSD within the last month.
Depression Self-Rating Scale	Birleson (1981)	8- to 14-year-olds	18-item scale to measure childhood depression.
*Child and Adolescent Functional Assessment Scale (CAFAS)	Hodges and Wong (1996)	7- to 17-year-olds	*This scale is to be used by a *trained clinician*. It assesses child functioning over the prior 3 months in school, home, community, behavior toward others, behavior toward self, mood, substance abuse, and thinking. Scale also assesses strengths. Caregiver strengths and problems can also be assessed,
Pictorial Pediatric Symptom Checklist (PPSC)	Jellinek and Murphy (PPSC) (n.d.)	4–16 year-olds	35 item pictorial and text descriptions. Question options: 0 = never, 1 = sometimes, 3 = often. Total scores range from 0 to 70 with a score of 28 or higher indicative of psychosocial impairment. Adequate validity. See Chapter 4.

Source: Birman, D. & Chan, W. (2008). Screening and assessing immigrant and refugee youth in school-based mental health programs. Center for Health and Health Care in Schools (Issue Brief #1). Retrieved from www.healthinschools.org; Caballero, T.M., De Camp, L.R., Platt, R.E., Shah, H., Johnson, S.B., Sibinga, E.M., & Polk, S. (2017). Addressing the mental health needs of Latino children in immigrant families. Clinical Pediatrics, 56(7), 648–658.

and psychosocial assessment are the purview of the pediatric or family APRN. These APRNs can improve care of immigrant, refugee, displaced, and culturally vulnerable children through awareness of risk factors for mental health disorders, integration of evidence-based screening instruments into their practice, advocacy for culturally relevant mental health resources, and advocacy for increasing the workforce available and appropriately trained to work with this population. Ciaccia and John (2016) and Seery et al. (2015) provide a structured overview of assessment considerations specific to refugee and immigrant youth for the primary care APRN. With the complex presentations of these youngsters, additional in-depth and evidence-based psychosocial and psychiatric assessments may be warranted, followed by brief or long-term psychiatric supportive interventions. Psychiatric-mental health APRNs are trained to provide these services. Given the issues of loss, trauma, and transitions that many immigrant children deal with, we support a healthcare model based on collaboration between practitioners and community care providers who work together over time to meet the changing medical, psychosocial, and cultural needs of youth.

Specific strategies for both primary care and psychiatric-mental health APRNs include active listening to the child and parents, an open and respectful interaction style, an awareness of community resources to support changing needs, and valuing and providing continuity of care. In addition, this population may need assistance with transitions, which may need to begin at the point of assessment with clear planning and education. Lastly, APRNs working with immigrant youth must recognize the critical role both parents (and significant adults) and school play in the development, socialization, and self-concept formation of these youths. Within school-based health centers, the pediatric or family APRN may be part of an interdisciplinary team that works to meet the educational, social, cultural, and psychological needs of these children. The APRN can foster communication between school and parents, support development of positive parenting skills and knowledge of normal child and adolescent development, teach the importance of healthy parent–child communication and relationship development, and endorse the importance of cultural partnerships (Gopalkrishnan 2018).

The Robert Wood Johnson Foundation has been active in supporting programs that have developed strategies aimed at engaging families, schools, youth, community programs, and mental health agencies in supporting healthy development of immigrant, refugee, displaced, and culturally vulnerable children. Caring Across Communities, a national initiative of the Robert Wood Johnson Foundation, works to implement school-connected mental health programs for immigrant and refugee children in 15 communities across the United States. School-based treatment programs have been endorsed as one effective strategy to meet the complex needs of immigrant, refugee, displaced, and culturally vulnerable youth (Graves et al. 2017; McNeely et al. 2017; Schapiro et al. 2018). Schools provide access to these youth and an opportunity to coordinate and place multiple needed services within the school.

Research, Education, and Practice Implications

Mendoza (2009) described three priority areas for research with immigrant youth that APRNs can and should pursue in order to develop the science on effective healthcare and outcomes for this population. These include developing and testing strategies to improve access to care, describing components of quality healthcare for individuals with complex needs, and understanding cultural factors that support positive development and health outcomes. Additional areas for research include comparison of behavioral and psychiatric presentations of stress associated with migration, acculturation, and trauma, immediate, short-term and long-term effects of social disruption, immigrant strengths across age groups, methods to improve early and accurate identification of immigrant mental health needs, and behavioral outcome comparison in youth across types and duration of parental involvement in schools. Nursing research should consist of qualitative, quantitative, and longitudinal studies.

Personal education efforts to develop skills working with immigrant, refugee, displaced, and vulnerable populations should include immersion in the cultural activities of the immigrant group and curiosity and openness to learning about the other. The American Academy of Child and Adolescent Psychiatry (AACAP) identified 13 practice parameters for clinicians aimed at improving their cultural competence (Pumariego et al. 2013). Several of these include conducting the evaluation in the language in which the child and family are proficient, being aware of cultural biases that may be barriers to clinical judgment, providing treatment in familiar settings within the community, assessing for immigration-related loss or trauma, and incorporating cultural strengths and child/family active participation in the treatment. Nursing education can make it a priority to include more opportunities for students to work with a variety of immigrant and vulnerable groups in public health, offering community-based learning experiences and supporting cultural immersions abroad.

APRNs are in a unique position to develop culturally informed practice skills by virtue of their increased interaction with a variety of children, adolescents, and families from multiple countries who have emigrated to the United States. As stated earlier, there have been dramatic increases in the number of immigrant and refugee youth, and this contact provides opportunities for nurses at all levels to learn about other cultures and cultural practices while developing person-specific care interventions in collaboration with the youth and parent to ensure respect and acknowledgment of cultural values.

Conclusion

This chapter has described factors that APRNs need to know about the unique and complex experiences of immigrant, refugee, displaced, and culturally vulnerable children and families to better understand their mental health and behavioral presentations and needs. The pervasive, far-reaching, and complex impacts of culture and acculturation have been explored to provide a context for this understanding. In addition, the need for the APRN provider to explore his/her implicit biases, become aware of cultural factors impacting mental health and clinical presentations in youth and families, and practice strategies to promote a more inclusive practice are discussed. The importance of providing care using a collaborative model that embraces continuity of care, youth and family inclusion in the development of care, and respect for the values of the immigrant, refugee, displaced, and/or vulnerable child or adolescent has been provided. The chapter ended with identifying areas of research for nurse scientists that would provide immense contributions to knowledge development and evidence-based practice with this population.

Resources

American Psychological Association. (2017). *Addressing the mental health needs of racial and ethnic minority youth: A guide for practitioners.* Available at http://www.apa.org/pi/families/resources/mental-health-needs.pdf.

Annie E. Casey Foundation. www.aecf.org.

Chaudry, A., Capps, R., Pedroza, J. et al. (2010). *Facing Our Future.* Urban Institute: *Children in the Aftermath of Immigration Enforcement* Available at https://www.urban.org.

Fletcher, S.E. (2015). *Cultural Sensibility in Healthcare.* Indianapolis, IN: Sigma Theta Tau.

Holtz, C. (2010). Global health issues. *Journal of Transcultural Nursing* 21 (Suppl. 1): 14S–38S.

Howard, P. and El-Mallakh, P. (eds.) (2010). Mental health across the lifespan. *Nursing Clinics of North America* 45 (4): 501–660.

Lopez, M., Hofer, K., Bumgarner, E., & Taylor, D. (2017). *Developing culturally responsive approaches to serving diverse populations: A resource guide for community-based organizations.* National Research Center on Hispanic Children & Families.

National Institute on Minority Health and Health Disparities (NIMHD). htpp://http://www.nimhd.nih.gov.

PEW Hispanic Foundation. http://www.pewhispanic.org.

Reach Institute, Culturally Responsive Mental Health Screening Tools. Available at https://www.thereachinstitute.org/newsletters/151-culturaay-responsive-mental-health-screening-tools.

Robert Wood Johnson Foundation. www.rwjf.org.

Suarez-Orozco, C., Suarez-Orozco, M., and Teranishi, R. (2016). *Pathways to Opportunities: Promising Practices for Immigrant Children, Youth & Their Families.* Globalization & Education: Institute for Immigration.

Urban League. www.urban.org.

References

Abraido-Lanza, A., Echeverria, S., and Florez, K. (2016). Latino immigrants, acculturation, and health: promising new directions in research. *Annual Review of Public Health* 37: 219–236.

Achenbach, T.M. (1991). *Manual for Child Behavioral Checklist.* Burlington, VT: University of Vermont.

Achenbach, T. (2015). *ASEBA DSM-5 oriented scales.* Available at http://www.aseba.org/research/ASEBA DSM-5orientedscales.htm (accessed 11 november 2019).

Adair, J.K. (2015). *The impact of discrimination on the early schooling experiences of children from immigrant families.* Washington, DC: Migration Policy Institute.

American Academy of Pediatrics, Council on Community Pediatrics (2013). Providing care for immigrant, migrant, and border children. *Pediatrics* 131: e2028–e2034.

American Psychiatric Association (2013). Cultural Formulation. In: *Diagnostic and Statistical Manual of Mental Disorders*, 5e, 750–759. Washington, DC: American Psychiatric Association.

Anderson, N., Andrews, M., Bent, K. et al. (2010). Culturally based health and illness beliefs and practices across the life span. *Journal of Transcultural Nursing* 21 (Suppl. 1): 152S–235S.

Andrews, M., Backstrand, J., Boyle, J. et al. (2010). Theoretical basis for transcultural care. *Journal of Transcultural Nursing* 21 (Suppl. 1): 53S–136S.

Atewologun, D. (2018). Intersectionality theory and practice. *Oxford Research Encyclopedia Business and Management.* doi: 10.1093/acrefore/9780190224851.013.48

Barber, C. and Vega, L. (2011). Conflict, cultural marginalization, and personal costs of filial care giving. *Journal of Cultural Diversity* 18 (1): 20–28.

Berry, J. (1997). Immigration, acculturation and adaptation. *Applied Psychology* 46: 5–34.

Berry, J.W. (2005). Acculturation: living successfully in two cultures. *International Journal of Intercultural Relations* 29: 697–712.

Berry, J.W. (2015). Acculturation. In: *Handbook of Socialization Theory and Research* (eds. J.E. Grusec and P.D. Hastings), 520–538. Guilford Press.

Betancourt, T.S., Newnham, E.A., Birman, D. et al. (2017). Comparing trauma exposure, mental health needs, and service utilization across clinical samples of refugee, immigrant, and US-origin children. *Journal of Trauma Stress* 30 (3): 209–218.

Birleson, P. (1981). The validity of depressive disorder in childhood and the development of a self-rating scale: a research report. *Journal of Child Psychology and Psychiatry* 22: 73–88. Available at http://dx.doi.org/10.1111/j.1469-7610.1981.tb00533.x.

Birman, D. & Chan, W. (2008). *Screening and assessing immigrant and refugee youth in school-based mental health programs.* Center for Health and Health Care in Schools (Issue Brief #1). Available at www.healthinschools.org.

Bronfenbrenner, U. (1994). Ecological models of human development. *International Encyclopedia of Education* 3: 1643–1647.

Bronfenbrenner, U. (2005). *Making Humans Beings Human: Bioecological Perspectives on Human Development.* Thousand Oaks, CA: Sage.

Caballero, T.M., De Camp, L.R., Platt, R.E. et al. (2017). Addressing the mental health needs of Latino children in immigrant families. *Clinical Pediatrics* 56 (7): 648–658.

Campinha-Bacote, J. (1998). *The Process of Cultural Competence in the Delivery of Healthcare Services*, 3rde. Cincinnati, OH: Transcultural C.A.R.E. Associates.

Center for Health and Health Care in Schools. (2019). *Improving vulnerable children's health and school success*. Available at http://healthinschools.org/our-work/vulnerable-populations.

Child Trends (n.d.). *Immigrant demographics*. Available at www.childtrends.org.

Ciaccia, K.A. and John, R.M. (2016). Unaccompanied immigrant minors: where to begin. *Journal of Pediatric Health Care* 30 (3): 231–240.

Crea, T.M., Lopez, A., Taylor, T., and Underwood, D. (2017). Unaccompanied migrant children in the United States: predictors of placement stability in long term foster care. *Children and Youth Services Review* 73: 93–99.

Crenshaw, K. (1989). *Demarginalizing the intersection of race and sex: A Black feminist critique of antidiscrimination doctrine, feminist theory and antiracist politics*. University of Chicago Legal Forum, Issue 1, Article 8. Available at http://chicagounbound.uchicago.edu/uclf/vol1989/iss1/8.

Cross, T., Bazron, B., Dennis, K., & Isaacs, M. (1989). *Towards a culturally competent system of care: A monograph on effective services for minority children who are severely emotionally disturbed*. Washington, DC: CAASP Technical Assistance Center, Georgetown University Child Development Center.

Downes, E.A. and Graham, A.R. (2011). Health care for refugees resettled in the US. *Clinician Reviews* 21 (3): 25–31.

DuPont-Reyes, M., Villatoro, A., Phelan, J. et al. (2019). Adolescent views of mental illness stigma: an intersectional lens. *American Journal of Orthopsychiatry* 90: 201–211. https://doi.org/10.1037/ort0000425.

Evans, C.R. and Erickson, N. (2019). Intersectionality and depression in adolescence and early childhood: a MAIHDA analysis of the national longitudinal study of adolescents to adult health, 1995-2008. *Social Science & Medicine* 220: 1–11.

Falicov, C. (2007). Working with transnational immigrants: expanding meanings of family, community and culture. *Family Process* 46: 157–171.

Fernandes-Alcantara, A.L. (2018). *Vulnerable youth: Background and policies*. Congressional Research Service, 7-5700. Available at www.crs.gov.

Fuligni, A. (1998). The adjustment of children from immigrant families. *Current Directions in Psychological Science* 7: 99–103.

Gomez, S. and Castaneda, H. (2019). "Recognizing our humanity": immigrant youth voices on health care inn Arizona's restrictive political environment. *Qualitative Health Research* 29 (4): 498–509.

Goodman, R. (1999). The extended version of the strengths and difficulties questionnaire as a guide to child psychiatric caseness and consequent burden. *Journal of Child Psychology and Psychiatry* 40: 791–799.

Gopalkrishnan, N. (2018). Cultural diversity and mental health: considerations for policy and practice. *Front Public Health* 6: 179. https://doi.org/10.3389/fpubh.2018.00179.

Graves, S.L., Herndon-Sobalvarro, A., Nichols, K. et al. (2017). Examining the effectiveness of culturally adapted social-emotional intervention for African-American males in an urban setting. *School Psychology Quarterly* 32 (1): 62–74.

Greene, M.C., Jordans, M.J.D., Kohrt, B.A. et al. (2017). Addressing culture and context in humanitarian response: preparing desk reviews to inform mental health and psychosocial support. *Conflict and Health* 11: 21. https://doi.org/10.1186/s13031-017-0123-z.

Hall, W.J., Chapman, M.V., Lee, K.M. et al. (2015). Implicit racial/ethnic bias among health care professionals and its influence on health outcomes: a systematic review. *American Journal of Public Health* 105 (12): e60–e76.

Hamilton, H., Noh, S., and Adlaf, E. (2009). Adolescent risk behaviours and psychological distress across immigrant generations. *Canadian Journal of Public Health* 100: 221–225.

Hightower, A., Cowen, E., Spinell, A., and Lotyczewski, B. (1987). The child rating scale: the development of a socioemotional self-rating scale for elementary school children. *School Psychology Review* 16: 239–255.

Hodes, M. and Vostanis, P. (2019). Practitioner review: mental health problems of refugee children and adolescents and their management. *Journal of Child Psychology and Psychiatry* 60 (7): 716–731.

Hodges, K. and Wong, M. (1996). Psychometric characteristics of a multidimensional measure to assess impairment: the child and adolescent functional assessment scale. *The Journal of Child & Family Studies* 5: 445–467.

International Organization for Migration. (2019). *IOM Glossary on Migration*. Available at http://migrationdataportal.org.

ISSOP (2018). Migration working group. ISSOP position statement on migrant child health. *Child: Care, Health & Development* 44 (1): 161–170.

Jellinek, M.S. & Murphy, J.M. (n.d.). Pictorial Pediatric Symptom Checklist. Available at www.massgeneral.org.

Jellinek, M.S. and Murphy, J.M. (1988). Screening for psychosocial disorders in pediatric practice. *American Journal of the Diseases of Children* 142: 1153–1157.

Jellinek, M.S., Murphy, J.M., Robinson, J. et al. (1988). Pediatric symptom checklist: screening school-age children for psychosocial dysfunction. *Journal of Pediatrics* 112: 201–209.

Kagan, P.N., Smith, M.C., and Chinn, P.L. (2014). *Philosophies and Practices of Emancipatory Nursing: Social Justice as Praxis*. New York: Routledge.

Kagawa-Singer, M., Dressler, W., & George, S. (2015). Culture: The missing link in health research. *Social Science &n Medicine*, 170, 237–246.

Keesing, R.M. and Strathern, A. (1998). *Cultural Anthropology: A Contemporary Perspective*. Belmont, CA: Wadsworth/Thompson Learning.

Kim, S. (2004). The experiences of young Korean immigrants: a grounded theory of negotiating social, cultural, and generational boundaries. *Issues in Mental Health Nursing* 25: 517–537.

Kirmayer, L.J. and Bhugra, D. (2009). Culture and mental illness: social context and explanatory models. In: *Psychiatric Diagnosis: Challenges and Prospects* (eds. I. Sallorum and J. Mezzich), 29–40. Wiley.

Kleinman, A. (1988). *The Illness Nnarratives: Suffering, Healing & the Human Condition*. New York, NY: Basic Books.

Kleinman, A. and Benson, P. (2006). Anthropology in the clinic: the problem of cultural competency and how to fix it. *PLoS Medicine* 3 (e294): 1673–1676.

Kwak, K. and Rudmin, F. (2014). Adolescent health and adaptation in Canada: examination of gender and age aspects of the healthy immigrant effect. *International Journal for Equity in Health* 13 (1) https://doi.org/10.1186/s12939-014-0103-5.

Leinaweaver, J. (2010). Outsourcing care: how Peruvian migrants meet transnational family obligations. *Latin American Perspectives* 37 (5): 67–87.

Liboro, R.M. (2018). Racial minority immigrant acculturation: examining Filipino settlement experiences in Canada utilizing a community-focused acculturation framework. *Community Psychology in Global Perspective* 4 (1): 66–84.

Linton, J.M., Choi, R., and Mendoza, F. (2016). Caring for children in immigrant families. *Pediatric Clinics of North America* 63: 115–130.

Llabre, M. and Hadi, F. (2009). War-related exposure and psychological distress as predictors of health and sleep: a longitudinal study of Kuwaiti children. *Psychosomatic Medicine* 71: 776–783.

Lopez-Class, M., Castro, F., and Ramirez, A. (2011). Conceptions of acculturation: a review and statement of critical issues. *Social Science & Medicine*. https://doi.org/10.1016/j.socscimed.2011.03.011.

Macksoud, M. (1992). Assessing war trauma in children: a case study of Lebanese children. *Journal of Refugee Studies* 5: 1–15.

Marion, L., Douglas, M., Lavin, M. et al. (2016). Implementing the new ANA standard 8: culturally congruent practice. *Online Journal of Issues in Nursing* 22 (1).

Martinez, S. (2018). Today's Migrant Flow Is Different. *The Atlantic*, June 26.

McDermott-Levy, R. (2009). Acculturation: a concept analysis for immigrant health. *Holistic Nursing Practice* 23: 282–288.

McNeely, C.A., Morland, L., Doty, B. et al. (2017). How schools can promote healthy development for newly arrived immigrant and refugee adolescents: research priorities. *Journal of School Health* 87: 121–132.

Mendoza, F. (2009). Health disparities and children in immigrant families: a research agenda. *Pediatrics* 124: S187–S195.

Miller, A. (1998). Child fosterage in the United States: signs of an African heritage. *The History of the Family an International Quarterly* 3 (1): 35–62.

Park, J.Y. (2017). Responding to marginalization: language practices of African-born Muslim refugee youth in an American urban high school. *SAGE Open* https://doi.org/10.1177/2158244016684912.

Passel, J. (2011). Demography of immigrant youth: past, present, and future. *The Future of Children: Immigrant Children* 21: 19–41.

Patel, V., Flisher, A., Hetrick, S., and McGorry, P. (2007). Mental health of young people: a global public health challenge. *Lancet* 369: 1302–1313.

Patel, S.G., Clarke, A.V., Eltareb, F. et al. (2016). Newcomer immigrant adolescents: a mixed-methods examination of family stressors and school outcomes. *School Psychology Quarterly* 31 (2): 163–180.

Perreira, K. and Ornelas, I. (2011). The physical and psychological well-being of immigrant children. *The Future of Children: Immigrant Children* 21: 195–218.

Perreira, K.M., Marchante, A.N., Schwartz, S.J. et al. (2018). Stress and resilience: key correlates of mental health and substance use in the Hispanic community health study of Latino youth. *Journal of Immigrant and Minority Health* 21: 4–13.

Phinney, J.S., Berry, J.W., Vedder, P., and Liebkind, K. (2006). The acculturation experience: attitudes, identities, and behaviors of immigrant youth. In: *Immigrant Youth in Cultural Transition* (eds. J.W. Berry, J.S. Ohinner, D.L. Sam and P. Vedder), 71–116. Mahwah, NJ: Lawrence Erlbaum Associates.

Portes, A. and Rivas, A. (2011). The adaptation of migrant children. In the future of children. *Immigrant Children* 21: 219–246.

Pumariega, A.J., Rothe, E., Mian, A. et al. (2013). Practice parameter for cultural competence in child and adolescent psychiatric practice. *Journal of the American Academy of Child Adolescent Psychiatry* 52 (10): 1101–1115.

Pynoos, R., Rodriguez, N., Steinberg, A., Stuber, M., & Frederick, C. (1998). *Reaction index-revised*. Unpublished psychological test, University of California Los Angeles.

Reynolds, C. and Kamphaus, R. (1992). *Behavior Assessment System for Children*. Circle Pines, MN: American Guidance Service.

Schapiro, N.A., Gutierrez, J.R., Blackshaw, A., and Chen, J.L. (2018). Addressing the health and mental health needs of unaccompanied immigrant youth through an innovative school-based health center model: successes and challenges. *Children and Youth Services Review* 92: 133–142.

Seery, T., Boswell, H., and Lara, A. (2015). Caring for refugee children. *Pediatrics in Review* 36 (8): 323–340.

Siemons, R., Raymond-Flesh, M., Auerswald, C.L., and Brindis, C.D. (2017). Coming of age on the margins: mental health and wellbeing among Latino immigrant young adults eligible for Deferred Action for Childhood Arrivals (DACA). *Journal of Immigrant Minority Health* 19: 543–551.

Smokowski, P.R., Rose, R.A., and Bacallao, M. (2010). Influence of risk factors and cultural assets on Latino Adolescents' trajectories of self-esteem and internalizing symptoms. *Child Psychiatry & Human Development* 41 (2): 133–155. https://doi.org/10.1007/s10578-009-0157-6.

Suárez-Orozco, C. & Carhill, A. (2008). Afterword: New directions in research with immigrant families and their children. In H. Yoshikawa & N. Way (Eds.), Beyond the family: Contexts of immigrant children's development. *New Directions for Child and Adolescent Development*, 121, 87–104.

Suarez-Orozco, C. and Todorova, I. (2003). The social worlds of immigrant youth. In: *New Directions for Youth Development: Understanding the Social Worlds of Immigrant Youth*, vol. 100 (Winter) (eds. C. Suarez-Orozco and I. Todorova), 15–24. Jossey-Bass.

Suarez-Orozco, C., Rhodes, J., and Milburn, M. (2009). Unraveling the immigrant paradox: academic engagement and disengagement among recently arrived immigrant youth. *Youth & Society* 41: 151–185.

Suarez-Orozco, C., Bang, H., O'Connor, E. et al. (2010). Academic trajectories of newcomer immigrant youth. *Developmental Psychology* 46: 602–618.

Tienda, M. and Haskins, R. (2011). Immigrant children: introducing the issue. *The Future of Children: Immigrant Children* 21: 3–18.

United Nations High Commissioner for Refugees. (2018). *Displaced individuals*. Available at http://globalcitizen.org.

US Department of Homeland Security. (2012). *Secretary Napolitano announces deferred action process for young people who are low enforcement priorities*. Washington, DC: DHS Press Office.

Walden, J. (2017). Refugee mental health: a primary care approach. *American Family Physician* 96: 81–84.

Whitfield, L. (2017). *Culturally specific interventions to support adolescent immigrant and refugee mental health*. Sophia, St. Catherine University repository. Available at https://sophia.stkate.edu/msw_papers/811.

World Health Organization (2004). *The global burden of disease: 2004 update*. Geneva: World Health Organization.

Wu, Q., Ge, T., Emond, A. et al. (2018). Acculturation, resilience and the mental health of migrant youth: a cross-country comparative. *Public Health* 162: 63–70.

Yayan, E.H. (2018). Post-traumatic stress disorder and mental health states of refugee children. *Archives of Psychiatric Nursing* 32: 885–889.

Yearwood, E.L. (1998). *'Growing up' children: Current child rearing practice among immigrant Jamaican families*. Doctoral dissertation. Available from ProQuest Dissertations and Theses database. UMI No. 9907831.

Yearwood, E.L. & DeLeon Siantz, M.L.D. (2010). Global issues in mental health across the life span: Challenges and opportunities. In P. Howard & P. El-Mallakh (Eds.) [Special Issue], *Mental Health Across the Lifespan. Nursing Clinics of North America*, 45, 501–519. Elsevier.

Yearwood, E.L., Crawford, S., Kelly, M., and Moreno, N. (2007). Immigrant youth at risk for disorders of mood: recognizing complex dynamics. *Archives of Psychiatric Nursing* 21: 162–171.

Zayas, L.H., Brabeck, K.M., Heffron, L.C. et al. (2017). Charting directions for research on immigrant children affected by undocumented status. *Hispanic Journal of Behavioral Sciences* 39 (4): 412–435.

31

Conducting Behavioral Health Research with Children and Using Research Methods

Elizabeth Burgess Dowdell[1] and Judith Fry-McComish[2]

[1]M. Louise Fitzpatrick College of Nursing, Villanova University, Villanova, PA, USA
[2]Wayne State University, Detroit, MI, USA

Objectives

After reading this chapter, advanced practice registered nurses (APRNs) will be able to:

1. Discuss the roles of APRNs as consumers, collaborators, and initiators of research.
2. Describe the characteristics and use of quantitative, qualitative, and mixed methods research designs that can be used in nursing research or evidenced-based practice.
3. Identify sources of funding for APRNs who wish to conduct behavioral health research.
4. Describe the ethical responsibilities of the APRN, as an investigator or research team member, when conducting research or evidence-based practice projects with human participants.

Introduction

Injury-related incidents such as motor vehicle accidents (occupants and pedestrians), homicides, suicides, malignant neoplasms, and congenital anomalies are the leading causes of death in children and adolescents aged 1 to 24 years (Centers for Disease Control and Prevention [CDC] 2018a). Many risky health-related behaviors that contribute to morbidity and mortality begin in childhood and adolescence. The 2017 Youth Risk Behavior Survey (YRBS) reported the most common risky behaviors of teens and young adults were unintentional injuries and violence, tobacco use, alcohol, and other drug use, sexual behaviors that contribute to unintentional pregnancy and sexually transmitted infections including human immunodeficiency virus (HIV) infection, unhealthy dietary intake, distracted driving, and physical inactivity (CDC 2018b). Although these risk behaviors occur across all adolescent groups, some populations such as minorities or those from underrepresented groups are disproportionately affected.

Health behavior research seeks to describe the prevalence of a health-related behavior in a specific population, compare patterns across groups, and examine factors that promote or inhibit the occurrence of risky or protective health behaviors. The ultimate goals are to understand why individuals engage in behaviors that place them at risk for adverse health consequences and identify the individual-, family-, and community-level

Child and Adolescent Behavioral Health: A Resource for Advanced Practice Psychiatric and Primary Care Practitioners in Nursing, Second Edition. Edited by Edilma L. Yearwood, Geraldine S. Pearson, and Jamesetta A. Newland.
© 2021 John Wiley & Sons, Inc. Published 2021 by John Wiley & Sons, Inc.
Companion website: www.wiley.com/go/Yearwood

factors that contribute to these risk behaviors in order to design interventions to prevent health risk behavior, change behavior, and reduce adverse health outcomes. This chapter will discuss the different roles of advanced practice registered nurses (APRNs) in research and the process of conducting health behavior research with at-risk children and adolescents.

APRNs as Research Consumers, Contributors, and Collaborators or Investigators

With a graduate-level education, training, and leadership roles as healthcare providers and coordinators of care, APRNs are the frontline practitioners at the intersections of behavioral health practice and research with at-risk children, adolescents, and families. APRNs frequently assume one or more of three primary roles in relation to research: consumers of research, contributors to ongoing research endeavors, and/or collaborators or generators of research studies.

Research Consumers

As consumers of research, APRNs review and critically evaluate current research and findings in the nursing and behavioral health literature in order to guide evidence-based practice (EBP) in their work settings (LoBiondo-Wood and Haber 2014). Readers are referred to Chapter 29 for a thorough discussion of EBP.

Research Contributors

In addition to being informed consumers of nursing and behavioral science research, and promoting the dissemination and use of EBP, APRNs often work in clinical sites and agencies where clinical trials and other research studies with children, adolescents, and families are being conducted. These APRNs are able to contribute to the generation of new knowledge through their participation as research team members. However, APRNs must be very clear about what their roles and responsibilities are on a research project and be knowledgeable about the rules and regulations that are associated with each research team role. For example, research team members who are involved in recruiting participants, completing informed consent procedures, and collecting data from research participants must complete training and certification on the ethical conduct of research and the protection of human subjects. Online training/certification programs are available through most universities and major medical centers as well as through the National Institutes of Health (NIH; www.nih.gov).

In addition to ensuring that they have completed any required individual training, APRNs who are asked to participate as team members of research studies should first verify that the study has been reviewed and approved by the appropriate authorities. All research studies that involve human subjects require approval by the institutional review board (IRB) of the university, medical center, or other community institution where the study is being conducted. Depending on the level of risk to patients or participants that is associated with participation in the study, the IRB may grant the study "exempt" status, conduct an expedited review, or conduct a full-board review. If information from a patient's medical record is being obtained, the rules governing confidentiality of patient information must also be observed. Such studies must comply with the regulations of the Health Insurance Portability and Accountability Act of 1996 (HIPAA; https://www.hhs.gov/foia/privacy/index.html).

Research Collaborators and Investigators

Beyond being research consumers and team members, there is a growing need for APRNs themselves to collaborate and initiate research studies to examine research questions that are of significance and relevance to nursing. Many of the most important research questions are derived from experience, observations from practice, and knowledge of the population with whom one works. As research investigators, APRNs can further the development of nursing science and promote nursing's voice in the development of interdisciplinary science to promote positive health behaviors among at-risk children, adolescents, and families. With nursing's longstanding commitment to health promotion and prevention, APRNs are qualified to assume a leading role in interprofessional healthcare provision and research.

How does one initiate a research study? It all begins with a question. As previously mentioned, research questions often come from practice and clinical observations. From personal observations in practice, it may "seem" to the APRN that certain youth are more likely to engage in a certain behavior, X, than other youth. Likewise, the APRN may question the best way to intervene with a specific ethnic or cultural group. A first step is to search the published literature and determine what is already known. If there are gaps in the literature, or if little is known about a question of interest that is significant to nursing and health, research on the question may be warranted. See the National Institute of Nursing Research (NINR) priorities (https://www.ninr.nih.gov/sites/files/docs/NINR_StratPlan2016_reduced.pdf) and Healthy People 2020 priorities (US Department of Health and Human Services [USDHHS], https://health.gov/healthypeople/objectives-and-data/leading-health-indicators).

This is not to say that the APRN with no research experience (and a full-time job) should "go it alone." Research can be time-consuming and demanding. It is easy for an inexperienced researcher to become mired down in the time and work required for any research study. It is also easy to overlook potential problems and flaws in study design. In order to be worthwhile, research needs to be rigorous and methodically executed. An experienced researcher can anticipate study flaws and confounds, and assist in the development of the best possible study to answer the research question. A practicing APRN with a researchable question should identify experienced researchers who could serve as potential collaborators and develop a research team. Collaboration is an excellent way to capitalize on many people's individual expertise and distribute the workload. Thus, roles and responsibilities need to be made very clear from the start. Every research team should include at least one member who is an expert in research design (quantitative, qualitative, or mixed methods) and an expert in data analysis. If you are planning a quantitative study in which data will be statistically analyzed, a statistician should be consulted from the outset.

Conducting Health Behavior Research with At-risk Children, Adolescents, and Families

Health behavior research seeks to describe patterns of health behavior and understand why individuals engage in behaviors that place them at risk for adverse health consequences. Ultimately, information gathered is used to design interventions to change behavior, support behavior change, and reduce adverse health outcomes. However, health behavior is complex. For example, most adolescents and young adults "know" the facts about smoking; they are knowledgeable about the adverse effects of cigarette smoking on their health. So why do adolescents smoke cigarettes? Similarly, why do adolescents drink alcohol? Exhibit unhealthy eating behaviors (e.g. overeating, anorexia, bulimia)? Engage in unprotected sex? Because health behavior is complex and knowledge alone does not determine behavior, simplistic interventions that seek to change behavior by increasing knowledge are unlikely to succeed, and studies examining use of interventions designed to change knowledge alone are equally unlikely to be funded.

Research Methods Used by APRNs

When an APRN is a principal investigator (PI) or a co-investigator (Co-I) on a research team, they will be involved in the design of the research study to be conducted. The most important issues to consider when planning the conduct of a research study are the research problem and, more specifically, the research question or questions to be answered. The research question guides the research design and methodology of the study, and the composition of the research team. For example, if the research question asks about the frequency or prevalence of a mental health diagnosis among children and adolescents, it would be appropriate to use a quantitative design. Conversely, if the research question asks about the personal life experience of an adolescent who is experiencing depression for the first time, a qualitative design would be appropriate (Brown 2014; LoBiondo-Wood and Haber 2014; Melnyk and Fineout-Overholt 2019; Norwood 2010; Polit and Beck 2016).

Quantitative Research Methods

Quantitative research aims to provide information that is generalizable to a population and can be used to demonstrate causality or make predictions (Norwood 2010; Polit and Beck 2016). Quantitative research is used to *quantify* the problem, i.e. to quantify attitudes, opinions, behaviors, and other defined variables. The goal is to generalize results from a sample to the population from which the sample was drawn. In general, quantitative studies focus on the frequency of a condition, the strength of a relationship between or among variables, the strength of an outcome, or the amount of difference between groups (LoBiondo-Wood and Haber 2014; Norwood 2010; Polit and Beck 2016).

Quantitative researchers use numerical data to answer the research question, and data collection methods include various forms of questionnaires or surveys (e.g. paper, online, or using mobile devices) and/or systematic observation. The studies can involve one-time data collection or multiple data collection sessions (e.g. repeated measures or longitudinal data collection). For example, if the research question is, "How do depressed adolescents relate to their peers in social situations?" the data might be collected using a questionnaire that asks the adolescent to rate their level of comfort in a social situation. One question might be, "In general, how comfortable do you feel when interacting with a friend at a party?" with response options ranging from (1) not at all comfortable to (5) extremely comfortable. Studies that use quantitative research methods have been the most common type of published research in nursing and healthcare journals (Melnyk and Fineout-Overholt 2019; Polit and Beck 2016).

One major characteristic of quantitative research is an attempt to maintain objectivity by controlling as many extraneous variables as possible that could influence study outcomes. This is especially important in experimental studies such as those that test a nursing intervention.

In intervention studies and randomized controlled trials, the goal is to administer the intervention in a consistent manner to all participants and reduce outside influences as much as possible. A data collection plan is delineated prior to implementation and is carefully followed throughout the study, and data analysis typically does not take place until all data collection is completed. Data are analyzed using statistical methods such as descriptive statistics (frequency, mean, standard deviation, percent), chi-square, t-tests, analysis of variance (ANOVA) or covariance techniques, and correlational or regression analyses. These methodological features of quantitative research studies are designed to maintain control over extraneous variables so that study results can be considered valid and reliable (Brown 2014; LoBiondo-Wood and Haber 2014; Melnyk and Fineout-Overholt 2019; Norwood 2010; Polit and Beck 2016). Reliability and validity of the study results are important elements of quantitative research design. Reliability is the *consistency* with which study instruments measure the construct under consideration and validity is the extent to which the study instruments *accurately* measure the construct being investigated (Norwood 2010; Polit and Beck 2016). To assess reliability and validity, study findings are evaluated using a variety of statistical techniques that produce estimates of reliability (e.g. internal consistency is assessed with Cronbach's alpha) and validity (e.g. construct validity is assessed with factor analysis) (Kellar and Kelvin 2013).

Quantitative research can be nonexperimental or experimental. Experimental studies are considered stronger than nonexperimental studies because there is more control over extraneous variables (factors that could influence the study results). Common experimental designs used in nursing studies are quasi-experimental and true experiments. Intervention studies in nursing often use quasi-experimental designs because of the difficulty of using true random assignment to an intervention or control group. Common types of nonexperimental research designs used by nurses include descriptive, correlational, and cohort studies.

Experimental Research Designs

Quasi-experimental and experimental research studies both examine differences between groups. True experiments are considered the strongest designs for examining the effectiveness of an intervention because these designs provide the most stringent control over the variables being studied as well as control over extraneous variables.

The key characteristics of a true experimental design are:

1. Researcher manipulates the independent variable (the intervention).
2. The control group does not receive the intervention.

3. Participants are randomly assigned to the experimental (intervention) or control (comparison) group.

Quasi-experimental studies can also examine the effectiveness of an intervention. However, these studies lack either randomization or a control group. This occurs in situations where randomization is not feasible (no comparison group is available) or ethical (not ethical to withhold a promising treatment from some patients) (LoBiondo-Wood and Haber 2014; Norwood 2010; Polit and Beck 2016). Common types of quasi-experimental research reported in nursing journals are nonequivalent pretest-posttest design and one-group repeated measures designs. Common types of experimental research reported in nursing publications are equivalent (two-group) posttest only, equivalent groups pretest-posttest, Solomon four-group, and one-group cross-over designs. Studies using factorial designs are also common. All these designs and the types of statistical tests used to analyze data are described in more detail in nursing research and statistics textbooks such as Polit and Beck (2016) and Kellar and Kelvin (2013), and are reviewed in textbooks on EBP such as Brown (2014) and Melnyk and Fineout-Overholt (2019).

Quantitative Nonexperimental Research Designs

While studies that use nonexperimental designs are not considered as strong as experimental designs for determining cause and effect, quantitative nonexperimental research is useful for addressing many nursing research problems. Types of nonexperimental research designs used by nurses are descriptive, correlational, and cohort designs (Brown 2014; Melnyk and Fineout-Overholt 2019; Norwood 2010; Polit and Beck 2016).

Nurses conduct descriptive studies to gain more information about a specific situation or phenomenon. They use a descriptive design to describe what is observed or to document characteristics of a situation, phenomenon, or group of people (Norwood 2010). Descriptive research can be used to document children's responses to traumatic events. For example, a nurse researcher may conduct a descriptive study to describe anxiety levels, school phobia, or coping strategies among children exposed to gun violence in school (e.g. children present at Sandy Hook elementary in Connecticut or a high school in Park City, Florida). Researchers using descriptive designs are concerned with extraneous variables that may obscure the true characteristics of the groups or phenomenon under consideration. Threats to validity in a descriptive study are controlled through sampling strategies, providing explicit operational definitions of the variables under study, and carefully designed data collection protocols that are implemented in a consistent manner (Norwood 2010).

In descriptive research, surveys, questionnaires, or interviews are common forms of data collection and are used to assess things like attitudes, behavior, perceptions, healthcare needs, and satisfaction with care (Brown 2014; Norwood 2010). In some cases, descriptive studies are used to obtain preliminary data to establish a knowledge base and generate hypotheses for correlational, quasi-experimental or experimental studies. Case studies describe one patient or a small group of patients and are used to provide in-depth descriptions of the experiences or outcomes of individual patients who have received an intervention, or for whom the outcomes are in some way different than expected (Norwood 2010; Polit and Beck 2016).

Correlational research is conducted to examine relationships among variables that are present in a single group (Brown 2014; Norwood 2010; Polit and Beck 2016). While correlational research cannot provide evidence for cause and effect, relationships between important variables can identify patterns in multiple studies over time that can present compelling evidence that an intervention is needed. For example, many studies on long-term cigarette use and the incidence of lung cancer have provided sufficient evidence to indicate that cigarette smoking should be avoided, especially by children and adolescents.

Cohort studies also examine relationships between variables, in this case exposure to some risk factor that may result in a health problem. In cohort studies, nurse researchers follow two groups of people over time, those with a risk factor for a health problem and those without it, to determine if the health problem occurs (Brown 2014; LoBiondo-Wood and Haber 2014; Melnyk and Fineout-Overholt 2019). For example, two groups of children (those with and without mothers with a diagnosis of major depression) are followed to see if and at what age the children of mothers with depression are themselves more likely to be diagnosed with major depression.

Qualitative Research Designs

Qualitative research is often exploratory research. It is used to gain an understanding of underlying reasons, opinions, and motivations. It provides insights into the problem or helps to develop ideas or answers to questions about a "lived" experience. Research questions asked in qualitative studies differ from those of quantitative studies and vary based on the research tradition chosen for the study. Qualitative research is a general term that refers to the use of several research designs that generate narrative findings for the purpose of providing in-depth description and promoting deeper

understanding of a phenomenon or a group of people (Melnyk and Fineout-Overholt 2019; Norwood 2010; Polit and Beck, 2016). Common research traditions used by nurses to guide data collection and analysis in qualitative research are ethnography, grounded theory, and phenomenology (Brown, 2014; Melnyk and Fineout-Overholt, 2019; Norwood, 2010; Polit and Beck, 2016). Qualitative data collection methods vary and use unstructured or semi-structured techniques. In qualitative research, data are frequently collected in a naturalistic setting (e.g. the participant's home) using interview, focus group, or participant observation techniques (Norwood, 2010; Polit and Beck, 2016). Data are narrative rather than numerical (e.g. transcripts of in-depth interviews or observations, historical documents) and are analyzed using some form of content or thematic analysis (Norwood, 2010; Polit and Beck 2016). In general, for analysis, raw data are typically read by one or more members of the research team, initial codes are developed that describe concepts that emerge from the data, and themes are derived which describe broader interpretations of the data. Discrepancies that arise in interpretation of the codes and themes are commonly resolved through consensus among research team members (Palinkas 2014; Polit and Beck 2016). Ensuring the validity of data and study findings (i.e. ensuring that the study is accurately measuring or reflecting the phenomenon under investigation) is paramount in both quantitative and qualitative research.

In qualitative research, the term "trustworthiness" is used to connote the concept of validity. Several criteria are used to evaluate the study's trustworthiness: credibility, transferability, confirmability, and dependability (LoBiondo-Wood and Haber 2014; Melnyk and Fineout-Overholt 2019; Polit and Beck 2016). Confirmability refers to objectivity and involves member checks (checking back with the participants to see if they agree with the interpretation of the data) (Melnyk and Fineout-Overholt 2019; Polit and Beck 2016). For example, in a study designed to describe domains of postpartum doula care, McComish et al. (2004, 2009) observed and recorded mother–infant and mother–toddler interactions, as well as interactions of infants and toddlers with a doula. One finding of the study was that doulas facilitated infant–mother attachment. Data collection occurred over a 12-week period with six in-home visits and used prolonged engagement to obtain data from both mothers and their postpartum doulas about their newborn infants and toddlers. Triangulation was used by collecting data from both interviews and observations during those visits. Analysis of data also included member checks to confirm that the participants agreed with the researchers' interpretation of the data.

Dependability is demonstrated by careful documentation of the way in which the research process was carried out, with special attention to the way that decisions were made in interpreting the study data (e.g. resolving disagreements about data interpretation through consensus) and using an audit trail to document the processes used in data collection and analysis (Melnyk and Fineout-Overholt 2019).

Credibility refers to ensuring that the data represent the viewpoint of the study participants, not the biases of the researchers. Credibility is achieved using several strategies including, but not limited to, prolonged engagement with the participants (multiple interviews or observations over time), saturation of the data, and documentation of and reflection on investigator biases. Triangulation, another strategy for achieving credibility, involves collection of data from several sources in order to obtain multiple perspectives. If the multiple perspectives agree, credibility is enhanced. Transferability refers to the potential for applying the study findings in other settings (Polit and Beck 2016) or the potential of the findings being meaningful to people in similar situations (Melnyk and Fineout-Overholt 2019).

Ethnography focuses on cultural traditions, grounded theory focuses on social processes and structures, and phenomenology focuses on obtaining in-depth information about life experiences. Examples of research questions in these types of studies include the following:

Ethnography: What are the cultural norms that guide parents in dealing with children diagnosed with an autism spectrum disorder in an unstructured school situation?

Grounded theory: How do parents make the decision about whether to enroll their child diagnosed with an autism spectrum disorder into a specialized school program or keep them mainstreamed in a public school?

Phenomenology: What is it like to be the parent of a child diagnosed with an autism spectrum disorder, especially as it relates to the child's attendance and interactions in school?

An advantage of qualitative research is that it contributes to in-depth understanding of phenomena that arise in provision of care to vulnerable populations such as children experiencing severe mental illness. A disadvantage is that data collection and analysis are often time-consuming and expensive. While there are several computer programs available to assist with data analysis, ultimately the research team must make decisions about the themes that emerge from the data, and this takes considerable time related to being immersed in the data and

conducting member checks to make sure participants confirm interpretation of the data (Polit and Beck 2016). APRNs can find more in-depth discussions of the many types of qualitative designs in nursing research textbooks such as Polit and Beck (2016) and EBP textbooks such as Melnyk and Fineout-Overholt (2019).

Mixed-methods Research

Reports of mixed-methods research are becoming more common in nursing and healthcare journals (Bressan et al. 2016; Chiang-Hanisko et al. 2016; Kettles et al. 2011; Palinkas, 2014). Mixed-methods research is an approach that combines the strengths of quantitative and qualitative research to obtain a richer and deeper understanding of the phenomenon under consideration than could be obtained with either approach alone, in either a single study or a series of related studies (Kettles et al. 2011; Zhang and Creswell 2013). The use of mixed methods has long been advocated as a useful strategy for addressing the complexity of the research questions that are needed to solve healthcare problems (Bressan et al. 2016; Sandelowski 2000).

Nurses have been combining quantitative and qualitative methods in research studies for many years. Chiang-Hanisko et al. (2016) described three approaches to using mixed-methods research in nursing studies: parallel mixed methods, sequential mixed methods, and conversion mixed methods. With the parallel mixed methods approach, both types of data are collected and analyzed concurrently, but separately. Results and inferences from each type of data are reported separately, and then synthesized during final interpretation of the results.

With the sequential mixed-methods approach, the qualitative and quantitative methods occur in two separate time-ordered phases, and collection and analysis of one type of data follows and is dependent on the collection and analysis of the other type of data. The design can be sequential exploratory (qualitative followed by quantitative) or explanatory (quantitative followed by qualitative). In research studies that use the sequential exploratory design, interview data might be gathered in the qualitative phase. Themes derived from the interviews can be used to create questionnaire items for data collection in the quantitative phase.

In the conversion mixed methods approach, data collection can begin with either qualitative or quantitative data. In the analysis process, qualitative data are converted to numbers or quantitative data are converted to words. These processes are sometimes referred to as quantitizing or qualitizing (Chiang-Hanisko et al. 2016; Sandelowski 2000). Refer to Chiang-Hanisko et al. (2016) for detailed examples of the use of all three mixed-methods approaches: parallel, sequential, and conversion. Although these examples do not use children or adolescents as participants, they provide an excellent overview of the use of these mixed-methods research approaches. Zhang and Creswell (2013) describe a similar use of these approaches to mixed methods design using the terms integration, connection, and embedding, and the APRN nurse researcher may want to consult this reference. Polit and Beck's (2016) well-known nursing research textbook also includes a discussion of mixed-methods research.

Building a Research Team

When APRNs are PIs or Co-Is of a research team, they are responsible for making sure that each team member understands the nature of the research project and the implications of participating. Important questions to answer when developing a research team include:

- What is the research question to be answered?
- What type of data will be collected? How and by whom?
- How will the data be analyzed and by whom?
- Who will be the lead or PI?
- Who will be the Co-I and other research team members?
- What will be each person's contribution to the project?
- Who will receive credit and be included in publications or presentations of research results? (Who will be first author, second author, etc.?)

Potential research collaborators may already be present in the clinical practice site. Many large medical centers have research centers and research directors or a director of nursing research. These individuals may be able to provide direct assistance or refer an APRN who is a new investigator to experienced researchers who may be of assistance. Other clinicians, practitioners, physicians, administrators, and leaders within the clinical site may be interested in participating in a research team. While these individuals may be valuable research team members who are able to provide both clinical expertise and access to patient populations, they may not be experts in research design and data analysis. In order to be successful, the research team needs to have members who are experienced researchers and methodological experts. If there are experienced researchers present in the clinical setting, they may be ideal choices as collaborators. These persons bring an additional benefit as they are likely to be knowledgeable about the procedures and approvals needed to conduct a research study in that specific clinical practice site.

A local university may also be a source for identifying research collaborators, particularly if it is a research-intensive university. Many universities have faculty web pages that provide an overview of the faculty members' research interests and experience. Another way to identify potential collaborators is through reviewing published research reports in nursing and interdisciplinary journals and by attending research conferences. Since research collaborators do not have to be located in the same city or state, experienced researchers who have similar interests may be willing to serve as Co-Is or consultants for your project. Whether or not they are local, experienced researchers may be familiar with how to best answer the questions of interest. They may know of reliable and valid instruments or how to use qualitative methods to measure the phenomenon of interest. Experienced researchers may have research staff and may be able to identify statisticians or others who can help plan and execute data analysis. Finally, if the focus of the research study is to develop and/or test an intervention, the team should consult or include an experienced intervention researcher on the team.

Collaboration on research teams frequently includes nurses who hold a PhD or a Doctor of Nursing Practice (DNP). Accepted as the terminal degree in almost all professions, PhD-prepared APRNs are educated to be nurse scientists who conduct research that is intended to generate external evidence that can be generalized/applied to the larger population from which the sample was selected (Edwardson 2010; Grey 2013; Melnyk 2013). In contrast, the DNP-prepared APRN has been identified by the American Association of Colleges of Nursing (AACN) as the entry level for advanced practice nursing (Edwardson 2010; Grey 2013; Melnyk 2013). Since 2004, there has been an acceleration in the number of programs that are graduating DNP-prepared nurses for advanced practice. DNP-prepared APRNs are educated to be expert clinicians who focus on EBP, that is, evaluating and implementing research evidence in the practice setting to improve quality of care and patient outcomes (Edwardson 2010; Glanz et al. 2008a,b; Melnyk 2013). In general, their involvement in research is to generate data at the local level and conduct EBP, quality improvement, or outcomes management projects (Melnyk 2013). Data in these projects are used to solve practice problems within a unit, institution, or local regional area (Edwardson 2010; Glanz et al. 2008a,b; Melnyk 2013).

DNP-prepared APRNs often work as health system or hospital leaders who collaborate with nurse researchers to implement new innovations in practice (Trautman et al. 2018). Working together, PhD- and DNP-prepared APRNs can identify areas of concern that are appropriate for examination at the local level. Following that, they may identify other important aspects of the problem that are appropriate for more sophisticated research designs, including use of experimental designs (e.g. studies that compare effectiveness of two or more treatments currently used in practice) or translational research. This collaboration has the potential to decrease the timeline for nursing research findings to be implemented in practice (Trautman et al. 2018).

Sources of Research Funding for Nurses

In addition to building a research team, it is necessary to identify other resources needed to conduct a research study. For the APRN in primary care or behavioral or mental health, key questions include:

- What other resources (time, personnel, equipment, space) are needed to conduct the study?
- Will research grant funding be needed? If so, how much money is needed? Where might the needed funding be obtained?
- How will a researcher gain access to the population of interest?

For more than 20 years, the NINR has been one of the primary funders of nursing research in the United States. The research priorities of the NINR include health promotion, disease prevention, enhancing wellness, developing personalized treatments and self-management strategies for chronic conditions, and end-of-life care. There are also a number of other NIH institutes and centers that have missions and priorities that focus on areas that may be of interest to APRNs who focus on child and adolescent mental health, including:

- National Cancer Institute (NCI)
- National Institute on Alcohol Abuse and Alcoholism (NIAA)
- National Institute of Allergy and Infectious Diseases (NIAID)
- Eunice Kennedy Shriver National Institute of Child Health and Human Development (NICHD)
- National Institute on Drug Abuse (NIDA)
- National Institute of Mental Health (NIMH)
- National Institute on Minority Health and Health Disparities (NIMHD).

Many other federal and nonfederal agencies, foundations, and private organizations also fund research that is consistent with their particular mission. The CDC awards millions of dollars in research grants every year to enhance understanding of the mechanisms of disease and health-risk behaviors.

Other organizations fund research in their particular areas of interest. Most have websites or publications that describe their research grant programs, funding cycles, and eligibility requirements. While most NIH research grants require that the PI hold a doctorate or other terminal degree, many foundations, specialty organizations, and regional research foundations accept research grant applications from APRNs with a masters or DNP degree. Nongovernment organizations that frequently fund nursing research include:

- State nurses' associations and local specialty nursing organizations
- Robert Wood Johnson Foundation (RWJF)
- American Nurses Foundation (ANF)
- Sigma Theta Tau International (STTI) and local chapters of STTI
- International Society of Psychiatric-Mental Health Nurses (ISPN)
- American Psychiatric Nurses Association (APNA)
- American Academy of Nurse Practitioners (AANP)
- American Association of Critical Care Nurses (AACCN)
- National Association of Pediatric Nurse Associates and Practitioners (NAPNAP)
- Association of Women's Health, Obstetric, and Neonatal Nurses (AWHONN)
- Academy of Neonatal Nursing (ANN).

Ethical Issues Related to Conduct of Mental Health Research with Children and Adolescents

There are several ethical issues that are important in the conduct of research with children, adolescents, and their families who may have or be at-risk for behavioral or mental health problems. Three priority issues are validity of study data and results, scientific misconduct, and human rights/informed consent. Protection of human rights and informed consent are issues that are commonly considered important in the conduct of research. However, other factors are important considerations in conducting research in an ethical manner.

Validity of Study Data and Results

Nurse researchers ensure that study data and results are valid in several ways: by using the most appropriate study design for answering the research question, by decreasing the threats to validity, and by assessing psychometrics of instruments used to collect the data. Ensuring the validity of study data and results is accomplished through attention to detail in design and implementation of a study and rigorous methodology regardless of whether the study is quantitative or qualitative.

In quantitative studies, this is especially important when a study is designed to test the effectiveness of an intervention, for example when one group of depressed adolescents receives an intervention that includes meditation (treatment group) and another group does not receive meditation as part of the intervention (comparison group). In this case, it is important that threats to validity are controlled through sampling strategies, explicit operational definitions of the two treatment conditions, and carefully designed data collection protocols that are implemented in a consistent manner (Norwood 2010; Polit and Beck 2016).

In qualitative studies, validity of data and results is accomplished in two major ways. First, it is imperative that the research team carefully implements the study design in a way that is consistent with the qualitative tradition that is being used to guide the study (e.g. ethnography, grounded theory, or phenomenology). Second, evidence of validity and reliability are enhanced through strategies that ensure the trustworthiness of the data: credibility, transferability, confirmability, and dependability (Melnyk and Fineout-Overholt 2019; Norwood 2010; Polit and Beck 2016). These strategies are described in more detail in the section on qualitative research designs.

Research Misconduct

Research misconduct is defined as "fabrication, falsification, or plagiarism in proposing, performing, or reviewing research, or in reporting research results" (USDHHS 2019). While research misconduct is rare, the problem is so prevalent that in 1989 the Office of Research Integrity (https://ori.hhs.gov) was formed to develop policies and provide oversight in detection, investigation, and prevention of research fraud (Norwood 2010). The most commonly reported types of research misconduct involve misrepresenting study data so that the results favor the hypotheses proposed by the research team (Norwood 2010). Other forms of misconduct include enrolling research participants without clearly delineating the risks associated with study procedures, falsely reporting results in publications, or misrepresenting one's qualifications or involvement in a study as an investigator or author of a publication (Norwood 2010). All types of misconduct are monitored by the Office of Research Integrity and can result in penalties for the researcher or the institution in which the researcher is employed. When research misconduct includes plagiarism or publication fraud, the researcher is usually required to make a public retraction or withdraw the findings, and that publication cannot be cited by other researchers (Norwood 2010).

Increasingly, nurses and other healthcare professionals who conduct research are under great pressure to publish the results of their studies. Historically, studies that show statistically significant results are more likely to be published. Even though studies that find no difference between intervention and comparison groups may report findings that are vital to the health of society, those studies are less likely to be accepted for publication. Hence, some researchers are tempted to be less stringent in the way in which they report results. Traditionally, the significance level of $p \leq 0.05$ is considered the standard for stating that a result is statistically significant, indicating a reportable difference between two groups. However, there is some precedence for reporting results with a significance level between 0.05 and 0.10 as "a trend toward significance." While this practice does not constitute blatant research misconduct, it is an example of how researchers can be tempted to exaggerate the implications of their study results when interpreting and discussing the implications of their study for application to clinical practice. In nursing, the rule of thumb has been that a researcher who is being conservative will not report any result higher than 0.05 as significant (Polit and Beck 2016).

Informed Consent with Children and Adolescents Involved in Mental Health Research

APRNs who participate as PI, Co-I, or as a research team member should understand that collecting data from human subjects can be a complicated process. Although much of nursing research differs from medical treatment, many mental health nursing research studies involve a behavioral intervention as part of the research protocol. When recruiting subjects to participate in a research project, researchers must do a thorough assessment of the risk/benefit ratio in any one of several domains, including physical, emotional, and privacy (Norwood 2010). Institutional protocols and state and national laws require that all individuals be provided with detailed information prior to participating in any research project or study (Norwood 2010; Polit and Beck 2016). All data collection is governed by ethical principles on how human beings must be treated during the research process. In 1978, the Belmont Report, which was generated by the National Commission for the Protection of Human Subjects of Biomedical and Behavioral Research, identified three ethical principles, beneficence, respect for human dignity, and justice/fair treatment, that have formed the basis for ethical standards in the conduct of research since that time, including the code of scientific conduct of the American Nurses

Association (ANA) (Griffin and Titler 2015) and the ethical regulations of the USDHHS known as Title 45 Part 46 of the Code of Federal Regulations (Office for Human Research Protections [OHRP] 2010, 2019).

Beneficence involves protection of research participants from harm. This includes protection from physical, psychological, social, or economic harm, and from exploitation. Furthermore, the benefits of the research should outweigh the risks of participation, meaning that all proposed research must be assessed to ensure that the benefits to society are greater than the risks to those who agree to participate (Mandal et al. 2011; Morrow et al. 2015; Norwood 2010). Making sure that the members of the research team are qualified and that they use an appropriate research design helps to ensure that beneficence is maintained. *Respect for human dignity* includes the right of any study participant to self-determination (Mandal et al. 2011; Morrow et al. 2015; Norwood 2010) and their right to full disclosure (Norwood 2010). These rights are addressed through informed consent and protection from coercion, either in the form of pressure from those in authority or from excessive monetary incentives for participation. *Justice* includes the right to fair treatment (Mandal et al. 2011; Norwood 2010) and privacy (Norwood 2010). Fair treatment in research is concerned with who is invited to participate and how they are treated during a study. Selection of participants should be based on inclusion criteria that are essential to answer the research question(s), and while the study is being conducted all participants should be treated equitably and should have the option to withdraw from the study for any reason without negative consequences. All participants must have the right to privacy (Norwood 2010). To protect participants' privacy, researchers use one of two strategies, anonymity or confidentiality. When anonymity is used, there is no way of linking an individual participant with their data, meaning that names or other identifying information is not available to the researcher. When confidentiality is used, participants can be linked to their responses on a questionnaire or to biological specimens, but the data are protected. This is typically accomplished by assigning an identification number for data from each participant and keeping data in a secure location, either physically or electronically. In qualitative studies that use group interviews such as focus groups, confidentiality may also include a pledge of confidentiality from group members (Norwood 2010).

Prior to beginning any research study or project, approval from the IRB that governs the research setting must be obtained. The IRB pays particular attention to the process of informed consent. Informed consent has evolved over time and is now universally accepted as a significant part of sample recruitment and data collection (Polit and Beck 2016). Informed consent must include notifying participants of the following:

- They may choose to participate or not participate in the study.
- They may change their mind and withdraw from the study at any time without harm or consequences.
- What the study is and what participation in the study entails.
- What the potential benefits of participating in the study are.
- What potential risks (physical, emotional, economic, social, or legal) may occur as a result of participating in the study.

Informed consent must be written in simple language. If participants cannot read, forms should be read to potential participants by a member of the research team. Many studies may include participants who identify English as a second language; consent form(s) for these individuals should be written in their native language or read and clearly explained by an interpreter. Finally, persons who are approached and invited to participate in a research study should have sufficient time to carefully think about whether to participate.

Children's Ability to Provide Informed Consent

The question of including children and adolescents, especially young children or vulnerable children, as participants in research studies is one that has been debated for years and is coupled with the concern of whether a child can provide an informed consent for their own participation. The researcher must assess the developmental and cognitive capacity of the child or adolescent to ensure the individual has the ability to understand and evaluate the risk, benefits, and requirements of participation in the study before agreeing or declining to consent (Cheah and Parker 2014). In 2005, the USDHHS in its Policy for the Protection of Human Subjects in subpart Section 46.402 defined a child as "a person who has not attained the legal age for consent to treatments or procedures involved in the research, under the applicable law of the jurisdiction in which the research will be conducted" (USDHHS 2005, p. 12). In 2016, NIH changed its policy on Inclusion of Children to define children as "individuals under 18 years old," which is typically considered the age of consent (OHRP 2016). An additional policy related to inclusion of participants in research went into effect on 25 January 2019. This policy, "Inclusion of Individuals across the Lifespan as Participants in Research Involving Human Subjects," requires inclusion of individuals of all ages, including children and older adults, a requirement to provide justification for excluding participants based on age, and provision of data on participant age at enrollment for all federally funded projects (OHRP 2017).

In both law and ethics, children and adolescents have been presumed to lack the capacity to provide informed consent; a child is considered a "developing person" (OHRP 2016). Depending on where the child or adolescent is in his or her development or chronological age, she or he may not be considered to be intellectually, emotionally, or cognitively capable of providing legal informed consent. It is the immaturity of his or her cognitive development that may be in question, or the lack of experiences in situations similar to what she or he is being asked to do regarding participation in the research study. The Common Rule (USDHHS Title 45 CFR 46 Subparts A, B, C, and D) is the baseline standard of ethics to which any government-funded research in the United States is held (OHRP 2010, 2019). The Common Rule and the Revised Common Rule requires parental permission and assent from children generally aged 7 or older for federally regulated research in the United States (OHRP, 2010, 2019).

Child Assent

In addition to obtaining parental consent, most studies that involve children and adolescents under the age of 18 must also obtain child assent. Child assent refers to a child's affirmative agreement to participate in a research study; assent is not the same as failure to object (Cheah and Parker, 2014; Morrow et al. 2015; ORHP 2019). In order to obtain child assent, the child must be provided with the same basic information given during the process of informed consent. This information may need to be simplified or limited depending upon the child's comprehension level and ability to make decisions (Cheah and Parker 2014; OHRP 2019). IRB guidelines vary with regard to documentation of assent, and researchers should be certain they understand the requirements of their own IRBs. Some IRBs require children above age 12 or 14 years to sign a separate youth consent/assent form (ORHP 2019). For children and adolescents, the language used in an assent form must be at a developmentally appropriate level (Cheah and Parker 2014; Morrow et al. 2015). Recent research has examined this issue and has concluded that decisions about child assent, parental consent, and/or child consent should be considered in the context of the geographic and societal situation in which the child lives. In the United States and in geographic areas with high economic status, children may not have engaged in the same level of responsibility as children in areas with poorer economic status (Cheah and Parker 2014). In some areas

of the United States and in low-income countries, children take on more responsibility for caring for younger siblings (and in some cases their own children) before the age of 18. These children may be able to provide informed consent for themselves (Cheah and Parker 2014). In addition, in many cultures, the elders in the family make decisions for the entire family and it is inappropriate to seek consent from the child's parents (Cheah and Parker 2014). As more people from a broader range of cultures become participants in research studies in the United States, it will become more important to think of informed consent in a broader context and make decisions about informed consent or assent based on the maturity of children and adolescents or their cultural context (Cheah and Parker 2014; Morrow et al. 2015).

Emancipated Minors

Emancipation is a formal legal action in which an adolescent can petition to basically free him/herself (minor child) from the supervision of his or her adult parent(s). All states have laws dealing with the "emancipation" of minors, that is, laws that specify when and under what conditions children become independent of their parents for important legal purposes. Emancipated minors can assume most of the legal rights of adulthood, including the right to enter into contracts and the ability to consent to medical care, if they are able to provide court documents to verify their status (Legal Information Institute [LII] 2017). The provisions that permit a minor to be considered emancipated vary from state to state and may depend upon the specific circumstances. For example, a minor can be considered emancipated for one specific purpose (e.g. for obtaining birth control) but not for others such as consenting to surgery or entering into a legal contract (LII 2017). A suggested guideline for use with adolescents who state that they are emancipated is to request a copy of the emancipation order prior to enrollment into the research study and/or check with the IRB at your institution.

Thought Questions

1. What do you want to study and why is this study important?
2. What benefits could potentially be derived from this project?
3. What are the strengths/weaknesses of the research question and design?
4. What are the ethical implications for the potential participants?
5. Can findings from this project be used in a different setting or with different children or adolescents?

Exemplar of a Research Study

A quantitative, nonexperimental research study was conducted to survey high school students about their internet and health risk behaviors, with the aim of developing a descriptive profile of a student who participates in high-risk internet behaviors (Dowdell 2014). The overarching goal for this study was to build on knowledge specific to risky internet behaviors by examining high school students' internet risk behaviors, self-exploitation (sexting), and electronic aggression (bullying). The study employed a cross-sectional, survey research design, collecting data via paper and pencil.

Findings are based on a sample of 5437 high school students in grades 9–12 from six public, private, or parochial (faith-based) high schools in Pennsylvania and Texas. Four of the six schools offered a variety of curricula that included courses identified as college track or college/honors/advanced placement track. Two of the schools offered both of these tracks and a vocational track. Fifty-six percent of the sample was female, 22% identified as nonwhite, and over 93% reported using social networking sites on a regular basis (Dowdell 2014).

Data were collected at each high school on a designated day during one school period or class. Survey distribution was dependent upon the school, with the majority of surveys given in an extended homeroom session. However, in two schools the surveys were given out in an English, technology, or health class. The paper and pencil surveys (questionnaire) used in this study were the Youth Internet Safety Survey (YISS) developed by Mitchell et al. (2001) and the Youth Risk Behavior Surveillance System (YRBSS) that addressed health-risk behavior, developed by the CDC in 1990 (CDC 2020). The YISS, which in its original form was a telephone survey, was adapted for use with paper and pencil by eliminating open-ended questions. A socio-demographic data sheet that identified areas such as age, ethnicity, and family background was also used to collect basic information from students.

Since some questions elicited sensitive information, we went to great lengths to ensure that the students' responses were anonymous and strictly confidential, hoping, of course, to increase truthful responding. As approved by the IRB, high schools were asked to electronically post several documents and also send them home to parents/guardians and students. These documents, authored by the PI, included an information sheet and letter that described the purpose of the study, the data collection process, steps taken to maintain student confidentiality, and an internet tip sheet. Anonymity was protected by having no identifying information (e.g. name, date of birth, student school id number, homeroom number, name of school, name of city, etc.)

requested or placed on the questionnaire. Confidentiality was protected by not supplying specific information to school administration or personnel, such as student names, individual classroom survey response rate, or total numbers of completed surveys from different teachers or sections. Also, all data shared with administration were reported as aggregate.

Prior to beginning the survey, each classroom teacher was asked to read both the consent form and a script that listed the students' rights (e.g. skipping a question if they chose). The script informed students that their responses would be kept confidential from school administration, personnel, and from other students. A student's willingness to start the survey was their implied assent to participate in the study. The estimated time to complete the survey was 20 minutes, which is based on the reading level of the survey as well as time taken to complete a similar survey with more questions during a previous study. Within 24 hours of students completing the survey, the PI securely transported the paper surveys back to her office, where they were locked in file cabinets. For the schools in Texas, the surveys were delivered, collected, and mailed to the PI by the Texas contact person, a forensic APRN. The PI then oversaw transportation of completed surveys to statistical support offices, where the data entry process was closely monitored and a review of a random selection of surveys was conducted to assure accuracy of data entry. In data analysis, frequencies were run on all variables and a series of Pearson correlations were used to determine a relationship or interaction between variables. If there was an interaction between variables, a cross-tabulation was used to determine significance. When determining the level of significance for results, a significance level (p value) of 0.05 was used. Chi-square analysis was also conducted on all dichotomous variables, and ANOVA was used for all continuous variables to determine any significant group differences.

This study had eight general conclusions: (i) internet risk-taking behaviors clustered, (ii) electronic aggression was often combined with other forms of bullying (traditional) and could include sexual material, (iii) electronic aggression and online harassment increased with each grade promotion, with students who used the internet to harass or threaten others online being more likely to also report being in trouble at school, in trouble with the police, being in physical fights, being a victim of cyber bullying, and/or sending sexts, (iv) sexting was a behavior that also increased with age and grade, electronic aggression, communication with online strangers, viewing sexually explicit material online, and health risk behaviors, (v) students who had online relationships with strangers also reported experiences with electronic aggression, sexting, and viewing sexually explicit materials, (vi) students who met online strangers at offline meetings reported experiencing violent acts, (vii) students who met online strangers at offline meetings were more likely to report having experience with electronic aggression and sexting, and (viii) viewing sexually explicit materials online correlated with electronic aggression, sexting, and relationships with online strangers (Dowdell 2014).

Every day, high school students interact with a variety of professionals for a multitude of reasons that include school troubles or concerns, alcohol use, aggression, victimization, health, and wellbeing. In this study, three behaviors, electronic aggression, viewing sexually explicit material online, and sexting, were associated with almost all of the other risk-taking behaviors and were the ones that clustered with health risks. There are a significant number of media tools and sites that can be used to disseminate electronic aggression, view pornography, and send photos. As technology, namely hand-held data devices such as cell or smartphones, improve with faster service, more memory, and more storage, adolescents will have greater, unsupervised access to the internet. While the majority of adolescents reported participation in some risk taking, there did appear to be a small but growing group of adolescents who were harmed as well as victimized by their participation on the internet. Overall, this study described the clustering of risk-taking behaviors (electronic aggression, sexting, viewing sexually explicit materials) with other internet risk behaviors (online relationships, sharing personal information online, unsafe posting) and with risk-taking health behaviors (smoking and alcohol) (Dowdell 2014). Risk-taking behaviors are not new to this generation but the technology available is new and changing, with more students participating in electronic aggression and self-exploitation behaviors on the internet and within their personal relationships. APRNs, other providers, and persons in schools can use these findings to develop plans and policies to address issues of electronic aggression and internet risk in schools. In addition, these findings can be used to design prevention strategies to keep youth safer on the internet.

Summary

In conclusion, APRNs who work in primary care or psychiatric-mental health settings must be knowledgeable about research. In their roles as direct care providers and leaders, APRNs should, at the very least, be informed consumers who use research findings to guide EBP. APRNs who are involved in the design and conduct of research have many research approaches and designs from which to choose to answer the research question(s). The research problem and question(s) always guide selection of the research approach. However, for many research problems, the research team can choose to use either a qualitative or a quantitative approach, or to use a mixed-methods approach that includes elements of both quantitative and qualitative design. Whatever approach is selected, the quality of the research product can be strengthened by using techniques which enhance the reliability and validity of the study findings. It is incumbent upon all APRNs who interact with research participants to be aware of their responsibilities regarding the ethical conduct of research and treatment of research participants, especially children and adolescents. As research team leaders, such as Co-Is and collaborators, APRNs can initiate research projects that help build nursing science and advance our knowledge of behavioral interventions for children and adolescents who are at risk for mental health problems.

References

Bressan, V., Bagnasco, A., Giuseppe, A. et al. (2016). Mixed-methods research in nursing – a critical review. *Journal of Clinical Nursing* 26: 2878–2890. https://doi.org/10.1111/jocn.13631.

Brown, S.J. (2014). Evidence-Based Nursing: The Research-Practice Connection, 3e. Burlington, MA: Jones & Bartlett Learning.

CDC (2018a). Ten Leading Causes of Death and Injury. National Center for Injury Prevention and Control, Centers for Disease Control and Prevention. Available at https://www.cdc.gov/injury/wisqars/LeadingCauses.html.

CDC. (2018b). *Youth Risk Behavior Surveillance – United States, 2017.* MMWR, 67 (No. SS-8). Centers for Disease Control and Prevention. Available at https://www.cdc.gov/healthyyouth/data/yrbs/pdf/2017/ss6708.pdf.

CDC. (2020). *Youth Risk Behavior Surveillance System (YRBSS) overview.* Available at https://www.cdc.gov/healthyyouth/data/yrbs/overview.htm.

Cheah, P.Y. and Parker, M. (2014). Consent and assent in paediatric research in low-income settings. *BMC Medical Ethics* 15: 1–10. https://doi.org/10.1186/1472-6939-15-22.

Chiang-Hanisko, L., Newman, D., Dyess, S. et al. (2016). Guidance for using mixed methods design in nursing practice research. *Applied Nursing Research* 31: 1–5. https://doi.org/10.1016/j.apnr.2015.12.006.

Dowdell, E.B. (2014). *Self-Exploitation and Electronic Aggression: High Risk Internet Behaviors in Adolescents.* Award No. 2010-MC-CX-0002. Washington, DC: Office of Juvenile Justice and Delinquency Prevention, Office of Justice Programs, US Department of Justice.

Edwardson, S.R. (2010). Doctor of philosophy and doctor of nursing practice as complementary degrees. *Journal of Nursing Practice* 26 (3): 137–140. https://doi.org/10.1016/j.profnurs.2009.08.004.

Glanz, K., Rimer, B., and Viswanath, K. (eds.) (2008a). Health Behavior and Health Education: Theory, Research and Practice, 4e. San Francisco, CA: Wiley.

Glanz, K., Rimer, B., and Viswanath, K. (2008b). The scope of health behavior and health education. In: Health Behavior and Health Education: Theory, Research and Practice, 4e (eds. K. Glanz, K. Rimer and K. Viswanath), 3–22. San Francisco, CA: Wiley.

Grey, M. (2013). The doctor of nursing practice: defining the next steps. *Journal of Nursing Education* 52 (8): 462–465. https://doi.org/10.3928/01484834-20130719-02.

Griffin, E. and Titler, M. (2015). Using evidence through collaboration to promote excellence in nursing practice. In: Evidence-Based Practice for Nurses: Appraisal and Application of Research, 3rde (eds. N.A. Schmidt and J.M. Brown), 43–68. Sudbury, MA: Jones & Bartlett Publishers.

Kellar, S.P. and Kelvin, E.A. (2013). Munro's Statistical Methods for Health Care Research, 6e. Philadelphia, PA: Lippincott Williams & Wilkins.

Kettles, A.M., Creswell, J.W., and Zhang, W. (2011). Mixed methods research in mental health nursing. *Journal of Psychiatric and Mental Health Nursing* 18: 535–542. https://doi.org/10.1111/j.1365-2850.2011.01701.x.

Legal Information Institute (2017). Emancipation of Minors. New York: Cornell Law School Available at https://www.law.cornell.edu/wex/emancipation_of_minors.

LoBiondo-Wood, G. and Haber, J. (2014). Nursing Research: Methods and Critical Appraisal for Evidence-Based Practice, 8e. Philadelphia, PA: Mosby.

Mandal, J., Acharya, S., and Parija, S.C. (2011). Ethics in human research. *Tropical Parasitology* 1: 2–3. https://doi.org/10.4103/2229-5070.72105.

McComish, J.F. and Visger, J.M. (2009). Domains of postpartum doula care and maternal responsiveness and competence. *Journal of Obstetric, Gynecologic, and Neonatal Nursing* 38: 148–156. https://doi.org/10.1111/j.1552-6909.2009.01002.x.

McComish, J.F., Campbell-Voytal, K., and Rowland, C. (2004). Postpartum doula care: Content and process. *International Doula* 12 (4): 22–25.

Melnyk, B.M. (2013). Distinguishing the preparation and roles of doctor of philosophy and doctor of nursing practice graduates: national implications for academic curricula and health care systems. *Journal of Nursing Education* 52 (8): 442–448. https://doi.org/10.3928/01484834-20130719-01.

Melnyk, B.M. and Fineout-Overholt, E. (2019). Evidence-Based Practice in Nursing & Healthcare: a Guide to Best Practice, 4e. Philadelphia, PA: Wolters Kluwer.

Morrow, B.M., Argent, A.C., and Kling, S. (2015). Informed consent in paediatric critical care research – a South Africa perspective. *BMC Medical Ethics*: 1–13. https://doi.org/10.1186/s12910-015-0052-6.

National Commission for the Protection of Human Subjects of Biomedical and Behavioral Research (1978). The Belmont Report: Ethical Principles and Guidelines for the Protection of Human Subjects of Research. Bethesda, MD: The Commission, Department of Health, Education and Welfare Available at https://www.hhs.gov/ohrp/regulations-and-policy/belmont-report/index.html.

NIH. (2017). *Revision: NIH policy and guidelines on the inclusion of individuals across the lifespan as participants in research involving human subjects*. National Institute of Health. Available at https://grants.nih.gov/grants/guide/notice-files/NOT ().

Norwood, S.L. (2010). Research Essentials for Evidence-Based Practice. Upper Saddle River, NJ: Pearson Education.

OHRP. (2010). *Policy guidelines for the Common Rule: Title 45 CFR 46 (Public Welfare)*. Office for Human Research Protections, US Department of Health and Human Services. Available at http://www.hhs.gov/ohrp/researchfaq.pdf.

OHRP. (2016). *Special protections for children as research subjects. Office for Human Research Protections*. Available at https://www.hhs.gov/ohrp/regulations-and-policy/guidance/special-protections-for-children/index.html.

OHRP. (2017). *Revised common rule*. Available at https://www.hhs.gov/ohrp/regulations-and-policy/regulations/finalized-revisions-common-rule/index.html.

OHRP (2019). *The Revised Common Rule Compliance Dates and Transition Provision (45 CFR 46.101(l))*. Office for Human Research Protections, US Department of Health and Human Services. Available at https://www.hhs.gov/ohrp/regulations-and-policy/requests-for-comments/draft-guidance-revised-common-rule-compliance-dates-transition-provision-45-cfr-46-1011/index.html.

Palinkas, L.A. (2014). Qualitative methods in mental health services research. *Journal of Clinical Child and Adolescent Psychology* 43 (6): 851–861. https://doi.org/10.1080/15374416.2014.910791.

Polit, D.F. and Beck, C.T. (2016). Nursing Research: Generating and Assessing Evidence for Nursing Practice, 10e. Philadelphia, PA: Wolters Kluwer.

Sandelowski, M. (2000). Combining qualitative and quantitative sampling, data collection, and analysis techniques in mixed-methods studies. *Research in Nursing & Health* 23 (3): 246–255. https://doi.org/10.1002/1098-240x(200006)23:3<246::aid-nur9>3.0.co;2-h.

Trautman, D.E., Idzik, S., Hammersla, M., and Rosseter, R. (2018). Advancing scholarship through translational research: the role of PhD and DNP prepared nurses. *The Online Journal of Issues in Nursing* 23 (2), Manuscript 2. doi: https://doi.org/10.3912/OJIN.Vol23No02Man02.

USDHHS. (2005). *Public Welfare: Protection of Human Subjects*. US Department of Health and Human Services. Available at https://www.hhs.gov/ohrp/regulations-and-policy/guidance/guidance-on-407-review-process/index.html.

USDHHS. (2019). *Definition of Research Misconduct*. Office of Research Integrity, US Department of Health and Human Services. Available at https://ori.hhs.gov/definition-misconduct.

Zhang, W. and Creswell, J. (2013). The use of "mixing" procedure of mixed methods in health services research. *Medical Care* 51 (8): e51–e57. ISSN: 0025-7079/13/5108-0e51.

32

Advanced Practice Registered Nurses Interfacing with the School System

Melissa M. Gomes[1] and Naomi A. Schapiro[2]

[1] Hampton University School of Nursing, Hampton, VA, USA
[2] University of California, San Francisco, San Francisco, CA, USA

Objectives

After reading this chapter, advanced practice registered nurses (APRNs) will be able to:

1. Discuss historical premise and rationale for behavioral health promotion within the school environment for students with emotional or behavioral presentations.
2. Review federal legislation and special education mandates responsible for inclusion of in-school support services for students in need.
3. Present evidence-based collaborative practice models for use in the school system.
4. Describe the school-based health center model of care and how it has the potential to improve access to behavioral health services, student success, and improved behavioral outcomes.
5. Identify APRN roles and responsibilities for collaboration within the school community.

Introduction

According to the World Health Organization (WHO), half of all mental illnesses begin before the age of 14, with an estimated 10–20% of youth worldwide experiencing a mental illness (WHO 2018). The mental and psychosocial health of youth is of great concern because it directly impacts their ability to develop a healthy trajectory. Without effective intervention, mental health problems can hinder normal development, academic success, and self-concept, accounting for the leading cause of disability among youth (WHO 2018). Therefore, effective prevention measures and early identification

of mental illness are imperative and the advance practice nurse, especially those working in and with schools is vital in this measure.

School, as part of the student's developmental framework, is the predominant setting for the daily experiences of children and adolescents – interactions with teachers, peers, and classmates, enactment of roles and responsibilities, and of course engagement in academics. Cooperation, working within a structure, and learning are major expectations of the student attending school. Inability or decreased ability to function in school is often an early sign of an underlying health, emotional, behavioral, or psychological issue. As an important

Child and Adolescent Behavioral Health: A Resource for Advanced Practice Psychiatric and Primary Care Practitioners in Nursing,
Second Edition. Edited by Edilma L. Yearwood, Geraldine S. Pearson, and Jamesetta A. Newland.
© 2021 John Wiley & Sons, Inc. Published 2021 by John Wiley & Sons, Inc.
Companion website: www.wiley.com/go/Yearwood

factor within the childhood experience, school can impact children positively or negatively based upon their personal interactions. With children and adolescents spending an average 6.65 hours in the school setting, this time serves as a prime opportunity to intervene on their behalf (National Center for Education Statistics n.d.) using prevention methods and interventions to support healthy psychosocial development.

The Need for an Integrated Response to the Mental Health Needs of Children and Adolescents

The WHO developed the Mental Health Action Plan 2013–2020 which advocates for all, including youth, and calls for an expansion of services in order to promote greater efficiency of resources There are four major tenets of the plan: (i) strengthen leadership to provide equal care for mental illness, (ii) provide care that is without silos and that provides easy access in community-based settings, (iii) develop crucial interventions/strategies to promote wellness and prevent mental illness, and (iv) provide evidenced-based care grounded in mental health research (WHO 2013). This plan has been accepted as an integral component of the effort to implement "a lifecycle approach" to meeting the mental health needs of children and adolescents which will require intersecting efforts of policy makers, practitioners, parents, and youth. Advance practice registered nurses (APRNs) are integral in this cross-sectional development.

This chapter will explore the tenets of the WHO Mental Health Action Plan, while outlining contextual factors which are integral to a positive mental health and academic trajectory. A presentation of common behavioral issues of youth seen in schools will be reviewed in combination with evidence on the effectiveness of collaborative models, and the leadership and advocacy role of APRNs in school-based practice models. We will highlight and present a case exemplar illustrating how school-based programs can meet the mental health needs of youngsters.

An Exploration of the Strength of Leadership to Provide Equal Care for Mental Illness

Mental Health in the Education System

Education, although federally legislated, is implemented on the state level. There are several levels between federal legislation and school implementation. State boards of education implement and enforce the mandates set forth by the federal government and state legislature, while their designees (local school districts) dispense regulations guiding practices in schools that will then be evaluated.

Local school boards, or local educational agencies, interpret state mandates and manage operating funds that are allocated by state-level entities and, in some cases, physical and capital resources from federal, state, and local sources. School boards determine distribution of funds at the local level in many cases; however, there are districts whose budgets must be approved by a local populous vote. A superintendent, who serves as a chief executive officer, hired by local school boards, usually serves as the head of the school district. Schools with their administrators, faculty, and support staff are, in turn, charged with the implementation of directives from federal, state, and local authoritative bodies (US Department of Education n.d.). School nurses may be hired by school districts, departments of health, universities, or by the individual school. In 2017, the National Association of School Nurses (NASN) conducted a survey and found that only 39% of schools have a full-time school nurse, with multiple schools within districts sharing a nurse. This review of educational legislation's "trickle down" is intended to provide a summary of the authorities involved with implementing the federal mandates. Because of differing state and municipal laws and policies, APRNs are advised to become familiar with the relevant governing principles of the school districts in the areas that they serve.

No longer is the task of education concerned only with the mastery of academics. Schools have more recently been recognized as the primary environment and home community for enrolled students, thereby making significant contributions to child socioemotional development. The centrality of school in the life of children and adolescents provides a natural opportunity for onsite delivery of services that support the biopsychosocial needs of children. Special education history seems to have evolved full circle from including and supporting children with disability or special needs in contained environments to requiring that all other options and supportive interventions and/or teaching methods be utilized to keep special needs students in mainstream environments.

Attention to the health, safety, and developmental needs of children in schools is historically linked to federal education legislation and, more directly, federal mandates for special education, which are shown in Table 32.1. The US education system is a federal, state, and local partnership mandated to serve the educational needs of all children. Schools play a major role in any comprehensive system of care for children, with 98 271 public schools educating 50 million school-age youth across the United States in 2013 (National Center for Education Statistics n.d.). The Office of Special Education and Rehabilitative Services (OSERS) of the US Department of Education further estimates that there were approximately 7.2 million children in 2016 who were receiving special education services for physical,

Table 32.1 History of special education

Civil Rights Act Title VI of the Elementary and Secondary Education Act. Created a Bureau of Education for the Handicapped.

- 1973: Section 504 of the Rehabilitation Act. Protects qualified individuals from discrimination based on their disability.

- 1974: Family Educational Rights and Privacy Act (FERPA). Allows parents to have access to all personally identifiable information collected, maintained, or used by a school district regarding their child.

- 1975: The Education for All Handicapped Children Act (EAHCA).
  - 1975: Mandated all school districts to educate students with disabilities.
  - 1977: The final federal regulations are enacted at the start of the 1977–1978 school year; provides a set of rules to which school districts must adhere when providing an education to students with disabilities.

- 1986: The EAHCA is amended with the addition of the Handicapped Children's Protection Act. Clarifies that students and parents have rights under EAHCA and Section 504.

- 1990: The Americans with Disabilities Act (ADA). Adopts the Section 504 regulations as part of the statute; "504 Plans" for individual students have become more common in school districts.

- 1990: The EAHCA is amended and renamed the Individuals with Disabilities Education Act (IDEA). School districts are now required to look at outcomes and assist students with disabilities in transitioning from high school to postsecondary life.

- 1997: IDEA. Is reauthorized and requires students with disabilities to be included in state- and district-wide assessments. Regular education teachers are required to be a member of the individualized education plan team.

- 2001: No Child Left Behind Act (NCLB). Sets the goal that all students, including students with disabilities, are to be proficient in math and reading by the year 2014. Waivers granted in 2012 to increase flexibility.

2004: IDEA. Requires more data on outcomes to assure greater accountability at the state and local levels; school districts must provide adequate instruction and intervention for students to help keep them out of special education.

2015: Every Student Succeeds Act (ESSA). Maintains commitment to higher academic standards and equity, with more state and local flexibility, replaces NCLB.

Source: Developed from ESSA (https://www.ed.gov/essa) and Peterson (2007, Timeline of special education history, retrieved from https://media.timetoast.com/timelines/petersonj-july-17-2007-a-timeline-of-special-education-history-in-undefined-retrieved-may-1-2013-from-httpadminfortschoolsorgpupilservicesstaffinfoa20timeline20of20special20education20historyhtm - https://mi022.k12.sd.us/History.htm (n.d.); US Department of Justice (2005). A guide to disability rights laws. Available at http://www.ada.gov/cguide.htm.

emotional, behavioral, or psychological disabilities (OSERS 2018), of whom only 5.5% were identified as having an "emotional disturbance."

Advocates for school-based health and mental health services argue that the school should be a major site in which behavioral healthcare is implemented because school is the one constant environment that most youth attend (Arenson et al. 2019; Bains and Diallo 2016; Institute of Medicine 2009; Minier et al. 2018). The requirement to add intervention and instruction to prevent students from needing segregated special education services must be inclusive of all students, including those with emotional and behavioral disorders (EBD). This caveat has opened the doors to expanding support services in the school environment, and led to school systems collaborating with other domains to enrich the school community. These efforts serve to facilitate functioning and readiness to learn in the children and adolescents who attend.

In 2019, the Substance Abuse and Mental Health Services Administration and the Center for Medicare and Medicaid issued a joint statement on treatment efforts for students in school with mental health and substance use disorders. They identified best practice treatment models, Medicaid benefits available to cover treatment costs, and treatment strategies for use in schools (McCance-Katz and Lynch 2019).

However, with many of the stressors and traumas children face, teachers and administrators may be ill-equipped to handle the multifactored presentation of behavioral health problems in our school settings. APRNs have demonstrated the ability to lead and coordinate behavioral health treatment for children with mental health challenges and this model should be more widely implemented in schools. APRNs specializing in mental health can provide the needed leadership role based on training and expertise.

An Exploration of the Provision of Care Without Silos to Facilitate Easy Access in Community-based Settings

There is a need to reduce the time from presentation of symptoms to sustained, planned, targeted interventions. Historically, students who present with undiagnosed or ineffectively treated mental health challenges are often late in accessing treatment and are further challenged in finding adequate assistance due to provider shortages and a lack of knowledge on additional strategies for accessing resources. According to an analysis of data from the 2016 National Survey of Children's Health (Whitney and Peterson 2019), 16.5% of children had at least one mental health disorder, and over 49% of these did not receive needed care from a behavioral health clinician. Prevalence gaps in care vary widely from state to state, and it is likely that parental reluctance, poor insurance coverage, and lack of access to appropriate mental health clinicians are all implicated. The unique role of the APRN serves to fill the gap between behavioral presentation and immediate intervention. The APRN practicing in a community-based school setting can mitigate this with their ability to diagnose, prescribe effective pharmacotherapeutic regimens, and implement integrated treatment options in real time.

An Exploration of the Development of Crucial Interventions/Strategies to Promote Wellness and Prevent Mental Illness

Description of the Issue

Historically, keeping kids safe often meant expelling those who were disruptive and potentially dangerous to the school setting through behaviors, words, and actions that could potentially be deemed dangerous. While school suspensions as a means of removing disruptive youth helped to prevent a potential danger risk, it set up a cascading effect on the individual who was removed, often resulting in cumulating removals. According to Zhang et al. (2016), during the 2011–2012 school year 3.45 million students nationwide were given out-of-school suspension in an effort to create a safe school environment. Black males accounted for 48% of suspensions and black females accounted for 29% of the suspensions, which was twice the average of their white counterparts, who received 21% and 9%, respectively. The data indicated that black youth were getting removed from the school system in disproportionate numbers, often for minor disruptive offenses.

Removal from the academic environment is often a result of behaviors that are deemed disruptive and disorderly. However, consistent research shows that African American and Latinx students receive harsher punishments for the same infractions than white students, and that African American students were particularly likely to be sent out of class for subjective infractions such as "disrespect" or "loitering" (Skiba et al. 2011, p. 88). Although the focus is often excessive discipline of boys, African American girls are six times more likely to be suspended than white girls (versus three times more

likely for boys) (Williams Crenshaw et al. 2015). Skiba et al. (2011) found that even when controlled for socioeconomic status, racial disparities in amount and severity of discipline persisted. This subjective approach leads to inconsistent standards for behavior which are confusing to youth who may already be subjected to life uncertainty and may want to take control in their own small way of their behavior. A qualitative analysis of open-ended questions revealed that students had less school connectedness when they felt that school discipline was inequitable, there was an overreaction to small offenses, and there was no action taken when bullying was reported to administration (Thomas and Smith 2004). Other researchers found that suspensions are greater for black and minority youth even though deviant attitudes and a regard for disruptive behavior was not significantly higher among black students. In fact, it was higher among white students, who the researcher identified as having more favorable attitudes toward deviant behavior at a younger age (Huang 2018). This further compounds the question, why are black and minority students suspended at twice the rate? To prevent confusion and bias, and in an effort to mitigate harsher discipline practice, suggestions have been made to increase teacher cultural competency and sensitivity to decrease an overmonitoring of behaviors that are subjectively described as more disorderly. Changing from subjective discipline practices could change the perception of the environment for the student and lead to a greater sense of connection and academic performance, and serve as a protective mechanism for a student with at-risk factors such as living in a single-parent home (Huang et al. 2017). Other efforts such as increasing student involvement and working on factors that could be tailored to the student's likes and dislikes also helped to engage the student to align with school expectations. With this, family connectedness and optimism could be protective for youth disconnected from school (Stoddard et al. 2011).

The impact of suspensions on lack of ability to develop prosocial attachments is an important aspect of the negative effect suspensions have on youth. When a youth is suspended it is particularly difficult for them to develop positive peer attachments as they are removed from the positive social supports offered in a structured setting. This potentially makes them more at risk for criminalized behavior, with a resulting increase in referrals to the juvenile justice system (Cuellar and Markowitz 2015).

For the majority of students who present with persistent behavioral problems in the academic setting, school suspension does nothing to help replace the problem behaviors warranting suspension. It is rather a way of hoping that the consequence of getting removed from the setting will better inform future decision making, but it does not provide opportunities for the learning of replacement behaviors, especially if the youth is going to sit at home without a proper resource structure to teach them what is appropriate (Mowen and Brent 2016). In contrast, many teachers and administrators have tried to use a positive approach to discipline, and a trauma-informed approach to classroom management, to create a classroom atmosphere that minimizes triggers for behavioral outbursts, as discussed below. One randomized controlled test of an online intervention to teach empathic discipline to middle school students resulted in cutting suspensions by half in the intervention schools (Okonofua et al. 2016). Other approaches to reduce suspensions involve targeted use of behavioral health services (Kang-Yi et al. 2018).

An Exploration of the Call for Evidenced-based Care Grounded in Mental Health Research

In addition to special education legislation, there have been other contributors to the movement for in-school support of children with special needs. The division of Adolescent and School Health at the Centers for Disease Control and Prevention (CDC) has been the leading advocate for health promotion and delivery of services in schools using the eight components of the Whole School, Whole Community, Whole Child Framework. The components are a coordination ring, health education, health services, counseling, psychological and social services, social and emotional climate, family engagement, and community involvement (CDC 2018).

Two academic centers, the School Mental Health Project (n.d.) at the University of California, Los Angeles, and the Center for Health and Health Care in Schools (n.d.) at George Washington University, have been instrumental in developing resources and models for improving academic outcomes in youth with mental health conditions. Using a combination of research, policy development, and funding of community initiatives, both organizations work to improve health outcomes for vulnerable populations and decrease health and educational inequities by helping schools address behavioral health barriers that impede youth learning and school engagement.

Community-based collaborations, such as school-based health centers (SBHCs) and school-linked health centers, provide mental health services to students (Bains and Diallo 2016). These formulations usually involve APRN providers. In a recent position paper, the National Association of School Nurses (2017) asserted that "behavioral health, which encompasses mental health, is as critical to academic success as physical well-being" and noted that school nurses, because of training and location in schools, have the expertise to identify, advocate for, and facilitate treatment for children with behavioral and mental health conditions. School nurses are an important part

of the team to aid in early recognition of symptoms and can be an integral component in prevention efforts that support emotional wellness (Ravenna and Cleaver 2016). On the occasion that a school health services team includes both school nurses and APRNs, school nurses can assist in primary interventions for students at risk for emotional and behavioral problems and can develop and implement secondary interventions for students identified with behavioral health problems. The school nurse can serve as a referral source to primary care (PC). APRNs and psychiatric-mental health APRNs provide treatment to students with health and mental health issues.

School-based Health Centers

Over the past 30 years, schools partnering with community-based health and mental health organizations and individuals have become the largest providers of mental health services to children. Among those children who receive mental health services, up to 80% access care at school. While many of these children and adolescents receive services by participating in special education programs or from mental health clinicians hired by school districts, an increasing number are getting help through one of the SBHC models. As of 2014, there were 2315 SBHCs serving youth and communities in 49 states and the District of Columbia (School Based Health Alliance [SBHA] n.d.). Table 32.2 illustrates the services provided by SBHCs across the country (SBHA n.d.)

SBHCs located within the school or on school grounds can be operated by the school or a county health department, or can be affiliated with an outside community health agency or hospital. The SBHC personnel consist of both medical and mental health providers. Of the 2.6 million employed nurses in 2010, 2.76% were school nurses and of that number approximately 3% were APRNs (NASN 2007; US Department of Health and Human Services 2010).

Research and evaluations have demonstrated that SBHCs greatly enhance children's access to healthcare. In the state of Connecticut, during 2007–2009, mental health visits accounted for almost a third of the visits to an SBHC. Rates peaked at 8 and 13 years of age, and the authors suggest that the increased utilization for these age groups could coincide with incidences of increased academic demands. The uptick in usage demonstrates the utility of the SBHC in meeting the mental health needs of youth facing a variety of changes during fundamental periods of growth and development (Baines et al. 2017). A recent analysis of the 2010–2011 census data from the School Based Health Alliance (SBHA) found that SBHCs that had been open longer, had more students, and received more state funding were more likely to offer mental health services (Larson et al. 2017).

Table 32.2 Services provided by SBHCs

Types of service provider	Percentage	Number of SBHCs responding
Primary care	100%	1737
Behavioral health	62.7%	1737
Health educator	12.4%	1737
Nutritionist	16.8%	1737
Nursing or other clinical support	69.3%	1737
Services provided		
Immunizations (any)	86.2%	1541
Screenings for depression	76.1%	1683
Screenings for anxiety/nervousness/phobias	71.2%	1683
Screenings for attention/concentration/ADHD	67.7%	1683
Social skills/relationship issues/conflicts	71.5%	1683
Individual counseling for substance use	79.7%	1391
Individual counseling for suicide prevention	76.0%	1391
Individual counseling for violence prevention	75.8%	1391

ADHD, attention deficit hyperactivity disorder.
Source: Data from School-Based Health Alliance (SBHA) (n.d.). School-based health centers: National census school year 2013–2014. Retrieved from https://www.sbh4all.org/school-health-care/national-census-of-school-based-health-centers/.

SBHC have demonstrated effectiveness in caring for a wide variety of students. Research has indicated that there are varying models related to the needs of the student population. One study argued that the majority of SBHCs have used a collaborative model for care but have mainly used APRNs in a PC role and have used school psychologists and counselors for mental healthcare. This suggests that an expansion of the model may be needed to provide real-time services for youth with the highest risk/need of mental health treatment, as psychiatric nurse practitioners are able to diagnose, prescribe, and intervene with youth who present with more critical mental health needs (Larson et al. 2017).

Etiology of Behavioral Health in Schools

The Individuals with Disabilities Education Act (IDEA 2004), first enacted in 1990 and then amended in 1997 and 2004, is the current federal policy relevant to children with disabilities, including children with EBD, that assures "special education" in the least restrictive environment possible following development of an Individual Education Plan (IEP) (US Department of Education 2000). For each child deemed eligible, schools must convene a multidisciplinary team of educators,

specialty providers, family members, and, when appropriate, the student, to develop an IEP that meets the student's learning and emotional needs in the least restrictive environment possible. The program should be designed to provide all additional health and related services necessary to allow that student to fully participate in his or her education.

The IEP describes the goals the team sets for a child during the school year, as well as any special support needed to help the child achieve the identified goals. Students struggling in school may qualify for support services, allowing them to be taught in a need-specific and individualized way, for reasons such as learning disabilities, emotional disorders, mental retardation, autism, hearing or visual impairment, speech or language impairment, and/or developmental delay. Children who are eligible for services under IDEA are also protected under Section 504. However, if the disability *does not adversely affect educational performance*, the child is *not* eligible for services under IDEA and can be vulnerable to neglect of disability needs.

Section 504 of the Rehabilitation Act enables qualified students with a disability (not otherwise qualified under the IDEA) to receive the accommodations needed to enable them to participate in school programs to the same extent as their nondisabled peers. To be eligible for protections under Section 504, the child must have a physical or mental impairment that *substantially limits* at least one major life activity (i.e. walking, seeing, hearing, speaking, breathing, learning, reading, writing, performing math equations, working, caring for oneself, and performing manual tasks). Under Section 504 and Title II of the Americans with Disabilities Act, school systems must accommodate the needs of students with disabilities. Modifications can include changing rules, policies or practices, removing architectural or communication barriers, modifying testing and homework parameters, and/or providing aids, services, or assistive technology (Lipkin et al. 2015; Understood for Learning and Attentional Issues n.d.; US Department of Education 2008).

Students with EBD present with behaviors which are described as noncompliant, disruptive, labile, and aggressive. Presentation of such behaviors can result in problems with establishing interpersonal connections. Social isolation can be a problem as stigma associated with the externalizing behaviors makes it difficult to find support systems and harness relationships within the community and school (Mann and Heflinger 2016).

Historically, schools have educated children diagnosed with an EBD within special education environments and Section 504 designations, without significantly involving families and other organizations in the community. The special education and school support staff provided services to the special education population, and often the PC provider in the community would be aware of the special education services, but further coordination or communication is rare and limited to prescriptive notations on school forms for specialized services. More recently, this isolationist view has dissipated, as evidence supports the interconnectedness of the child, family, and community environments and a greater emphasis is placed on serving all children with mental health needs and collaborating with outside agencies (Atkins et al. 2017). Changes in service philosophy, including increased emphasis on providing care in the least restrictive setting, greater attention to involving families in service planning, and a focus on building on existing strengths, as opposed to the traditional deficit-based approaches, have provided impetus for collaboration and locating community-based services in schools (Brueck 2016). Eighty-three percent of schools report providing case management for students with behavioral or social problems and nearly half of all schools contract with or make other arrangements

with a community-based organization to provide mental health services to students (Center for Health and Health Care in Schools 2011). The movement toward integrating mental health services in SBHC services has come to mean that comprehensive education services include the provision of case management and coordination of support services for students in need. Case management and care coordination are usually carried out by a designated school staff member who serves as the liaison between school, family, and community resources.

The School Team

School support personnel are a critical component of the school team, which includes school nurses or allied health professionals, guidance counselors, school social workers, school psychologists, and parent outreach/support workers. Other members of the community, such as legal advocates, legal guardians, and representatives from the department of social services, may also be involved in the support of an individual child. Engaged parents or caretakers who are advocates for their children should be kept informed at all times by the team and included in planning and decision-making meetings.

These professionals are the core to any school support collaboration and are likely already known to the student and family. This sense of affiliation and familiarity may augment the collaborative process and facilitate entry of the APRN new to the school community, student, or family. The school nurse or allied health staff are generally engaged in routine health surveillance and in-school management of treatments for students in need. The nurse may be in daily contact with at-risk students and have experience in the school support team processes and thus can serve as a liaison for the APRN collaborating on students' behalf. APRNs who are not a part of a school or SBHC should obtain consent from parents and assent from older children and adolescents if they wish to communicate with school personnel.

School counselors, sometimes known as guidance counselors, are often best known by students and are the first layer of support outside of the classroom; these individuals are excellent resources for the APRN interfacing with schools. The school counselor may have first-hand experience with the processes involved in responding to the special requirements of the student experiencing an emotional or behavioral disorder. Although the level of counseling is usually more academically focused and less clinical, it is not uncommon for students to become accustomed to using the guidance office for counseling support. The school social worker is the next level of support, with the social worker role varying from school to school but usually involving counseling, academic and developmental testing, and some level of case management for an identified caseload. The school psychologist may have a part-time presence and is often only involved in assessment with a very limited clinical or interventionist role.

In many cases school support focuses on special education and Section 504-related assessments and evaluation. Increasingly, community agencies provide mental healthcare in schools, which is not limited to children with IEP or 504 plans (Atkins et al. 2017). When no school-based health or mental healthcare is available, the recommendations for nonacademic follow-up, assessment, counseling, and intervention are placed in the hands of parents and guardians, but great care needs to be taken to ensure they have the knowledge base to understand illness presentation and what to do once they recognize a problem exists. Acquisition of additional community-based medical, mental health, or developmental support services may be hindered by lack of availability within the region, parent or guardian inability to take time off from work to meet with outside providers, and/or lack of coverage for the cost of needed care.

When school-based treatment is not an option, the structure and process of case management become paramount. Although ongoing case management and coordination may be absent from the infrastructure of most schools, the school's willingness to partner with community providers and establish processes has the potential to eliminate gaps between needs and service provision.

APRN Collaboration

School nurses are certified at the state level, with a minimum requirement of a baccalaureate degree (NASN 2011). However, many school nurses have additional educational credits, up to a Masters' degree, and some have been prepared in advanced practice roles. APRNs comprise the majority of PC clinicians in SBHCs. Collaborative and integrated models of primary and behavioral healthcare have become more prevalent in school-based and community settings. Under the Affordable Care Act, PC providers have been increasingly given the responsibility for assessing and beginning treatment of mild to moderate behavioral health conditions (Mechanic and Olfson 2016). The American Academy of Pediatrics has developed guidelines for PC assessment and treatment of attention deficit hyperactivity disorder (Subcommittee on Attention-Deficit/Hyperactivity Disorder et al. 2011), depression (Zuckerbrot et al. 2007, 2018), and substance abuse (Levy et al. 2016). Collaboration between primary care (PC) APRN and psychiatric mental health (PMH)

APRNs has demonstrated effectiveness in meeting multiple needs in children with limited access to PC as well as mental health interventions across prevention and treatment domains (Burka et al. 2014). The PC-APRN can provide initial assessment and management of mental health services, including prescribing, and is a referral source for children and adolescents with more complex needs. Some pediatric nurse practitioners (who are also APRNs but with a pediatric focus) have attained an additional certificate as a primary mental health specialist (Hawkins-Walsh and Van Cleve 2019). The PMH-APRN is an appropriate consultant when children require additional assessment, complex psychotropic medications, and treatment for serious mental health issues. In addition to providing services to individuals, PMH-APRNs serve as school resources around such diverse issues as violence, post-traumatic stress disorder, trauma and adverse childhood experiences, and the impact on overall student academic functioning, mental, and physical health.

Concerns have been voiced about the lack of evidence-based school mental health interventions. In response, nurses and others have started to develop and study the impact of programs with special regard to vulnerable and medically underserved populations in schools. Stephan et al. (2015) have developed a framework for providing prevention and youth development services to all students. Their framework recognizes the diversity of individual student needs and includes elements such as conflict resolution, peer support, and after-school programming, and the most intensive services for youth with the highest symptom levels and/or greatest functional difficulties. Cummings et al. (2010) compared racial and ethnic differences in mental health service use among adolescents. While no differences were found in school-based use of mental health services, significant differences were noted in clinical settings, indicating that schools may be critical avenues for reducing the unmet need for mental health services among racial/ethnic minorities. Other researchers have noted that school-based mental health services can be a link to specialized care in the community for youth with the greatest needs (Tegethoff et al. 2014).

One intervention for youth exposed to trauma is cognitive behavioral interventions for trauma in schools (CBITS) (Jaycox et al. 2018), a manualized group intervention that can be delivered by APRNs and other mental health professionals. In a study of statewide implementation of CBITS, one study found 90% retention rate, 42% decrease in symptom levels, 25% decrease in problem severity, and statistically significant improvement in functioning (Hoover et al. 2018).

Linkage with Behavioral/Psychiatric Profile of the Child and Adolescent

APRNs caring for children and adolescents with an EBD should be able to advise their client's families of special education resources and school supports that facilitate their child's functioning within their primary environment, the school. APRNs involved in the care and treatment of youth with emotional health needs are often called upon by parents to participate in a dialogue with school staff and administrators as part of the parental request for special education and in school supportive or adaptive services. In effect, the provider is asked to "prescribe" or "validate" considerations that are not academic in nature but are imperative for the optimal functioning of the individual child in the school setting. This can be accomplished by ensuring that a full assessment is done to explore antecedents to behaviors which may be identified as trigger points that may warrant alternative coping strategies or the education of teachers, administration, and the student to prevent an exacerbation of symptoms. These range from validating indications for less restrictive settings, facilitating the administration of treatments necessary for safe and comfortable functioning in the school environment, and developing behavioral and logistical plans for adapting to stressors that may arise within the school environment. In most instances, the input of the APRN will be provided through correspondence or by attendance and participation at the IEP or other student support team meetings. Parents concerned with their ability to be heard as advocates for their children may seek support from community-based advocates and mental health navigators.

Many students experiencing emotional and behavioral health issues are not identified by the school system as special needs, although their diagnoses may clearly impact their ability to learn and, therefore, in most states they are eligible for specialized accommodations and services. When these students are not serviced through special education and remain within the mainstream population, they struggle and often fail. These students may be the patients of APRNs practicing in the community, in a school-based or school-linked health service, or recently discharged from an inpatient facility. The task of any APRN is to consider the elements of school participation as part of the treatment planning for management of the individual child in order to promote both optimal health and academic success. There is a role for the APRN to assist students and their families in obtaining the school-related supports entitled to them and related to their functional disability or diagnosis through the implementation of a 504 plan or an IEP, when warranted.

The APRN Role in School Collaboration

First and foremost, the APRN must be knowledgeable of the medical and behavioral health resources already available within the school and the community. Assessment of school functioning is part of the comprehensive health assessment for school-age and adolescent youth. When establishing a plan of care, school-related issues and supports should be a natural consideration for this age group. Not all cases call for in-school collaboration; however, for the child who is struggling socially or exhibiting behavioral or emotional issues, the incorporation of school support through direct consultation or through facilitation of the parent role as advocate through education, documentation, or consultation is an appropriate intervention. The APRN or other providers collaborating with the school system whether from the outside community or from within a school-linked/school-based service arrangement must, together with school administration, work in the spirit of mutual respect and consideration in developing guidelines for the collaborative processes involved with the service.

The increase in school-based support programs and the expansion of school mental health services have created unique professional opportunities for APRNs to be employed directly or through subcontracts within the school environment. This role may be endorsed through employment in the role of school nurse or mental health provider, as a PC provider or mental health provider of an SBHC, or as a provider/employee of a PC or mental health practice linked with a school through subcontract for the provision of support services to school students. Depending on the level of integration of the health services, the APRN may be positioned to be a key player in the development of team processes and planning that promote stability and consistency of approach in facilitating the treatment and support of the student with an EBD. School nurses might be the point of entry for students whose somatic and behavioral complaints suggest a mental health condition (NASN 2018). Consistent with the NASN Framework for 21st Century School Nursing Practice, they may participate in IEP meetings, refer, case manage, and advocate for more behavioral health services, meet with children who return to school after hospitalization, and participate in teacher training and staff wellness (Maughan et al. 2016).

In any of these circumstances, the role of the APRN is directed by professional standards of care and scope of practice requirements of the State Board of Nursing. School policies about information sharing in the academic milieu are equally rigid and are mandated by the Family Educational Rights and Privacy Act of 1974 (FERPA), which provides protection against sharing students' personally identifiable information just as the

Health Insurance Portability and Accountability Act (HIPAA) regulations protect patients' privacy related to identifiable healthcare information. APRNs should clearly understand their role and responsibility in the care of students and ensure adequate protective measures and permissions are in place prior to commencing the communication process. These requirements should be explained initially and reinforced throughout the process of interfacing with the school staff and administration so that professional requirements related to scope of care and communication are better understood and tolerated within the collaborative process. Empirical evidence has suggested that given the intense levels of service required, care should be taken to avoid the insertion of stigma to prevent negative mental health outcomes related to underreporting of symptoms and underutilization of services (Mann and Heflinger 2016).

Participation as part of a team or network of school administrators, educators, and health service providers can be both challenging and rewarding. The collective impact of these endeavors is potentially much farther reaching than what is possible when providing services without collaboration. When school-based or school-linked arrangements exist, the APRN working within the school system has a unique perspective from the shared experience of the school environment. Socialization with school staff and administrators as well as integration as a community member through roles in various school-wide activities, planning meetings, or committee participation can be instrumental in promoting credibility as a collaborator. Additionally, the experience provides first-hand understanding of the systems at work in the coordination of student-focused services.

The school-based model of care has important advantages for treatment planning for students in need. Scheduled appointments at a school or school-based health center may increase treatment plan adherence; parents may be engaged via telehealth platforms or telephone contact, alleviating the stress of missed work or transportation issues. Referral and consultation with affiliates of the professional staff providing care in the school enhance access to specialty providers and other resources through that agent's network.

Parents and guardians are the gatekeepers in the process of interfacing with schools; their consent is critical to outsiders' entry and access to school records and strategy sessions. The APRN's knowledge, experience, and ability to assist parents and family members in understanding the complex issues regarding etiology and course of treatment of their child's condition are great assets to the process of achieving comprehensive services through school and community services. The APRN serves as advocate and mentor; parents and guardians, empowered by the information and resources from the APRN, are better prepared to advocate for their children. The parents' improved understanding of the clinical issues, combined with their knowledge of what works for their child, assists them in informing others of their child's special needs and considerations. Once collaborating with "in-school" support persons, it is imperative that the APRN serves as a liaison between school professionals and the family, helping to ensure a completeness of understanding of the needs and treatment plan implementation.

Evidence-based Implications for Practice, Research, and Education in Child and Adolescent Behavioral Health in Primary Care

Several reviews of school-based mental health services have shown that they provide increased access to care (Atkins et al. 2017; Lai et al. 2016), yet research on mental health outcomes of school-based interventions is lacking (Arenson et al. 2019). One evidence-based program of note, which identifies the application of overall system guidance and directed intervention for behavioral concerns in the school setting, is the School Wide Positive Behavioral Interventions and Supports (SW-PBIS) program. SW-PBIS is a multifaceted intervention that merges decades of research on effective instruction, behavior management, and systemic school change. Initially developed and disseminated at the University of Oregon by Drs. Horner and Sugai (2015), SW-PBIS encourages schools to take a proactive approach aimed at promoting socially appropriate behavior and preventing problem behavior.

The goal of SW-PBIS is to create systems in schools that infuse best practices in behavior management throughout the school. Using a three-tiered prevention model, primary prevention is available to 100% of the school and 80% of the school population is expected to be successful behaviorally. The remaining students in the top two tiers are those who do not successfully respond to the primary system and require additional interventions and supports to be successful. These two tiers of students are matched with interventions that will effectively meet their behavioral support needs. Secondary prevention includes specialized groups for students with at-risk behaviors, whereas tertiary prevention group interventions are more intensive and include matching interventions to address unique individualized needs (Pace et al. 2014).

The care and treatment of the two tiers of students identified as needing more supports form the priority group that schools usually focus on, either through structured programs for early identification and intervention or by natural course as the at-risk child self-identifies or is "picked up" through the intuition or experience of school support personnel. In both cases, once it is apparent that a higher level of care is required to support student academic function, collaboration with clinical service providers is needed to help formulate a plan of action based upon the student's identified academic, behavioral, and emotional needs, diagnosis, and level of functioning.

The format of the PBIS plan has a prescriptive value that affords easy delineation of roles for the APRN operating within this system. Primary prevention, assessment, education, and promotion may be carried out by both the pediatric and mental health focused-APRN (PMH-APRN); assessment of behavioral and emotional health risk is part of each provider's routine assessment whether completed individually or through a schoolwide screening. Both types of APRNs may run health education and social support type groups for a school's general population and for high-risk students. This service acts as a supportive measure for the child with EBD who is seen by an outside provider as a means to augment other behavioral or medication components of her or his plan of care. Tertiary care, whether individualized or delivered as a group intervention, is within the domain of the PMH-APRN alone as the specific knowledge and skills required for behavioral intervention, counseling, and psychopharmacology fall within the domain of that practice. The supportive functions in this domain include routine follow-up of medication management/compliance and periodic laboratory assessment for symptoms and side effects. The PMH-APRN is vital to the translation of diagnoses and treatment plan needs which serve to inform the development of tailored IEPs based upon the functional and emotional needs of the student.

Best practices associated with successful school collaborations concerning the provision of mental health include, but are not limited to:

Developing procedures for the identification, referral, and disposition of students needing assistance.
Communicating with students, teachers, and families to obtain views on problems and concerns and their suggestions for addressing them.
Coordinating, as available, the provision of prevention and intervention programs.
Collaborating with school support teams, updating on treatment plans, based upon the demonstrated emotional and behavioral presentation of the student.
Developing a "reentry" plan of care for students who are returning from treatment for an EBD in an inpatient or partial hospitalization setting.
Developing educational programs for teachers and school staff on EBD and how to manage youth in both the community and at home (Paulus et al. 2016).

When considering *identification and referral procedures* it is best to be clear about what level of support the APRN is able to offer. If the APRN is already the PC provider or the mental health provider overseeing the behavioral health treatment plan for the child with EBD, the identification is more of an introduction of self to school personnel as an established support with an interest in coordination of all aspects of the individual student's care. In this model the provider, with the parent's consent, attempts to collaborate with in-school supports in order to share information, consult on interventions, and coordinate services to ensure augmentation of all available resources on the patient's behalf. For instance, the APRN in the community may contact school support via telephone, e-mail, or letter to request the further evaluation of a potential learning disability, share information regarding any organic entities that may be related to the child's school function, or request support in the day-to-day management of a student's established treatment plan. This approach may require only brief interface initially with a plan for periodic communication of progress and review or revision of planned strategies.

APRNs working within the school or SBHC or contracted through schools may be instrumental in the schoolwide establishment of procedures for identification and referral of students that exhibit a need for support, as well as planning for student-specific interventions. Clear referral and communication policies should be established at the onset of the collaborative relationship and carried out in a consistent manner.

Communicating with the school community and family usually means the APRN would go to the family, visit the school, and hold forums or focus groups as part of a school community offering. Providers based in schools and providers from the surrounding community can gain an introduction through parents' associations. In the case where the group of interest is intrinsic to the school community, the principal or their designee may act as the central mediator of passage within the school walls and for access to staff. It is important to identify the key stakeholders within an individual school – those individuals who have the power to make decisions and promote change. There are a number of staff meetings and enrichment offerings over the course of a school year where an APRN from in-house or the community may seek a forum to reach school staff, provide education, and request support or feedback. These opportunities can also be used as an arena to gain referral and promote the available services of the APRNs and affiliated programs.

Coordination of services is at the heart of the nursing process. After carefully assessing the child or adolescent, a nursing diagnosis and treatment plan are formulated; these often include other services and supports for the student who is central to the encounter. Understanding the individual needs for services and assuring that services are provided in a timely manner with a focus on quality care are core to that process. Often the APRN is the most aptly informed about the progress and involvement of support services. The APRN may ensure this role as coordinator, liaison, and organizer of services directed at the success of the centrally placed student/patient. The school-based model may include the APRN's assumption of additional roles that promote consultation and/or education regarding a schoolwide behavioral intervention.

Participation in school-based meetings concerning the student being served is a forum for collaboration considered key to success. The APRN's participation can range from correspondence to attendance at IEP meetings. In the case of the community-based APRN provider, it is advised that a format for collaboration be decided after consultation with the school-based support liaison or the coordinator of special education services. In the case of providers who share space in the school or who are contracted for referral directly from the school, a more routine presence in this team process may be expected and planned for as the APRN or other provider may be utilized in a consultative manner for the schoolwide management of this process.

Developing a reentry plan should be incorporated as part of discharge planning for the student returning to school from inpatient or partial hospitalization. Students should be aware of additional supports or plans to alleviate the stress of reentry to the school milieu. School staff can benefit from understanding that the absence was related to a health issue so that their plans and expectations regarding makeup assignments and remediation should be assistive to the student's reentry. Generally, this communication need not be too specific or revealing about the nature of the absence but should be clear to eliminate the possibility of overwhelming the student with academic expectations relative to making up the work. Hospitalizations and inpatient treatment stays may result in a revised treatment plan. Health and behavioral professions should also plan for the student's reentry, which may include additional sessions, assessments, and advocacy for the newly returned student.

Developing educational programs for teachers and school staff on EBD may include providing staff development offerings of an educational nature to provide insight and overview of the issues involved in EBD in the school setting, or informally where the provider offers self as a resource to staff who may be struggling through classroom management issues generally or related to EBD students. The time required to meet this goal may make this level of involvement unrealistic for the collaborating community-based provider but can be configured as part of the in-kind contribution of a school-based provider.

Developing and providing educational programs for students is a crucial health promotion and disease prevention role of the APRN. The following are topics that are particularly applicable in the school environment:

- trauma
- adverse childhood experiences
- bullying awareness and prevention
- stigma
- depression and anxiety
- respectful communities
- preventing violence
- coping skills
- identifying and communicating feelings
- physical and emotional effects of substance use.

It is relevant to note that evidenced-based treatment protocols for the care and management of a variety of EBDs in the child and adolescent population have been developed and tested. The problems and disorders for which evidence-based treatments now exist encompass the concerns that bring the great majority of children and adolescents into clinical care. Tested treatments have now been developed to address multiple internalizing conditions within the anxiety–depression spectrum, multiple externalizing conditions ranging from chronic disobedience and aggression to the disruptive behavior disorders, autism, and related developmental disorders. Psychosocial strategies such as behavioral parent training, behavioral classroom management, behavioral peer interventions, and organizational skills training have shown promise as alternative strategies to medication (Schoenfelder and Dasser 2016). Among students in middle adolescence, strategies which promote mutual respect and the desire to attain social position can serve to motivate and sustain positive behavior change (Yeager et al. 2018). Restorative practices using perspective taking and peer mediation is a process that does not solely focus on blame but rather is based on exploring the varying sides of the problem issue to gain perspective and an exploration of feelings. This helps to engage the youth in the development of strategies that move beyond the symptoms of externalizing behavior to examine the root cause (Rasmussen et al. 2018).

Summary

The APRN engaged in the care of the child/adolescent with behavioral health needs is in a unique position to facilitate child/adolescent assessments, management, reentry, transition, and stabilization to the school environment. Nursing's core roles of advocate, educator, and liaison are instrumental in formulating a plan of care that is considerate of the child/adolescent's primary environment, the school.

Although the practitioner and the school administrators and counselors may agree to work in the best interest of the child and their mental health and educational needs, it must be recognized that these types of collaborations are a new concept and engender potential complications, many of which are at the communication level. Concerns tend to occur around levels of disclosure, specificity of roles, systems for access, consultation, and consistency in adhering to treatment plans.

Promoting an understanding of the role and intention of the APRN in the care of students experiencing emotional behavioral disorder can be invaluable to the APRN in the process of school collaboration; putting the student centrally in the process gives all participants a chance to contribute to the overall outcome of student success. APRNs should take the time to explain their role and the nature of the advanced practice classification in order to clarify the professional conduct expectations and distinguish the client-centered focus of care that drives their participation with school and community in the care of the individual student. Keeping the focus on the common goal of the successful student allows all participating team members to envision their contribution to the process and can keep the tone of the collaboration positive and proactive.

Resources

Bright Futures/Mental Health. Information on early recognition and intervention for specific mental health problems and mental disorders. Provides a tool kit for use in screening, care management, and health education. http://brightfutures.org/mentalhealth/pdf/tools.html.

Center for Health and Health Care in Schools. http://healthinschools.org/#sthash.rwBPL6Ga.dpbs.

Council for Exceptional Children, Understanding the Differences Between IDEA and Section 504,

Education of All Handicapped Children Act of 1975, Pub. L. No. 94–142 § 689 Stat. 773 (1975).

Educators for Social Responsibility. www.esrnational.org.

Individuals with Disabilities Education Improvement Act of 2004 (IDEA), Pub. L. No. 108–446, 118 Stat. 2647 (2004) [Amending 20 U.S.C. §§ 1400 et seq.].

Do Something. Website for children. www.dosomething.org.

KidPower. Website for kids. http://kidpower.org/SERVICES/Children.html.

Massachusetts General Hospital School Psychiatry Program. Help for clinicians, educators, and parents to meet the needs of young people with depression, bipolar disorder, attention deficit/hyperactivity disorder, autism spectrum disorders, and anxiety disorders, including panic disorder and obsessive–compulsive disorder. https://www.massgeneral.org/children/child-psychiatry.

Mental health care for youth. Who gets it? How much does it cost? Who pays? Where does the money go? RAND Health. Santa Monica, CA. 2002. https://www.rand.org/pubs/research_briefs/RB4541.html.

National Assembly of School-Based Health Care, general website resources on school based health. https://www.sbh4all.org.

National Association of State Boards of Education. www.nasbe.org.

National Center for Learning Disabilities, Section 504 and IDEA comparison chart. https://ncld.org/get-involved/learn-the-law/adaaa-section-504/.

National Institute of Mental Health. http://www.nimh.nih.gov/topics/topic-page-children-and-adolescents.shtml.

National Association of School Nurses. www.nasn.org.

National Center for Learning Disabilities Navigator. https://www.charitynavigator.org/index.cfm?bay=search.summary&orgid=6730.

National Dissemination Center for Children with Disabilities. www.nichcy.org.

SAMHSA's National Mental Health Information Center. https://www.samhsa.gov.

School-Based Health Alliance. www.sbh4all.org.

Teaching Tolerance (Southern Poverty Law Program). https://www.splcenter.org/teaching-tolerance.

University of Maryland's Center for School Mental Health. Offers prepared Power Point presentations, classroom education material, and other clinical references for clinicians. https://www.umms.org/ummc/health-services/psychiatry/services/child-adolescent/outpatient/school-mental-health.

US Department of Health and Human Services, The Center for Mental Health Services and the National Institute of Mental Health. Contains mental health information related to health and human services research programs, policies, and media campaigns and highlights the latest research findings and policy efforts. See Mental Health: The Cornerstone of Heath. http://www.mentalhealth.org/cornerstone,

References

Arenson, M., Hudson, P.J., Lee, N., and Lai, B. (2019). The evidence on school-based health centers: a review. *Global Pediatr. Health* 6: 2333794x19828745. https://doi.org/10.1177/2333794x19828745.

Atkins, M.S., Capella, E., Shernoff, E.S. et al. (2017). Schooling and children's mental health: realigning resources to reduce disparities and advance public health. *Annu. Rev. Clin. Psychol.* 13: 123–147.

Baines, E., Blatchford, P., and Kutnick, P. (2017). Promoting Effective Group Work in the Primary Classroom: A Handbook for Teachers and Practitioners. Routledge.

Bains, R.M. and Diallo, A.F. (2016). Mental health services in school-based health centers: systematic review. *J. Sch. Nurs.* 32 (1): 8–19. https://doi.org/10.1177/1059840515590607.

Brueck, M.K. (2016). Promoting access to school-based services for children's mental health. *AMA Journal of Ethics* 18 (12): 1218–1224. https://doi.org/10.1001/journalofethics.2016.18.12.pfor1-1612.

Burka, S.D., Van Cleve, S.N., Shafer, S., and Barkin, J.L. (2014). Integration of pediatric mental health care: an evidence-based workshop for primary care providers. *J. Pediatr. Health Care* 28 (1): 23–34. https://doi.org/10.1016/j.pedhc.2012.10.006.

Center for Health and Health Care in Schools. (2011). *Children's mental health needs, disparities, and school-based services: A fact sheet.* Available at http://healthinschools.org/issue-areas/school-based-mental-health/background/fact-sheet/#sthash.mVxcjSOl.dpbs.

CDC. (2018). *Whole, School, Whole Community, Whole Child (WSCC).* Centers for Disease Control and Prevention. Available at https://www.cdc.gov/healthyschools/wscc/index.htm.

Cuellar, A.E. and Markowitz, S. (2015). School suspension and the school-to-prison pipeline. *Int. Rev. Law Econ.* 43: 98–106.

Cummings, J.R., Ponce, N.A., and Mays, V.M. (2010). Comparing racial/ethnic differences in mental health service use among high-need subpopulations across clinical and school-based settings. *J. Adolesc. Health* 46: 603–606.

Hawkins-Walsh, E. and Van Cleve, S.N. (2019). A job task analysis of the expanding role of the pediatric mental health specialist and the nurse practitioner in pediatric mental health. *J. Pediatr. Health Care* 33 (3): e9–e17. https://doi.org/10.1016/j.pedhc.2018.11.001.

Hoover, S.A., Sapere, H., Lang, J.M. et al. (2018). Statewide implementation of an evidence-based trauma intervention in schools. *Sch. Psychol. Q.* 33 (1): 44–53. https://doi.org/10.1037/spq0000248.

Horner, R.H. and Sugai, G. (2015). School-wide PBIS: an example of applied behavior analysis implemented at a scale of social importance. *Behav. Anal. Pract.* 8: 80–85.

Huang, F.L. (2018). Do black students misbehave more? Investigating the differential involvement hypothesis and out-of-school suspension. *J. Educ. Res.* 111 (3): 284–294.

Huang, F.L., Eklund, K., and Cornell, D.G. (2017). Authoritative school climate, number of parents at home, and academic achievement. *Sch. Psychol. Q.* 32 (4): 480–496.

Individuals with Disabilities Education Act of 2004 (HR 1350). (2004). Available at https://sites.ed.gov/idea/.

Institute of Medicine (2009). Preventing Mental, Emotional, and Behavioral Disorders Among Young People: Progress and Possibilities. Washington, D.C.: National Academies Press.

Jaycox, L.H., Langley, A.K., and Hoover, S.A. (2018). CBITS: Cognitive Behavioral Intervention for Trauma in Schools, 2nd (revised) edn. Santa Monica, CA: Rand Corporation.

Kang-Yi, C.D., Wolk, C.B., Locke, J. et al. (2018). Impact of school-based and out-of-school mental health services on reducing school absence and school suspension among children with psychiatric disorders. *Eval. Program Plann.* 67: 105–112. https://doi.org/10.1016/j.evalprogplan.2017.12.006.

Lai, K., Guo, S., Ijadi-Maghsoodi, R. et al. (2016). Bringing wellness to schools: opportunities for and challenges to mental health integration in school-based health centers. *Psychiatr. Serv.* 67 (12): 1328–1333. https://doi.org/10.1176/appi.ps.201500401.

Larson, S. (2016). *School-based health centers: A model of care to meet the behavioral and mental health needs of children and adolescents.* PhD Dissertation, University of California, San Francisco.

Larson, S., Spetz, J., Brindis, C.D., and Chapman, S. (2017). Characteristic differences between school-based health centers with and without mental health providers: a review of National Trends. *J. Pediatr. Health Care* 31 (4): 484–492. https://doi.org/10.1016/j.pedhc.2016.12.007.

Levy, S.J., Williams, J.F., and Committee on Substance Abuse and Prevention (2016). Substance use screening, brief intervention, and referral to treatment. *Pediatrics* 138 (1): e20161210. https://doi.org/10.1542/peds.2016-1210.

Lipkin, P.H., Okamoto, J., and Council on Children with, D., & Council on School, H (2015). The Individuals with Disabilities Education Act (IDEA) for children with special educational needs. *Pediatrics* 136 (6): e1650–e1662. https://doi.org/10.1542/peds.2015-3409.

Mann, A.K. and Heflinger, C.A. (2016). Community setting-specific and service-seeking stigma toward children with emotional and behavioral doisorders and their families. *J. Community Psychol.* 44 (2): 199–213.

Maughan, E.D., Duff, C., and Wright, J. (2016). Using the framework for 21st-century school nursing practice in daily practice. *NASN Sch. Nurse* 31 (5): 278–281. https://doi.org/10.1177/1942602x16661558.

McCance-Katz, E. & Lynch, C. (2019). *Guidance to states and school systems on addressing mental health and substance use in schools.* Joint Information Bulletin School Based Services, SAMHSA and CMS.

Mechanic, D. and Olfson, M. (2016). The relevance of the affordable care act for improving mental health care. *Annu. Rev. Clin. Psychol.* 12: 515–542. https://doi.org/10.1146/annurev-clinpsy-021815-092936.

Minier, M., Hirshfield, L., Ramahi, R. et al. (2018). Schools and health: an essential partnership for the effective care of children with chronic conditions. *J. Sch. Health* 88 (9): 699–703. https://doi.org/10.1111/josh.12671.

Mowen, T. and Brent, J. (2016). School discipline as a turning point: the cumulative effect of suspension on arrest. *J. Res. Crime Delinq.* 53 (5): 628–653. https://doi.org/10.1177/0022427816643135.

NASN. (2018). *The school nurse's role in behavioral/mental health of students.* Position Statement, National Association of School Nurses. Silver Spring, MD: Author.

NASN. (2007). *Coordinated school health programs.* Position Statement, National Association of School Nurses. Silver Spring, MD: Author. Available at www.nasn.org.

NASN. (2011). *The role of the school nurse and school-based health centers.* Position Statement, National Association of School Nurses. Silver Spring, MD: Author. Available at www.nasn.org.

NASN. (2017). *The role of the 21st century school nurse.* Position Statement, National Association of School Nurses. doi: https://doi.org/10.1177/1942602X17716449

NASN. (2018). The school nurse's role in behavioral/mental health of students. Position Statement, National Association of School Nurses. Silver Spring, MD, Author. Available at https://higherlogicdownload.s3.amazonaws.com/NASN/3870c72d-fff9-4ed7-833f-215de278d256/UploadedImages/PDFs/Position%20Statements/2018-ps-behavioral-health.pdf.

National Center for Education Statistics (n.d.) Available at https://nces.ed.gov

OSERS. (2018). *40th annual report to Congress on the implementation of the Individuals with Disabilities Education Act, 2018.* Alexandria, VA: US Department of Education. Available at https://www2.ed.gov/about/reports/annual/osep/2018/parts-b-c/40th-arc-for-idea.pdf.

Okonofua, J.A., Paunesku, D., and Walton, G.M. (2016). Brief intervention to encourage empathic discipline cuts suspension rates in half among adolescents. *Proc. Natl. Acad. Sci. USA* 113 (19): 5221–5226. https://doi.org/10.1073/pnas.1523698113.

Pace, R.T., Boykins, A.D., and Davis, S.P. (2014). A proactive classroom management model to enhance self-efficacy levels in teachers of adolescents who display disruptive behaviors. *J. Psychosoc. Nurs. Ment. Health Serv.* 52 (2): 30–37.

Paulus, F.W., Ohmann, S., and Popow, C. (2016). Practitioner review: school-based interventions in child mental health. *J. Child Psychol. Psychiatry* 57 (12): 1337–1359.

Peterson, J. (2007). *A timeline of special education history.* Available at https://media.timetoast.com/timelines/petersonj-july-17-2007-a-timeline-of-special-education-history-in-undefined-retrieved-may-1-2013-from-.

Rasmussen, H.F., Ramos, M.C., Han, S.C. et al. (2018). *J. Adolesc.* 62: 70–81.

Ravenna, J. and Cleaver, K.P. (2016). School nurses' experiences of managing young people with mental health problems: a scoping review. *J. Sch. Nurs.* 32 (1): 58–70.

Schoenfelder, E.N. and Dasser, T. (2016). Skills versus pills: psychosocial treatments for ADHD in childhood and adolescence. *Pediatr. Ann.* 45 (10): e367–e372. https://doi.org/10.3928/19382359-20160920-04.

School Mental Health Project, UCLA (n.d.) http://smhp.psych.ucla.edu.

SBHA. (n.d.). *School-based health centers: National census school year 2013–2014.* School Based Health Alliance. Available at https://www.sbh4all.org/school-health-care/national-census-of-school-based-health-centers.

Skiba, R.J., Horner, R.H., Choong-Geun, C. et al. (2011). Race is not neutral: a National Investigation of African American and Latino disproportionality in school discipline. *Sch. Psychol. Rev.* 40 (1): 85–107.

Stephan, S.H., Sugai, G., Lever, N., and Connors, E. (2015). Strategies for integrating mental health into schools via a multitiered system of support. *Child Adolesc. Psychiatr. Clin. N. Am.* 24 (2): 211–231. https://doi.org/10.1016/j.chc.2014.12.002.

Stoddard, S.A., McMorris, B.J., and Sieving, R.E. (2011). Do social connections and hope matter in predicting early adolescent violence? *Am. J. Community Psychol.* 48 (3–4): 247–256. https://doi.org/10.1007/s10464-010-9387-9.

Subcommittee on Attention-Deficit/Hyperactivity Disorder, Steering Committee on Quality Improvement and Management (2011). ADHD: Clinical Practice Guideline for the Diagnosis, Evaluation, and Treatment of Attention-Deficit/Hyperactivity Disorder in Children and Adolescents. *Pediatrics* 128 (5): 1007–1022. https://doi.org/10.1542/peds.2011-2654.

Tegethoff, M., Stalujanis, E., Belardi, A., and Meinlschmidt, G. (2014). School mental health services: signpost for out-of-school service utilization in adolescents with mental disorders? A nationally representative United States cohort. *PLoS One* 9 (6): e99675. https://doi.org/10.1371/journal.pone.0099675.

Thomas, S.P. and Smith, H. (2004). School connectedness, anger behaviors, and relationships of violent and nonviolent American youth. *Perspect. Psychiatr. Care* 40 (4): 135–148. https://doi.org/10.1111/j.1744-6163.2004.tb00011.x.

US Department of Education. (2000). *A guide to the individualized education program (IEP).* Available at www2.ed.gov.

US Department of Education. (n.d.). *Mission and federal role in education.* Available at http://www2.ed.gov/about.

US Department of Education Office of Civil Rights. (2008). *Protecting students with disabilities.* Available at www2.ed.gov.

US Department of Health and Human Services. (2010). *The registered nurse population: Findings from the 2008 national sample survey of registered nurses.* US Department of Health and Human Services, Health Resources and Services Administration. Available at http://bhpr.hrsa.gov/healthworkforce/rnsurvey/2008.

US Department of Justice. (2005). *A guide to disability rights laws.* Available at http://www.ada.gov/cguide.htm.

Understood for Learning and Attention Issues (n.d.) *The difference between IEP and 504 Plans.* Available at https://www.understood.org/en/school-learning/special-services/504-plan/the-difference-between-ieps-and-504-plans.

White, J.A. and Wehlage, G. (1995). Community collaboration: if it is such a good idea, why is it so hard to do? *Educ. Eval. Policy Anal.* 17 (1): 23–38.

Whitney, D.G. and Peterson, M.D. (2019). US national and state-level prevalence of mental health disorders and disparities of mental health care use in children. *JAMA Pediatr.* 173 (4): 389–391. https://doi.org/10.1001/jamapediatrics.2018.5399.

Williams Crenshaw, K., Ocen, P., & Nanda, J. (2015). *Black girls matter: Pushed out, overpoliced and underprotected.* Available at https://static1.squarespace.com/static/53f20d90e4b0b80451158d8c/t/54dcc1ece4b001c03e323448/1423753708557/AAPF_BlackGirlsMatterReport.pdf.

WHO. (2004). *The World Health Organization's information series on school health.* Geneva: World Health Organization.

WHO. (2018). *Adolescent mental health.* Geneva: World Health Organization. Available at https://www.who.int/mental_health/maternal-child/child_adolescent/en/.

WHO. (2013). *Mental Health Action Plan 2013–2020.* Geneva: World Health Organization. Available at https://apps.who.int/iris/bitstream/handle/10665/89966/9789241506021_eng.pdf?sequence=1.

Yeager, D.S., Dahl, R.E., and Dweck, C.S. (2018). Why interventions to influence adolescent behavior often fail but could succeed. *Perspect. Psychol. Sci.* 13 (1): 101–122.

Zhang, A., Musu-Gillette, L., and Oudekerk, B.A. (2016). Indicators of School Crime and Safety: 2015 (NCES 2016-079/NCJ 249758). Washington, DC: National Center for Education Statistics, US Department of Education, and Bureau of Justice Statistics, Office of Justice Programs, US Department of Justice.

Zuckerbrot, R.A., Cheung, A.H., Jensen, P.S. et al. (2007). Guidelines for Adolescent Depression in Primary Care (GLAD-PC): I. Identification, assessment, and initial management. *Pediatrics* 120 (5): e1299–e1312.

Zuckerbrot, R.A., Cheung, A., Jensen, P.S. et al. (2018). Guidelines for Adolescent Depression in Primary Care (GLAD-PC): part I. Practice preparation, identification, assessment, and initial management. *Pediatrics* 141 (3): e20174081. https://doi.org/10.1542/peds.2017-4081.

33

Child and Adolescent Mental Health Policy

Sally Raphel[1] and Eileen K. Fry-Bowers[2]

[1]University of Maryland School of Nursing Emerita, Johns Hopkins University School of Nursing Emerita, Baltimore, MD, USA
[2]Hahn School of Nursing and Health Science, University of San Diego, San Diego, CA, USA

> The mentally sound child works well, plays well, feels well, loves well, copes well and hopes well.
>
> Anthony and Cohler (1987)

Objectives

After reading this chapter, advanced practice registered nurses will be able to:

1. Describe the history of children's rights.
2. Identify current major policy areas related to child and adolescent mental health.
3. Explore partnerships within nursing to expand the focus on child and adolescent mental health promotion.
4. Propose collaborative advocacy for child and adolescent mental health policy implementation in primary care settings.

Introduction

Fostering social, emotional, and mental health in children as a part of healthy child development was named a national priority at the start of this century (US Department of Health and Human Services [USDHHS], US Public Health Service, Office of the Surgeon General 2000). Even so, it has not been a policy priority since that time. At the time of this writing, the 115th Congress, 2017–2018, had considered at some level 1027 health bills (seven signed into law), 211 Mental Health Bills (eight signed into law), and 12 Child Mental Health bills (one signed into law). The one notable legislative success for child health was the Protect Our Children Act, (US Senate Resolution 782 2017c), signed into law on 2 November 2017, which reauthorized the National Internet Crimes Against Children Data System and the National Strategy for Child Exploitation Prevention and Interdiction through fiscal year 2022 (Raphel 2019). Yet, statistics reveal that the need remains unreasonably high, with disparities evident among specific populations (e.g. children of color and low-income children). In the United States alone, 15 million children need mental health services of some kind; however, it is estimated that only 20% (3 million) receive any type of help. Of that number, only 20% are treated by clinicians actually trained in child mental health (Child Welfare League of America 2018). Policy development is key to meeting these mental health needs, yet mental health policy formation has been slow to gain traction in the United States. As such, strong, sustained advocacy is required to

Child and Adolescent Behavioral Health: A Resource for Advanced Practice Psychiatric and Primary Care Practitioners in Nursing,
Second Edition. Edited by Edilma L. Yearwood, Geraldine S. Pearson, and Jamesetta A. Newland.
© 2021 John Wiley & Sons, Inc. Published 2021 by John Wiley & Sons, Inc.
Companion website: www.wiley.com/go/Yearwood

promote change around children's mental health, with a focus on continued modification of public policy based on evolving needs and resources (Longest 2015). The public policymaking process and results are influenced by many factors. It is critical to first identify the problem(s). For example, heightened awareness of health, limited access to care, runaway costs, and quality factors add impetus to policy development at a national level, but often policy responses are influenced by politics rather than the best evidence at the point in time.

Mental health is recognized as a critical component of children's wellbeing and overall general health but actions to promote it are lacking. Insurance coverage and payment for mental health services are often a barrier to access. Many experts agree that children with mental health issues, especially from low-income families, are not able to access needed care due to gaps, flaws, and general uncertainty in state Medicaid and Children's

Health Insurance Programs (CHIP), as well as shortcomings inherent in the Paul Wellstone and Pete Domenici Mental Health Parity and Addiction Equity Act of 2008 (MHPAEA) (US House Resolution 6983 2008). Moreover, limitations imposed by the Supreme Court's decision (*National Federation of Independent Business v. Sebelius 2012*) regarding the Medicaid expansion provisions of The Patient Protection & Affordable Care Act of 2010 (ACA) and recent state and federal government actions that further limit Medicaid have resulted in differential access to care, even in the post ACA era (Alker et al. 2018; Rawal and McCabe 2016). Although the Children's Health Insurance Program (CHIP) originally called the State Children's Health Insurance Program or SCHIP has enjoyed bipartisan support, reauthorization has not been easy. Table 33.1 describes the lengthy struggle to get action for the CHIP.

Table 33.1 Timeline of CHIP reauthorization 2018

1997: The Balanced Budget Act of 1997 (BBA 97; US House of Representatives 1997) established the State Children's Health Insurance Program (SCHIP), a block grant to states that allowed them to cover uninsured children who were not eligible for Medicaid and whose family income was generally below 200% of the federal poverty level (FPL). The SCHIP program expired on 30 September 2007.

2007: During the summer of 2007 in anticipation of expiration of SCHIP on 30 September 2007, the House of Representatives and the Senate passed separate SCHIP reauthorization bills that would have significantly expanded funding and coverage for children. On 3 October 2007, President George W. Bush vetoed HR 976, the Children's Health Insurance Program Reauthorization Act of 2007, which had passed Congress with strong bipartisan support. On 12 December 2007 he again vetoed a subsequent version of the legislation, HR 3963. On 21 December 2007, President Bush signed into law the Medicare, Medicaid, and SCHIP Extension Act of US Senate 2007 as a temporary reauthorization of CHIP and extension of the program through April 2009.

2009: On 4 February 2009, President Obama signed into law HR 2, the Children's Health Insurance Program Reauthorization Act (CHIPRA) of the US House of Representatives 2009, which was one of the first pieces of legislation passed by the 111th Congress and which extended CHIP through 2013.

2010: The Patient Protection and Affordable Care Act (ACA; US House of Representatives 2010) PL 111–148 was signed into law by President Obama on 23 March 2010. It extended CHIP funding through 30 September 2015. The ACA also increased CHIP federal matching rates and required states to maintain eligibility standards through 30 September 2019.

2015: Prior to expiration of funding in 2015, the Medicare Access and CHIP Reauthorization Act (MACRA; US House of Representatives 2015) was passed and signed into law on 16 April 2015. MACRA further extended CHIP funding through 30 September 2017.

2017: In anticipation of expiration of CHIP on 30 September 2017, two different bills were introduced, each of which would have reauthorized the CHIP program:

- Keep Kids' Insurance Dependable and Secure Act of 2017 (Hatch/Wyden) (S. 1827, US Senate 2017b)
  - Introduced 18 September 2017 referred to Senate Finance Committee
  - 21 co-sponsors
- Related bill: HEALTHY Kids Act (Burgess) (H.R. 3921)
  - Introduced 23 October 2017 on calendar
  - No co-sponsors

Neither bill advanced in its respective chamber due to extended partisan disagreement regarding the federal budget negotiations.

2018: On 22 January 2018, President Donald J. Trump signed into law a 6-year reauthorization of CHIP as part of H.R. 195, the Federal Register Printing Savings Act of 2017 (US Senate 2017a), including Extension of Continuing Appropriations Act, 2018 (US House of Representatives 2018b), which passed by the House, by a vote of 266–150, and by the Senate, by a vote of 81–18.

Weeks later, on 9 February 2018, Congress voted to extend CHIP for an additional 4 more years, on top of the current 6-year extension, as a part of the Bipartisan Budget Act of 2018 (Senate, 71–28; US House of Representatives 2018a, 240–186). President Trump signed the budget act into law and the authorization of CHIP is presently extended through 2027.

Nevertheless, Medicaid remains a significant source of funding for behavioral healthcare, including mental health and substance use disorder services and supports, for children and youth in the United States. In fact, from 2005 to 2011, the percentage of children in Medicaid who used behavioral healthcare increased from 9.6% to 11.2%, a 17% increase, with most of that increase occurring between 2008 and 2011 (Pires et al. 2018). The increased rate was driven by a 19% increase in the percentage using behavioral health services and a 16% increase in the percentage of children using psychotropic medication. More specifically, in 2011, 8% of children in Medicaid or over 2.5 million children used behavioral health services, up from 6.7% in 2005. In 2011, 6.7% of children in Medicaid or over 2 million children used psychotropic medication, up from 5.8% in 2005 (Pires et al. 2018). Of note, however, almost half of children receiving psychotropic medications in 2011 did not receive accompanying behavioral health services, a finding similar to 2005. Even more disconcerting is that while the rate of service use has increased, the nationwide 8% rate of use is actually low given that a number of studies indicate that approximately 20% of children and youth have a diagnosable mental health condition and need behavioral health services (Pires et al. 2018). Significant regional differences in access to care also persist, especially for low-income children and children of color (Boyd-Barrett 2018).

Implementation of the ACA created new opportunities for expanding the capacity of child and adolescent mental health systems to meet these persistent and increasing needs. Beginning on January 1, 2014, coverage of mental health conditions and substance use disorders became a required part of the broad package of "essential benefits" services that qualified health insurance plans sold through the state marketplaces under the ACA and had to be covered. In addition, guaranteed issue and community rating requirements prevented insurers from refusing to sell insurance to people with preexisting conditions, including mental health or substance use disorders, and from setting premiums higher for people with behavioral health conditions. Moreover, coverage for behavioral healthcare must be at parity with coverage for medical/surgical care, based on the parity protections defined previously by the MHPAEA. These changes in coverage requirements were intended to expand the scope of coverage for behavioral health treatment and increase the availability of behavioral health coverage for people purchasing plans in the individual and small-group markets, which could potentially improve access to services (Cowell et al. 2018).

Unfortunately, the underdeveloped state of children's mental health services across the United States hindered the ability to capitalize on improved access to services (Behrens et al. 2013). Management and delivery of mental health services for children are far less robust than services that address children's physical health needs. Adoption of effective evidence-based interventions for preventing and treating behavioral health disorders in children has been slow, and serious shortages of pediatric mental health providers exist across the United States. These factors have led to decreased utilization of needed treatment, long wait times, and long distances traveled to care (Olsen 2017). In addition, major service systems, such as education, social service, physical health, housing, income support, and juvenile justice, are "siloed," and as a result do not support an integrated approach to care. Finally, although demonstration programs at the community and state levels that expand child and youth mental health services have produced positive outcomes (Mann and Hyde 2013), support for children's mental health services has not been high on the public or political agenda (Behrens et al. 2013). This chapter reviews historical and current child and adolescent mental health policy issues that influence nursing care provided in primary care and psychiatric settings.

Children's Rights

For centuries, children were seen as property rather than as individuals. Some societies viewed them as resources of the state, or disposed of them due to infirmity or gender. Children were not identified by society as vulnerable and in need of protection until the beginning of the twentieth century with the enactment of the first children's laws in Western countries (Yarrow 2009). Child protection laws identified the child as vulnerable and in need of societal protection. In time, child protection shifted to a focus on the children's rights movement. The child was no longer seen as powerless and without responsibility, but as an autonomous being with the right to participate in society (Abrams et al. 2015). The importance of the child rights movement has been keenly felt in the area of child and adolescent mental health. Advanced practice registered nurses (APRNs) need to be prepared to consider including children's rights, an undertheorized domain of social science and research efforts, particularly as they relate to mental health treatment (Huntington and Scott 2015).

The changing status of children in society has led to a change in family dynamics, and support of children's rights can conflict with the rights of the parents (Huntington and Scott 2015). The APRN's keen assessment of family dynamics can provide a family-centered approach leading to early assessment and treatment. Parent and family bias specific to mental health stigma needs to be explored while respecting the rights of both child and parent.

The United Nations (UN n.d., 1989 Declarations document) members declared 1979 the International Year of the Child (IYC), and in 1989 the UN General Assembly adopted an expanded version to its own 1959 Declaration of the Rights of the Child, broadening the original to include protocols for food, shelter, lodging, health, and education:

1. The child must be given the means requisite for its normal development, both materially and spiritually.
2. The child that is hungry must be fed, the child that is sick must be nursed, the child that is backward must be helped, the delinquent child must be reclaimed, and the orphan and the waif must be sheltered and succored.
3. The child must be the first to receive relief in times of distress.
4. The child must be put in a position to earn a livelihood, and must be protected against every form of exploitation.
5. The child must be brought up in the consciousness that its talents must be devoted to the service of its fellow men (United Nations International Children's Emergency Fund [UNICEF] https://www.unicef.org/).

Subsequently, the UN issued a Convention on the Rights of the Child (CRC). All of the CRC goals were expressed with respect to a child's age and evolving capacities, with the child's best interests always the paramount concern. The convention repeatedly emphasized the primacy and importance of the role, authority, and responsibility of parents and family. In general, the convention called for:

- freedom from violence, abuse, hazardous employment, exploitation, abduction, or sale
- adequate nutrition
- free compulsory primary education
- adequate healthcare
- equal treatment regardless of gender, race, or cultural background
- the right to express opinions and freedom of thought in matters affecting them
- safe exposure/access to leisure, play, culture, and art (UNICEF, https://www.unicef.org/child-rights-convention).

The CRC was the first legally binding international treaty to give universally recognized norms and standards for the protection and promotion of children's rights, and came into force on 2 September 1990 (Convention on the Rights of the Child 2018a). Currently 196 countries have ratified it, including every member of the UN except the United States (Convention on the Rights of the Child 2018b).

Although President Clinton's Administration signed the treaty, it never submitted it to the Senate for its advice and consent to ratification because of strongly stated personal opposition led by the then-Senate Foreign Relations Committee Chairman, Jesse Helms, due to concerns regarding sovereignty of state as well as the primacy of parental rights. Although the United States signed the treaty in 1995 after a significant delay, to date, no US President has submitted the treaty to the US Senate for ratification (Convention on the Rights of the Child 2018a).

Certainly, the tenants of the CRC promote the mental health of growing children with each having a right to be wanted, be born healthy, live in a healthy environment; have basic needs met, experience continuous loving care, and acquire the cognitive skills needed for life. While treatment of illness and behavioral problems is an urgent need, it is now known that prevention is equally important. A 2004 World Health Organization (WHO) report found that since the days of mental hygiene in the early twentieth century, many ideas have been offered to prevent behavioral problems and mental disorders in children. The document states "Some experimental programs were instituted in primary health care and schools; however, systematic development of science-based prevention programs and controlled studies to test their effectiveness did not emerge until 1980" (p. 7). The evidence points out that for people in positions of authority to significantly influence a change in primary prevention and early intervention . . . "it is only possible through successful collaboration between multiple partners involved in research, policy and practice, including community leaders and consumers" (p. 7). Stroul (2007) observed, "Based on current clinical evidence, the time has come and passed to integrate the training and practice of pediatricians and other clinicians with mental health professionals" (p. 2). Enhanced communication between mental health and primary care practitioners advances the effectiveness, efficiency, and sustainability of care, and ultimately improves the health and wellness of children and families dealing with mental health challenges (Substance Abuse and Mental Health Services Administration-Health Resources Services Administration [SAMHSA-HRSA] 2014).

Policy Formation

Policy and mental health policy makers in particular establish the vision, values, and principles of the issue. Policy craftsmanship is very important, and the need for policy is initiated by several means: public stimulus, research substantiation, or governmental/organizational request. The process requires backing up the information gathered and forecasting. Incorporating a cost–benefit analysis is necessary to determine whether the policy can produce the results that are envisioned. Likewise, an attempt to answer what action is morally right is warranted. Consideration of affected societal groups (e.g. children, parents, their support systems, providers) or constituent wishes becomes a crucial part of the process. Policy vision sets what is desirable for the mental health of a country's citizens and what is possible according to available resources and technology. Values and principles should be the basis of governmental objectives and goals, and from these flow strategies and courses of action.

Examples of values and principles in mental health policies include psychological wellbeing, mental health as indivisible from general health, community care and participation, cultural relativism, protection of vulnerable people, accessibility, and equity. A few accompanying principles are that mental health promotion should be integrated (i) into social and educational services, (ii) into the general health system, (iii) with a least restrictive form of care, and (iv) with intersectoral collaboration and linkages with community development (WHO 2004).

The main areas for action in all mental health policy are human rights, organization of services, financing, collaboration (of providers/agencies), human resources and training for caregivers/clinicians, promotion, prevention, treatment and rehabilitation, essential drug (medication) procurement and distribution, advocacy, quality improvement, information systems, research, and evaluation of policies and services. Adequate financing is one of the most critical global factors in the implementation of mental health policy. Integral to the field of mental health policy is a strong support for human rights legislation (WHO 2013).

Legislation is essential to guarantee that the dignity of people with mental disorders is preserved and protected. In the United States, childhood mental illness and behavioral problems, including substance use, must be approached on parity with medical health problems and expanded to nontraditional settings (home, school, community, clinics) (Mental Health America [MHA] 2018). With the passage of the landmark 2008 MHPAEC introduced by Senators Paul Wellstone and Pete Domenici, mental health coverage was mandated (US House of Representatives 2008). The Act was intended to end health insurance benefits inequity in the United States and required that group plans of 51 or more employees be no more restrictive than the predominant requirements and limitations placed on substantially all medical/surgical benefits, authorized services were to include a continuum of health promotion and illness prevention services, and least restrictive

interventions were to be employed. Yet, since plans covering fewer than 50 employees and group plans that did not offer any mental healthcare coverage at all were exempt from the MHPAEA, the Act did not create access where none existed. The ACA (US House of Representatives 2010), however, included mental health and substance use disorder care as an "essential health benefit" (EHB) for "non-grandfathered individual and small group plans" which effectively included smaller plans under the MHPAEA. Even so, insurance parity has only led to small increases in mental health service use among children, and reduction in out-of-pocket expenditures appears to be too small in magnitude to have a meaningful impact on families' financial burden (Barry et al. 2013; Kennedy-Hendricks et al. 2018).

Why is Policy Important?

The statistics concerning psychiatric problems among children and adolescents are alarming. The Global Burden of Disease Study indicates that by 2020, childhood neuropsychiatric disorders will increase by more than 50% internationally to become one of the five most common causes of morbidity, mortality, and disability among children in the world. Although the number of children receiving care has doubled in the last decade, the extent of unmet needs is still great (National Alliance on Mental Illness 2018). It is well established that without treatment, psychological problems disrupt the child's social, academic, and emotional development and result in family turmoil. Also 7.5 million parents are affected by depression every year. This puts at least 15 million children at risk for a wide range of problems (Institute of Medicine [IOM] 2009). Additional past policy reports from the Office of the Surgeon General on Youth Violence (USDHHS 2001b), Suicide Prevention (USDHHS 2001a), and Risk of Drinking (USDHHS 2007) have each spotlighted grave concerns and offered action plans.

In 2010, Merikangas et al. published the first comprehensive prevalence data on the range of *Diagnostic and Statistical Manual of Mental Disorders IV* (DSM-IV) mental disorders with and without severe impairment, comorbidity across broad classes of disorder, and sociodemographic correlates in a nationally representative sample of US adolescents. The overall prevalence of disorders with severe impairment and/or distress was 22.2%, or more than one in five adolescents being affected (11.2% with mood disorders, 8.3% with anxiety disorders, 9.6% behavior disorders). The median age of onset for disorder classes was 6 years for anxiety, 11 years for behavior, 13 years for mood, and 15 years for substance use disorders (Merikangas et al. 2010). Merikangas

(2018) noted that ongoing collective data analyses is not reported partially because of "lack of coordination of sampling and methods across agencies that support these studies" (p. 307). Even so, additional research finds that among youths with more severe impairment, fewer than half accessed services in 2010–2012 (Olfson et al. 2015). Recent estimates indicate that the annual cost of such disorders among American youth and their families may be close to a quarter of a trillion dollars, highlighting the importance of mental health policy for American youth (O'Connell et al. 2009). Failure to provide effective and timely care has serious personal and societal consequences, as the evidence supports.

Focusing on importance, a study funded by the USDHHS (2009) published in *Children and Youth Services Review* found that 45% of youth with prior involvement with the child welfare system had at least one mental health problem as they transitioned to adulthood. The study sampled over 5000 children from 92 child welfare agencies across the country. More than a quarter of the youth were in the clinical range for depression. The study also examined the youths' surrounding life circumstances, finding that at least 60% lived in households at or below the national poverty line and only about a quarter lived with one or more parent. The study's authors called for policymakers, researchers, clinicians, and service system administrators to acknowledge these extreme needs and work better with this vulnerable population (USDHHS 2009).

Nearly 10 years later, mounting evidence supports the relationship between adverse childhood experiences (ACEs), substance use disorders, and behavioral and mental health problems. Exposure to chronic stressful events disrupts pediatric neurodevelopment, resulting in impairment in a child's cognitive functioning or ability to cope with negative or disruptive emotions. In response, the child may adopt negative coping mechanisms, including substance use or self-harm, which often manifest during adolescence (SAMSHA 2018). Evidence indicates that these poor coping mechanisms contribute to disease, disability, and social problems well into adulthood, are linked to higher health costs across the life course, and may contribute to health inequities (Merrick et al. 2018; Purewal et al. 2016).

Timeline of Existing Policy Development

Nursing has been at the forefront of policy development for mental health in a formal way since the 1990s. The strong impetus for policy in this area came from the Nursing's Agenda for Health Care Reform (American

Nurses Association [ANA] 1991), in the policy document *Health Care Reform: Essential Mental Health Services* (Krauss 1993), and in the strong voices of nurse leaders (Raphel 2017). Nursing's plan addressed the need for reform in areas such as primary-mental health service delivery, universal access to a basic mental health benefits package, and structure and financing of the public mental-health system for continuous care (Krauss 1993). Children and adolescents were one of the life span target groups. The belief was stated that primary care clinics, school health clinics, community health centers, and pediatric offices were the most likely places where children and adolescents would receive care. This included services for those with behavioral, emotional, and mental health concerns. Nursing's policy statement proposed the integration of mental health promotion and mental illness prevention into existing primary care settings using nurses already in the system to conduct routine mental health assessments and refer to child mental health APRNs for treatment. The vision in this policy was that funding would be directed to the local central authority, making the authority responsible for delivery of services, thus creating an organized system for continuous community-based care. Krauss (1993) presented childhood risk factors and extrinsic and intrinsic protective factors pivotal to developmental mental health to make the case for comprehensive care.

Government policy bodies have taken steps to provide for children's mental health, as one can see in Box 33.1. In 1999, the Surgeon General of the United States released the landmark first national US mental health policy document *Mental Health: A Report of the Surgeon General* with a major section dedicated to children and adolescents (USDHHS 1999). The overarching themes in the policy report were to take a life span approach, to use a public health perspective, to stress that mental disorders were disabling, to promote mind and body as inseparable, to acknowledge that effective treatments existed, and consumer and family movements were critical to advocacy. In Chapter 3 (Children and Mental Health) specific concerns and issues were laid out. The first major point of the conclusions was that there was a wide range of normal for children. Efficacious psychosocial and pharmacologic treatments existed, and primary care and schools were major settings for recognition and treatment of mental disorders. The text went further to state that multiple problems associated with serious emotional disturbance required a systems approach, cultural differences exacerbated problems of access, and families were essential partners in the treatment process.

Box 33.1 Decades of mental health policy statements

- *Health Care Reform: Essentials of Mental Health Services.* Nursing's Mental Health Policy Statement
- *Mental Health: A Report of the Surgeon General* published with a major section dedicated to children and adolescents
- *Children's Mental Health: A National Action Plan* released by Dr. David Satcher
- *Youth Violence: A Report of the Surgeon General* was released
- *A National Strategy for Suicide Prevention: Goals and Objectives for Action* Surgeon General
- *Crossing the Quality Chasm: A New Health System for the 21st Century.* Institute of Medicine Committee on Quality of Health Care in America
- *Achieving the Promise: Transforming Mental Health Care in America.* Report of the President's New Freedom Commission on Mental Health
- *Prevention of Mental Disorders: Effective Interventions and Policy Options.* Report of WHO Department of Mental Health and Substance Abuse
- *Improving the Quality of Health Care for Mental and Substance-use Conditions* from the Institute of Medicine Quality Chasm Series
- *The Surgeon General's Call to Action to Prevent and Reduce Underage Drinking* was released

In 2000, an important policy delineation of children and mental health came from Surgeon General David Satcher in the form of a Report of the Surgeon General's Conference on Children's Mental Health: A National Action Agenda (USDHHS 2000). The overarching vision was that mental health was a critical component of children's learning and general health. Fostering social and emotional health in children as a part of healthy child development must be a national priority. Both the promotion of mental health in children and the treatment of mental disorders were identified as major public health goals (USDHHS 2000). To achieve these goals, the National Action Agenda had as guiding principles a commitment to:

1. Promoting the recognition of mental health as an essential part of child health.
2. Integrating family-, child-, and youth-centered mental health services into all systems that serve children and youth.
3. Engaging families and incorporating the perspectives of children and youth in the development of all mental health care planning.
4. Developing and enhancing a public-private health infrastructure to support these efforts to the fullest extent possible (pp. 5–6).

Goals for policy implementation by government and agencies followed. These were to:

1. Promote public awareness of children's mental health issues and reduce stigma associated with mental illness.
2. Continue to develop, disseminate, and implement scientifically proven prevention and treatment services in the field of children's mental health.
3. Improve the assessment of and recognition of mental health needs in children.
4. Eliminate racial/ethnic and socioeconomic disparities in access to mental healthcare services.
5. Improve the infrastructure for children's mental health services, including support for scientifically proven interventions across professions.
6. Increase access to and coordination of quality mental healthcare services.
7. Train frontline providers to recognize and manage mental health issues, and educate mental healthcare providers about scientifically proven prevention and treatment services.
8. Monitor the access to and coordination of quality mental healthcare services (p. 6).

This was a clear message to the nation that children and adolescents were important. The national focus on vulnerable children and adolescents was maintained by a number of subsequent government policy statements, including A National Strategy for Suicide Prevention: Goals and Objectives for Action (USDHHS 2001a) and Youth Violence: A Report of the Surgeon General (USDHHS 2001b). Although a national dialogue about evidence-based practice and empirically validated treatments for children had been ongoing for a decade, youth and families continued to suffer because of missed opportunities for prevention of psychiatric disorders and early interventions in behavioral problems. Mental health professionals identified culturally relevant clinical standards and implementation guidelines as needing to be included in the dialogue on child and adolescent mental health (USDHHS 2000).

In 2002, the President's New Freedom Commission on Mental Health identified policies that could be implemented by federal, state, and local governments to maximize the use of existing resources, improve coordination of treatments and services, and promote successful community integration for children with serious emotional disturbance. They reported the current system "a patchwork relic—the result of disjointed reforms and policies . . . with barriers that often add to the burden of mental illness for individuals, their families and our communities" (New Freedom Commission 2003, p. 4).

They identified that services remained fragmented, disconnected, and inadequate. To address some of these issues, a special coalition was formed entitled the Annapolis Coalition on Behavioral Health Workforce Education to address training issues. This was a collaborative effort to identify a set of core or common competencies as a key strategy for advancing behavioral health education, training, and workforce development initiatives. The Annapolis Coalition received grant funding from the SAMHSA to commission a series of position papers and to convene a body of experts in a summit to develop competencies.

Building on *Crossing the Quality Chasm: A New Health System for the 21st Century* (IOM 2001), additional gaps in treatment knowledge were defined by the IOM. Evidence-based clinical practice guidelines were unavailable for many mental/substance use problems and illnesses, especially for individuals at both ends of the age continuum, children, and older adults (IOM 2006). This policy document put forward an agenda for change with strategies for filling knowledge gaps and actions needed for quality improvement at all levels of the healthcare system. The failures to treat persist (IOM 2006); this is especially true from data reported for gaps in effective treatment for children and adolescents. The IOM policy work group labeled the critical features of an ideal system of care for depressed parents and their children as (i) multigenerational, (ii) comprehensive, (iii) available across settings, (iv) accessible, (v) integrative, (vi) developmentally appropriate, and (vii) culturally sensitive. The goals from mental health policy for treating depression would be to provide hope, foster resilience, and promote health, general/mental, and recovery (Evans 2009; IOM 2009).

In 2006, after more than a decade, the key concepts for policy change were again reported to include comprehensive identification of needs and strengths, family driven, individualized care in the least restrictive setting, family voice, choice, and engagement, local systems' partnerships, accountability, and overall health status monitoring in the context of mental health treatment. Identification of a level of care for each child in need, outreach through ongoing case managers and healthcare managers, and interventions with an integrated plan and quality measures were recommendations from the Georgetown Institute Forum (Stroul 2007). More recently, proceedings from the National Academies of Sciences, Engineering, and Medicine, addressed the continued need to improve behavioral outcomes for children and noted that the number of trained clinicians is limited and contributes to access barriers to effective treatment options. Areas of specific focus of the proceedings included (i) behavioral health promotion and

risk prevention through multigenerational surveillance, (ii) incorporating exposure to evidence-based practices into the content and assessment of training programs focused on the need for changing systems to support implementation, (iii) fostering integrated, interprofessional care, (iv) training the future child healthcare workforce to meet the needs of children with disabilities and chronic medical conditions, (v) engaging patients and parents in co-promotion of behavioral health to improve care, (vi) enhancing training through the power of accreditation, certification, and credentialing, (vii) enhancing training for healthcare professionals to improve the behavioral health of children, youth, and families involved in other child-serving systems, and (viii) how current reimbursement for training and clinical care impacts the focus on behavioral health for children, youth, and families (Olson 2017).

Contemporary legislative activity includes the passage of the 21st Century Cures Act (US House Resolution 34 2016a), which was signed into law by President Obama on 13 December 2016. This package of healthcare bills contained many mental health, substance use, and criminal justice provisions taken from the Helping Families in Mental Health Crisis Act (US House Resolution 2646 2016b), the Mental Health Reform Act of 2016 (US Senate Resolution 2680 2016b), the Mental Health and Safe Communities Act (US Senate 2002 2015a), and the Comprehensive Justice and Mental Health Act (US Senate Resolution 993 2015b) and marked progress toward reform of the mental healthcare system in the United States. Most recently, the 115th Congress passed sweeping legislation to address substance use in the form of the Support for Patients and Communities Act (US House Resolution 6 2017b) and the Opioid Crisis Response Act (US Senate Resolution 2680 2017d), which includes provisions to improve access to addiction treatment, as well as many other interventions to stem an ongoing opioid use epidemic, from law enforcement efforts against illicit drugs to combating the over-prescription of opioids. Even so, bipartisan government employees assert that legislation will not result in more money and resources being distributed in all areas of need during the opioid crisis (Bipartisan Policy Center 2019).

Child and Adolescent Mental Health Promotion

Policy Statements are Useless without Action Plans and Implementation!

Because policy formation includes input from vested groups, key stakeholders, and child advocates, the opportunities for partnerships between public (government)-private partnerships should follow. For example, public policy integrating mental health into primary care settings is getting considerable and deserved attention. It is agreed that children and adolescents are the populations with unique service needs, requiring specialized planning and coordinated service delivery approaches. As far back as 1995, the American Psychiatric Association (APA) published the *Diagnostic and Statistical Manuel of Mental Disorders – Primary Care* (DSMMD-PC) in collaboration with 10 national organizations for primary care providers (APA 1995). Chapter 7 of that manual addresses disorders usually first diagnosed in infancy, childhood or adolescence, noting that the primary care presentation can be extremely diverse. Consideration of developmental variation is key to accurate identification. One should refer to the appropriate section based on presenting symptoms for the suggested algorithm (p. 176). This work led to collaboration between the American Academy of Pediatrics (AAP) and APA for a *Diagnostic and Statistical Manuel of Mental Disorders – Primary Care (DSMMD-PC) Child and Adolescent Version* (AAP 1996) released October 1996. The manual is a compendium that blends developmental, behavioral, and primary care pediatrics for diagnosing and assessing mental health issues in primary care.

In 2006, the Georgetown University Training Institute developed recommendations for policy and technical assistance to support communities implementing effective mental health service delivery in primary care settings. Experts facilitated discussion focusing on strategies for policy, services, financing, advocacy, information development/dissemination and training, and technical assistance. They called for policy implementation through specific actions, such as (i) providing consultation to primary care clinicians on behavioral health issues, (ii) increasing the role of primary care clinicians in identifying and addressing behavioral health needs, (iii) co-locating mental health specialists in primary care settings for increased access and consultation to primary care clinicians, (iv) implementing a medical home approach to ensure mental health, physical care, dental, eye care, etc. are accessible, and (v) providing health and mental health services through school-based clinics (Stroul 2007, p. 6).

In past decades, we slowly have moved from policy to action plans and implementation, as various collaborative primary care-mental health promotion constituent models have been put forward. Nurses through the National Association for Pediatric Nurse Practitioners (NAPNAP) stepped up with the Keep Your Children Safe and Secure (KySS) (Melnyk et al. 2001). This

prevention program was based on the philosophy that comprehensive healthcare that includes prevention efforts and early recognition and treatment of mental health problems in children will result in an optimal level of functioning and development as a foundation for productive adult years. KySS partners included: Society of Pediatric Nurses (SPN), Sigma Theta Tau International Honor Society of Nursing, the National Assembly of School Based Health Care (NASBHC), and the National Youth Anti-Drug Media Campaign. A key issue explored was primary care and specialty referrals for mental and physical health. Through efforts to raise awareness, disseminate information, educate health professionals, teachers, and the public and continued development of effective partnerships, the hard work of this core group received recognition. One southwestern university was awarded a grant for a national KySS Fellowship for nurse practitioners (NPs) in underserved United States (Raphel 2012, p. 528). This was a collaborative endeavor between Arizona State University College, Healthcare Innovation, and NAPNAP's KySS Program. Another example of enactment of policy related to training and education programs for primary care NPs and other nurses was the publishing of mental health curriculum for pediatric nurses in the primary care setting.

The Children's Mental Health Campaign (CMHC) started in 2006 with a collaboration between Boston Children's Hospital and the Massachusetts Society for the Prevention of Cruelty to Children. Now six major organizations representing parent and professional advocacy, mental health, healthcare policy, a children's hospital, health law advocacy, and prevention have partnered together. The mission of CMHC is to "advocate for policy, systems, and practice solutions to ensure all children in Massachusetts have access to resources to prevent, diagnose, and treat mental health issues in a timely, effective, and compassionate way." They focus on access to care, court-involved youth, school-based behavioral health, substance use prevention, and infant and early childhood mental health (https://childrensmentalhealthcampaign.org/about). Today CMHC works within a network of more than 200 other organizations across the state.

The Minnesota Association for Children's Mental Health (MACMH) is an organization with a mission to promote positive mental health for infants, children, adolescents, and their families. They offer training, events, and publications to educate families, caregivers, and communities (https://macmh.org/). Included in their resources is an educator's guide, *An Educator' Guide to Children's Mental* Health.

On the federal level, a group the National Council for Behavioral Health introduced Mental Health First Aid to the United States in 2008; more than 1 million Americans from all walks of life have been trained, from teachers, police officers and first responders to veterans, politicians and national sports figures. The partnership with Boys and Girls Clubs of America extends the reach of this potentially lifesaving program (National Council for Behavioral Health 2018). Other advocacy groups such as MHA have disseminated eight position papers on Children's Mental Health, specifically numbers 42–49 (MHA 2018).

Collaborative Advocacy

Nursing has a professional, ethical, and social directive to advocate as part of the nursing process (Schlairet 2009). Typically, nurses see this as part of their job and one of the primary reasons they entered the profession. Although advocacy is considered a part of daily clinical nursing practice, the concept is not well defined in measurable terms and is often vague. The *Oxford Dictionary of Nursing* (McFerran 2003) defines advocacy as an integral part of the professional healthcare practitioner's role. The ANA includes advocacy within nursing's Social Policy Statement, stating that nurses provide "advocacy in the care of individuals, families, communities, and populations" (ANA 2015a, p. 23).

Advocacy is also included in the ANA Code of Ethics for Nursing (ANA 2015b). The Code of Ethics Provision 7.3 states contributions through nursing and Health Policy Development involve, "the nurse participates as advocate . . . in civic activities related to health care with informed perspective on nursing and healthcare policy" and "The nurse promotes, advocates for, and strives to protect the health, safety and rights of the patient, and the nurse collaborates with other health professionals and the public in promoting community, national, and international efforts to meet health needs" (Fowler 2015, pp. 28, 29). Advocacy is also recognized in almost all major nursing professional organizations, with a separate committee, division, or special interest group for advocacy, healthcare policy, or government affairs.

Although nursing advocacy behaviors, such as analyzing, counseling, and responding, have been identified in the literature, there was not an instrument that measured the nursing advocacy process especially as it impacted the role of the advocate, advocate activities, and outcomes, and the perspective of the nurse and patient (Vaartio et al. 2009). The literature supported that when nurses advocated, they could experience loss of control and self-determination, as well as conflict. But there was limited research on the behaviors and the time nurses advocated during their daily practice (Vaartio et al. 2009).

APRNs need to understand and practice advocacy behaviors that result in positive professional and clinical outcomes, as well as the policy that shapes them. Further research into the understanding of nursing advocacy education and implementation will provide APRNs with empiric data supporting the influence of nursing as a change agent in healthcare. The concept of "Leading the Way" (Cohen et al. 1996) applies to political involvement but also applies to all areas of professional and clinical practice where nursing initiates change. Mason et al. (2016) prepare students to be politically active in leadership roles in the workplace, government, professional organizations, and the community. The APRN can use these behaviors and strategies in many different roles within healthcare delivery and conduct research regarding the resulting outcomes.

Advocacy has a wide range of definitions and use in nursing. Advocacy can occur at the bedside as the APRN empowers the child or family to gain information or influence. Advocacy can relate to professional goals and advancement. Advocacy also can occur within a social or political context. The following five types of nurse advocacy can be used to develop a foundation for incorporating short- and long-term goals into a professional and clinical advocacy strategy (Kubsch et al. 2004):

1. legal advocate
2. moral-ethical advocate
3. spiritual advocate
4. substitutive advocate
5. political advocate.

Advocacy knowledge and behaviors are necessary both clinically and politically to effect change. APRNs can no longer be passive and attempt to effect change at the distal end of the health policy system, where frustrations can lead to negative consequences such as conflict with colleagues, poor communication, reprimand, loss of professional control, and, for some nurses, pressure to resign or a decision to leave the profession.

Advocating beyond the bedside and into the public and political environment will lead to improved patient outcomes, enhanced professional empowerment, and professionalism. In the United States, healthcare has become a political issue. Politics and policy drive healthcare coverage, healthcare organization regulation, and clinical practice policies. Mason, Leavitt, and Chaffee, in their chapter Policy and Politics: A Framework for Action (2007), state, "Nursing is concerned with health; therefore, every action and decision that influences health and the health system should be important to nurses" (p. 3). In order for APRNs to be seen as healthcare leaders, they must politically advocate for the APRN role regarding nursing image, clinical privileges, and reimbursement. Once the APRN achieves heightened visibility and clinical practice, impact on child and adolescent mental health services will be easier to achieve.

Professional nursing organizations are also active in policy advocacy, with a separate branch usually devoted to professional and public healthcare goals. The ANA Membership Assembly and Board of Directors work together to chart the best course for nursing's future (https://www.nursingworld.org/ana/leadership-and-governance/). APRNs should be members of the ANA and members of specialty organizations that support child and adolescent health issues and mental health agendas. Professional nursing organizations participate in policy development through collective membership, and both psychiatric and primary care APRNs can be actively engaged in current advocacy and policy discussions.

NAPNAP was established in 1973; its mission is to promote optimal health for children through leadership, practice, advocacy, education, and research. The organization has championed many child health causes, including gun safety, access for contraception to avoid pregnancy, and access for children with special needs Although the organization does not specifically address mental health issues, it created a special interest group on Developmental and Behavioral Health (DBHSIG) "to provide a networking opportunity for pediatric and family APRNs working in developmental-behavioral pediatrics, child and adolescent psychiatry, and those in primary care who have a strong interest in the developmental, behavioral and mental health needs of young children, school-age children, adolescents and their families" (para 1). The DBHSIG focus is on prevention, early recognition, treatment, and referral of these needs and it provides a forum to share resources and information for practice, research, and advocacy (NAPNAP 2018). In addition, NAPNAP utilizes its membership to speak to global issues related to child healthcare needs and is an excellent example of a specialty nursing organization where united primary care APRNs and psychiatric APRNs can achieve collaborative goals.

On 5 October 2010, the IOM released a groundbreaking report, *The Future of Nursing: Leading Change, Advancing Health*. The report recommended overcoming practice barriers that prevent nurses from responding to a rapidly changing healthcare system.

More specifically, it states the following:

- Nurses should practice to the full extent of their education and training.
- Nurses should achieve higher levels of education and training through an improved education system that promotes seamless academic progression.

- Nurses should be full partners, with physicians and other healthcare professionals, in redesigning health care in the United States.
- Effective workforce planning and policy making require better data collection and information infrastructure (p. 4).

This report, equally applicable to child and adolescent primary care and psychiatric practitioners, has the potential to be a springboard for policy changes as healthcare transforms and changes. The report points out that responsibility for these changes rests on government, business, healthcare, and insurance agencies, as well as the profession of nursing. Nursing is poised to initiate and participate in policy changes that will advance nursing practice (IOM 2010).

Psychiatric mental health nurses are putting action to words by joining with colleagues from all aspects of nursing in a coalition. The Nursing Community Coalition (NCC) supports the following core principles:

- Nurses are an integral part of the healthcare team, are involved in every aspect of care, and are committed to the patient, their families, and the community.
- The contributions made by the practice and science of nursing are critical to the delivery of high-quality, life-saving, preventive, and palliative healthcare across all care settings, geographic areas, and social determinants of health.
- Nursing involvement is essential to the development of all aspects of new healthcare policy, legislation and information technology infrastructure. Presently, NCC includes 61 nursing groups working toward advocacy for substantial legislation. Through monthly conference calls, they draft Nursing's response to Capitol Hill activities and keep an eye on government at the Federal level (https://www.thenursingcommunity.org/). It has a very busy agenda.

An Exemplar: Policy Can be Toxic

At the time of this writing, we have a premiere example of US public policy without forethought or planning. The US Attorney General announced a new "zero tolerance" policy of referring all border crossings for federal criminal prosecution, which led to children being separated from their families as their parents are sent to jail (NPR 2018). What the Department of Justice called a "new" plan to curtail "illegal immigration" or migration of undocumented persons in April 2018 quickly raised concern (US Department of Justice 2018). Many were appalled at the separation of children from their parents at the US/Mexico border from 19 April through 31 May 2018.

Children as young as 3 years were taken from parents and housed in warehouses with no consideration for care or comfort or plan for reunification. Overall, nearly 1995 immigrant children were separated from their parents during a 6-week period according to the Department of Homeland Security. The separation of children from their parents at the border brought widespread and bipartisan condemnation of the act, from nurses' groups, politicians, activists, celebrities, and parents. One official said the policy is a "moral humanitarian crisis." "Every parent who has ever held a child in their arms, every human being with a sense of compassion and decency, should be outraged" (Clinton 2018). The children were and are being held in facilities run by the Office of Refugee Resettlement within the USDHHS, in facilities such as a converted Walmart in Texas. While laws and case precedent govern how undocumented children are to be treated at the border, none mandates the separation of children from their parents. Under a 1997 legal agreement known as the Flores Settlement, children can be detained no longer than 20 days and the government is required to release them from immigration detention without unnecessary delay to their parents, other adult relatives, or licensed programs (Kandel 2017). By mid-June of 2018, a total of 11 786 children under age 18 were detained, with 2322 children 12 years old or younger (Luthra and Taylor 2018). With regard to public sentiment, a contemporaneous Quinnipiac University poll (2018) found that 66% of Americans opposed the policy while 27% supported it. Given our current understanding of the evidence regarding parent–child separation and exposure to prolonged and highly stressful experiences, this policy will result in short- and long-term physical and mental health consequences for these children.

Summary

Fifteen million children need mental health services of some kind; only 20% (3 million) receive any type of help. Of that group, only 20% are treated by clinicians actually trained in child mental health (Stroul 2007). A recent 2016 secondary analysis of data from the 2016 National Survey of Children's Health (Ghandour et al. 2019) found that for children 3–17 years of age, the estimated prevalence of three mental health disorders was 7.1% (4.4 million) for current anxiety problems, 7.4% (4.5 million) for behavioral/conduct problems, and 3.2% (1.9 million) for current depression. Of these children the percentages for treatment for behavioral problems, anxiety, and depression were 53.5%, 59.3%, and 80%, respectively. One limitation of this study, however, was that the data were parental report. The researchers conclude that treatment gaps for mental health among children and adolescents

still exist. Health policy statements for child and adolescent mental health exist and must be applied. Parity legislation has established equity between health and mental health care in the United States. The most urgent and difficult part of child mental health policy action and implementation still faces global healthcare systems. In this country, there are pockets of excellent mental healthcare. Many more are needed to meet the critical access problems that exist. It is decreed in multiple policy documents that primary care is the site for child and adolescent mental healthcare. Collaborations of all kinds are needed to effect changes in the current resource poor environment. Models have appeared at the state and county levels using coordination of dozens of agencies but funding methods are often uncertain or insufficient. Advocacy is needed to make it happen. All policies are not positive. Stakeholder nursing groups such as primary care and psychiatric APRNs are well poised to lead the way.

Critical Thinking Questions

1. What role can APRNs play in child mental health policy formation?
2. How would you start to design a collaborative plan for policy advocacy for a current child mental health issue?
3. How does policy become legislation for mental health care?

References

Abrams, D., Ramsey, S., and Mangold, S. (2015). Children and the Law in a Nutshell, 5e. St. Paul, MN: West Academic.

Affordable Care Act. (2010). Retrieved Oct. 3, 2018 from https://www.kff.org/health-reform/fact-sheet/summary-of-the-affordable-care-act

Alker, J., Jordan, P., Pham, O., and Wagnerman, K. (2018). How Mississippi's Proposed Medicaid Work Requirement Would Affect Low-Income Families with Children. Washington, D.C.: Georgetown University Health Policy Institute, Center for Children and Families Available at https://ccf.georgetown.edu/wp-content/uploads/2018/08/Propsed-Medicaid-Work-Requirement-Mississippi.pdf.

AAP (1996). Diagnostic and Statistical Manual for Primary Care: Child and Adolescent Version (DSM-PC). Washington D.C: American Academy of Pediatrics.

ANA (1991). Nursing's Agenda for Health Care Reform. Washington, DC: ANA Publishing.

American Psychiatric Association (1995). Diagnostic and Statistical Manual of Mental Disorders: Primary Care Version. Washington, DC: APA Publishing.

ANA (2015a). Guide to Nursing's Social Policy Statement. Silver Spring, MD: Author.

ANA (2015b). Guide to the Code of Ethics for Nurses, 2e. Silver Spring, MD: Author.

Anthony, E.J. and Cohler, B.J. (1987). The Invulnerable Child. New York, NY: Guilford Press.

Barry, C.L., Chien, A.T., Normand, S.T. et al. (2013). Parity and out-of-pocket spending for children with high mental health or substance abuse expenditures. *Pediatrics* 131: e903–e911. https://doi.org/10.1542/peds.2012-1491.

Behrens, D., Lear, J.G., and Price, O.A. (2013). Improving Access to Children's Mental Health Care: Lessons from a Study of Eleven States. Washington, D.C: George Washington University, The Center for Health and Health Care in Schools Available at https://hsrc.himmelfarb.gwu.edu/sphhs_centers_chhcs/8.

Bipartisan Policy Center (2019). Tracking federal funding to combat the opioid crisis. Washington, DC: Bipartisan Policy Center Available at https://bipartisanpolicy.org/wp-content/uploads/2019/03/Tracking-Federal-Funding-to-Combat-the-Opioid-Crisis.pdf.

Boyd-Barrett, C. (2018). *Few low-income children get mental health care in California, despite need.* California Health Report. Available athttp://www.calhealthreport.org/2018/07/18/low-income-children-get-mental-health-care-california-despite-need.

Child Welfare League of America. (2018). *The nation's children 2018.* Available at https://www.cwla.org/wp-content/uploads/2018/03/National-Childrens-Factsheet-2018-.pdf.

Children's Mental Health Campaign. (2018). *Children's mental health campaign.* Available at https://childrensmentalhealthcampaign.org.

Clinton, H. (2018). *Hillary Clinton on family separation: Every human being with a sense of compassion and decency should be outraged.* Availableathttps://www.vox.com/2018/6/18/17476268/hillaryclinton-family-separation-border-immigration.

Cohen, S., Mason, D., Kovner, C. et al. (1996). Stages of nursing's political development: where we've been and where we ought to be. *Nursing Outlook* 44: 20–23.

Convention on the Rights of the Child. (2018a). *How does the United States ratify treaties?* Available at http://www.childrightscampaign.org/why-ratify/how-does-the-united-states-ratify-treaties.

Convention on the Rights of the Child. (2018b). Participating countries. Available at http://www.childrightscampaign.org/what-is-the-crc/participating-countries.

Cowell, A.J., Prakash, S., Jones, E. et al. (2018). Behavioral health coverage in the individual market increased after ACA parity requirements. *Health Affairs* 37: 1153–1159. https://doi.org/10.1377/hlthaff.2017.1517.

Evans, M.E. (2009). Prevention of mental, emotional, and behavioral disorders in youth: the Institute of Medicine report and implications for nursing. *Journal of Child and Adolescent Psychiatric Nursing* 22: 154–159.

Fowler, M.D.M. (ed.) (2015). Guide to the Code of Ethics for Nurses, 2e. Silver Springs, MD: American Nurses Association.

Ghandour, R.M., Sherman, L.J., Vladutiu, C.J. et al. (2019). Prevalence and treatment of depression, anxiety, and conduct problems in US children. *Journal of Pediatrics* 206: 256–267. https://doi.org/10.1016/j.jpeds.2018.09.021.

Huntington, C. and Scott, E. (2015). Children's health in a legal framework. *The Future of Children* 25: 177–197.

IOM (2001). On Crossing the Quality Chasm: A New Health System for the 21st Century. Washington, DC: National Academies Press.

IOM (2006). Improving the Quality of Health Care for Mental and Substance-Use Conditions: Quality Chasm Series. Washington, DC: National Academies Press Available at https://www.nap.edu/catalog/11470/improving-the-quality-of-health-care-for-mental-and-substance-use-conditions.

IOM (2009). Depression in Parents, Parenting and Children: Opportunities to Improve Identification, Treatment and Prevention [Report Brief. Washington, DC: National Academies Press Availableathttps://www.nap.edu/catalog/12565/depression-in-parents-parenting-and-children-opportunities-to-improve-identification.

IOM (2010). The Future of Nursing: Leading Change, Advancing Health. Washington, DC: National Academies Press Available at http://books.nap.edu/openbook.php?record_id=12956&page=4.

Kandel, W. (2017). Unaccompanied Alien Children: An Overview. Washington, D.C.: Congressional Research Service Available at https://fas.org/sgp/crs/homesec/R43599.pdf.

Kennedy-Hendricks, A., Epstein, A.J., Stuart, E.A. et al. (2018). Federal parity and spending for mental illness. *Pediatrics* 142 (2): e20172618. https://doi.org/10.1542/peds.2017-2618.

Krauss, J.B. (1993). Health Care Reform: Essentials of Mental Health Services. Washington, DC: American Nurses Publishing.

Kubsch, S.M., Sternard, M.J., Hovarter, R., and Matzke, V. (2004). A holistic model of advocacy: factors that influence its use. *Complementary Therapies in Nursing Midwifery* 10 (1): 37–45.

Longest, B.B. (2015). Health Policymaking in the United States, 6e. Chicago, IL: Health Administration Press.

Luthra, S. & Taylor, M. (2018, June 21). 1 in 5 immigrant children detained during 'zero tolerance' border policy are under 13. *Huffpost.* Availableathttps://www.huffingtonpost.com/entry/1-in-5-immigrant-children-detained-during-zero-tolerance_us_5b2bbc0be4b00b9b51c42115.

Mann, C. & Hyde, P.S. (2013). *Joint CMCS and SAMHSA informational bulletin: Coverage of behavioral health services for children, youth, and young adults with significant mental health conditions.* Available at https://www.medicaid.gov/federal-policy-guidance/downloads/CIB-05-07-2013.pdf.

Mason, D.J., Leavitt, J.K., and Chaffee, M.W. (eds.) (2007). Policy and politics: a framework for action. In: Policy and Politics in Nursing and Health Care, 5e, 1–18. St. Louis, MI: Saunders Elsevier.

Mason, D.J., Gardner, D.B., Outlaw, F.H., and O'Grady, E.T. (eds.) (2016). Policy & Politics in Nursing and Health Care, 7e. St. Louis, MO: Elsevier.

McFerran, T.A. (2003). Oxford Dictionary of Nursing, 4e. Oxford: Oxford University Press.

MHA. (2018). *Position statements.* Mental Health America. Available at https://www.mhanational.org/position-statements.

Merikangas, K.R. (2018). Time trends in the global prevalence of mental disorders in children and adolescents: gap in data on US youth [Editorial]. *Journal for the American Academy of Child and Adolescent Psychiatry* 57: 306–307. https://doi.org/10.1016/j.jaac.2018.03.002.

Merikangas, K.R., He, J.P., Burstein, M. et al. (2010). Lifetime prevalence of mental disorders in U.S. adolescents: results from the National Comorbidity Survey Replication--Adolescent Supplement (NCS-A). *Journal of the American Academy of Child and Adolescent Psychiatry* 49: 980–989.

Merrick, M.T., Ford, D.C., Ports, K.A., and Guinn, A.S. (2018). Prevalence of adverse childhood experiences from the 2011-2014 behavioral risk factor surveillance system in 23 states. *JAMA Pediatrics* https://doi.org/10.1001/jamapediatrics.2018.2537.

National Alliance on Mental Illness. (2018). *Mental health by the numbers.*Availableathttps://www.nami.org/Learn-More/Mental-Health-By-the-Numbers.

Melnyk, B.M., Moldenhauser, Z., Veenema, T. et al. (2001). Keep your children/yourself safe and secure [KySS] program: A national effort to reduce psychosocial morbidities in children and adolescents. *Journal of Pediatric Health Care* 15: 31A–34A. Available at https://www.jpedhc.org/article/S0891-5245(01)67853-2/fulltext.

National Council for Behavioral Health. (2018). *National council for behavioral health partners with boys and girls clubs of America to offer youth mental health first aid.* l Available at https://www.mentalhealthfirstaid.org/external/2018/09/boys-girls-clubs-of-america-partnership.

National Federation of Independent Business v. Sebelius. (2012). 567 US 519.

National Public Radio. (2018). *What we know: Family Separation and "Zero Tolerance" at the Border.* Available at https://www.npr.org/search?query=What%20we%20know%20%3A%20Family%20%20separationn&page=1.

New Freedom Commission on Mental Health (2003). Achieving the Promise: Transforming Mental Health in America. DHHS Pub No.SMA-03-3831 (ed. United States Department of Health and Human Services). Rockville, MD.

O'Connell, M.E., Boat, T., and Warner, K. (2009). Preventing Mental, Emotional, and Behavioral Disorders Among Young People: Progress and Possibilities, 2009. Washington, DC: The National Academies Press.

Olfson, M., Druss, B.G., and Marcus, S.C. (2015). Trends in mental health care among children and adolescents. *New England Journal of Medicine* 372: 2029–2038.

Olson, S. (Rapporteur), Division of Behavioral and Social Sciences and Education; National Academies of Sciences, Engineering, and Medicine. (2017). *Training the future child health care workforce to improve behavioral health outcomes for children, youth, and families. Proceedings of a workshop--in brief.* Washington, D.C.: National Academies Press. Available at https://www.nap.edu/catalog/24789/training-the-future-child-health-care-workforce-to-improve-behavioral-health-outcomes-for-children-youth-and-families.

Pires, S., McLean, J., and Allen, K. (2018). Faces of Medicaid Data Series: Examining Children's Behavioral Health Service Use and Expenditures, 2005–2011. Hamilton, N.J: Center for Health Care Strategies Available at https://www.chcs.org/media/Childrens-Faces-of-Medicaid-2018_072718-1.pdf.

Purewal, S.K., Bucci, M., Gutierrez Wang, L. et al. (2016). Screening for adverse childhood experiences (ACEs) in an integrated pediatric care model. *Zero to Three* 36 (3): 10–17.

Quinnipiac University. (2018). *Poll. Stop taking the kids, 66 Percent of US voters say, Quinnipiac University national poll finds; support for dreamers is 79 percent.* Available at https://poll.qu.edu/national/release-detail?ReleaseID=2550.

Raphel, S. (2012). Child psychiatric nursing. In: Principles and Practice of Psychiatric Nursing, 10e (ed. G.W. Stuart), 669–691. St. Louis, MO: Elsevier Mosby.

Raphel, S. (2017). Policy in times of chaos. *Archives of Psychiatric Nursing* 31: 327–328.

Raphel, S. (2019). US policy for children's mental health. *Archives of Psychiatric Nursing* 33: 307–310. https://doi.org/10.1016/j.apnu.2019.01.013.

Rawal, P. and McCabe, M.A. (2016). Health Care Reform and Programs that Provide Opportunities to Promote Children's Behavioral Health: A Discussion Paper (ed. National Academy of Medicine). Washington, DC: Available at https://nam.edu/wp-content/uploads/2016/07/Health-Care-Reform-and-Programs-that-Provide-Opportunities-to-Promote-Childrens-Behavioral-Health.pdf.

SAMHSA-HRSA (2014). Advancing Behavioral Health Integration within NCQA Recognized Patient-Centered Medical Homes. Rockville, MD: SAMHSA-HRSA Center for Integrated Health Solutions Available at https://commed.umassmed.edu/sites/default/files/publications/Behavioral_Health_Integration_and_the_Patient_Centered_Medical_Home_FINAL.pdf.

Schlairet, M. (2009). Bioethics mediation: the role and importance of nursing advocacy. *Nursing Outlook* 57 (4): 185–193.

Stroul, B.A. (2007). *Integrating mental health services into primary care settings.* Summary of the Special Forum, National Tech Assistance Center for Children's Mental Health. Washington, DC: Georgetown University Center for Child & Human Development.

United Nations. (n.d.). *Children: Declaration of the rights of the child.* Available at https://www.un.org/en/sections/issues-depth/children/.

USDHHS. (2001a). *A national strategy for suicide prevention: Goals and objectives for action.* Rockville, MD: Centers for Disease Control and Prevention, National Center for Injury Prevention and Control, Substance Abuse and Mental Health Services Administration, Center for Mental Health Service, National Institutes of Health, National Institute of Mental Health, US Department of Health and Human Services.

USDHHS. (2001b). *Youth violence: A report of the surgeon general.* Rockville, MD: Centers for Disease Control and Prevention, National Center for Injury Prevention and Control, Substance Abuse and Mental Health Services Administration, Center for Mental Health Service, National Institutes of Health, National Institute of Mental Health, US Department of Health and Human Services.

USDHHS (2009). National Survey of Child and Adolescent Well-Being (NSCAW), 1997–2010. Rockville, MD: Administration for Children & Families, US Department of Health and Human Services.

USDHHS, US Public Health Service, Office of the Surgeon General (1999). Mental Health: A Report of the Surgeon General. Rockville, MD: US Department of Health and Human Services, US Public Health Service, Office of the Surgeon General.

USDHHS, US Public Health Service, Office of the Surgeon General (2000). Children's Mental Health: A National Action Plan. Rockville, MD: US Department of Health and Human Services, US Public Health Service, Office of the Surgeon General.

USDHHS, US Public Health Service, Office of the Surgeon General (2007). The Surgeon General's Call to Action to Prevent and Reduce Underage Drinking. Rockville, MD: US Department of Health and Human Services, US Public Health Service, Office of the Surgeon General.

US Department of Justice. (2018). *Attorney general announces zero-tolerance policy for criminal illegal entry.* Available at https://www.justice.gov/opa/pr/attorney-general-announces-zero-tolerance-policy-criminal-illegal-entry.

US House of Representatives. (1997). *The Balanced Budget Act of 1997.* H.R. 2015 (105th Congress). Available at https://www.congress.gov/bill/105th-congress/house-bill/2015?q=%7B%22search%22%3A%5B%22balanced+budget+act+of+1997%22%5D%7D&s=7&r=1.

US House of Representatives. (2008). Paul Wellstone and Pete Domenici Mental Health Parity and Addiction Equity Act of 2008. H.R. 6983 (110th Congress). Available at https://www.govtrack.us/congress/bills/110/hr6983.

US House of Representatives. (2009). Children's Health Insurance Program Reauthorization Act (CHIPRA) of 2009. H.R. 2 (111th Congress). Available at https://www.congress.gov/bill/111th-congress/house-bill/2?q=%7B%22search%22%3A%5B%22Children%27s+Health+Insurance+Program+Reauthorization+Act+of+2009%22%5D%7D&s=2&r=1.

US House of Representatives. (2010). The Patient Protection & Affordable Care Act. H.R. 3590 (111th Congress). Available at https://www.congress.gov/bill/111th-congress/house-bill/3590?q=%7B%22search%22%3A%5B%22Patient+Protection+and+Affordable+Care+Act+2010%22%5D%7D&s=2&r=54.

US House of Representatives. (2015). Medicare Access and CHIP Reauthorization Act (MACRA) of 2015. H.R. 2 (114th Congress). Available at https://www.congress.gov/bill/114th-congress/house-bill/2/text.

US House of Representatives. (2016a). 21ˢᵗ Century Cures Act. H.R. 34 (114th Congress). Available at https://www.congress.gov/bill/114th-congress/house-bill/34?q=%7B%22search%22%3A%5B%22hr+34%22%5D%7D&s=3&r=1.

US House of Representatives. (2016b). Helping Families in Mental Health Crisis Act. H.R. 2646 (114th Congress). Available at https://www.govtrack.us/congress/bills/114/hr2646.

US House of Representatives. (2017a). Healthy Kids Act. H.R. 3921 (115th Congress). Available at https://www.congress.gov/bill/115th-congress/house-bill/3921?q=%7B%22search%22%3A%5B%22hr3921%22%5D%7D&s=1&r=1.

US House of Representatives. (2017b). Support for Patients and Communities Act. H.R. 6 (115th Congress). Available at https://www.congress.gov/bill/115th-congress/house-resolution/1099?q=%7B%22search%22%3A%5B%22H.R+6+SUPPORT+for+Patients+and+Communities+Act%22%5D%7D&s=4&r=1.

US House of Representatives. (2018a). Bipartisan Budget Act of 2018. H.R. 1892 (115th Congress). Available at https://www.congress.gov/bill/115th-congress/house-bill/1892?q=%7B%22search%22%3A%5B%22bipartisan+budget+act+of+2018%22%5D%7D&s=8&r=1.

US House of Representatives. (2018b). Extension of Continuing Appropriations Act of 2018. H.R. 195. (115th Congress). Available at https://www.congress.gov/bill/115th-congress/house-bill/195?q=%7B%22search%22%3A%5B%22extension+of+continuing+appropriations+act+of+2018%22%5D%7D&s=5&r=2.

US Senate. (2007). Medicare, Medicaid, and SCHIP Extension Act of 2007. S. 2499 (110th Congress). Available at https://www.congress.gov/bill/110th-congress/senate-bill/2499?q=%7B%22search%22%3A%5B%22medicare+medicaid+SCHIP+extension+act+of+2007%22%5D%7D&s=4&r=1.

US Senate. (2015a). Mental Health and Safe Communities Act of 2015, S. 2002 (114th Congress). Available at https://www.congress.gov/bill/114th-congress/senate-bill/2002.

US Senate. (2015b). The Comprehensive Justice and Mental Health Act of 2015. S. 993 (114th Congress). Available at https://www.congress.gov/bill/114th-congress/senate-bill/993.

US Senate. (2016). Mental Health Reform Act of 2016. S. 2680 (114th Congress). Available at https://www.congress.gov/bill/114th-congress/senate-bill/2680?q=%7B%22search%22%3A%5B%22S2680.%22%5D%7D&s=4&r=3.

US Senate. (2017a). Federal Register Printing Savings Act of 2017. S. 1195 (115th Congress). Available at https://www.congress.gov/bill/115th-congress/senate-bill/1195?q=%7B%22federal+register+printing+savings+act+of+2017%22%5D%7D&s=3&r=1.

US Senate. (2017b). Keeping Kids Insurance Dependable and Secure (KIDS) Act of 2017 (115th Congress). Available at https://www.congress.gov/bill/115th-congress/senate-bill/1827?q=%7B%22search%22%3A%5B%22s1827%22%5D%7D&s=5&r=1.

US Senate. (2017c). Protect Our Children Act. S. 782 (115th Congress). Available at https://www.congress.gov/bill/115th-congress/senate-bill/782/all-actions?overview=closed.

US Senate. (2017d). The Opioid Crisis Response Act. S. 2680 (115th Congress). Available at https://www.congress.gov/bill/115th-congress/senate-bill/2680/all-info.

Vaartio, H., Leino-Kilpi, H., Suominen, T., and Puukka, P. (2009). Nursing advocacy in procedural pain care. *Nursing Ethics* 16: 340–362.

WHO (2004). Promoting Mental Health. Concepts, Emerging Evidence, Practice. A Summary Report. Geneva, Switzerland: World Health Organization Available at http://www.who.int/mental_health/evidence/en/promoting_mhh.pdf.

WHO (2013). Comprehensive Mental Health Action Plan for 2013–2020. Mental Health Strengthening our Response. Geneva, Switzerland: World Health Organization.

Yarrow, A.L. (2009). History of US Children's Policy, 1900–Present. Washington, DC: First Focus Available at https://firstfocus.org/wp-content/uploads/2014/06/Childrens-Policy-History.pdf.

Index

Child and Adolescent Behavioral Health: A Resource for Advanced Practice Psychiatric and Primary Care Practitioners in Nursing,
Second Edition. Edited by Edilma L. Yearwood, Geraldine S. Pearson, and Jamesetta A. Newland.
© 2021 John Wiley & Sons, Inc. Published 2021 by John Wiley & Sons, Inc.
Companion website: www.wiley.com/go/Yearwood